588

Scientific Foundations of Anaesthesia

The basis of intensive care

Fourth edition

Scientific Foundations of Anaesthesia

The basis of intensive care

Fourth edition

Edited by

Cyril Scurr
CBE, LVO, FRCS, FFARCS, HonFFARCS(I)
Honorary Consulting Anaesthetist, Magill Department of Anaesthesia, Westminster Hospital, London

and

Stanley Feldman
BSc, MB, BS, FFARCS
Professor of Anaesthesia, Magill Department of Anaesthesia, Charing Cross and Westminster Medical School; Honorary Consultant Anaesthetist, Westminster Hospital, London

and

Neil Soni
FFARACS/(Endorsed in Intensive Care)
Senior Lecturer, Magill Department of Anaesthesia, Charing Cross and Westminster Medical School; Director of Intensive Care Unit and Honorary Consultant Anaesthetist, Westminster Hospital, London

Published simultaneously by:

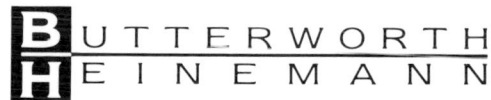

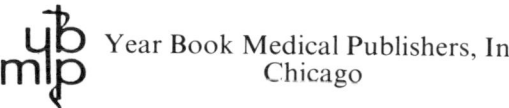

Year Book Medical Publishers, Inc
Chicago

Butterworth-Heinemann Ltd
Linacre House, Jordan Hill, Oxford OX2 8DP

 PART OF REED INTERNATIONAL BOOKS

OXFORD LONDON BOSTON
MUNICH NEW DELHI SINGAPORE SYDNEY
TOKYO TORONTO WELLINGTON

First published 1970
Second edition 1974
Third edition 1982
Reprinted 1983, 1984, 1987
Fourth edition 1990
Reprinted 1991

British Library Cataloguing in Publication Data
Scientific foundations of anaesthesia. – 4th ed.
    1. Medicine. Anaesthesia
    I. Scurr, Cyril. II. Feldman, Stanley A. (Stanley
    Anthony), 1930 – III. Soni, Neil
    617′.96

ISBN 0 7506 0462 X UK
      0 8151 7796 8 USA

Published in the United States of America by
Year Book Medical Publishers Inc
200 North LaSalle Street, Illinois 60601, USA

CHICAGO LONDON BOCA RATON

Printed in Great Britain by Bookcraft (Bath) Ltd.

PREFACE TO THE FIRST EDITION

> ... the relations of etherization to medical science or physiology ... is a tempting field of research ... which cannot be without its influence on the progress of our knowledge of disease.
>
> J. SNOW, London, 1847

John Snow's prophecy that research in anaesthesia would influence our understanding of medicine and disease, has been amply fulfilled. This book is largely concerned with this increase in our knowledge and our expanding appreciation of the physiological processes that maintain life and which may be affected by disease.

No attempt has been made to teach the practical, technical aspects of anaesthesia. Our objective has been to complete a volume which covers the scientific foundations upon which are based the clinical practice of anaesthesia, resuscitation and the care of acutely ill patients in intensive care units. We have tried, not merely to illustrate 'what happens', but also to explain 'why' and 'how'. In order to do this it is necessary to have some knowledge of physics, mathematics and measurement techniques. We have therefore included chapters on the relevant aspects of these subjects.

Although it was originally intended to present the text as short and simple chapters, it soon became evident that these objectives were frequently incompatible with our main aim. In many instances this approach was bound to lead to a superficial, unscientific presentation. We have therefore encouraged authors to present a more detailed coverage of some of the less well appreciated aspects of the subject.

It has been our intention that each chapter should be complete in itself and to this end limited repetition has been unavoidable. Authors have been requested to give a list of key references for further reading that might be of value to anaesthetists, in addition to the usual bibliography. In this way we have tried to present a series of up-to-date chapters reviewing the salient features of the scientific foundations of anaesthesia.

We are most grateful to our many contributors for their co-operation, to members of Magill Department of Anaesthetics of Westminster Hospital for their help with the preparation of proofs and to Mr. Owen Evans of Heinemann Medical Books Ltd., for his advice and assistance.

July, 1970

C.F.S.
S.A.F.

PREFACE TO THE FOURTH EDITION

In the 10 years since the last edition of this book there have been enormous advances in our understanding of the scientific basis of physiology and in the way in which disease may influence normal function. The advent of the fourth edition of *Scientific Foundations of Anaesthesia* has given the editors a chance to expand the coverage of the book to include those areas where new knowledge is producing exciting changes in the conceptual approach to management. Much of this has been in the realm of cell function, and the response of the body to injury at a cellular, humoral and immunological level. This new material, together with the sciences involved in physiology and pharmacology and the principles of measurement, is not only the basis of anaesthesia but also the foundation of intensive care. As a result the book also covers much of the science involved in the application of intensive care. Whilst this coverage is not exhaustive the nature of this expansion is indicated by the inclusion of *Intensive Care* in the title.

In order to keep the size of the book within reasonable bounds the editors have had to decide upon the priorities of subjects for inclusion in this new edition. Less topical subjects have been dropped and the coverage of others curtailed to reflect the contemporary thought. All chapters have been reviewed and revised extensively. About one half of the book is completely new and just under one third are new subject titles. We have been fortunate to have had assistance in the preparation of this edition from leading contributors in the field not only from the UK, but also from the USA and Australia who between them have produced a very complete review of the basic science underlying the practice of anaesthesia. Because each section review has to be complete in itself it is inevitable that certain common ground will be covered in complementary chapters but this has been kept to a minimum consistent with a clear comprehension of each chapter.

Because of the international nature of the contributors and the world wide readership of the book, variations in the use of units of measurements are inevitable. Whenever the editors have thought it helpful the SI equivalent unit has been included.

The editors have endeavoured to produce a book that is up-to-date in the information contained and topical in the subject matter included. A book of this size concerning anaesthesia inevitably involves an enormous amount of work and the editors would like to thank Heinemann Medical Publishers for their assistance.

Cyril Scurr
Stanley Feldman
Neil Soni

CONTENTS

LIST OF CONTRIBUTORS

A. P. Adams, PhD, FCAnaes
  Professor of Anaesthetics, University of London,
  Guy's Hospital Medical School, London;
  Honorary Consultant Anaesthetist, Lambeth,
  Southwark, Lewisham Area Health Authority
  (Teaching)

John L. Atlee III, BA(Biology), MS(Pharmacology),
  MD, FACA
  Professor of Anesthesiology, Medical College of
  Wisconsin, Milwaukee County Medical Complex,
  Milwaukee, WI, USA

J. M. Baden, BSc, MRCP, FFARCS
  Associate Professor of Anesthesia, Stanford
  University School of Medicine and Veterans
  Administration Medical Centre, Palo Alto,
  California, USA

Paul G. Barash, MD
  Professor and Chairman, Yale University School
  of Medicine, New Haven, CT, USA

J. P. Blackburn, MA, FFARCS, DIC
  Consultant Emeritus. Formerly Consultant in
  Clinical Measurement, Westminster Hospital

Margaret E. Bone, FFARCS
  Senior Registrar in Anaesthesia, St Bartholomew's
  Hospital, London

William Cameron Bowman, PhD, DSc, FRSE, Hon
  FFARCS
  Professor of Pharmacology and Vice Principal of
  the University, University of Strathclyde, Glasgow

Warren E. Bruce, FFARACS
  Staff Specialist Anaesthetist, Department of
  Anaesthetics and Resuscitation, Westmead
  Hospital, Sydney, Australia

Keith Budd, FFARCS
  Consultant in Anaesthesia and Pain Relief, Royal
  Infirmary, Bradford

John A. Bushman, MBCS, FInst MC
  Acting Director, Research Department of
  Anaesthetics, Royal College of Surgeons; Senior
  Lecturer LHMC; Honorary Consultant Newham
  District

Bart Chernow, MD, FACP
  Associate Professor of Anaesthesia (Critical Care)
  Harvard Medical School; Co-Director, Henry K.
  Beecher Memorial Anaesthesia Laboratories;
  Associate Director, Respiratory-Surgical ICU
  Massachusetts General Hospital, USA

P. Cliffe, BSc, PhD, FInstP
  Former Director, Department of Clinical
  Measurement, Westminster Hospital, London

Michael J. Cousins, MD(Syd), FFARCS,
  FFARACS, FCAnaes
  Professor and Chairman, Department of
  Anaesthesia and Intensive Care, Flinders Medical
  Centre, Flinders University of South Australia,
  Bedford Park, SA 5042 Australia

Benjamin G. Covino, PhD, MD
  Chairman, Department of Anaesthesia, Brigham
  and Women's Hospital; Professor of Anaesthesia,
  Harvard Medical School, Boston, Massachusetts,
  USA

N. J. H. Davies, DM, MRCP, FFARCS
  Senior Lecturer in Anaesthesia, Department of
  Clinical Physiology, Brompton Hospital, London

David Denison
  Professor of Clinical Physiology, National Heart
  and Lung Institute; Director, Lung Function Unit,
  Brompton Hospital, London

A. H. Dickenson, BSc(Hons), PhD
  Lecturer in Pharmacology, University College,
  London

Charles Cook, MD
  Clinical Associate in Anesthesia, Massachusetts
  General Hospital, Instructor in Anesthesia,
  Harvard Medical School

H. B. Fairley, FFARCS, FRCPC
  Professor and Chairman, Department of
  Anesthesia, Stanford University School of
  Medicine, Stanford, California

S. A. Feldman, BSc, FFARCS
  Professor of Anaesthesia, Charing Cross and
  Westminster Medical School; Honorary
  Consultant Anaesthetist, Westminster Hospital

Malcolm M. C. D. Fisher, MD(Otago), FFARACS
  Head of Intensive Therapy Unit, Royal North
  Shore Hospital of Sydney, St Leonards, Australia

Michael D. Frye, MD
  Assistant Professor of Medicine, Director of
  Respiratory Therapy, East Tennessee State
  University College of Medicine; Veterans
  Administration Hospital, Mountain Home,
  Tennessee, USA

David G. Gadian, MA, DPhil
  Professor in Physics in Relation to Surgery,
  Hunterian Institute, Royal College of Surgeons of
  England, Lincoln's Inn Fields, London

M. M. Ghoneim, MD
  Professor, Department of Anesthesia, College of
  Medicine, University of Iowa, Iowa City, Iowa

W. J. Glover, FFARCS
  Consultant Anaesthetist, Hospital for Sick
  Children, London

W. M. Gray, BSc, PhD
  Principal Physicist, West of Scotland Health
  Boards, Department of Clinical Physics and Bio-
  Engineering, Glasgow

Betty L. Grundy, MD
Professor of Anesthesiology, University of Florida
College of Medicine, Chief of Anesthesiology
Service, VA Medical Centre, Florida

C. D. Hanning, BSc, FFARCS
Senior Lecturer in Anaesthesia, Leicester General
Hospital, Leicester

Merel H. Harmel, BA, MD, FFARCS
Professor Emeritus Anesthesiology, Duke
University Medical Center, Durham, North
Carolina, USA

Felicity H. Hawker, FFARCS
Specialist in Intensive Care, Royal Prince Alfred
Hospital, Camperdown, New South Wales,
Australia

Thomas L. Higgins, MD, FACP
Medical Director, Cardiothoracic I.C.U. Cleveland
Clinic Foundation, Ohio, USA

Ken Hillman, FFARCS, FFARACS
Director of Anaesthetics, Intensive Care and
Coronary Care, The Liverpool Hospital, Sydney,
Australia

A. J. W. Hilson, MSc(Nucl. Med), FRCP
Consultant in Nuclear Medicine and Honorary
Clinical Senior Lecturer, Royal Free Hospital and
School of Medicine, London

Roberta L. Hines, MD
Assistant Professor of Anaesthesia, Yale
University; Director of Cardiothoracic Intensive
Care Unit, Yale New Haven Hospital, New Haven

Carol A. Hirschman, MD
Professor of Anesthesiology and Environmental
Health Sciences at the Johns Hopkins University,
Baltimore, USA

William E. Hoffman, PhD
Director of Research Laboratory, Department of
Anesthesiology, Michael Reese Hospital and
Medical Center, Chicago, Illinois

C. J. Hull
Professor of Anaesthesia, Department of
Anaesthesia, Royal Victoria Infirmary, Newcastle
upon Tyne

James P. Isbister, BSc(Med), FRACP, FRCPA
Head of Department of Haematology, Royal
North Shore Hospital of Sydney, St Leonards,
Australia

D. C. O. James, MD, MSc, FRCPath, BPharm,
FIBiol
Formerly Consultant Pathologist (Blood
Transfusion and Transplantation Immunology),
Westminster Hospital, London

D. J. Jenkinson, BA, MSc, PhD
Professor of Pharmacology, Department of
Pharmacology, University College, London

J. Gareth Jones, MD, FRCP, FFARCS
Professor of Anaesthesia, University of Leeds

Joan J. Kendig, PhD
Professor of Biology in Anesthesia, Department of
Anesthesia, Stanford University School of
Medicine, Stanford, California

Nguyen D. Kien, PhD
Assistant Adjunct Professor, Department of
Anesthesiology, School of Medicine, University of
California, Davis, California

Richard J. Kitz, MD
Henry Isaiah Dorr Professor, Anesthetist-in-chief,
Massachusetts General Hospital, Boston,
Massachusetts

Greg Koski, PhD, MD
Assistant Professor of Anesthesia, Harvard
Medical School; Director K. Beecher Memorial
Research Laboratories; Department of Anesthesia,
Massachusetts General Hospital, Boston,
Massachusetts

Wolfgang J. Kox, MD, PhD
Senior Lecturer, Department of Anaesthetia,
Charing Cross and Westminster Medical School;
Honorary Consultant Anaesthetist (Director ICU),
Charing Cross Hospital

Henry B. Kram, MD
Assistant Professor of Surgery, Drew University;
Attending Surgeon, M. L. King Jr. Hospital, Los
Angeles, California

Kenneth R. LaMantia, MD
Assistant Professor, Department of
Anesthesiology, New Haven, Connecticut, USA

A. F. Lant, PhD, FRCP
Consultant Physician, Westminster Hospital;
Professor of Therapeutics, Westminster Medical
School, London

Harry A. Lee, BSc, FRCP, MRCS
Professor of Renal Medicine, University of
Southampton; Consultant Physician, Portsmouth
Group of Hospitals; Titular Head of Infectious
Diseases Department, St. Mary's Hospital,
Portsmouth

J. M. Leigh, MD, FFARCS
Director, Intensive Care Unit, Royal Surrey
County Hospital, Guildford, Surrey

John B. Leslie, MD
Assistant Professor of Anesthesiology, Duke
University Medical Centre, Durham, North
Carolina

Piers J. A. Lesser, FFARCS
Consultant Anaesthetist, Royal Halifax Infirmary,
Halifax, Yorkshire

Edward Lowenstein, MD
Professor of Anesthesia, Harvard Medical School;
Anesthetist-in-chief, Department of Anesthesia and
Critical Care, Beth Israel Hospital, Boston,
Massachusetts

J. N. Lunn, MD, FFARCS
Reader in Anaesthetics, University of Wales, College of Medicine, Heath Park, Cardiff

Rosemary Macdonald, PhD, FFARCS
Consultant Anaesthetist, St James's University Hospital, Leeds

Vincent Marks, MA, DM, FRCP, FRCPath
Professor of Clinical Biochemistry and Consultant Chemical Pathologist, Department of Biochemistry, University of Surrey, Guildford GU2 5XH

Ian Neering, PhD
Senior Lecturer in Physiology and Pharmacology, School of Physiology and Pharmacology, University of New South Wales, Sydney, Australia

J. Norman, PhD, FFARCS
Professor of Anaesthesia, University of Southampton

Gerald N. Olsen, MD, FACP, FCCP
Professor of Medicine, Director Division of Pulmonary and Critical Care Medicine, University of South Carolina School of Medicine, Columbia, South Carolina

Brian L. Partridge, MD, DPhil
Assistant Professor of Anesthesiology, University of California, San Diego VA Medical Center, San Diego, CA 92161

G. D. Parbrook, MD, FFARCS
Senior Lecturer, University Department of Anaesthesia, University of Glasgow and Consultant Anaesthetist, Glasgow Royal Infirmary, Glasgow

K. S. Pearson, MD
Assistant Professor, Department of Anesthesia, College of Medicine, University of Iowa, Iowa City, Iowa

Ian Power, BSc, FCAnaes
Lecturer in University Department of Anaesthesia, Royal Infirmary, Edinburgh

John A. Reitan, MD
Professor of Anesthesiology, University of California Medical School, Davis, California

Reid Rubsamen, MD, AB (Biochemistry and Computer Science), MS (Computer Science)
Assistant in Anesthesia, Massachusetts General Hospital, Instructor in Anesthesia, Harvard Medical School

William C. Shoemaker, MD
Professor of Surgery UCLA; Vice Chairman, Department of Surgery King-Drew Medical Center, Los Angeles, California

George A. Skowronski, MB, BS(Hons), MRCP(UK), FRACP
Senior Staff Specialist, Intensive Care Unit, Flinders Medical Centre, Bedford Park, South Australia

N. Ty Smith, MD, DPhil
Professor of Anesthesia, University of California, San Diego; VA Medical Center, San Diego, CA 92161

Neil Soni, FFARCS (endorsed in intensive care)
Senior Lecturer, Magill Department of Anaesthesia, Charing Cross and Westminster Medical School, Director of Intensive Care Unit, Westminster Hospital, London

A. A. Spence, MD, FCAnaes, FRCP(Glas)
Professor of Anaesthetics, Royal Infirmary, Edinburgh, EH3 9YW

T. W. Stone, BPharm, PhD, DSc
Professor of Pharmacology, University of Glasgow, Glasgow

D. A. P. Strickland, BSc
Deputy Director, Department of Clinical Measurement, Westminster Hospital

L. Strunin, MD, FFARCS
Professor and Chairman, Department of Anaesthesia, University of Calgary, Alberta, Canada

M. K. Sykes, MA, FFARCS, Hon FFARACS, Hon FFA(S.A.)
Nuffield Professor of Anaesthetics, University of Oxford, Fellow, Pembroke College, Oxford

Thomas A. Torda, MD, FFARACS
Associate Professor, Head, Department of Anaesthesia and Intensive Care, Prince Henry Hospital, Sydney, Australia

D. Trenchard, BSc, PhD
Senior Investigator Cardiothoracic Unit, Cardiothoracic Institute, formerly Midhurst Branch

James R. Trudell, PhD
Associate Professor of Chemistry in Anesthesia, Department of Anesthesia, Stanford University School of Medicine, Stanford, California

Bryan Walton, FFARCS
Consultant Anaesthetist, The London Hospital, London

John B. West, MD, PhD, DSc, FRCP, FRACP
Professor of Medicine and Physiology, School of Medicine, University of California, San Diego, La Jolla, California

Christine M. Williams, BSc(Hons) Nutrition, PhD Medicine
Lecturer in Human Nutrition, Division of Nutrition and Food Science, Department of Biochemistry, University of Surrey, Guildford, Surrey

B. A. Willis, PhD, FFARCS
Senior Registrar in Anaesthetics, University Hospital of Wales, Heath Park, Cardiff

CONVERSION TABLE

mmHg → kPa

mmHg	kPa	mmHg	kPa	mmHg	kPa	mmHg	kPa	mmHg	kPa	mmHg	kPa
1	0·133	36	4·80	71	9·46	112	14·9	182	24·3	252	33·6
2	0·267	37	4·93	72	9·60	114	15·2	184	24·5	254	33·9
3	0·400	38	5·07	73	9·73	116	15·5	186	24·8	256	34·1
4	0·533	39	5·20	74	9·86	118	15·7	188	25·1	258	34·4
5	0·667	40	5·33	75	10·0	120	16·0	190	25·3	260	34·7
6	0·800	41	5·47	76	10·1	122	16·3	192	25·6	262	34·9
7	0·933	42	5·60	77	10·3	124	16·5	194	25·9	264	35·2
8	1·07	43	5·73	78	10·4	126	16·8	196	26·1	266	35·5
9	1·20	44	5·87	79	10·5	128	17·1	198	26·4	268	35·7
10	1·33	45	6·00	80	10·7	130	17·3	200	26·7	270	36·0
11	1·47	46	6·13	81	10·8	132	17·6	202	26·9	272	36·3
12	1·60	47	6·27	82	10·9	134	17·9	204	27·2	274	36·5
13	1·73	48	6·40	83	11·1	136	18·1	206	27·5	276	36·8
14	1·87	49	6·53	84	11·2	138	18·4	208	27·7	278	37·1
15	2·00	50	6·67	85	11·3	140	18·7	210	28·0	280	37·3
16	2·13	51	6·80	86	11·5	142	18·9	212	28·3	282	37·6
17	2·27	52	6·93	87	11·6	144	19·2	214	28·5	284	37·9
18	2·40	53	7·07	88	11·7	146	19·5	216	28·8	286	38·1
19	2·53	54	7·20	89	11·9	148	19·7	218	29·1	288	38·4
20	2·67	55	7·33	90	12·0	150	20·0	220	29·3	290	38·7
21	2·80	56	7·47	91	12·1	152	20·3	222	29·6	292	38·9
22	2·93	57	7·60	92	12·3	154	20·5	224	29·9	294	39·2
23	3·07	58	7·73	93	12·4	156	20·8	226	30·1	296	39·5
24	3·20	59	7·86	94	12·5	158	21·1	228	30·4	298	39·7
25	3·33	60	8·00	95	12·7	160	21·3	230	30·7	300	40·0
26	3·47	61	8·13	96	12·8	162	21·6	232	30·9		
27	3·60	62	8·26	97	12·9	164	21·9	234	31·2		
28	3·73	63	8·40	98	13·1	166	22·1	236	31·5		
29	3·87	64	8·53	99	13·2	168	22·4	238	31·7		
30	4·00	65	8·66	100	13·3	170	22·7	240	32·0		
31	4·13	66	8·80	102	13·6	172	22·9	242	32·3		
32	4·27	67	8·93	104	13·9	174	23·2	244	32·5		
33	4·40	68	9·06	106	14·1	176	23·5	246	32·8		
34	4·53	69	9·20	108	14·4	178	23·7	248	33·1		
35	4·67	70	9·33	110	14·7	180	24·0	250	33·3		

kPa → mmHg

kPa	mmHg	kPa	mmHg
1	7·50	21	158
2	15·0	22	165
3	22·5	23	172
4	30·0	24	180
5	37·5	25	188
6	45·0	26	195
7	52·5	27	202
8	60·0	28	210
9	67·5	29	218
10	75·0	30	225
11	82·5	31	232
12	90·0	32	240
13	97·5	33	248
14	105	34	255
15	112	35	262
16	120	36	270
17	128	37	278
18	135	38	285
19	142	39	292
20	150	40	300

cmH_2O → kPa

cmH_2O	kPa	cmH_2O	kPa
1	0·098	21	2·06
2	0·196	22	2·16
3	0·294	23	2·26
4	0·392	24	2·35
5	0·490	25	2·45
6	0·588	26	2·55
7	0·686	27	2·65
8	0·784	28	2·74
9	0·883	29	2·84
10	0·981	30	2·94
11	1·08	31	3·04
12	1·18	32	3·14
13	1·27	33	3·24
14	1·37	34	3·33
15	1·47	35	3·43
16	1·57	36	3·53
17	1·67	37	3·63
18	1·76	38	3·73
19	1·86	39	3·82
20	1·96	40	3·92

Reproduced with permission from *The SI for the Health Profession* (1977). World Health Organisation, Geneva.

SECTION 1
PHYSICAL BASIS OF THE SCIENCE OF ANAESTHESIA

1. SI Units
D. A. P. Strickland

The establishment of the International System (SI) of units had the following beneficial results:

1. Achievement of unification across a wide range of scientific disciplines.
2. Simplification of a very large number of equations and relationships
3. Decimalization—the progressive discouragement of such units as the Imperial system with their mixed radices (such as 12 inches, 3 feet, 22 yards, 10 chains and 8 furlongs)
4. A long overdue rationalization of many aspects of nomenclature and symbols.

This does not mean that that are no other systems of units legitimately in use in special scientific and other fields. It does not even mean that measures based on factors other than 10 have no merit; a ten-fingered species did not produce so many 12 and 60 based systems without reason. The number 10 with its two factors, 2 and 5, has no advantages for carpentry, typographical design or the packing of eggs.

In what follows, important terms will be clarified first; then the subject of physical quantities and units will be discussed sufficiently to give the reader confidence in using SI units and, importantly, in interpreting new or unfamiliar ones in the forms in which they are met in modern texts.

Formality in the Use of Symbols

It is a mistake to assume that precision in the use of symbols is merely a pedantic mannerism. The correct methods of writing unit symbols, and consequently of reading them, are described here for two quite practical reasons. The first is that casual departure from internationally agreed techniques in these matters has in the past caused unnecessary confusion—not always suspected by those guilty of it. The second is that attention to this aspect of the subject is repaid by providing rapid and concentrated insight into many other aspects.

QUANTITIES, UNITS, AND SYMBOLS

In this context *quantity* means any physical quantity, such as mass, time, energy or pH, which may be measured in science. The result of a measurement is described by a number and a unit: for example, a pressure of 20 pascals. This involves a *quantity name* (pressure here) and a *unit name* (pascal). A physical quantity has an associated *quantity symbol* (or more than one, depending on the context) and a *unit symbol*. For example if we write: $p = 20$ Pa the quantity symbol is p and Pa is the unit symbol.

Quantity names may vary between disciplines for various reasons. For example, 'volume' in one context may become 'vital capacity' or 'displacement' in others. Variations in *quantity symbols* occur because the same text may involve different quantities having the same initial letter (such as temperature and time), or because a physical quantity may exist in different forms in a particular discipline—such as the many versions of volume used in respiratory physiology but quite unknown outside that field.

In contrast, *unit names* and *unit symbols* are rapidly becoming standardized by international and interdisciplinary agreement, but there are commonsense reasons for certain variations in unit symbols. One concerns typesetting and layout, for which there are officially recognized alternatives such as m/s or m·s⁻¹; another allows for choice where one form has more meaning than another in a given context, such as when joule per litre (J/L) is more informative than kilopascal (kPa). Such flexibility is not the same as the use of local laboratory jargon or the pet symbols of individuals which lead to inconsistency and to incomprehension across disciplines.

An Important Aspect of Unit Symbols

A useful way of interpreting a result such as $p = 20$ Pa is to put into words: 'the quantity (p) is the product of the number (20) and the unit (Pa)'. This is like reading an algebraic equation such as $x = 3y$. It makes the point that Pa is not merely an abbreviation, it is a *symbol* and is *handled as such*. Growing practices which illustrate this are the heading of tables and annotating the axes of graphs with dimensionless quotients such as $p/$Pa. For example an entry of 20 means that the measured pressure (p) is in the ratio 20 to the stated unit. Treating a unit symbol like an algebraic entity is also particularly helpful when establishing

TABLE 1.1

NAMES AND SYMBOLS FOR SI BASE AND SUPPLEMENTARY UNITS

Physical quantity	Name of unit	Unit symbol
Base		
length	metre	m
mass	kilogram	kg
time	second	s
electric current	ampere	A
thermodynamic temperature	kelvin	K
luminous intensity	candela	cd
amount of substance	mole	mol
Supplementary		
plane angle	radian	rad
solid angle	steradian	sr

Notes for Table 1.1
Thermodynamic temperature was called Absolute temperature.
Amount of substance is sometimes abbreviated, as in the term substance concentration.

conversions between units and for understanding (or refuting) those made by other people.

SI Base and Supplementary Quantities and their Units

Science is in no way remarkable in being based on a limited number of fundamentals—concepts which are used in the precise definitions of others, but which can only themselves be described by extended discussion. In science these are called *base quantities*, and currently SI recognizes seven, shown as the first group in Table 1.1. They are regarded as independent of one another rather as are the three dimensions in space. All other quantities are defined in terms of them and are called *derived quantities*.

Two quantities called *supplementary* are added to these: *plane angle* and *solid angle*. The first concerns such matters as rotation and orientation; the second occurs in derived quantities which describe the way such things as light, gravity and radiations are directionally distributed in space.

Since all readers will be familiar with at least some of the SI base units, and because the less familiar ones are fairly complicated, their definitions are removed to the Appendix for convenience of reading.

Derived Quantities

Built up from the seven base and two supplementary quantities is the whole structure of derived quantities, such as area, speed, mass, density and others which are defined as their need becomes apparent. Their units: square metres (m^2), metres per second (m/s), kilograms per cubic metre (kg/m^3), are based on conventions resulting from considerable intelligent thought. Before summarizing these, the basic arsenal of nine has to be augmented as shown in Tables 1.2 and 1.3.

NON-SI UNITS ACCEPTED IN ASSOCIATION WITH SI (TABLE 1.2)

The first six items in Table 1.2 are there because they are, for excellent reasons, universally established. The litre (redefined as exactly one cubic decimetre in 1964) and the tonne are there because enough people intend to continue using them. The litre is unique in having alternative symbols: the upper case L is admitted where the lower case (l) and the number 1 might be confused.

It is unusual to find the raised symbols ° ′ and ″ joined to SI symbols. If they need to be, they are best set in brackets: (°) etc.

TABLE 1.2

NON-SI UNITS ACCEPTED FOR GENERAL OR SPECIALIZED USE

Physical quantity	Name of unit	Symbol	Value in SI units
For general use			
time	minute	min	60 s
time	hour	h	3600 s
time	day	d	86 400 s
plane angle	degree	°	$(\pi/180)$ rad
plane angle	minute	′	$(\pi/10\ 800)$ rad
plane angle	second	″	$(\pi/648\ 000)$ rad
volume	litre	l, L	0.001 m^3 ($= 1$ dm^3)
mass	tonne	t	1000 kg
Specialized fields			
mass	unified atomic mass unit	u	$1.660\ 54 \times 10^{-27}$ kg
energy	electronvolt	eV	$1.602\ 18 \times 10^{-19}$ J
length	astronomical unit	AU	$1.496\ 00 \times 10^{11}$ m
length	parsec	pc	3.0857×10^{16} m

Note for Table 1.2
This table is complete to assure the reader that nothing which *might have* concerned his work has been edited out.

These eight accepted non-SI units are all exact by definition. The last four are included so that the reader knows that there are no others which *might* have concerned him. The atomic mass unit may be met in physical chemistry texts and the electronvolt concerns radioactivity and radiation. Their values (rounded here) are experimentally derived; adjusted values are periodically published by the Committee on Data for Science and Technology (CODATA) of the International Council of Scientific Unions.

SI UNITS GIVEN SPECIAL NAMES (TABLE 1.3)

Certain derived units are given names because they occur so often; it is more convenient to speak of a newton of force than a metre kilogram per second squared. Where these are based on the names of scientists the convention is to use lower case initial (newton, joule, ohm etc.) for the full name, but to restore the upper case (N, J, Ω) for the unit symbol.

Any of the names and symbols in the left hand column of Table 1.3 may be used as parts of more complex SI derived units. Also, it will be seen from the third column that derived units involving other special named units may have alternative forms useful in different contexts. The examples here are representative.

Conventions Intended to Avoid Ambiguity

Ambiguity and error are completely avoidable if certain conventions are observed. In this text they are highlighted as numbered conventions in related groups so that they can be referred to easily. For each group the reasons are stated at the end of its section.

Convention 1. With the single exception of the litre (l or L) *no variation* is accepted for the unit symbols listed here:

Table 1.1	m	kg	s	A	K	cd	mol	rad sr
Table 1.2	min h	d	t	u	eV	l		
Table 1.3	C	°C	F	H	Hz	J	lm	lx N Ω
	Pa	S	T	V	W	Wb	Bq	Gy Sv

Convention 2. All unit symbols are printed in roman (upright) type.

Convention 3. Unit symbols *never* take the pluralizing s, and are not punctuated (unless they end a sentence). Thus: 3 kg (*not* 3 kg. and *not* 3 kgs).

Reason 1. Despite the fact that some units use the same letter as a decimal prefix (e.g. m for milli and d for deci) these unit symbols are always identifiable by their *position* in a statement. For example in $x = 30$ m,

TABLE 1.3
SI DERIVED UNITS GIVEN SPECIAL NAMES

Unit-name and Symbol		Physical quantity	In terms of other units
General science			
coulomb	C	Electric charge; quantity of electricity	s·A
degree Celsius [a]	°C	Celsius temperature	K
farad	F	Capacitance	C/V
henry	H	Inductance	Wb/A, V/(A/s)
hertz [b]	Hz	Frequency	s^{-1}
joule	J	Energy; work; quantity of heat	N·m
lumen	lm	Luminous flux	cd·sr
lux	lx	Illuminance	lm/m^2
newton	N	Force	$m·kg/s^2$
ohm	Ω	Electric resistance	V/A
pascal	Pa	Pressure; stress (mechanical)	N/m^2, J/m^3
siemens	S	Electric conductance	A/V, Ω^{-1}
tesla	T	Magnetic flux density	Wb/m^2
volt	V	Electric potential; electromotive force	W/A, J/C
watt	W	Power; radiant flux	J/s
weber	Wb	Magnetic flux	V·s
Health and safety			
becquerel [b]	Bq	Activity (radionuclide)	s^{-1}
gray	Gy	Absorbed dose (radiation); kerma; specific energy imparted	J/kg
sievert	Sv	Dose equivalent	J/kg

Notes for Table 1.3
(a) Special name replacing kelvin when stating Celsius temperature. Temperature *differences* may be expressed in either kelvins or degrees Celsius.
(b) Special names for inverse second: becquerel for rate of discrete radioactive events; hertz for continuous periodic phenomena in general. Currently (1987) there are 19 entries in this table; all are given here to assure the reader that nothing which *might have* concerned his work has been edited out.

the symbol m can only mean metre because 'thirty milli' is unacceptable jargon. To someone who had not met the millimetre, the first m in 25.4 mm must mean milli and the second one mean metre because mm is not in the list of Convention 1. The point becomes more apparent when one meets unfamiliar examples, such as fl (femtolitre has been cited for cell volumes) and mlx (millilux). It is for such *practical* reasons that the international authorities deprecate abuses such as using K instead of k for kilo. Decimal prefixes are dealt with fully in Table 1.4 below.

Reason 2. This avoids confusion with *quantity symbols* which are always in italic (sloping) type. Thus although *N* can represent a number of molecules, N can only mean newton, the unit of force.

Reason 3. Despite often having originated as abbreviations, unit symbols are *not abbreviations by nature*, so they need neither the s nor the period (.). Moreover, they *must not* take the s because this is the symbol for the second, nor the period (.) since that is an alternative symbol-multiplication sign where the raised dot (·) is not available.

Accepted Representation of Other Derived Unit Symbols

Derived units based on multiples or quotients of those collected as in Convention 1 have symbols formed as follows.

Convention 4. *Products* are shown in any of three ways. For example, for the product pascal second:

Pa·s *or* Pa.s *or* Pa s (note the small space)

Convention 5. *Quotients* use either the horizontal quotient-line or the solidus (/) or negative exponents coupled with any of the three forms of product. Thus for millimole per kilogram:

$$\frac{mmol}{kg} \; or \; mmol/kg \; or \; mmol \cdot kg^{-1} \; or \; mmol.kg^{-1}$$
$$or \; mmol \; kg^{-1}$$

Convention 6. More than one solidus must not be used unless brackets are used to remove all doubt as to what is meant. For example to express the number of millimoles of a substance entering unit mass of tissue each second, the following are unambiguous:

mmol/(kg·s) *or* (mmol/kg)/s *or* mmol·kg^{-1}·s^{-1}
Note: mmol/kg/s should *never* be used.

Reason 4. In the context of unit symbols, groups of letters *without* space or delineating sign (dots or /, the solidus) represent either plain units (e.g. cd, mol, rad, min) or units modified by a prefix (e.g. kPa, mm, MHz). Therefore some delineation is essential for products. The point on the line (.) is used where the raised point (·) is not available. The small space is best

not used where hasty reading (or printing) might encourage confusion of, say m for milli and m for metre. (See later, Table 1.4 and associated conventions.)

Reason 5. Valid alternatives serve different requirements of print spacing and style (the horizontal line is sometimes used on graphs). Negative indices throughout are often used for complicated cases, especially when their nature is to be made clear between disciplines.

Reason 6. Expressions like x/y/z are deprecated in *all* scientific contexts. For example, there is no way of knowing whether 2/3/5 is supposed to mean a fifth of 2/3 (= 2/15) or 2 divided by 3/5 (= 10/3). To a restricted circle the meaning of mmol/kg/s may seem obvious, but such practice invites unsuspected error (especially when adjusting ranges of units) and misunderstanding outside such circles.

Decimal Prefixes used with SI (Table 1.4)

The conventions associated with these prefixes, and their reasons, clarify many features of the correct use of SI symbols in general.

Convention 7. There are no exceptions to these symbols (nor their *typographic case*).

Convention 8. Prefix symbols are in upright type, as are the unit symbols they modify.

Convention 9. They must *always* be followed by a unit symbol; this must be *without space or punctuation*. Examples are:

ns, μm, mmol, MHz (nanosecond, micrometre, millimole, megahertz).

Convention 10. Multiple prefixes should *not* be used. E.g. use nm (nanometre), *not* mμm.

Convention 11. An exponent used with a prefixed unit refers to the *entire unit*. For example km^2 means (km)^2, *not* 1000 m^2.

TABLE 1.4
PREFIXES FOR SI UNITS

Prefix and symbol		Factor	Prefix and symbol		Factor
deci	d	10^{-1}	deca	da	10^1
centi	c	10^{-2}	hecto	h	10^2
milli	m	10^{-3}	kilo	k	10^3
micro	μ	10^{-6}	mega	M	10^6
nano	n	10^{-9}	giga	G	10^9
pico	p	10^{-12}	tera	T	10^{12}
femto	f	10^{-15}	peta	P	10^{15}
atto	a	10^{-18}	exa	E	10^{18}

Convention 12. For historical reasons one SI unit, the kilogram, incorporates a prefix in its name. Its symbol (kg), when unmodified, is treated as an entity. However, decimal multiples and fractions are formed by attaching the appropriate prefix to the symbol g (*not* to kg) despite the fact that the gram is not a base unit for SI. So 10^{-6} kg is written mg, *not* μkg, and it follows that 10^{-3} kg is written g, *not* mkg. The appearance of gram or g is therefore perfectly valid when the context requires it, even with SI.

Convention 13. In a unit involving quotients any prefix is better in the numerator, as with kilometre per second rather than metre per millisecond.

Convention 14. A prefix symbol should never stand alone (see also Convention 9) either to represent a number or, worse still, a unit.

Reason 7. The precise form must be used so that a prefix symbol can instantly be recognized from its (invariable) position immediately leading a known unit symbol. Note especially that kilo uses k, not K.

Reason 8. Italic type is used for *quantity symbols*, so using upright type avoids confusing, for example, m for metre or milli with *m* as the symbol for a mass.

Reason 9. Products of units may be indicated either by a dot *or by a space* (Convention 3). Thus m N and m·N can both mean the product of the metre and the newton; but mN can only mean millinewton.

Reason 10. Consider two examples, each of which might be unfamiliar to some readers: mmol·kg^{-1} s^{-1}, and klm/m^2. The blocks preceding any multiplying or dividing sign are: mmol and klm. Neither of these are on the list of plain unit symbols, so each must start with a prefix (milli and kilo here). The remainders (mol for mole and lm for lumen) must therefore be unit symbols. Relaxation of this convention by *ad hoc* stringing together of letters carries a strong risk of ambiguity of which the perpetrator may be unaware.

Reason 11. This has always been so; scientific convention agrees with common usage here.

Reason 12. The alternative has all the potential disadvantages of multiple prefix symbols, and it would strike most people as absurd.

Reason 13. This creates uniformity of notation and facilitates comparison of results across disciplines. However this convention is sometimes relaxed if it renders a unit unfamiliar or artificial in context; it should conform to the usual practice in the discipline concerned. The fact that the density of water is about 1 Mg/m^3 does not require that everyone should quote it that way.

Reason 14. As in ordinary speech, floating prefixes are ambiguous ('He is an anti'). Moreover, several prefix symbols are the same as unit symbols which can stand alone (or as numerators) *in their own right*. For example, m/s legitimately means metre per second; it would be eccentric to use it for thousandths of a reciprocal second (10^{-3}/s, or once every 1000 s). Also, although such usage as k for kilohm (kΩ) and μ for micrometre (μm) are ineradicable in laboratory jargon, it may happen that the person who reads or hears 'k' may assume 1000 of something not intended, perhaps with dangerous results.

CONVERSION FACTORS TO SI FROM OTHER UNITS (TABLE 1.5)

Purpose. This table is to assist the reader when referring to older texts using systems such as the CGS (centimetre gram second), FPS (foot pound second) and Imperial units. A selection is given in alphabetical order within alphabetically arranged groups. The symbols are those likely to be met in the more recent of such texts. They are given for ease of reference, and although most have international status, many variants were used in the past, such as p.s.i. for lbf/in^2.

Guidance Values. These values are given to sufficient precision for many purposes and with prefixed units that make the numerical values easily understood. For example, since the foot is commonly thought of as about 30 cm, the square foot is expressed as 929 cm^2 rather than 0.0929 m^2 or 9.29 dm^2.

Greater Precision Column. Having noted the order of size, this column can be used for adjusting to whatever prefixed unit is required and for working to greater precision if needed. In *this* column, exact values are indicated by bold-faced least significant digit; rounded-off values are generally given to six figures and in customary scientific notation.

Pressure Units. The ones which refer to water or mercury are those known as *conventional units*. They are based on standard gravity (free-fall acceleration of 9.806 65 m/s^2) and standard liquid densities which are, for water and mercury respectively, 1000 kg/m^3 and 13 595.1 kg/m^3 exactly. The torr was defined as the exact fraction 1/760 of a standard atmosphere, and differed trivially from the mmHg (at the eighth significant figure).

Anglo-Saxon Units. Where units based on the FPS are met, care should be taken when they differ across the Atlantic. Not only do the UK and US gallons differ in definition and value but the UK fluid ounce is a different fraction (1/160) of its gallon from the fraction (1/128) used by its US counterpart for which logical powers of 2 extend further down the scale. Also, in the US the ton (2240 lb) is called the long ton, there being a short ton (2000 lb).

TABLE 1.5
EXAMPLES OF CONVERSION FACTORS FROM OTHER UNITS TO SI UNITS
(See main text for comments)

Name of unit	Symbol	Value for guidance	Value to be used for greater precision	
Area				
are	a	100 m²	1.0	× 10² m²
square foot	ft²	929 cm²	9.290 30	× 10⁻² m²
square inch	in²	6.45 cm²	6.4516	× 10⁻⁴ m²
square yard	yd²	0.836 m²	8.361 27	× 10⁻¹ m²
Density				
gram per cubic centimetre	g/cm³	1 kg/L	1.0	× 10³ kg/m³
pound per cubic foot	lb/ft³	16.0 kg/m³	1.601 85	× 10¹ kg/m³
pound per gallon (UK)	lb/gal	99.8 kg/m³	9.977 64	× 10¹ kg/m³
Energy				
British thermal unit	Btu	1.06 kJ	1.055 06	× 10³ J
calorie, at 15°C	cal₁₅	4.19 J	4.1855	J
erg	erg	100 nJ	1.0	× 10⁻⁷ J
foot poundal	ft·pdl	42.1 mJ	4.214 01	× 10⁻² J
foot pound–force	ft·lbf	1.36 J	1.355 82	J
horsepower–hour	hp·h	2.68 MJ	2.684 52	× 10⁶ J
kilogram–force metre	kgf·m	9.81 J	9.806 65	J
kilowatt hour	kW·h	3.6 MJ	3.6	× 10⁶ J
litre atmosphere	l·atm	101 J	1.013 25	× 10² J
therm	therm	106 MJ	1.055 06	× 10⁸ J
Force				
dyne	dyn	10 µN	1.0	× 10⁻⁵ N
kilogram–force	kgf	9.81 N	9.806 65	N
poundal	pdl	138 mN	1.382 55	× 10⁻¹ N
pound–force	lbf	4.45 N	4.448 22	N
ton–force (UK)	tonf	9.96 kN	9.964 02	× 10³ N
Length				
ångström	Å	0.1 nm	1.0	× 10⁻¹⁰ m
foot	ft	30.5 cm	3.048	× 10⁻¹ m
inch	in	2.54 cm	2.54	× 10⁻² m
mile (statute)	mile	1.61 km	1.609 34	× 10³ m
yard	yd	0.914 m	9.144	× 10⁻¹ m
Mass				
dram	dr	1.77 g	1.771 85	× 10⁻³ kg
grain	gr	64.8 mg	6.479 89	× 10⁻⁵ kg
hundredweight (UK)	cwt	50.8 kg	5.080 23	× 10¹ kg
ounce, avoirdupois	oz	28.3 g	2.834 95	× 10⁻² kg
pound, avoirdupois	lb	454 g	4.535 92	× 10⁻¹ kg
stone (UK)	stone	6.35 kg	6.350 29	kg
ton (UK)	ton	1020 kg	1.016 05	× 10³ kg
tonne	t	1000 kg	1.0	× 10³ kg
Power				
British thermal unit per hour	Btu/h	293 mW	2.930 71	× 10⁻¹ W
foot poundal per second	ft·pdl/s	42.1 mW	4.214 01	× 10⁻² W
foot pound–force per second	ft·lbf/s	1.36 W	1.355 82	W
horsepower, British	hp	746 W	7.457 00	× 10² W
kilogram–force metre per second	kgf·m/s	9.81 W	9.806 65	W
Pressure, mechanical stress				
bar	bar	100 kPa	1.0	× 10⁵ Pa
dyne per square centimetre	dyn/cm²	0.1 Pa	1.0	× 10⁻¹ Pa
foot of water	ftH₂O	2.99 kPa	2.989 07	× 10³ Pa
inch of mercury	inHg	3.39 kPa	3.386 39	× 10³ Pa
inch of water	inH₂O	249 Pa	2.490 89	× 10² Pa

TABLE 1.5—*contd.*

Name of unit	Symbol	Value for guidance	Value to be used for greater precision	
Pressure, mechanical stress—contd.				
kilogram–force per square metre	kgf/m²	9.81 Pa	9.806 65	Pa
millimetre of mercury	mmHg	133 Pa	1.333 22	$\times 10^2$ Pa
millimetre of water	mmH$_2$O	9.81 Pa	9.806 65	Pa
poundal per square foot	pdl/ft²	1.49 Pa	1.488 16	Pa
pound–force per square foot	lbf/ft²	47.9 Pa	4.788 03	$\times 10^1$ Pa
pound–force per square inch	lbf/in²	6.89 kPa	6.894 76	$\times 10^3$ Pa
standard atmosphere	atm	101 kPa	1.013 25	$\times 10^5$ Pa
ton–force per square foot (UK)	tonf/ft²	107 kPa	1.072 52	$\times 10^5$ Pa
torr	Torr	133 Pa	1.333 22	$\times 10^2$ Pa
Radioactivity quantities				
curie	Ci	37 GBq	3.7	$\times 10^{10}$ Bq
curie per gram	Ci/g	37 TBq/kg	3.7	$\times 10^{13}$ Bq/kg
erg per gram	erg/g	100 µGy	1.0	$\times 10^{-4}$ Gy
rad	rad	10 mGy	1.0	$\times 10^{-2}$ Gy
rem	rem	10 mSv	1.0	$\times 10^{-2}$ Sv
röntgen	R	258 µC/kg	2.58	$\times 10^{-4}$ C/kg
röntgen per second	R/s	258 µA/kg	2.58	$\times 10^{-4}$ A/kg
Surface tension				
dyne per centimetre	dyn/cm	1 mN/m	1.0	$\times 10^{-3}$ N/m
poundal per foot	pdl/ft	454 mN/m	4.535 92	$\times 10^{-1}$ N/m
pound–force per foot	lbf/ft	14.6 N/m	1.459 39	$\times 10^1$ N/m
Velocity				
foot per second	ft/s	30.5 cm/s	3.048	$\times 10^{-1}$ m/s
inch per second	in/s	25.4 mm/s	2.54	$\times 10^{-2}$ m/s
kilometre per hour	km/h	27.8 cm/s	2.777 78	$\times 10^{-1}$ m/s
mile per hour	mile/h	44.7 cm/s	4.470 40	$\times 10^{-1}$ m/s
Viscosity, dynamic				
centipoise	cP	1 mPa·s	1.0	$\times 10^{-3}$ Pa·s
poise	P	0.1 Pa·s	1.0	$\times 10^{-1}$ Pa·s
Viscosity, kinematic				
centistokes	cSt	1 mm²/s	1.0	$\times 10^{-6}$ m²/s
stokes	St	1 cm²/s	1.0	$\times 10^{-4}$ m²/s
Volume, capacity				
cubic foot	ft³	28.3 L	2.831 68	$\times 10^{-2}$ m³
cubic inch	in³	16.4 ml	1.638 71	$\times 10^{-5}$ m³
cubic yard	yd³	0.765 m³	7.645 55	$\times 10^{-1}$ m³
fluid ounce (UK)	fl oz	28.4 ml	2.841 30	$\times 10^{-5}$ m³
fluid ounce (US)	fl oz	29.6 ml	2.957 35	$\times 10^{-5}$ m³
gallon (UK)	gal	4.55 L	4.546 09	$\times 10^{-3}$ m³
gallon (US)	gal	3.79 L	3.785 41	$\times 10^{-3}$ m³
pint (UK)	pt	568 ml	5.682 61	$\times 10^{-4}$ m³
pint (liquid) (US)	liq pt	473 ml	4.731 76	$\times 10^{-4}$ m³

Units Based on Weight. In modern terms these have the word *force* (rather than *weight*) in their names. Their origin is practical; they derive from the use of physical weights as simple sources of force in early mechanical devices and in much ergometric apparatus. Irrespective of *where* such devices were used, the force units are defined in terms of standard gravitational acceleration (exactly 9.806 65 m/s²; approxim-ately 32.174 ft/s²). This explains why units involving the kilogram–force are about 9.81 times the corresponding SI unit, and why units involving the pound–force are about 32.2 times those using the poundal. The poundal and the newton are called *absolute* in contrast to *gravitational* units.

Litre-based Units. The reader may detect small discrepancies in conversion factors involving the litre (such as the litre atmosphere energy unit). The definition of the litre was changed in 1964 (12th Conférence Générale des Poids et Mesures: CGPM) from an experimentally determined value (1.000 028 dm³) to exactly 1 dm³.

Such differences have little practical effect (other than eroding confidence in quoted numbers), but it is important to know that from time to time aspects of even the SI may change. Fortunately, changes still to come are unlikely to affect medical measurements greatly. For example, a recent change takes the speed of light as reference and, to nine significant figures, leaves the metre to be determined in terms of it and the second. Readers need not be disturbed by this apparently arbitrary basis for so basic a unit; from before the 1000 paces of the Roman legionary, units have always been defined in terms of what has to be done, in principle, to demonstrate them.

APPENDIX AND GUIDE TO REFERENCES

Definitions of the SI Base Units

Many people are surprised to find that base *quantities*, as such, are not defined. This is because for generations, people have been taught that the act of defining is important and that everything is susceptible to this. To repeat that 'mass is the measure of the quantity of matter in a body' is acceptable provided it is recognized to be no more than a rather inadequate synonym. A better one is that it is *one* measure of the amount of matter, appropriate for discussing inertia and gravitational effects. It is better because it excludes measures such as volume or number of atoms.

In contrast the base *units* have precise and official definitions, which are included here for completeness. These definitions are adjusted occasionally in Resolutions of the Conférence Générale des Poids et Mesures (CGPM).

metre The metre is the length of the path travelled by light in vacuum during a time interval of 1/299 792 458 of a second. (17th CGPM, 1983.)

kilogram The kilogram is the unit of mass; it is equal to the mass of the international prototype of the kilogram. (3rd CGPM, 1901.)

second The second is the duration of 9 192 631 770 periods of the radiation corresponding to the transition between the two hyperfine levels of the ground state of the caesium 133 atom. (13th CGPM, 1967.)

ampere The ampere is that constant current which, if maintained in two straight parallel conductors of infinite length, of negligible circular cross-section, and placed 1 metre apart in vacuum, would produce between these conductors force equal to 2×10^{-7} newton per metre of length. (9th CGPM, 1948.)

kelvin The kelvin, unit of thermodynamic temperature, is the fraction 1/273.16 of the thermodynamic temperature of the triple point of water. (13th CGPM, 1967.)

mole 1. The mole is the amount of substance of a system which contains as many elementary entities as there are atoms in 0.012 kilogram of carbon 12.
2. When the mole is used, the elementary entities must be specified and may be atoms, molecules, ions, electrons, other particles, or specified groups of such particles. (14th CGPM, 1971.)

candela The candela is the luminous intensity, in a given direction, of a source that emits monochromatic radiation of frequency 540×10^{12} hertz and that has a radiant intensity in that direction of (1/683) watt per steradian. (16th CGPM, 1979.)

Definitions of the Radian and Steradian

These are included for completeness. The steradian in particular may be unfamiliar; it helps to quantify the degree to which phenomena such as radiations are directionally concentrated. Both have a clear purpose however: they simplify formulae for those who use them.

radian The radian is the plane angle between two radii of a circle which cut off on the circumference an arc equal in length to the radius.

steradian The steradian is the solid angle which, having its vertex in the centre of a sphere, cuts off an area of the surface of the sphere equal to that of a square with sides of length equal to the radius of the sphere.

SI as a Coherent System

Coherent unit systems have only one unit for each physical quantity and the relationships between units involve multiplication and division with no numerical factor *other than the number one* (1). For example the unit of speed is 1 metre divided by 1 second, and the unit of energy is 1 unit of force (newton) multiplied by 1 metre. There are therefore no awkward scaling factors to be committed to memory. Since all equations between physical quantities have precisely the same form as those between their numerical values the number of relationships to be remembered is greatly reduced.

An example of non-coherence is the use of millimetre of mercury for pressure and litre for volume. Their product yields a work unit of approximately

133.3 millijoules which is inconvenient even if noticed to be *about* 4/30 J. In the past such situations have led to the evolution of special units such as (here) the litre–millimetre of mercury and the analogous litre–atmosphere. The argument against this solution is that the evolved unit may be unknown outside a particular field and correspondence with other work may be obscured. There is also a subtle educational danger when (as here) the awkward factor is seen to be approximated by some simple fraction: the progression from inconvenient factor to a supposed exact relationship and thence to a putative natural law is almost inevitable. Most dangerous of all are those happy accidents which produce factors *close to unity*; these can lead to the false impression that the quantities so related as essentially *identical*.

Warning on the Use of the Litre

Although the litre is accepted for use in association with SI this is on the understanding that it is *no more* than as the special name for the cubic decimetre, which is exactly one-thousandth of the cubic metre, the SI unit.

For example, in anaesthetic applications, the litre and the kilopascal (which is one thousand times the SI unit) are often used together. The product of pressure and volume has the same dimensions as energy (as does the work involved in breathing), and the product $kPa \cdot L$ is exactly the same as $Pa \cdot m^3$: both yield the joule. However if the litre is used in conjunction with some unprefixed SI unit, a factor of 1000 can slip in unnoticed. For example, the density of room air is of the order of one SI unit, say $1.2 \, kg/m^3$. If we retain the kg but use the litre the value is $0.0012 \, kg/L$, which is $1.2 \, g/L$. Notice that the 1.2 reappears because both numerator and denominator are thousandths of the SI unit. The particular danger occurs when using a formula intended for physicists or engineers and unthinkingly substituting numerical values familiar to habitual litre-users. Such errors are more insidious than, for example, translating between flow rates based on minutes and those using seconds; the factor of 60 is less easily obscured.

A similar source of error involving a factor of 1000 is carried over from early teaching of 'molecular weight' (relative molecular mass). On changing to SI it would have been chaotic to redefine the mole substantially. Although it is comforting to know that, for example, a mole of substance of relative molecular mass 12 still has a mass of 12 grams, if we substitute into a formula which 'expects' base SI units this is $0.012 \, kg$.

The Naming of Compound Units

This is best understood from representative examples. There are two sensible conventions: the avoidance of unacceptable phrases such as 'cubic second' and 'square ampere', and the absence of confusing repeti-tions of the word 'per' (as for the solidus; *see* Convention 6).

dynamic viscosity	$Pa \cdot s$	pascal second
metabolic heat production	W/m^2	watt per square metre
acceleration	m/s^2	metre per second squared
specific volume	m^3/kg	cubic metre per kilogram
molar heat capacity	$J/(mol \cdot K)$	joule per mole kelvin
Avogadro constant	mol^{-1}	reciprocal mole
number density of molecules	m^{-3}	reciprocal cubic metre

Guide to References for the Chapter

References for this subject serve three main purposes. In the first they present the essential facts about base and supplementary units, special names and symbols and the formalities of writing these; all references naturally quote the ultimate international scientific authority on these matters. The second purpose embraces an extension to all possible derived units, for which offical recommendations include some degree of reasonable flexibility within clearly defined limits. The third concerns the reasons which underlie official decisions and draws on the historical development of SI. No one reference covers all aspects equally well so the following quide to some which have authoritative status is offered here.

1. Bell R. J., Goldman David T., eds. (1986). *SI The International System of Units*. London: HMSO.
   This is the translation, approved by the Bureau International des Poids et Mesures (BIPM), of its publication *Le Système International d'Unités* (SI). In addition to the usual definitions of SI base and supplementary quantities and related tables, it gives a clear historical account of the relevant decisions made by CGPM and CIPM and outlines the organization and functions of CGPM and of the CIPM and its various Consultative Committees. Its main merit lies in the broad view of the subject it presents.
2. Lowe D. Armstrong (1975). *Progress in Standardization*: 2. *A Guide to International Recommendations on Names and Symbols for Quantities and on Units of Measurement*. Geneva: WHO.
   This also gives an account of SI and information on prefixes and printing and has various technical appendices, but its two major sections present symbols and units for an extremely wide range of quantities and conversion factors to SI for a very large range of units. The view is taken that there is virtually no limit to the current and potential applications of the physical to the biological sciences. Despite some changes in SI since this was published, it is still a useful broadly based reference.

3. BS 350 *Conversion Factors and Tables*: Part 1: 1974 (1983) *Basis of tables, conversion factors.*
   This covers a wide range of conversion factors and is particularly clear and authoritative on the subject of Imperial and some US measures. As with many British Standards it is widely available in major public libraries in the UK.
4. BS 5555: (1981) *SI Units and Recommendations for the Use of their Multiples and of Certain Other Units.*
   This corresponds to the *International Standard* ISO 1000–1981. It deals with base and supplementary units, decimal prefixes, special units associated with SI, and rules of printing. It also lists suggested decimal multiples and submultiples of SI and some other units for a wide range of derived quantities. In this respect it gives a fairly broad view and is best used in conjunction with the next reference; but see also Reference 6.
5. BS 5775: *Quantities, Units and Symbols.*
   This is in fourteen parts all of which are equivalent to the corresponding parts of the *International Standard* ISO 31. The first (called Part 0) is devoted to general principles. It deals clearly with quantities, units, prefixes, notations and printing conventions; it also clarifies the proper use of technical terms such as coefficients, factors and parameters and others such as specific, density, linear, surface, molar and concentration. Despite its formality it is very readable. Part 11 is devoted to mathematical signs and symbols, and Part 12 deals with dimensionless parameters (of which the Reynolds number is most likely to be known by anaesthetists).

The other Parts (1 to 10 and 13) are concerned with various branches of physical science, giving tables of quantities, quantity symbols, identifying definitions and remarks. Facing these are corresponding units, their symbols, definitions and important conversion factors and other information (including annexes on FPS and other units).

6. *ISO Standards Handbook: 2 Units of Measurement* (1982) 2nd edn. Geneva: International Organization for Standardization.
   This is a convenient collection of the international standards referred to in (4) and (5): ISO 1000–1982(E) and the fourteen sections of ISO 31 (various dates). It is reduced only in page size.

Updated Numerical Values

When several sources of data on conversion factors and Universal constants are consulted, small discrepancies may be detected, fortunately usually in low significant figures. For conversion factors, the values given by the ISO (and thence by BSI) are to be preferred; they are periodically amended, and the fact of amendment recorded in the BSI and ISO catalogues. The ultimate authority for Universal constants is the International Council of Scientific Unions Committee on Data for Science and Technology whose interdisciplinary committee (CODATA) issues bulletins, published by Pergamon Press, on this and many other topics. In 1987 the appropriate CODATA bulletins were Number 11 (1973) adjusted by Number 63 (1986).

2. Physical Principles
D. Strickland

Mechanical quantities
  Base quantities
  Displacement, speed, velocity and
    acceleration
  Force
  The triangle of vectors
  Resolution of vectors
  Work and energy
  Momentum
  Rotation of bodies
  Angular velocity and moment of inertia
  Centrifugal and centripetal force
  Power
  Pressure
  Temperature
  Pressure, volume and temperature of gases
  Types of problem involving the gas laws

The laws of Boyle and Charles
Avogadro's hypothesis
Partial pressure (Dalton's Law)
The gas laws for real gases
Specific heats of gases
Specific heat ratio
Adiabatic and isothermal changes
Solubility of gases in liquids
Bunsen and Ostwald solubility coefficients
Diffusion of gases—some preliminaries
The Fick diffusion equation
Krogh's diffusion coefficient
Diffusion capacity of the lung
Graham's law of gaseous diffusion
Vapours, evaporation and saturation vapour
  pressure
Mixtures of gases and vapours
Cooling due to evaporation
Boiling and latent heat of vaporization
Humidity
Condensation and dew-point
Viscosity

MECHANICAL QUANTITIES

In this chapter basic mechanical quantities are defined and discussed. It is helpful when considering physical science, to look for some underlying pattern. It is natural to think in terms of linear relationships between cause and effect, and this aspect will be stressed.

The historical order of the subject will not be adhered to, since revision is often made more efficient by taking as a starting-point some fact or concept which is now well-established. For example, when dealing with the equations of state of gases, the Kinetic Theory definition of temperature is taken as basic, and mercury and other thermometers are regarded as imperfect measuring instruments. Reference to Chapter 4 can then be made for detailed explanation of temperature as a problem of measurement.

In accordance with current practice the SI system of units (Système Internationale d'Unités) will be used in this chapter, but reference will be made to other units which are still in common use.

Base Quantities

Mechanical science has developed in terms of certain base quantities, including *mass*, *length* and *time*, which are regarded as analogous to the fundamental axioms of mathematics. It is not easy to produce satisfactory definitions of these quantities, since it is in the nature of definitions that they should refer new concepts back to ones which are already understood. Statements such as 'mass is the measure of the quantity of matter in a body', or 'time is the measure of separation of events' lack the precision of other definitions, e.g. 'velocity is the rate of change of displacement with time' for exactly this reason.

It is profitable, however, to extend the discussion of mass by considering how we are aware of it. We do not assess mass by counting atoms and estimating the 'quantity of matter' in one atom. Our immediate awareness of mass is due to the inertial opposition we sense when we shake an object. Again, the fact that we evolved on the surface of a planet makes us aware that the more massive a body is (in the sense of offering inertial opposition to shaking), the more strongly it is pulled towards the centre of the planet. This has sometimes led to confusion between mass and *weight*, a confusion reinforced by the unfortunate use of the same or similar units to measure two quite different quantities.

Whether mass is assessed by inertial opposition to change of motion or by the local earth-surface convenient technique of weighing, it becomes clear that mass is a scalar quantity. By a scalar quantity, we mean one which is fully described by a number and a unit. If one walks two miles the distance covered is described entirely by the number '2' and the unit 'mile'. In contrast a *vector* quantity requires a statement of *direction*. For example, when navigating a ship it is important to know the direction as well as the magnitude of the ship's motion, since 2 miles south is not equivalent to 2 miles north in a crowded shipping lane. To return to mass, two bodies which are separately assessed to have the same mass as the standard kilogram will, when together, produce twice the observed effects (of opposition to motional change, or of weight on the earth's surface) as each separately. Unlike mass, weight is a *vector* quantity requiring, in addition to number and unit, the specification of direction.

Unit lengths, such as the metre, were also primarily defined by reference to some standard separation, such as that between two marks on a specially constructed and preserved object. Greater precision and greater trust in constancy was achieved (at the expense of less direct apprehension) by taking the wavelength of some specific light emanation as standard. More recently the metre has been defined in terms of the distance travelled by light in a specified time (*see* Chapter 1). Similarly, although the second was originally defined in terms of astronomical observations on the motion of our slightly wobbling and slowing-down planet, it is now compared to the periods of oscillation of identifiable atomic events.

Displacement, Speed, Velocity and Acceleration

The speed of a moving object is the time-rate at which it covers distance along its path, and this exemplifies a human tendency to define new quantities as the rates of change of more familiar ones. Experience shows that there are differences in both result and techniques between running in circles and running in straight lines. The distinction hinges on the extension of the scalar concept of distance (which is applicable to paths straight or crooked) to the vector concept of *displacement*. Displacement is distance measured in a specified direction, and a circular tour leaves no resultant displacement despite the distance covered. When direction is associated with speed, we use the specially committed term *velocity* (time-rate of change of displacement) to describe the derived vector quantity. The need for this distinction becomes clear when we consider how vector quantities combine, by the well-known triangle of vectors.

When we are moving we are aware of velocity by observations on other objects which we recede from or approach, or whose apparent spatial disposition changes by parallax. Our awareness of *acceleration* (time-rate of change of velocity) is much more direct, due to the jolts and shakings our bodies experience when their velocities *change*. A car-driver may sense an acceleration of less than 1 metre per second in each second ($1\,\mathrm{m\,s^{-2}}$), while being completely unaware of his velocity of (say) 30 thousand metres per second towards Jupiter. Another aspect of acceleration that justifies its formal incorporation into our descriptive terminology is that to achieve acceleration on a flat surface, an unaided human being must exert some thrust. This is particularly clear when skating, because a velocity, once achieved, requires negligible effort to maintain.

Force

The abundance of lay terms relating to the activity of pushing, thrusting, lifting and hauling inert objects testifies to its relevance to our way of describing the physical world. The word *force* has been selected for formal definition, and should (in scientific discussion) be precisely used. What a force does depends on where it is applied. For example, it may

1. Compress a resilient object—effecting a *displacement*
2. Keep a body moving on a frictional surface—maintaining a *velocity*
3. Change the velocity of a body—effecting an *acceleration*

Any reproducible and measurable effect could have been taken as the basis of definition, and as an interim measure we will consider the acceleration phenomenon. The most obvious definition of unit force is that, freely applied, it gives unit mass unit acceleration in the direction of application. Consequently, the obvious metric unit is the kilogram (kg) times the metre per second per second. The urges to abbreviate and to celebrate have contracted the obvious ($1\,\mathrm{kg\,m\,s^{-2}}$) to the *newton* (N). It must be admitted that we all forget the meaning of such compressed unit-names from time to time, and it is a useful discipline to associate the name with both the quantity defined and with its true meaning. Thus one newton (of force) gives one kg (of mass) an acceleration of $1\,\mathrm{m\,s^{-2}}$. Similarly the CGS unit, the dyne, gives $1\,\mathrm{g}$ mass an acceleration of $1\,\mathrm{cm\,s^{-2}}$. Conversion factors become obvious in terms of true meanings. Thus, since $1\,\mathrm{N}$ gives $1000\,\mathrm{g}$ an acceleration of $100\,\mathrm{cm\,s^{-2}}$, it is obviously 100 000 times as large as the dyne. A newton is the order of force necessary to support a large cup of coffee.

Gravitational Units

In the past, complications have been introduced due to parochialism, not only with national units such as the FPS system, but also with the local terrestrial-surface gravitational units. Due to the universal attraction between bodies, our local large body (the Earth) forces us continuously towards its centre, countered by the resilience of objects that we deform by standing on them. In Fig. 2.1, a body E in England is being pulled towards a body P in Peru. By symmetry, there will be some comparable body J somewhere around Java exerting an equal force at E which will in consequence be affected as if by the two strings of a catapult. The resultant force passes through the Earth's centre, and the same will be true for all such pairs—in fact this defines the gravitational centre of the Earth. The total force on E depends on its mass (m, say), and removing any support under E exposes it to an unopposed force W, or

$$W = km$$

where k depends on the mass of the Earth and on its radius. This force W is the *weight* of the body, at the surface of the Earth. Since force is mass multiplied by acceleration, the factor of proportionality k is the

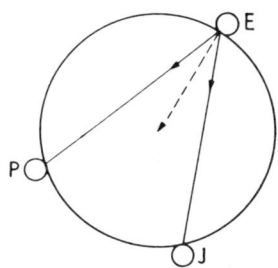

Fig. 2.1

acceleration measured when objects fall at the Earth's surface. Usually this is denoted by g, the (local) gravitational acceleration of 9.81 m s^{-2} (to three significant figures). Hence the formula

$$W = mg$$

is a special example of the more general law

$$F = ma$$

Other Aspects of Force

Complex systems, such as air flowing in the lungs, involve forces which fulfil different functions according to where they occur. Friction, such as in viscous drag, demands an applied force to maintain even an unchanging velocity, while elastic recoil of tissue and the compression of gases demand forces to maintain displacements. These requirements are in addition to the demands of acceleration when the velocities of gases and tissues are changed. In the simplest cases, and in approximations to real situations, there are *linear* laws similar to Newton's $F = ma$. The simplest frictional law is

$$F = rv$$

where v is the velocity and r gives a measure of resistance (frictional force required per unit velocity maintained), just as m measures inertia as inertial force required per unit acceleration achieved.

For resilient systems the simplest (linear) law is

$$F = sx$$

where x is the displacement caused by force F. Here the factor of proportionality, s, is the force of compression needed per unit displacement caused, and it assesses the stiffness of the system. Where interest centres on pressure rather than force and on volume rather than linear displacement, analogous relationships can be proposed and their validity investigated. Such analogous relationships illustrate the tendency to look for linear relationships and to define new quantities as ratios of previously defined ones. Lung compliance is an example of this.

The Triangle of Vectors

If a body is displaced (Fig. 2.2) from A to B, and then to C it is obvious that the result is the same as if it had gone direct from A to C. We are distinguishing between *distance* (path ABC is obviously greater than path AC) and the vector *displacement*. Having left A and arrived at C by any path, such as P, the net displacement is still n units of length in the direction A-to-C. The vector displacements A-to-B and B-to-C add according to the triangle rule to give A-to-C. This addition can be regarded as calculation by means of a map.

Mapping is used by navigators to obtain resultant velocities, since velocity is rate of change of displace-

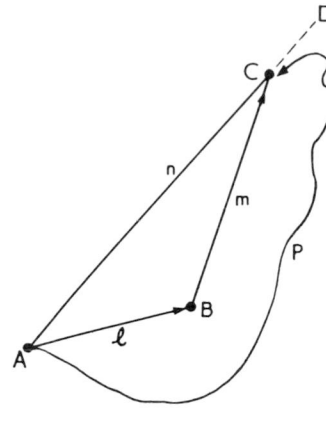

Fig. 2.2

ment. For example, suppose that the body moves with velocity l/t in the direction A-to-B, and that simultaneously it is given a velocity m/t parallel to BC. In time t it will arrive at C and the effect will be the same as a single velocity n/t along direction A-to-C. Consequently the same 'map', with a scale interpreted in terms of velocity, can be used to add velocities. Similarly, accelerations, being rates of change of velocities can be mapped and added, while forces, being proportional to accelerations yield to the same technique. The parallelogram of forces (or any vectors) is merely an alternative construction (Fig. 2.3) in which the vector

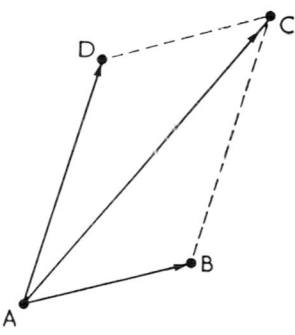

Fig. 2.3

arrows (AB, AD) are for convenience located at the same starting-point on the map, and the resultant is represented in magnitude and direction by the diagonal AC from the same starting-point.

Resolution of Vectors

In Fig. 2.4, J represents a joint and interest is focussed on the thrust F_1, towards it. This is called the component of the total force F in the direction shown, and F_1 is one of the pair of forces F_1, F_2 such that if they were applied simultaneously the effect would be indistinguishable from the single force F. The inverse process to combining vectors to obtain their resultant

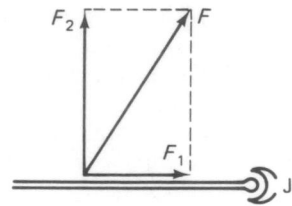

Fig. 2.4

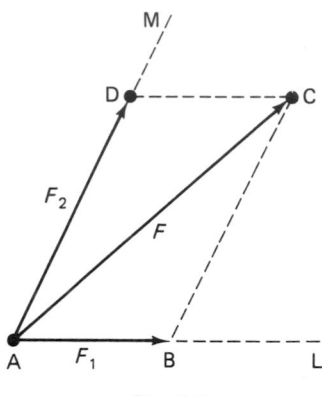

Fig. 2.5

Consequently the formulae

$$F_1 = F \cos \theta$$

$$\text{and} \quad F_2 = F \sin \theta$$

for such situations are frequently used and regarded as obvious.

Work and Energy

To define the *work* done by a system, and its *energy* (capacity for doing work) requires some refinement of the intuitive and often vague lay concepts from which the terms were borrowed. Energy is manifested in many forms, such as mechanical, electrical, thermal, chemical, nuclear and electromagnetic. In addition, there are lay terms such as 'fatigue' to confuse the issue since one can certainly become 'fatigued' leaning against a wall. When it was realized that energy is conserved when converted from one form to another, it became clear that a definition in terms of mechanical events would serve as a basis.

Other units, such as the calorie, can be related to mechanical units by experimental determination.

In Fig. 2.7 a force is applied to a body and moves it

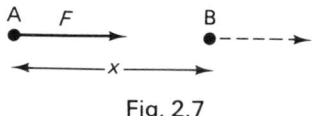

Fig. 2.7

a distance x from A to B. Intuitively one feels that more work is done if the necessary force F is greater, and that more is done the larger x becomes. Accordingly, the work done is defined as

$$\text{Work} = Fx$$

The unit of work is therefore the work done when unit force moves its point of application unit distance *in its own direction*. The specification of direction is necessary, as is clear in Fig. 2.8. Here a body is being

is called *resolving* them into components. In Fig. 2.5 we wish to know the forces which, acting along two directions AL, AM would produce the same effect as F. The parallelogram constructed with a diagonal proportional to F and with sides parallel to AL, AM yields components F_1, F_2 whose magnitudes can be measured (or calculated by trigonometry) from this map, or 'vector diagram'.

Often the selected directions are perpendicular to one another for the excellent reason that a force along AY (Fig. 12.6) has no influence on motion along AX,

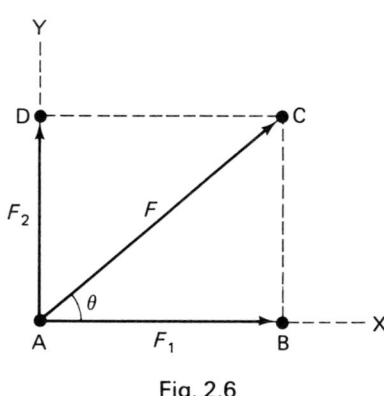

Fig. 2.6

so that the resulting perpendicular motions can be analysed separately. For this special case, F_1 and F_2 can easily be calculated, since

$$\text{AB/AC} = \cos \theta$$

$$\text{and} \quad \text{BC/AC} = \sin \theta$$

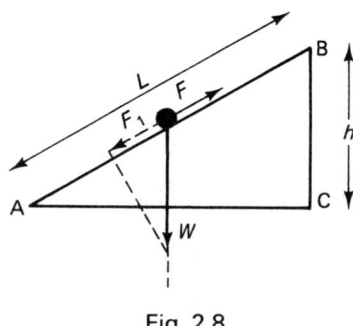

Fig. 2.8

pulled up a well-lubricated ramp. Ramps, like gears and levers, are constructed so that a given amount of work can be performed by application of a restricted force, albeit acting over a greater distance. If the body had been raised directly through height h, the work done would have been the large force (W) multiplied by the small distance (h). With the ramp, it is the relatively small force F which is needed to overcome the component F_1 of W in the direction shown. The work done is this smaller force multiplied by the correspondingly greater distance L in the direction of that force. Since h is the same fraction ($\sin \theta$) of L as F is of W, the work done is the same, with or without the ramp, for

$$Wh = FL$$

It is important to distinguish between useful work done by a machine or a human and the non-productive work done maintaining muscle tone when the human applies force to an unmoving object. Such work involves chemical activity and is difficult to measure, but of course this is no reason why it should not be expressed in mechanical units.

The SI unit of work is the newton (of force) multiplied by the metre, and is abbreviated to the joule (J). The CGS unit is the *erg* of work, being that done by a dyne of force moving its point of application through 1 cm in its own direction. Since the newton is 100 000 dynes and the metre is 100 cm,

$$1\,J = 10^7\,\text{erg}$$

The joule is a convenient unit for measuring the work done by human beings performing simple every-day activities such as raising moderately large drinks from table to lip. Work is as obviously scalar in nature as is volume of liquid.

Potential and Kinetic Energy

Since the energy of a system is its capacity for doing work, the same units are involved. Energy units include various versions of the calorie, all of the order of 4.2 joules, but the current trend is to express all energies in terms of joules.

When dealing with mechanical energy it is usual, as a matter of convenience, to distinguish between kinetic energy (k.e.) and potential energy (p.e.). If, relative to some point regarded as fixed, a body initially at rest is given a velocity, work has to be done

since force must be applied over a distance in order to accelerate the body. This work is in effect stored as kinetic energy, and may in principle be recovered by arranging that the body passes on its energy to whatever stops it. Apart from interchange between mass and energy in nuclear events, energy is simply conserved during interchanges.

The kinetic energy of a body of mass m moving with velocity v with respect to the fixed point (reference frame) is given by

$$\text{k.e.} = \tfrac{1}{2}mv^2$$

This formula, with one factor squared, has many counterparts in energy calculations, and it is instructive to consider it in more detail. It is reasonable that the energy is proportional to the mass, since doubling the mass would, for a given history of acceleration leading up to the velocity v, require double the force over the same path. To appreciate the v^2 term, imagine a man pushing a car from rest. Suppose that he exerts a constant force, and that by the time v is $1\,\text{m s}^{-1}$ he has travelled $10\,\text{m}$. Since the average velocity is $0.5\,\text{m s}^{-1}$ this part of the operation would take 20 seconds. If he continues until v becomes $2\,\text{m s}^{-1}$, since the force, and hence the acceleration, is constant he will have pushed for 40 seconds. The overall average velocity being $1\,\text{m s}^{-1}$, the total distance would be 40 m. He therefore applies the force over *four times* the distance required to reach $1\,\text{m s}^{-1}$ in order to produce *double* this velocity. Consequently four times as much energy is expended. These results are summarized in Fig. 2.9. Notice that the v^2 term is justified by the need to quadruple the distance while doubling the velocity. The factor $\tfrac{1}{2}$ in the formula can be explained by investigating the detail. The work done by force F acting over distance x is

$$\text{Work} = Fx$$

If the time taken is t, the acceleration is v/t, so

$$\text{Work} = m(v/t)x$$

Since the average velocity is $\tfrac{1}{2}v$, the distance x is

$$x = (\tfrac{1}{2}v)t$$

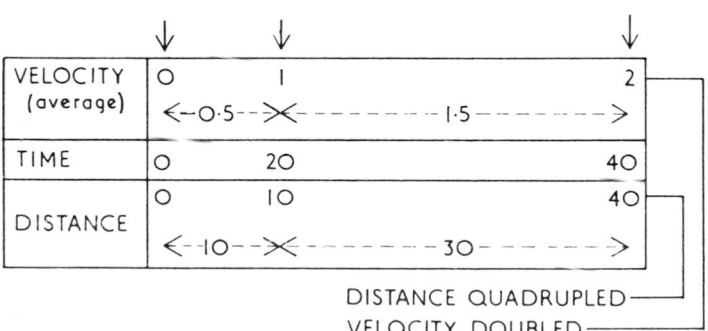

Fig. 2.9

and substitution yields

$$\text{Work} = \tfrac{1}{2}mv^2$$

A further point to note is that, in terms of velocity, this formula is non-linear in contrast with the linear relationships we are pre-disposed to seek. This is solely a consequence of our decision to relate the k.e. to the velocity, rather than to the path-length x, to which the k.e. is linearly related. This decision is a rational one however, since the k.e. is a function of the velocity no matter how this velocity was achieved. We have chosen the application of a constant force in order to derive the result simply. The same result can be obtained with a varying force by application of the calculus.

It will be seen later that the equation of the state of a perfect gas ($P = RT/V$) involves a non-linear relationship between the parameters P and V by which we elect to describe the state of the gas, although this is based on a linear relationship between mean molecular kinetic energy and the absolute temperature of the sample.

Potential Energy. The energy possessed by a mechanical system by virtue of its present geometrical configuration (as opposed to its state of motion) is exemplified by springs which are distorted against the tendency for the molecules to retain their original layout, and by bodies poised under the influence of a gravity. When a body is raised against gravity, work must be done; the body and the Earth somewhat resembling a spring that is being stretched. To raise a mass m through a height h where the gravitational acceleration is g (that is, the weight is mg) demands mgh units of work to be done, or

$$\text{p.e.} = mgh$$

Here the energy is linearly related to the height, and height is the obvious parameter to measure.

The simplest spring requires a force F to stretch it a distance x given by

$$F = sx$$

At the beginning of stretching ($x = 0$) the force is zero, so the average is $\tfrac{1}{2}F$. This gives the result

$$\text{p.e.} = \tfrac{1}{2}Fx$$
$$= \tfrac{1}{2}sx^2$$

which is analogous to the k.e. formula.

Momentum

When a body is about to collide with another and give up all its energy, for example in the form of heat, the parameter that best describes the moving body is its k.e. ($\tfrac{1}{2}mv^2$). In contrast, in a perfectly *elastic* collision there is no wasted energy, and the best parameter to describe the oncoming body in those circumstances is

known as its momentum, mv. A vivid distinction between

$$\text{k.e.} = \tfrac{1}{2}mv^2$$

and

$$\text{momentum} = mv$$

is provided by the invention of the elastic-recoil jewellers' window, which returns bricks to would-be robbers. Whereas a conventional window shatters with production of heat and sound and the rupture of the bonds between particles of glass, and leaves a motionless brick in the wreckage, the more sophisticated window reverses the sense of the velocity of the brick. During this operation the brick exerts a force on the window (and *vice versa*) just as in the case of a gas molecule rebounding from the wall of the container. This force is equal to the *rate of change of momentum*, since,

$$F = ma$$

where a = rate of change of v,

so F = rate of change of mv.

This relationship is in fact a more general definition of force than the interim one given earlier, since it covers cases in which the mass is changing as well as the velocity, as for example when a rocket consumes its fuel.

When dealing with kinetic theory of gases, use will be made of momentum. If one is concerned with heat exchange, kinetic energy is the relevant parameter, but when considering pressure it is the reversal of momentum that is important. Like velocity, momentum is a vector quantity, and corresponding to the conservation of energy in a closed system there is a law of conservation of momentum in collisions. This law states that, measured in any direction, the algebraic sum of the products of mass and velocity of colliding bodies is unchanged by the collision. At first sight a mathematically inclined criminal might be surprised to see his brick returned with its momentum reversed, but precise measurement would reveal that the jeweller's shop and the Earth had gained momentum in the opposite direction immediately after the impact. The associated velocity change would be exceedingly small because the mass in the Earth is so large. However, astronauts and people in punts do well to avoid throwing massive objects.

Although we shall mainly discuss perfectly elastic collisions, the law of conservation of momentum is quite general. Two extreme examples are: (a) two perfect billiard balls colliding head-on and then recoiling with equal and *opposite* velocities, and (b) two flaccid cushions meeting with equal and opposite velocities and simply stopping. In each case the *total* momentum in any direction is unchanged. In the latter case all the k.e. is converted to heat.

Moments

Figure 2.10 illustrates a force applied to a lever, caus-

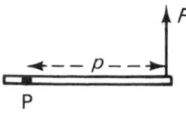

Fig. 2.10

ing it to rotate about P. It is a common experience that the effectiveness of such a force in imparting twist depends both on the magnitude of the force and on the distance p perpendicular to the line of action. The measure of twist-effectiveness is called the *moment* or *torque* and is defined as the product

$$\text{moment} = Fp$$

Although this has the same dimensions as work (both involving force multiplied by distance) it is an important distinction that p is a purely geometrical factor and is measured at right-angles to the line of action. If the lever moves, work will be done, but this will be the product of F and the distance moved by F *along* its line of action. To maintain this distinction the terms newton and metre are not combined into the joule, and the SI unit of torque is the newton-metre (N m). Another important distinction between work and torque is that the former is a scalar while the latter requires specification of sense of rotation.

The two most common classes of problem involving moments concern equilibrium (prevention of rotation) and rotary motion as such. Figure 2.11 shows an equilibrium situation. The clockwise moment due to the large force F' applied less effectively (smaller p')

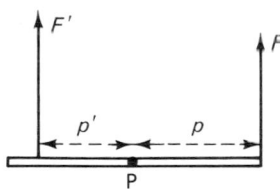

Fig. 2.11

equals the counter-clockwise product of the smaller force F and the larger p, or

$$F'p' = Fp$$

Similarly in Fig. 2.12 F' is necessarily larger than F. Figure 2.13 illustrates the price paid for the convenience of exerting a smaller force, since arranging that p'

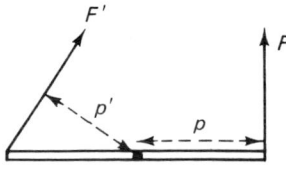

Fig. 2.12

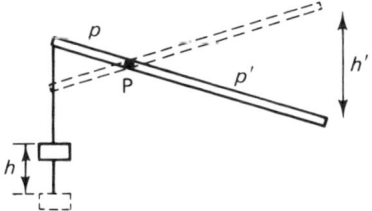

Fig. 2.13

is greater than p requires the user to push for a greater distance *along* the line of action when the lever is used. Geometrically, h' is greater than h by the same factor as p' is greater than p. As in the case of the ramp, the work done is exactly the same whether the lever is used or not. Levers and gears (continuous levers) are examples of transformer-like devices in which one factor (force for example) is in effect traded for another (displacement) to satisfy a requirement of matching a load to a source of energy which has limitations set to the manner in which it can supply energy. An interesting example is the lever formed by the forearm which trades the large force available by small displacement muscles for the relatively small force but large displacement requirements of the moving hand in human actions such as throwing.

Rotation of Bodies

The application of a single force can produce a torque, but will tend to cause linear (i.e. translational) as well as rotational motion, as can be seen when one tries to spin a top with one finger. The application of two equal and opposite forces (as when using finger and thumb) produces rotation only, and since this technique has the effect of producing twist without wear on bearings it merits the special name *couple*. The moment (torque) of a couple is simply the sum of the moments due to the two forces.

The structure of laws and formulae that describe translational motion is exactly mirrored in the field of rotary motion. Just as force can change linear momentum and impart kinetic energy of translation, so a torque can give angular momentum and establish rotational kinetic energy. Figure 2.14 shows a small body constrained to move in a circular path. In

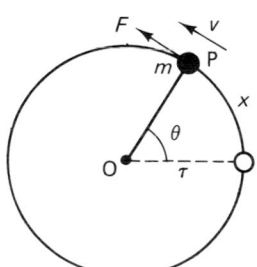

Fig. 2.14

general this body might be a particle within a solid object, but to establish some new ideas we will consider it separately and imagine that it is provided with a force F that continuously adjusts its line of action so as to be always perpendicular to OP. The torque τ, applied is

$$\tau = Fr$$

and we enquire how much work is done in moving round the arc x. The result

$$\text{Work} = Fx$$

is true but unrealistic, since in an extended body each particle has its own value of x, the particles nearer O travelling smaller distances x than those further out. However, we feel intuitively that more work is done if we have to apply larger torque, so substituting τ/r in place of F we see that

$$\text{Work} = \frac{\tau x}{r}$$

In radian measure, the angle θ is *defined* as the ratio of the arc x to the radius r, so

$$\text{Work} = \tau\theta$$

Notice that the angle θ is common to all particles of a rotating extended body, so θ is a sensible parameter to involve in calculations. The self-evident result, that the work done is proportional to the torque applied and to the angle turned shows an excellent reason for the existence of radian measure, since the formula is exactly analogous to the translational formula.

$$\text{Work} = Fx$$

Had θ been expressed in degrees the formula would have been

$$\text{Work} = \frac{2\pi}{360}\tau\theta$$

which is less obviously analogous.

Angular Velocity and Moment of Inertia

When the particle in Fig. 2.14 has been set into motion, the kinetic energy is $\frac{1}{2}mv^2$, but v is just as unrealistic a parameter as x. However all particles in a rotating body share the same rate of sweeping out angle round the axis, and this *angular velocity* is usually denoted by ω. Suppose that having reached a steady state the period of rotation is T seconds, then

$$\omega = \frac{2\pi}{T} \text{ radians per second}$$

Now in T seconds the particle covers a path $2\pi r$, so

$$v = \frac{2\pi r}{T}$$

Comparing these results shows that

$$v = r\omega$$

This enables us to express kinetic energy more realistically as

$$\text{k.e.} = \frac{1}{2}(mr^2)\omega^2$$

By using the special symbol I for the term in parenthesis we obtain two analogous formulae:

$$\text{k.e.} = \frac{1}{2}mv^2 \text{ (Translational)}$$

$$\text{k.e.} = \frac{1}{2}I\omega^2 \text{ (Rotational)}$$

In all results for rotary motion the measure of inertia (analogous to mass in the translational case) is I, the *moment of inertia*.

In Fig. 2.14, $I = mr^2$, while for for an extended body I is the sum of all the contributions mr^2 for all the particles. For storing energy of rotation, the effectiveness of a mass depends on the square of its distance from the axis. This is appreciated by ballet dancers entering a pirouette with arms outstretched, and known in detail by designers of recording galvanometers. The modern long thin galvanometer is intended to have low moment of inertia, in contrast with the fly-wheel which has as much of its mass as possible concentrated at its rim.

Figure 2.15 gives some of the analogous quantities and relationships for translational and rotational motion.

SOME TRANSLATORY QUANTITIES	THEIR ROTATORY EQUIVALENTS
MASS _ _ _ _ _ _ _ _ _ _ _ _ _ _ m	MOMENT OF INERTIA _ _ _ _ $I (= \Sigma mr^2)$
DISTANCE _ _ _ _ _ _ _ _ _ _ x	ANGLE _ _ _ _ _ _ _ _ _ _ _ _ θ
VELOCITY _ _ _ _ _ _ _ _ _ _ $v (= \dot{x})$	ANGULAR VELOCITY _ _ _ _ $\omega (= \dot{\theta})$
ACCELERATION _ _ _ _ _ _ _ $a (= \dot{v})$	ANGULAR ACCELERATION _ $\dot{\omega}$
FORCE _ _ _ _ _ _ _ _ _ _ _ F	TORQUE _ _ _ _ _ _ _ _ _ _ _ τ
LINEAR MOMENTUM _ _ _ _ _ mv	ANGULAR MOMENTUM _ _ _ $I\omega$
KINETIC ENERGY _ _ _ _ _ _ $\frac{1}{2}mv^2$	KINETIC ENERGY _ _ _ _ _ _ $\frac{1}{2}I\omega^2$
ACCELERATION LAW _ _ _ _ $F = ma$	ACCELERATION LAW _ _ _ _ $\tau = I\dot{\omega}$
LINEAR SPRING _ _ _ _ _ _ _ $F = Sx$	ROTATING SPRING _ _ _ _ _ $\tau = k\theta$
ENERGY IN SPRING _ _ _ _ _ $\frac{1}{2}Sx^2$	ENERGY IN SPRING _ _ _ _ $\frac{1}{2}k\theta^2$

Fig. 2.15

Centrifugal and Centripetal Force

If a body such as the mass in Fig. 2.16 is swinging round on the end of a string, even if its speed is constant, the other aspect of velocity, that is *direction*,

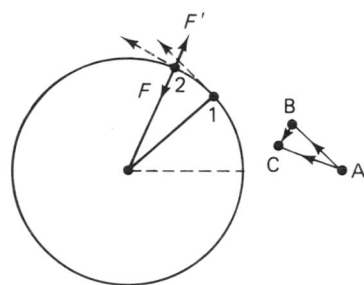

Fig. 2.16

is changing continuously. A vector diagram mapping the velocities at two instants close together shows AB representing the velocity at point 1 and CA that at point 2. The difference between these velocities maps as BC, and it is seen that for small time interval this difference is directed towards the centre of curvature of the path. Now an acceleration consistently directed at right-angles to the path requires a force to maintain it. This force (F) is the *centripetal force* provided by the restraining string. The *centrifugal force* (F') exerted on the string is merely an example of Newton's action and reaction law. It can be shown that

$$F = \frac{mv^2}{r}$$

where v is the magnitude of the velocity (speed) and r is the radius of the orbit. The appearance of v^2 is due to the fact that doubling v not only doubles the velocity being altered, but halves the time taken to alter it. Similarly, halving r halves the time scale of the motion, which therefore demands greater acceleration.

Power

The lay term *powerful,* which is applied to people or devices capable of doing considerable work in a short time, is the basis for the formal definition of the power developed by a system as the rate at which it does work. The unit is the joule of work per second, and is abbreviated to the *watt* ($1 \text{ W} = 1 \text{ J s}^{-1}$). The watt is not the exclusive property of the subject of electricity, and it is perfectly valid to speak of the power developed by the muscles of the heart in terms of watts. Other units, such as the horse-power, can be expressed in terms of the watt.

Pressure

When a surface is bombarded by molecules and the momentum of the molecules (normal to the surface) is reversed, the surface experiences a force. The effective-ness of this force, as far as production of local strain is concerned, depends on the area over which it is distributed. The force per unit area is called the pressure, and may be measured in newtons (N) per square metre; 1 N m^{-2} is equivalent to 10^5 dynes distributed over 10^4 square centimetres, so

$$1 \text{ N m}^{-2} = 10 \text{ dyn cm}^{-2}$$

In our natural environment, we are bombarded by molecules of air of a particular density (about 1 kg m^{-3}) and of a particular order of temperature (and hence of kinetic energy). The resulting 'atmospheric pressure' is clearly important to us, and measurement shows this to be of the order of 10^5 N m^{-2} (10^6 dyn cm^{-2}). The reason why the air around us is compressed to the extent that it causes this order of pressure is that the air at the Earth's surface is supporting the weight of air stacked vertically above, and, like a pile of cushions, the lower layers are compressed more than the upper ones.

A column of liquid is similarly compressed, but liquids being far less compressible than gases, the variation of density up the column is very small. This suggests a convenient method of producing known pressures at will, and by balancing such pressures against unknown pressures provides us with a method (the liquid column manometer) of measuring the latter. Since a column of liquid of height h, cross-sectional area A and density ρ has a mass $\rho h A$, its weight (a force) at the surface of the Earth is $\rho h A g$. Consequently the pressure exerted at the base is $\rho h A g / A$, or

$$P = \rho g h$$

For a chosen liquid (e.g. mercury) and chosen planet (e.g. Earth), ρ and g are known, so the pressure produced is proportional to the height of the column. The simplicity and convenience of this technique led to the short-hand reference to the height of a liquid column as a measure of pressure, and the unit '1 mmHg' of course means the pressure caused by a column of mercury 1 mm high at the Earth's surface.

Classes of Problem Involving Pressure Measurement
When considering the flow of fluids through vessels (blood in arteries or air in air-ways) we are concerned with the *differences* in pressure between two ends of a vessel. If the pressures at both ends are increased by (say) 50 mmHg, the pressure difference is unaltered. In such problems the actual baseline from which pressure is referred is irrelevant. There is an important distinction between problems involving pressure differences and those involving absolute measure of pressure. For example, when considering the solution of gases in a liquid or the compression of gases in a cylinder, the important measure is the actual force per unit area— that is the result of actual bombardment to which the sample is subjected. To clarify this distinction, consider a mercury manometer (Fig. 2.17) being used to measure a pressure in a liquid (communicating at A),

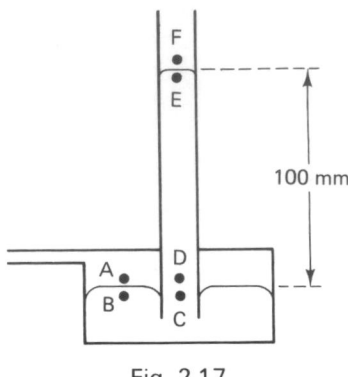

Fig. 2.17

the measurement taking place on the Earth's surface, with the end (F) open to the atmosphere. Suppose that molecules at A bombard those at B, the pressure to be measured being P. Once equilibrium has been reached, mercury no longer moves, so molecules at C are known to be subjected to the same pressure environment (that is bombardment giving rise to the same rate of momentum reversal over unit area) as those at B. The measurement problem has therefore been transferred to assessing the pressure at C. Now this pressure results from the act of supporting the column of mercury (D to E) plus the effect of the bombardment of molecules at E by air molecules at F. For example, suppose the mercury column to be 100 mm high, and the effect of air molecules bombarding E to be the same as would have been caused by an extra column of mercury 760 mm high with no atmosphere above it (atmospheric pressure = 760 mmHg at the time of the measurement). From the point of view of molecules at C (and hence at B and therefore at A), the pressure would be 860 mmHg. If there were oxygen molecules at A and the far end of the tube connected to the manometer were sealed, then this would be the relevant pressure as far as the resulting compression of the oxygen is concerned. This becomes doubly clear if we express the pressure in fundamental terms—i.e. in $N\,m^{-2}$. We obviously should not ignore the fact that our measuring instrument does not cease at the top (E) of the tube, when describing the number of newtons per square metre to which the oxygen is subjected.

In contrast, suppose that this manometer were measuring an arterial pressure via a catheter or needle, and that another was being used for venous pressure measurement, with a column showing 4 mm. If our interest lay in the difference between arterial and venous pressure it would be correct (but unusual) to quote the arterial pressure as 860 mmHg and the venous pressure as 764 mmHg. By convention we take the baseline value (atmospheric pressure) as understood, and give the results as 100 mmHg and 4 mmHg respectively. It is interesting (and revealing of the state of our understanding) to consider the length of the arterial pressure manometer column in quite different circumstances. Suppose the patient to be in a hyper-

baric enclosure in which the density of his local atmosphere had been artificially increased, and that a state of equilibrium had been established. It is unusual to think in terms of the density of the local atmosphere (although the object of the exercise is in fact to present tissues with more oxygen molecules bombarding unit area than is normal outside), and we will enquire what pressure in *excess of* atmosphere was necessary to create this situation. It is important to know what is meant when reference is made to the pressure inside a hyperbaric enclosure, since 2 atmospheres in excess of the outside pressure is not the same thing as 2 atmospheres total. Suppose that, unambiguously, the pressure inside was 1000 mmHg above that outside. If the open end of the manometer lay inside the enclosure, the column would still be 100 mm high. The absolute measure of pressure at A would be 100 mmHg due to the action of the heart, plus the 1760 mmHg due to the local atmosphere with which the patient's tissues are in equilibrium. However, the top of the column would be subjected to the same 1760 mmHg giving 1860 mmHg at A and 1760 mmHg at E, which accounts for the support of a 100 mm column. If the open end of the manometer had been outside, the column would have needed to be 1100 mm high since the air at F would have only contributed 760 mmHg pressure. This agrees with the fact that the patient's arterial pressure would be 100 mmHg above the pressure in the enclosure, or 1100 mmHg above outside atmospheric pressure. To appreciate fully the meaning of pressure measurements taken this way it is instructive to observe that were it not for the opening to the atmosphere at F the column would need to be 1100 + 760, or 1860 mm high to back-off the pressure existing in the environment of the patient's artery, and that this figure in turn reflects the fact that we are using mercury on the Earth's surface. On the Moon, where weights are one-sixth of Earth-surface values, and where there is no atmosphere the column would be 6 × 1860, or 11 160 mm high. The corresponding length for venous pressure measurement would be 6 × (4 + 1760), or 10 584 mm. An arterial pressure quoted as 11 160 mmHg absolute and a venous pressure of 10 584 mmHg absolute lacks the ring of familiarity, but as far as the patient's haemodynamic status is concerned this represents a pressure difference of 576 mmHg (Moon gravity), or 96 mmHg (Earth gravity).

Although few anaesthetists are likely to be involved with patients in hyperbaric enclosures on the Moon, it is important to appreciate the following facts:

1. That the mercury pressure scale arose from the convenience of observing a length when measuring a pressure.
2. That, no matter what units are used, fluid dynamics calculations are concerned with pressure differences, so that baselines or reference levels are often tacitly omitted.
3. That as far as the environment of molecules at a

particular site is concerned, the essential question is how many molecules are concentrated there and how much momentum is involved during collisions over a given area. Since we rarely know (or measure) the density of molecules or their momenta, we relate our observations to the quantity we can measure, that is pressure. For problems of compression the important measure is absolute pressure.

Other Pressure Symbols and Units

Where there is a serious possibility of ambiguity the word 'absolute' may be added to denote pressures referred to true zero (that is, compared with no molecular collisions), and the word 'gauge' is added to denote pressures measured above atmospheric. Accordingly the abbreviations 'a' and 'g' were met, as in $N\,m^{-2}a$ or $lbf\,in^{-2}g$. The abbreviation p.s.i. for pounds-weight per square inch is becoming less often met. In cases where the unit is still used, the modern terminology is 'pounds-force' (lbf) per square inch.

The newton per square metre is given the special name *pascal* in SI ($1\,Pa = 1\,N\,m^{-2}$). The meteorological *bar* is exactly $100\,000\,Pa$ ($100\,kPa$), and the *standard atmosphere* (atm) is now *defined* as exactly $101.325\,kPa$. Since this corresponds to $760\,mmHg$ it follows that, to three significant figures $1\,mmHg$ equals $0.133\,kPa$ ($133.322\,Pa$). A useful approximation to remember is $7.5\,mmHg$ for $1\,kPa$ to better than 1 part in $10\,000$.

Pressure Related to Work

Figure 2.18 illustrates a syringe being used to eject fluid at a pressure P (absolute), so the force being exerted on the plunger is given by

$$F = PA$$

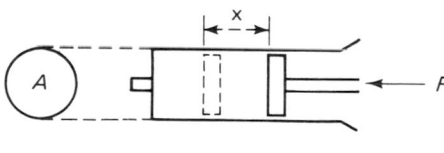

Fig. 2.18

If the plunger moves some distance (x), work will be done, given by

$$Work = Fx$$
$$= PAx$$

Now Ax is the volume ejected (V, say), so

$$Work = PV$$

We see from this that we can define pressure either as force per unit area or as work per unit volume. This is made doubly clear by writing

$$Pressure = \frac{FORCE \times DISTANCE}{AREA \times DISTANCE}$$

since cancelling DISTANCE gives the usual definition, while not cancelling it gives the alternative definition.

It is clear that by a 'strong' pump we mean one capable of exerting a large pressure. Similarly, a 'strong' pump is capable of doing a considerable amount of work with each unit volume it ejects. It is as legitimate to measure pressure in joules (of work done) per m^3 (of fluid ejected) as by newtons (of force exerted) per m^2 (of area involved). The simplicity of physicists' calculations of work done by pumps is disguised in medicine by the use of special units. The use of mmHg for pressure spoils the simplicity of

$$Work = PV$$

More generally, if the pressure changes during the ejection, the work is found by summing the products of pressure and increments of volume ejected, or

$$Work = \int P\,dV$$

The litre and its symbol (L) are officially incorporated into SI. The 12th Conférence Générale des Poids et Mesures (1964) rescinded the earlier definition of $1.000\,028\,dm^3$, and the litre is now the special name for exactly one cubic decimetre. This being $1/1000$ of a cubic metre shows that the joule can be equated to the kilopascal-litre, which is more suitable to us than working in terms of the (rather small) pascal together with the cubic metre. The symbol L is accepted as alternative to lower case l where the latter could be confused with the numeric 1.

Temperature

Our main concern with temperature here will be its relevance to the kinetic theory of gases. It is known that heating a body raises the average kinetic energy of its molecules. However, temperature is primarily a lay concept (as a human perception of 'hotness'), and like force and energy, awaited formal definition. Unfortunately the invention of imperfect thermometers preceded the development of kinetic theory. Suppose that scientists had instead developed an instrument for measuring mean molecular kinetic energy. Over the range of human perception a good correlation would have been noted between lay 'temperature' and measured kinetic energy. It would have seemed obvious to *define* temperature as proportional to mean molecular kinetic energy, and to extend the definition beyond the human range, as in Fig. 2.19. Four important consequences would have been:

1. The existence of an absolute zero of temperature would have been more obvious.
2. The relationship

   Temperature = Constant × Mean Molecular k.e.

   would have been regarded as a mere definition (not a natural law).
3. A decision would have been awaited to set the temperature scale—i.e. to choose the factor of proportionality.

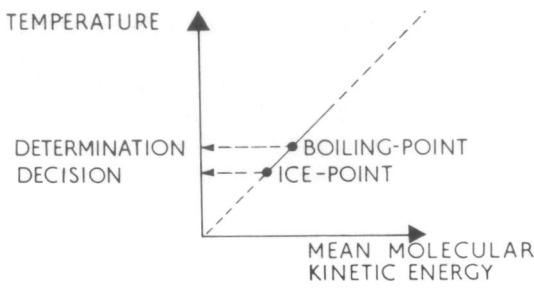

Fig. 2.19

4. There being no thermometers, as we know them, there would have been no preconceived opinion on setting the scale.

To set the scale, suppose that the melting of ice had been chosen as a reproducible phenomenon. Some reasonable number, such as 1000, might have been selected for the point marked DECISION on the figure. This choice would have given reasonable steps in temperature for most medical, domestic and meteorological purposes, and certainly the suggestion of 273 would have been regarded as eccentric. After the scale had been set, the determination of other temperatures (such as that of boiling water) would have been purely a matter of experiment (*see* DETERMINATION on the figure).

The invention of the mercury-in-glass thermometer, for which the convenient end-points (melting-point of ice and boiling-point of water) would have already been decided, would have been seen as making available a cheap instrument. The imperfections of its scale would have been noted as an example of imperfect linearity, rather as some ECG recorders are known to be non-linear. Gas thermometers would have been greeted as instruments of better linearity and precision, and all subsequent experimentation based on thermometers would have been regarded as limited in precision by the imperfections of the measuring instruments.

In contrast, we have inherited a system of temperature scales based on the behaviour of actual thermometers, and the historical order of the subject introduces complications analogous to the assumption that the first recorded ECG traces were definitive and that voltage is only associated with the ECG in some rather esoteric way.

From the point of view of anaesthetists, temperature *differences* between actual and normal, and between one site and another, are equally well measured in any agreed scale. For temperature *differences* the SI unit of thermodynamic temperature, the kelvin (K) and the degree Celsius (°C) are interchangeable. The relationship between thermodynamic temperature T and Celsius temperature t is given exactly by $T = t + 273.15$, but for much work the familiar '273' is adequate.

Pressure, Volume and Temperature of Gases

In a sample of gas at a known temperature, the molecules are continually interchanging momentum by collisions, and consequently have a spread or spectrum of kinetic energies distributed about an average which is specific for that temperature. In Fig. 2.20 we imagine that a molecule has been removed from the sample at an instant when its kinetic energy was equal to the average, and transferred to a small box. When a molecule rebounds from the surface of a container, occasions will arise when its reception will have been more vigorous than at others, since the agitation of the molecules of the container is also subject to a spread. On average, the fact that the container is in temperature equilibrium with the gas enables us to simplify the situation in Fig. 2.20 by

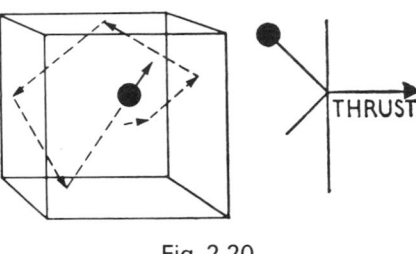

Fig. 2.20

assuming that the molecule rebounds without loss or gain of kinetic energy. Our intention is to regard this molecule as undergoing average experiences and to confine our attention to results that would be unchanged if all the molecules in a sample underwent these experiences.

At each impact, the component of the momentum of the molecule perpendicular to the face is exactly reversed in this simplified model, and the trajectory for one of the collisions is shown in side elevation to the right of the figure. If the container were sufficiently small, the collisions would be frequent enough for each face to experience a pressure due to continual reversals of momentum. Just as we discuss temperature (rather than kinetic energy) because we possess thermometers, so we introduce pressure into our description of the gas because it is measurable and has been correlated with factors of interest to us, both in physics and in medicine. Clearly the molecule rebounds from six faces, and it is necessary to take into account the angles of impact at each face to calculate pressure. Suppose that the molecule had been trapped when it happened to be travelling perpendicular to one face (Fig. 2.21). Rebounding between two of the six faces, it will exert pressure on one-third of the six. When allowance has been made for the angle of impact and for the longer times between impacts for the six-face rebound (Fig. 2.20), it is found that the pressure experienced in the two-faced situation is three times as great as when all six faces are involved.

In Fig. 2.21, if t is the time between impacts on one face

$$t = 2x/v$$

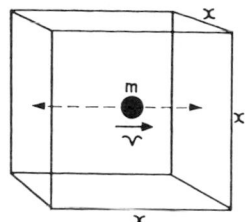

Fig. 2.21

Since the momentum is reversed on impact, the force (rate of change of momentum) is

$$F = 2(mv)/t$$

$$= mv^2/x$$

Since the area of the face is x^2, the pressure is

$$P = F/x^2$$

$$= mv^2/x^3$$

When allowance is made for this pressure being three times as large as when all faces are affected, the result becomes

$$P = \tfrac{1}{3}mv^2/x^3$$

or, denoting the volume (x^3) by V,

$$PV = \tfrac{1}{3}mv^2$$

Notice that this result is proportional to the kinetic energy of the molecule.

If the rest of the molecules are introduced into the box, and the total number in the sample is N_s, the result becomes

$$PV = \tfrac{1}{3}(N_s m)v^2$$

where v^2 is called the 'mean value of the squares of the velocities'. Notice in passing that this is not the same as saying that v is the mean velocity. For comparison if we had three square pieces of paper with sides 1, 2 and 3 cm, the mean area would be one-third of $14\,cm^2$. This would correspond to a square of 2.16 cm side, not 2 cm.

Having shown that the product PV is proportional to the number of molecules and their mean kinetic energy, we introduce temperature by reference to the absolute (kinetic theory) scale. For a given *sample* of a given gas (that is given N_s and m) this is usually done by noting that PV is proportional to the kinetic energy and hence to the temperature and writing

$$PV = R_s T$$

where the factor of proportionality R_s is called the *gas constant for that sample.*

The contribution per molecule is expressed by the gas constant per molecule, which is known as Boltzmann's constant (k), so

$$PV = N_s kT$$

Comparing this with

$$PV = \tfrac{1}{3}N_s mv^2$$

gives another interpretation of Boltzmann's constant, since

$$kT = \tfrac{1}{3}mv^2$$

shows that k is two-thirds of the kinetic energy change per molecule corresponding to 1 kelvin change of absolute temperature.

It is a matter of individual preference which of the many formulations of the ideal gas law (equation of state) is regarded as basic. One scheme is illustrated in Fig. 2.22. If we imagine the contribution of *one*

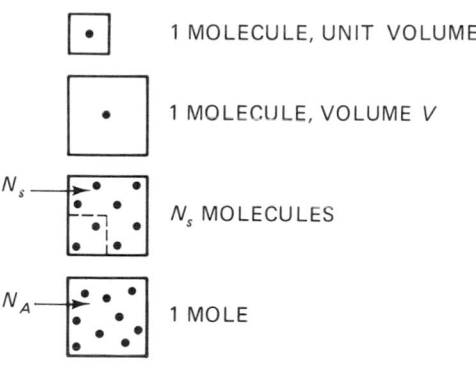

Fig. 2.22

(average experience) *molecule* to the pressure in a *unit volume* to be

$$P_1 = kT$$

we need remember that only the temperature of the sample can affect what this molecule does in the unit volume box. Increasing the volume will reduce the rate of collisions and increase the area involved, and the smaller pressure is

$$P = \frac{kT}{V}$$

Increasing the number of molecules to N_s (any number) gives

$$P = \frac{N_s kT}{V}$$

This reveals that P is proportional to T, and that (at a given temperature) depends only on the number of molecules per unit volume. For a 1 mole sample the number of molecules is called the Avogadro constant N_A (*see* later), so for 1 mole

$$P = \frac{N_A k T}{V}$$

The product $N_A k$ is called the *molar gas constant* (R) and, like N_A and k, is one of the fundamental physical constants. For 1 mole

$$PV = RT$$

Finally, for any sample of n moles the general result is

$$PV = nRT$$

Types of Problem Involving the Gas Law

The choice of formula depends on the problem concerned, and it is convenient to divide the problems into two classes. When the gas or gases are in fixed quantities and where we are concerned only with their redistribution, the simplest formula is usually

$$PV = N_s k T$$

It is not necessary to know the actual number or the value of k, since these factors cancel in calculations. For example, suppose that a sample of N_1 molecules in a volume V_1 at pressure P_1 and temperature T_1 are mixed with another sample of N_2 molecules originally at P_2 and T_2 in a volume V_2, so that they occupy the total volume ($V_1 + V_2$). If the temperature equilibrates to T_3, the pressure P_3 is given by

$$P_3(V_1 + V_2) = (N_1 + N_2)kT_3$$

but $\qquad P_1 V_1 = N_1 k T_1$

and $\qquad P_2 V_2 = N_2 k T_2$

Substituting for the quantities $N_1 k$ and $N_2 k$ gives

$$P_3(V_1 + V_2) = T_3\left(\frac{P_1 V_1}{T_1} + \frac{P_2 V_2}{T_2}\right)$$

The advantage of working in terms of numbers of molecules is that molecules do not vanish in physical processes such as mixing, diffusion and entering into solution. Their numbers must therefore be accounted for at all stages in the calculations.

When the problem is to establish the PVT relationships for a specific sample (such as a given mass) we must, in effect, become 'aware' of the numbers of molecules involved. It would be absurd, however, to calculate the number of molecules and look up the value of Boltzmann's constant, and it is more usual to resort to the form

$$PV = nRT$$

The Laws of Boyle and Charles

In experiments with gases Boyle discovered that at constant temperature a sample of given mass dis-

played an approximately inverse relationship between pressure and volume, or

$PV = $ constant (given mass and given temperature).

Later work by Charles and by Gay-Lussac showed experimentally that several common gases, when allowed to expand under constant pressure as the temperature was raised, expanded approximately equally for equal temperature increments. In terms of temperature $t°C$, this relationship is approximately

$$\frac{V}{273 + t} = \text{constant (given mass and pressure)}$$

which, in terms of absolute temperature T reduces to

$$V = \text{constant} \times T$$

These experimentally determined laws are clearly accounted for by the theoretical relationship

$$PV = nRT$$

by restricting the variables PV and T to vary in pairs.

Avogadro's Hypothesis

For a perfect gas (that is a theoretical material exactly obeying the simple gas law $PV = N_s k T$), Avogadro's hypothesis states that, at a given temperature and pressure, the number of molecules per unit volume would be independent of the gas concerned. It is instructive to express this another way. If we confine ourselves to pressure, temperature and volume measurements alone (which we often do, since these are measurable quantities with which we become familiar), there can be no way of knowing which gas is in a container. To illustrate this with simple numbers, imagine that one side of the container of Fig. 2.20 is free to move, and that, under the impression that a molecule of mass m is trapped, we are holding this side in position. Now suppose that the original sample had contained a trace of heavier gas (for example one having molecules of mass $4m$), and that by chance one of these had been selected on the basis of possessing the average kinetic energy. Now we were expecting a molecule of mass m and velocity v, whose kinetic energy would be

$$\text{k.e.} = \tfrac{1}{2}mv^2$$

It is easy to see that a molecule of mass $4m$ having this kinetic energy would have velocity $\tfrac{1}{2}v$, since substituting $4m$ and $\tfrac{1}{2}v$ in the expression for kinetic energy gives

$$\text{k.e.} = \tfrac{1}{2}(4m)(\tfrac{1}{2}v)^2$$
$$= \tfrac{1}{2}mv^2$$

Having half the expected velocity, this molecule takes *twice* as long between impacts, but we find its momentum to be *twice* the expected value mv, since

$$\text{momentum} = \text{mass} \times \text{velocity}$$
$$= (4m)(\tfrac{1}{2}v)$$
$$= 2mv$$

Now the force on the wall equals the rate of change of momentum, and since both the momentum and the time lapse between impacts are doubled, the force is exactly the same as the expected molecule would have produced.

We have illustrated this with simple ratios which can be easily visualized, but the result

$$PV = \tfrac{1}{3}mv^2 N_s$$

shows that for $\tfrac{1}{2}mv^2$ constant the result is independent of m because of compensating adjustment of v.

In summary, we see that pressure measurements cannot distinguish between the 'expected' gas and the interloper, which agrees with Avogadro's hypothesis. For a specified volume (1 cm^3) at standard temperature (0°C) and pressure (1 atmosphere) the number of molecules is of the order of 2.69×10^{19}, which is Loschmidt's number. Another aspect of this is that a mole sample, which contains rather more than 22 400 times as many molecules will, at standard temperature and pressure, occupy a volume of the order of 22.4 litres.

The Mole; Avogadro's Constant

Physical chemistry evolved in a manner which resulted in our inheriting a somewhat arbitrary, though useful, standard 'packet' of matter, the *mole*. In retrospect, it is obvious that atoms combine chemically in integer proportions. For work on a macroscopic scale any sufficiently large number (say 10^{20}) could be regarded as a convenient packet, both from the point of view of measurability and because (unlike, say, a dozen) such a huge number can accommodate the integer proportions involved in even highly complex molecules.

Again, traditionally, we think of the mass of a given type of atom in terms of (as a ratio of) the mass of some standard particle, as is evident by the use of such terms as 'atomic (and molecular) weight', although it is perhaps unfortunate that the word 'weight' slipped into the terminology at this point. In the past there has been discussion on which particle should be used as reference. Had the universe been tidier in the sense that the masses of all atoms had been exact multiples of the mass of the hydrogen atom, there would have been no discussion. However, even if isotopes having different masses for the same element did not exist, the fact remains that atoms are not multiples of hydrogen atoms, and there are arguments to be made in favour of different reference masses. Essentially the best choice would result in as many of the ratios as possible being near to whole numbers, so that, for approximate work, we effect a 'data reduction' by remembering these numbers for elements of importance to our work. It is also desirable that the reference particle should be unambiguous and not to depend on some local terrestrial accident such as the proportion of different isotopes in a 'naturally occurring' sample of some element. Currently references are still found to the chemical scale based on a reference mass of one-sixteenth of that of the average atom in a sample of naturally occurring oxygen, and the physical scale based on one-sixteenth of the mass of isotope oxygen–16. More recent references have become unified to the scale in which a value of exactly 12 is assigned to the isotope carbon–12.

Recognizing that the small differences between these scales are relevant for more accurate work, we can simplify the picture by regarding the mole as a sample consisting of a standard number of molecules so selected that we can state the mass of the sample (in grams) to whatever precision we compute the molecular weight. This number, the Avogadro constant, is approximately 6.02×10^{23}. The *order* of this number is consequent on the original decision to take the gram as the basic unit of mass, and its *precise value* depends on the atomic weight scale concerned, as well as on the precision of the current best estimate, of course.

Clearly, the importance of the mole is due to its reference to a specified number of molecules. Quantities such as the gas constant per mole and specific heats per mole are listed and may be regarded as constants for a numerically specified sample. Boltzmann's constant is similarly a constant for a specified sample, in this case a sample of one molecule. As such, it is convenient for theoretical work concerning individual molecules and as a parameter in the statistical analysis of macroscopic groups.

Partial Pressure (Dalton's Law)

Since pressure measurements cannot distinguish between different molecules in a mixed sample, the contribution to total pressure made by a given constituent is in proportion to the number of molecules of that constituent. If all others were removed, then provided that the only influence between constituents had been the random momentary collisions, the remaining molecules would continue with the same average kinetic energy. They would therefore maintain their same contribution (now the only one) to the pressure. The original total pressure must therefore have been the sum of the pressures each constituent produces alone, and these contributions depend only on the number of molecules present, for a given temperature. The simplest form of the gas law, $PV = N_s kT$ illustrates this. If there are two gases, for which we use the suffices 1 and 2, and there are N_1 molecules of gas 1 and N_2 of gas 2, then

$$PV = (N_1 + N_2)kT$$

because there is no way of distinguishing between molecules as far as PV and T measurements are concerned. Taken in isolation the partial pressures would be given by

$$P_1 V = N_1 kT$$
$$P_2 V = N_2 kT$$

The factors V and kT, being common, cancel to give

$$\frac{P_1}{N_1} = \frac{P_2}{N_2} = \frac{P}{N_1 + N_2}$$

This states that the partial pressures and the total pressure are in the same ratios as the separate and combined numbers of molecules. Although we do not normally think in terms of numbers of molecules we usually either know the masses (and the molecular 'weights') of the constituents, or their original separate volumes at given pressure and temperature, or we know their relative abundance in a given mixture. It will be noted that any statement concerning partial pressures in a mixture of gases is merely another way of making a statement of their relative *numerical* abundance, provided that their interactions involve only mutual interchange of kinetic energy in collisions.

The Gas Law for Real Gases

In Fig. 2.23 molecule A is approaching the wall of a

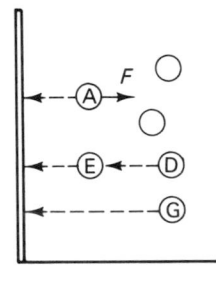

Fig. 2.23

container. The simple kinetic theory of gases assumes that, apart from momentum interchange on collision, there is no interaction between molecules. In a real gas there are forces of attraction between molecules, so that when A reaches the wall it is doing so against the small force F tending to pull it back into the body of the gas. As a result the pressure actually *measured* will be less than *predicted* by the simplified theory. Van der Waals allowed for this error by replacing P by

$$P + \frac{a}{V^2}$$

where a is a constant for the sample. It will be noted that (for a given number of molecules) the larger the volume the smaller this correction becomes.

Another assumption is that the molecules are of negligible size, so that a molecule such as D colliding with another E can be regarded as indistinguishable from a single molecule G covering the whole distance to the wall. Clearly, when we considered the time taken between collisions with the walls, we should have allowed for the fact that molecules have finite size, and that the distance travelled by molecules D

and E is less than it would have been had they been infinitesimally small. This principle is well-known to drivers of shunting engines. Since we measure volume of the container and pressure at its walls, both factors must be corrected, and van der Waals' equation of state is of the form

$$\left(P + \frac{a}{V^2}\right)\left(V - b\right) = RT$$

where b corrects for the volume error. Although these corrections are small for gases at room temperature, they become important as the liquid phase is approached. In particular, plotting P versus V for low temperatures gives a curve such as A in Fig. 2.24, which shows (in contrast to the approximately inverse relationship of curve C) a region over which pressure would be constrained to decrease as the volume decreases. In fact the broken line from L to M is traversed, as part of the sample passes into the liquid phase, and the remainder continues to obey the equation of state. Van der Waal's equation (and other similar empirical equations) also indicates the

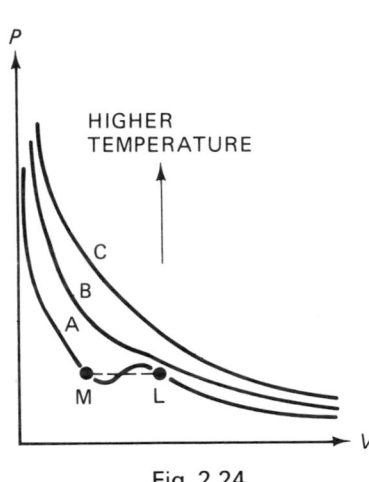

Fig. 2.24

existence of a critical temperature (for curve B) above which the liquid phase is not entered. For curve B the unstable section just does not occur.

In physical terms, liquefication by compression results when the intermolecular attractive forces overcome the random thermal motions, so the substance must be compressed enough *and* at low enough temperature. For such a case as curve A, to the left of point M the entire sample is liquefied.

The distinction between gases and vapours, which is related to the critical isothermal curve (B), is taken up later in this chapter.

Specific Heats of Gases

The definition of specific heat of a solid or liquid as the energy required to raise the temperature of unit mass by one degree presents little conceptual difficulty. When energy is absorbed it is shared among the molecules, and we can expect to account fully for the energy supplied. Some will be manifested by an increase of kinetic energy of motion of the molecules, and some may cause increase in rotational or vibrational energy in molecules more complex than those of the ideal gas.

Suppose that a sample of matter is totally enclosed in a container, so that as the sample expands it must push back the restraining walls of the container. Some of the energy supplied is expended in deforming the container, so less energy is available to be taken up by the sample. Consequently, even when allowance has been made for raising the temperature of the container, more energy is needed to raise the temperature of the sample than would have been required had the expansion not occurred. Now it is important to take into account external constraints. Depending on the circumstances, heating a gas sample may involve anything between the two extremes of complete freedom to expand and complete restraint. It is obviously unsatisfactory to have an infinite number of answers to the question 'what is the specific heat of this gas?', so we define two specific heats corresponding to the two extreme cases.

The specific heat at constant volume (c_p) is the energy required to raise the temperature of unit mass of gas by one degree, expansion being permitted under conditions of constant pressure. This energy is therefore shared between the 'internal' process of raising the energy of the gas molecules and the process of forcing back whatever surfaces are maintaining the constant pressure environment. For unit mass and unit temperature rise we may express this as

$$c_p - \text{Energy gained by gas molecules} + P\Delta V$$

where ΔV = increase of volume

and P — maintained pressure (constant).

The specific heat at constant volume (c_v) is the energy required to produce unit temperature rise in unit mass when the volume is not allowed to increase. Here the container is not pushed back, so

$$c_v = \text{Energy gained by gas molecules}$$

Since the temperature rise and the number of molecules are the same for both cases, the internal energy (that taken up by the gas) is the same, so we have

$$c_p = c_v + P\Delta V$$

This accords with our understanding that whatever energy is demanded by the process of expansion against constraint is not available for the gas molecules. It remains only to assess this energy deficit. For a perfect gas, a unit mass will have the equation of state

$$PV = R_1 T$$

where R_1 is the gas constant for the unit mass concerned. If the pressure remains at P and the temperature is raised to $T + 1$ the volume will be given by

$$P(V + \Delta V) = R_1(T + 1)$$

so

$$P\Delta V = R_1$$

Consequently, the two specific heats are related by

$$c_p = c_v + R_1$$

The term 'specific heat' is giving way to 'specific heat capacity', particularly in physics and chemistry literature. The SI unit (in place of the cal g^{-1} °C^{-1}) may be written as either $J\ kg^{-1}K^{-1}$ or $J\ kg^{-1}$ °C^{-1}, because for temperature *changes* the kelvin and the degree Celsius are identical.

When the sample is 1 mole instead of unit mass, the corresponding quantities (symbols C_p and C_v) are called the *molar heat capacities*, their SI unit being $J\ mol^{-1}\ K^{-1}$. As will be seen, for ideal gases each is exactly related to the molar gas constant R, which is a fundamental physical constant. Its value is just over $8.314\ J\ mol^{-1}\ K^{-1}$.

Specific Heat Ratio, γ

For the perfect monatomic gas, all the energy taken up by the gas (sometimes called 'internal' energy) appears as kinetic energy of translation. If we compare the two formulations of the equation of state for a given sample,

$$PV = \tfrac{1}{3}N_s m v^2$$

$$PV = nRT$$

we see that the internal energy is

$$N_s(\tfrac{1}{2}mv^2) = \tfrac{3}{2}nRT$$

The specific heat at constant volume is the energy supplied to raise the temperature from T to $T + 1$, so for a 1 mole sample

$$C_v = \tfrac{3}{2}R$$

Combining this with the result

$$C_p = C_v + R$$

gives

$$C_p = \tfrac{5}{2}R$$

Thus the ratio of C_p to C_v is given by

$$\gamma = \tfrac{5}{3}$$

This value agrees reasonably with measured values for monatomic gases such as helium, but for diatomic gases the value is nearer to 1.4, which leads us to a further distinction between real gases and the ideal gas. It has been supposed that energy interchange between molecules is restricted to the distribution of kinetic energy, with three degrees of freedom corresponding to purely translatory motion. When vibrational and rotational energy are taken into account we see that only some of the energy taken up when gas is heated at constant volume appears as kinetic energy in the equation of state. This invalidates the result

$$C_v = \tfrac{3}{2}R$$

which is seen to be a low estimate. Attempts to relate values of γ to models of real gases met with little success until the limitations of classical mechanics stimulated the development of quantum-mechanics. However, it is clear that disparities between the behaviour of real gases and the predictions for ideal gases, both in relation to heat transfer and to the equation of state can be anticipated in terms of the simplifying assumptions we have made.

Adiabatic and Isothermal Changes

In general, changes of pressure or volume or both are accompanied by both energy transfer and temperature change. It is convenient to consider one factor being fixed. For example, an isothermal change may be approximated by compressing a gas sufficiently slowly to permit the temperature to remain in equilibrium with the surroundings. Under these circumstances the energy supplied by the source of compression is lost to the surroundings. For a perfect gas the equation predicts that the result of decreasing the volume will be an increase of pressure (due to more frequent bombardment of the walls), and for a real gas one of the empirical equations of state can be used to determine the pressure-volume relationships. For an adiabatic change (approximated by sudden volume changes), the energy supplied (in the case of compression) is contained within the sample, and is manifested by a temperature change. Since all three parameters ($P V$ and T) are changing, the problem is to find how any pair (P and V for example) vary during the change, since knowing this enables us to find the third by using the equation of state. For example, suppose that a sample of perfect gas initially occupies a volume V at pressure P and temperature T, and is allowed to expand suddenly to occupy a larger volume LV ($L > 1$). Because the gas does work against the restraining container or surroundings, its temperature will be lower. Suppose that the pressure falls to P_a during the adiabatic expansion, and that the new volume is held constant while the gas absorbs energy from the surroundings, and that when the temperature is back to T the pressure has risen to P_i (corresponding to an isothermal change). For a perfect gas, we know that

$$P_i(LV) = PV$$

or
$$P_i = \frac{P}{L}$$

We expect to find that P_a is less than this, and in fact the result is

$$P_a = \frac{P}{L^\gamma}$$

where γ (the ratio of specific heats) is greater than unity. This result is established as an exercise in the use of differential calculus in text-books on heat, and is usually expressed as

$$PV^\gamma = \text{constant}$$

for adiabatic changes. It is important to note that this is not in conflict with the statement that PV is constant if the temperature does not change.

Surface Tension

Cohesive forces between molecules of a liquid may be sufficiently noticeable at surfaces as to give the impression of a 'skin' under tension. Just as pressure is defined as force per unit area perpendicular to a surface within a volume, so by analogy the force per unit length perpendicular to a line within a surface describes surface tension effects. In Fig. 2.25, we

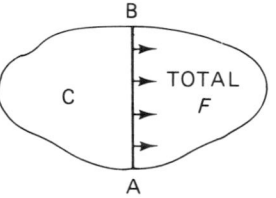

Fig. 2.25

imagine a surface being maintained across a line AB by distributed forces. Those shown may be thought of as preventing the surface at the side C from breaking away. If $AB = l$, the surface on tension is defined as

$$\sigma = \frac{F}{l} \ \text{N m}^{-1}$$

Just as pressure can be thought of in terms of energy change per unit change of volume (joules per m^3) as an alternative to force per unit area (newtons per m^2), so surface tension may be related to energy per unit area (joules per m^2) instead of as newtons per metre.

If a surface (Fig. 2.26) is stretched to cover a larger area, the energy required is Fx, or σlx. Hence

$$\sigma = \frac{\text{Energy change } (Fx)}{\text{Area change } (lx)}$$

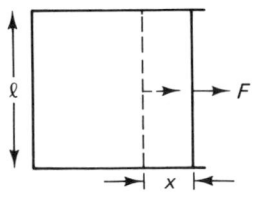

Fig. 2.26

This reasoning is extended when surface tension is treated thermodynamically, since on changing its area a surface requires energy changes, just as does a gas when changing its volume. Thus when a surface suddenly enlarges without energy from outside (that is, adiabatically) the temperature drops as the surface energy can increase only at the expense of the internal energy of the liquid.

There are a number of formulae relating surface tension to specific problems. For example, the pressure inside a bubble of gas within a liquid must be such as to maintain its structural integrity. If we imagine the bubble to be halved and fitted with a disk-shaped cap, the thrust on the cap (pressure multiplied by area, or $P\pi r^2$) must exactly equal the total thrust originally maintained by surface tension acting round the periphery.

Consequently

$$P\pi r^2 = \sigma 2\pi r$$

or

$$P = \frac{2\sigma}{r}$$

To this result must be added any hydrostatic pressure due to the bubble being beneath the surface of the liquid.

Solubility of Gases in Liquids

There is no simple way of anticipating how soluble a given gas will be in a liquid, although in general the more easily liquefied gases tend to be the more soluble. With increase of temperature—and thus of molecular agitation—the general tendency is for a liquid to reject gas molecules, but this is not absolutely invariable, especially where chemical reactions become involved.

The influence of pressure is expressed by *Henry's law*, which states that for most gases, provided that the pressures are not too high nor the temperatures too low, and provided chemical reactions are not involved:

the mass of a gas dissolved by a given volume of solvent, at a given constant temperature, is proportional to the partial pressure of the gas in equilibrium with the solution.

It is useful to envisage this law as stating that the number of gas molecules dissolved into unit volume of the liquid is proportional to the partial pressure. The factor of proportionality is a function of the gas, the liquid, and the temperature.

Bunsen and Ostwald Solubility Coefficients

These two frequently met measures of solubility are defined here in such a way that the features they share are stressed by identical wording, while differences are indicated by use of italics:

For a given gas dissolved in a given liquid at a stated temperature:

1. The *Bunsen* solubility coefficient (α) is, numerically, the amount dissolved in unit volume of the liquid in equilibrium with the gas at a partial pressure of *one standard atmosphere* (760 mmHg, or 101.325 kPa), the amount being expressed as the volume the gas would occupy when brought to *standard temperature and pressure dry* (s.t.p.d.), i.e. 0°C and 1 atm.

2. The *Ostwald* solubility coefficient (λ) is, numerically, the amount dissolved in unit volume of the liquid in equilibrium with the gas at the partial pressure *actually pertaining*, the amount being expressed as the volume the gas would occupy dry when at the *temperature and partial pressure actually pertaining*.

Examination of these definitions reveals that although they refer to different pressures, within each definition *itself* the same pressure is specified for the act of dissolving and for the assessment of the gas volume. If the gas obeys Henry's law, an increase (for example) of partial pressure will increase the number of gas molecules going into solution, but if it obeys Boyle's law, the same increase in the pressure to which the volume is referred will compress the gas correspondingly. As a result, for such gases the essential difference between the two coefficients concerns the temperature only, the Bunsen coefficient referring the gas to standard temperature and the Ostwald coefficient leaving it at the actual temperature of the act of solution. For gases which also obey the law of Charles the relationship is:

$$\lambda = \alpha\left(1 + \frac{t}{273}\right)$$

where t is the Celsius temperature of the solution.

Since, in general, heating liquids tends to drive out dissolved gases, both coefficients are functions of temperature, quite apart from the above relationship. Other facts to note are as follows:

(i) The coefficients are now often regarded in terms of amount dissolved in unit liquid volume *per* unit pressure, rather than *at* a specified pressure. This makes them readily adaptable to changes of units, the only underlying assumption being that Henry's law holds over the pressure range of interest. For example, it is found that about 0.51 L of CO_5, assessed at s.t.p.d., dissolves in 1 L of a certain liquid when the partial pressure of the CO_2 is 1 atm. This can be translated into SI terms and in terms of mmHg by using:

$$1\,\text{atm} = 760\,\text{mmHg} = 101.325\,\text{kPa}$$

Clearly the (s.t.p.d. assessed) volumes dissolved *per* kPa or *per* mmHg follow by dividing the figure of 0.51 by 101.3 or by 760 respectively.

(ii) Sometimes the amount of gas is expressed in moles ('amount-of-substance') rather than as a volume. For many purposes the ideal-gas molar volume ($22.4\,L\,mol^{-1}$) is used. In this example the 0.51 L corresponds to about 23 millimole.

(iii) It is important to ascertain what is meant when a numerical value is quoted for a solubility coefficient. There are currently different pressure units in use, and some practices (such as expressing volume ratios as 'ml/100 ml' or as 'volumes percent') are still met, although now deprecated by the International Organization for Standardization, the World Health Organization and other official bodies. It is possible that the eventual unambiguous use of either mass or amount-of-substance (in moles) for both solvent and solute will introduce order into the subject, for reference purposes and for communication between disciplines.

Diffusion of Gases—Some Preliminaries

Diffusion is the process whereby a substance spreads through the space available to it, by random molecular motion (as opposed to bulk movement such as is caused by convection). Important situations involving diffusion as a concept include:

1. Redistribution within a simple enclosure, in response to spatial differences of concentration.
2. Diffusion across membranes or porous barriers, in response to concentration differences between compartments so separated.

Diffusion flux density is the name given to the rate of passage (with respect to *time*) of material across unit cross-sectional area perpendicular to the direction of diffusion. For this discussion the symbol J will be used, and the SI unit is mole-per-second per square metre ($mol\,s^{-1}\,m^{-2}$). It is almost invariably better to work in terms of *amount of substance* (in moles), and to convert to volumes if necessary later.

Concentration (c) is likewise expressed as amount of substance (gas etc.) per unit volume of space, and will be quoted here in moles per cubic metre ($mol\,m^{-3}$).

Concentration gradient (dc/dx) expresses the rate of change of concentration with distance. Here 'x' is taken as distance measured in the direction in which diffusion is being considered to take place. Since diffusion proceeds from higher to lower concentration regions, the gradient is negative (i.e. 'downwards') in the direction of diffusion. We will express the gradient in terms of moles-per-cubic-metre per metre, or $mol\,m^{-4}$. In this context 'gradient' is being used in its strict sense—i.e. rate of change with respect to distance. Four aspects of diffusion will now be considered:

1. The Fick diffusion equation, and Diffusion coefficient.
2. Krogh's diffusion coefficient.
3. Diffusion capacity of the lung.
4. Graham's law.

The Fick Diffusion Equation

This expresses the fact that the rate of diffusion of material across unit area (the diffusion-flux density) is greatest where the concentration changes most rapidly with respect to distance, or briefly:

diffusion-flux density is proportional to concentration gradient

Expressed symbolically this becomes:

$$J = -D\frac{dc}{dx}\,mol\,s^{-1}\,m^{-2}$$

The negative sign merely formalizes the observation made above, that dc/dx is negative in the direction of diffusion. The factor of proportionality, D, is called the *coefficient of diffusion*. It is seen here to mean the diffusion flux density caused by unit concentration gradient. The SI unit of D is as follows:

$$\frac{mol\,s^{-1}\,m^{-2}}{mol\,m^{-4}} \quad or \quad m^2\,s^{-1}$$

Spoken aloud as 'square metres per second' this is an excellent example of a unit which, although impeccably correct, is the result of cancelling out meaningful terms. It also reveals that provided we are consistent in choosing the same measure of quantity in diffusion-flux density and concentration gradient (both involving moles, or both involving volumes specified appropriately) the result is independent of this choice. In earlier literature, values of D are given in $cm^2\,s^{-1}$ or $cm^2\,min^{-1}$. For example, CO_2 diffusing in air has D of the order of $0.14\,cm^2\,s^{-1}$, or $1.4 \times 10^{-5}\,m^2\,s^{-1}$. In water D for CO_2 is of the order $15 \times 10^{-4}\,cm^2\,min^{-1}$, or say $0.25 \times 10^{-4}\,cm^2\,s^{-1}$.

Krogh's Diffusion Coefficient

For a given gas diffusing through a given liquid, Krogh's diffusion coefficient (K) links the general diffusion coefficient (D) with the Bunsen solubility coefficient (α). In comparison with

$$J = -D\frac{dc}{dx}$$

we have

$$J = -K\frac{dP}{dx}$$

That is, *Krogh's diffusion coefficient is the diffusion-flux density per unit pressure-gradient.*

To visualize this, consider a region of high partial pressure (P_1) and high concentration (c_1) separated from a region where they are low (P_2 and c_2) by distance x. From the definition of the Bunsen coefficient,

$$(c_1 - c_2) = \alpha(P_1 - P_2)$$

Hence the concentration gradient (numerically, ignoring the sign) is

$$\frac{c_1 - c_2}{x} = \alpha\left(\frac{P_1 - P_2}{x}\right)$$

Generalizing this—that is taking small changes of distance

$$\frac{dc}{dx} = \alpha\frac{dP}{dx}$$

So

$$K = \alpha D$$

Diffusion Capacity of the Lung

A cautionary observation on the use of the word 'gradient' is desirable here. Even in everyday English the word has the connotation of a ratio—the ratio of height climbed to distance travelled. Similarly in general scientific use, ratios are almost invariably implied, and we meet potential gradient (volts per metre), temperature gradient (kelvins per metre) as well as velocity gradient (as in viscosity). In this section, concentration gradient and pressure gradient have been used in their strict scientific sense. However, in medicine there are occasions when the word is used somewhat more loosely—it being assumed that the context is clear to workers in the particular field. One such example is met in the common definition of *diffusion capacity of the lung* as:

$$\frac{\text{net rate of gas transfer (ml min}^{-1})}{\text{partial pressure 'gradient' (kPa)}}$$

The denominator is, of course, a pressure *difference*. Naturally a pressure gradient does exist across the alveolar membrane, but this concerns the diffusion coefficient of the membrane *per se*.

It will be observed that diffusion capacity is a measure of a flow-type 'effect' per unit driving 'cause'. There are other scientific quantities of this nature, the best known of which is the electrical conductance of a *specimen* of conducting material. This is given by

$$\text{conductance} = \frac{\text{current flow (amperes)}}{\text{potential } \textit{difference} \text{ (volts)}}$$

and is of the reciprocal of resistance. It should also be noted that the electrical quantity

$$\frac{\text{current density (amperes per square metre)}}{\text{potential } \textit{gradient} \text{ (volts per metre)}}$$

also exists, and is called the *conductivity* of a *material*. This is analogous to diffusion coefficient.

Graham's Law of Gaseous Diffusion

This states that the rates at which different gases diffuse is *inversely proportional to the square-roots of their molecular masses*, other factors being kept constant. This is easily understood by imagining two different gases in identical environments. Being at the same temperature, their mean molecular kinetic energies will be the same. As a result, the product of molecular mass and the square of the velocity will be the same for 'average' molecules in both gases. Hence, in general, the velocities of the molecules will be inversely proportional to the square-roots of their masses and it is molecular velocity which is primarily involved in diffusion processes.

Vapours, Evaporation and Saturation Vapour Pressure

Reference has already been made, under the heading of the Gas Laws for real gases, to the *critical temperature* of a substance. This is the temperature above which the substance cannot be liquefied by compression. Although the terms 'gas' and 'vapour' are sometimes used as if interchangeable, strictly speaking a substance is a gas when at a temperature above its critical value. Thus although oxygen is a gas at room temperatures, water does not become a true gas until above 400°C, and iron becomes one within the Sun's atmosphere.

Now it is possible for molecules to leave the surface of a liquid (evaporation) or a solid (sublimation) at temperatures below the critical value. The mechanism is that of random movement, whereby the more energetic molecules are able to break away from the attraction of those molecules they leave behind. Molecules so penetrating beyond the interface constitute what is called a *vapour*—that is, gaseous phase at a temperature below the critical value.

Vapours are encountered in two forms: *saturated* and *unsaturated*. A saturated vapour is one which exists in equilibrium with its own liquid, so that as many molecules are in the act of leaving the liquid surface as are returning to it, both processes being random. In such a situation a pressure is exerted by the vapour which is unique for that substance at that temperature. Thus any attempt to compress the vapour results in molecules returning to the liquid phase so that the same number per unit volume remain in the vapour phase. The pressure measured under these circumstances is called the *Saturation Vapour Pressure* (s.v.p.).

In contrast, in a container having too little of a substance in vapour form for there to be a 'reservoir' of liquid, the vapour is said to be unsaturated and behaves as a gas. In particular, compression at fixed temperature is accompanied by rise of pressure, until the s.v.p. is reached, after which condensation results in the maintenance of this steady pressure.

Another contrast between a saturated vapour and a gas concerns variation of pressure with temperature. For a given mass of gas in a fixed volume, the increase of pressure with temperature is approximately linear. For a saturated vapour, rise of temperature shifts the whole spectrum of energies of the liquid molecules upwards. This results not only in a greater chance of any given molecule having sufficient energy to cross the interface, but increases the number possessing the necessary minimum energy to do so. Figure 2.27 illustrates the progressively steepening graphs of s.v.p. versus temperature. The upper curve is for a more volatile substance (like ether), and the lower one for a less volatile one (like water). Based on the theoretical work of Clapeyron and Clausius there are empirical equations for these curves for various substances. However these are are not particularly easy to manipulate algebraically, but can be simply handled by computers. Tables and graphs of s.v.p. versus temperature are in more general use at the present time.

Mixtures of Gases and Vapours

In practice vapours are often produced in association with gases, such as air. An important example concerns saturated water vapour with air. The contribution to the total pressure made by the saturated vapour is unaffected by the presence of the other gases and (for example) is known to be 47 mmHg for water vapour at 37°C. Thus if a container has saturated water vapour at this temperature, as well as other gases, and if the total pressure is 760 mmHg, only 713 mmHg has to be accounted for by the gases. According to Dalton's Law of partial pressure the individual contributions due to the various gases (e.g. oxygen, nitrogen, CO_2) are in proportion to their relative abundances in that specimen. For comparison, the SI values corresponding to 47, 760 and 713 mmHg are respectively 6.3, 101.3 and 95 kPa.

Cooling due to Evaporation

When the more energetic molecules break away from a liquid surface during the process of forming a vapour, this leaves the less energetic ones behind and so lowers the temperature of the bulk of liquid remaining. If the molecules that break free are removed from the vicinity, they cease to belong to the liquid sample. This therefore cools until any further heat loss by this mechanism just balances heat replacement from other sources, such as conduction from warmer bodies in contact with the remaining liquid.

Boiling and Latent Heat of Vaporization

Boiling is the process of conversion from the liquid to the vapour phase, in which bubbles of the vapour form before it escapes from the surface. This means that there is a vapour pressure set up which just equals the external pressure, and the bubble formation can be thought of as if the external pressure has 'failed' to suppress the establishment of a small local saturated vapour region. It is for this reason that 'Boiling Point' of a liquid is not a uniquely determined temperature,

but decreases with reduction of externally maintained pressure. It follows that redrawing Fig. 2.27 with the temperature scale vertical gives graphs of boiling

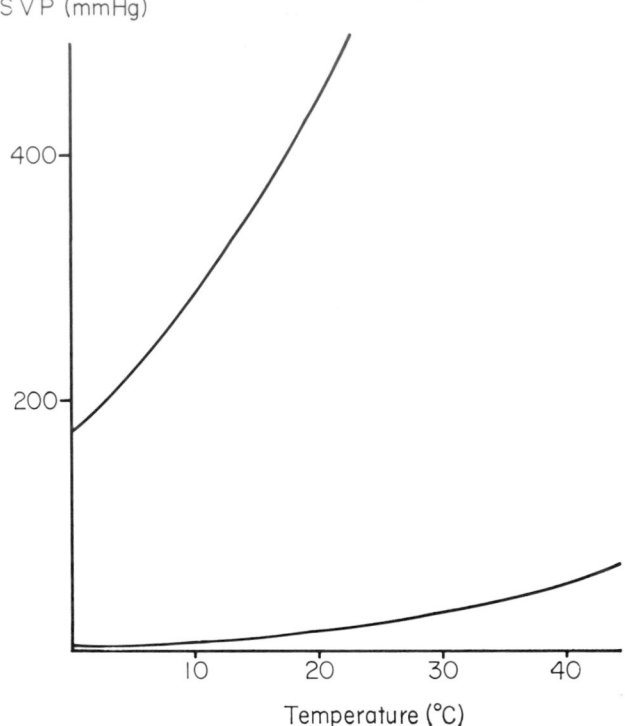

Fig. 2.27 Conversion: 1 mmHg = 0.1333 kPa (400 mmHg = 53.3 kPa).

point (temperature) versus ambient pressure. Where the context is unambiguous, 'boiling point' often implies the value at standard atmospheric pressure (the word 'normal' is progressively less often used in such contexts). Boiling is merely one situation (with more obvious activity taking place) in which molecules escape across the interface. One well-known aspect of boiling is the need to pressurize cooking-vessels at high altitude in order to reach the necessary temperatures for culinary purposes without losing all the water. An extension of this is the steam sterilizer in which this process is pursued to temperatures above 100°C by pressurizing beyond one atmosphere.

The *latent heat of vaporization* of a substance is the heat energy necessary to convert unit mass from the liquid to the vapour phase at constant temperature. It is usually specified under external pressure conditions of one atmosphere, and so at the standard boiling point of the liquid. The latent heat required is larger if the temperature at which vaporization is accomplished is reduced.

Humidity

In a sample of (undried) air, water molecules as

vapour share the *space* with other gas molecules. The mass of water per unit volume is called the *Absolute Humidity*. For each temperature there is a maximum absolute humidity corresponding to just the number of water molecules per unit volume of space that produces the s.v.p. at the temperature. Thus at 37°C, for which the s.v.p. is 6.3 kPa (47 mmHg), the maximum absolute humidity is about 50 grams per cubic metre (50 mg L^{-1}).

The ratio: *Actual water vapour pressure/saturation vapour pressure* is, to a good approximation, the same as the ratio: *actual absolute humidity/maximum absolute humidity* since the vapour pressure at a given temperature is proportional to the number of molecules (and hence the mass) per unit volume. Usually expressed as a percentage this ratio is called the *Relative Humidity* for the sample at that temperature. For example, a sample of air at 20°C, at which the s.v.p. is 2.4 kPa (18 mmHg) and for which the actual vapour pressure is 0.96 kPa (7.2 mmHg), has a relative humidity of 0.96/2.4 or 40%. If it were raised to 37°C (s.v.p. = 6.3 kPa or 47 mmHg) without addition of water, the relative humidity would fall to about 15% (0.96/6.3). Except for very precise work the relatively small rise of the actual (unsaturated) vapour pressure is usually ignored compared with the much greater increase of s.v.p. In this example such allowance would bring the answer nearer to 16% than 15%.

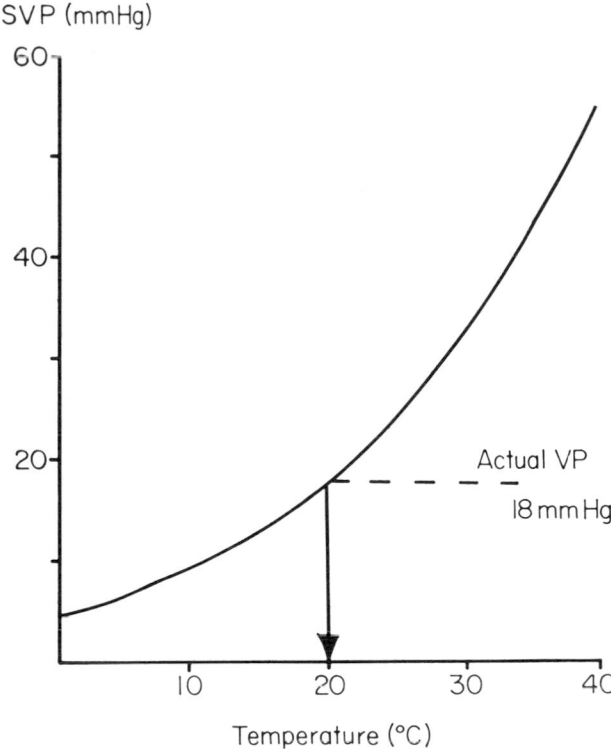

Fig. 2.28 Conversion: 1 mmHg = 0.1333 kPa (60 mmHg = 8.0 kPa; 18 mmHg = 2.4 kPa).

Condensation and Dew-point

If a sample of air cools until a temperature is reached where the actual vapour pressure equals the s.v.p., the relative humidity is 100%. This temperature is called the *Dew-point* for that air, and further cooling gives condensation. Figure 2.28 is for a sample unsaturated until 20°C is reached. The broken line indicating the actual vapour pressure would slope downwards to the left in a more exact treatment.

Viscosity

On an ideal motorway all vehicles would remain in lane, and for each lane there would be a speed exactly maintained by vehicles in that lane. This situation would be spoiled by vehicles drifting laterally, because (even discounting catastrophes) a mutual 'drag' effect would increase the resistance to flow of traffic. In a similar way, in fluid flow where velocity differentials occur laterally to the direction of flow (compare with adjacent traffic lanes), random lateral movements of particles inject 'out of lane' miscreants, resulting in friction between layers. In passing, it is appropriate that this effect is known as an example of 'transport' phenomena—those in which an effect is transported across a medium by motion of the particles.

Because of adhesion between fluid and the walls of tubes and other channels, it is common to find velocities varying from zero at walls towards maxima away from them. For a channel of a given size and

shape there is, for any given fluid, an upper limit of flow up to which 'lane discipline' is sufficiently well maintained, and motion proceeds as if in layers, constituting *laminar* (streamline) flow. Beyond such limits the flow is *turbulent*, and the lateral motions become macroscopic, producing eddies and swirling paths.

Newton's Law of Viscous Flow

For laminar flow the viscous drag between two adjacent layers having contact area A is a force F which increases in proportion to A. If the symbol v denotes the velocity within a given layer, we are concerned with the velocity gradient, or the rate at which v changes per unit distance across the layers. Denoting distance measured laterally by s (side-ways), the velocity gradient is written as dv/ds. To a good approximation F is found to be proportional to this, so

$$F = \eta A \frac{dv}{ds}$$

where η is a constant of proportionality for a given fluid. Often known in brief as the *viscosity*, its full name is the *coefficient of dynamic viscosity*. Examination of the defining equation shows that the meaning of η is the force per unit area tangential to the motion, per unit lateral velocity gradient.

Another way of expressing Newton's law of viscous flow is

$$\frac{F}{A} = \eta \frac{\mathrm{d}v}{\mathrm{d}s}$$

which is seen to be an example of the extremely common form

$$\text{effect} = \text{constant} \times \text{cause}$$

The cause, which we have called lateral velocity gradient is often referred to as the *shear rate*. The effect, which is the tangential force per unit contact area, is called the *shear stress*.

Units of Dynamic Viscosity

In SI units the shear rate is measured in metres per second (axially) per metre (laterally), or $\mathrm{m\,s^{-1}\,m^{-1}}$. Expressed as $\mathrm{s^{-1}}$ ('per second') this is correct, but scarcely informative. However it follows that the unit of dynamic viscosity is the newton of force divided by the square metre and then divided by 'per second', which reduces to newton seconds per square metre ($\mathrm{N\,s\,m^{-2}}$). The corresponding CGS unit is the dyne second per square centimetre ($\mathrm{dyn\,s\,cm^{-2}}$), better known as the poise (P) after Poiseuille. Since the dyne is one-hundred-thousandth of a newton and the square centimetre is one-ten-thousandth of a square metre

$$1\,\mathrm{P} = 0.1\,\mathrm{N\,s\,m^{-2}} = 0.1\,\mathrm{Pa\,s}$$

The modern tendency is to express dynamic viscosity in pascal-seconds, which unfortunately suppresses the distinction between pressure (force per unit area perpendicular to the force) and shear stress where the force is tangential to the relevant surface.

Temperature and Pressure Effects

Increase of temperature of a gas causes deeper lateral transport between 'lanes' because of the higher thermal velocities. This explains the general rise of viscosity with temperature increase observed in gases. Increase of pressure has little effect, because the consequent tighter packing has two conflicting results. The first is greater chance of collision; the second is less scope for lateral wandering.

The dominant factor in viscosity of liquids is the cohesions between passing molecules (they form short-term partnerships). Increase of temperature weakens these liaisons, and liquids generally are less viscous at higher temperatures.

Kinematic viscosity

In many circumstances the density of a fluid must be considered, as well as its viscosity. Examples include flow involving gravitational 'pressure heads' and flow in which accelerations take place. In both cases density enters into the problem since both weight and inertial opposition to acceleration are mass-dependent. In the mathematics of such studies it is found convenient to normalize equations encountered, by dividing throughout by the density and so reducing all relationships to a standard density basis.

The coefficient of kinematic viscosity is simply the ratio of the dynamic viscosity to the density of the fluid, or

$$v = \frac{\eta}{\rho}$$

The act of dividing $\mathrm{N\,s\,m^{-2}}$ by $\mathrm{kg\,m^{-3}}$ eventually yields the SI unit as the $\mathrm{m^2\,s^{-1}}$. The CGS unit is called the stokes (St).

Another important application of this ratio concerns turbulent flow. It is not surprising to find that increase of dynamic viscosity tends to reduce turbulence by damping out any disturbances in the flow pattern. The opposite effect is found when the density is increased. This is because any swirling disturbances that are set up tend to persist more when more dense material is involved, for the denser the material is, the more it is able to retain energy within eddies.

Reynolds Number (Re)

For a fluid flowing in a channel an empirical relationship is found to link the average velocity ($\bar{v}$) above which flow becomes turbulent, with the kinematic viscosity and with the dimensions of the channel. In particular, for a cylindrical tube of diameter D the *dimensionless* number.

$$Re = \frac{D\bar{v}}{v}$$

is found to have to be in excess of 2000 for turbulence to occur. In this context 'average' velocity means the average across the tube, not the time-average. To interpret this, imagine turbulence is just about to occur. An increase of velocity will obviously promote turbulence, and we have already argued that, as far as irregular motion is concerned it is the ratio known as kinematic viscosity which is important. An increase in D is able to promote turbulence simply by removing lateral constraints. However, it is very important to examine this from another point of view, since in medicine problems arise in which it is not so much that a given average velocity is involved, but that a given flow has to be considered within vessels of varying diameters.

Re-casting Reynold's number in terms of volume flow ($\dot{Q}$) and also in terms of the data most likely to be well-known gives:

$$Re = \frac{4\rho\dot{Q}}{\pi D\eta}$$

This states that, for a *given flow rate*, turbulence is most likely to occur for dense fluids of low dynamic viscosity in narrow tubes. Naturally this does not contradict the implication suggested by the first formulation of *Re*, that for a given average *velocity* turbulence is more likely if the diameter is large. An example makes this clear: with a *given volumetric flow*, halving the diameter reduces the cross-section area of the vessel 4-*fold*. This quadruples the average velocity, so whereas the *D* in the numerator of $D\bar{v}/v$ is halved, this is more than offset by quadrupling the $\bar{v}$. This is an example of the need for care when interpreting a formula: it is essential that the correct conditions are imposed when judging the effects of various terms.

Non-newtonian Fluids

Gases and simple liquids are often quoted as being 'newtonian' fluids. This means that for them Newton's law of viscous flow holds. This in turn implies that their dynamic viscosities (η) are not affected by the motion itself, and can be taken as constants. *Non-newtonian* fluids do not obey this law because, for them, η alters as the shear rate alters. Although blood is a non-newtonian fluid, for much work it is treated as sufficiently near newtonian to simplify models of blood flow, for which there are more than enough complications anyway.

Poiseuille's Equation

For laminar flow of a newtonian fluid along a cylindrical tube of radius *R*, the Poiseuille equation gives the *volume flow* as:

$$\dot{Q} = \frac{\pi}{8} \cdot \frac{P}{L} \cdot \frac{R^4}{\eta}$$

Here *P* is the pressure drop along a length *L* of tube, so the term *P/L* means the *axial pressure gradient*. Setting aside the purely numerical term $\pi/8$, the volume flow depends:

1. Directly on the pressure gradient, which may reasonably be thought of as the *cause*.
2. Inversely on the viscosity. This is reasonable, since for a given geometry and velocities, increase of viscosity means increased drag.
3. On the fourth power of the radius.

This third factor (R^4) is very significant, as can be seen by imagining a tube to be replaced by one of half the radius. This would result in considerable increase of opposition to flow, since R^4 would be reduced 16-*fold*. This will be elaborated later.

Velocity Profile

Fluid velocity varies from zero at walls towards maxima away from them. It is found experimentally, and can be confirmed mathematically, that although velocity is greatest down the centre of a tube, it varies

most rapidly near the walls. A graph of velocity at various positions, versus distance from the axis of a cylindrical tube is shown in Fig. 2.29, superimposed on a diagram showing representative particle paths

Particle paths

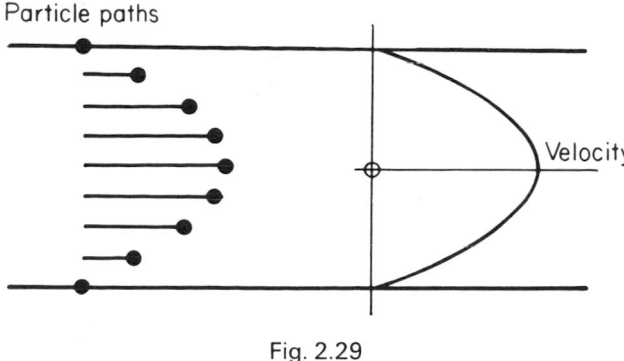

Velocity

Fig. 2.29

over unit time. For laminar flow of a newtonian fluid driven by a *steady* pressure gradient, this shape is found to be a *parabola*. From our point of view it is important that the velocity falls off most rapidly as the wall is approached. However, although the actual velocities are greatest near the centre, the edges are not to be neglected in assessment of total flow, since the low velocities are offset by the relatively larger circumferences than near the central core. Analysis shows that the average velocity is exactly half the maximum, in the parabolic profile case. In this context 'average' velocity $\bar{v}$ means that velocity which, had it applied all across the tube would have given the same flow as actually occurs. In fact it is found that:

$$\text{Maximum velocity} = \frac{P}{4L\eta} \cdot R^2$$

$$\text{Average velocity} = \frac{P}{8L\eta} \cdot R^2$$

It follows that

$$\dot{Q} = \bar{v}\pi R^2$$

$$= \frac{\pi P R^4}{8L\eta}$$

Although Poiseuille's equation is a useful qualitative guide, more complicated velocity profiles are met with alternating flows. These are due to acceleration and deceleration effects which, being different between the different velocity layers, break up the simple pattern with over-shoot and under-shoot effects. With *turbulent* flows the relatively large-scale lateral movements tend to even out the flow profile. The flatter profiles resulting are reminiscent of toothpaste coming from a tube. The higher opposition to flow associated with turbulent flow is related to the very steep velocity profiles, or high shear rates, near the vessel walls.

Qualitative Appreciation of Poiseuille's Equation

Returning to Poiseuille's equation, it is instructive to explore the dependence on the fourth power of the radius, by taking a simple example. Consider the consequences of choosing a *smaller* tube (say by halving R), while increasing the pressure to maintain the same volume flow. The steps in the argument are:

1. Halving the radius reduces the cross-section area to a quarter, and so enforces a 4-*fold* increase in all velocities if the same flow is maintained.
2. Because of the smaller radius, the lateral changes of these velocities are cramped into half the space. Consequently the velocity gradients are increased 8-*fold*
3. Considering the moving mass of fluid as a whole, there is only a quarter of the area over which the applied pressure can develop the thrust required to move the fluid past the vessel wall. At first sight this would seem to worsen the situation a further four times, requiring a 32-*fold* increase of pressure.
4. However, because the actual surface area of wall in contact with the fluid is halved (having the radius halves the circumference), the necessary increase of pressure is not 32-*fold* but is 16-*fold* as predicted by the equation.

This is of considerable importance, not only in the flow of fluids in vessels but also in the recording of remote pressures, such as blood-pressures monitored along catheters.

Resistance of a Tube

For a given length of circular tube passing a steadily flowing newtonian fluid without turbulence, Poiseuille's equation can be written as:

$$\frac{\text{Pressure}}{\text{Flow}} = \frac{8L\eta}{\pi R^4} = \text{Constant}$$

By analogy with Ohm's law for the relationship between potential difference and current (electric flow), as is discussed later in the chapter, it is convenient to think of this constant as the resistance of the given tube to flow of the stated fluid.

Where turbulence is set up, either due to generally increased flow or to localized eddies at discontinuities, the resistance ceases to be constant. As with the description of other non-linear effects, various algebraic relationships are met for particular fluids over different flow ranges for a variety of tubes, orifices etc. These are essentially no more than the result of fitting power-series and other algebraic equations to empirical data. One of the simplest is for fully turbulent gas flow through a pipe, for which the resistance is itself roughly proportional to flow. This may be met as:

$$\text{Pressure} = \text{Constant} \times \text{Flow}^2$$

or as $\quad\quad \text{Flow} \propto \sqrt{\text{Pressure}}$

All such empirical approximations are to be regarded as being restricted to known and established situations, and not taken as universal.

ELECTRICAL QUANTITIES

The rest of this chapter has two objectives. The first is to extend the list of physical quantities dealt with so far by introducing some of the more useful electrical and magnetic quantities and their associated units. As concepts related to this aspect of science are discussed, important relationships will be detected between electrical quantities, which are analogous to relationships between the more familiar mechanical ones. For example, it is much easier to understand inductive reactance when the underlying concept is recognized as strictly analogous to the opposition experienced when shaking a medicine-ball.

The second objective is to discuss topics, such as linearity, distortion and equivalent circuits, which are of particular use in the understanding of electrical circuits. Electrical and communications engineers have enjoyed a considerable advantage in the past, because their subjects lend themselves to greatly simplifying concepts which allow very rapid assessment of the essentials of apparently complex devices and systems. Because of the strong analogous relationships between the various branches of science, these concepts, theorems and problem-solving strategems are not restricted to electrical circuits but are of considerable general interest.

Electric Charge

The earliest observations on the effects of electricity involved the production of what was called 'static electricity' by friction, as when two materials (such as glass and silk) are rubbed together. It was found that two pieces of glass so treated then repelled one another, as did two pieces of silk. In contrast, it was found that a piece of the glass and a piece of the silk attracted one another. It was therefore conceived that these materials had been 'charged' by something which existed in two distinct forms. These ideas were expressed by saying that 'like charges (of electricity) repel one another' and 'unlike charges attract one another.' It only remained to observe that when two bodies oppositely charged come together they could become inert, to justify calling the two forms *positive* and *negative*, implying that they neutralize one anothers' effects. As to which should be called positive— the decision was essentially as arbitrary as the decision of the British to drive on the left. The subsequently discovered *electron* was found to fall into the 'negative' category, while the atomic nuclei were found to be 'positive.'

The quantity of electricity associated with a body is called the *electric charge*. Various units have been defined, but we are here concerned with the coulomb (C). It is advantageous as an interim measure to regard electric charge as basic, and for the moment we will picture the coulomb in terms of the electric charge associated with some measurable amount of ionized material. In fact, an early definition took it as the charge associated with the electrolytic deposition of 0.001 118 gram of silver from silver nitrate solution.

Electric Current

When sources of *moving* electric charge were developed by analogy with the current of a flowing fluid (litres per minute, or more appropriately cubic metres per second) *electric current* was defined as the rate of passage of electric charge. On this basis we would expect current to be measured in *coulombs per second* $(\mathrm{C\,s^{-1}})$. The urges to abbreviate and to celebrate tend to obscure the obvious by calling this unit the ampere $(1\mathrm{\,A}=1\mathrm{\,C\,s^{-1}})$.

Using the familiar symbols, Q for charge and I for current, we see that a steady current of I amperes (coulombs per second) flowing for t seconds involves the passage of Q coulombs, given by

$$Q = It$$

For various reasons, it has been decided to take the ampere as the SI defined unit, and to regard the coulomb as the charge deposited when one ampere flows for one second.

Electromotive Force (EMF)

All sources of electric current (cells, generators, etc.) are capable of creating at their terminals (*see* A, B in Fig. 2.30) excess positive and excess negative charge:

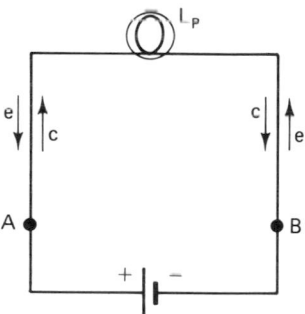

Fig. 2.30 Note conventional symbol for a cell and for a lamp. Electron flow is indicated by arrows e, conventional current by arrows c.

that is, they cause separation of charges in otherwise neutral material. When a conducting device (such as a lamp, shown symbolically in the figure) is connected between the terminals, it is the attraction between opposite charges which causes the flow of current. In describing the 'strength' of a pump we have already seen that an important interpretation of pressure is work done per unit quantity of fluid driven by the pump. By analogy the 'strength' (electromotive force) of an electrical generator is the work done when it drives unit quantity of electric charge round an external circuit. For example, if in driving 1 coulomb the source does 240 joules of work, we say that the EMF is 240 joules per coulomb. The joule per coulomb is abbreviated to the volt $(1\mathrm{\ V}=1\mathrm{\,J\,C^{-1}})$, but it is worth thinking in terms of what it means. Thus a 6 volt battery of cells will do 6 joules of work with every coulomb passed, just as a 6 newton per square metre pressure source does 6 joules of work for each cubic metre of fluid pumped.

'Conventional' Current Flow

Although both positive and negative charge carriers (ions) can exist in electrolytes and ionized gases, in metals only the loosely bound outer electrons are free to move. Consequently, the flow of electricity may involve the passage of different charges moving in opposite directions in some situations, while in the system of Fig. 2.31 charges of one sign only (electrons)

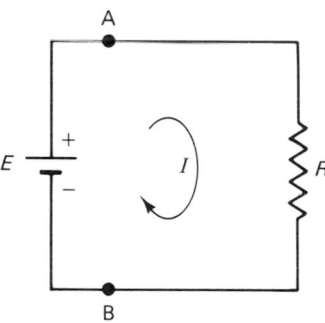

Fig. 2.31 The zig-zag symbol represents any circuit element offering resistance to current. *I* indicates conventional sense of current.

flow away from the electron-repelling electrode B towards the positive electrode A. Before the discovery of electrons it was decided *quite arbitrarily* (but of course consistently) to label electrodes positive and negative, and it was postulated that the (unseen) electric current flowed from the one called positive to the one called negative. For many applications it is irrelevant which way the actual charge carriers flow, and it is very common to encounter a diagram such as Fig. 2.31 in which R represents some circuit element or device in which it is of academic interest whether negative or positive ions or both are involved.

Resistance to Flow of Electricity

When electrons or ions move through a material under the action of an electric 'field' (region of attraction one way and repulsion the other for a given charged particle), collisions occur. This has two important consequences:

1. The material becomes heated as energy is imparted to the molecules affected.
2. These collisions constitute resistance to the flow of current.

Such resistance is analogous to the resistance of an airway to the extent that it imposes a restriction on the current that can be forced through by a given EMF. In his famous experiments Ohm quantified the concept of resistance and we would say that a resistance of R units restricts the current from a source of EMF E volts to I amperes, where

$$I = \frac{E}{R}$$

The unit of R is thus the volt per ampere, which is abbreviated to the ohm ($1\,\Omega = 1\,V\,A^{-1}$).

Potential Differences

In an anaesthetic circuit pressure differences exist between various points due to the resistances to flow caused by tubing, bends, joints, etc. Similarly no electrical circuit consists of a single resistance, since there is always at least the 'internal' resistance of the source, due to material imperfections. Consequently electrical circuits consist of at least two parts, such as r and R in Fig. 2.32, which has two elements in series. For

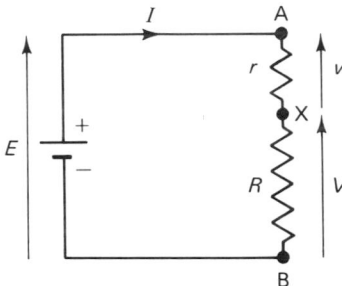

Fig. 2.32 The addition of potential differences v and V to equal the applied EMF E. Following from the scalar nature of energy.

example, R might represent an obvious 'load,' such as a lamp and r might represent the internal resistance of the source.

For every coulomb of charge passing between A and B, the work done is E joules, because the EMF is E joules per coulomb. Some of this is dissipated as heat in R and the rest within r. The number of joules per coulomb dissipated between X and B is called the potential difference (V volts), or the potential of X relative to B. This compares directly with the pressure difference between two points in a fluid flow system. Ohm showed that this potential difference is

$$V = IR$$

and we similarly find that for AX

$$v = Ir$$

Now energy is not only conserved, but is scalar, so the total energy delivered by the source for each coulomb passed, must equal the sum of the energies dissipated in the circuit. For this reason we find that potential differences in series are simply additive, or

$$E = V + v$$

It therefore follows that

$$E = I(R + r)$$

In words, this means that resistance in series are additive.

The analogy between electrical and fluid resistances is important. A resistive circuit element is one which dissipates energy when flow takes place, and it is this energy dissipated, for unit charge passed, that we call potential difference in the electrical case. In fluid systems this corresponds to pressure difference, given by energy dissipated per unit volume passed.

Power Related to Electric Current

By definition of the volt (joule per coulomb), if Q coulombs pass between terminals X and B across which a potential difference of V volts exists, VQ joules of work is done. If it takes t seconds to do this, the power (rate of doing work) is

$$W = VQ/t \text{ joules per second}$$
or
$$W = VI \text{ watts}$$

It is mainly due to the non-coherent units of pressure and flow encountered in medicine that this simple relationship is better known than its fluid flow counterpart:

$$\text{Power} = \text{Pressure difference} \times \text{Flow}$$

For example, a flow of 6 litres per minute (10^{-4} cubic metres per second) occurring with a pressure difference of $12\,kNm^{-2}$ (90 mmHg) requires the pump to develop a power of

$$W = 12\,000 \times 10^{-4}$$
$$= 1.2 \text{ watts}$$

Electrical Components other than Resistance

In mechanical systems we encounter four common classes of component:

1. *Dissipative components* such as frictional resistance.
2. *Potential energy storage components* such as springs.
3. *Kinetic energy storage components* such as flywheels, and
4. Components which *transform*, or adjust the level of mechanical thrusts and motions, such as levers and gears.

Similarly in electrical circuits we meet

1. *Resistive* elements which dissipate energy.
2. *Capacitors* which store energy electrostatically.
3. *Inductors* which store energy electromagnetically, and
4. *Transformers* which adjust levels of voltage and current.

The concepts underlying these are important, not only for the understanding of electrical apparatus, but also for appreciating the problems of electrical safety and reduction of electrical interference (*see also* Chapter 3).

Capacitance

In Fig. 2.33 X and Y represent two conducting bodies

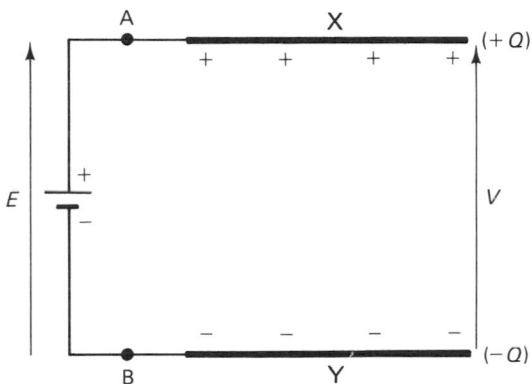

Fig. 2.33 Charging a capacitor.

separated from one another by an insulating (or dielectric) gap, and connected to a source of EMF. Because like charges repel one another, some of the excess electrons at terminal B avail themselves of the opportunity to spread out on Y, *temporarily* constituting a current in YB. Although these electrons are unable to cross the gap, their arrival repels some electrons from X, and these electrons are attracted to the positive terminal A anyway. Consequently a transient current flows, conventionally along AX and YB, completing the circuit. This leaves the pair XY in a 'charged' state, manifested in two ways:

1. A potential difference V is associated with the separated charges: this rises to equal the EMF E, at which point the process stops.
2. An 'electric field'—a region in which attraction in a specific direction is experienced by any charged body—is set up in the gap.

If, during the transient flow, Q coulombs of negative charge arrive at Y and leave X (as shown by the excess positive charge $+Q$ remaining), it is found that the charge Q is proportional to the potential difference V, or

$$Q = CV$$

The factor of proportionality C is constant for a given pair of conducting bodies XY. It is the charge in coulombs established per volt of potential difference set up. This is reminiscent of compliance, defined as volume taken up per unit change of pressure difference set up, and C is known as the capacitance of the system. The unit is essentially the coulomb (of charge stored) per volt (of potential difference necessarily set up), and is abbreviated to the farad, so

$$1 \text{ F} = 1 \text{ coulomb per volt}$$

Aspects of Capacitance

Although some applications of capacitance involve the energy storage aspect, it is more important that during transient conditions and in cases where sources of EMF are alternating, the action across the insulated gap discussed above can give rise to current flow *without* direct connection. This is deliberately used in electrical circuits involving capacitors (devices made to exhibit known capacitance). Such devices have capacitances in the range of picofarads (1 pF = 10^{-12} F) to thousands of microfarads. However, capacitance can exist between any two separate conducting bodies, such as a patient and an electrical cable, or an anaesthetist and his patient. (This matter is discussed in Chapter 3.) Three factors determine the capacitance between two bodies. Capacitance increases if the area of the bodies is increased, since this gives more opportunity for the charges to spread. Similarly, decreasing the distance between the bodies intensifies the field and permits more electrons to arrive at one and repel electrons from the other. Finally the introduction of an insulating material, in place of a vacuum or air, can increase capacitance by a factor depending on the material used.

Some Aspects of Magnetism

Magnetic fields are regions in which certain types of phenomena are observed, including:

1. The attraction and repulsion of magnets and magnetizable pieces of metal.
2. Interaction with current-carrying conductors, as in meters and motors.
3. The induction of EMFs, as in electrical generators and transformers.

The magnetic effects near permanent magnets, due to electron movements at the molecular level can be thought of as similar to those produced near conductors by the gross movement of electrons. It is the second and third categories of phenomena which are relevant here and to assist in the visualization of these, some aspects of 'magnetic flux' will be recapitulated. Although in the historical development of the subject, magnetic flux came relatively late, our present purposes are better served by taking over this concept as a starting point.

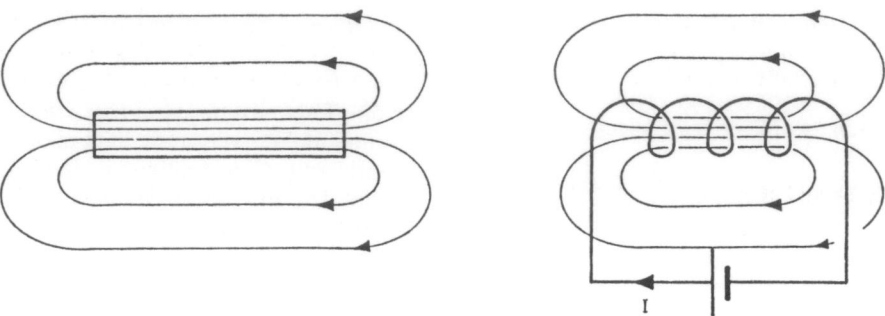

Fig. 2.34 Magnetic flux due to a bar magnet and due to a current-carrying coil. As far as observed effects are concerned, the source is irrelevant.

Magnetic Flux

The phenomena of electromagnetism are visualized— a first step towards explanation—by imagining lines indicating the presence of these phenomena, as illustrated in Fig. 2.34. Here, within and around both a permanent magnet and a conductor (in the form of turns of wire) carrying current, the closed loops drawn are representative of lines of magnetic flux. In passing, the reason for coiling the conductor is simply to arrange more of it to lie close to the region where the effects are desired to be produced. The term 'flux' suggests that, in the absence of human sensory awareness, early workers supposed that some form of influence (possibly even a substance) actually flowed around magnetic circuits. These lines are drawn so as to be most densely packed where the observed effects are most pronounced. In addition, at any point the direction associated with these lines coincides with the direction in which a north-seeking pole would be attracted. Of course, these convenient lines are simply an aid to visualization just as are lines of longitude, contour lines and isobars.

Electromagnetic Induction

Figure 2.35 represents a conductor AB, either as a single 'turn' or more generally a number (N) of turns, lying within a region of magnetic flux. It is found that an EMF can be induced within the conductor if its relationship to the flux is made to vary either by:

1. Moving the conductor or the magnetic circuit producing the flux, relative to one another, so that a different amount of flux threads (or 'links' with) the conductor, or

2. Altering the amount of flux, without moving the conductor or the flux source. The easiest way of doing this is to *produce* the flux by passing current through some other conductor and simply varying this 'magnetizing' current.

Whatever the mechanism, it is found that *the more rapid the change, the larger is the EMF.*

Induction of an EMF in this way enables us to quantify magnetic flux. The unit is the weber (Wb), and it is defined so that flux linkage changing at the *rate* of 1 weber per second (in one turn) causes an EMF of 1 volt to appear. Thus if ϕ webers of flux link with N turns, and ϕ is changing, then the resulting EMF is N multiplied by $d\phi/dt$, in volts. Notice that the observed phenomenon is the appearance of an EMF, and we imagine changing flux linkage to visualize this process, rather as a meteorologist feeling a strong wind might picture this in terms of a region of high isobar density having moved across the weather map.

Flux Density

Since the packing density of lines of flux is imagined as representing the local concentration of observed effects, we formalize this by defining *flux density* (usual symbol B) as the number of flux lines passing through

One turn N turns

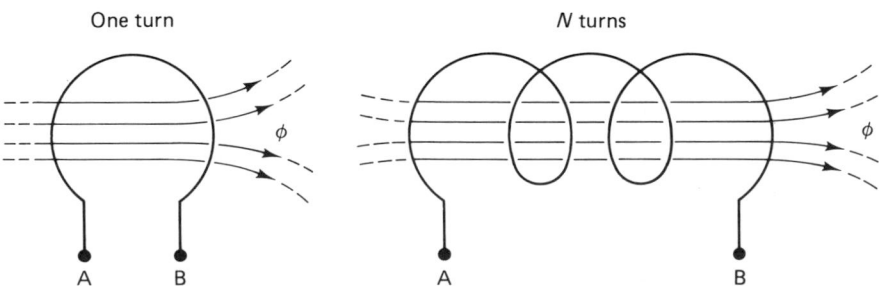

Fig. 2.35 Flux linking with a conductor with one or more 'turns'. EMF is induced if the linkage *changes*.

unit cross-sectional area—i.e. per unit area normal to their direction. The unit of flux density is therefore the weber per square metre, abbreviated to the *tesla*:

$$1 \text{ T} = 1 \text{ Wb m}^{-2}$$

The Motor Effect and the Moving Coil Meter

Figure 2.36 illustrates a section of a conductor carrying a current I amperes, and lying perpendicular to

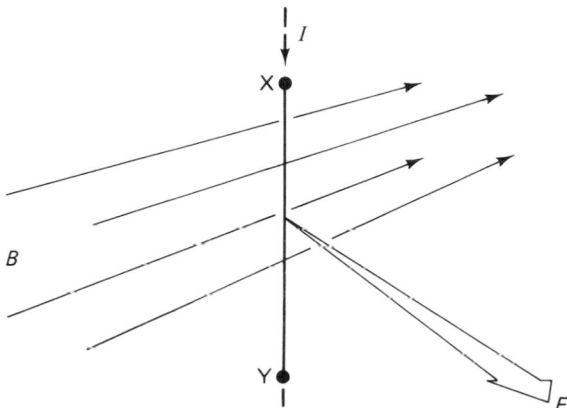

Fig. 2.36 Force on a conductor carrying a current within a region of magnetic flux—the Motor Effect.

magnetic flux of density B teslas. If the length XY is L metres it is found that a force F newtons acts as shown, mutually perpendicular to the flux and to the conductor. F is larger for stronger flux density, for greater current and for greater length of conductor, i.e.

$$F = BIL \text{ newtons}$$

Recording devices based on the moving coil meter movement rely on this effect. If the rectangular coil ABCD in Fig. 2.37 is arranged always to lie in the same plane as the magnetic flux as shown, then a current I

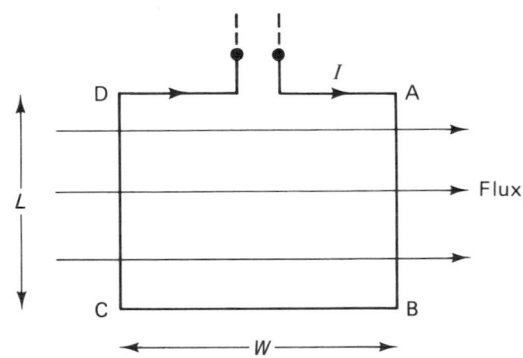

Fig. 2.37 The rectangular coil—basis of moving-coil meters.

to be measured causes a force BIL to pull the side AB out of the plane of the diagram, and an equal force to push CD into that plane. The coil will be twisted by a torque given by $WBIL$ newton metres, and measurement of this torque permits I to be measured. To do this the coil (which usually has many turns—say N) is pivoted and allowed to twist against a restoring spring for which the opposing torque is proportional to the angle of rotation θ. Hence the rotation ceases when

$$NBWL.I = S\theta$$

S being the stiffness coefficient of the spring. Figure 2.38

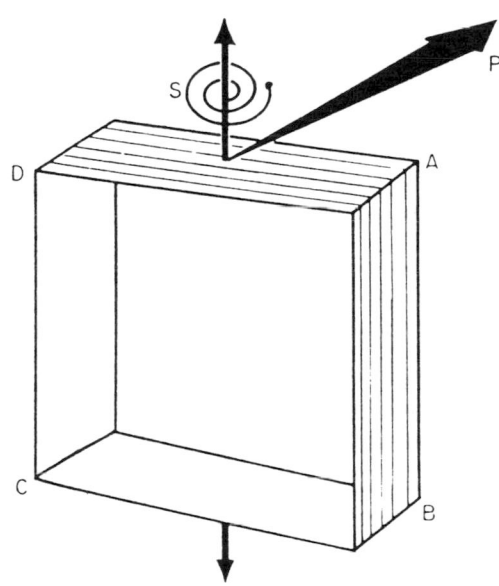

Fig. 2.38 Arrangement of restoring spring S and pointer P. Several turns are wound on a frame A B C D.

illustrates the arrangement, showing the rectangular pivoted frame on which the turns are wound, the restoring spring S and a pointer P fixed to the frame. To ensure that, even as it rotates, the coil always lies coplanar with the flux and that B is constant, curved pole pieces NS (shown in Fig. 2.39) are used, with a fixed soft iron cylinder C to concentrate the flux and make it radial as required. The coil is mounted coaxially with C and its sides swing within the gaps NC and CS.

Electromagnetic Induction and the Generation of Electricity

If a coil is rotated in a magnetic field the effect is the reverse of the motor effect, and an EMF is generated. One of the simplest examples is when a rectangular coil rotates in a uniform (as opposed to radial) field. Here the flux linkage alternates from maximum when the plane of the coil is at right-angles to the flux, through zero when they are coplanar and to max-

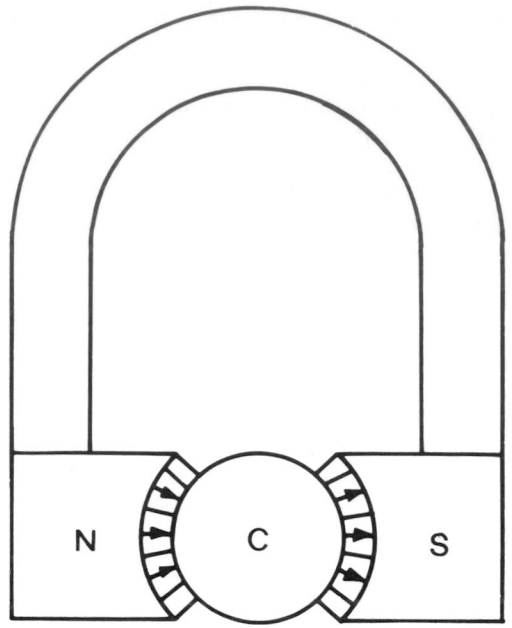

Fig. 2.39 Obtaining a radial uniform magnetic flux.

imum in the reverse direction after 180 degrees rotation. This gives rise to a sinusoidally varying EMF, such as is encountered with the alternating current (a.c.) mains electricity supply. The advantages of a.c. supplies include:

1. Ease of transmission.
2. Greater flexibility from the point of view of the user.

These both depend on the fact that 'transformers' can increase or decrease the size of an alternating EMF as required. For transmission of power it is easier to work at very high voltages (with correspondingly low currents in the cables), the voltage being brought down to safer values before handing over to the consumer. Within apparatus the 240 volt public supply may be stepped up for some purposes and down for others.

Certain 'geometrical' aspects of the sinusoidally alternating waveform are of importance. In Fig. 2.40 the

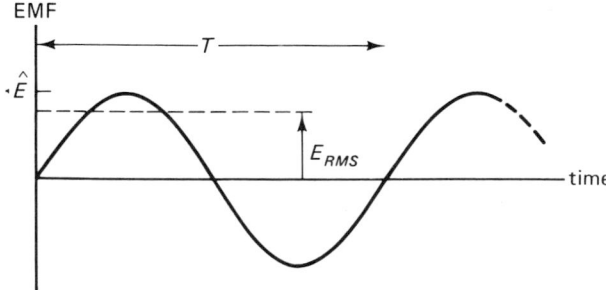

Fig. 2.40 The sinusoidal waveform, showing period (*T*), peak amplitude (*Ê*) and RMS measure.

time *T* for a complete cycle of alternation is called the period, or periodic time. The number of cycles per second is known as the frequency (*f*) and

$$f = 1/T$$

Until recently the unit of frequency was called the cycle per second (c/s) but it is now called the hertz (Hz). Thus if *T* is 20 milliseconds, *f* is 50 Hz.

The peak amplitude reached is shown as $\hat{E}$, but it is usual to specify sinusoidal EMFs by the steady value which would produce the same heating effect. Since a high value of *E* causes a proportionally high value of current *I* in a load, the power delivered, being given by *EI* depends on the *square* of *E*. As a result the effective equivalent steady value is often called the RMS (square root of the mean of the squares) value, E_{RMS}. This value gives more prominence to the higher excursions of *E* than the intermediate values and may be shown to be

$$E_{RMS} = \hat{E}/\sqrt{2}$$

It is this value which is actually quoted, so the 240 volt a.c. mains actually alternates with a peak value of $240\sqrt{2}$, or 340 volts.

Mutual- and Self-induction

In Fig. 2.41 current I_1 from an alternating supply

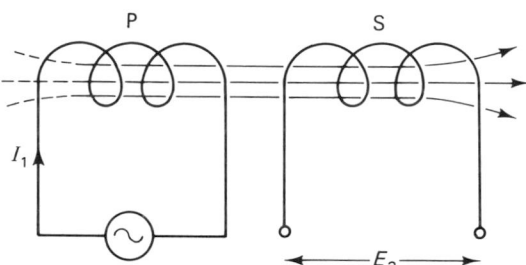

Fig. 2.41 Mutual induction: when the current (I_1) in P changes, the resulting changing flux induces an EMF (E_2) in S.

(represented by the circuit symbol shown) causes magnetic flux which also alternates. An EMF E_2 is consequently induced in a conductor such a S linked by changing flux due to the current I_1. The magnitude of the EMF induced in the 'secondary' circuit S is found to be proportional at all times to the rate of change of flux linkage, and hence of the current in the 'primary' circuit causing this flux. Symbolically

$$|E_2| \propto \frac{dI_1}{dt}$$

$$= M \frac{dI_1}{dt}$$

The factor of proportionality *M*, which gives the

secondary EMF caused by unit rate of change of primary current is called the coefficient of mutual inductance. Its unit is the henry (H), which is short for the volt per ampere-per-second.

Mutual inductance is deliberately created in devices known as transformers, but is also important in explaining some forms of electrical interference, as will be seen in Chapter 3.

In transformers the use of very tight coupling, by winding P (primary) and S (secondary) on top of one another, often on cores of ferromagnetic materials which encourage the establishment of flux, makes it possible to create efficiently an alternating EMF in the secondary circuit, the energy being transferred by magnetic linkage with the primary circuit. If the secondary winding has more turns than the primary, the induced EMF can be larger than the supply EMF, and vice versa if the secondary has fewer turns. This enables, for example, the mains supply to be transformed up in EMF for some requirements, and down for others.

Self-inductance, as the name suggests, concerns EMF induced in a circuit due to a changing current flowing in the circuit itself, in contrast to current in an adjacent circuit. In Fig. 2.42 an electrical source causes

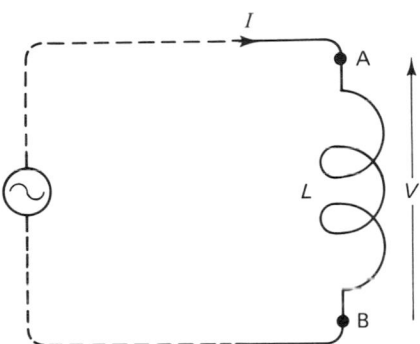

Fig. 2.42 Self-induction: here the alternating flux is caused by the a.c. *I*. (The broken lines are to suggest that the circuit causing the current is not under discussion.)

changing current *I* to flow in a circuit represented by the coil AB. The consequent changing flux links the circuit itself, and an EMF is induced between the terminals AB just as truly as if the flux had been caused by some other source. In this case the number of volts induced by unit rate of change of current is called the (coefficient of) self-inductance, or simply the inductance, of the circuit. The common symbol is *L*, and the unit is the henry, as for mutual inductance.

Electrical and Mechanical Analogues

In the simplest law of sliding friction the force (*F*) of opposition experienced is approximately proportional to the velocity of the moving surface (*v*), or

$$F = rv$$

corresponding to Ohm's Law for electrical resistance

$$V = RI$$

The simplest spring opposes a movement (displacement, *x*) by a force

$$F = Sx$$

where *S* expresses the stiffness. This can be re-written as

$$x = CF$$

C is the reciprocal of *S*, a measure of compliance. This is seen to be analogous to the capacitance low

$$Q = CV$$

This analogy also is *consistent* with that for resistance, because if charge *Q* is taken as analogous to displacement *x*, this agrees with current *I* (rate of change of charge) being analogous to velocity *v* (rate of change of displacement).

Inductance is found to be analogous to mass, because if we denote by *V* the potential difference induced between the terminals of a circuit exhibiting inductance *L* henries, measured in the sense of *opposing* a rate of change of current d*I*/d*t* we find

$$V = L \, dI/dt$$

This is precisely analogous to the result

$$F = ma$$

for a mass *m* being accelerated, since

$$a = dv/dt$$

These analogous quantities are listed, together with consequent extensions in Table 2.1. They enable us to relate the less familiar concepts of electrical circuits to events such as accelerations, displacements, thrusts

TABLE 2.1

Mechanical concept, etc	
Displacement	x
Velocity	$v = dx/dt$
Force	F
Friction resistance law	$F = rv$
Compliance law	$F = x/C$
Inertia law	$F = m \, dv/dt$
Work definition	work $= Fx$
Power law	Power $= Fv$
Kinetic energy	K.E. $= \frac{1}{2}mv^2$
Potential Energy	P.E. $= \frac{1}{2}CF^2$
Electrical analogue	
Charge	Q
Current	$I = dQ/dt$
Potential difference p.d.	V
Electrical resistance law	$V = RI$
Capacitance law	$V = Q/C$
Inductance law	$V = L \, dI/dt$
P.D. definition	Work $= VQ$
Electrical power	Power $= VI$
Energy in inductance	Energy $= \frac{1}{2}LI^2$
Energy in capacitance	Energy $= \frac{1}{2}CV^2$

and so on which we experience with our own bodies and the many simple mechanical devices encountered every day. In this table, the compliance C refers to $1/S$ for a simple spring. This is itself analogous to volume compliance, as met by anaesthetists. Also, to preserve the obvious similarity between p.e. and energy in a capacitance, the former is expressed as $\frac{1}{2}CF^2$, but substitution yields the more familiar $\frac{1}{2}Sx^2$.

Impedance and Phase Concepts

If one's hand is moved to and fro under water, with a sinusoidal motion (fastest in the centre, slowing towards the extremes), the frictional resistance force is felt to be maximal when the velocity is maximal, and zero when the velocity is zero. In the same way, the potential difference across a resistor is found to be 'in phase with' the current through it.

In contrast, if a heavy object is shaken from side to side, the inertial opposition forces are felt to be greatest at the instants when the velocity is zero (at the lateral extremes of the shaking), and zero when the velocity is maximum (in the middle of the shake). This is expressed by saying that the force is a quarter of a cycle out of phase with the velocity, or that they are 'in quadrature.' Figure 2.43 illustrates the analogous phenomenon for the inductor. Since V depends on the rate of change of I it is maximal when I changes most rapidly—on coming through zero.

Not only are V and I in quadrature, but it is found that for a given current amplitude the peak value of V is larger the more rapidly I changes—that is, the higher the frequency. The ratio of the peak value of V to that of I is (to distinguish the phenomenon from resistance) called the *reactance* of the inductor (X). X is obviously greater for larger inductance (L), since the larger L is for a given peak current, the more it opposes the changing current. In fact it is found that

$$X = 2\pi f L \text{ ohms}$$

Notice that this opposition to a.c. is in no way due to resistance. Even a copper conductor an inch thick will oppose and set a limit to a *changing* current.

Capacitance also exhibits quadrature phase relationship between current and potential difference, the only distinction being that, because it takes time for a capacitor to establish a p.d. when a current flows, the p.d. lags a quarter of a cycle behind the current. With the inductor the 'inertia-like' opposition to changing current results in the latter lagging behind the potential difference. It is also found that the reactance (size of V divided by size of I) varies with frequency, but since a higher frequency provides less time for the capacitor to charge before the current reverses it is found that the reactance *falls* as frequency increases. Also, since a large capacitance means one that can take on a relatively large charge before the opposing p.d. becomes appreciable, it is not surprising to find that the reactance falls with larger capacitance. It is found that, for a capacitor

$$X = \frac{1}{2\pi f C} \text{ ohms}$$

The appearance of 2π in the formulae for reactances of inductors and capacitors is a simple consequence of the geometry of the sinusoid. Whether measured graphically or deduced by using the differential calculus, it is found that the steepest rate of rise, had it been maintained would have caused peak amplitude to be reached in the fraction $1/2\pi$ of a cycle.

As in mechanical systems, the two electrical energy storing devices (L and C) behave differently from one another as frequency is changed, one increasing its opposition to a.c., the other lowering it. In general, circuits may have mixtures of components, resistive and reactive, and the opposition to a.c. is not simply proportional or inversely proportional to frequency as with pure reactances, but varies in a more complicated way. For mixed circuits the term *impedance* is used to suggest opposition. Thus

$$\text{impedance } (Z) = \frac{\text{size of p.d. across circuit}}{\text{size of current through it}}$$

R (resistance) and X (reactance) are thus special cases of Z (impedance), R being used for purely dissipative components, and X for purely energy-storing ones.

It is important to appreciate, even if only in quite general terms, that for circuits in general, impedances and the phase relationships between current and potential difference can vary with frequency. Reference will be made to this in discussions of applications of electrical circuitry and devices.

Resonance

By pressing down gradually on the roof of a car, the opposition developed by the springs when given time to act can be easily felt. In contrast, to become aware of the inertia of the car it is necessary to press down sharply, because inertial opposition depends on

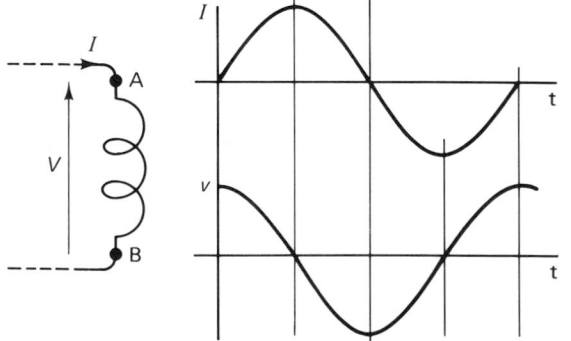

Fig. 2.43 Inertia-like behaviour of an inductor, V is maximal when I is changing most rapidly, and zero when I passes through its peak.

acceleration instead of displacement. By pressing up and down at the frequency at which the car shakes 'naturally,' the inertial opposition and the stiffness opposition can be made to cancel one another. For example, the moment when the springs are most compressed and pushing upwards most strongly is the moment when the mass is undergoing greatest deceleration. Similarly, half a cycle later the springs are pulling down most forcibly at the instant when the tendency to overshoot requires to be controlled by downwards acceleration. With the inertial and compressional forces fighting one another, the man rocking the car at the correct rate merely has to overcome the third physical component, the frictional resistance. It should be noticed that, as in other analogous oscillatory systems, a mass and spring continuously interchange energy between two forms—kinetic and potential here. In electrical resonant circuits, inductance and capacitance correspond to mass and spring.

Resonance is the general term for phenomena in which two mechanisms that oppose changes of condition nullify each other's effects at some special frequency, so permitting much greater oscillatory changes than either would alone. When such a system oscillates freely after some initial impulse, the resonance is said to be natural, or free. Forced resonance merely refers to the response of such a system to a maintained sinusoidal excitation.

Stray and Unseen Components

Mechanical devices have unavoidable limitations, due to the requirements of physical materials and structures. Examples include the irreducible mass of a moving pointer, the springiness of a connecting-rod and the friction in a bearing. Electrical devices have similar limitations, of which the most obvious is the self-resistance every component has because it is made of real matter. Less obviously, because every circuit passing a current is linked by its own magnetic flux, each component has some self-inductance. Even though such inductance may be very small compared with that of a purpose designed inductor, its effect may become important at high enough frequencies.

At frequencies encountered in most electro-medical work, capacitance is more significant. Between any two parts of any device, when potential differences occur, capacitance effects are produced. When a.c. is involved, such *self-capacitances* give rise to current flow across gaps, just as real as are met with manufactured capacitors. Particularly important examples of such effects are the *stray* capacitance between pairs of leads, the capacitance between parts of the wiring of apparatus, and the capacitances involving patients, electrical apparatus and anaesthetists discussed in Chapter 3.

The Importance of Parallel (Shunt) Impedances

Many of the phenomena associated with electronic

devices cannot be adequately understood without knowledge of how components behave in parallel with one another, as are the resistances *A* and *B* in Fig. 2.44. Just as two roads in parallel act as by-passes to one another and oppose the flow of traffic less than either alone, so the combined resistance (*R*, say) of this

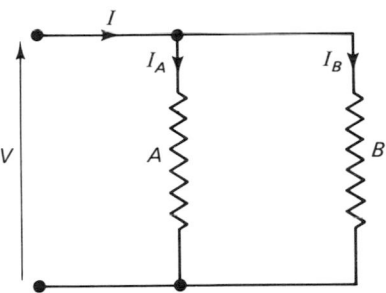

Fig. 2.44 Resistances in parallel. Since each current is proportional to *V*, they are simply additive.

circuit will be less than either *A* or *B*. Since the total current *I* is the sum of the two currents shown,

$$I = I_A + I_B$$

Now the two resistances share the same potential difference *V*, so

$$I = \frac{V}{A} + \frac{V}{B}$$

A single equivalent resistance *R* taking the same total current, given the same p.d. would require that

$$I = \frac{V}{R}$$

$$\frac{1}{R} = \frac{1}{A} + \frac{1}{B}$$

In words, *the reciprocals of parallel resistances are additive.* Obviously the reciprocal of *R* is larger than either reciprocal, being the sum of the two, so *R* is smaller than either *A* or *B*, as anticipated. The result is sufficiently important to have available in the following more convenient form:

$$R = \frac{AB}{A + B}$$

The ideas introduced above can be extended to cover parallel reactances, and (most generally) impedances. A particularly important situation, in which one of two parallel components is capacitive, is shown in Fig. 2.45. This covers cases where *C* is stray, as well as where *C* is deliberately introduced. Such a deliberately introduced capacitor is often called a *decoupling* capacitor, intended to divert unwanted alternating currents from some circuit, represented here by *R*. It is instructive to see how the action of such a circuit can be argued without recourse to mathematics.

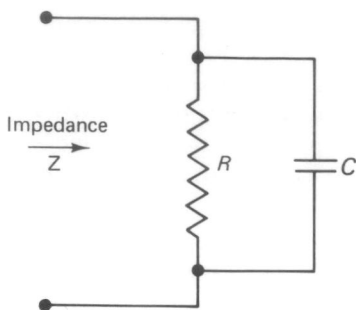

Fig. 2.45 Resistance and reactance in parallel. The effect of the capacitor, compared with that of the resistor, depends on frequency.

1. For currents at frequencies high enough for the reactance ($1/2\pi f C$) to be small compared with R, most of the current flows through C. R may be thought of as being short-circuited, in effect, by the low reactance of C. Clearly the impedance will fall towards zero as the frequency is raised indefinitely.

2. At frequencies low enough for the reactance of C to become very large compared with R, in particular as d.c. is approached, little current flows through C, which becomes less and less important. The impedance therefore tends towards R as the frequency is decreased.

3. Notice that at both extremes *it is the smaller impedance that dominates a parallel combination*, by accepting the major part of the current. This is the opposite effect to that met with series components, where the larger one dominates by imposing the main restriction on the current, and by taking the major share of the available p.d. across its terminals. To the motorist it is self-evident that with a high impedance road in series with a wide one, the minor road dominates the situation. With a by-pass it is the better road that dominates, provided of course that traffic divides according to the ease of the roads, and not by some mass act of malevolent stupidity on the part of the other motorists.

Equivalent Circuits

Knowledge of the operation of individual electrical components is only one aspect of understanding circuits, and the same observation applies to the study of mechanical, hydro-dynamic and other analogous systems such as are met in acoustics and in the many models of physiological systems currently being investigated. There are certain extremely powerful analytical tools available to the electrical and electronic engineers, and these are being more and more widely used in other analogous fields. A simple example is the concept of there being, for a given complex circuit, one or more simpler circuits which are to stated extents and under defined circumstances equivalent to the actual circuit. A very simple example of this is often taken as so obvious that it is often not formally stated: the assumption that circuit elements can be regarded as 'lumped' between two terminals each. Reflecting on the fact that all components have self-resistance and inductance 'distributed' throughout their structures, and capacitance distributed over their parts, reveals that the simple series and parallel components shown on diagrams are simplifications. In fact, at higher frequencies than those for which a given lumped equivalent circuit can be regarded as a good enough approximation, either more elaborate equivalent circuits have to be postulated, or full acceptance has to be made of the distributed nature of components. This is not only true in electronics, but extends to such topics as cardiovascular and respiratory models. However, at any stage in an investigation it may become possible to imagine some simplified model which is equivalent to a complex system to some acceptable degree.

Two of the most profoundly important concepts used routinely by engineers are linked together and will be discussed next. Although they have mathematical aspects which are important to the engineer, the underlying ideas are common-sense ones, and are as important to the non-mathematically oriented reader as to the engineer who uses the associated mathematics intelligently rather than by rote.

Linear Components and Devices

A linear device is one which produces some measurable effect which is simply proportional to some measurable quantity regarded as the cause. Simple examples that have been met include mass, for which acceleration is proportional to applied force, resistance for which current is proportional to p.d. and capacitance with p.d. proportional to charge stored. Similarly, provided they do not employ ferromagnetic cores so permeated by flux that they have become saturated, transformers yield secondary EMFs proportional to the rates of change of their primary currents. Sometimes devices are accepted as being only approximately linear in their behaviour, often over some restricted range. An example is lung-compliance. If pressure change is regarded as cause and volume uptake as effect, the extent to which it is useful to regard the relationship between these as linear is well-known to respiratory physiologists.

The really important aspect of linear devices is expressed as the *Principle of Superposition*. This states that the response of a linear device to the sum of simultaneous and different stimuli is the same as the sum of the responses to the stimuli taken one at a time. For example, no matter how complicated an electrical circuit is, provided it is made up of linear components, its response to a complex signal made up of a mixture of d.c. and alternating currents of different frequencies can be understood by taking the signal components one at a time, finding how the circuit responds to each and then adding together these responses to get the total response. To understand how a stethoscope modifies the characteristics of a heart sound, or how an amplifier affects a signal to be recorded or how a bed of rock transmits an earthquake wave, the same processes are involved:

1. Determine if the system concerned is linear.
2. If so, find how it treats any given signal component in isolation.
3. Sum the individual responses to individual components of the signal.

When a system or device is *non-linear*, either it must be treated as a complex of linear approximations, or its response to specific stimuli must be argued in detail for those stimuli. Sometimes this process is simple—a ratchet screwdriver is non-linear in its response to alternating twists of the user's wrist, but its action can be understood by thinking about the nature of a typical 'input' twist and the precise nature of the device. However, with really complicated non-linear systems the behaviour of each part may depend on the current state of its response and detailed prediction of behaviour may become a matter for computer-assisted analysis. A very obvious example of a non-linear system concerns the flow of fluid along a tube for which the elastic properties depend on the extent to which it is stretched. Clearly the flow response to some small pressure component will be different if this is superimposed on a small standing (mean) pressure than it will if the mean pressure is so large as to stretch the tube to near its limit.

Thévenin's Equivalent Circuit Concept

The object here is to investigate a way of thinking about complicated circuits that reduces them (conceptually, as well as mathematically) to the trivially simple circuit of Fig. 2.47. The concept is contained in a theorem of the same name, and it applies to electrical circuits, acoustic, mechanical, hydrodynamic and other analogous assemblages, and indeed to all systems existing or yet to be evolved, provided that they consist of components which are linear in the sense described above. Stated for electrical circuits:

Any assemblage of linear components, no matter how complex, can be replaced as far as its effect at two terminals AB are concerned, at any stated signal frequency, by a single source of EMF in series with a single impedance connected to AB.

For engineers the theorem also tells how the EMF and the impedance can be calculated, but it is more important here to discuss the idea further. Figure 2.46 shows an arbitrarily selected circuit with more than one source and several linear components. They are linear in that for each of them any change in the magnitude of the current through it would produce a proportional change in p.d. across it. The sources are

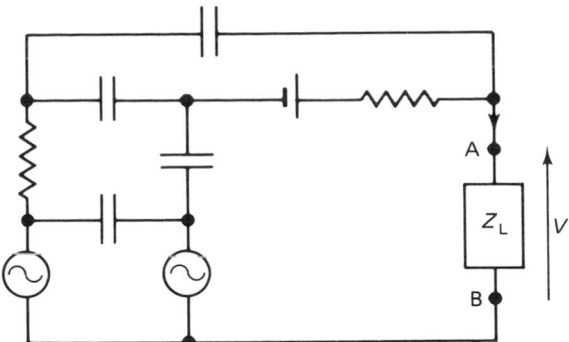

Fig. 2.46 This circuit is (arbitrarily) complicated. However, it is possible to think simply about it when the concern is with what happens at some external 'load' Z_L.

also assumed to have linear internal impedances, simply included with the other components. The box marked Z_L (denoting 'load' in this context) takes a current (I) when connected across AB. It is almost trite to say that there could be an infinite number of possible circuits which, if connected across AB would send the same current through Z_L. It is even true that there are, given a free hand in choosing the EMF and impedance, an infinite number as simple as that in Fig. 2.47. Obviously if some circuit did not quite do this, adjustment of its EMF, the nature and size of the impedance, or both, could always be made on an *ad hoc* basis until the result was just right. However, Thévenin was being more subtle. His object was not merely to derive an equivalent circuit delivering the correct current into some particular load, but to choose E and Z so that the equivalence holds *no matter what value of Z_L happens to be connected*. This restricts the choice, but increases the usefulness of the exercise, for we wish to be able to think of any linear circuit as replaced by an easily visualized equivalent that holds no matter what circuit is attached to follow it. The uniqueness of the equivalent can easily be appreciated by the following argument. To hold for the extreme case where Z_L is an open-circuit, E must

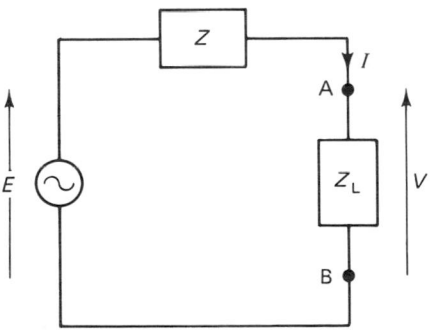

Fig. 2.47 Thévenin's equivalent in a simple circuit. E and Z are chosen so that Z_L is treated as it was in the complex original circuit.

be equal to whatever p.d. appears across AB when Z_L is removed. This fixes E. At the other extreme, with Z_L a short-circuit, the equivalent circuit gives a current of E/Z. Since this must equal the short-circuit current delivered by the original circuit, this in turn fixes Z. The full statement of the theorem shows that:

1. E must be made equal to the open-circuit p.d. that would appear across the terminals.
2. Z must equal the impedance which would be measured looking back into AB with all internal EMFs 'switched off,' but with their internal impedances remaining. It is a relatively easy matter, for those interested, to show that this impedance is the same as gives the short-circuit current when divided into E.

Although to the engineer this theorem is important for answering specific problems, the really important idea is that of *legitimately* regarding some complex device as if it had been much simpler. It is perfectly reasonable to ask, in connection with a new blood-pressure transducer, or a new physiological signal amplifier, 'What is the equivalent source circuit that represents this device at its output terminals?' An engineer will be able to calculate these from knowledge of the contents, but all users can enquire about and subsequently think in terms of the Thévenin equivalent circuit.

Input and Output Impedances

Much human activity consists of connecting devices together, so that the output of one device provides the input to the next. Thévenin has shown that for linear devices a circuit can be simplified in the imagination, as far as the current delivered to the following circuit is concerned. Thévenin's equivalent series impedance (Z) is sometimes known as the *source impedance* and sometimes as the *output impedance* of the circuit, as seen by a circuit connected across AB. The *input impedance* of a circuit is the impedance which, connected across the previous circuit, demands the same current as does the actual circuit at its input terminals.

With this in mind, it is easy to see that the trivial-looking circuit in Fig. 2.47 is really quite important. If Z_L is the input impedance of a device or circuit, and if E and Z are the Thévenin EMF and output impedance of the previous circuit, then these three quantities (E, Z and Z_L) are all that is required for determining the signal passed on to the second device from the first. This is quite general, and so it is worth examining and interpreting the result for V, the p.d. passed on in this otherwise apparently unimportant-looking circuit. For this exercise Z and Z_L will be treated as resistances. Similar considerations apply in more general cases of impedances, with differences which become more important as the subject is dealt with in greater detail.

Ohm's law, applied to Z_L gives

$$V = IZ_L$$

while, applied to the whole circuit it gives

$$I = \frac{E}{Z + Z_L}$$

Consequently

$$V = \frac{EZ_L}{Z + Z_L}$$

If this result is (merely typographically) rearranged to look as follows:

$$V = \left(\frac{Z_L}{Z + Z_L}\right) . E$$

its interpretation at once becomes clear, especially when expressed in words:

The output terminal p.d. (V) is the same fraction of the total EMF as the 'load' resistance (Z_L) is of the total resistance.

To illustrate the simplicity of this, if an electromanometer transducer with an output impedance of 1 kΩ is connected to an amplifier with an input resistance of 100 kΩ, the fraction of the source EMF passed on will be 100/101. In contrast, if an electrode with a resistance of 50 kΩ were connected to the same amplifier, only the fraction $\frac{2}{3}$ would go on to be amplified.

Attenuators and Potential Dividers

An *attenuator* is a circuit for reducing a signal, usually by splitting an applied p.d. into fractions and rejecting what is not required. The simplest form consists of two resistors such as A and B in Fig. 2.48(a). The output voltage is given by the fraction $B/(A + B)$ of the input. More complicated circuits are made when special additional properties are wanted, in particular when it is vital to present constant resistance to both the previous and the following circuits even when attenuation is altered.

The term *potential divider* is applied to the simple circuit. Potential dividers may be fixed, stepped

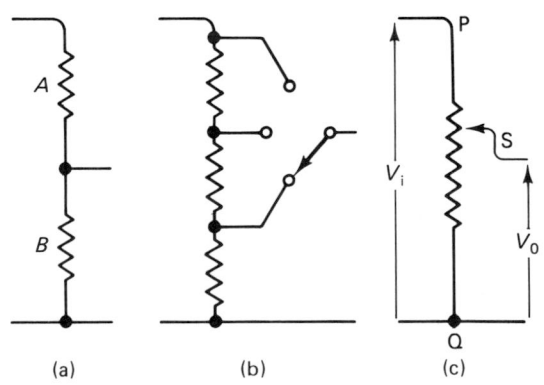

Fig. 2.48 (a) Fixed (b) switched and (c) continuously variable potential dividers.

variable or continuously variable. Stepped variable attenuators (Fig. 2.48(b)) enable overall amplification in such equipment as ECG recorders and cathode-ray oscilloscopes to be altered in calibrated steps, by switching different resistors in as needed. Continuous variable potential dividers are typified by the volume controls on radio receivers, and by the 'preset' screwdriver adjustments found on many equipments. These latter are no different in principle from the others; they are simply adjusted infrequently.

The simplest form of continuously variable potential divider uses a resistor manufactured with a sliding contact that can ride from one end to the other. The circuit symbol is shown in Fig. 2.48(c), where an adjustable fraction of the applied p.d. is being selected. If the resistance between S and Q is x ohms and the total between P and Q is r ohms, the fraction

$$\frac{V_0}{V_i} = \frac{x}{r}$$

is variable between 0 and 1 as x is varied from 0 to r by sliding S from the end Q towards P. The term *potentiometer* has become associated with such potential dividers because an early method of measuring a potential difference involved comparing it with a tapped fraction of a known EMF. Another word still encountered is *rheostat*. This relates to one particular use of a variable resistance inserted in series with a circuit whose resistance alters, in order to keep the current constant by compensating for resistance changes. A potential divider such as that shown can be used as a simple variable resistance by connecting between S and Q (or S and P). As the slider is moved towards the other end that is connected, the resistance between them decreases. Used as a rheostat this would compensate for an increase in the resistance of the circuit with which it was in series.

Wheatstone's Bridge as Two Potential Dividers

The following circuit was invented to solve a particular problem—that of finding an unknown resistance in terms of known ones. The same circuit configuration appears in many applications, and since it illustrates several ideas it is worth treating as an example.

In Fig. 2.49 two potential dividers are energized by the same source of EMF. The potential difference (V) between the terminals A B is to be regarded as an output to a following circuit: in the original use this was a sensitive meter for establishing a null condition ($V = 0$). For convenience, the conductor marked X is taken as a reference for potentials, just as sea-level can be taken as a reference for heights. Denoting the potential of A with respect to X by V_{AX} (and similarly for V_{BX}), it follows that

$$V = V_{AX} - V_{BX}$$

This is precisely analogous to saying that the difference between the heights of two camps A and B on

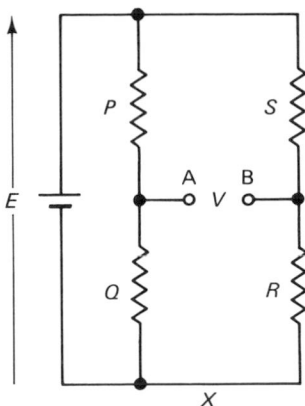

Fig. 2.49 The Wheatstone Bridge circuit. To assess V, AX is regarded as the output terminals of one potential divider and BX those of another.

Everest equals the height of A above sea-level minus that of B, also referred to as sea-level.

Now each of V_{AX} and V_{BX} can be written as a fraction of E, so

$$V = \left(\frac{Q}{P + Q}\right). E - \left(\frac{R}{R + S}\right). E$$

Two aspects of this result are important. When Q is the same fraction of $P + Q$ as R is of $R + S$ the bridge is said to be *balanced*, and V is zero. This is often expressed as follows:

$$\frac{Q}{P + Q} = \frac{R}{R + S}$$

so

$$QR + QS = PR + QR$$

or

$$QS = PR$$

This enables (say) R to be found in terms of the other three. The second important aspect is that alterations in one or more of the 'arms' of the bridge, provided that the changes are small in relation to the starting values of the resistances, give rise to an output V that is reasonably linearly related to the resistance changes. This principle is used in very many circuits and devices.

The Concept of Filtering

As is known by musicians and was established as a celebrated theorem by Fourier, any repetitive waveform can be analyzed into component sinusoids, the lowest frequency-components (the fundamental) repeating at the same rate as the signal, and the others being whole multiples (harmonics) of this. The complete theorem goes on to show how the amplitudes and relative phases of the various components of a given waveform can be calculated.

More advanced versions of this theorem established that any waveform, even if non-repetitive, can be considered in terms of sinusoidal components, although not harmonically related unless the waveform is repetitive. Children 'listening to the sea' in shells are actually selecting from random background noise those frequency-components to which the shell-ear cavities are broadly tuned.

Circuits involving reactive components, such as the simple resistor by-passed by a capacitor, resonant circuits, and even ostensibly resistive circuits at frequencies at which stray capacitances and inductances are noticeable, affect the various frequency-components of complex signals to different extents. When such variations of the signal passed on are unwanted, they are regarded as *amplitude/frequency* distortion. This is normally accompanied with variations of relative phases of different components, as between input and output, known as *phase/frequency distortion.*

Filters are circuits in which the transmission of signals in some bands of frequency and rejection of others is deliberate. The principles and processes are the same as for distortion—only the intention is different. Filters vary in complexity, being more so the more stringent the conditions placed on

1. the sharpness required—i.e. the rapidity of transition between frequencies passed and those attenuated,
2. constancy of impedance presented to the circuits to which they are attached, with variation of frequency.

Discussion of such circuits is inappropriate here, but the description of the behaviour of two simple circuits having crude filter characteristics is justified by the useful ideas that emerge and by the frequency with which these circuits occur in electronic devices.

Single CR Low and High Pass Circuits

In Fig. 2.50, R is either an actual resistor or the

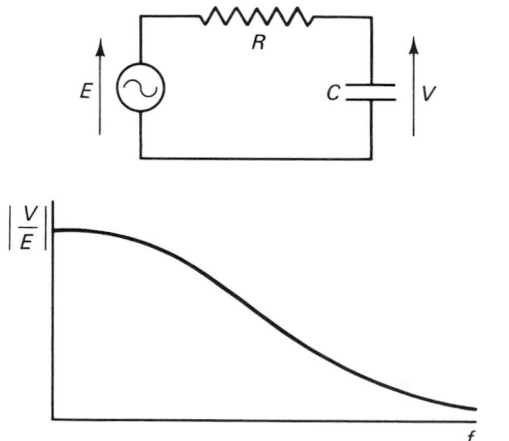

Fig. 2.50 Illustrating low-pass filtering. The ratio of the output V to the input E decreases as the reactance of the capacitor falls.

Thévenin equivalent source resistance for a more complicated circuit. C may be an actual capacitor, or some stray capacitance as discussed earlier. The circuit acts as a frequency-dependent potential divider. At frequencies high enough to make the reactance of C small compared with R, the p.d. across the capacitor becomes a very small fraction of E. As the frequency is decreased C begins to dominate the circuit and the p.d. across R becomes trivial. Briefly, at high frequencies C tends towards a short-circuit, and V tends towards zero. At low frequencies C tends towards an open-circuit, making the current through R and thus the fraction of E lost across R negligible. The ratio of the size of V to that of E is plotted, the graph being called the *amplitude/frequency response curve* of the circuit.

Figure 2.51 is an example of an a.c. *coupling circuit* often met in electronic circuits, and particularly

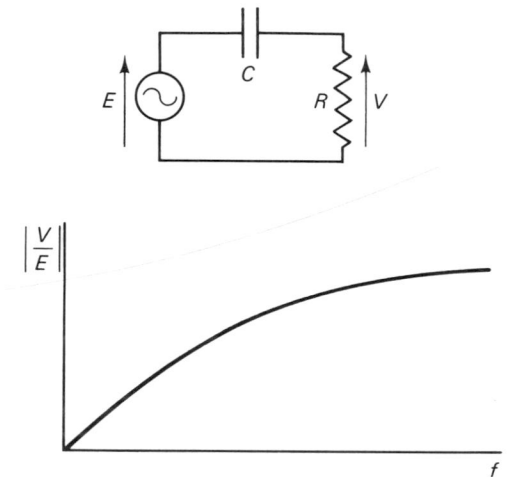

Fig. 2.51 Illustrating high-pass filtering. Here the output is greater when less voltage is dropped across C.

noticeable in ECG amplifiers. It is a crude high-pass filter, being obviously the converse of the previous circuit. Here it is the p.d. across R which is passed on and that across C discarded. Strictly speaking it rejects 'very low' frequencies (such as polarization effects from skin electrodes), where 'low' means frequencies for which $1/2\pi f C$ is large compared with R. It is often loosely stated to 'block d.c.', although examination of the response curve shows that d.c. is merely the ultimate low frequency.

Exponential Waveforms

Exponential decay is an important phenomenon in many diverse branches of science. In electronic circuits the simple CR combination just discussed is the most common circuit exhibiting exponential effects, when energized with d.c. If a direct voltage E (Fig. 2.52) is suddenly switched across a capacitor and resistor at

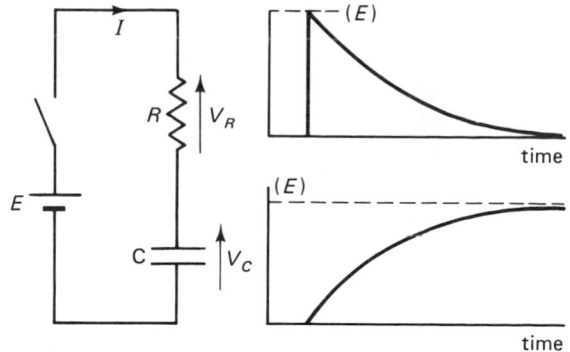

Fig. 2.52 Exponential waveforms.

a time when the capacitor is discharged ($V_C = 0$), all of E is momentarily developed across R. As the capacitor charges, the rise of V_C makes V_R fall (since their sum must always equal E). By Ohm's law the current falls proportionally, from the initial E/R towards zero. Since smaller current means less rapid establishment of charge Q, the p.d. across the capacitor *rises less rapidly the more the process continues*. The fall of I illustrates precisely what an exponential decay is—one for which the rate of change decreases as the quantity falls. The time-constant is the time taken for the fall to reach 36.8% (i.e. 1/e) of the starting value. For the CR circuit it can be shown to be given by

$$\text{Time constant} = CR$$

the result being in seconds when the capacitance is in farads and the resistance is in ohms. Obviously a larger capacitance takes more charge and a larger resistance reduces the charging current. A time constant of a few seconds is often encountered with the input circuits of ECG recorders, and the exponential decay curve can be seen in the recovery from a step calibration signal.

Similar exponential decay of current is met when a charged capacitor is discharged through a resistor. The effect is analogous to the gradual closing of a door with a spring and a hydraulic damper.

FURTHER READING

The basic quantities of mechanical science are covered clearly at elementary level in *Applied mathematics made simple* by Patrick Murphy (London: W. H. Allen Ltd.). A well-illustrated and well-written book with some vivid examples is *Force, matter and energy* by D. J. Williams (London: English Universities Press Ltd.). In this book the background mathematics is also developed in a helpful way. A witty and informative book covering a wide range of topics is *The world of measurements* by H. Arthur Klein (London: George Allen and Unwin Ltd.). This discusses the meaning and background history of physical quantities and units in an unusually refreshing manner.

For a more formal treatment of symbols and matters concerning the use of SI units, see the references in the appendix to Chapter 1 on SI units.

Basic electrical quantities are well-described with examples, in *Principles of electricity* in SI units by A. Morley and E. Hughes (London and New York: Longman Group Ltd.).

3. Biological Electrical Signals and Patient Safety

J. P. Blackburn

In this chapter we consider sources of biological electrical potentials, the electrodes required to detect them, and the amplifiers and recorders used to display the signals. Problems of electrical interference and safety are discussed. Finally there is a short section on surgical diathermy.

BIOLOGICAL ELECTRICAL SIGNALS

Electrical potentials can be detected in almost all parts of the body and it is well known that the inside of a cell is about 80–90 mV negative with respect to the outside, because of the differences in ionic composition between the inside and the outside of the cell. Changing potentials are associated with the depolarization of 'excitable tissues' and may be recorded from the central and peripheral nervous systems, the sense organs and skeletal, smooth or cardiac muscle. Electrical signals of interest to the anaesthetist are recorded from the heart, the central nervous system and the neuromuscular system.

THE ELECTROCARDIOGRAM

In spite of the complexities of different lead systems the electrocardiogram is essentially a measurement of the potential difference between two points. These may be two points on the body, as in the standard leads I, II and III, or with the chest leads the potential difference is measured between the chest lead and a 'central terminal' obtained by combining signals from the right and left arms and the left leg in such a way as to derive their average.

The use of the conventional 12 lead electrocardiogram (ECG) is well established for diagnostic purposes, while for arrhythmia detection in the intensive therapy unit a single lead is commonly employed. In addition, the electrical changes in the heart may be recorded rather more efficiently and in more detail using an orthogonal vector system. An array of eight electrodes is placed on the patient in such a way that the electrical signals originating from the heart are recorded in three planes at right angles. These three signals contain at least as much information as the 12 lead ECG because they are recorded simultaneously, so that phase information between the leads is not lost. The problems of maintaining an array of electrodes on the patient limits the usefulness of the system for long term studies.

When recorded from the surface of the body, the ECG has a peak amplitude of about 1 mV and frequencies in the range of 0.05–100 Hz are usually recorded. The sensitivity of the recorder is set so that 1 mV produces a pen deflection of 1 cm.

THE ELECTROENCEPHALOGRAM

This is a complex electrical signal conventionally recorded using a large array of electrodes. However during surgery or in the postoperative period a pair of electrodes is often adequate.

The electrical signal is about 50–200 μV in amplitude and for descriptive purposes the frequency range of the electroencephalogram (EEG) is divided as follows:

Delta waves	0–4 Hz
Theta waves	4–8 Hz
Alpha waves	8–13 Hz
Beta waves	13 Hz and above

The EEG may be a useful guide to the adequacy of cerebral perfusion during open heart surgery and has also been used to determine and control the depth of anaesthesia. Its use is still being evaluated (see Chapter 28). Changes associated with reduced cerebral perfusion, hypoxia or hypothermia are non-specific. Initially slow wave activity becomes more marked and increases in amplitude, then the electrical signals are reduced and finally no electrical activity is seen. It is now accepted that brain death should be diagnosed on clinical grounds (Conference of Medical Royal Colleges, 1976), but an isoelectric EEG over several days may be useful supportive evidence of brain death.

Signals free from artefact and interference may be difficult to record under clinical conditions, and the signals may require expert analysis. However the cerebral function monitor (CFM) (Prior, 1980) is considerably easier to use and the records can be readily interpreted. The EEG signal is recorded using two electrodes, band-pass filtered between 2–15 Hz to eliminate interference, amplitude-limited and rectified. The output is displayed on a slow-speed recorder as a smooth line drawn through the peaks of the compressed signal. A second channel is used to indicate the state of the electrodes and to record when the amplifier has been overloaded. Alterations in the amount or character of cerebral activity are easily visible (Fig. 3.1), but focal disturbances cannot be

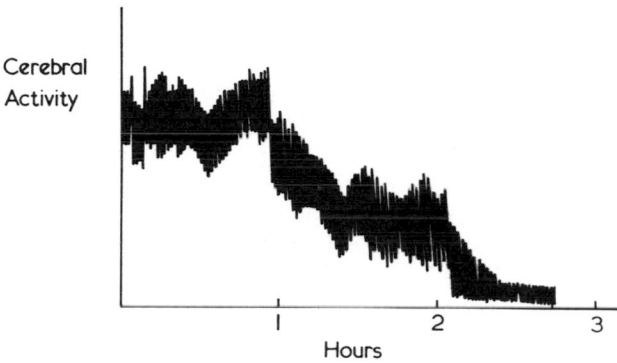

Fig. 3.1 Trace of cerebral activity, showing reduction in activity following hypotension and cardiac arrest.

detected. The CFM has been used for the detection of neurological damage during open heart surgery. In addition, the CFM may have a place in assessing the depth of anaesthesia, particularly the problems of awareness during anaesthesia and recovery after short anaesthetic procedures (Dubois et al., 1978a, b).

THE ELECTROMYOGRAM

As applied to anaesthesia, electromyography is still regarded primarily as a research tool for investigating various neurological conditions and determining the site and duration of action of muscle relaxants, although it is the most practical method of recording evoked motor activity in certain situations, especially in neonates. For clinical purposes, assessment of the type and intensity of neuromuscular block is made by observing the muscle contractions which occur when the appropriate motor nerve is stimulated. This is usually done by applying supramaximal twitch or tetanic stimuli to the ulnar nerve with surface electrodes (Goat, 1979) and measuring the contraction of the hypothenar muscles or adductor pollicis (Feldman, 1974). Tetanic stimuli are painful in conscious patients and four supramaximal stimuli may be delivered at 2 Hz after a rest period. The 'train of four' is potentially more useful, as the ratio of the fourth to

the first twitch amplitude is used to indicate the degree of non-depolarizing neuromuscular blockade. Train of four nerve stimulators which also display the ratio of the fourth to the first twitch amplitude are commercially available.

Electromyographic studies are used for a more detailed assessment of neuromuscular conduction. Again, a supramaximal stimulus is applied to a motor nerve and the electrical activity of a group of muscle fibres is recorded using surface or needle electrodes. One nerve fibre typically supplies 100–300 muscle fibres which make up a 'motor unit', so when the nerve is stimulated a large number of muscle fibres are activated.

The response from a single muscle fibre is biphasic and lasts about 1 ms, while the response from a motor unit is more complex and has a duration of 5–10 ms. The amplitude of the response from a motor unit varies between 100 µV and 1.5 mV depending on the size of the unit and the position of the electrodes. It should be noted that signals of this type change too rapidly to be displayed by a pen recorder. Cathode-ray oscilloscopes can record such signals without distortion.

The display of an integrated electromyograph can also be used to evaluate neuromuscular function. The principle relies on the reasonable correlation that exists between the integrated EMG of a muscle and the number of muscle fibres exhibiting a propagated action potential in response to nerve stimulation. The Datex Relaxograph (TM) applies a standard train of four stimulus patterns to a suitable peripheral nerve using a supramaximal stimulus which is sought automatically and records the resultant electrical activity of the stimulated muscle. This integrated electromyograph is displayed in the form of a bar chart analogous to a record of muscle twitch tension. The device is easy to use and clinically useful. However the correlation between twitch tension and integrated EMG although generally good is affected by variables such as skin temperature and skin impedance so that measurement of twitch tension is preferred for research purposes.

A more detailed account of the changes which occur with neuromuscular blockade has been given by Miller (1978).

ELECTRODES

Electrical signals may be detected with intracellular electrodes, extracellular electrodes placed near the structure of interest, or most commonly using surface electrodes, such as those required for recording the ECG or the EEG. The main purpose of these electrodes is to detect biological electrical potentials from various sources, but in practice when a metal electrode is in contact with an electrolyte a number of electrochemical potentials are generated which may interfere with the signal of interest. These potentials often contain slowly fluctuating components, but the effects can be greatly reduced by suitable filtering when, as with the ECG, a.c. coupled amplifiers can be used. Artefacts produced by the electrodes may be troublesome when small signals requiring d.c. coupled amplifers are investigated.

Electrode Potential

The most obvious electrical effect occurring at the electrode is the electrode potential. This is the potential difference between the metal of the electrode and the solution (tissue fluid, electrode jelly, etc.) surrounding it. In order to measure this voltage some method of making electrical contact with the solution must be found, as the potential of a single electrode (half-cell) cannot be measured in isolation. Electrode potentials are measured with respect to a standard electrode. The standard hydrogen electrode is used as a reference and is arbitrarily assumed to be at zero potential, although a calomel reference electrode is often more convenient to use. This has an electrode potential of about $+0.3$ V with respect to the hydrogen electrode, so allowance can be made for its contribution to the EMF of the cell.

If a metal electrode is immersed in an electrolyte, which may be electrode jelly in the case of ECG or other surface electrodes, or tissue fluid electrodes placed in or near cells being investigated, there is a tendency for the metal to go into or come out of solution, depending on its position in the electrochemical series. Metals with negative electrode potentials (such as zinc, iron or tin) tend to ionize and pass into solution, leaving the electrode negatively charged with respect to the electrolyte, while the reverse reaction occurs with metals which develop positive electrode potentials.

Thus taking a silver electrode as an example:

$$Ag \rightleftharpoons Ag^+ + e^-$$

Metallic silver forms silver ions in solution, leaving electrons on the electrode. Also, silver ions in solution combine with these electrons, leaving the electrode positively charged. In practice the equilibrium is over to the left in the equation shown above and silver ions tend to come out of solution with the result that the electrode is about 0.8 V positive to the electrolyte.

Ideally, when two identical electrodes are used in the same electrolyte, the potentials developed by the two half-cells will be identical and should cancel when the electrodes are used together, although in practice small differences remain. Potential differences varying between a few microvolts and tens of millivolts have been described, depending on the type of electrode and the conditions under which the electrodes are prepared and used. In addition, the potential difference may not be stable, but may show marked fluctuations. If dissimilar metals are used for the two electrodes then there will be a potential difference between them which will depend on the positions of the metals in the electrochemical series. The electrode potential will

also be affected by the composition and concentration of the electrolyte.

Liquid-junction Potentials

When different electrolytes are in contact with each other without mixing, a liquid-junction potential is developed at the interface between the two solutions. This arises when the solutions have different concentrations and ionic mobilities. If the ions diffuse at different rates there will be a net separation of charges and a potential difference between the two solutions will result. If a solution of sodium chloride at 37°C is in contact with a similar solution which is ten times more concentrated, then a junction potential of 12.7 mV is produced, because of the differing mobilities of the sodium and chloride ions. If potassium chloride solutions are used instead of sodium chloride then the junction potential is only 1.1 mV because the mobilities of potassium and chloride ions are almost identical. Potassium chloride solution is used to connect the calomel electrode to the system under investigation, so the junction potential will be small. When electrolytes containing many different ions are in contact the liquid junction potential is very difficult to calculate, so where possible this situation is avoided by using a potassium chloride 'salt bridge' to connect different solutions.

Polarization Effects

When recording electrodes are connected to an amplifier, the current which flows depends on the potential difference between the electrodes and the input characteristics of the amplifier. This current causes a chemical reaction or a change in concentration at the interface betwen the electrode and the electrolyte. The change in composition may result in the deposition of metal or the formation of gas bubbles at the electrodes and the chemical reaction produces an EMF which opposes that of the cell. Under these conditions the electrodes are said to be polarized and the potential difference which should exist between them as a result of the physiological process is reduced because of electrochemical events at the electrodes. Under some circumstances the current may be limited by the availability of ions at the electrode. This effect is used to advantage in the polarographic oxygen electrode.

Non-polarizable (or reversible) electrodes are used whenever possible and can be made by keeping the metal electrode in contact with a solution of one of its own salts. Chemical changes still occur at the interface between the electrode and the electrolyte, but charge is carried freely by the common ions so electrochemical events at the electrodes should not limit the current which can be drawn from the system.

The commonest reversible system for physiological use is the silver/silver chloride electrode. Only small currents can be taken as silver chloride is virtually insoluble, but the electrode has the advantage that it is relatively non-toxic.

$$Ag \text{ (on electrode)} + Cl^- \leftrightharpoons AgCl \text{ (on electrode)} + e^-$$

Charge is carried freely by the chloride ions from the electrolyte to the electrodes. At one electrode, ions combine with metallic silver to form silver chloride and free electrons, while the opposite reaction occurs at the other electrode, where silver chloride dissociates into chloride ions and metallic silver. If heavier currents are to be passed, a soluble salt must be used. Salts of mercury or zinc can be employed, but are highly toxic to the tissues.

ELECTRICAL CHARACTERISTICS OF THE SOURCE OF SIGNALS AND THE AMPLIFIER

When recording electrical changes, the source of signals should have as low an impedance as possible, while the amplifier should have a high input impedance to minimize the current drawn from the preparation. The resistance of dry skin may be more than $1\,M\Omega$, but the skin impedance can be reduced to about $2000\,\Omega$ by using electrode jelly. Alternatively the high impedance stratum corneum is breached using needle electrodes or multiple puncture electrodes. In practice it is important that the impedances are approximately equal at the various electrodes when recording the ECG. Unequal skin impedance may cause distortion of the signal, particularly when the augmented limb leads or chest leads are recorded. For instance when a chest lead is recorded, the potential difference between the chest electrode and the 'central terminal' (made up of contributions from the left and right arms and left leg) is measured. The average of the limb potentials will actually depend on conditions at the individual electrodes and distortion of the signal may result if large differences are present.

Capacitive electrodes, associated with suitable amplifiers, have been developed for long term use. When this arrangement is used, the electrode does not make contact with the skin directly but is insulated from it, so the body beneath the electrode forms one plate of a capacitor and the electrode forms the other plate. The advantage of the system is that no skin preparation is needed and electrode jelly is not used.

It is important to use an amplifier with an input impedance which is high in comparison with the signal source. If the input impedance of the amplifier is low, not only may an unacceptably large current be taken from the preparation leading to electrode artefacts, but also the voltage recorded by the amplifier will not be the true voltage which exists at the electrodes under open circuit conditions. Consider the case of a d.c. voltage generator (for simplicity), where the source resistance representing the tissue and total skin resistance is S and the resistance presented by the amplifier is R (Fig. 3.2). If the voltage developed by the generator is E volts, this will also be the potential

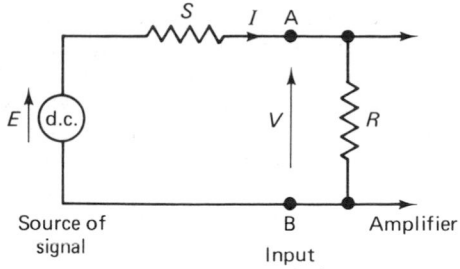

Fig. 3.2 Simple circuit showing the effect of source impedance S and amplifier input impedance R. (For details *see* text.)

difference at two points A and B on the surface of the skin under open circuit conditions. When the amplifier is connected, however, a current I will flow in the circuit.

$$I = \frac{E}{S + R}$$
$$V = IR$$
$$\therefore \quad V = \frac{R}{S + R} \cdot E$$

Where V is the voltage across the input terminals of the amplifier (this is discussed fully in Chapter 2). For example, if the source resistance equals the amplifier input resistance, the input voltage to the amplifier is half the source voltage.

Amplifiers

Suitable amplifiers must have adequate sensitivity, must remain stable and should have a suitable frequency response so that the input signal can be amplified without distortion. The importance of a high input impedance has already been stressed. ECG amplifiers, for instance, have input impedances ranging from 1–$50\,M\Omega$. Amplifiers may be 'single-ended' in which case one of the connections is made to the 'active' input of the amplifier while the other input lead is connected to a reference, usually earth. This simple arrangement is adequate when signals of several volts are being considered and where one side of the input can be earthed, but electrical interference may be a problem when signals such as the ECG and EEG are being recorded. This problem will be discussed later.

More complex amplifiers may have two active inputs which are symmetrically arranged with respect to an earth or other reference connection. Differential amplifiers of this type are commonly used to record biological electrical potentials. Electrical signals applied as differences of voltage between the active inputs are amplified, but the amplifier does not respond appreciably to electrical changes affecting both inputs equally with respect to the reference. This feature is known as 'common mode rejection', and the common mode rejection ratio of a typical amplifier might be 10 000:1, meaning that a signal applied to both input terminals equally, would need to be 10 000 times larger than a signal applied between them for the same change in the output. This technique is used to reduce a potent cause of electrical interference, because mains 'hum' affecting both inputs equally with respect to a reference connection will not appear at the output.

Details of amplifiers will not be considered, but in general, amplifiers capable of amplifying d.c. or slowly changing signals operate in one of two ways. They may either be directly coupled, or they may convert their d.c. input into an a.c. signal which can then be amplified in a conventional a.c. coupled amplifier. This conversion is achieved either by 'chopping' the input signal using a relay or a solid state switch, or by modulating the input as in a so-called carrier amplifier. An amplified version of the original signal must be resynthesized at the output.

RECORDING DEVICES

Once the signal has been amplified it must be displayed. One of the most useful general purpose displays is the cathode ray oscilloscope. In this instrument a beam of electrons is focussed onto a fluorescent screen and the beam is deflected by applying voltages to plates inside the oscilloscope tube (Fig. 3.3). The electrons can be deflected very rapidly,

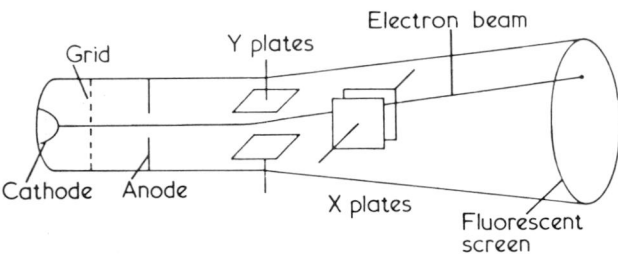

Fig. 3.3 Simplified diagram of cathode ray tube. The X and Y plates constitute the deflection system.

so the instrument has a high frequency response, but permanent records are inconvenient to obtain as the trace has to be photographed. Storage oscilloscopes, where the trace may be stored on the tube and examined at leisure have been developed. Memory oscilloscopes are also available where the data is stored in digital form within the instrument. The information is scanned and displayed rapidly so that the trace remains bright on the screen even though a slow sweep speed is used, such as when displaying ECG or blood pressure waveforms. The trace can often be 'frozen' if needed and the stored information may be 'dumped' onto a pen recorder if a permanent record of the trace is required.

Other types of recorder include photographic instruments, where mirror galvanometers deflect white or ultraviolet light onto suitably sensitized paper (Fig. 3.4). Pen recorders are commonly

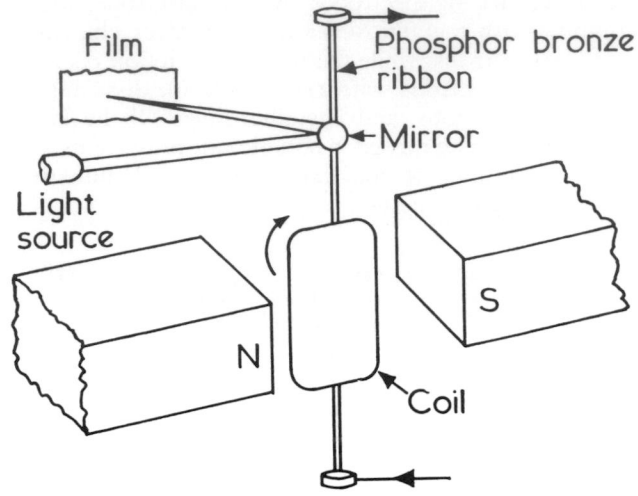

Fig. 3.4 Mirror galvanometer system.

employed (Fig. 3.5) and may use an ink system with pens or an ink jet (which has a higher frequency response), or thermal instruments which write with a heated stylus on specially prepared paper (as in most ECG machines).

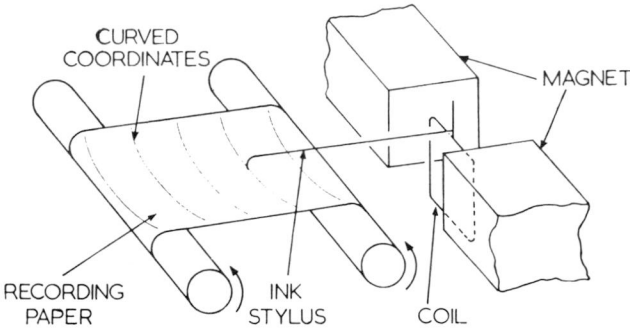

Fig. 3.5 Pen recorder, showing curvilinear distortion.

A pen attached to a galvanometer will normally sweep out an arc on the paper as it is deflected. The curved lines on the trace make timing of events difficult and the signals look distorted. With thermal recorders the paper is usually drawn over a knife edge on which the stylus rests, so that the trace is always at right-angles to the paper (Fig. 3.6). The same effect may also be achieved by mechanically lengthening the pen as it is deflected so that it writes in rectilinear coordinates. These techniques produce amplitude distortion in the records, but this can either be corrected electrically in the amplifier or mechanically in the pen system.

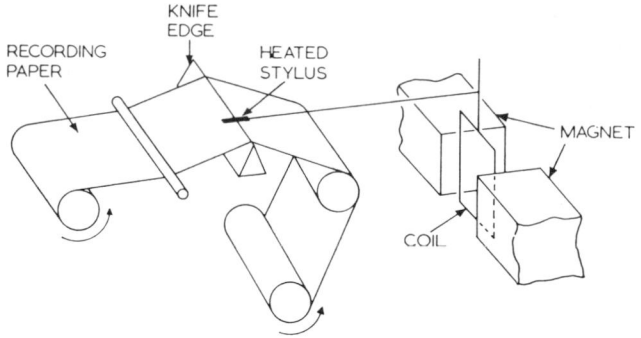

Fig. 3.6 Thermal recorder for rectilinear recording.

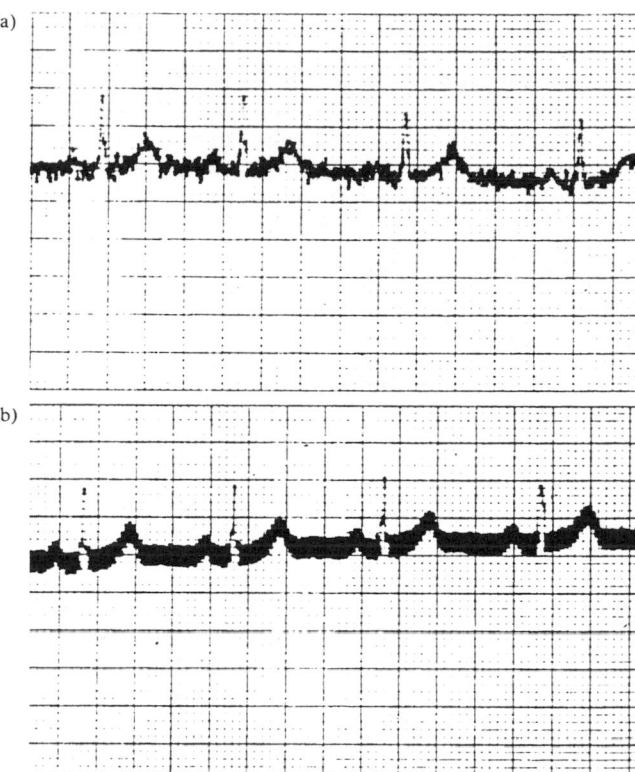

Fig. 3.7 Electrocardiogram showing (a) skeletal muscle potential; (b) 50 Hz mains interference.

The galvanometer and pen arm behaves as a complex mass-spring system which will resonate at a specific frequency and will overshoot if a step change is applied to it, in the same way as the catheter manometer system considered in Chapter 5. Optimal damping should be applied to reduce overshoot and provide the best frequency response. This may be achieved electrically or by using oil as the damping medium.

Although cathode ray oscilloscopes are capable of recording physiological signals without distortion (the frequency response is limited by the amplifiers and may be in the MHz range), pen recorders will only respond satisfactorily up to about 100 Hz and then only over a restricted range of amplitude. Ink jet recorders may be used up to about 1 kHz, while mirror galvanometers may respond to frequencies of up to 3 kHz.

ELECTRICAL INTERFERENCE

Biological electrical potentials may be contaminated by electrical interference produced by the patient or by external sources, usually the alternating current mains. Interference produced by the patient is caused by skeletal muscle action potentials which arise associated with movement or shivering. The trace has a characteristic appearance (Fig. 3.7a) and the ECG signal may be completely obscured by the interference. Slow base-line wander on the ECG is usually associated with changes at the electrodes themselves.

Mains frequency interference, often called 'hum', may be troublesome during ECG or EEG recording, particularly in an environment where mains operated equipment is in use, such as an operating theatre or intensive therapy unit. Unlike small electronic components which can be 'screened' from some forms of mains interference, patients are physically large, unscreened conductors, often in an environment in which electrical interference is present.

SOURCES OF ELECTRICAL INTERFERENCE

Capacitively Coupled Interference

Interference arises because of capacitive coupling between the source of interference and the patient from whom the signals are obtained, as shown in Fig. 3.8. The interference originates from a source of alternating EMF such as mains power cables. Often only one side of the mains supply is 'live' and the neutral line is at nearly the same potential as the local 'earth'.

The mains live conductor L acts as one plate of the capacitor C, while the patient is the other plate. The other side of the mains is connected to earth through an impedance Z_1 which usually has a low value. The

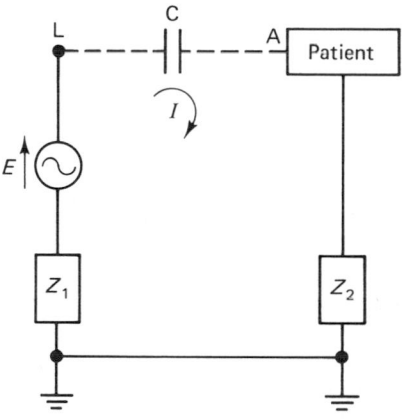

Fig. 3.8 Electrical interference produced by capacitive coupling.

patient is also connected to earth through the imped-ance Z_2. The size of Z_2 will depend very much on local conditions. It will be large if the patient is iso-lated from earth (for instance lying in bed) or may be very low if the patient is connected to earth (for in-stance by an earthed diathermy plate). When L goes positive with respect to earth, negative charges will be attracted towards the surface A and positive ones re-pelled. When E reverses in polarity, negative charges will be repelled at A and positive ones attracted. Thus a mains frequency current I flows through the patient, even though there is no direct electrical connection between the patient and the mains. Interference of this type can also be picked up by signal leads and elec-trical components in the amplifier.

Capacitively coupled interference can be reduced by moving the patient away from the source of interfer-ence (in other words reducing C) and by 'screening' as much of the equipment as possible. The source of interference is surrounded by a conductor connected by a low resistance pathway to earth as shown in Fig. 3.9. C_1 and C_2 represent the capacitance between L and the screen and between screen and the patient,

output from E via C_1, from the point of view of the patient. The screen can be a thin sheet of metal foil, a metal box, or may be wire mesh when flexibility is necessary, as with screened cables. Sources of interfer-ence should be screened as far as possible and signal leads and amplifiers should also be screened.

Electromagnetically Induced Interference

As discussed in Chapter 2, when a magnet is moved in a coil an EMF is generated. Also when a current flows through a conductor, such as a mains lead, it gener-ates a magnetic flux around the conductor and if 50 Hz mains alternating current is flowing the flux will change in time with the mains supply. If other con-ductors, such as the patient or the signal leads to the amplifier, lie in the changing magnetic flux, then vol-tages will be induced in the conductors. A simple cir-cuit is shown in Fig. 3.10, where 'hum' is induced in the signal lead to the amplifier.

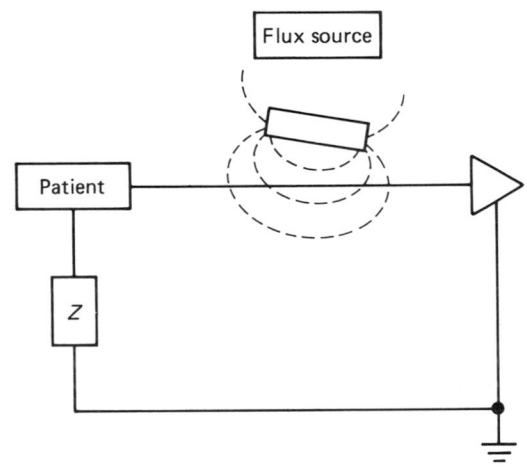

Fig. 3.10 Electromagnetically induced interference, showing a source of alternating magnetic flux which induces an alternating voltage in the signal lead between the patient and the amplifier.

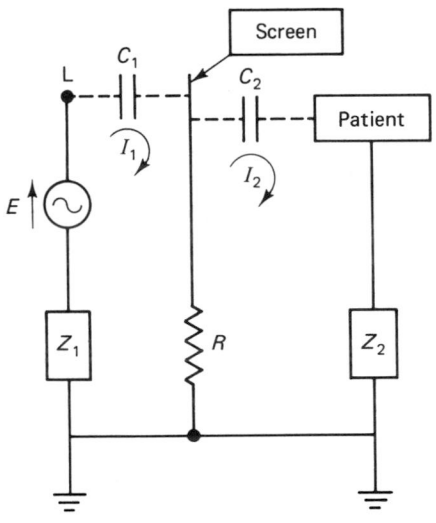

Fig. 3.9 Screening used to reduce capacitively coupled interference.

and R respresents the low resistance of the screen and the wire connecting it to earth. For greater generality the impedances Z_1 and Z_2 (which may be anything from direct connections to the high reactances of small stray capacitances) have been left in the circuit. A current I_1 flows from the source through the screen and there will thus be a potential difference across resistance R. As far as the patient is concerned this small p.d. becomes the source instead of E, and con-sequently the lower R is made the less p.d. appears across the patient. Notice that connecting the screen to earth does no more than virtually short circuit the

'Hum' can also be induced in the earth wiring and this may cause trouble as shown in Fig. 3.11. Lead I of the ECG is recorded using a differential input ampli-fier and the ECG machine has a reference connection made to the right leg (to assist common mode rejec-tion by the amplifier). The patient is also connected to mains earth at points A and B. These connections may be deliberate, such as through the earthed electrode of a diathermy apparatus (the machine is represented by C in the diagram), or accidental where the patient is touching some earthed equipment, bedside lamp or water pipe for instance. An 'earth loop' ABCDE has been produced and as part of the earth wiring lies alongside mains power cables it is inevitable that the earth conductors will be cut by changing electro-magnetic flux and that a current will flow in the earth

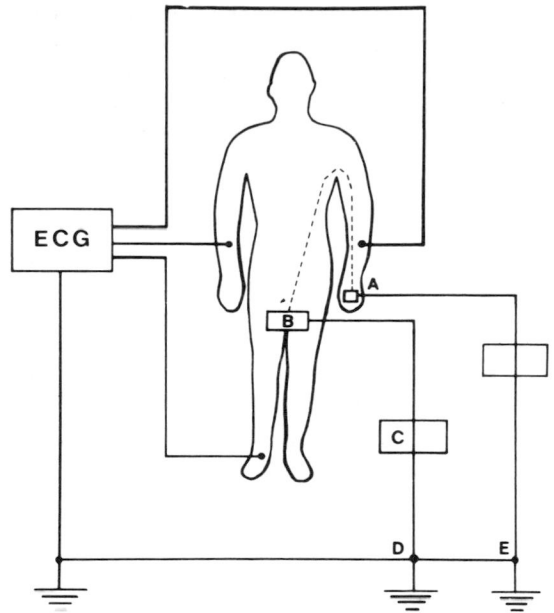

Fig. 3.11 Earth loop ABCDE involving the patient, producing electromagnetically induced interference.

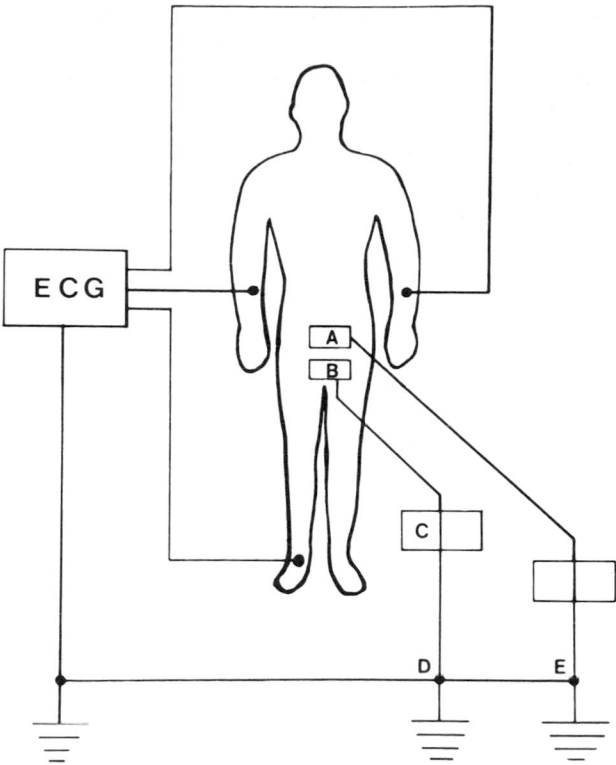

Fig. 3.12 Electromagnetically induced interference in the earth loop ABCDE. Current no longer flows through the patient.

loop. This mains frequency current flows through the patient, as shown by the dotted line, and it is highly unlikely that it will affect the left and right arm electrodes equally. In other words, it will present a signal which will be amplified by the differential input amplifier.

The situation is improved considerably if the two earth connections are made to the same place on the patient as shown in Fig. 3.12. Although current still flows in the loop ABCDE as before, no mains induced current flows through the patient.

Electromagnetically induced interference is generated in the same way as the effects produced in a transformer, where the source of interference represents the primary of the transformer and the patient, signal leads and earth connections take the place of the secondary winding. We have already discussed one technique for reducing this type of interference, by avoiding multiple earths on the patient, so that earth loops involving the patient are not formed. Other methods involve deliberately making the transformer as inefficient as possible. Sources of interference should be kept as far away from the patient and associated equipment as is practicable. It is often impossible to screen the source as large amounts of soft iron would have to be used to confine the flux. The area of the secondary winding should be reduced by keeping the leads close together and twisting the leads helps to cancel out induced voltages.

In spite of various precautions to reduce interference as much as possible, we are still left with a physically large and only partially screened conductor, comprising the patient, signal leads and amplifier, in a 50 Hz environment. In addition, this environment will not be constant as people and appar-

atus move about. As a result there will almost certainly be some interference present.

In Fig. 3.13, I represents the current flowing through the patient as a result of this electrical interference. The current flows to earth through the impedance Z and will produce a potential difference between electrodes A and B (a differential signal), which will be amplified along with the ECG, and mains hum will be seen on the trace unless the 'hum' signal is small compared with the ECG signal.

In addition the whole patient will be varying in potential with respect to earth by $V = IZ$ volts. This

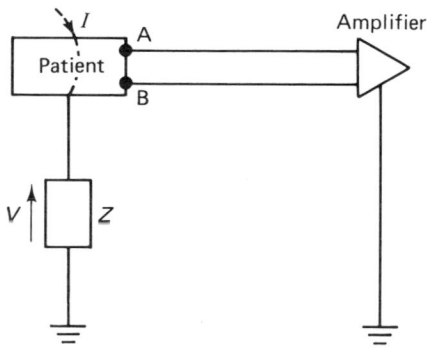

Fig. 3.13 Patient connected to differential input amplifier to illustrate common mode and differential signals.

common mode signal (affecting both A and B equally) may be ten or a hundred times larger than the 1 mV ECG signal, but should not cause interference provided that the amplifier has good common mode rejection.

In summary, the reduction of electrical interference depends on:

1. Careful electrode and signal lead technique.
2. Correct screening and earthing.
3. Well designed equipment, e.g. high common mode rejection ratio.

ELECTRICAL SAFETY OF PATIENTS

As more and more electrical equipment is used at the bedside or connected to the patient, it is important that doctors and nurses are aware of the electrical hazards which may arise (Loughman and Watson, 1971; Hull, 1978; Chambers and Saha, 1979; Hahn, 1980).

Electric Shock

When a voltage is applied between contacts placed on the surface of the body, a current will flow depending on the impedance of the pathway. The resistance between the surface of the skin and the underlying tissue varies between several megohms and tens of kilohms depending on the local conditions. As already mentioned, when electrode jelly is used to reduce the skin resistance it usually falls to about 2 kΩ, but may be as low as 300 Ω. The resistance of the underlying tissues is likely to be a few hundred ohms. It is important to note the variability of these figures, which makes dogmatic assertions suspect.

Mains frequency currents (50 Hz) are particularly effective in producing ventricular fibrillation and if the source is applied externally, for instance between the two arms, the following effects are found:

Threshold of feeling	0.5–2 mA
Muscular contraction	15–100 mA
Ventricular fibrillation	50 mA–2 A

The frequency of the stimulating current is important. If direct current is used, about five times the current is required, while when the diathermy is used, large high frequency currents pass through the body without ill effect (Fig. 3.14).

Depolarization of excitable tissue depends on the current density (the current flowing per unit area) across the cell membrane. Current density is difficult to measure in practice and so the total current flowing between the electrodes is usually quoted. When surface electrodes are applied to the limbs, only about 1/1000th of the current flows through the heart because of the multiplicity of available pathways.

In order to appreciate the ways in which electrocution can arise, we must first consider the mains power supply (Dobbie, 1972a). The single phase 240 V

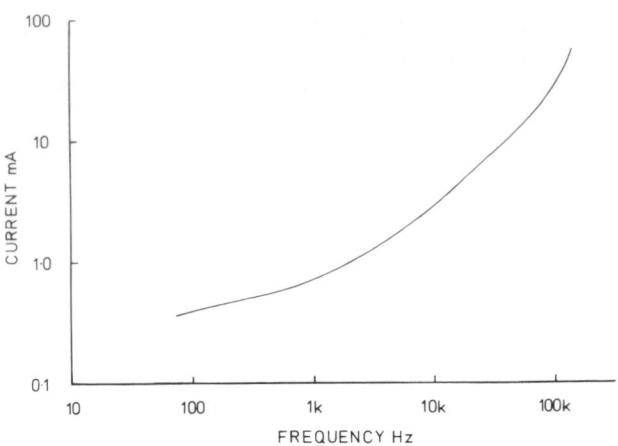

Fig. 3.14 Effect of frequency on threshold of sensation.

a.c. mains supply normally provided at socket outlets (Fig. 3.15) consists of:

1. A 'live' wire (L) which alternates at approximately 240 V with respect to local 'earth'.
2. A 'neutral' wire (N) carrying the return load current, and which is near 'earth' potential.
3. An 'earth' wire (E), not always present, which should be at local earth potential. This earth

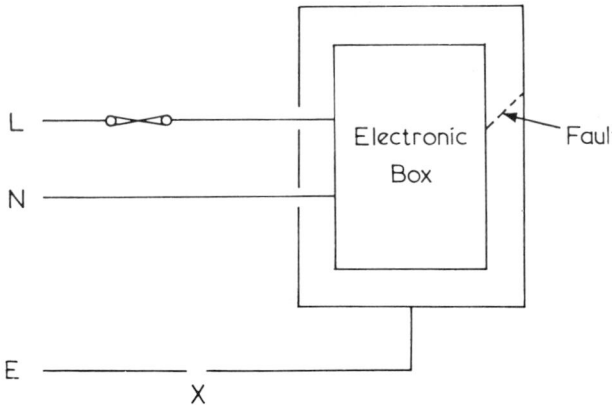

Fig. 3.15 Dangerous situation, showing broken earth lead X and live connection from electronics to outer metal case.

wire provides a return path for what are known as 'leakage currents' arising in the instrument. These are always present, because of capacitive and inductive coupling, between live and earthed parts of the instrument. In addition, the earth wire is normally connected to the metal case of the instrument so that if, under fault conditions, some live part of the instrument comes in contact with the case, the earth wire can carry a large current and the case will remain near earth potential. Eventually if the current is large enough the fuse or circuit breaker will operate.

A current, limited by the resistance of the pathway and the rating of the fuses, will flow through the patient if he completes the circuit between the live and neutral or the live and earth wires.

It is possible for a current to reach the patient through the ECG or EEG electrodes if faults develop within the instrument, but equipment faults which endanger the patient in this way are very rare and usually two or more faults have to be present before the patient is at risk.

Manufacturers of electro-medical equipment in the UK are guided by publications and regulations of professional and official bodies, including the British Standards Institution (1979). The provision of mains earth connection for reasons of safety relies on the mains plug being inserted into a three-pin mains socket. Even if patients are not involved, it is potentially dangerous for the user to ignore this requirement. In addition, the earthing serves as the first line of defence against capacitively coupled mains interference. One of the commonest electrical faults in mains operated equipment is disconnection of the earth wire. Usually the equipment will operate apparently normally in this condition so the operator is unaware that a potentially hazardous situation exists. However, if a second fault now develops, the case or other accessible parts of the instrument may become 'live' and constitute an electrical hazard both for the patient and the operator as shown in Fig. 3.15.

The current which can flow between the neutral and earth wires is likely to be much smaller but may endanger the patient under some circumstances. The potential difference between the local earth and the mains supply neutral is likely to be a few volts because the latter, which completes the mains supply circuit, cannot be guaranteed to be at earth potential at all points along its length.

One way of improving the situation is to isolate the electrical supply to the equipment from earth by using an isolating transformer as shown in Fig. 3.16.

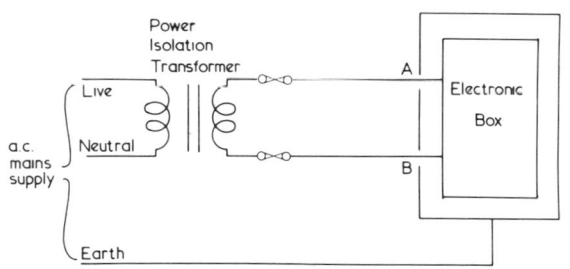

Fig. 3.16 Use of an isolating transformer.

Although 240 V is present between the supply wires A and B, the current which flows between A and Earth or B and Earth is very small (usually less than 0.5 mA) and exists only because of the leakage within the transformer. In general however, isolating transformers are not used because they are expensive items of equipment which require leakage current monitors to establish that they are working effectively, and because they contribute only marginally to improved patient safety.

Microelectrocution

A more subtle cause of electrocution can arise when intracardiac electrodes are used or when a saline filled catheter forms a conducting pathway within the heart. When an intracardiac electrode is used all the current passes through the myocardium and the current density depends on the size and position of the electrode. A small electrode in contact with ventricular muscle will have the lowest threshold for the production of ventricular fibrillation. A wide range of currents have been quoted. Green et al. (1972) found that the threshold for ventricular fibrillation in dogs with an electrode catheter in the right ventricle was never less than 200 µA and often a current of 1 mA was required. In a further study Raftery et al. (1975a) showed the threshold for minimal rhythm changes was 60 µA, while transient pump failure occurred with a current of 100 µA. In addition, ventricular fibrillation could not be produced with an atrial electrode using currents of up to 10 mA. Similar thresholds have been found in man. However, the most susceptible individual fibrillated when a current of about 80 µA passed across the ventricular wall (Watson et al., 1973; Raftery et al. 1975b). A study by Roy et al. (1976), using small electrodes, reported lower fibrillation thresholds. However an analysis by Hull (1978), using the data of Watson et al. (1973), suggests that currents of less than 44 µA are unlikely to produce ventricular fibrillation in man.

Small currents which can endanger the patient may occur even when equipment is working normally and may be difficult to detect. The possibility of microelectrocution should always be considered when there is a catheter or other connection in the ventricle, particularly if arrhythmias occur in association with gross electrical interference on the ECG.

Hazards Arising from Earth Connections

Ideally, two or more pieces of earthed equipment should be at the same potential. In practice, however, there may be significant differences in potential between earth connections even in the same room. A current flowing down the mains earth conductor will alter the potentials of the earth sockets around the room, simply because the earth wiring cannot have zero resistance. Small currents (less than 0.5 mA) flow normally as 'leakage currents' from mains operated equipment and larger 'fault currents' arising in faulty equipment will increase this effect. If earth leads from equipment earthed some distance away (for instance at a central monitoring station or computer) are applied to the patient together with locally earthed devices, then there may be several volts between the two earth points. Not only will there be large earth loops which may give rise to interference, but the patient may run the risk of microelectrocution (Fig. 3.17).

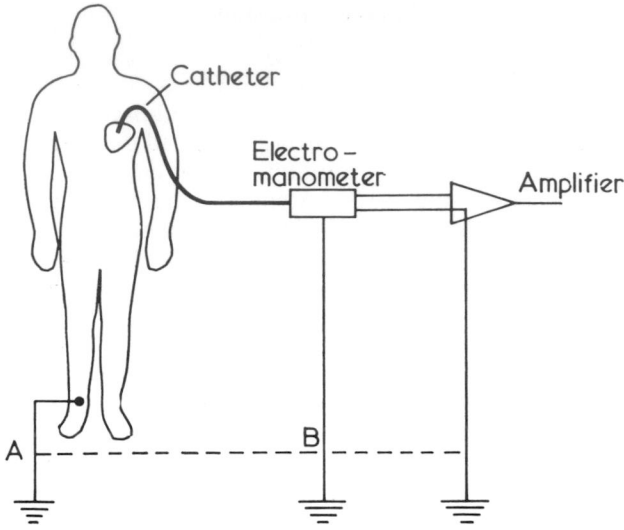

Fig. 3.17 Multiple earthing. If points A and B are at different potentials, then current will flow through the patient and across the myocardium.

Earth Points Having Different Potentials

It is almost impossible to ensure that all the earth connections which may be made to the patient deliberately or accidentally are at the same electrical potential. Thus it is recommended that the patient is isolated from earth, particularly when there are intra-cardiac electrical connections, to reduce the risk of microelectrocution. The absence of a low resistance pathway to earth will also help to safeguard the patient from electric shock should he happen to touch faulty electrical equipment.

SAFETY PRECAUTIONS

The patient and other personnel must be adequately protected from electric shock and the patient may also need protection from microelectrocution. Measures which increase patient safety will also reduce electrical interference.

The Mains Supply

1. Hospital engineering staff are responsible for the maintenance of the mains supply and test procedures are well established.
2. Isolation transformers have already been considered and the scheme is shown in Fig. 3.16. Contact between either of the floating supply wires and earth will not result in appreciable current flow. The leakage capacitance in the transformer and

associated wiring will result in a current of less than 0.5 mA flowing if one side of the isolated supply is short circuited to earth. If one wire of the isolated supply becomes accidentally grounded the system reverts to that of the conventional mains supply. A line isolation monitor measures the impedance of both the isolated power lines to earth and triggers an alarm if the impedance drops below a pre-set level (such as 25 kΩ). Line isolation transformers are expensive and it is important to establish that such a system is justified in practice (Dobbie, 1972b).

Equipment

1. Mains operated equipment must be effectively earthed for reasons already stated. When possible, all equipment associated with a patient should be plugged into a single group of power sockets sharing a common earth. If necessary other metal objects within reach of the patient should also be connected to this earth point. This ensures that the accessible parts of electrical apparatus in the vicinity of the patient are as nearly as possible at the same electrical potential.
2. Battery operated instruments should not be earthed and must be insulated to prevent accidental earth connections.
3. Connections between equipment and the patient should be isolated from earth. Isolated pacemakers are used routinely and isolated ECG machines, pressure transducers, flow meters and other equipment are readily available (Fig. 3.18). These may

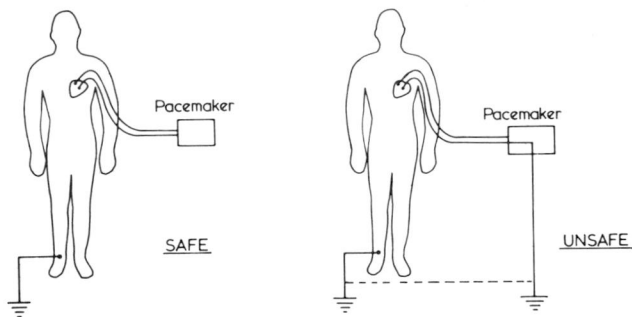

Fig. 3.18 Isolated equipment should be used and direct earth connections avoided, particularly if a conducting pathway to the myocardium exists.

be battery driven, or special circuitry involving transformer or optical coupling will effectively isolate the patient leads from mains earth. Patient monitoring equipment must be capable of withstanding the voltages produced by surgical diathermy and defibrillation equipment and still maintain efficient isolation. Where a diathermy with an earthed indifferent electrode is used, the plate should be connected to earth through a capacitor of about 0.01 μF. This will have a reactance of about 300 kΩ at 50 Hz and less than 20 Ω at 1 MHz (approximately diathermy frequency). British Standards Institution (1979) recommendations specify that equipment used in association with intra-cardiac connections, where there is a risk of microelectrocution, should not allow mains frequency current of more than 10 μA (50 μA under fault conditions) to flow between any patient connections or between connections to the patient and earth. Equipment used with external electrodes only can pass up to 100 μA (500 μA under fault conditions) between the electrodes and earth. The d.c. current which can flow between connections to the patient should be less than 10 μA, otherwise electrolytic skin reactions are likely to occur.

4. Maintenance of equipment. The commonest undetected fault in mains operated equipment is disconnection of the earth wire in the mains lead. This can often pass unnoticed until a second fault develops which may cause electrocution. Efficient maintenance of equipment is the only safeguard and needs consideration by those responsible for its use (Editorial, 1972; Monk and Shaw, 1975; North, 1975; Editorial, 1979).

The Patient

1. The patient should be isolated from earth as previously discussed (Pocock, 1972a,b). From the point of view of electrical safety, isolating the patient from earth means avoiding low impedance earth connections which may carry sufficiently large currents to cause electric shock or microelectrocution. Connections involving the use of antistatic rubber which is of relatively high impedance, to avoid the build up of static electricity in the anaesthetic breathing circuit, are of course desirable and will not increase the risk of electrocution.

2. When an earth connection to the patient is unavoidable, or occurs accidentally, it should be to a single point on the patient. This will eliminate earth loops involving the patient and will reduce electrical interference, as well as contributing to patient safety.

SURGICAL DIATHERMY

When the diathermy is in use a high frequency current (300 kHz–3 MHz) passes through the patient. In the simplest case the current flows between the active electrode and the indifferent (plate) electrode. The active electrode should make only a small area of contact with the tissue, so the current density is high and direct heating of the tissue occurs. This may be accompanied by charring or complete disruption of the cells if an arc is formed when the diathermy is used for cutting. The plate electrode makes a large area of contact with the patient and the current density is low,

so that no tissue damage is found (Mitchell et al., 1978; Whelpton, 1980).

In general, high frequency continuous oscillation is used for cutting, while bursts of lower frequency are preferred for coagulation. The current which flows through the patient is very variable, usually 200–400 mA flows during coagulation, but currents of up to 2 A may be used in urology. Originally spark gap oscillators were used and these are still considered very suitable for coagulation. Valve and transistor ('solid state') machines are now available.

The plate electrode may be connected within the machine in various ways.

1. One side of the generator and the indifferent electrode may be connected directly to earth. This was common practice until a few years ago, but had the disadvantage that a direct earth connection was made to the patient.

2. It was also recommended that a capacitor of about 0.01 μF was inserted between the plate lead and earth. This had a reactance of about 20 Ω at diathermy frequency, but more than 300 kΩ at 50 Hz. The risk of mains electrocution was thus reduced, as described above.

3. Isolated diathermy. Modern solid state machines may be effectively isolated from earth on both sides of the generator and virtually no current can flow through the patient unless both electrodes are connected to complete the circuit as shown in Fig. 3.19. If, however, the plate is inadvertently connected to earth, the diathermy is no longer isolated and may be hazardous in certain situations (Mitchell, 1979; Hahn, 1980).

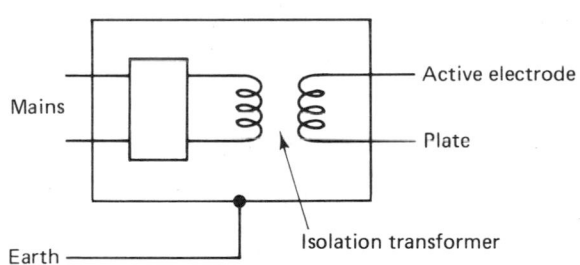

Fig. 3.19 Isolated diathermy.

When bipolar electrodes are used with an isolated diathermy the plate electrode is no longer used and the current flows directly between the two electrodes (such as the two blades of the diathermy forceps). This system has advantages for neurosurgery or during laparoscopy, as adjacent tissues cannot be damaged.

Diathermy Hazards

Fires and Explosions

The diathermy forms an electric arc with sufficient

energy to ignite flammable gas mixtures and flammable solutions used for preparing the skin.

Diathermy Burns

1. Under the plate. If the plate makes contact with the patient over too small an area, the current density will be high and a burn may result. Such lesions are characteristically small, deep and very painful. Metal foil electrodes may become crinkled with use and only make contact with the skin at a few places. Poor plate contact is likely to raise the impedance of the circuit. Thus the machine will not perform satisfactorily at its usual setting and the output of the generator will have to be increased if the surgeon is to obtain adequate power for co-agulation or cutting. This should alert the theatre staff to the possibility of a badly connected plate, or other fault in the equipment. The subject of lesions under the diathermy plate and elsewhere has been considered by Dobbie (1969, 1974) and Mitchell et al. (1978).

2. Other sites. Until recently, diathermy machines used to complete the circuit via an earth return. This meant that connections made to the patient would provide multiple pathways for current to flow and current would be distributed according to the impedances of the individual pathways (Fig. 3.20).

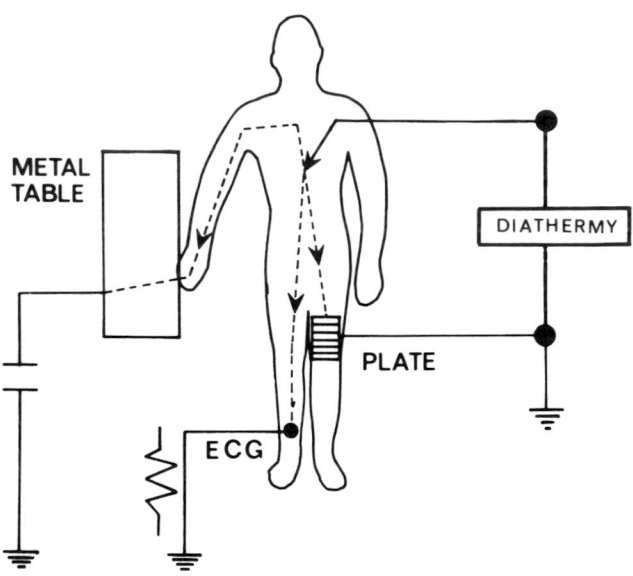

Fig. 3.20 Current from the earthed diathermy flows through multiple pathways.

If the plate is disconnected or makes poor contact, larger currents will flow along other routes and the current density may be sufficiently high to produce a burn. Needle electrodes for ECG or other monitors are particularly vulnerable in this

respect as they make good contact with the tissues over a small area and should not be used. Note that the patient leads of 'isolated ECG monitors' are only effectively isolated from earth at low frequencies (such as 50 Hz) and are effectively connected to earth at the high frequency at which the diathermy operates, because of capacitive coupling between the signal leads and the screens surrounding them. Similarly the operating table, even though not connected directly to earth, is a large metal object capacitively coupled to earth. Burns may thus occur if the patient touches the table, as the impedance of the operating table to earth is about 1000 Ω (Dobbie, 1969).

Mains Electric Shock and Microelectrocution

A directly earthed diathermy plate is undesirable, as discussed above.

Precautions against Diathermy Burns

1. Correct application of the diathermy plate, if possible close to the site of operation, is important. 'Plate monitor' circuits ensure that the plate is connected to the machine, but do not guarantee that the plate is connected to the patient.
2. The patient should not touch exposed metal on the operating table.
3. ECG cables for use in theatre should have 10 kΩ resistors in each lead close to the patient to reduce the current which can flow along these pathways (Becker et al., 1973; Bond, 1975).
4. Inadvertent operation of the diathermy may be hazardous, particularly during laparoscopy. There should be an audible indication that the machine is in operation.
5. Isolated diathermy machines, where the circuit is not completed via an earthed pathway, should be used.
6. Effective maintenance of the diathermy machine and all associated equipment is essential.

Diathermy burns, electrocution and other electrical mishaps have resulted from the use of obsolete and inadequately maintained equipment. The introduction of conducting devices within the heart has become relatively commonplace and thus it is possible to produce ventricular fibrillation with small currents which may endanger the patient both under fault conditions and when the equipment is operating normally. It is important that manufacturers of equipment and those responsible for its installation and use are aware of these hazards and are able to avoid them in practice.

REFERENCES

Becker C.M., Malhotra I.V., Hedley-Whyte J. (1973). The distribution of radio-frequency current and burns. *Anesthesiol.*, **38**, 106.

Bond W.H. (1975). Electrical hazards of disposable monitoring electrodes. *Lancet*, **i**, 852.

British Standards Institution. (1979). *Specification for safety of medical electrical equipment*. BS 5724, Part 1.

Chambers J.J., Saha A.K. (1979). Electrocution during anaesthesia. *Anaesthesia.*, **34**, 173.

Conference of Medical Royal Colleges. (1976). Diagnosis of brain death. *Br. Med. J.*, **2**, 1187.

Dobbie A.K. (1969). The electrical aspects of surgical diathermy. *Biomed. Eng.*, **4**, 206.

Dobbie A.K. (1972a). Electricity in hospitals. *Biomed. Eng.*, **7**, 12.

Dobbie A.K. (1972b). Is money for safety unlimited? *Med. Biol. Eng.*, **10**, 542.

Dobbie A.K. (1974). Accidental lesions in the operating theatre. *NAT News.*, **11**, 9.

Dubois M., Scott D.F., Savege T.M. (1978a). Assessment of recovery from short anaesthesia using the cerebral function monitor. *Br. J. Anaesth.*, **50**, 825.

Dubois M., Savege T.M., O'Caroll T.M. et al. (1978b). General anaesthesia and changes on the cerebral function monitor. *Anaesthesia.*, **33**, 157.

Editorial. (1972). Equipment maintenance. *Biomed. Eng.*, **7**, 219.

Editorial. (1979). *Anaesthesia.*, **34**, 145.

Feldman S.A. (1974). Measurement of neuromuscular block. In *Measurement in Anaesthesia*, p. 39. (Spierdijk J., Leigh J.M., Feldman S.A. eds.). The Hague, Boston: Leiden University Press.

Goat V.A. (1979). Peripheral nerve stimulators. *Br. J. Clin. Equip.*, **4**, 122.

Green H.L., Raftery E.B., Gregory I.C. (1972). Ventricular fibrillation threshold of healthy dogs to 50 Hz current in relation to earth leakage currents of electromedical equipment. *Biomed. Eng.*, **7**, 408.

Hahn C.E.W. (1980). Electrical hazards and safety in cardiovascular measurements. In *The circulation in anaesthesia.* (Prys-Roberts C. Ed.). Oxford: Blackwell Scientific Publications.

Hull C.J. (1978). Electrocution hazards in the operating theatre. *Br. J. Anaesth.*, **50**, 647.

Loughman J., Watson A.B. (1971). Electrical safety in Australian Hospitals and proposed standards. *Med. J. Aust.*, **2**, 349.

Miller R.D. (1978). Monitoring of neuromuscular blockade. In *Monitoring in Anesthesia.* (Saidman L.J., Smith N. Ty. eds.). New York: John Wiley.

Mitchell J.P., Lumb G.N., Dobbie A.K. (1978). *A Handbook of Surgical Diathermy* (2nd edn). Bristol: Wright.

Mitchell J.P. (1979). The isolated circuit diathermy. *Ann. Roy. Coll. Surgeons.*, **61**, 287.

Monk I.B., Shaw A. (1975). Medical equipment hazards—Practical experience in a large region. *Biomed. Eng.*, **10**, 132.

North R. (1975). Safety testing patient-connected electronic equipment. *Br. J. Clin. Equip.*, **1**, 29.

Pocock S.N. (1972a). Earth-free patient monitoring. Part I. *Biomed. Eng.*, **7**, 21.

Pocock S.N. (1972b). Earth-free patient monitoring. Part II. *Biomed. Eng.*, **7**, 67.

Prior P. (1980). Noninvasive monitoring of cerebral function. *Br. J. Clin. Equip.*, **2**, 54.

Raftery E.B., Green H.L., Gregory I.C. (1975a). Disturbances of heart rhythm produced by 50 Hz leakage currents in dogs. *Cardiovasc. Res.*, **9**, 256.

Raftery E.B., Green H.L., Yacoub M.H. (1975b). Disturbances of heart rhythm produced by 50 Hz leakage currents in human subjects. *Cardiovasc. Res.*, **9**, 263.

Roy O.Z., Scott J.R., Park G.C. (1976). 60 Hz ventricular fibrillation and pump failure thresholds versus electrode area. *IEEE Trans. Bio-Med. Eng.*, **23**, 45.

Watson A.B., Wright J.S., Loughman J. (1973). Electrical thresholds for ventricular fibrillation in man. *Med. J. Aust.*, **1**, 1179.

Whelpton D. (1980). Performance evaluation of surgical diathermy in different electrodes. *Clin. Physics and Physiol. Measurement.*, **1**, 59.

FURTHER READING

Sykes M.K., Vickers M.D., Hull C.J. (1981). *Principles of Clinical Measurement.*, Oxford: Blackwell Scientific Publications.

4. The Measurement of Temperature
P. Cliffe

Physical meaning of temperature
Clinical thermometers
Thermocouples
Platinum resistance thermometry
Thermistor thermometers
Dial thermometers

PHYSICAL MEANING OF TEMPERATURE

The physical definition of temperature can be established by considering the way in which information about it is obtained. In common with the measurement of any other physical quantity, a property of matter is chosen which varies with temperature; e.g. length of a metal, volume of a liquid, pressure or volume of a gas, pressure of a saturated vapour, colour of a substance, electrical resistance of a metal or semi-conductor, or the EMF developed across the junctions of dissimilar metals.

For illustration, consider Fig. 4.1, in which the length of a metal rod is chosen. The property of length defines the 'scale' of temperature. Now to give the scale quantitative significance, measure the value of the property (length of the rod) at two fixed temperatures, namely, that of pure melting ice and that of steam, at standard atmospheric pressure. The choice of a graduation system, e.g. 0–100 units on the Centi-

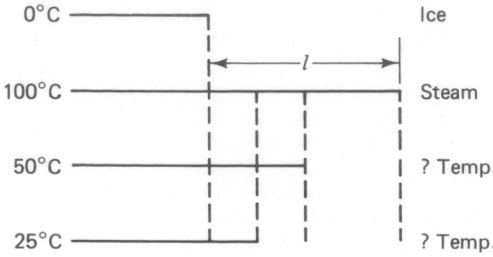

Fig. 4.1 Principles of scales of temperature.

grade graduation, then defines a temperature difference of 100°C. Alternatively, the choice of 32 and 212 units is made for the Fahrenheit graduation system.

For the temperatures at any other point on the 'scale' the assumption is made that increments in temperature are proportional to the corresponding increments in the measured property, i.e. temperature changes are defined in this example as being proportional to the changes in the length of a metal rod which they produce. Hence, the measurement of temperature is reduced to that of measuring the length of the rod. For example, 50°C is the temperature of the rod which has increased by $L/2$, and so on.

Clearly, the choice of another 'scale', such as a gas scale or resistance scale, would again require temperature by definition to vary linearly with the change in volume or pressure of the gas or the electrical resistance. As they are not closely related properties, the different scales would not agree.

In view of this apparently unsatisfactory nature of the definition of temperature, scientists in the last century sought means whereby a temperature scale may be defined independently of any material substance.

One approach involved the study of gas thermometers. For example, it would be possible arbitrarily to define temperature as proportional to changes in pressure in a constant volume hydrogen thermometer of specified design, with the pressure of the gas specified at the ice point. However, when gases other than hydrogen are used in such a gas thermometer, the measured values of temperature are found to differ slightly. If the pressure of gas at the ice point is infinitely reduced, it can be shown that at this limit all gases behave in the same way and have the properties of an 'ideal' gas. The ideal gas scale of temperature may thus be defined, as for the constant volume hydrogen scale, and by measurement of the properties of actual gases extrapolated to zero pressure, corrections may be made to the constant volume hydrogen scale. This can be done, although within the range of 0–100°C the corrections are only of the order of 0.003°C. The ideal gas scale turns out to be identical with another 'theoretical' scale, called the thermodynamic scale, defined in terms of the efficiency of an ideal heat engine.

The modern definition of temperature is related to the thermodynamic scale, and is essentially based on the accurate definition of fixed points such as the ice and steam points, but extended to cover a wide range of temperature from a fraction of a degree absolute to thousands of degrees centigrade. The present day specifications are laid down in 'The International Practical Temperature Scale of 1968' published by HMSO.

Application to Thermometers

In medicine, temperature measurements may be required in patients or in apparatus. Where the temperature of patients is required the usual thermometers are:

1. Mercury in glass (the clinical thermometer)
2. Thermocouple
3. Resistance (metal)
4. Thermistor (resistance of semi-conductor).

In scientific apparatus, the above types are also used, but frequently 'dial' thermometers are employed.

5. Dial thermometers—mercury in steel
   vapour pressure
   bimetallic elements

Clinical Thermometers

Within the limited accuracy (±0.1°C) required from a clinical thermometer, it probably remains the most satisfactory instrument for routine clinical use. Its disadvantages include:

1. Breakage
2. Slow response, due to relatively high thermal capacity
3. Unsuitability for remote reading
4. Unsuitability for recording
5. Difficulty of application to unconscious patients
6. Unsuitability for subcutaneous or intracavity temperatures, e.g. from sites in the oesophagus, nasopharynx, or rectum.

Electrical thermometry overcomes these disadvantages.

Another important use of the mercury thermometer relates to the calibration of electric thermometers. The mercury thermometer may be obtained in a wide variety of ranges and accuracies and these can be checked by the National Physical Laboratory by comparison with a standard. The resulting accuracy of calibration is usually adequate for most medical applications.

Thermocouples (Fig. 4.2)

When a circuit made of two dissimilar metals has the two junctions maintained at different temperatures, an electromotive force (EMF) is developed. The arrangement of metals is called a 'thermocouple' and the effect is called the Seebeck effect.

The relationship between the EMF developed and

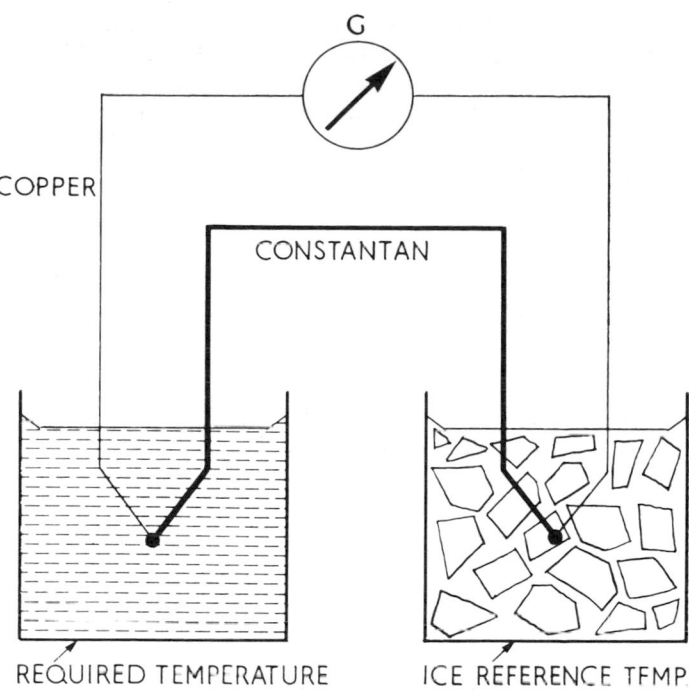

Fig. 4.2 The principle of the thermocouple.

In order to measure temperature it is necessary to maintain the temperature of one junction constant, the other can then be used to determine the required temperature provided the EMF of the thermocouple is measured. If the galvanometer, G, has a high resistance compared with the thermocouple so that there is negligible potential difference across the couple, then the potential difference across G is equal to the EMF and the current through G is proportional to the EMF.

This simple arrangement is associated with certain difficulties. From the practical standpoint the use of ice may be inconvenient. Furthermore, if the metal at the galvanometer terminals differs from that which terminates the thermocouple, then further thermojunctions are formed. If they differ in temperature they will produce thermo-EMFs. The law of intermediate metals states that, provided the temperature remains unchanged, any different metal may be placed in one part of the leads joining two thermojunctions, without changing the overall EMF. Clearly this requires no variation in temperature at the galvanometer terminals. These objections have been overcome in one commercial instrument as shown in Fig. 4.3.

The 'cold junction' is mounted in a small copper cylinder about 5 mm long and 5 mm in diameter. The junction is mounted very close to the terminals of a sensitive reflecting galvanometer of which the upper suspension is connected to a bimetallic spiral spring. Because of their close proximity within a small metal box, the junction, the bimetallic spring and the terminals, are at approximately the same temperature. This is further ensured by enclosing the instrument in a stout metal case, the conductivity of which encourages a uniform temperature inside.

As room temperature changes, the temperature of the junction changes, and this is compensated by the movement of the bimetal spring, so that the net effect is that of a constant reference temperature. The nonlinear relationship between galvanometer deflection

the temperature difference between the junctions is approximately parabolic in form, and may be represented by

$$E = At + Bt^2$$

Where E is the EMF developed for a temperature difference of $t°$C, while A and B are constants which depend on the metals forming the thermocouples. The effect of the non linear factor B varies with the metal pair. For copper and constantan (an alloy of copper and nickel) the maximum deviation from linearity between 0–100°C is between 2–3°C, although for other combinations it is less. In practice, the metal junctions are made by silver soldering or welding.

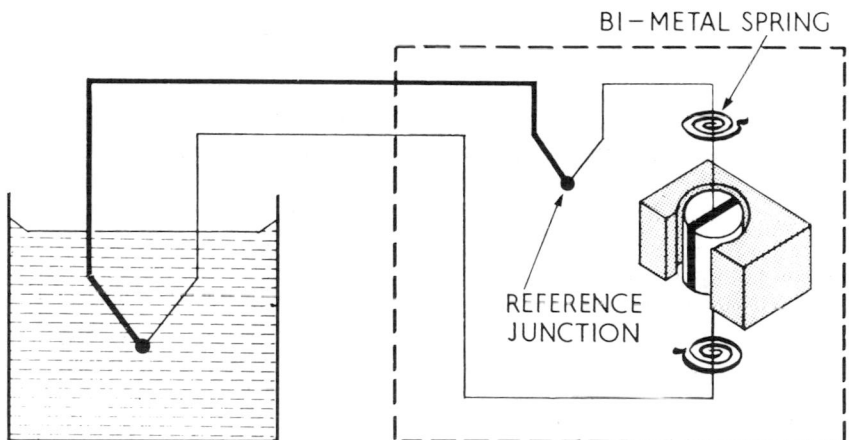

Fig. 4.3 Mechanical cold junction compensation in the thermo-electric thermometer.

and temperature is corrected by the use of a non-linear galvanometer scale. However, for the thermo-couples supplied the effect is small and only careful observation would reveal that the scale divisions are not equal.

This instrument is available in two models for reading 0–50°C or for 16–46°C (± 0.1°C). The thermo-junctions are of nichrome and constantan, which produce an EMF of 46.5 mV per °C. They are supplied in a large variety of forms: needles of approximately 22 gauge, as applicators for rectal and intraoesophageal use, as loops for attaching to the skin, etc. By a manually operated switching device up to 15 junctions may be read sequentially. The advantages of this type of instrument are as follows.

1. The junctions may be very small and versatile
2. The thermocouples respond rapidly on account of their low thermal capacity
3. The accuracy is adequate

Although a sensitive galvanometer is employed, no special levelling is required. The movement may be clamped so that the instrument can be carried about in a case without special precautions.

Recording with Thermocouples

Certain problems are encountered in recording from thermocouples, partly because the voltage output per degree centigrade is only about 50 mV and partly because the cold junction temperature has to be kept constant. While for laboratory use the cold junction may be maintained in melting ice in a vacuum flask, this procedure is often inconvenient in the operating theatre.

One very satisfactory method of overcoming the difficulty, is to use the principles embodied in Fig. 4.3. The galvanometer scale can be replaced by a double photoelectric cell. Light reflected from the galvanometer mirror is distributed between the cells as the coil is deflected, and the photocell output is proportional to the angular deflection. Correction circuits can linearize the EMF-temperature relationship and the amplified output is applied to a multipoint chart recorder.

Platinum Resistance Thermometry

The resistance of a metal varies with temperature according to the relation:

where $R_t = R_0 (1 + at + bt^2)$

      R_t = resistance at temperature t°C

      R_0 = resistance at ice temperature

a and b are constants which have been accurately determined for various metals.

For a 100 Ω coil of platinum, the resistance change near ice temperature is about 0.4 Ω per °C.

Knowing the values of a and b, if the resistance of a

coil is accurately measured at the ice point, an unknown temperature may be determined from the above relation if R_t is accurately measured. When used in this way a platinum resistance thermometer is capable of much higher accuracy than is usually required medically, e.g. a few thousandths of a °C. The practical arrangement is as in Fig. 4.4, which shows a modified Wheatstone bridge. The fixed arms P, Q and R of the bridge may be wound with constantan, which has a negligible temperature coefficient of resistance and is thus thermostable.

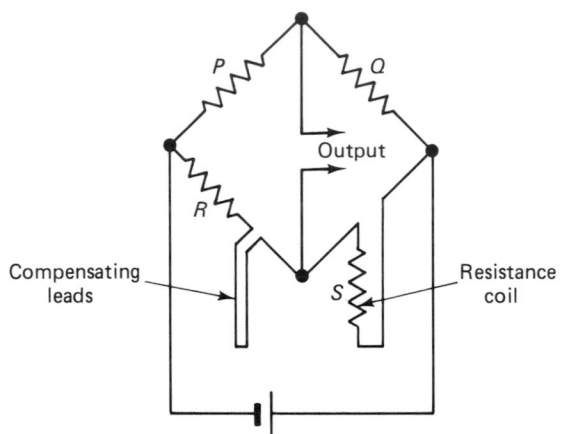

Fig. 4.4 Bridge circuit for a resistance thermometer.

In order that no resistance error is introduced by the connecting leads to the coil, a second pair of 'false' leads is included in the thermometer housing and these are connected into the opposite-fixed arm Q. Hence, the resistance of the actual leads is balanced out.

The current through the coil must be limited to avoid self-heating. For example, for a 100 Ω coil, the power dissipated should be limited to about 0.1 mW, so that the current through the coil should not exceed 1 mA. Thus a change of temperature of 1°C would produce a change of bridge output voltage of approximately 400 mV, compared with about 40 mV/°C for a thermocouple. Resistance coils may be made sufficiently reproducible as to be readily interchangeable.

For medical use the chief disadvantage has been the physical size of the coil and correspondingly slow response time. While the rectal and oesophageal thermometers have been produced commercially, smaller probes are not readily available.

Although high accuracy of temperature measurement is possible with bridge circuits if the resistance is measured by balancing the bridge, it is often desirable to have a direct reading instrument. This is possible, because as the thermometer coil resistance changes the bridge is unbalanced, and the resulting current may be related to temperature, and read directly from a suitable meter. Two problems arise with bridge circuits;

1. The resistance of the detecting element does not vary linearly with temperature. For platinum, between 0° and 100°C the maximum error arising from assuming a linear relationship is approximately 0.4°C.
2. If the resistance of one arm of a bridge is changed in equal steps, the corresponding steps of unbalanced current in the galvanometer will not be equal, i.e. the relation between resistance change in one arm and unbalanced current is non-linear. The problem may be resolved in three ways:

(a) *Non-linear scale*. As for the thermocouple, the resistance thermometer may be calibrated against a standard and a special non linear scale can be prepared for the galvanometer so that actual temperature and observed temperature are made equal.

(b) *Selection of bridge parameter*. Commercial galvanometers are normally supplied with linear scales. If one of these is used for the bridge, and the temperature range is restricted, e.g. to 20°C within the physiological range, it is possible to limit the non-linear error by the correct choice of bridge resistances. The principle is discussed below in the section on thermistors.

(c) *Electronic linearization*. By electronic circuits, using diodes, it is possible to correct the slope of any curved characteristic, piece by piece, until it becomes linear within specified limits. This technique can be applied to the outputs of bridge circuits.

Thermistor Thermometers

The thermistor is a semiconducting element consisting of a heavy metal oxide which has a large negative temperature coefficient of resistance. Oxides of manganese, nickel, cobalt, iron and zinc have been used. Thermistors are produced by compressing such oxides in powder form to beads, rods or discs, and sintering the mixture at high temperature into a solid mass. Electrodes are applied by firing on metal colloids, applied as paints or by fusing the material around wires.

For biological use, minute beads ranging in diameter from 0.015–0.25 cm are available, which may be sealed into the tip of hypodermic needles. Figure 4.5 shows a photomicrograph of such a bead (STC/U.23) compared with the head of a match. They have a very small thermal capacity and can respond to a change of temperature rapidly—in as little as 0.2 seconds. However, they are not as stable as metal resistance elements and most thermistors show an ageing as an increase of resistance with time over a period of months. In addition, they may exhibit hysteresis

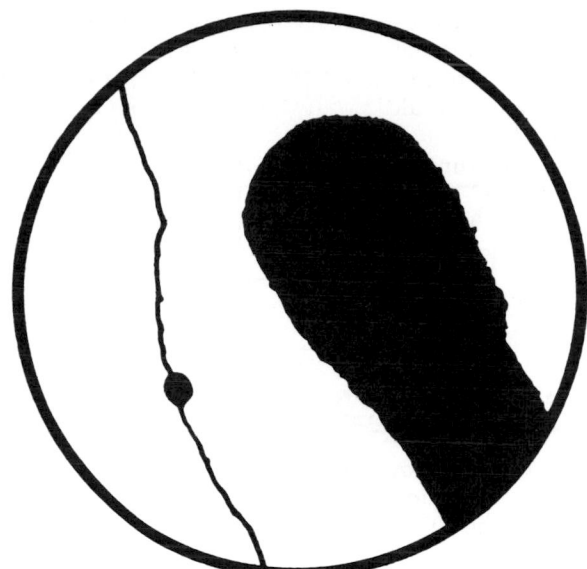

Fig. 4.5 Thermistor bead compared with a match.

effects if subjected to rapid, large temperature fluctuations and it is sometimes recommended that they be recalibrated if subjected to temperature changes of greater than 10°C per minute, or to greater changes than 50–60°C. Furthermore, variations occur from one to another of the same type so that individual calibrations are necessary, although matched pairs are now available.

The variations of resistance of EMF with temperature are non-linear for resistance thermometers and thermocouples, but the deviation from linearity is relatively small. This is not so for the thermistor where the resistance varies exponentially with the reciprocal of the absolute temperature. Compared with the metallic resistor the resistance change is large, e.g. the thermistor approximately halves its resistance for a 20°C increase in temperature. Because of this relatively large sensitivity the thermistor is well suited to the measurement of small temperature changes, such as that within the pulmonary artery during thermal dilution procedures for measuring cardiac output.

Thermistors are used in bridge circuits, but because of their relatively high resistance compared with metal coils, no special requirements are necessary regarding compensating leads. The problems of non-linearity are dealt with as described previously.

The principle of selecting bridge parameters to provide linear but limited ranges of temperature-resistance relations is shown in Fig. 4.6. The left hand curve (solid line) shows the variation of resistance of the thermistor with increasing temperature. Notice that the resistance decreases as shown when the temperature rises. Furthermore, the out of balance current is not proportional to the change of resistance but follows a curve. This is shown on the right hand side (dotted curve) of Fig. 4.6, where the temperature

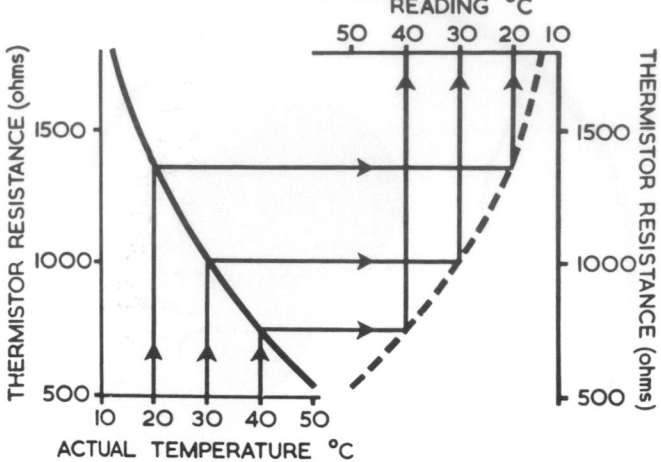

Fig. 4.6 Principle of linearizing thermistor characteristics when used in bridge circuits.

reading is, of course, the out of balance current suitably calibrated as a temperature. By arranging that the bridge constants are such that the shape of the right hand curve for the bridge is the same as the left hand curve for the thermistor, the reading will correspond with the actual temperature.

Dial Thermometers

Bimetallic. If a flat spiral spring is made up of two differing metal ribbons in contact, then on heating, the spring will tend to wind (or unwind) because of the difference in expansion between the metals. This movement may be transferred to a pointer.

Pressure Gauge Types. In the Bourdon gauge, the 'spring' consists of a hollow ribbon of metal which unwinds as the pressure inside it is increased and this movement causes a needle to rotate against a scale. Attached to the pressure gauge via a capillary is a steel tube filled with mercury, or a metal tube filled with a volatile liquid in the presence of its saturated vapour. The pressure changes produced by changing the temperature of the active elements may be calibrated so that the dial reads in temperature units. The accuracy is about $\pm \frac{1}{4}°C$ and the minimum range usually about 30°C.

5. The Measurement of Blood Pressure
G. D. Parbrook and W. M. Gray

GENERAL PRINCIPLES

Regardless of the technique of measurement, some general principles apply. Blood pressure is not constant but varies with the site of measurement. Fig. 5.1 illustrates the hydrostatic effect that arises because the

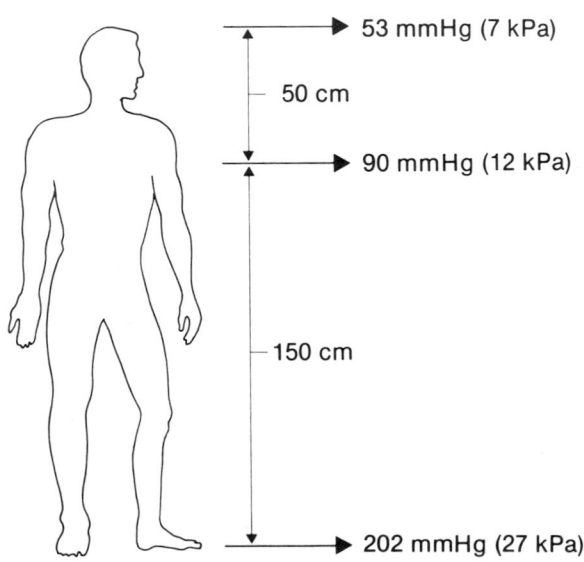

Fig. 5.1 Hydrostatic effects upon mean blood pressure. (From *Basic Physics and Measurement in Anaesthesia*, (1985). Heinemann Medical Books, with permission.)

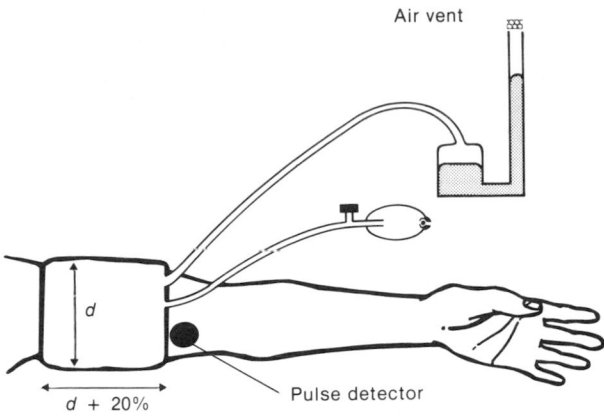

Fig. 5.2 Noninvasive measurement of blood pressure. (From *Basic Physics and Measurement in Anaesthesia*, (1985). Heinemann Medical Books, with permission.)

circulation is a system of tubes filled with liquid. In a tall man who is standing, the mean blood pressure could vary from 53 mmHg (7 kPa) at his head to 202 mmHg (27 kPa) at his feet, compared with a mean pressure of 90 mmHg (12 kPa) at his heart. This hydrostatic effect can be calculated from the difference in height in centimetres knowing that 7.5 mmHg (1 kPa) equals 10 cmH$_2$O pressure.

Unless it is stated to the contrary, blood pressure measurements will be assumed to be those at the level of the heart. The arm of a supine patient will normally be at this level but inaccuracies arise if posture is forgotten when blood pressure is taken at other positions particularly when the patient is on a tilted operating table. A false reading can also arise from the same cause during invasive measurement if the pressure transducer is not at the same horizontal level as the point at which the pressure is required.

In addition to these hydrostatic effects, the blood pressure also depends on the calibre of the vessel and its distance from the heart. Because there is a fall in pressure as liquid flows through a tube, it might be expected that the pressure in the arterioles would be lower than that in the arteries. This simple concept is complicated by the fact that blood pressure is pulsatile and changes in the wave pattern in different vessels alter the systolic pressures in them.

Blood pressure also shows a diurnal variation, being lower during sleep. Minor changes of pressure occur too during the respiratory cycle and more marked changes during intermittent positive pressure ventilation, when, in addition to cyclical changes, there may be a general reduction in blood pressure due to effects upon venous return. Anxiety raises the blood pressure, so readings on several separate occasions may be required to obtain a representative value. Finally the blood pressure varies with the cardiac cycle from the peak (systolic) to the lowest (diastolic) pressure. To obtain an accurate mean pressure an integration technique would need to be applied to an arterial pressure trace, but in clinical practice mean pressure is often taken as being diastolic pressure plus one third of the difference between diastolic and systolic pressure.

NONINVASIVE TECHNIQUES

Auscultation

The simplest noninvasive system for measuring blood pressure consists of an inflatable cuff connected to a mercury or aneroid manometer. The cuff is normally placed on the upper arm although the calf and thigh are sometimes used. The pressure at which the pulse returns after occlusion is identified by a detector system (Fig. 5.2).

The cuff must be positioned so that the centre of its bladder is on the medial side of the arm over the brachial artery. The width of the cuff should be 20% greater than the diameter of the arm ('*d*' in the figure).

The cuff with its tubing and connections should not leak. The mercury manometer must read zero correctly before use, and it should be used vertically unless it is of the type calibrated to be used at an angle. Partial blockage of the air vent or of the connecting tubes may lead to inaccurate or sluggish readings. Although aneroid gauges are more portable, their calibration requires frequent checking.

The cuff is inflated to a pressure above the expected systolic pressure and pressure is slowly released at a rate of 2–3 mmHg per second. The systolic pressure is indicated by the reappearance of the peripheral pulse at the detector, the simplest form of which is a hand palpating the radial artery. Auscultation over the brachial artery at the elbow allows recognition of the systolic pressure by detection of the first phase Korotkoff sound, i.e. the first sounds resulting from blood flow in the artery. The second phase Korotkoff sound is a slight muffling and the third a rise in volume of the auscultation sounds. The fourth phase is an abrupt fall in sound level and is sometimes taken as representing diastolic pressure, although the final loss of all sound (fifth phase) is more widely accepted as indicating diastolic pressure.

In anaesthesia, a pulse detector or pulse oximeter detector is often used on the patient's finger. This may then be used in conjunction with the blood pressure cuff though the apparent systolic pressure indicated may be lower than the true systolic pressure in this case.

Other more specialized detector systems can be used and microphone, ultrasonic detector and oscillometric systems are particularly suited to the automated techniques considered later.

Oscillometry

In the oscillometric technique the cuff is used both to detect the pulse and to measure the pressure. The 'Von Recklinghausen Oscillotonometer' is an example of an apparatus using this principle. This apparatus uses a double cuff and a sensitive bellows, D in Fig. 5.3, which detects pulse oscillations from the distal compartment of the double cuff. Bellows M measures the pressure from the proximal compartment of the

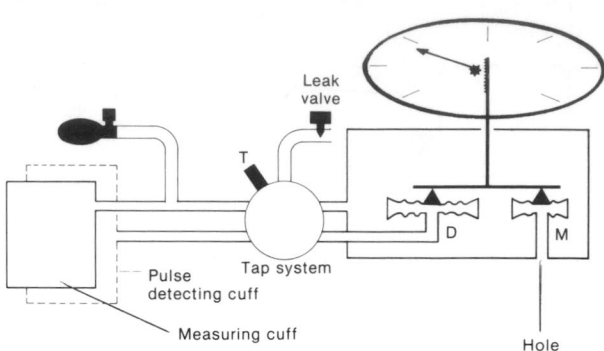

Fig. 5.3 The Von Recklinghausen Oscillotonometer. (From *Basic Physics and Measurement in Anaesthesia*, (1985). Heinemann Medical Books, with permission.)

cuff. To measure pressure, the user inflates the cuffs to above the expected systolic pressure, then adjusts the tap T to bring the bellows D into operation and to allow a slow leak through the leak valve. The point when oscillations commence is taken as indicating systolic pressure. The operation of the instrument is described in more detail by Sykes et al; (1981). The oscillotonometer provides a useful method of checking trends of systolic pressure but its accuracy is dependent upon several factors including the cuff deflation rate (Hutton and Prys-Roberts, 1982).

Automated Measurement

Automated techniques have the advantage that they free the anaesthetist from the tasks of cuff inflation and auscultation. In addition, the systems incorporate a timer to allow automatic control of the interval between measurements. Fig. 5.4 shows the principle of automated systems. A transducer senses the pressure

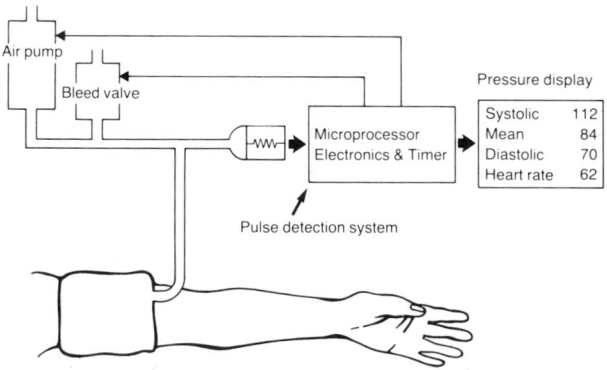

Fig. 5.4 The principle of automated noninvasive measurement of blood pressure.

and converts it to an electrical signal which can be electronically processed. An air pump inflates the cuff to a suitable high initial value, e.g. 160 mmHg, or, in repeated readings, to 25 mmHg above the previous systolic measurement. During a reading, the pressure is slowly released at the bleed valve at 2–3 mmHg per second until diastole is reached. A pulse detection system identifies the systolic, mean and diastolic pressures, which can then be displayed. Finally, the bleed valve allows rapid deflation of the cuff after the diastolic pressure has been reached.

The detection system can be of several types. In one type, a microphone in the cuff is positioned over the brachial artery and a microprocessor in the machine analyses the Korotkoff sounds to detect systole and diastole. Two other detection techniques, the ultrasonic and oscillometric, have been more commonly used and warrant more detailed description.

Ultrasonic Technique

In this technique, an ultrasonic transmitter and receiver are positioned over the brachial artery to detect arterial wall movement (Fig. 5.5). When the artery is either fully open or fully closed the ultrasound waves are reflected with very little change of frequency. However, during cuff deflation the arterial

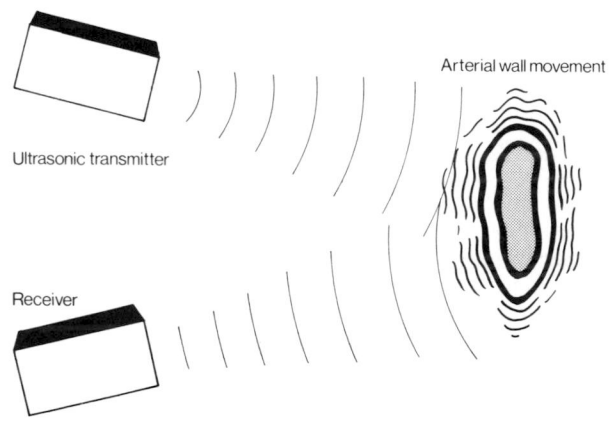

Fig. 5.5 The principle of the ultrasonic technique. (From *Basic Physics and Measurement in Anaesthesia*, (1985). Heinemann Medical Books, with permission.)

wall pulsates strongly between systole and diastole, and these movements cause Doppler shifts in the frequency of the ultrasound waves. An example of an instrument using this technique is the 'Arteriosonde', which gives reliable measurements for patients of all ages, including infants, provided that the detector is accurately positioned and an appropriate gel is used to give good contact with the skin. However, it can be difficult to position the detector correctly, and this has been a major factor in a move away from instruments like the Arteriosonde towards instruments with oscillometric detectors, which are not so critically dependent on positioning.

Oscillometric Technique

In contrast to the nonautomated form of this technique, a single cuff is normally used for both arterial occlusion and pulse detection. Movement of the arterial wall is transmitted to the cuff causing pressure changes which are detected by a transducer in the processing unit to which the cuff is connected. The principles are described in detail by Ramsey (1979). Popular models using this technique are the 'Dinamap' and the 'Accutorr'.

Above the systolic and below the diastolic pressure, the oscillations of pressure produced in the cuff by the movement of the arterial wall are negligible. As the cuff is deflated, the oscillations begin when systolic pressure is reached, increase to a maximum at the mean arterial pressure and then decrease until diastolic pressure occurs. Integrated circuits in the processing unit analyse the signals from the transducer and so enable systolic, mean and diastolic pressures to be displayed. The system gives reliable readings in adults and children provided the appropriate cuff size is used, but, in common with other noninvasive techniques, readings are less accurate if the patient has a dysrhythmia and the apparatus fails to record at low pressures e.g. below 50 mmHg.

Frequency of Cuff Inflation

The frequency of cuff inflation is limited by the time for the measurement process, and most automated systems only permit readings at a maximum rate of one per minute. Even this frequency may be too great for long-term use as it may cause impeded blood flow, which is both clinically undesirable and liable to produce inaccurate results, and a maximum frequency of every two minutes may then be preferable. To avoid these problems, an automated technique has been developed which measures pressure with a cuff and detector on the finger (van Egmond et al., 1985). The detector used is a photo-plethysmograph which measures infrared absorption at a wavelength specific for arterial blood and this system can give almost continuous noninvasive recording of blood pressure. A commercial version of this system, the 'Finapres', is now available and has been reported to function well even during peripheral vasoconstriction (Dorlas et al., 1985) but its eventual role in clinical practice remains to be established. In the meantime, for patients in whom rapid changes of blood pressure are likely, for example following sudden blood loss, during operation for phaeochromocytoma, or during controlled hypotension, the standard method of monitoring blood pressure is by invasive measurement.

INVASIVE MEASUREMENT

Invasive measurement of arterial pressure is used in preference to noninvasive methods when dysrhythmias are present, when rapid changes in blood pressure can occur or when information about the shape of the arterial waveform is required. Although invasive measurement is of wider applicability and capable of greater accuracy than noninvasive techniques, it is more complex to perform and its potential advantages can only be realized if the anaesthetist understands the principles of the method and takes appropriate precautions to obtain accurate measurements. In the following sections, after a brief description of the equipment used for invasive measurement, we will summarize the necessary theoretical background and will then show how this can provide practical guidelines for ensuring accurate pressure measurements.

Equipment

Invasive pressure measurement requires the use of an arterial cannula, a catheter and transducer, an amplifier and some means of displaying the pressure waveform, such as a visual display unit or a recorder. A typical arrangement is shown in Fig. 5.6. Pressure changes in the artery are transmitted through the saline in the catheter to the transducer, where they cause the flexible diaphragm to move. This movement is detected by means of a strain gauge, and the amount of movement taken as a measure of the change in arterial pressure. In most commercial trans-

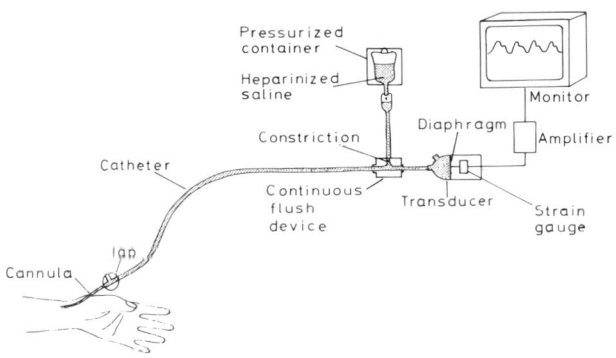

Fig. 5.6 Equipment required for invasive pressure measurement.

ducers, the strain gauge consists of an electrical resistor connected to the diaphragm, and the circuitry required to measure the change of resistance (known as a 'Wheatstone bridge') is incorporated in the transducer body. In some models the resistor and associated circuitry are built into a single silicon chip to form a 'semiconductor strain gauge' and this arrangement produces a rugged and reliable device.

For the purposes of analysis, it is necessary to consider the catheter and transducer as an integral system, which, for conciseness, we shall refer to as an 'arterial manometer'.

Cannulation Procedure

If possible, a peripheral artery, such as the radial or

ulnar artery, should be chosen for cannulation, so that the whole limb is not threatened if a clot or haematoma forms. To prevent clotting in the cannula, it is necessary to flush it with heparinized saline, and the most satisfactory way of doing this for long-term monitoring is by means of a continuous flushing system (e.g. the 'Intraflo'), as shown in Fig. 5.6. This provides a steady flow of about 4 ml/h to flush the catheter and cannula.

Potential Errors

It will be shown later that presently available catheter-transducer systems have to be operated at the limits of their capabilities to give accurate results, and this requires careful preparation, assessment and adjustment of the system. Fig. 5.7 illustrates the kind of

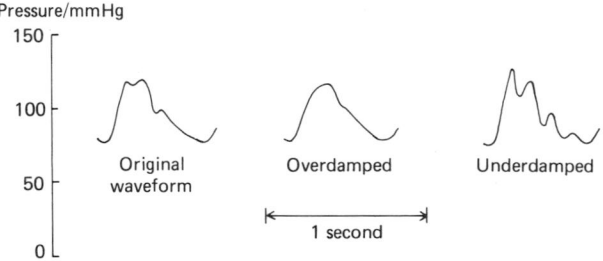

Fig. 5.7 Distortions of arterial pressure waveform caused by incorrect damping. In the underdamped waveform, the systolic pressure is overestimated by 14 mmHg (1.9 kPa) and the diastolic pressure underestimated by 2 mmHg (0.3 kPa). (Adapted from Gardner, 1981.)

distortions that can arise in incorrectly adjusted systems. The two distorted waveforms shown are described as being 'overdamped' and 'underdamped' respectively. (Damping will be discussed more fully later.) With both types of distortion, mean pressure will be correctly indicated, but diastolic and systolic pressures will be inaccurate. In the underdamped case, systolic pressure will be overestimated and diastolic pressure underestimated, while the opposite will be true in the overdamped case. Underdamped systems can lead to overestimation of systolic pressures by up to 30 mmHg (Gardner, 1981) and the consequences of a clinical decision being made on the basis of such erroneous readings could be potentially disastrous.

Arterial Manometer as a Measurement system

An arterial manometer is an example of a measurement system (Doebelin, 1983). In a measurement system, a physical quantity is detected and then undergoes processing and manipulation until it finally emerges in a form which is more easily displayed and comprehended than the original. The original quantity is known as the *input variable* and the final processed quantity as the *output variable*. In the case of

the arterial manometer, the input variable is arterial pressure and the output variable is volume displacement. (It would be equally valid to regard the output variable as being the electrical signal produced by the transducer, or even, if we extend the boundaries of the manometer system somewhat, the waveform produced on the monitor screen. However, as most of the potential distortion of the pressure measurements arises in the conversion to volume displacement, it is appropriate to treat the latter as the output variable for present purposes.) In an ideal measurement system, the waveform of the output variable would have exactly the same shape as that of the input variable, but in practice the measurement system introduces distortion in the waveform. The amount of distortion can be reduced both by good design and also by correct adjustment of the system. The fidelity with which a measurement system reproduces the input variable is indicated by its *input–output relations*, which depend upon the physical characteristics of the system.

The task of characterizing completely the behaviour of a particular measurement system is thus equivalent to describing its input–output relations for all possible input waveforms. At first sight, this would appear to be a formidable undertaking, because of the infinite variety of input waveforms that could occur. However, the task is greatly simplified for repetitive waveforms, such as the arterial pressure waveform, by the fact that they can be represented by the sum of simple standard waveforms, as we now discuss.

Fourier Series Representation of a Repetitive Waveform

In the early nineteenth century, the French mathematician Fourier showed that any repetitive waveform can be represented as a series consisting of a steady value together with a sum of sine waves of amplitudes, frequencies and phases that can be calculated from the form of the original waveform. (The meanings of 'amplitude', 'frequency' and 'phase' are illustrated in Fig. 5.8). A series representation of this type is known as a Fourier series and the individual sine waves are known as harmonics. The lowest frequency harmonic has the same frequency as the original wave, known as the fundamental frequency, and the other harmonics have frequencies that are integral multiples of the fundamental frequency. The higher frequency harmonics represent the more rapidly changing regions of the original waveform, and so the higher harmonics of a 'spikey' waveform will tend to be larger than the corresponding harmonics of a smooth waveform of the same frequency. Figure 5.9 shows how a complex waveform can be represented progressively more closely by adding increasing numbers of harmonics from its Fourier series.

The importance of Fourier series for the analysis of measurement systems lies in the fact that, for many systems, the effect of the system on any repetitive

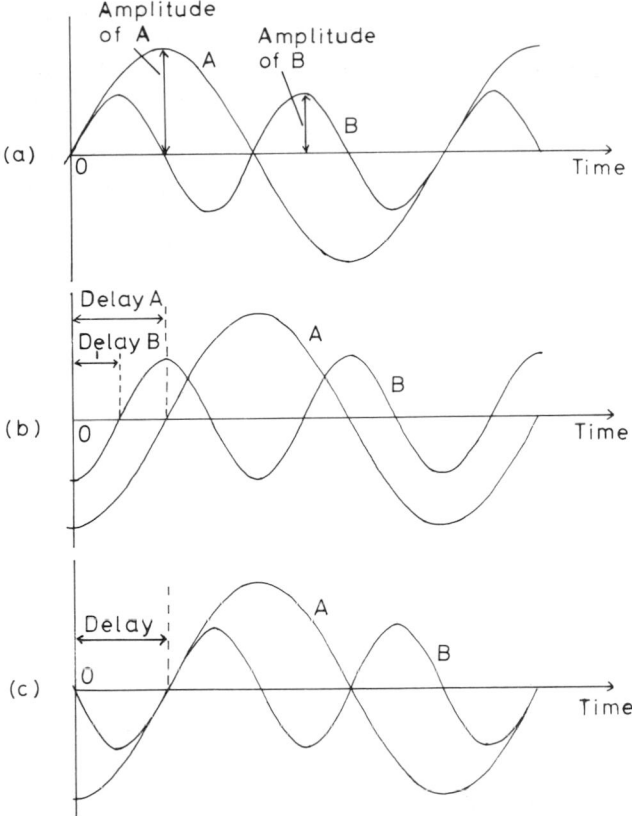

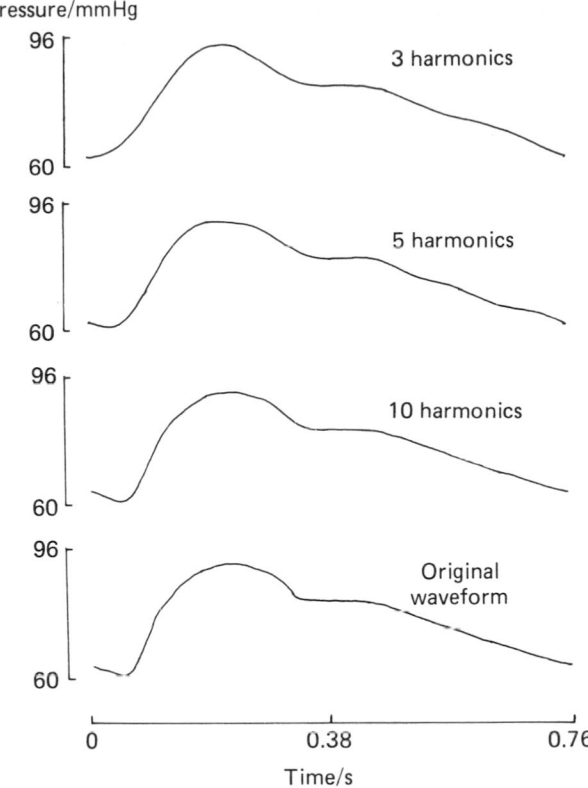

Fig. 5.8 Amplitude, frequency, and phase. Curves A and B are two sine waves. Wave B has twice the frequency of wave A. The phase indicates the fraction of a complete cycle which the wave has undergone and increases from 0°–360° throughout the cycle. In (a), both waves have a phase of 0° at time 0. In (b), both waves have experienced a phase shift of −90° with respect to (a), so that their phase at time 0 is −90°. However, compared to (a), wave A has experienced a *time* delay twice that of wave B. In (c), the phase shift of wave A is still -90°, but that of wave B is twice as great, at −180°. This produces the same time delay for both waves and restores the time relationship between the waves present in (a). The relative time shift seen in (b) would produce distortion, known as *phase distortion*, when the waves were summed, but no such distortion would occur in (c), where the phase shift is proportional to the frequency.

Fig. 5.9 The use of increasing numbers of harmonics of a Fourier series to achieve progressively closer approximations to the original waveform, in this case a pressure waveform from the ascending aorta. (Adapted from Patel et al., 1965.)

input waveform can be predicted by calculating its effect on each of the harmonics of the Fourier series for the waveform and then adding the resulting output harmonics. Thus, the problem of describing the effect of the system on the infinite variety of possible waveforms becomes reduced to that of describing its effect on sine waves of different frequencies. The input–output relations for input sine waves of different frequencies constitute the *frequency response* of the system. When the frequency response is known, the response to any repetitive waveform can be derived.

Requirements for a Measurement System

An ideal measurement device would deal with all the harmonics of the input waveform in an identical fashion, so that when the output harmonics were summed, they would produce a waveform which was an exact replica of the input waveform. The amplitudes of the output harmonics would then bear a constant ratio to the corresponding amplitudes of the input harmonics and there would be no phase difference between the output and input harmonics. However, there is one circumstance where no distortion of the waveform will occur even if the second condition is not met: if the amplitude response is constant but each harmonic suffers a phase shift proportional to its frequency, the output waveform will be undistorted, but delayed with respect to the input wave. This is illustrated in Fig. 5.8. This delay would be equivalent to less than one complete cycle of the original waveform, and would normally be acceptable. This is an important point, since it is rarely possible to design a measurement system with no phase shift, but relatively easy to achieve a phase shift proportional to frequency.

A properly designed measurement system should therefore produce minimal amplitude and phase distortion for the range of frequencies present in the input waveform. This does not require the absence of distortion at all frequencies, since the harmonic components of a waveform tend to be larger at the lowest frequencies and become progressively smaller at higher frequencies until they become indistinguishable from biological and instrumental noise. Patel et al. (1965) have demonstrated this pattern for the harmonics of pressure waveforms obtained from the heart and great vessels of man (see Fig. 5.9), and have shown that most of the important information is contained in the range 0–20 Hz. This indicates that a manometer with a flat amplitude response up to 20 Hz and a phase shift proportional to frequency in this range will be adequate for recording arterial pressures for most purposes.

Arterial Manometer as a Second-order System

When considered as a measurement system, the arterial manometer has two important properties: the elastic recoil of the diaphragm generates a *restoring force* that opposes the original pressure change, and there is *inertia* in the system (the mass of the saline and the diaphragm). These properties are characteristic of a large class of measurement systems, known as *second-order systems* because of the type of equation that describes their behaviour. These systems can exhibit the phenomenon of *resonance*, which is of crucial importance in determining their performance characteristics.

Properties of Second-order Systems

It is useful to investigate the properties of second-order systems by considering a simpler instrument of this type than the arterial manometer—the force-measuring spring scale.

Static Response

The spring scale is shown in Fig. 5.10a, while Fig. 5.10b shows how it can be modelled as a simple spring-mass system for the purposes of mathematical analysis. The input variable is the force F_I and the output variable is the displacement x. For a constant F_I, the spring is compressed until the restoring force generated by the spring balances F_I. If the spring obeys Hooke's Law, the restoring force is proportional to the displacement x, so that, at equilibrium,

$$F_I = Sx \qquad (1),$$

where S is the spring constant, or stiffness. The *static sensitivity* K is defined as the output/input ratio for a steady input, i.e. x/F_I in this case, and thus, from equation (1),

$$K = 1/S \qquad (2).$$

In practice, Hooke's Law will not hold exactly, and K will not be constant for different magnitudes of F_I. For a well designed balance, however, the variation in K will be small over the specified measuring range.

Dynamic Response

If F_I varies with time, then the relation between F_I and x becomes more complex. The reason is that now only part of F_I contributes to deflecting the spring, the remainder being required to overcome the inertia of the system (i.e. accelerate the moving parts) and overcome friction. The presence of inertia and friction means that the output x can not follow the input F_I instantaneously, and therefore there will be a time lag between x and F_I. The behaviour of a system for a varying input is known as the *dynamic* behaviour, in contrast to the *static* behaviour for a steady input. Mathematical analysis of the dynamic behaviour of the spring scale leads to a second-order differential equation, which has a solution consisting of two components, known as the *transient* and *steady-state responses*. The transient response has a time course characteristic of the system (not of the input) and is typically a short-lived oscillation, while the steady-state response represents the system's response to the driving force after the transient effects have died down.

Step Response and Damping

The transient response of the spring scale can be readily demonstrated by applying a fixed force until the deflection is steady and then suddenly removing this force. The scale will return to its equilibrium position ($x = 0$), not immediately but gradually, either by a damped oscillation (if the frictional force is small) or without oscillating (if the frictional force is large). These responses are illustrated in Fig. 5.11a. In the limiting case when friction is absent, the system oscillates indefinitely about the equilibrium position, with its *natural frequency* f_0, given by

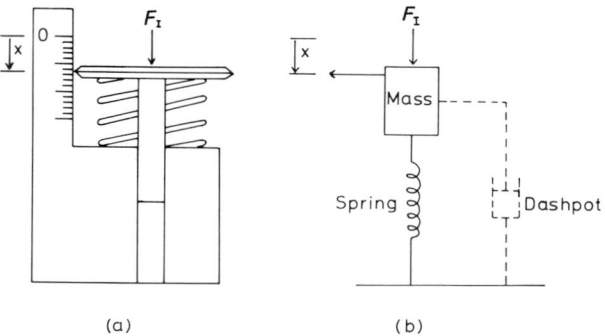

$$f_0 = \frac{1}{2\pi} \sqrt{\frac{S}{m}} \qquad (3)$$

where m is the mass of the moving parts. The oscillatory motion normally dies out because of friction and

Fig. 5.10 The force-measuring spring scale (a), and its representation as a mass-spring system (b). The dashpot shown in broken lines in (b) is added to increase the damping, as described in the text. (Fig. 5.10a adapted from Doebelin, 1983.)

this effect is known as *damping*. The degree of damping is indicated by the damping factor β, given by

$$\beta = \frac{R}{2\sqrt{mS}} \qquad (4)$$

where R is the frictional force per unit velocity (assumed constant). For small β, there is a large overshoot of the equilibrium position and the oscillation takes a while to die down, but, as β increases, the frequency of the oscillation decreases and its amplitude dies away more rapidly until, for $\beta > 1$, the oscillation is completely damped out and there is no overshoot of the equilibrium position. The value of β can in fact be determined from the amount of the initial overshoot (see Fig. 5.11b). The response of a measurement system to a change in input of this sort is known as the *step response*; step response tests provide a quick way of obtaining information about the system's behaviour, in particular allowing f_0 and β to be estimated.

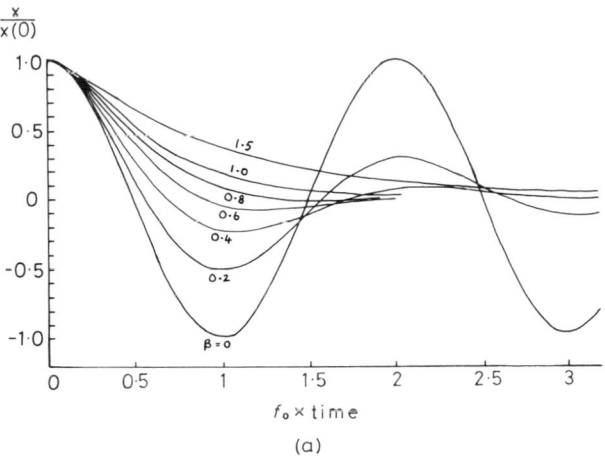

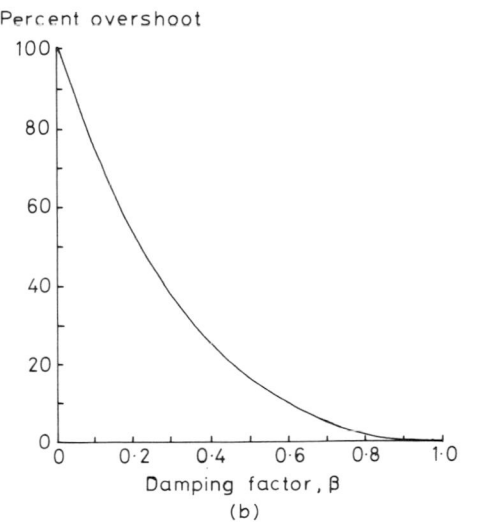

Fig. 5.11 Step response of a second-order system (a), and dependence of overshoot on damping factor (b). (Adapted from Doebelin, 1985.)

This example illustrates the difference between the transient and steady-state responses. The new steady level represents the steady-state response and the approach to the steady level represents the transient response. In general, the transient response arises because the initial conditions of the system (e.g. at rest in a position other than its equilibrium position) are not in harmony with the 'requirements' of the driving force. In the above example the driving force was zero, but in general it will change with time. In considering the input–output relations of an instrument, we are primarily interested in its behaviour after the transient response has died down, i.e. in its steady-state behaviour.

Frequency Response and Resonance

For a second-order instrument, the frequency response can be specified in terms of the dependence of the output/input amplitude ratio and phase difference upon the input frequency, as shown in Fig. 5.12. The curves illustrate the phenomenon of resonance when $\beta < 0.7$. Resonance is said to occur when the amplitude ratio increases and passes through a maximum value as the frequency is increased. The frequency at which the maximum ratio occurs is less than f_0 and is known as the *resonant frequency*. For all values of β, the amplitude ratio has a value of K at zero frequency. As zero frequency corresponds to a steady force, this is consistent with our previous definition of K as the static sensitivity. The shape of the amplitude ratio curve depends upon the value of β, and the resonant peak becomes less pronounced as β increases. At zero frequency, there is no phase lag between output and input signals, but as the frequency increases the phase lag becomes progressively greater. Again, the pattern of change depends upon the value of β, but the lag is always $90°$ for $f = f_0$ and tends towards $180°$ as f becomes large. The phenomenon of resonance occurs because the measurement system has an inherent natural frequency for vibration and it responds more strongly to an harmonic input the more closely the input frequency approaches this natural frequency.

For a measurement system, resonance is undesirable because it introduces amplitude and phase distortion. There are two approaches to avoiding this type of distortion, which can be used separately or together. The first is to arrange for the resonant frequency of the instrument to be well above the frequency of the highest significant harmonic in the input waveform, so that the system is operating on the flat initial region of the amplitude response curve. This approach also has the advantage that, because the initial region of the phase response curve is linear, the phase lag will be proportional to frequency, a condition that will avoid phase distortion, as was pointed out above. However, it is often not possible to increase the resonant frequency, and the second approach, which is to increase the damping, must be followed. It can be seen from Fig. 5.12 that, for

$\beta < 0.7$, increasing the damping lowers the height of the resonant peak and extends the flat region of the curve to higher frequencies. However, for $\beta > 0.7$, there is no resonant peak, and further increase of β causes the amplitude ratio to drop off at progressively lower frequencies. The value of β that produces the widest flat amplitude ratio is 0.64; for this β the ratio remains flat to within 2% for frequencies up to 67% of f_0. Moreover, as Fig. 5.12 also indicates, the phase lag is also linear over the widest frequency range when $\beta = 0.64$. Hence many commercial second-order instruments are designed to have β about 0.64.

Parallel Damping

One way of increasing the damping of a mass-spring system is to add a component known as a 'dashpot' in parallel with the spring, as shown in Fig. 5.10b. This device, which consists of a piston that slides inside a cylinder filled with oil, does not exert any force when the system is at rest, but exerts a viscous resistive force when the system is in motion. It therefore supplements the intrinsic resistance to motion of the system and so increases β (see equation (4)). As with any resistive element, the dashpot works by providing a

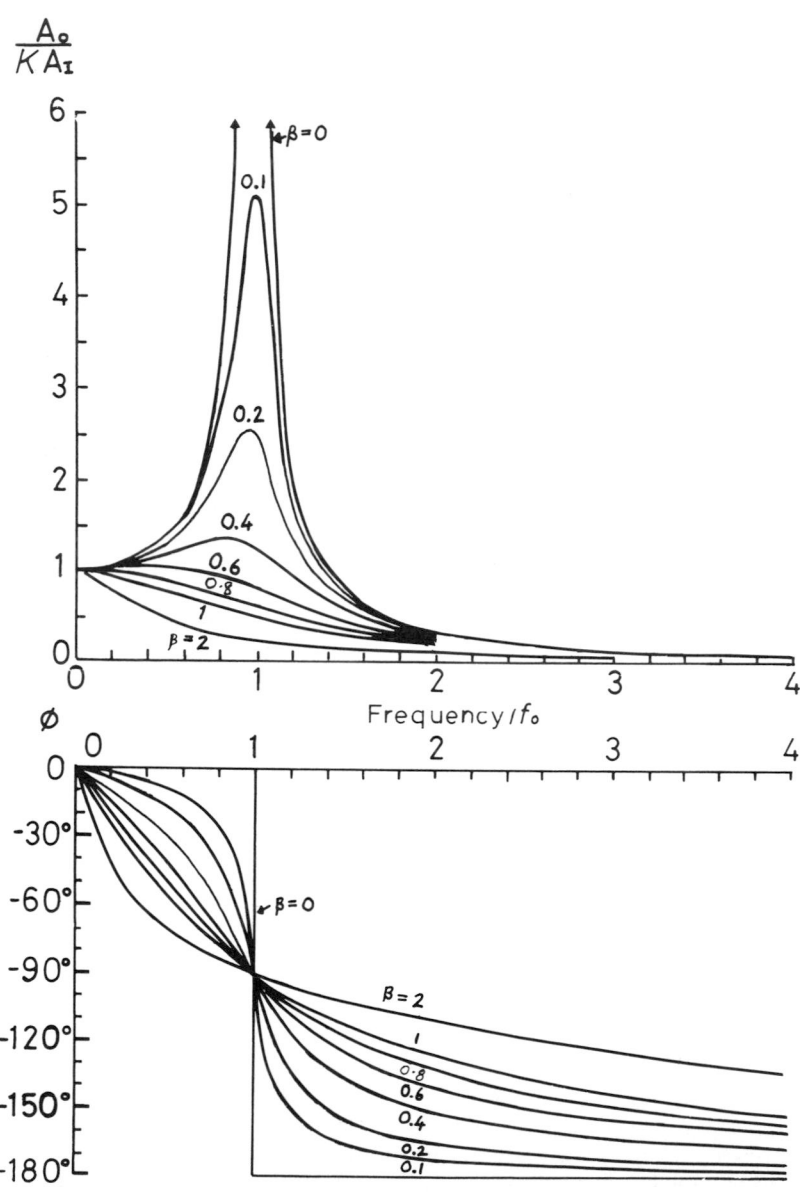

Fig. 5.12 Frequency response curves for a second-order instrument. A_I and A_0 are the amplitudes of the input and output signals, respectively; K is the static sensitivity and ϕ is the phase difference between the output and the input; negative values of ϕ indicate a phase lag. (Adapted from Doebelin, 1983.)

mechanism for the energy of the vibrations to be dissipated as heat.

So far, we have assumed that the mass of the vibrating system moves as a single entity under the action of the varying input force. However, in reality the energy of the vibrations travels up and down the mass in the form of waves, which are reflected alternately from the spring support at one end and from the top of the mass at the other end. While this elaboration of the model does not lead to any appreciable improvement in the accuracy of its numerical predictions, it does allow an alternative view of the operation of the dashpot which will be helpful when we consider the damping of manometer systems. In the absence of damping, a particular wave travels up and down the spring with undiminished amplitude. If the mass is being driven by an external force at the system's resonant frequency, the wave reflected at the top of the mass is in phase with the new wave being introduced by the force, and reinforces it. This leads to a progressive increase in the amplitude of the composite wave travelling up and down the spring, or in other words to the phenomenon of resonance. The introduction of the dashpot in parallel with the spring provides an alternative pathway down which some of the vibrational energy can flow and be dissipated, and so prevents the indefinite build-up of the wave amplitude that leads to large resonant peaks. In short, the dashpot operates by providing *parallel damping*.

Dynamic Behaviour of Arterial Manometer

As stated earlier, an arterial manometer can be considered as a measurement system in which the input variable is the pressure P and the output variable the volume displacement of the diaphragm V. If E is the volume elasticity of the diaphragm ($\Delta P/\Delta V$), then the static sensitivity K is given by

$$K = 1/E \qquad (2a).$$

Note that this is identical in form to equation (2), but has the spring constant S replaced by the volume elasticity E. Note also that the static sensitivity of the manometer is equal to the compliance of the transducer diaphragm C ($= \Delta V/\Delta P = 1/E$). Modern pressure transducers have a static sensitivity that is constant to within about 3% over their measuring range, so that variations in K for different magnitudes of input signal are not normally a major source of error.

Expressions for the resonant frequency and damping factor for an arterial manometer can be obtained by regarding it as a second-order system and solving the differential equation for the system. It might be thought that the natural frequency and damping factor could be obtained from equations (3) and (4) by substituting the appropriate expressions for the mass of liquid in the system and the frictional resistance to flow. However, there is an additional complexity in this system that does not exist in the simple mass-

spring system, and this arises from the fact that, for a given volume flow rate, the fluid velocity depends on the cross-section of the flow channel. The essence of any oscillatory motion is the interchange of energy between potential and kinetic forms. In the mass-spring system, the potential energy is associated with the deformation of the spring, while the kinetic energy is associated with the motion of the mass. Similarly, for the manometer system, the potential energy is associated with the deformation of the transducer diaphragm and the kinetic energy with the motion of the liquid in the tubing and the transducer dome. However, since the kinetic energy of a particular mass is proportional to the square of the velocity, there will be more energy associated with flow through a narrow tube than there will be associated with the same volume flow rate through a wide tube. This effect can be calculated by treating each mass element of the flowing liquid as if it has an effective mass equal to its actual mass divided by the square of the cross-sectional area of the tube. (This is equivalent to multiplying each mass element by a factor proportional to the square of its velocity.) For a tube of length l and radius r, containing liquid of density ρ, the true mass is $\pi r^2 \rho l$, and the effective mass is $\frac{\pi r^2 \rho l}{(\pi r^2)^2}$, or $\frac{\rho l}{\pi r^2}$. If this expression for the mass of liquid is substituted for m in equation (3), and if the spring constant S is replaced by the volume elasticity of the transducer diaphragm E, then the following relation is obtained for the resonant frequency f_0

$$f_0 = \frac{r}{2}\sqrt{\frac{E}{\pi \rho l}} \qquad (3a)$$

A more rigorous mathematical analysis of the system's behaviour confirms the correctness of equation (3a) (Hansen, 1950). (The derivation of equation (3a) involves the reasonable assumption that the kinetic energy of the liquid flowing in the transducer is negligible compared to that of the liquid flowing in the catheter, which is equivalent to saying that l/r^2 for the transducer is negligible compared to l/r^2 for the catheter).

Equation (3a) allows us to deduce how the physical properties of the manometer system effect the resonant frequency. Thus, taps, blood clots and kinks in the tubing will all cause a reduction in the effective radius of the catheter and will therefore decrease f_0. f_0 can be increased by using a shorter or wider catheter or by using a transducer with a stiffer diaphragm. It should also be noted that the presence of bubbles, which will increase the effective compliance of the system, will decrease E and hence decrease f_0.

Derivation of an expression for the damping factor requires knowledge of the nature of the liquid flow. An approximate expression for β can be obtained by treating the flow as laminar and applying Poiseuille's equation. (In fact Poiseuille's equation does not hold for oscillatory flow, but the errors introduced by assuming that it does are not large enough to affect the validity of the conclusions to be drawn (McDonald, 1974). It can then be shown (Hansen, 1950) that the damping factor β is given by

$$\beta = \frac{4\mu}{r^3} \sqrt{\frac{l}{\pi\rho E}} \qquad (4a)$$

where μ is the viscosity of the manometer liquid.

Thus it can be seen that those factors which tend to increase f_0 (large r, large E and small l) all tend to decrease the damping, and damping will be least for a short, wide catheter with no bubbles.

Because the behaviour of a second-order system is completely predictable if the static sensitivity, undamped natural frequency and damping factor are known, the frequency response and step response curves of Figs. 5.11 and 5.12, together with the discussion of the resonant behaviour of the spring scale, can be immediately extended to the manometer system.

Manometer as a Distributed System

The above treatment of manometer dynamics involved the implicit assumption that the manometer liquid was incompressible and the tubing completely rigid, so that the liquid moved as a single unit and the volume displacement was identical at all points in the system at a given time. This is physically impossible, since it implies that changes in arterial pressure are transmitted instantaneously, i.e. at infinite speed, to the transducer diaphragm. In reality, the manometer liquid is not incompressible and the tubing not completely rigid, and pressure waves travel with finite speed down the tubing (Fry, 1960; Gabe, 1972). At any given time, the volume displacement now varies continuously along the system, which is known as a *distributed system*, in contrast to the simpler rigid system, which can be described by a single value of the volume displacement and is known as a *single degree of freedom system*. As with the spring-scale, this more rigorous approach allows an alternative interpretation of resonance, which can now be viewed as arising from the superposition of direct and reflected waves at the transducer diaphragm. This does not affect materially the conclusions reached above on the effects of manometer properties on resonant behaviour, but does suggest the possibility of adjusting the damping by means of a parallel resistive element analogous to the mechanical dashpot.

Adjustment of Manometer Frequency Response

One way of obtaining a frequency response sufficiently wide for all clinical purposes is to adopt the first approach mentioned earlier and to use a manometer system with a high natural frequency. This is the rationale behind the use of catheter-tip tranducers, which can have an f_0 of up to 40 kHz. However, these transducers are expensive and fragile, and so anaesthetists generally use conventional catheter-transducer systems. As most transducers presently available have the same compliance (0.04 mm^3/mmHg), there is little scope for increasing f_0 by changing transducer models. Although these transducers can have an intrinsic natural frequency of more than 200 Hz, the addition of catheter, taps and arterial cannula lowers the natural frequency substantially, so that the value obtained in the theatre is unlikely to be greater than 30 Hz (Allan et al., 1988), and the figure will be considerably lower if care is not taken to eliminate bubbles from the system. Since a demanding pressure waveform may require a level frequency response of up to 20 Hz, it is apparent that damping has to be adjusted to give a β close to the optimum of 0.64, which will provide a level response up to about 20 Hz. As commonly used catheter-transducer systems are underdamped (Allan et al., 1988), correct adjustment requires a method for increasing β while leaving f_0 unchanged. Our earlier discussion showed that β could be increased by increasing the length of the catheter or decreasing its radius, but both of these changes would lower f_0. The solution is to provide parallel damping by using a device similar in principle to the mechanical dashpot.

The Accudynamic (Allan et al., 1988) is a commercially available device designed to allow β to be adjusted without affecting f_0. In this device, which is shown in Fig. 5.13, the needle valve constitutes a variable resistance and the 0.1 ml air bubble effectively acts as a compliance that couples the resistive element to atmospheric pressure for cyclic pressure changes, but blocks the passage of steady signals and thus prevents loss of liquid from the system. Thus, for the

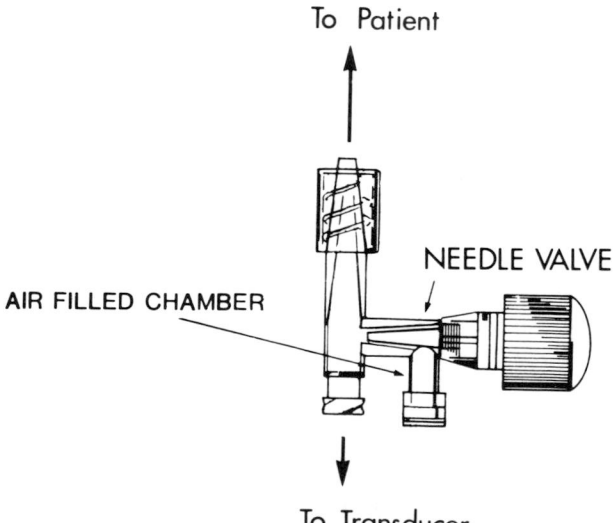

Fig. 5.13 The Accudynamic. The resistance of the passage leading to the air bubble depends on the setting of the needle valve, which is adjusted by the control knob. (Reproduced from Allan, Gray et al., 1988, with the permission of the authors and publishers.)

varying components of the arterial waveform, the device acts as a variable resistance in parallel with the transducer; it therefore provides a channel for the dissipation of some of the energy contained in the pressure waves flowing back and forth along the catheter, and adjustment of the needle valve allows β to be changed without affecting f_0.

It is necessary to assess the frequency response of a manometer system in theatre to check that the resonant frequency is sufficiently high and that the damping factor is optimum. One way of doing this is to carry out a step test by opening and then quickly releasing a fast flush device (Gardner, 1981). This will produce a trace similar to one of the family depicted in Fig. 5.11a. The resonant frequency can be estimated directly from the trace and the damping factor from the degree of overshoot. The damping should be adjusted until the overshoot is about 6%, which corresponds to optimal damping (Fig. 5.11b). The step signal should be applied so that it is 'seen' by the entire catheter-transducer system, and not just by the transducer; this can be done by connecting the continuous flush device to the proximal end of the catheter, for example at the tap connecting it to the arterial cannula (Fig. 5.6).

REFERENCES

Allan M.W.B., Gray W.M., Asbury A.J. (1988). Measurement of arterial pressure using catheter-transducer systems. Improvement using the Accudynamic. *Br. J. Anaesth.* **60**: 413.

Doebelin E.O. (1983). *Measurement Systems. Application and Design.* 3rd edn. London: McGraw-Hill.

Doebelin E.O. (1985). *Control System Principles and Design.* p. 87. Chichester: Wiley.

Dorlas J.C., Nijboer J.A., Butijn W.T., et al. (1985). Effects of peripheral vasoconstriction on the blood pressure in the finger, measured continuously by a new noninvasive method (The 'Finapres' R). *Anesthesiol.*, **62**, 342.

Fry D.L. (1960). Physiologic recording by modern instruments with particular reference to pressure recording. *Physiol. Rev.*, **40**, 753.

Gabe I.T. (1972). Pressure measurement in experimental physiology. In: *Cardiovascular Fluid Dynamics*, pp. 11–50. (Bergel D.H., ed.) London: Academic Press.

Gardner R.M. (1981). Direct blood pressure measurement—dynamic response requirements. *Anesthesiol.*, **54**, 227.

Hansen A.T. (1950). The theory for elastic liquid-containing membrane manometers. Special part. *Acta Physiol. Scand.*, **19**, 332.

Hutton P., Prys-Roberts C. (1982). The oscillotonometer in theory and practice. *Br. J. Anaesth.*, **54**, 581.

McDonald D.A. (1974). *Blood Flow in Arteries*, 2nd edn. pp. 174–208, 446–451. London: Arnold.

Patel D.J., Mason D.T., Ross J., et al. (1965). Harmonic analysis of pressure pulses obtained from the heart and great vessels of man. *Am. Heart J.*, **69**, 785.

Ramsey M. (1979). Noninvasive automatic determination of mean arterial pressure. *Med. Biol. Eng. Comput.*, **17**, 11.

Sykes M.K., Vickers M. D., Hull C. J. (1981). *Principles of Clinical Measurement.* 2nd edn. pp. 159–172. Oxford: Blackwell.

van Egmond J., Hasenbos M., Crul J.F. (1985). Invasive v. noninvasive measurement of arterial pressure. Comparison of two automatic methods and simultaneously measured direct intra-arterial pressure. *Br. J. Anaesth.*, **57**, 434.

6. Measurement of Blood Flow and Cardiac Output
N. T. Smith and B. L. Partridge

The term cardiac output implies mean total forward flow per minute. While most of the methods described in this chapter may be used to estimate cardiac output, the majority of techniques for measurement of cardiac output in humans use methods related to the Fick principle. These techniques include direct Fick and indicator-dilution methods (dye-dilution and thermal dilution).

In addition to these techniques, we shall discuss a number of other methods

1. Methods from which much of our knowledge has been obtained about the haemodynamic actions of anaesthetic and ancillary agents.
2. Methods which may provide the future clinical techniques for measuring cardiac output, particularly for monitoring surgical patients.

The former include the direct flowmeter techniques, ballistocardiography, and direct Fick techniques; the latter, pulse contour techniques, echocardiography including Doppler techniques, radionuclide angiocardiography, impedance cardiography, and systolic time intervals.

THE GOLD STANDARD

One of the major problems in evaluating methods for measuring cardiac output is defining the '*true standard*' used for comparison. Each of the techniques for measuring cardiac output has serious drawbacks, which will be discussed below. These drawbacks are serious enough that none truly deserves to be called the '*gold standard*' (*see* Wesseling et al., 1981). The first problem arises with the definition itself: Is *total forward* flow of blood what we want to measure? Cardiac output does not take into account regional and organ differences in blood flow. Cerebral, coronary and perhaps hepatic and renal blood flow are usually of greatest interest to the anesthetist, but these are measured indirectly, if at all, by cardiac output. Similar cardiac outputs may be produced but incur drastically different energy expenditures, depending on the heart's position on the Starling curve. Even what is meant by cardiac output is not clear in the presence of valvular lesions or intra and extra-cardiac shunts. Most techniques assume that right and left heart outputs are equal, but in the presence of major shunts this may not be the case. Which, then, is the true cardiac output?

Cardiac output may vary considerably during respiration or, particularly, during artificial ventilation. The degree of variation depends on many factors, however, including volume status, ventilatory parameters, position, blood pressure and chest compliance. Is the 'true' cardiac output one that averages respiratory cycles, or one where all measurements are made at one point in the cycle? If the latter is chosen, which point should be used? These issues confound comparisons of techniques, some of which measure beat-to-beat variation in cardiac output and some of which average the output over several cardiac and/or respiratory cycles. In addition, most studies comparing methods of estimating cardiac output report only correlations between results obtained by various methods. Absolute values are often omitted, and no regression equations are given. One should not be surprised that various methods of measuring cardiac output and blood flow show good correlations with one another; each method will detect when cardiac output increases, regardless of whether or not absolute changes are the same.

In light of these factors, perhaps the only accurate measurement of cardiac output is flow produced extracorporally with a roller pump. Even this approach has difficulties, since the various flow measuring techniques are affected in different ways by the use of pulsatile *versus* continuous flow.

FLOWMETERS

Cardiac output, or at least blood flow, may be measured directly by either implanted flowmeters or by extracorporal flow measurements.

Electromagnetic Flowmeter

All electromagnetic flowmeters use Faraday's Law of electromagnetic induction (Fig. 6.1). The strength of

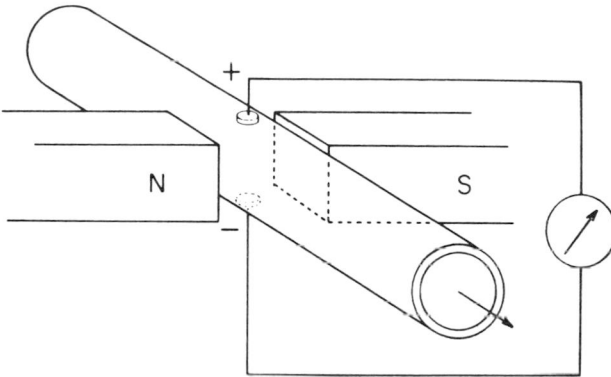

Fig. 6.1 Principle of the electromagnetic flowmeter. The blood vessel is placed between the poles of a magnet, which is illustrated by the bars N and S. Flow through the vessel induces a potential difference at right angles to the direction of flow and magnetic field. The potential difference is measured using the electrodes located on the external surface of the vessel wall. This voltage is amplified and recorded by the meter in the electrode circuit.

the induced field E is perpendicular to and proportional to the applied magnetic force and the flow velocity:

$$E = vB \sin \phi$$
$$\phi = \text{angle between field } B \text{ and velocity } v$$

The original d.c. flowmeters suffered from serious zero drift due to development of electrode-fluid potentials. The flow induced potentials could not be easily distinguished from the background electrochemical potentials.

These problems were overcome by using a.c. flowmeters with either sinusoidal or square wave excitation. Although this theoretically limits the possible rate of the sampling of flow, in practice it gives sufficiently high sampling rates for flows that occur under physiological circumstances. Since the sinusoidal current flowmeters are generally smaller and generate little heat, they can be used to measure blood flow in all but the smallest vessels. A variety of different sized probes which can be implanted into animals as part of long-term experiments are commercially available. However, these probes require exposure of the vessel under study thereby precluding easy application to clinical use.

With the earlier flowmeters neither the baseline nor the zero-flow level was predictable or stable regardless of the type of flowmeter used (Dobson et al., 1966). This resulted from the transformer effect, alignment problems, and the capacitive and resistive coupling between the electrodes and the magnet coils. Whatever the problem, the zero may be determined by assuming that the flow in the ascending aorta or the pulmonary artery is nil during the latter part of diastole, or alternatively by temporarily inducing cardiac arrest.

The disadvantages inherent in the earlier electromagnetic flowmeters were due to the necessarily high current of about 1 ampere; this made them unsuitable for use in the clinical environment. Grounding of the transducer was also a problem with chronically implanted flowmeters. Improvements in the signal-to-noise ratio have allowed development of battery operated electrodes with built-in isolators. The need for a ground electrode having been removed, the electrodes are generally safe for use in patients.

To avoid having to expose the vessel under study and having the transducer outside the vessel with the blood flowing through it, catheter-tip flow probes have also been developed (Mills, 1966; Bond and Barefoot, 1967; Mills and Shillingford, 1967). The same physical principles apply to these probes as to external probes. It is possible to have a pressure and flow probe mounted in a catheter that is only 2.3 mm diameter and hence suitable for introducing into the chambers of the heart or into major vessels.

Investigators have achieved various modifications, which principally reduce the heat produced by these flow probes, as well as further reduce their size while maintaining their accuracy. These modifications, however, necessitate increasing electronic refinement and expense.

Laser Doppler Flowmeters

Cutaneous blood flow may be measured noninvasively by the laser Doppler flowmeter. This apparatus uses the Doppler shift (*see* description in discussion on echocardiography). The frequency of light reflected off moving blood cells in the skin is used to estimate local blood volume. Several studies have examined its use in assessing microcirculation during plastic surgery (Power and Fraser, 1978; Katz et al., 1983) and in monitoring cardiac status in critically ill patients (Eyer et al., 1987, Waxman et al., 1987). As might be expected, poor correlation is seen between cutaneous flow and cardiac output in patients with very low outputs.

Ultrasonic Flowmeters

Ultrasonic flowmeters utilize the properties of sound waves travelling through a moving fluid. There are two types of ultrasonic flowmeters, utilizing either pulsed-transit time or Doppler shift. The former is rarely used clinically and will not be discussed in this chapter.

Doppler shift flowmeters have been one of the most useful innovations in cardiovascular physiology, with many applications in clinical medicine. The Doppler-shift phenomenon is familiar as the change in pitch (frequency) that occurs when a train passes by. The apparent pitch of the sound made by the train is increased as the train approaches, and decreased as it recedes, a phenomenon that occurs because sound waves are compressed and then expanded relative to the observer. This physical principle forms the basis of many ranging techniques. The Doppler effect also occurs when sound from a stationary source is reflected by a moving object. In the case of the Doppler velocity meter, sound is reflected by the moving red blood cells, and flow velocity can be estimated by the Doppler shift of the reflected sound.

The Doppler Flowmeter

Lead zirconate crystals are imbedded in the opposite sides of a cylindrical probe so that their acoustical axes are oriented at a 45° angle with the longitudinal axis of the probe. A 10 MHz signal is beamed from one crystal through the vessel wall into the blood stream. Part of the signal is back-scattered from the blood and excites the sensor crystal. This portion of the signal is amplified and detected. The difference between the transmitted and received frequencies, that is, the Doppler shift of backscattered sound, is a measure of the blood velocity.

If two sine waves of nearly identical frequency are superimposed, the resultant wave shows cyclical *beating* of amplitude and phase (Fig. 6.2). The rate of beating is equal to the difference in frequency of the two signals. One way of using Doppler instruments is to present the beat frequency (i.e. the difference, or f-f_0) directly as an audio output and to rely for interpretation on the ear of a trained observer; in effect this uses the instrument as an ultrasonic stethoscope. In a typical instrument, a change in flow velocity from 0–100 cm/s provides an audible signal with a frequency ranging from 0–3500 Hz. Alternatively, the beat frequency may be used to provide an output giving the blood velocity directly. This is the method of choice if one wishes to study pulse waveforms in individual blood vessels. Determination of the average Doppler frequency and the conversion of this signal into an electrical signal is usually performed with a zero-crossing meter, the output of which is proportional to the number of zero-crossings per unit of time. Note that unless phase shifting is taken into account, an increase in frequency (positive Doppler shift) will result in the same beat frequency as a decrease in frequency (negative Doppler shift). This is important when considering possible applications. One can purchase Doppler instruments which do not give the direction of the velocity. With directional Doppler flowmeters, forward and backward flow in arteries and veins, i.e. flow from and towards the crystals, can be recorded separately. In nondirectional systems, all movements of the red blood cells are added and represented as forward flow.

The Transcutaneous Doppler Velocity Meter

The Doppler frequency shift technique was developed further by Baker (1964) to detect blood flow transcutaneously by constructing a transducer assembly in which the transmitting and receiving ultrasound transducers were mounted side by side (Fig. 6.3). This is the instrument which has ultimately gained so many applications in clinical medicine.

Certain precautions are necessary with external ultrasonic probes to ensure optimal performance. Since ultrasound is almost completely reflected at any interface with air, it is necessary to provide an acoustic coupling medium between the transducer and the tissue in which measurements are being made. A variety of substances can be used, including olive oil,

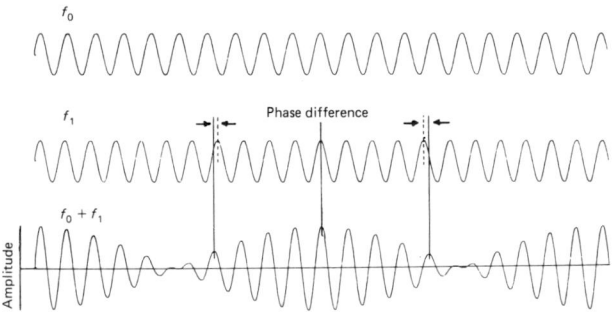

Fig. 6.2 Beating of two sine waves. When two sine waves of nearly identical frequency are added, the resultant wave shows cyclical variation in amplitude and phase. The frequency of the cycle is a function of the difference in frequency (f-f_0) of the two sine waves; the direction of phase shift depends upon whether f-f_0 is positive or negative.

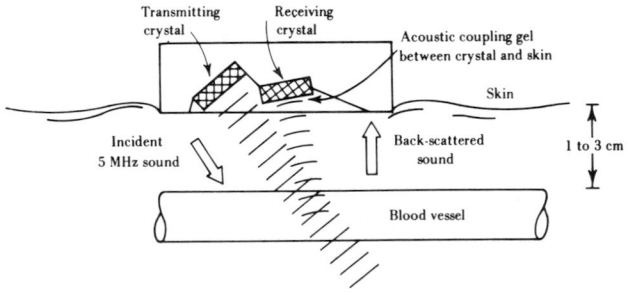

Fig. 6.3 The transcutaneous (noninvasive) Doppler velocity meter. The crystals are adjacent to, rather than opposite to each other as with the original Doppler velocity probe. The ultrasonic beam is directed diagonally through the skin and the vascular channel. Some ultrasound is reflected off blood cells, received by the second crystal, and processed as described in the text.

electrode paste and specially prepared water-soluble gels.

With Doppler flowmeters, ultrasound can be transmitted continuously (i.e. continuous wave, or CW Doppler) or intermittently (pulsed Doppler). With CW Doppler flowmeters, the ultrasonic beam is usually transmitted from one crystal and the backscattered ultrasound received by another. These systems are easy to build and to operate, but vessel wall motion artifacts are often difficult to eliminate, at least without the loss of flow velocity-induced frequencies. The high-amplitude, low-frequency signals due to vessel wall motion influence the shape of the frequency spectrum, and therefore, the accuracy of the determination of the average velocity. Moreover, with CW Doppler flowmeters, no information can be obtained about the diameter of the vessel, so that volume flow cannot be determined with transcutaneous devices. However, CW Doppler devices have found considerable clinical use in the detection of air bubbles in the vascular system resulting from venous air embolism during surgery.

Baker (1970) combined the pulsed and Doppler shift techniques into a single instrument that provided a velocity profile of blood flow across the diameter of an unopened artery. With pulsed Doppler flowmeters one single crystal, operating alternatively as transmitter and receiver, is usually used. The sound transmission is intermittent (pulsed) so that during the intervals between pulses the crystal receives the backscattered signals from the red blood cells at a given distance from the transducer. This makes it possible to assess vessel diameter and velocity profiles (Peronneau et al., 1971; Hagl et al., 1974) and to reduce vessel wall motion artifacts.

The major advantages of the pulsed ultrasound Doppler technique involve its possible applications in noninvasive measurements. Vessel diameter may be assessed transcutaneously, and, by multiplication by the flow rate estimated from the Doppler, the volume of blood flowing through a vessel may be estimated.

Transcutaneous Measurement of Cardiac Output

After the pioneering work by Light, who measured aortic blood flow velocity by a technique he called aortovelography (Light 1969, 1974, 1976; Sequeria et al., 1976), it has been tempting to try to measure cardiac output noninvasively via the Doppler technique. Although the problems are the same as with conventional transcutaneous Doppler measurements, the initial results have been promising and commercial devices have been available since 1982.

Calculation of cardiac output depends upon measurement of both the mean velocity of flow and the cross sectional area of the aorta. This is done by applying the Doppler equation

$$V = \frac{\Delta f c \cos \phi}{2f}$$

where V = blood velocity, Δf = the Doppler shift, c = speed of sound in tissue (1540 m/s), f = the original ultrasound frequency and ϕ = the angle of intersection of the ultrasonic beam with the direction of blood flow. If the angle equals zero, then $\cos \phi = 1$, simplifying the equation. In practice, angles of $< 18°$ are acceptable, since $\cos \phi > 0.95$. Thus Δf is proportional to blood velocity within 5% (Mehta et al., 1985). Estimation of stroke volume requires integration of mean flow rates over the entire cardiac cycle. To calculate cardiac output, a continuous wave Doppler is placed on the suprasternal notch, and the position and angle are adjusted until an optimal waveform is obtained (Mackay and Hechtman, 1975; Huntsman et al., 1983) (Fig. 6.4). Calculating flow re-

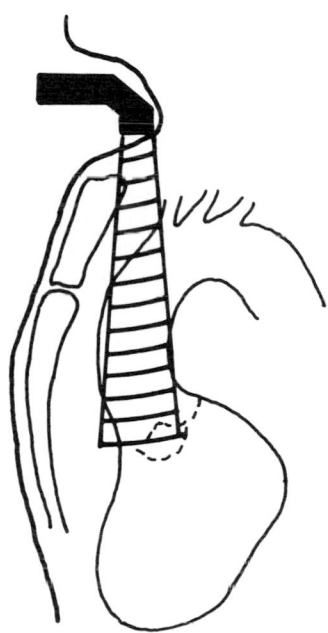

Fig. 6.4 Positioning of Doppler probe in the suprasternal notch. Angle of intersection between the Doppler beam and the descending aorta, Ø, must be less than 18° to keep the error due to positioning angle less than 5%. *See text.*

quires an estimate of aortic root diameter. This may be accomplished by M-mode echocardiography or from established nomograms. An alternative is to compute cardiac output by another method (e.g. thermal dilution) and then to back calculate an aortic root diameter for later use by the Doppler-based cardiac output computer. All of these techniques have pitfalls. Accuracy of the nomograms have been challenged, and if one needs to perform an invasive cardiac output estimation, the greatest advantage of noninvasive Doppler imaging is lost. Calculation of aortic root diameter by M-mode echocardiography requires a trained observer and access to the chest, which may not be possible intraoperatively. If one is interested only in relative changes in cardiac output, the technique has been found to be useful (Light et al., 1979).

In addition to the usual problems with the CW Doppler, which include difficulties in positioning and calibration, one has the uncertainty of measuring velocity or flow in the aortic arch, which may not be representative of true cardiac output. First, the Doppler model is based on flow through a rigid tube, and the human aorta is elastic, changing shape and diameter during pulsatile flow. Furthermore, diameter may change over very short periods of time if blood pressure, contractile force and volume status are not constant. Each of these factors is affected, of course, by anesthetics. Second, as noted previously, the transducer must be directed towards the back of the aortic arch so that the ultrasonic beam intersects the aortic axis at a shallow angle, or the amplitude of the Dopplershift will be underestimated (Huntsman et al., 1983). In spite of these considerations, Fisher et al. (1983) have demonstrated that errors are small over a clinically useful range of angles of intersection. Third, since the portion of the aorta where Doppler measurements are made occurs after take off of the coronary, carotid, and innominate arteries, Doppler measured cardiac outputs ignore flow to these areas. If flow in these arteries changes significantly, distal blood flow might be adequate despite a decrease in flow to the coronary or cerebral circulation. And this, unfortunately, may be the case during anaesthesia, when there are often marked shifts in regional blood flow. Fourth, the method assumes uniform flow across the cross-section of the aorta, a condition that does not exist. Rather, the technique measures a sample flow which is assumed to be representative of mean flow in the aorta. Nevertheless, the potential convenience of beat-to-beat estimation of cardiac output has resulted in considerable efforts to improve and validate this technique.

Numerous investigators have shown fair to excellent correlations between Doppler estimates of cardiac output and those computed by other means (Chandraratina et al., 1984; Darsee et al., 1980 a, b; Schuster et al., 1984). Fisher et al. (1983) found a correlation of 0.98 between pulsed Doppler measurements and roller-pump measurements in open-chest dogs. Standard error of measurement was 0.2 L/min. Steingart et al. (1980), found correlations of 0.74–0.96 in a similar preparation compared with electromagnetic flowmeters applied directly to the aorta. Colocousis et al. (1977) compared CW Doppler estimates with thermodilution cardiac outputs in closed-chest dogs and found a correlation of 0.95. Marquis et al. (1981) compared pulse-wave Doppler and phased-array Doppler and found a correlation of 0.99 for continuous flow and 0.86 for pulsatile flow in water tank models, and 0.83 for the correlation between pulsed Doppler and direct Fick estimations (*see below* for explanation) in 11 patients. More recently, Huntsman et al. (1983), demonstrated an excellent correlation between cardiac output calculated by a then proto-

type commercial pulsed Doppler versus the thermodilution technique, while Loeppky et al. (1984) found correlations of 0.91 between pulsed Doppler and direct Fick measurements. Haites et al. (1985), have used a commercially available Doppler device to measure velocity profiles in patients with various disease states and found that aortic velocity estimated with this device correlates well with thermodilution cardiac output even if no aortic root diameter is calculated. They were able to show reduction in aortic velocity with age and in disease states such as hypertension, atrial fibrillation and cardiac failure.

Zhang et al. (1985), have estimated cardiac output using calculated mitral orifice rather than aortic root diameter. Cardiac output was calculated by multiplying the corrected mitral orifice area by CW or pulsed Doppler estimation of maximum diastolic velocity, and the results were compared with the direct Fick method. Continuous wave Doppler consistently overestimated cardiac output. Correlation was only as high as 0.89, and as would be expected, there was considerable overestimation of cardiac output by the Doppler methods in patients with mitral regurgitation.

A major difficulty with this technique is that the mitral orifice varies considerably over the cardiac cycle, necessitating averaging over multiple cardiac cycles and making beat-to-beat measurements impossible. At least with present technology, this technique is unlikely to supplant Doppler cardiac output based upon aortic root diameter.

Daigle et al. (1975) combined the Doppler and echo techniques. An echo-ranging instrument measured aortic diameter, from which absolute volume flow—and thus stroke volume—could be measured. It is possible to incorporate the Doppler into an esophageal probe (Matsumoto et al., 1979; Colley and Martin, 1980). Unfortunately, aortic measurement by echocardiography does not necessarily correlate well with actual measurements at surgery (Mark et al., 1986), so the early commercially available Doppler echocardiographs frequently produced cardiac output measurements with a large fixed offset from those obtained from other methods (Freund and Padavich, 1985). More recent versions show a better relationship (Freund, 1986).

THE FICK PRINCIPLE

The Fick principle states that the size of a stream may be calculated by adding a substance to a stream and measuring the amount of substance that enters and leaves the stream and the concentration difference resulting from such entry or removal (Fig. 6.5). This is true whether the substance is oxygen (direct Fick method), a foreign gas such as nitrous oxide or acetylene, or an intravenously injected substance (indicator-dilution method).

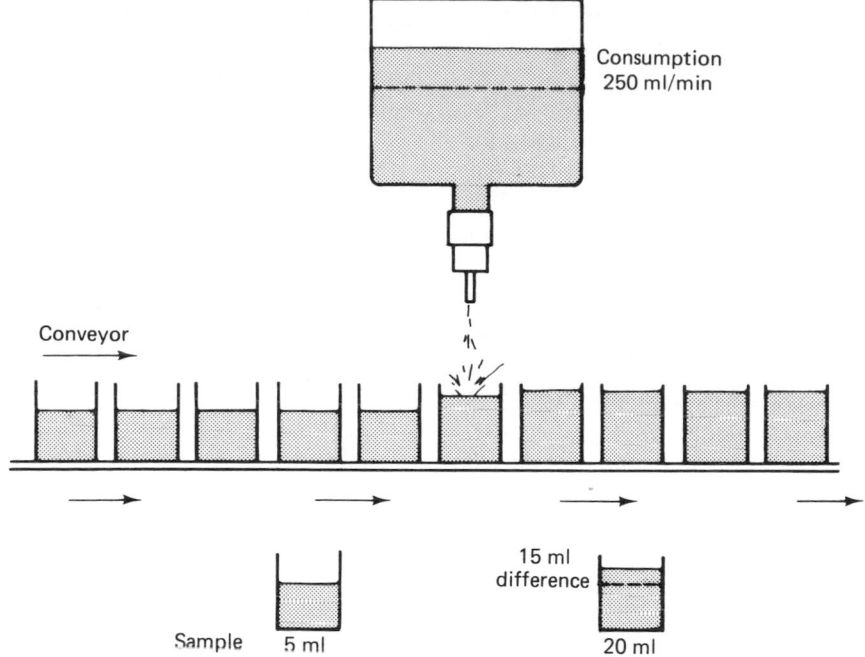

Fig. 6.5 *See* text. If each jar on the conveyor belt receives 5 ml of fluid, and the dispenser delivers 250 ml/min, 50 jars must pass the dispenser each minute to carry this quantity of fluid. Similarly, if each 100 ml of blood takes up 5 ml of oxygen from the lungs (the a_{O_2}-$\bar{v}_{O_2}$ difference), and if 250 ml of oxygen are consumed each minute, 50 jars of 100 ml (that is, 5000 ml) must have passed through the lungs each minute.

Direct Fick Method

The direct Fick method uses the relation:

$$CO\ (ml/min) = \frac{\dot{V}_{O_2}}{a_{O_2} - \bar{v}_{O_2}}$$

where CO = cardiac output, $\dot{V}_{O_2}$ = uptake of oxygen per minute, and $a_{O_2} - \bar{v}_{O_2}$ = arterial − mixed venous oxygen content difference. The method provides accurate estimates of cardiac output for research but at present, is too cumbersome for clinical use in the operating room.

To measure cardiac output by the direct Fick method, one needs to measure the uptake of oxygen by the lungs, plus the content of oxygen in arterial and mixed venous samples. To measure the uptake of oxygen, an accurate spirometer similar to that used in basal metabolic rate studies is sufficient. Measurement of oxygen content requires an accurate, stable oximeter. A mixed venous sample requires right ventricular or preferably pulmonary arterial catheterization. However, if the latter is done, it would be preferable to use the thermal dilution technique described below. Furthermore, to measure oxygen uptake, a circulatory steady-state period of 3–4 min is necessary. Nonetheless, this is a candidate for the 'gold-standard' of cardiac output measurement, since the effects of ventilation are built in by averaging over such a long period. Beat-to-beat variation in cardiac output, of course, cannot be calculated.

Indicator-Dilution Method

The indicator-dilution technique is derived from the Fick principle. Instead of measuring the concentration gradient produced by the endogenous addition or extraction of a substance, one measures the concentration gradient produced by injecting an exogenous substance, called an indicator. The initial concentration of the indicator is thus zero. Any indicator may be used, provided that it meets certain criteria:

1. is nontoxic
2. mixes rapidly with the blood
3. diffuses rapidly into the lungs during passage
4. is metabolized rapidly (30–60 min)
5. is easily and accurately measured with the measurement technique
6. is not influenced by haemoglobin concentration.

A number of indicators can satisfy these criteria, notably dyes, electrolytes, acids, cold, heat, and radioactive tracers. At present, dye-dilution, thermal dilution (cold), and radioactive tracer dilution have stood the test of time; each method has both advantages and disadvantages. Except with the thermal dilution technique, injection into the peripheral venous system is acceptable, but accuracy is improved if the indicator is injected into the right side of the circulation as close to the right ventricle as possible. The injection should be instantaneous and complete. The type of indicator used determines the instrument to be used for measuring it.

Dye-Dilution

The dye-dilution method was originally described by Stewart and Hamilton (Hamilton et al., 1948) for indocyanine green. Following injection of the dye, blood is continuously withdrawn at a convenient arterial site and the concentration of the indicator measured with a photodensitometer. An alternative, at least for research purposes, is to create a silastic shunt to allow photodensitometry without actually withdrawing blood (Boerboom and Boelkins, 1978). This technique has considerable appeal for research in small animals, when sampling of blood may affect cardiac output, although creating the shunt may itself alter cardiac output. The curve relating the concentration of dye to time elapsed is then plotted. A typical curve is shown in Fig. 6.6. Note that recirculation of the indicator occurs before the last portion has been measured.

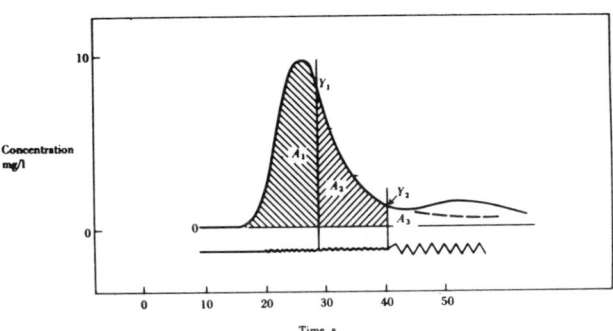

Fig. 6.6 A dye-dilution curve, as measured from an arterial cannula. Note the second hump, which represents recirculation. Extrapolation of this curve can be done as shown in Fig. 6.7, or as described in the text.

Next, one determines the total concentration of dye during the time interval represented by the curve. Ordinarily, this quantity could be derived by measuring the total area under the curve by planimetry. However, because early recirculation of dye is almost inevitable, some of the dye is measured twice. This redundancy error can be eliminated by manually replotting the curve on semilogarithmic paper, thereby using the exponential characteristics of the dye curve (Fig. 6.7).

Because replotting and planimetry are tedious and time-consuming, several simplifications have been proposed (Smith, 1969; Prys-Roberts, 1977; Blackburn, 1982). Some of these are shortcuts that compromise accuracy by measuring only a few selected points on the curve. Other formulae are better estimates but suffer from an important drawback: the exponential downslope is assumed but not tested. In fact, it

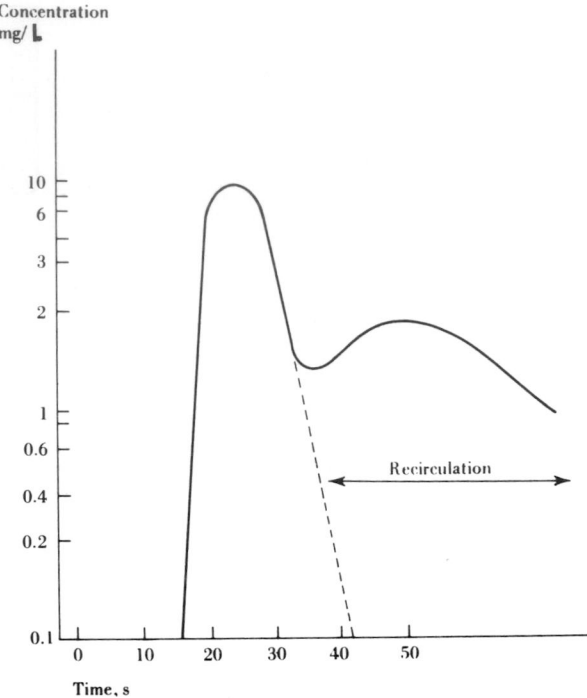

Fig. 6.7 Extrapolation of the dye-dilution curve by the semi-logarithmic method. If the concentration of dye passing the photodensitometer is replotted on semi-logarithmic paper, the descending portion of the first hump can be extrapolated to the base line as a straight line. The area under the initial curve can be used to derive the mean concentration of the dye during its first circulation. (Reproduced with permission from Bellville and Weaver, 1969).

is known that left-to-right shunts, valvular regurgitation, and other factors may affect the linearity of the semilogarithmic disappearance slope.

One of these techniques does not require a computer. It is a simple and reliable method for estimating the area under a dye curve and enables the estimation of cardiac output to be made on a simple calculator (Prys-Roberts, 1977). This effects a financial saving at little cost in accuracy.

A common solution to the recirculation problem is the use of forward triangulation. In Figs. 6.6 and 6.7 the area A under an exponentially decaying curve (to the right of Y_1) is given by:

$$A_{exp} = A_2 + A_3$$

The choice of about 60% of the peak value for Y_1 and about 40% for Y_2 locates two points which will very probably fall on the exponential portion of the curve. Although some inaccuracies arise from these compromises, they contribute only a small part of the error inherent in any indicator-dilution technique.

The electronic solution of these calculations, particularly integration, yields considerable savings in time. To this end, several special-purpose cardiac output computers have been developed. All of these systems are capable of integrating the dye curve. They differ mainly in their modes of extrapolating the curve. For example, a computer may integrate the curve in a linear fashion until 60% of the peak has been reached on the down-slope (Y_1, Fig. 6.6). A comparator then switches in a constant multiplication factor, usually 2 or 3. This augmented integration continues until 30 or 40%, respectively, of the peak is reached (Y_2, Fig. 6.6).

While dye-dilution is still used clinically and has the advantage that it may be used in patients with only a peripheral arterial line and a central venous catheter, the widespread application of flow-directed balloon-tipped pulmonary artery catheters (Ganz et al., 1971) has resulted in the near abandonment of this technique in favor of the thermal dilution technique.

Thermal Dilution

The thermal dilution method for estimating cardiac output (Fegler, 1954) has nearly supplanted other methods in clinical situations. Detection in the pulmonary artery after right atrial injection of indicator is usually preferred over other injection and detection sites; proper mixing of the indicator over the short distance is achieved by the mechanical action of the right ventricle. Thus any factor such as valvular lesion or intra-cardiac shunt that might decrease intraventricular mixing or result in streaming of blood/indicator will result in an over or underestimation of cardiac output. For example, Lipkin and Poole-Wilson (1985) measured 'cardiac outputs' of up to 30 L/min by thermodilution in patients who developed tricuspid regurgitation during excercise. In these instances, direct Fick measurements are more reliable. Otherwise, excellent correlations are seen between direct

Fick and thermodilution cardiac output measurements.

The principle of this method is similar to that described for dye-dilution, the indicator being either hot or cold injected fluid, and the sensor of temperature change being an intravascular thermistor probe (Branthwaite and Bradley, 1968; Olsson et al., 1970; Ganz et al., 1971). The application of this method in clinical monitoring requires a special catheter in which a thermistor bead is located at or slightly behind the tip of a balloon-tipped catheter (Ganz et al., 1971), which is floated into the pulmonary artery and inscribes a temperature/time dilution curve (Fig. 6.8). For excellent reviews of the complications associated with placement and use of flow-directed pulmonary artery catheters, *see* Damen and Bolten, 1986, Davies et al., 1986.

The basic Stewart-Hamilton formula applies to thermal dilution determinations. However, because of the unique problems involved, several correction factors must be incorporated. These factors account for a scale factor: the specific gravity of injected fluid, the specific heat of the fluid, the specific gravity of blood, the specific heat of blood, the volume of injected fluid, initial blood temperature, and the initial temperature of the injected fluid.

The thermal dilution method has several advantages: the indicator is relatively safe; preparation of 'cold' indicator solution is simple; the solution is stable; withdrawal of blood is not necessary; only one venous cannulation site is used; rapid dissipation of heat and the short distance between injection and sampling site decrease recirculation problems and permit rapid, repeatable determinations; and since dissipation of the cold indicator is rapid and complete, a background tracer concentration does not build up.

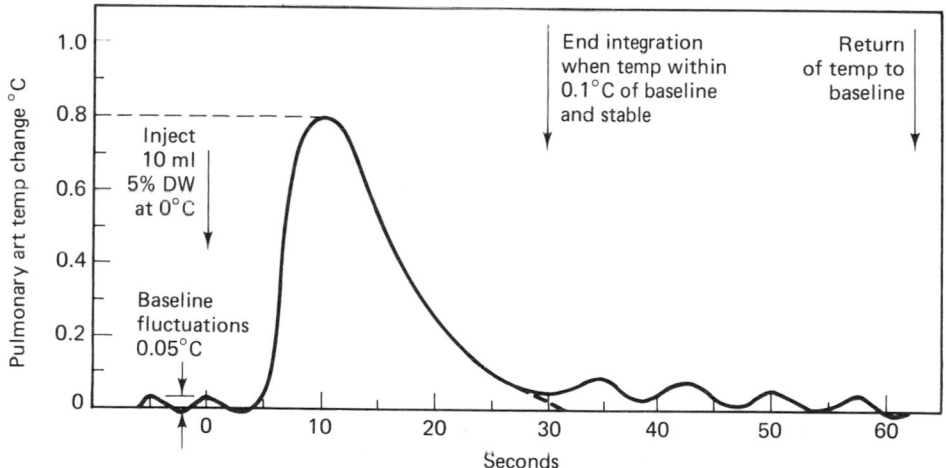

Fig. 6.8 An idealized reconstruction of a thermal dilution curve. Note the temperature fluctuations in the baseline. These fluctuations can be relatively magnified by the many conditions outlined in the text. This particular computer, the Instrumental Laboratory computer, attempts to compensate for this problem by ending integration when the temperature is within 0·1°C of baseline and stable. (Reproduced with permission from Berger, 1976).

Although the thermal dilution technique eliminates many of the problems involved with dye-dilution, its use only converts one set of problems to another. The rapid loss of heat requires that the injection and measuring sites be placed close together. Even with iced saline injectate, rapid injection necessary for the technique, may result in dysrhythmias due to the sudden distension of the ventricle and the sudden change in temperature. Operationally, the method as it is usually executed, involves several poorly controlled variables. Very accurate control of the volume of injected fluid and its temperature is required for the injection of a perfectly defined and reproducible bolus (Normann, 1976; Reiniger, 1976). Respiratory-related fluctuations in pulmonary arterial temperature and blood flow can create many problems; sometimes the fluctuations approach the injection-induced change in temperature (Jansen et al., 1982; Snyder and Powner, 1982).

Heat transfer in the syringe and the catheter and differences in the rate of injection constitute the most serious errors of the open-system manual thermal dilution method. There is a definite transfer of 'cold' from the fluid injected to the catheter wall and surrounding blood. Several factors influence this transfer, including the intra and extracorporal catheter length, rate of injection, and temperature difference between injectate and blood. An error of 1°C introduced for either temperature of blood or injected fluid will alter the cardiac output determination by approximately 3% over the range of cardiac outputs from 3–7 L/min. Errors are progressively greater for lower cardiac outputs (Runciman et al., 1981).

Attempts have been made to correct the problems associated with the thermal dilution method. The influence of the periodic cardiac and respiratory fluctuations is diminished but not eliminated by performing measurements at end expiration (Snyder and Powner, 1982), by electronic averaging and by the use of an iced (0°C) indicator that produces a relatively large temperature change, enhancing the 'signal-to-noise' ratio. Loss of cold from the injection fluid into the catheter wall and surrounding blood is compensated for by applying an empirical correction factor or by measuring temperature at the proximal end of the catheter (Runciman et al., 1981). Unfortunately, errors associated with heat loss are not linear and are greatest, reaching values of up to 20%, at very low cardiac outputs of 1.0 L/min or less. With most thermal dilution cardiac output computers, when an iced fluid is used the fluid should be used promptly and the syringe not handled to minimize potential rewarming errors. Many clinicians inject one syringe of cold solution into the catheter before measuring cardiac output to cool the catheter and reduce this error. The development of closed systems for preparing and delivering injectate has simplified this process as well as reduced the risk of catheter contamination and resultant bacterial sepsis.

The absence of indicator storage within the body, which allows for repeating the determinations within a short time, and the absence or near absence of recirculation, make it tempting to calculate cardiac output directly from the integral of the temperature-time function without extrapolation or correction and to use a simple analogue computer to deal with this calculation. This straightforward approach, however, is not without pitfalls. For example, the tail of the temperature-time function can be considerably distorted due to several causes: release of indicator from fluid remaining inside the catheter lumen after injection (i.e. absorption of heat), delayed arrival of indicator at the detection site, or slow washout of 'cold' from the myocardium and endothelial surfaces. These problems require the computer to carefully scan the baseline. Most of the other problems are approached with the forward triangulation method used for dye-dilution.

Commercially assembled cardiac output computers can average baseline fluctuations, integrate the indicator-dilution curve, incorporate the catheter correction factor, and digitally display the cardiac output in less than one minute after the injection. With all these features, cardiac output estimation by the thermal dilution technique is simple and rapid.

Six thermal computers were extensively tested by Powner and Snyder, 1978. All six appeared similar in accuracy and reproducibility. Other factors must therefore influence the selection of an individual system to meet a particular clinical or research need.

1. Cost of the unit and system components
2. Unit size and weight
3. Availability of dual dye and thermal dilution capability
4. A separate grounded battery power source, isolation of the electrical circuitry, or both
5. Adaptability of the computer to more than one brand of catheter
6. Integration with special-function catheters for pacing or intracardiac ECG monitoring
7. Availability and cost of an accessory recorder
8. System operation during hypothermia
9. Availability of a closed injection system
10. Presence of internal system checks such as separate injectate and body temperature readouts and thermistor continuity tests
11. Availability of an injectate temperature probe
12. Temperature sensing at the site of injectate
13. Automatic pulmonary arterial temperature sensing and entry to the computer, as opposed to separate entry of the patient's body temperature
14. Ease of calibration
15. Ease with which correction factors may be changed or the unit calibrated
16. Handling of baseline drifting and fluctuations
17. Handling of the delayed return to baseline
18. Handling of abnormal and hence inaccurate curves.

Recent development of thermistors with response

times of as little as 50 ms has allowed measurement of beat-to-beat temperature variation and hold the prospect of evaluation of ejection fraction measurements by thermodilution (Kay et al., 1983).

With both dye and thermal dilution techniques, one major problem remains unsolved; the interpretation of the indicator-dilution curve. So many errors can occur that no currently available inexpensive computer interprets or compensates for all of them. The best way to cope with the situation is to record the curve on paper or on a screen each time and validate it visually. The display of problem curves and the methods for dealing with them are, unfortunately, too extensive for this chapter.

Thermal Dilution Measurement of Ventricular Volumes

The original technique used in clinical practice for measuring ventricular volumes was a thermal dilution technique. The subject's own cooled blood or iced saline was injected into the ventricle. As the cooled blood washed out of the ventricle, a step-function, exponential with respect to time, was recorded by a fast responding temperature sensor placed in the root of the aorta. This allowed calculation of several types of ventricular volume (Rappaport et al., 1965).

Radioactive Tracer Techniques

The use of a radioactive indicator and precordial counting allows a relatively noninvasive estimation of stroke volume (SV), by the indicator-dilution method. The technique also eliminates the difficulties of repeated sampling. Some problems include the position of the patient, a selective detector to avoid the extra cardiac radioactivity, and the choice of an adequate indicator to improve the counting statistics.

The curve resulting from the precordial counting of radioactivity has two components, one for the right and one for the left ventricular output. Although this complicates matters, it allows comparison of right and left heart outputs. The computation of cardiac output can be made using the Stewart-Hamilton principle.

Indirect Fick Method

The indirect Fick method attempts to estimate cardiac output by the measurement of the content of one of the blood gases, usually CO_2. Essentially the lungs act as an aerotonometer to measure the tension of mixed venous blood, and hence its gas content. For this technique the patient must rebreathe, or hold in the lungs, gas mixtures, the concentrations of which do not change on being exposed to lung blood. Such mixtures could be made up by trial and error. A simpler way is to repeatedly rebreathe O_2 at 15 second intervals until the CO_2 tension of the rebreathed mixture reaches a constant figure, which is supposed to be that of mixed venous blood. Usually this plateau is reached after 3–

4 intervals of rebreathing. If the tension reached by this plateau is that of the mixed venous blood, and the tension of an end-tidal sample during nonrebreathing is the tension of arterial blood, we have established an a-v̄ CO_2 tension difference from which the a-v̄ content can be derived. (Wilmore et al., 1982).

Another approach to measuring indirect Fick cardiac outputs is the single-breath, constant expiratory technique proposed by Elkayam et al. (1984). This technique makes use of the fact that pulmonary blood flow is proportional to the relationship between absorption of an inert gas, acetylene (C_2H_2), from alveolar gas and the rate of change of lung volume during constant expiratory flow (Fig. 6.9). Provided

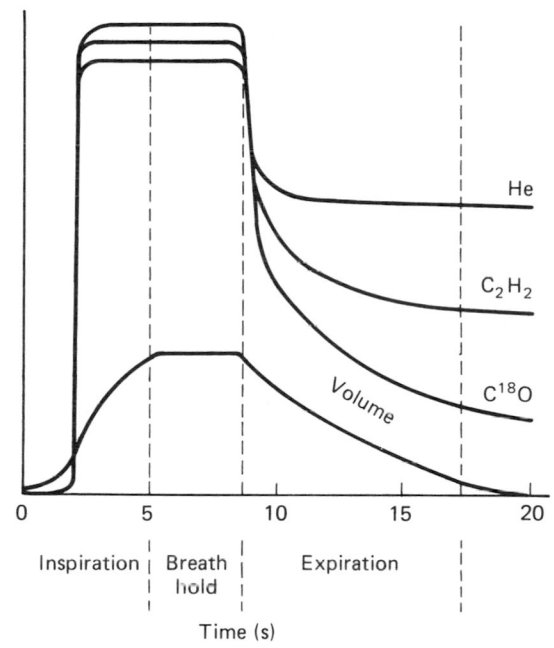

Fig. 6.9 Diagrammatic representation of raw data used to calculate pulmonary artery blood flow by single breath expiratory technique of Elkayam et al. (1984). He = helium concentration, C_2H_2 = acetylene concentration, $C^{18}O$ = labeled carbon monoxide.

that the patients do not have marked lung disease ($FEV_1/FVC > 60\%$), and large breaths are used to overcome small V/Q mismatch, results are promising. Mean difference between cardiac output calculated by this technique and by thermodilution was 0.031 L/min in twenty patients (Elkayam et al., 1984).

Whether by a single-breath technique or by a rebreathing technique, however, overall results have been variable (Heneghan and Branthwaite, 1981). One of the major problems is that the 'A-V difference' diminishes at different rates, depending on the duration of the rebreathing period. In addition, the optimal duration depends on the circulation time. Finally, as suggested above, pulmonary disease markedly influences the results.

CARDIAC OUTPUT FROM ARTERIAL PRESSURE

In spite of the conveniences offered by the indicator-dilution cardiac-output computers, cardiac output is still relatively difficult to measure, compared with blood pressure. The direct Fick and the indicator-dilution techniques have several disadvantages in the operating room. These techniques require skilled personnel, careful execution, sophisticated equipment, and elaborate calibration procedures. Each requires steady-state conditions, which usually do not exist. Even during ostensibly steady-state conditions, there are almost always breath-to-breath variations in stroke volume and cardiac output. Except with the newer noninvasive Doppler methods, the practising anesthetist can measure cardiac output only about every 1–2 min. To perform this measurement, he must either divert his attention from the patient for each measurement or have technical assistance. In contrast, blood pressure measurements are continuous, relatively simple to obtain and easy to calibrate.

What anesthetists need is a simple, inexpensive, reliable method for measuring cardiac output on a beat-to-beat basis. In addition to Doppler cardiac output computers, the most clinically promising of the methods thus far explored uses the blood pressure pulse contour. Investigators have been trying since the 19th Century to extract blood flow information from the arterial pulse. Otto Frank developed the Windkessel concept for this purpose. One of the earliest and most simple attempts used the pulse pressure to estimate stroke volume. In spite of various modifications, the method never became accurate enough for widespread use.

Several pulse contour methods have been tried, including the statistical approach (Starr et al., 1954) the pressure-gradient technique, the pressure-derivative method, the Windkessel appoach (Osborne et al., 1968), and the characteristic impedance method (Kouchoukos et al., 1969, 1970). Most of the earlier methods have not lived up to their initial expectations.

The pressure-gradient technique (Greenfield and Fry, 1965; Snell et al., 1965) is the only pressure-based technique which has been successfully used to compute instantaneous blood velocity. Other factors remaining constant, the pressure difference between two points in a tube determines the flow velocity between these points. The technique does present problems, however. Most of them relate to the fact that small errors in measurement are magnified to large errors in the results. In addition, the double-lumen catheter employed is 6.5 Fr in diameter and requires a large catheter sheath or an arterial cutdown for insertion.

The Characteristic Impedance Approach: The Wesseling (TNO) Method

This method works on the principle of Ohm's Law, i.e. that pressure and flow in arteries are related to each other, as are current and voltage or force and displacement. Thus, just as $I = E/R$, or current = voltage divided by resistance, so CO = AP/SVR, or cardiac output = mean arterial pressure divided by vascular resistance. Ohm's law holds even for pulsatile flow, at every instant of time. For R, we substitute Z_0, the characteristic impedance. Impedance is analogous to resistance, but more complex. To determine Z_0 directly is very difficult, although it can be calculated indirectly by measuring cardiac output by a standard method (Fig. 6.10).

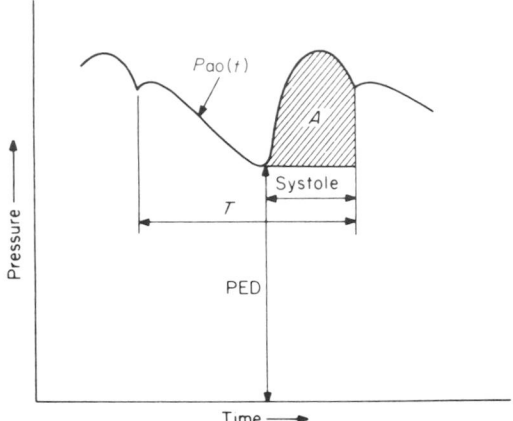

Fig. 6.10 The method of stroke volume computation by the COC is based on integration of the shaded area A. Divided by a patient constant Zo, the characteristic empedance, it yields stroke volume $Pao(t)$ = aortic pressure curve, T = cardiac cycle time, PED = end-diastolic pressure. (Reproduced with permission from Wesseling et al. (1974).)

The method was developed from transmission-line theory and tested extensively on an analogue computer model of the circulation. It was then examined thoroughly in dogs using an electromagnetic flowmeter (Wesseling et al., 1974a,b), healthy volunteer subjects using dye-dilution techniques (Smith et al., 1974), and patients in an intensive care unit using thermal dilution (Wesseling et al., 1976). Among other things, these studies have determined that Z_0 is remarkably constant in dogs, but changes with changes in heart rate and mean arterial pressure in man. A correction factor, adjusted for age, has been incorporated into the calculations and has improved the accuracy of the method. Studies in volunteers also demonstrated the feasibility of using a peripheral wave form, such as that from a radial artery. Since pulse contour methods were previously limited to the aorta, this observation opens many possibilities for the use of the method in monitoring.

The TNO method is simple enough that it can be implemented in a small, inexpensive computer. The computer method can perform no better than the information given it, however, emphasizing the fact that a good arterial pulse wave form is required for any of the pulse-contour methods.

Noninvasive, Beat-to-Beat Cardiac Output

Perhaps the most exciting future possibility for the pulse-contour method is that of a simple to use, noninvasive technique. Smith (1978) reported a series of patients in whom cardiac output was calculated from both direct and indirect arterial pressure tracings. The direct pressure was obtained via a conventional system, the indirect pressure was recorded from a commercially available, noninvasive tonometer placed on the skin over the radial artery. Throughout the sometimes precipitous changes produced during induction of anesthesia, arterial pressure, stroke volume, and cardiac output obtained via the tonometer managed to faithfully follow those obtained directly. Because of the difficulties in obtaining and maintaining a good signal, this tonometer did not reach routine use in the operating theatre.

Even more promising are techniques developed to measure a continuous pulsatile blood pressure from a finger pulse. This pulse is then modified by the arterial-tree model described above to produce a pulse which resembles that which would be recorded in the aorta, and the simulated aortic pulse is used to calculate stroke volume by the TNO method. The attraction of this method lies in its potential for obtaining a large number of important cardiovascular variables (blood pressure, stroke volume, heart rate, and all of the calculated variables) continuously and noninvasively.

IMAGING TECHNIQUES

The use of imaging techniques to measure stroke volume and thence cardiac output has increased markedly in the past several years. Usually, however, with these techniques, V is a byproduct of what are considered more important measurements (end-systolic and diastolic volumes and ejection fraction). Ejection fraction, however, can be measured without directly calculating absolute ventricular volumes. Frequently this simpler and less expensive measurement has replaced the calculation of absolute volumes (*see* Green and Bacharach, 1986).

The imaging techniques currently used are radiographic contrast ventriculography, echocardiography, and radionuclide angiocardiography. The first of these is definitely invasive, the second, noninvasive, and the third, arguably noninvasive.

Radiographic Contrast Ventriculography

Ventriculography is important to the anesthetist in at least two ways.

1. It is the source of much of the preoperative information for the cardiac surgery patient.

2. It is often the *standard* used to evaluate other techniques, especially other imaging techniques.

Ventriculography involves the rapid injection of a radiopaque dye directly into one of the ventricles, usually the left. The image is recorded onto rapidly moving X-ray film (usually at 60–80 frames/s) and the resulting image is analysed for ventricular volume. The image may be recorded in one or two planes. Single-plane ventriculography (SPV) is simpler and less expensive, but definitely less accurate than biplane ventriculography (BPV). The former is therefore more widely used clinically; the latter, however, should be used when an absolute standard is required.

Although more accurate than echocardiography, volume determination by ventriculography is beset by many of the same problems. The most troublesome problem remains the calculation of volume from diameters (much less from areas). These problems are discussed more fully in the section on echocardiography. In general, the volumes are determined by comparing a geometric model (e.g. oblate spheroid, ellipsoid of rotation, multiple cylinders) with angiographic ventricular outlines in single or orthogonal views. Neither the left nor the right ventricle is easily described by a simple geometric model, and, more importantly, each changes shape during the cardiac cycle. In spite of the difficulties, application of geometric models to single-plane and biplane angiocardiograms remains the accepted *standard* of left ventricular volume and EF measurements.

Even skilled observers, while able to detect abnormal motion in imaged patterns are frequently unable to agree on the exact borders of chambers in the displayed image. This results from two factors. The first is simply the noise in any measurement system and the precision of measurement. Defining the appropriate diameter to measure or recognizing the borders of the chamber to be measured entail judgements on the part of the observer. For a spheroid model of the ventricle, a measurement error of 5% could result in a 10–15% error in the calculated volume.

The second source of error stems from the projection of a three-dimensional ventricle onto a two-dimensional image plane. The amount of image material, whether it be contrast dye, radioactive counts or echoes returning from blood cells in the ventricle, is least at the edge of the ventricle, since there is least blood volume at the edge (Green et al., 1986). (Consider an ink-filled sphere projected onto a plane: the resultant circle will be darker in the center than at the edges due to the greater depth of the sphere and hence the greater amount of ink at that point.)

Radionuclide Angiocardiography

Some of the more promising methods to appear in recent years incorporate radionuclide imaging techniques to measure certain indicators of cardiac performance, such as cardiac output, left and right ventricular ejection fraction, and the magnitude and direction of intracardiac shunts. These radionuclide procedures are not entirely noninvasive, since peripheral intravenous injection is required. They do, however, offer certain advantages over more conventional invasive methods. In contrast to cardiac catheterization, the radionuclide techniques are safe and repeatable, do not induce measurable haemodynamic changes, and can be performed in most nuclear medicine laboratories with relatively little additional expense for specialized equipment.

There are two radionuclide methods useful for measuring stroke volume. With the 'first-pass' method, the initial transit of an intravenously injected radioactive bolus through the cardiac chambers is recorded. The technique is analogous to dye-contrast angiography, but less invasive. A second approach, the gated-cardiac blood-pool scan, uses radioactive substances that remain evenly distributed throughout and confined to the vascular space ('blood pool'), including the cardiac chambers, thereby providing an opportunity to examine both ventricles simultaneously when 'equilibrium' (complete mixing) has been reached (Strauss et al., 1971; Zaret et al., 1971). This is analogous to injecting a contrast dye which remains in the heart, instead of quickly passing out in a few beats.

Each technique has advantages and disadvantages. To repeat studies with the first pass method requires repeated injections of radioactive material. On the other hand, the gated-pool techniques must cope with a background of accumulated radiation around the heart; but following a single injection, studies can be repeated for up to about four hours (Green et al., 1986).

First Pass Radionuclide Angiography

Prior to study, a small catheter is inserted into a peripheral vein. The patient is then positioned before the detector of the camera, which may be a computerized, multi-crystal gamma camera. Data are typically recorded at 50 ms intervals for a 1 minute period following a discrete bolus injection of 15–20 µCi of technetium-99m pertechnetate which produces 150 keV gamma rays. Processing of data recorded over the left ventricle permits determination of left ventricular volume changes within each cardiac contraction. Left ventricular volume changes during a single average cardiac contraction are obtained by adding data from several individual contractions recorded at the time when the tracer was maximal within the chamber.

Counts from each of the individual images can be displayed as a motion study on a black and white or colour screen, and photographs of each portion of the study are obtained. Ventricular volumes and ejection fraction may be obtained by applying standard angiographic equations to the traced images. One can also obtain a ventricular time-activity curve, a plot of counts (activity) against time during initial transit of activity through the left ventricle. At slow sampling rates (e.g. two samples per second), the time-activity curve may closely resemble a typical indicator-dilution curve. Figure 6.11 shows a typical time-activity curve as printed out by a computer. Note the resemb-

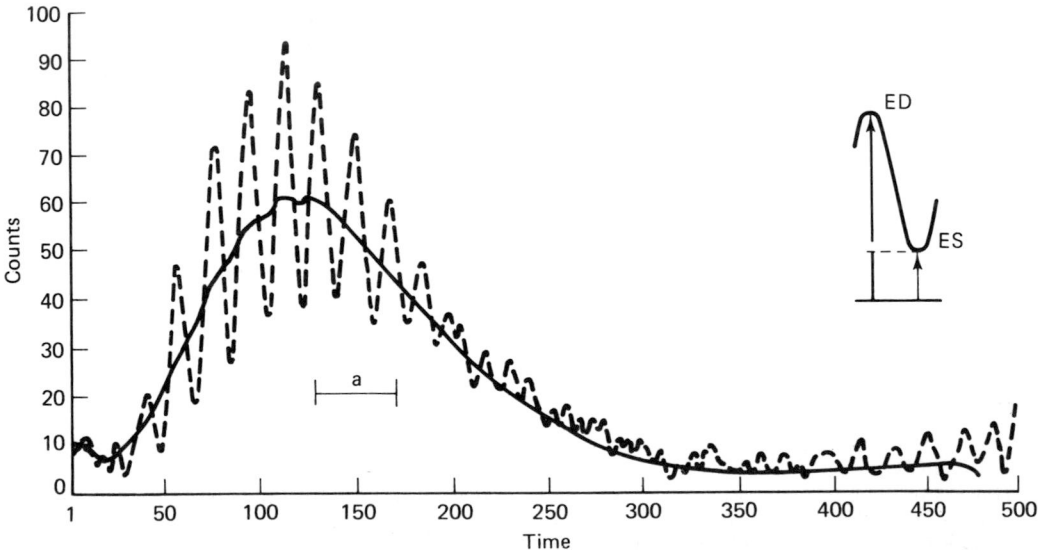

Fig. 6.11 Computer printout of a typical left ventricular time-activity curve. Each point represents data collected for 40 ms (25/s). Peaks correspond to end-diastole (ED), valleys to end-systole (ES). The average curve is superimposed as a fine dotted line. For analysis, a 2 s time period (line a) on the early down slope is used to calculate ejection fraction and in this example includes approximately 2.5 cardiac cycles. (Reproduced with permission from Schelbert et al., 1975).

lance to a dye or thermal dilution curve, but with fluctuations representing cardiac emptying and filling. The upper portion of each fluctuation represents end-diastole and the lower portion end-systole. Fig. 6.12a shows a simplified time-activity curve. Figure 6.12b shows a volume curve constructed from the counts in Fig. 6.12a.

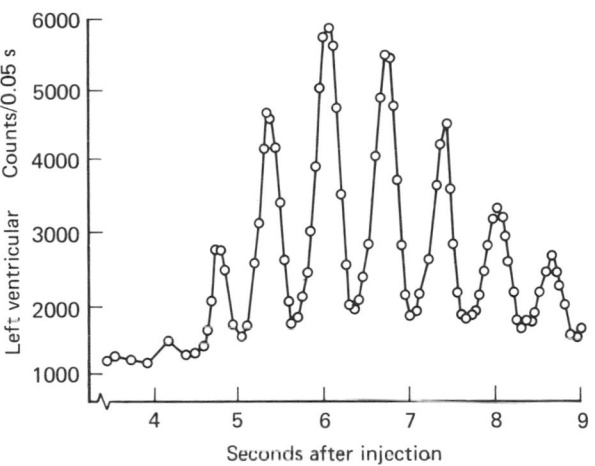

Fig. 6.12a These counts were recorded over the left ventricle. Counts fluctuate with each individual cardiac contraction as the tracer bolus moves through the changer. (Reproduced with permission from Jones, 1979).

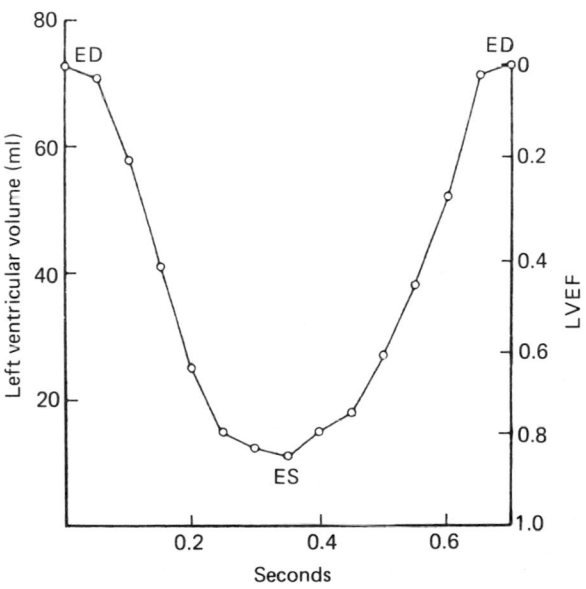

Fig. 6.12b This curve of an average cardiac cycle reflects volume changes within the left ventricle and measures the ejection fraction during the entire cardiac cycle. Moreover, using the end-diastolic image and volumetric analysis to obtain end-diastolic volume, the left ventricle volume is determined in millilitres throughout the cardiac cycle. (Reproduced with permission from Jones et al., 1979).

The Gated-Cardiac Blood-Pool Scan

After intravenous administration of a blood pool tracer such as technetium-99m labelled human serum albumin or red blood cells, the tracer is allowed to equilibrate in the vascular compartment. The scintillation camera is triggered (gated) by the patient's cardiac cycle during sequential 10–50 ms periods throughout the cycle. The data from many cycles are summed onto a single film to produce a high resolution image of at least 300 000 counts, all recorded during a specific portion of the cardiac cycle. In addition to visualization of the movement of the ventricular walls, the method produces a left ventricular time-activity curve. To permit calculation of left ventricular volumes and ejection fraction, images are recorded at assumed end-systole and end-diastole. Stroke volume, then, equals EDV-ESV. Averaging beats can eliminate minor inconsistencies or random errors. Other problems arise, however, because of the long time required for sample averaging, especially if there is patient motion, marked change in heart rate, or cardiac dysrhythmia.

Stroke volumes obtained by gated-cardiac blood-pool scanning correlate well with those from contrast angiography (Strauss et al., 1971; Kostuk et al., 1973; Garrett et al., 1985).

Characteristically, gated-blood-pool studies are carried out with a large, static, gamma camera and require moving the patient to the nuclear medicine suite. A new alternative is to employ an inexpensive portable nonimaging nuclear probe to measure rates of counts over a small portion of the chest (Lahiri et al., 1984). Lahiri et al., reported that such a probe, utilizing either a NaI or HgI$_2$ probe has excellent stopping power for gamma rays emitted by technetium-99. By gating the detector to the ECG they were able to plot beat-to-beat ventricular volume data. Correlations of 0.94 between ejection fraction calculated from the nuclear probe and from conventional gamma cameras were reported for 40 patients. Although Lahiri et al., found no difference between the two types of probes, both consistently overestimated ejection fraction by about 6.6% compared with the conventional gamma camera. Note that this method does not provide absolute cardiac output measurements, although it has the potential to provide beat-to-beat information about relative ventricular volumes.

Echocardiography

In clinical practice, ultrasonic echocardiography is becoming more common and may soon supplant radionuclide imaging for estimation of ejection fraction. Unlike the radionuclide techniques, it is totally noninvasive and does not require the injection of radioactive isotopes, whose cost, availability, and disposal may present problems.

Basic Background

To record the echogram, an ultrasonic transducer is placed on the chest wall. The transducer generates short bursts of sound (2–5 MHz), which travel along a finite path through the chest. At each interface between tissues with different densities a portion of the sound is reflected back to the transducer, and the remainder continues on, to be reflected by subsequent echo-producing interfaces. The instrument calculates the distance from transducer to each reflecting interface by measuring the time interval from sound transmission to reception of echoes. These depth readings through the thorax are repeated 1000 times per second. At this sampling rate, structures that move during the cardiac cycle can be tracked on an oscilloscope, and the pattern of motion of each interface can be analysed. Experience has led to clear identification of all cardiac structures represented on the echocardiogram, and standardized methods of directing the sound beam through the heart have been developed. The two ways of displaying the echo are the B, or brightness, mode and the M, or motion, mode. (B-mode echocardiography is rarely used now.) Watching the B-mode is like watching an ECG which is not moving in time. Moving the B-mode display over an oscilloscope screen or moving recording paper past the B-mode display produces the M-mode. The conventional M-mode echocardiogram displays the motion of the interventricular septum and left ventricular posterior wall through the cardiac cycle (Fig. 6.13).

To estimate the absolute size or volume of the left ventricle (LV) from one dimension, one must assume an idealized geometric model of the ventricle, so that the dimensions of the model can be directly related to the single dimension measured echocardiographically. For the 'normal' sized and shaped LV, the ellipsoid of revolution with a ratio of long axis (L) to a minor axis (M) of 2:1 is accepted (Fig. 6.14a). It is further

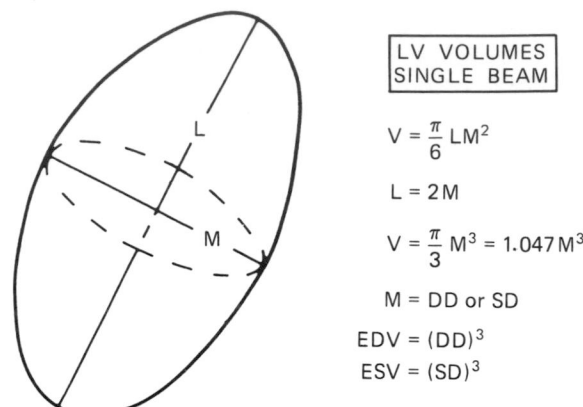

LV VOLUMES SINGLE BEAM

$$V = \frac{\pi}{6} LM^2$$

$$L = 2M$$

$$V = \frac{\pi}{3} M^3 = 1.047 M^3$$

$$M = DD \text{ or } SD$$

$$EDV = (DD)^3$$
$$ESV = (SD)^3$$

Fig. 6.14a Ellipsoid of revolution used as a model for calculating the volume of the left ventricle from one echocardiographic LV dimension. The short or minor axes (M) are equal and the long axis (L) is twice as long as the short axis. The formula for calculation of the volume of this model is shown. (Reproduced with permission from Roeland, 1977).

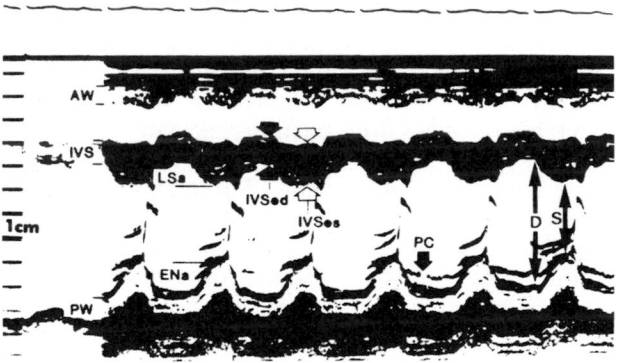

Fig. 6.13 Echocardiogram of the ventricle over several cardiac cycles. Depth calibration (1 cm) is in a portion of the record with low amplification of returning echoes. This portion (left) helps locate the fine pericardial signal near the posterior ventricular walls (PW). The posterior-wall endocardial amplitude (ENa), and left septal amplitude (LSa) are indicated by horizontal lines. Thickness of the inter-ventricular septum (IVS) at end-diastole (IVSed) and end-systole (IVSes) is measured as shown by the short arrows. Diastolic (D) and systolic (S) left ventricular dimensions are measured at the points shown by the longer vertical arrows. EKG denotes electrocardiogram. AW right ventricular anterior wall, and PC posterior chordae. (Reproduced with permission from Popp, 1977).

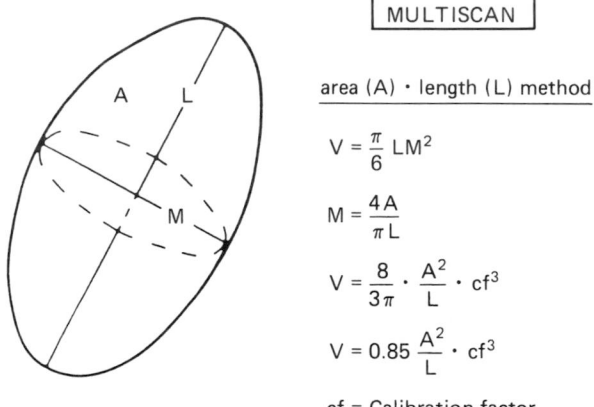

LV VOLUMES MULTISCAN

area (A) · length (L) method

$$V = \frac{\pi}{6} LM^2$$

$$M = \frac{4A}{\pi L}$$

$$V = \frac{8}{3\pi} \cdot \frac{A^2}{L} \cdot cf^3$$

$$V = 0.85 \frac{A^2}{L} \cdot cf^3$$

cf = Calibration factor

Fig. 6.14b Area-length formula applied to the prolate ellipse model of the left ventricle to calculate volumes from angiographic and multiscan (2-D) echocardiographic images. A = surface area of cross section: L = long axis, M = minor axis, V = volume. (Reproduced with permission from Roelandt, 1977).

assumed that the perpendicular short axes of the ellipsoid are equal and that these ratios remain constant through LV contraction, that is, that the LV walls contract uniformly. Since L = 2M, estimated volumes can be related to M^3.

Two-dimensional Echocardiography

Since the M-mode records in only one dimension over time, most modern machines record the echo in two dimensions, similar to an angiogram. Early methods for recording in two dimensions used a standard B-scan echograph. An electrocardiogram triggered the oscilloscopic image so that only diastole or systole was recorded. The cross-sectional image was then a composite of multiple cardiac cycles. Although the B-scan approach did provide more than a single dimension by which to estimate ventricular volumes, it had several limitations, most notably the difficulty in discerning the edges of structures.

Real-time, cross-sectional echocardiographic images are obtained by sweeping a beam back and forth in an arc, either electronically steering the ultrasonic beam, mechanically driving the transducer, or rapidly and sequentially firing transducers in a multi-element system. Each system produces an angiogram-like, real-time examination of the heart.

The use of cross-sectional images allows one to apply formulae widely tested in single-plane angiography to measure ventricular volumes. The common formula is an area-length formula based on the prolate ellipse model (Fig. 6.14b). Ultrasonic LV long-axis cross-sections in end diastole and end systole and the principle of determining the long-axis and surface area are shown in Fig. 6.15. As with angiography, accuracy depends upon the operator's ability to discern the cardiac silhouette and the assumptions made about three-dimensional ventricular shape and how this varies during the cardiac cycle. Image resolution, and hence accuracy and precision, has improved remarkably in recent years.

A newer technique, biplane echocardiography, may have a slight advantage over single-plane angiography when both are compared with traditional biplane angiography. The echo technique is, of course, non-invasive.

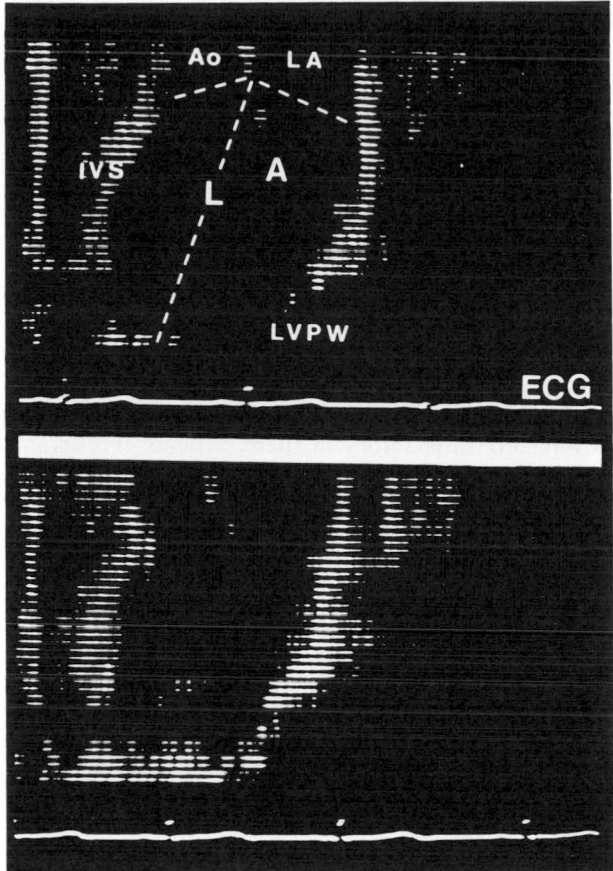

Fig. 6.15 End-diastolic (upper panel) and end-systolic (lower panel) sagittal long axis cross sections obtained from a normal subject. The outer contours of the LV can be traced and their motion pattern analysed. The outline area (A) can be measured by planimetry and the long axis (L) measured directly. The area-length formula is then applied to calculate the LV volumes. (*See* Fig. 6.12), Ao = aorta, IVS = inter-ventricular septum: LA = left atrium: LVPW = left ventricular posterior wall. (Reproduced with permission from Roelandt, 1977).

Problems with Echocardiography

Echocardiography has not reached the reliability, accuracy, or precision of contrast ventriculography. There are several reasons for this. With a 1.5 MHz signal, maximum resolution is only 1 mm. Although the size of the ventricle seems to make little difference, difficulties are accentuated in patients with emphysema, or those who are obese or for whatever reason have an exceptionally thick anterior chest wall, which absorbs ultrasonic energy. Sound does not travel through air as well as it does through soft tissue, and many patients with increased anteroposterior dimensions of the chest have very small areas of direct contact between the chest wall and the anterior heart wall. Thus the window for ultrasonic examination is limited and may not provide the standard dimension through the ventricle. In patients with subcutaneous emphysema, it may not be possible to visualize the heart at all with transthoracic echocardiography because of reflections from the subcutaneous air.

Two questions regarding volume measurement arise in the clinical situation where hearts may assume different shapes.

1. Should the same volume formula which is applied to a normal heart be used for an enlarged heart?
2. What errors are introduced by localized disorders in wall motion?

The 2:1 ratio assumed for the prolate ellipse is not constant, particularly as the heart dilates and becomes more spherical. Regression equations have been used with partial success, to allow for a change in shape with the change in size. However, the geometric complexities of the intact heart and the changes in shape that occur during contraction would seem to make derivation of stroke volume difficult (Smith, 1980). Under normal circumstances, M-mode echocardiography is a reasonably accurate method of estimating left ventricular volume, but its reliability is considerably compromised by segmental dysfunction. This results in a poor correlation between M-mode volumes and angiography in coronary disease (Schiller et al., 1979). Coronary artery disease constitutes the largest group of patients in cardiological practice (at least 60%). This is a serious disadvantage, since these are the very patients in whom accurate assessment of cardiac output and ventricular function is needed. The use of single-plane, two-dimensional echocardiography improves the accuracy, while bi-plane improves it further. However, no technique is completely satisfactory in these patients. Techniques taking several tomographic-like slices offer the best results, and gated CT or MRI scanning offers hope for future techniques (Garrett et al., 1985, Lipton et al., 1986).

Thus, the list of patients in whom standard formulae or methods are useless is long and includes the following.

1. Abnormal shape of the LV (e.g. asymmetric septal hypertrophy)
2. Segmental LV disease (e.g. coronary artery disease)
3. Conduction disturbances altering LV wall motion (e.g. left bundle branch block)
4. Abnormal motion patterns of the LV wall (e.g. atrial septal defect)
5. Small (e.g. mitral stenosis) and enlarged (e.g. cardiomyopathy) ventricles.

Several major problems confront the anesthetist before he can use echocardiography, namely: the relatively low percentage of patients providing useful recordings under the best of circumstances, (50–90%, the latter in children), the sensitivity of the recording to the placement and angle of the transducer, the position of the patient, the need to optimize the recording by examining it and readjusting the transducer, the need for operator skill and experience, the need for continuous physician interaction while recording with the two-dimensional technique, the difficulty in obtaining quantitative information, and the lag between presentation of the echocardiogram and the presentation of quantitative information.

Transesophageal Echocardiography (TEE)
Many of the techniques discussed in this chapter are adaptable to a probe which can be inserted into the esophagus. An esophageal probe is particularly attractive, since it is useful for monitoring surgical patients. The esophagus lies close to the aorta and the heart, and is usually 'out of the way' of the surgical procedure, although easily accessible to the anesthetist. In addition, obtaining several measurements from a single esophageal probe and cable would help relieve the clutter of the operating theatre. For example, one could measure temperature, the ECG, breath sounds, and heart sounds, as well as incorporate the continuous wave Doppler, pulsed Doppler or echocardiographic transducer—or any combination. In practice, TEE is usually added to those monitors already in use, and its expense has prevented routine adoption in the operating room.

Although there are many advantages to esophageal probes, there are also problems. Foremost of these is the size of the probe which almost precludes use in awake patients. The anesthetist thus does not have information about cardiac performance prior to or during induction of anesthesia, the time when he may need it most! In addition, one frequently encounters difficulty in placing the esophageal probe at the correct position and angle, although recently marketed probes have a wider angle of view, making their placement somewhat easier. Placement becomes easier with a two-dimensional echo system, since heart structures may be more easily identified as the probe is manipulated. Additional difficulties with esophageal probes are encountered when patients are positioned other than supine. Perhaps the worst position is the right lateral decubitus position, since the esophagus tends to fall away from the heart and obtaining an adequate signal can be very difficult. The advantage of esophageal probes, in addition to ease of use is that the sound wave travels through considerably less tissue than it does with the conventional echo (Fig. 6.16). The lack of lung tissue is especially important. Cardiac output measured with this device correlates fairly well with the CO obtained from the dye-dilution technique. Since the tracing is an M-mode tracing, it is subject to most of the problems inherent with that signal. However, devices such as this may represent the future in monitoring surgical patients. As currently configured, however, TEE requires an additional operator in the room to run the machine and interpret the signal.

ALTERNATIVE APPROACHES

Impedence Plethysmography
Impedance cardiography (ICG), a noninvasive technique, has undergone waves of enthusiasm and disillusionment. To measure the ICG, electrodes placed around the neck and abdomen are excited by a 100 kHz current, and the resulting voltage (impedance) changes are monitored from a second pair of electrodes around the patient's neck and chest.

Electrical impedance depends upon the volume and composition of material between the current generating electrodes. The rib cage describes a fairly rigid container made up of a core of incompressible material and fluid and two cylinders of partially air filled tissue, the lungs. These will change volume and orientation with the respiratory and cardiac cycles. Electrical impedance does not very much in the solid tissues of the thorax, although resistance within the

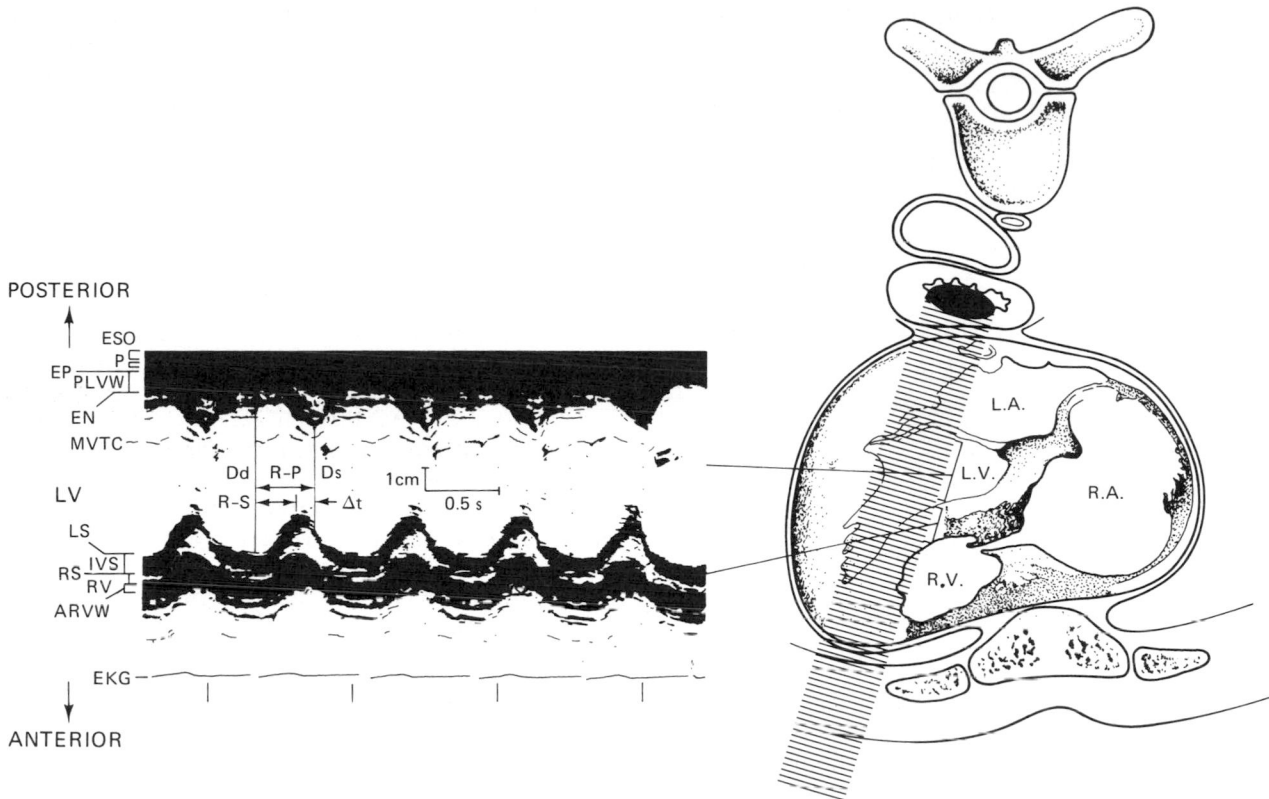

Fig. 6.16 M-mode Echocardiogram Recorded from the Transesophageal Probe. Note that this represents a mirror image of an echocardiogram recorded using the parasternal technique. (*See* Fig. 6.10) (Reproduced with permission from Oka et al., 1980).

air/fluid filled lungs varies as air and blood enter and leave them. It is this change in resistance, assumed to be proportional to changes in blood volume, which impedence cardiology measures. Multiple assumptions about chest dimensions, composition and physiology have to be made. Analysis of the waveform of resistance over several cardiac cycles allows estimation of the initial rate of pulmonary flow, and this is extrapolated over the entire cycle to estimate cardiac output (Kubicek et al., 1966).

The ICG has been tested against every 'gold standard' available: dye-dilution, thermal dilution, direct Fick, and the electromagnetic flowmeter. The results have been mixed, some investigators obtaining good results, but most obtaining mediocre or poor results. With early machines there may have been several reasons for these discrepancies. The most important are now listed.

1. The commonly used simple equation for stroke volume did not take into account changes which occur in the distribution of signal current within the thorax of patients having pathology of the lung or heart (Cooley, 1972), and significant errors can occur in these patients (Harley and Greenfield, 1968).
2. There was difficulty and inconsistency in reading

the wave form. More recent versions of the equipment have partially solved these problems, and commercially available machines provide correlations with thermodilution ranging from 0.74 to 0.95 (Tremper et al., 1986, 1987).

Some authors have disputed the assumptions of Kubicek et al., (1966) about the appropriate shape of the thorax (Bernstein, 1986 a,b) and the effect of ventilation, changes in blood volume, and changes in respiratory mechanics seen with pregnancy (Davies et al., 1986; de Swiet and Talbert 1986; Milsom et al., 1983).

One machine is currently being marketed commercially to measure cardiac output by impedence cardiography and has been used clinically to predict patients at risk for intraoperative cardiac dysfunction (Appel et al., 1986, Wong et al., 1987). However, it cannot give true beat-to-beat values, and is not reliable when the cardiovascular system is changing. Although it tracked manipulated changes in cardiac output regardless of whether mean arterial pressure was simultaneously raised or lowered, the machine was unable to measure cardiac output at very low levels of 1.4–1.7 L/min in dogs (Tremper et al., 1986). Whether or not this will become a useful clinical tool awaits further validation studies.

Systolic Time Intervals

The systolic time intervals (STI) are described elsewhere in this book. They are useful mainly for assessing ventricular function. Cardiac output and stroke volume have been correlated with the STI primarily to help understand the STI, not to look for a method of measuring CO. Nevertheless, there is a commercial device which claims to measure CO via the STI.

The ratio *PEP/LVET* has been chosen as the number from which to estimate stroke and cardiac index. However, although early results were encouraging, it is now clear that, while the STI are almost always abnormal when cardiac index (CI) is reduced, it is not uncommon to find an abnormal *PEP/LVET* in the face of a normal CI. Perhaps modifiers of the estimation of CI, such as arterial pressure, will improve the accuracy of the STI in this area.

In spite of these problems, it is important to realize that the STI, along with independent information about CO and SV, can constitute a valuable tool for the continuous assessment of cardiac function.

Ballistocardiography

The ballistocardiogram (Bcg) is best defined as a recording of the movement of the body caused by movements of blood within the body. These body movements can be registered as displacement, velocity or acceleration. Although the Bcg has been replaced as a technique for estimating cardiac output, it was used some time ago in one rather unusual set of circumstances. It was used to estimate cardiac output and stroke volume in what is probably the largest animal ever recorded, a young Californian grey whale. The whale's weight was calculated as 4500 kg. Her stroke volume was 7150 ml, while her cardiac output was 308 L/min (Smith and Smith, 1976). The cardiac output predicted by Iberall's formula, $CO = OW^{0.842}$, was 302 L/min. They did not, however, perform a dye-dilution cardiac output as a 'gold standard'; it would have required 13 bottles of green dye for one determination!

Sonomicrometry

A rather different approach to estimating stroke volume and hence cardiac output is to measure heart muscle contraction during systole. Expanding upon a technique first reported by Rushmer et al. (1956), Moores et al. (1985) have demonstrated that piezoelectric crystals implanted in the heart during surgery, a technique known as sonomicrometry, can provide instantaneous measurements of myocardial contractility as opposed to myocardial compliance. Standard research piezoelectric pulsed-transit ultrasonic transducers are implanted in the left ventricle to allow evaluation of pressure-geometry relationships and to serve as a continuous measure of myocardial function postoperatively. Moores et al. demonstrated

correlations of 0.954 between end-diastolic length as measured by the crystals and stroke volumes calculated from thermodilution. In addition, a negative correlation was seen between filling pressures and end-diastolic length. While the technique is promising, it has the drawback of possible myocardial injury during insertion or removal of the crystals, although this is probably no greater than that seen with routine insertion of ventricular pacing wires (Haasler and Spotnitz, 1983). This technique may find use for postoperative monitoring of patients undergoing cardiac surgery.

FUTURE DIRECTIONS

Thermodilution cardiac output has clearly become the standard, if not the 'gold standard', of clinical measurement of cardiac output. The two noninvasive measures of cardiac output currently being marketed heavily, namely Doppler echocardiography and impedence cardiography will likely become more common in the operating room despite their inherent problems because of their ease of use and low risk to the patient. Neither provides information about cardiac filling pressures, however, so it is not necessarily clear what therapy to employ when cardiac output is low or falling (e.g. is an inotrope necessary or is the patient hypovolemic?). If noninvasive cardiac output monitoring becomes ubiquitous, it is not clear whether this will actually affect the anesthetic outcome in the majority of cases, just as routine placement of pulmonary artery catheters in healthy patients would probably not benefit the majority of patients. None the less, the inherent risks of pulmonary artery monitoring, the difficulty of measuring direct Fick cardiac outputs and the impracticality of employing nuclear medicine techniques in the operating room all should act to encourage further refinements and developments in the noninvasive measurement of cardiac output and blood flow.

REFERENCES

Appel P.L., Kram H.B., Mackabee J. et al. (1986). Comparison of measurements of cardiac output by bioimpedance and thermodilution in severely ill surgical patients. *Crit. Care Med.* **14**, 933.

Baker D.W. (1964). A sonic transcutaneous blood flow-meter. *Proc 17th Ann. Conf. Med. Biol. Eng.*, **76**.

Baker D.W. (1970). Pulse ultrasonic Doppler's blood flow sensing. *IEEE Trans Sonics Ultrasound.*, **SU.17**, 170.

Bernstein D.P. (1986a). A new stroke volume equation for thoracic electrical bioimpedance: Theory and rationale. *Crit. Care Med.*, **14**, 904.

Bernstein, D.P. (1986b). Continuous noninvasive real-time monitoring of stroke volume and cardiac output by thoracic electrical bioimpedance. *Crit. Care Med.* **14**, 898.

Blackburn J.P. (1982). Computers and the anaesthetist. In *Scientific Foundations of Anaesthesia*, 3rd edn. p. 626. (Scurr C., Feldman S., eds): Oxford: Heinemann Medical Books.

Boerboom L.E., Boelkins J.N. (1978). Dye-dilution cardiac output without blood withdrawal in the conscious rabbit. *Am. Physiol. Soc.*, H258.

Bond R.F., Barefoot C.A. (1967). Evaluation of an electromagnetic catheter tip velocity sensitive blood flow probe. *J. Appl. Physiol.*, **23**, 403.

Branthwaite M.A., Bradley R.D. (1968). Measurement of cardiac output by thermal dilution in man. *J. Appl. Physiol.*, **24**, 434.

Chandraratina P.A., Nanna M., McKay C. et al. (1984). Determination of cardiac output by transcutaneous continuous wave ultrasonic Doppler computer. *Am. J. Cardiol*, **53**, 234.

Colley P.F., Martin R.W. (1980). Transesophageal Doppler monitoring of air embolism. *Anesthesiology*, **53**, S120.

Colocousis J.S., Huntsman L.L., Curreri P.W. (1977). Estimation of stroke volume changes by ultrasonic Doppler. *Circulation*, **56**, 914.

Cooley W.I. (1972). The calculation of cardiac stroke volume from variations in transthoracic electric impedance. *Bio-Med Eng.*, **1**, 316.

Daigle R.E., Miller C.W., Histand M.B. et al. (1975). Nontraumatic aortic blood flow sensing by use of an ultrasonic esophageal probe. *J. Appl. Phy.*, **38**, 1153.

Damen J., Bolton D. (1986). A prospective analysis of 1400 pulmonary artery catheterizations in patients undergoing cardiac surgery. *Acta Anaesthesiol. Scand.*, **30**, 386.

Darsee J.R., Mikolich J.R., Walter P.F. et al. (1980a). Transcutaneous method of measuring Doppler cardiac output—I. Comparison of transcutaneous and juxta-aortic Doppler velocity signals with catheter and cuff electromagnetic flowmeter measurements in closed and open chest dogs. *Am. J. Cardiol*, **46**, 607.

Darsee J.R., Walter P.F., Nutter D.O. et al. (1980b). Transcutaneous Doppler method of measuring cardiac output—II. Noninvasive measurement by transcutaneous Doppler aortic blood velocity integration and M-mode echocardiography. *Am. J. Card.*, **46**, 614.

Davies G.G., Jebson P.J., Hess D.R. (1986). Continuous Fick cardiac output compared to thermodilution. *Crit. Care Med.*, **14**, 881.

Davies G., Hess D., Jebson P. (1987). Continuous Fick cardiac output compared to continuous pulmonary artery electromagnetic flow measurement in pigs. *Anesthesiology*, **66**, 805.

Davies P., Francis R.I., Docker M.F. et al. (1986). Analysis of impedance cardiography longitudinally applied in pregnancy. *Br. J. Obstet. Gynaecol.*, **93**, 717.

de Swiet M., Talbert D.G. (1986). The measurement of cardiac output by electrical impedance plethysmography in pregnancy. Are the assumptions valid? *Br. J. Obstet. Gynaecol.*, **93**, 721.

Dobson A., Sellers A.F., McLeod F.D. (1966). Performance of a cuff-type blood flowmeter *in vivo*. *J. Appl. Physiol.*, **21**, 1642(A).

Dorlas J.C., Nijboer J.A. (1985). Photo-electric plethysmography as a monitoring device in anaesthesia. *Br. J. Anaesth.*, **57**, 524.

Elkayam U., Wilson A.F., Morrison J. et al. (1984). Noninvasive measurement of cardiac output by a single breath constant expiratory technique. *Thorax*, **39**, 107.

Eyer S., Borgos J., Strate R.G. (1987). Laser Doppler flowmetry and cardiac output in critically ill surgical patients. *Crit. Care Med.*, **15**, 778.

Fegler G. (1954). Measurement of cardiac output in anaes- thetized animals by a thermodilution method. *J. Exp. Physiol.*, **39**, 153.

Fisher D.C., Sahn D.J., Friedman M.J. et al. (1983a). The mitral valve orifice method for noninvasive two-dimensional echo Doppler determinations of cardiac output. *Circulation*, **67**, 872.

Fisher D.C., Sahn D.J., Friedman M.J. et al. (1983b). The effect of variations of pulsed Doppler sampling site on calculation of cardiac output: an experimental study in open-chest dogs. *Circulation*, **67**, 370.

Freund P.R. (1986). Modifications in the transesophageal Doppler: comparison with thermodilution measurement during cardiac output (sic) in anesthetized man. *Anesthesiology*, **65:3A**, A144.

Freund P.R., Padavich C.A. (1985). A comparison of cardiac output techniques: transesophageal Doppler versus thermodilution cardiac output during general anesthesia in man. *Anesthesiology*, **63**, A191.

Ganz W., Donoso R., Marcus H.S. et al. (1971). A new technique for measurement of cardiac output by thermodilution in man. *Am. J. Cardiol.*, **27**, 392 (B-29).

Garrett J.S., Lanzer P., Jaschke W. et al. (1985). Measurement of cardiac output by cine computed tomography. *Am. J. Cardiol.*, **56**, 657.

Green M.V., Bacharach S.L. (1986). Functional imaging of the heart: methods, limitations, and examples from gated blood pool scintigraphy. *Prog. Cardiovasc. Disease*, **28**, 319.

Greenfield J.C. Jr., Fry D.L. (1965). A critique: relationship of the time derivative of pressure to blood flow. *J. Appl. Physiol.*, **20**, 1141 (A).

Haasler G.B., Spotnitz H.M. (1983). Limitations of epicardial ultrasound crystals for studies of left ventricular function demonstrated by two-dimensional echocardiography in dogs. *Surg. Forum.*, **34**, 285.

Hagl S., Messmer K., Pfau B. et al. (1974). Influence of stenosis on the velocity profile analyzed by a pulsed Doppler ultrasonic flowmeter. In *Cardiovascular Applications of Ultrasound*, p. 216. (Reneman R.S. ed.). Amsterdam: North-Holland Publishing Company.

Haites N.E., McLennan F.M., Mowat D.H.R. et al. (1985). Assessment of cardiac output by the Doppler ultrasound technique alone. *Br. Heart J.*, **53**, 123.

Hamilton W.F. et al. (1948). Comparison of the Fick and dye-injection methods of measuring the cardiac output in man. *Am. J. Physiol.*, **153**, 309.

Harley A., Greenfield J.C. (1968). Cardiac output measurement by impedance plethysmography. *Aerosp. Med.*, **39**, 248.

Heneghan C.P.H., Branthwaite M.A. (1981). Noninvasive measurement of cardiac output during anaesthesia. An evaluation of the soluble gas uptake method. *Br. J. Anaesth.*, **53**, 351.

Huntsman L.L., Gams E., Johnson C.C. et al. (1975). Transcutaneous determination of aortic blood flow velocities in man. *Am. Heart J.*, **89**, 605.

Huntsman L.L., Stewart D. K., Barnes S.R. et al. (1983). Noninvasive Doppler determination of cardiac output in man. Clinical validation. *Circulation*, **67**, 593.

Jansen J.R.C., Schreuder J.J., Bogaard J.M. et al. (1982). Thermodilution technique for measurement of cardiac output during artificial ventilation. *J. Appl. Physiol.*, **584**, 91.

Katz J. (1984). Skin blood flow after axillary brachial plexus block. Use of laser Doppler flowmetry. *Regional Anesth.*, **9**, 68.

Katz J.D., Cronau L.H., Barash P.G. et al. (1977). Pulmonary artery flow-guided catheters in the perioperative period. Indications and complications. *JAMA*, **237**, 2832.

Kay H.R., Afshari M., Barash et al. (1983). Measurement of ejection fraction by thermal dilution techniques. *J. Surg. Res.*, **34**, 337.

Konstam M.A., Kahn P.C., Curran B.H. et al. (1984). Equilibrium (gated) radionuclide ejection fraction measurement in the pressure or volume overloaded right ventricle. Comparison of three methods. *Chest*, **86**, 681.

Kostuk W. J., Ehsant A., Karliner J.S. et al. (1973). Left ventricular performance after myocardial infarction assessed by radioisotope angiocardiography. *Circulation*, **47**, 242.

Kouchoukos N.T., Sheppard L.C., McDonald D.A. et al. (1969). Estimation of stroke volume from the central arterial pressure of postoperative patients. *Surg. Forum*, **20**, 180.

Kouchoukos N.T., Sheppard L.C., McDonald D.A. (1970). Estimation of stroke volume in the dog by a pulse contour method. *Circ. Res.*, **26**, 611.

Kubicek W.G., Karnegis J.N., Patterson R.P. (1966). Development and evaluation of an impedance cardiac output system. *Aerospace Med.*, **37**, 1208.

Lahiri A., Crawley J.C.W., Jones R.I. et al. (1984). A non-invasive technique for continuous monitoring of left ventricular function using a new solid state mercuric iodide radiation detector. *Clin. Sci.*, **66**, 551.

Lang-Jensen T., Berning J., Jacobsen E. (1983). Stroke volume measured by pulsed ultrasound Doppler and M-mode echocardiography. *Acta Anaesthesiol. Scand.*, **27**, 454.

Light L.H. (1969). Non-injurious ultrasonic technique for observing flow in the human aorta. *Nature*, **224**, 1119.

Light L.H. (1974). Initial evaluation of transcutaneous aortovelography—a new noninvasive technique for hemodynamic measurements in the major thoracic vessels. In *Cardiovascular Applications of Ultrasound*, p. 325. (Reneman, R.S. ed.). Amsterdam: North-Holland Publishing Company.

Light L.H. (1976). Transcutaneous aortovelography. A new window on the circulation? (Editorial). *Br. Heart J.*, **38**, 433.

Light L.H., Sequeira R.F., Cross G. et al. (1979). Flow-oriented circulatory patient assessment and management using transcutaneous aortovelography, a noninvasive Doppler technique. *J. Nucl. Med. Allied Sci.*, **23**, 137.

Lipkin D.P., Poole-Wilson P.A. (1985). Measurement of cardiac output during exercise by the thermodilution and direct Fick techniques in patients with chronic congestive heart failure. *Am. J. Cardiol.*, **56**, 321.

Lipton M.J., Brundage B.H., Higgins C.B. et al. (1986). Clinical applications of dynamic computed tomography. *Prog. in Cardiovasc. Dis.*, **28**, 349.

Loeppky J.A., Hoekenga D.E., Greene E.R. et al. (1984). Comparison of noninvasive pulsed Doppler and Fick measurements of stroke volume in cardiac patients. *Am. Heart J.*, **107**, 339.

Mackay R.S., Hechtman H.B. (1975). Continuous cardiac output measurement: aspects of Doppler frequency analysis. *IEEE Trans. Bio. Med. Eng. BME*., **22**, 346.

Matsumato M., Oka Y., Lin T.Y. et al. (1979). Transesophageal echocardiography for assessing ventricular function. *New York State J. Med.*, **79**, 19.

McLeod F.D. (1967). A directional Doppler flowmeter. *Digest of Seventh Intl. Conf. Med. Biol. Eng.* Stockholm., 213.

Mehta N., Iyawe V.I., Cummin A.R.C. et al. (1985). Validation of a Doppler technique for beat-to beat measurement of cardiac output. *Clin. Sci.* **69**, 377.

Mills C.J. (1966). A catheter tip electromagnetic velocity probe. *Physics Med. Biol.*, **11**, 323.

Mills C.J., Shillingford J.P. (1967). A catheter velocity probe and its evaluation. *Cardiovas. Res.*, **1**, 263.

Milsom I., Forssman L., Biber B. et al. (1983). Measurement of cardiac stroke volume during caesarean section: a comparison between impedance cardiography and the dye-dilution technique. *Acta Anaesthesiol. Scand.* **27**, 421.

Mohr R., Rath S., Meir O. et al. (1986). Changes in systemic vascular resistance detected by the arterial resistometer: preliminary report of a new method tested during percutaneous transluminal coronary angioplasty. *Circulation*, **74**, 780.

Moores W.Y., LeWinter M.M., Long W.B. et al. (1984). Sonomicrometry: its application as a routine monitoring technique in cardiac surgery. *Ann. Thorac. Surg.*, **38**, 117.

Normann N.A. (1976). Thermodilution technique for cardiac output. *N. Engl. J. Med.*, **295**, 48.

Oka Y., Matsumoto M., Orkin L.R. et al. (1980. *Am. J. Cardiol.*, **46**, 95.

Olsson B., Pool J., Vandermoten P. et al. (1970). Validity and reproducibility of determination of cardiac output by thermodilution in man. *Cardiology.*, **55**, 136.

Osborn J.J., Russell J.A.G., Beaumont J. et al. (1968). The measurement of relative stroke volume from aortic pulse contour or pulse pressure. *Vasc. Dis.*, **5**, 165.

Peronneau P.A., Pellet M.M., Xhaard M.C. et al. (1971). Pulsed Doppler ultrasonic blood flowmeter. Real-time instantaneous velocity profiles. In *Flow, its Measurement and Control in Science and Industry.* vol. 1, p. 1367. (Dowdell R.B., ed.). Pittsburgh Instrument Society of America.

Power E.W., Fraser W.W. (1978). Laser Doppler measurement of blood flow in microcirculation. *Plast. Reconstruct. Surg.*, **11**, 250.

Powner D.J., Snyder J.V. (1978). *In vitro* comparison of six commercially available thermodilution cardiac output systems. *Med. Instrum.*, **12**, 122.

Prys-Roberts C. (1977). Monitoring of the cardiovascular system. In *Monitoring in Anesthesia*. (Saidman L.J., Smith N. Ty. eds.). New York: John Wiley.

Reiniger E.J. (1976). Error in thermodilution cardiac output measurement caused by variation in syringe volume. *Cathet. Cardiovasc. Diag.*, **2**, 415.

Runciman W.B., Ilsley A.H., Roberts J.G. (1981). Thermodilution cardiac output—a systematic error. *Anaesth. Intens. Care.*, **9**, 135.

Rushmer R.F., Franklin D.L., Ellis R.M. (1956). Left ventricular dimensions recorded by sonocardiometry. *Circ. Res.*, **4**, 684.

Schiller N.B., Acquatella H., Ports T.A. et al. (1979). Left ventricular volume from paired biplane two-dimensional echocardiography. *Circulation*, **60**, 547 (10E).

Schuster A.H., Nanda N.C. (1984). Doppler echocardiographic measurement of cardiac output: comparison with a non-golden standard. *Am. J. Cardiol.*, **53**, 257.

Sequeira R.F., Light L.H., Cross G. et al. (1976). Transcutaneous aortovelography. A quantitative evaluation. *Br. Heart J.*, **38**, 443.

Smith N. Ty. (1969). Cardiac function evaluation. In *Techniques in Clinical Physiology—A Survey of Measurements in Anesthesiology.* p. 125–176. (Bellville, J.W., Weaver C. eds.) New York: Macmillan.

Smith N. Ty. (1978). Noninvasive beat-to-beat blood pressure and cardiac output. *Sci. Abstr. Annu. Meet. Am. Soc. Anesthesiol.* p. 31.

Smith N. Ty. (1980). Myocardial function and anaesthesia. In *The Circulation and Anaesthesia*, p. 57–114. (Prys-Roberts C. ed.). Oxford: Blackwell.

Smith N. Ty., Smith P.C. (1976). The BCG for measuring cardiac output in Californian grey whale. *Biblio. Cardiol.*, **35**, 129.

Smith N. Ty., Wesseling K.H., Weber J.A.P. et al. (1974). Preliminary evaluation of a pulse contour cardiac output computer in man. Feasibility of brachial or radial arterial pressures. *Proc. San Diego Biomed. Symp.*, **13**, 113.

Snell R.E., Clements J.M., Patel D.J. et al. (1965). Instantaneous blood flow in the human aorta. *J. Appl. Physiol.*, **20**, 691 (A).

Snyder J.V., Powner D.J. (1982). Effects of mechanical ventilation on the measurement of cardiac output by thermodilution. *Crit. Care Med.*, **10**, 677.

Starr I., Schnabe R.G., Askovitz S.E. et al. (1954). On the relation between pulse pressure and cardiac stroke volume, leading to a clinical method of estimating output from blood pressure and age. *Circulation*, **9**, 648.

Steingart R.M., Melker J., Barovick J. (1980). Pulsed Doppler echocardiography: measurement of beat-to-beat change in stroke volume in dogs. *Circulation*, **62**, 542.

Strauss H.W., Zaret B.E., Hurley P.F. et al. (1971). A scintiphotographic method for measuring left ventricular ejection fraction in man without cardiac catheterization. *Am. J. Cardiol.*, **28**, 575.

Tremper K.K. (1987). Continuous noninvasive cardiac output: are we getting there? Editorial. *Crit. Care Med.*, **15**, 278–9.

Tremper K.K., Hufstedler S.M., Barker S.J. et al. (1986). Continuous noninvasive estimation of cardiac output by electrical bioimpedance: an experimental study in dogs. *Crit. Care Med.*, **14**, 231.

Waxman K., Formosa P., Soliman H. et al. (1987). Laser Doppler velocimetry in critically ill patients. *Crit. Care Med.*, **15**, 780.

Wesseling K.H., Purschke R., Smith N.T. et al. (1976). A beat-to-beat cardiac output computer for clinical monitoring. In *Real Time Computing in Patient Management*. p. 32–112 (Payne J.P., Hill D.W. eds.). Stevenage: Peter Peregrinus Ltd.

Wesseling K.H., Smith N. Ty., Nichols W.W. et al. (1974a). A small beat-to-beat cardiac output computer. *Proc. San Diego Biomed. Symp.*, **13**, 107.

Wesseling K.H., Smith N. Ty., Nichols W.W. et al. (1974b). Beat-to-beat cardiac output from the arterial pressure pulse contour. In *Measurement in Anaesthesia*. p. 150–164. (Feldman S.A., Leigh J.M., Spierdijk J. eds.). Leiden: Leiden University Press.

Wesseling K.H., Smith N. Ty., Purschke R. et al. (1981). The pulse contour cardiac output computer is probably as accurate as the clinical Fick indicator-dilution methods. *Acta d' Anesthesiolgie.* In press.

Wilmore J.H., Farrell P.A., Norton A.C. et al. (1982). An automated, indirect assessment of cardiac output during rest and exercise. *Am. Physiol. Soc.* 1493.

Wong D.H., Tremper K.K., Hadjuczek J. et al. (1987). Noninvasive preoperative cardiovascular assessment and intraoperative hypotension. *Anesth. Analg.*, **66**, S1–S189.

Zhang Y., Nitter-Hauge S., Ihlen H. et al. (1985). Doppler echocardiographic measurement of cardiac output using the mitral orifice method. *Br. Heart J.*, **53**, 130.

7. The Measurement of Gas Flow and Volume
B. A. Willis and J. N. Lunn

THEORETICAL CONSIDERATIONS

This chapter considers some of the principles and methods used in anaesthesia to measure gas volume and volume flow rate. The methods are considered for convenience in the same sequence as the anaesthetic gases flow, i.e., from Boyle's machine to patient and from patient to atmosphere. Several initial points should be considered before the methods of measurement are discussed.

Units

The Système Internationale unit of volume is the cubic metre (m^3), that of time the second (s) so that $m^3 s^{-1}$ is the SI unit of volume flow rate. In anaesthesia volumes are conventionally and conveniently measured in litres (L) and millilitres (ml), time in minutes and volume flow rates in L/min or ml/min respectively. There are 1000 L in 1 m^3.

Pressure is conventionally measured in mmHg or cmH$_2$O, the SI unit being newton/m² or pascal (Pa). When converting one unit to another remember that:

1 Atmosphere (100%) = 101 kPa
                    = 1000 cmH$_2$O
                    = 760 mmHg.

So that (to within 1%) 1 kPa = 1%
                               = 10 cmH$_2$O
                               = 7.6 mmHg.

Velocity and Flow Rate

Consider the flow of gas along a uniform tube of cross-sectional area A, the flow rate being constant (Fig. 7.1). The quantum of gas, which was at point X

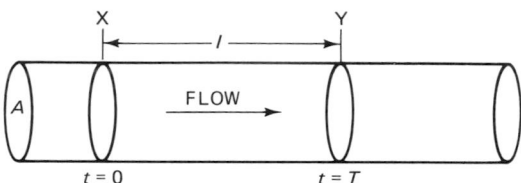

Fig. 7.1 Flow through a uniform tube.

at time $t = 0$, reaches point Y, a distance l along the tube at time, T. The velocity of the gas along the tube is l/T whereas the volume flow rate is the volume of gas which has passed X in unit time.

$$= \frac{lA}{T} = \frac{V}{T}$$

where $V = lA$ and is the volume of tube between X and Y.

Volume is usually represented by the symbol V and volume flow rate, which is a rate of change of volume, by $\dot{V}$ or dV/dt.

Laminar and Turbulent Flow

The velocity vector profiles for laminar and turbulent flows through uniform tubes are shown in Figs. 7.2a and 2b respectively. Under laminar flow conditions the velocity is zero at the walls and maximum axially.

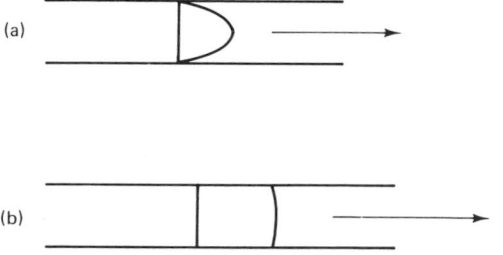

Fig. 7.2 Velocity vector profiles for laminar and turbulent flows.

Flow occurs according to the Poiseuille equation:

$$\dot{V} = \frac{\pi r^4 \Delta P}{8 \eta \, l}$$

Where $\dot{V}$ = volume flow rate
  ΔP = pressure difference across a length l of uniform tube, radius r
  η = viscosity coefficient

which means that for a given tube the volume flow rate increases linearly with the applied pressure (note the analogy between laminar flow and Ohm's law).

Under turbulent flow conditions Poiseuille's Law no longer applies. The Reynolds number is a dimensionless quantity whose magnitude gives some indication of whether flow is likely to be laminar or turbulent.

$$Re = \frac{\text{mean velocity} \times \text{density} \times \text{diameter}}{\text{viscosity}}$$

Re < 2000, flow is likely to be laminar
Re > 2500, flow is likely to be turbulent

Turbulent flow may be initiated by changes in diameter of the tubing, as in corrugated tubing, or by changes in direciton of flow, as in suction tracheal tube connectors and, once initiated, turbulence continues downstream.

Flow Through an Orifice

In contrast to laminar flow through a tube which is dependent on the viscosity of the gas flowing, flow through an orifice (which may be considered to be a special form of tube whose radius is much greater than its length) depends on the square root of the density of the gas, as well as on the area of the orifice and the square root of the applied pressure. It is, however, relatively independent of viscosity.

The Relationship between Volume and Volume Flow Rate

If a constant gas flow of 6 L/min occurs for 5 min, it is a simple calculation that a total volume of 30 L is released. Graphically this constant flow may be represented by the line ab in Fig. 7.3 and the product of

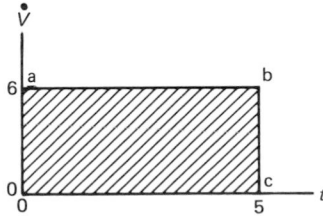

Fig. 7.3 Example of flow rate *vs* time graph.

6 L/min and 5 min (= ab × bc) is represented by the shaded area. In a similar manner any graph of flow versus time may be used to calculate the volume of gas which has flowed. If the flow rate is a continuously varying function of time, the area may be calculated by a variety of methods, some of which are outlined in Chapter 6.

Mathematically the relationship is expressed as:

$$V = \int \dot{V} \, dt$$

or

volume = sum (or integral) × time products
of all the flow rate   under the curve.

In a similar way if a gas source produces 10 L of gas in 2 min, it is an elementary calculation that the average flow rate is 5 L/min.

This may be represented graphically (*see* Fig. 7.4) showing a graph of volume *vs* time, where

point p represents $V = 0$ at $t = 0$ min, and
point q represents $V = 10$ at $t = 2$ min

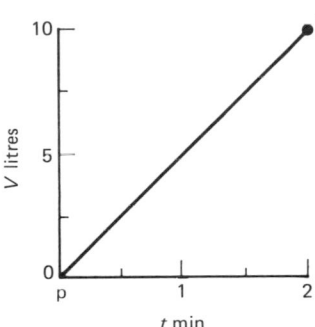

Fig. 7.4 Example of volume *vs* time graph.

The intuitive solution that the flow rate is 5 L/min is the slope or gradient of the line pq, i.e. pq = 10/2 L/min. If the volume is not a linear function of time then the volume flow rate is the gradient of a line drawn as a tangent to the curve at the relevant time. Mathematically this is expressed as:

$$\text{Volume flow} = \dot{V} = \frac{dV}{dt}$$

GAS FLOW INTO THE BREATHING SYSTEM—CONTINUOUS FLOW

Flowmeters are devices which measure volume flow rate either directly or indirectly, i.e., they have an output dependent on volume flow rate. The majority of the commonly used flowmeters take indirect readings and so accurate calibration is essential. Most flowmeters may be classified as being either constant pressure or constant orifice devices.

Constant Pressure Flowmeters
(sometimes called variable orifice).

The most commonly encountered examples of this group are the Rotameters found on the Boyle's machine (Fig. 7.5). The bobbin, with fluted edges to

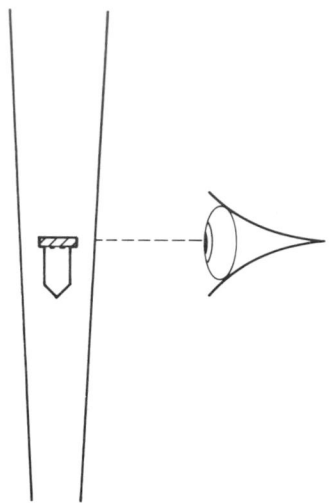

Fig. 7.5 The Rotameter constant-pressure flowmeter.

encourage rotation is supported by the gas flow through a glass tube whose bore is wider at the top than at the bottom. The greater the flow, the higher the bobbin is forced up the tube, though the pressure difference across the bobbin remains constant. This is because the bobbin has constant mass and therefore has a constant gravitational force acting on it.

Gas flow through a Rotameter may be laminar or turbulent. When at low flows, the bobbin is at the lower end of the tapered tube, the area of the annulus around the bobbin is relatively small compared with the length of the annulus (i.e., the length of the bobbin) and flow is predominantly laminar and therefore dependent on the viscosity of the gas. When the bobbin is at the upper end of the tapered tube at high flows the annulus around the bobbin has a greater area compared with its length, approximating to flow through an orifice and is therefore density dependent. (Most Rotameter tubes have two different tapers so that precision at low flows remains compatible with an ability to measure large flow rates.)

This explanation is grossly oversimplified and ignores the turbulence which occurs immediately above the bobbin at all flows, but does explain why a flowmeter calibrated under specified conditions of temperature and pressure for one gas may not be used with any degree of accuracy for a different gas or under different conditions due to differences in viscosity and density.

Other factors which may render Rotameters inaccurate are listed as follows.

1. Non vertical mounting which may result in the bobbin tilting to touch the walls of the tube.
2. Dirt within the Rotameter tube which may cause the bobbin to stick.
3. Static electricity which may cause the bobbin to adhere to the wall of the tube or stop rotating. (Clutton–Brock, 1972). Modern conducting tubing obviates this problem on Boyle's machine but the plastic O_2 flowmeters used on wards may be inaccurate due to static charge (Richardson and Shaw, 1986).
4. Leaks within the flowmeter due to cracked tubes or faulty joints between tube and Rotameter block.
5. Back pressure due to the flow from the Rotameter being used to drive a ventilator, humidifier or nebulizer. The indicated volume flow rate is reduced although the actual volume flow rate at atmospheric pressure is affected minimally.
6. Translocation of flowmeter tubes during routine service (Bird, 1985).

On modern Boyle's machines the flowmeters are stated to have an accuracy of $\pm 5\%$ of the indicated flow $\pm 0.5\%$ of the maximum flow rate.

Constant Orifice Flowmeters
(sometimes called variable pressure)

In this type there is a progressive increase in pressure drop, with increasing rates of flow, across a restriction in a tube. Pressure gauges (Bourdon) or water manometers (Foregger) are calibrated to indicate flow rate. The restriction is either a long narrow tube (Fig. 7.6a) so that the pressure drop is proportional to flow rate, or an orifice (Fig. 7.6b) in which case the pressure drop is proportional to the square of flow rate. The magnitude of this pressure difference can be shown to be related to the ratio between the diameters of the tubes and of the constriction (Ower and Pankhurst, 1966).

The pressures generated by a constant orifice flowmeter may be measured with relatively insensitive instruments, e.g., a water manometer, whose slow response time is no disadvantage if a constant flow rate is to be monitored.

The venturi tube (Fig. 7.6c) can be regarded as a

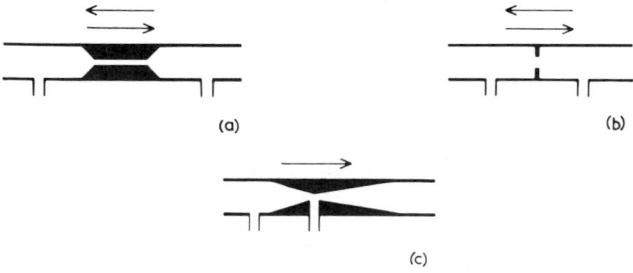

Fig. 7.6 Diagram of the airflow resistances of constant-orifice flowmeters: (a) Tube; (b) Orifice; (c) Venturi.

compromise between the tube and orifice type of airflow resistance. The acceleration of gas molecules through the throat of the venturi results in a loss of pressure which is compared with the pressure upstream from the constriction of the venturi tube. In a perfect venturi, the downstream pressure is equal to the upstream pressure.

Other Flowmeters

An alternative, and earlier version of a constant-pressure flowmeter (Coxeter, Fig. 7.7a) is one in which

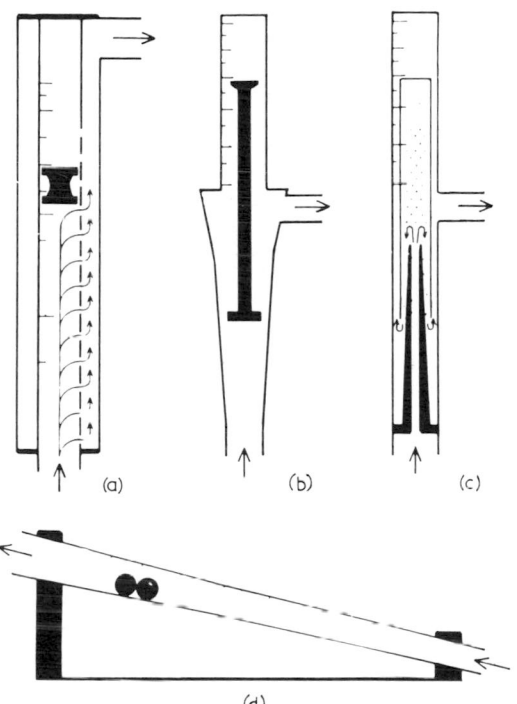

Fig. 7.7 Diagram of constant-pressure flowmeters (a) Coxeter; (b) Heidbrink; (c) McKesson; (d) Connell.

the escape of gas from the measuring tube is through a series of holes. The tube has parallel sides and, in this case, the bobbin rises up the tube to the point which reveals the appropriate number of holes to allow the gas to escape. This arrangement results in the bobbin being forced up the tube at fixed increments of flow and precludes precise measurement of flow between any two points.

Other flowmeters (Heidbrink; McKesson, Figs. 7.7b and c) have been manufactured whose internal dimensions change rapidly. This means that a wide range of flows can be metered by one tube albeit with some loss of precision. In another design (Connell, Fig. 7.7d) the tube is inclined and gas flow is indicated by the position of two ball-bearings. It was originally claimed that the second ball-bearing eliminated oscillation but in modern incline-flowmeters the

single ball-bearing does not oscillate noticeably. The Water-sight flowmeter Fig. 7.8a is both a variable pressure and a variable orifice device. A tube with a series of holes dips into water. As flow increases, the pressure in the tube increases and the number of orifices through which gas flows increase. The number of holes in use approximately indicates the volume flow rate; the extent of the error of this flowmeter can be seen in Fig. 7.8b.

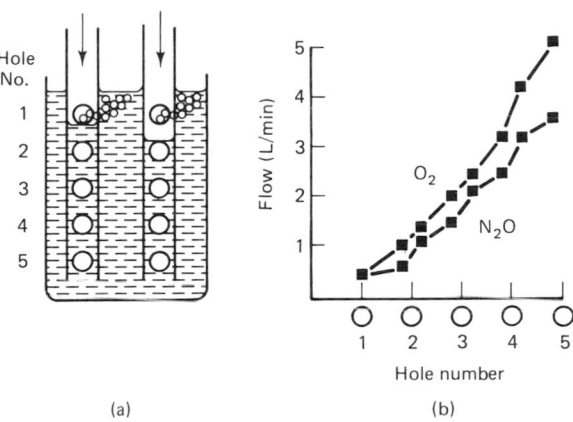

(a) (b)

Fig. 7.8 (a) The watersight flowmeter showing the variation of flow rate possible at one indicated flow rate. (b) Calibration curve for watersight flowmeter.

There are many different forms of airflow resistance. An orifice may be either a hole in a flat plate or a nozzle with tapering sides. The orifice may be prolonged into a tube or the nozzle and tube may be combined in a venturi. Other forms of airflow resistance are mentioned in connection with pneumotachography. Details of design, including the sites and sizes of points for pressure sensing in relation to the airflow resistance, are beyond the scope of this chapter: minimal standards have been published by the British Standards Institution.

GAS FLOW WITHIN THE BREATHING SYSTEM—INTERMITTENT FLOW

In intermittent flow the volume flow rate is changing rapidly and therefore a fast-response system is essential if the changes are to be followed faithfully.

Pneumotachography

A pneumotachograph is a fast-response measuring system based on a form of constant-orifice flowmeter It consists of a pneumatic resistance, across which a pressure difference is generated when gas flow occurs, and a means of measuring that pressure difference.

There are a number of designs of airflow resistance which are suitable. Most of these are essentially bundles of small bore tubes placed longitudinally in the gas flow. These provide a linear resistance so that pressure drop varies directly with flow rate, in accordance with the Poiseuille Law.

In one design (the Fleisch pneumotachograph Fig. 7.9) two corrugated strips of metal foil are wound

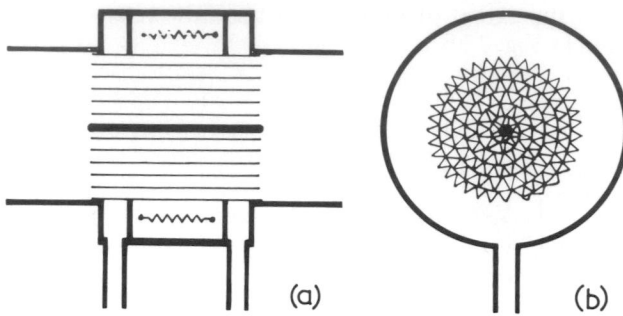

Fig. 7.9 Diagram of Fleisch pneumotachograph airflow resistance: (a) longitudinal section; (b) transverse section through the pressure sensing connection.

coaxially around a central rod producing a large number of linear pneumatic resistances in parallel. The pressure difference across the net resistance is measured using a differential pressure transducer and is dependent on flow rate. The purpose of the heating element in this particular instrument is to prevent water condensation which would change the sensitivity of the instrument in an unpredictable manner. Another design is a single orifice plate which causes a pressure drop proportional to the square of the flow rate. Mesh screens are also used as linear airflow resistances.

In pneumotachographs, which can be, and often are, connected to the patient's airway, care is taken to keep the pressure drop as small as possible. This not only helps to maintain laminar flow, but also avoids imposing additional airway resistance upon the patient.

The pressure drop increases linearly as the flow increases at first, but later, due to turbulence, non-linearity occurs. The useful range of airflow resistances is therefore limited at low flows by the small pressure differences and at high flows by non-linearity. Pneumotachographs have therefore to be constructed specifically for the particular range of flows to be measured. The wider the range of flows the greater the departure from exact proportionality and, even within the designated range, each airflow resistance becomes marginally non-linear at the higher flowrates. Any distortion of the resistance by condensate, damage or dirt will of course further alter this relationship. The requirement to select an appropriate airflow resistance for all anticipated flow rates is clear. It is important to remember in this selection that the highest, or peak, rate of flow is much greater than the average flow. In sinusoidal flow, the peak flow is

about three (π) times the average flow, taken over the complete cycle. In measuring a flow rate which declines exponentially (expiratory flow) the rate is initially at least ten times the average flow.

The airflow resistance in the expired gas pathway is at a temperature close to that of room temperature and is cooler than the warm moist gas that passes through, so that condensation occurs unless preventive measures are taken; the increase in pressure drop caused by condensation is particularly troublesome with metal screens, but the use of plastic has reduced this effect. Wide mesh screens also reduce the effect of condensation particularly when provision is made for drainage. Commercial airflow resistances are usually calibrated in terms of pressure drop per unit flow rate by the manufacturer, but this calibration should be repeated under the conditions of use if any meaningful measurements are to be made.

The pressure difference created by the airflow resistance is usually very small, of the order of 1–2 mm H_2O (0.01–0.02 kPa) and is sensed by a differential pressure transducer whose electrical output is then amplified and displayed. The differential pressure transducer should be selected carefully and matched with the pneumatic resistance in order that signal distortion is minimized.

Errors as great as 25–50% of the flow signal may occur during intermittent positive pressure ventilation of neonates with grossly abnormal lungs (Kafer, 1973). A similar error occurs when screens which buckle are used as airflow resistances during intermittent positive pressure ventilation.

In order to use a pneumotachograph for the measurement of volume, integration, either by electronic or graphic means, must be performed.

Other Flowmeters for Use during Intermittent Flow

Flow measuring devices utilizing a venturi to cause a measurable pressure difference can be used in reciprocating flow to record volumes in both directions (Ventigrator). Unfortunately this system generates turbulent flow and the small pressure drop at the lower flow rates gives low sensitivity but the large pressure differences at high flow rates increase sensitivity (Nunn and Ezi-Ashi, 1962). In addition, changes in the density of the gases affect the pressure drop considerably.

The rate of cooling (during inspiration) or warming (during expiration) of a thermistor has been used in a respiration monitor, particularly for small children (Millar et al., 1963) but this has not been made quantitative. The current required to maintain the temperature of the thermistor constant varies with the rate of flow which passes through it. One device, based on this phenomenon, was reported to have gross over-reading errors at small tidal volumes and the reverse at large tidal volumes: this is potentially very unsafe (Visick et al., 1971).

A thermistor is also used in the fluidic spirometer

(Fig. 7.10). This is a measuring instrument which has no moving parts and utilizes the Coanda effect. Gas entering the device escapes through either Channel A or B and the Bernouilli effect causes a subatmospheric pressure at the orifice of the small contralateral control channel so that there is no difference in pressure between points C and D. Gas flow occurs in the control channel which is sensed by the thermistor. Gas then escapes through the other channel (A or B) and the small flow in the control channel reverses. The volume of gas which passes through the main channel sufficient to cause oscillation in the control channel is, according to the manufacturers, constant at 17 ml. It is claimed that neither the nature of the gas nor the presence of water vapour affects the accuracy of this device which is also claimed to be better than 5% (Hedenstierna et al., 1976).

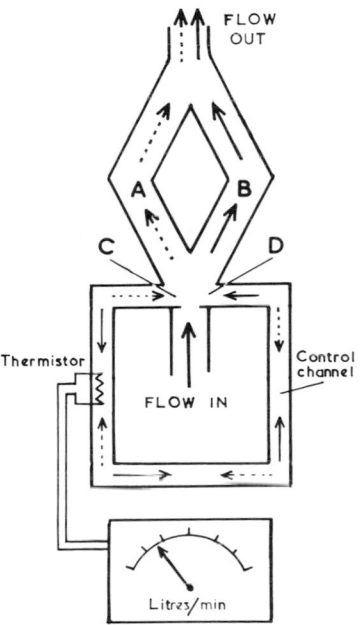

Fig. 7.10 The Fluidic spirometer (*see* text). When gas flow passes through channel A the flow follows the dotted arrow pathway in the control channel because the pressure at D is less than at C.

The speed of transmission of sound between a fixed transmitter and fixed receiver is dependent upon the velocity of air passing between them, this is the basis of an ultrasonic flowmeter which is incorporated into a system for lung function testing (Biomedical Engineering, 1969). This is unaffected by the pressure of the gas flow and less affected than other instruments by the composition of the gas mixture.

Anemometers

These are devices which are used in meteorology to measure wind speed and also to indicate direction.

There are many different designs for example, the cup, the swinging plate, the Pitot tube and the vane. The cup anemometer is bulky; it has three or four cups mounted so that they are filled sequentially with gas and cause the rotation of an indicator. The swinging plate anemometer is mounted vertically on knife edges and is deflected by the current of gas—the angle of inclination of the plate being proportional to the speed of gas flow. Neither of these two anemometers is known to have been applied to anaesthesia. The vane anemometer (c.f. windmill) has a number of flat plates attached to radial rods. These rods cause a spindle to rotate which carries a pointer to indicate rate of rotation.

Anemometers are commonly placed in anaesthetic or breathing systems to measure minute volume in situations where reciprocating flow is occurring although they may only respond to flow from one direction, e.g., the Wright respirometer.

Wright Respirometer

This is a modified vane anemometer; a single plate or vane is mounted on a rotor between jewelled bearings. A stator is necessary to direct the gas onto the vane (Fig. 7.11). It is cylindrical in shape and has a number

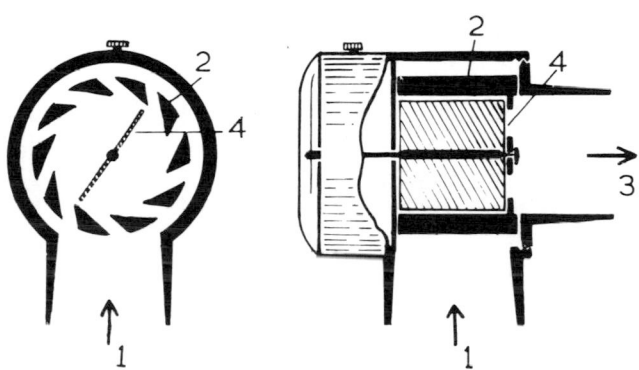

Fig. 7.11 Diagram of the Wright Respirometer. (1) Gas inlet; (2) Stator with slots; (3) Gas outlet; (4) Vane. (Reproduced with permission from W. W. Mushin et al. (1980). *Automatic Ventilation of the Lungs*, 3rd edn., p. 46. Oxford: Blackwell Scientific Publications.)

of slots cut through it; these have the effect of directing the gas onto the periphery of the vane. The rotation of the vane is transmitted through a system of gears to pointers moving over the dials. This latter mechanism is protected from moisture by a mercury seal which is vulnerable to damage. The vane does not move in response to flow in the reverse direction because there is no stator to deflect the gas. Vanes of this type respond to wind speed or velocity and therefore the volume displayed is dependent upon factors which alter velocity. When the gas passes through the slots in the stator its velocity changes. The velocity here bears a relationship, though not necessarily a linear one, to the volume which has passed.

There is 'slippage' at low flow rates and the vane is guaranteed to begin to rotate at less than 2.5 L/min. It is calibrated by the manufacturers by continuous flows of air (16 and 60 L/min). Thus, if the ventilation volumes which are to be measured are small, the respirometer under-reads the volume. Conversely, when the flow rates are great, inertial effects cause the vane to continue to rotate after the flow of gas has ceased and the respirometer over-reads.

A paediatric version of the Wright meter is available which reduces errors at low tidal volumes.

Changes in the composition of gas mixtures, in humidity, in instantaneous rates of gas flow and damage by rough handling (not to say dropping), all impose limitations on the accuracy of this device (Nunn et al., 1962; Lunn et al., 1970). Nevertheless for clinical purposes its use is justifiably widespread. The Dräger volumeter (Fig. 7.12) responds to flow in two

light shining upon the photoelectric cell is intermittently interrupted by the vane as it rotates producing a square-wave output whose frequency depends on the gas flow rate and the total number of square waves depends on the volume of gas passing through the meter. The output of the cell is processed electronically and either tidal volume or minute volume may be displayed. The vane has been strengthened by corrugations in order that, it is claimed, flows between 1.5 litres per minute and 300 litres per minute may be detected (Cox et al., 1974). The electronic anemometer is calibrated by sine-wave flow of air at a frequency of 20 cycles/min; it tends to under-read at frequencies below this and over-read at higher frequencies. An overall accuracy in clinical use of within 2% ± 1% of full scale deflection is claimed.

Another vane anemometer (Spiroflo, Fig. 7.13)

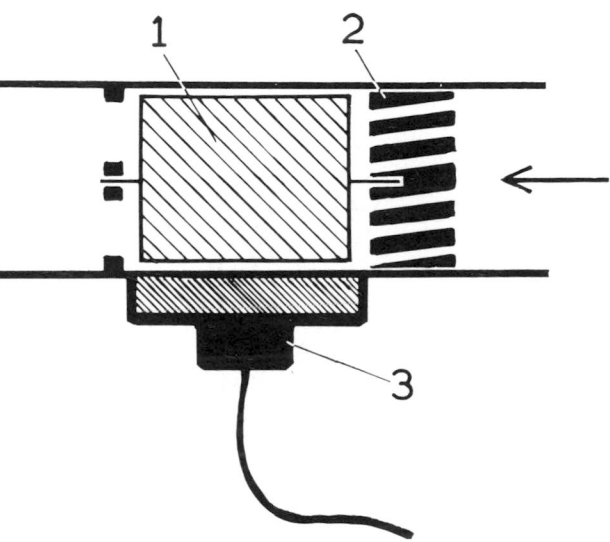

Fig. 7.13 Diagram of the Spiroflo. (1) vane; (2) stator (swirlplate); (3) transducer.

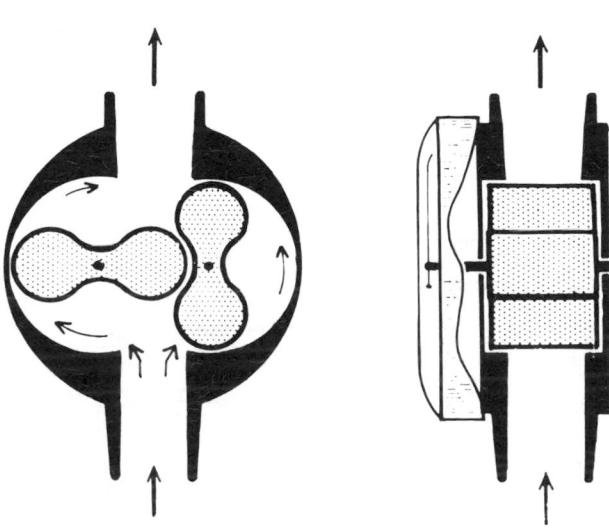

Fig. 7.12 Diagram of the Dräger Volumeter. (Reproduced with permission from W. W. Mushin et al. (1980). *Automatic Ventilation of the Lungs*, 3rd edn., p. 47. Oxford: Blackwell Scientific Publications.)

directions and consists of two rotors which interlock. Although this instrument is more accurate and larger than the respirometer, it is also more expensive and is affected by moisture.

Electronic Anemometers

Graphical recording of ventilation is impossible with either of the two anemometers described. In order to minimize some of the disadvantages mentioned above and to provide this facility, recent improvements in design have been made. In electronic versions of the Wright respirometer detection of the rotation of the vane is achieved by means of a photoelectric cell. The

with a stator which causes the gas to swirl onto the vane mounted in the axis of the gas flow uses a different method of detection. In this case the electrical output of a capacitance transducer is proportional to flow rate and tidal or minute volume can be displayed. It is this device which was found within the Cape 2000 ventilator.

It is claimed for both these electronic anemometers that they are not only less vulnerable to physical damage but also less affected by moisture than the non-electronic versions. Both instruments can be battery-operated and provide facility for graphical recording; in addition the necessity, during minute volume determinations, for independent timing is removed.

General Problems of Flow Measurement

Some of the sources of inaccuracy have already been

considered in relation to specific instruments but there are others which have a more general interest and importance. One of the major factors is whether the flow is laminar or turbulent. The calculation of Reynolds number which estimates which type of flow is likely to occur under specified conditions has already been mentioned.

In laminar flow the pressure drop, and therefore the indicated flow rate, is influenced by the viscosity of the gas. Viscous forces are those shearing forces within a moving column of air or other fluid. When exerted against the boundaries of a tube it is as if these forces were causing the air to adhere to the walls. Thus under laminar flow conditions if two gases have similar viscosities, e.g., helium and oxygen, approximately equal flowrates will be recorded. Under turbulent flow conditions the effect of density predominates and equal flowrates of gases with differing densities will not be recorded as being equal. This is the factor which prevents flowmeters being interchanged and produces errors should a flowmeter be used for anything but the designated gas. The density of a gas is affected by ambient temperature and pressure; viscosity is affected by the former only. Bobbin flowmeters are calibrated at designated temperatures (usually 15°C or 20°C) and pressures; in precise work, corrections are made to allow for variations in temperature or ambient pressure.

Under hyperbaric conditions the difference between indicated and actual flow through a bobbin flowmeter becomes clinically important because the density of gas is increased (McDowall, 1964). (The actual flow of gas at 2 atm is 71% of that indicated).

An increase in temperature of 1°C, between 20°C and 40°C, increases the viscosity of a gas by about 0.2% (Grenvik et al., 1966); this is unlikely to be important clinically but is important in investigations which use pneumotachography to measure the differences between inspired and expired volumes (Smith, 1964; Hobbes, 1967). Some bobbin flowmeters (gap meters) are scaled without reference to a particular gas and calibration charts are available for different gases.

GAS FLOW IN THE BREATHING SYSTEM— VOLUME

Measurement of the minute volume ventilation of anaesthetized patients is carried out conventionally on the expired gases. Were such measurements to be made on the inspiratory gases, leaks between the site of measurement and the patient would result in the minute-volume being overestimated, in addition leakage from the expiratory limb of the anaesthetic system is likely to be less than from the inspiratory limb, which is at a higher pressure. An underestimate of expiration is less hazardous clinically than an overestimate of inspiration.

In the laboratory, measurement of gas volumes may be made to a high degree of accuracy by the use of water displacement from calibrated vessels. For obvious reasons this method is not used in anaesthetic practice but it remains of fundamental use. Gas has first to be collected into air tight containers such as a Douglas bag. The contents can then be passed from the bag through a variety of gas meters or spirometers. Corrections must be applied for atmospheric conditions (water vapour, barometric pressure and temperature) and for losses through the walls of such bags which, in the case of a polyvinyl chloride bag (60 cm²; 0.25 mm thick), may amount to 200 ml/h of a mixture of 80% nitrous oxide in oxygen (Cooper, 1959).

Spirometers

The general design of these (Fig. 7.14) is a double walled cylindrical chamber, containing water in the space between the walls, with a light-weight cylinder bell inverted over it so that the water forms an airtight seal for the contents of the bell. The weight of the cylinder is balanced by a counter-weight or weights suspended over a pulley system. A pen may be used to make a recording on a rotating drum.

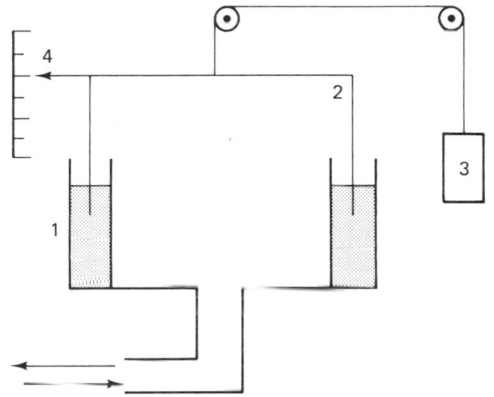

Fig. 7.14 The Spirometer showing: (1) cylindrical chamber; (2) cylinder bell; (3) counter weight; (4) pen.

Systems which have mechanical parts are prone to inaccuracy from inertia. Smoothly running pulleys are essential and many ingenious methods are used to overcome this problem. Once moving, the bell may fail to stop at the instant at which gas ceases to enter it, and an overestimate of volume will be recorded or the bell may oscillate. A significant depression of the water level can occur with high rates of gas inflow which will cause the gas to be exposed to a positive pressure. A further problem is the correct, leak-free, function of all valves in the system.

There are a number of different spirometers each of which has a special use but, in general, spirometers are of limited value during anaesthesia because of the need to supply fresh anaesthetic gases to the system and to absorb carbon dioxide. The traditional bag-in-box system has been adapted (Nunn, 1956) so that spirometers can be used satisfactorily in anaesthetic systems during spontaneous ventilation; an equivalent volume to the fresh gas flow is removed from the measuring system by continuous suction.

Volume of expired gas can be collected readily from the expiratory ports of automatic ventilators and there is no absolute need for complex apparatus at this point of application. Plastic bags can be used to collect gas and when these are filled to an appropriate extent it can be shown that their calibration, which relates their length to their volume, can be sufficiently satisfactory for repeatable measurements to be made (Cooper and Pask, 1960). It is of course also possible to pass this gas through dry gas meters.

Dry Spirometers

These are much more convenient to use but demand the highest standards of construction. The gas collection vessel is often a wedge-shaped bellows with plastic sides. These bellows must be light enough to allow a rapid response and also to avoid an increase in pressure within the system (back-pressure). The maximum back-pressure should not exceed 0.15 kPa in order to avoid errors in volume determinations (Cotes, 1966).

Special-purpose Spirometers

Special adaptations of these spirometers exist which incorporate timing devices so that forced expiratory volumes within specified times can be recorded. It is clearly essential that inertia be low and it is suggested that movement of the bellows should commence after 100 ml has entered them (Cotes, 1966). Movement of the pen carriage is triggered by movement of the bellows. One such spirometer is the Vitalograph (Fig. 7.15a), which, is spite of having a high inertia and failing to meet minimal requirements regarding

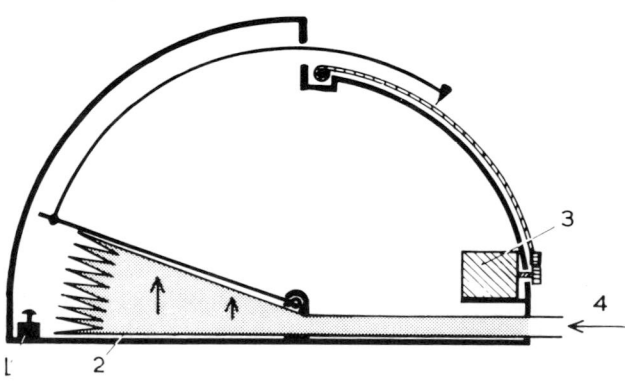

Fig. 7.15a Diagram of the Vitalograph. (1) switch released by movement of the bellows; (2) book bellows; (3) motor which drives the chart; (4) gas inlet into the book bellows.

back-pressure (Drew and Hughes, 1969), is widely used. There is another spirometer (McDermott) which meets these specifications (Collins et al., 1964).

However, it must be freely admitted that precision instruments, which are more costly, may not be justified in clinical work. Assuming that vital capacity is measured with the same instrument as is used for forced expiratory volume in one second (FEV_1) then the clinically useful relationship of FEV_1 as percentage of vital capacity (VC) will be less serious in error.

Note. In the interpretation of the Vitalograph output (Fig. 7.15b) the recording showing the maximum FEV_1 and FVC should be used since this is

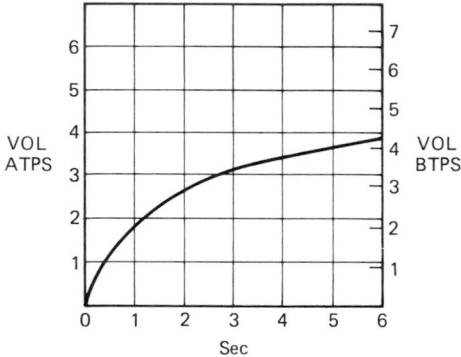

Fig. 7.15b The Vitalogram.

likely to approximate most closely to the physiological state of the individual being assessed. In calculating the ratio FEV_1 to FVC, both measurements of volume must be taken from the same vertical scale.

(The volumes at ATPS and BTPS are given on the left and right vertical scales respectively). The ratio will be the same for a given individual whichever scale is used, but errors will arise should the measurements be taken from different scales.

Peak Flow Measurement

Peak expiratory flow may be measured using a calibrated pneumotachograph, but for convenience in the ward the Wright peak flowmeter (Fig. 7.16) is preferred (Wright and McKerrow, 1959). The vane is forced around on its horizontal axis by the expiratory flow and a gradually increasing pathway is opened up for the expired gas to escape to the atmosphere through an annular slot. The vane carries with it the brake disc and its rotation is resisted by the slight tension of a spiral spring. After the reading has been made, the brake disc is released by a push button whose action is to dislodge the floating disc so that the vane and the pointer are returned to the zero stop by the spiral spring. The miniature Wright peak flow-

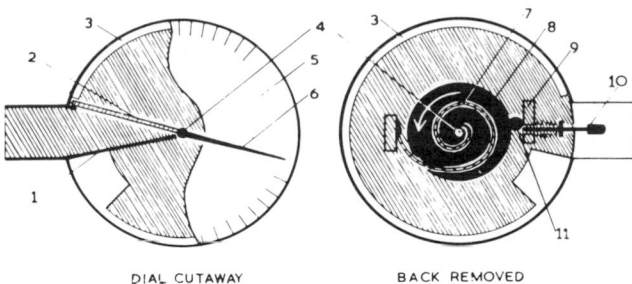

Fig. 7.16 Diagram of the Wright peak flowmeter. (1) fixed plate to direct gas; (2) vane; (3) annular slot; (4) shaft; (5) dial; (6) pointer; (7) spiral spring; (8) brake disc; (9) fixed block; (10) push button zeroing knob; (11) floating disc.

meter (Wright, 1978) (Fig. 7.17) is a less cumbersome version of the Wright peak flowmeter. It consists of a light spring loaded piston mounted coaxially within a tube having a longitudinal slot as the variable orifice. Expired gases blown into the instrument are able to escape by moving the piston and passing through a length of the slot which depends on the flow rate. The

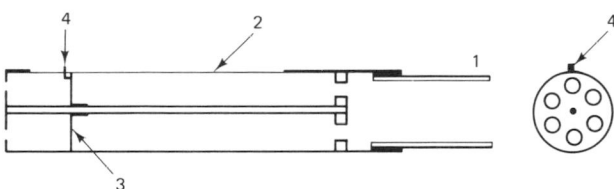

Fig. 7.17 The miniature Wright Peak flowmeter showing: (1) mouth piece; (2) linear slot; (3) light piston; (4) indicator.

piston carries an indicator which runs in the slot and so measures peak flow indirectly on an external scale. Fisher and Shaw (1980) performed calibration studies on conventional and miniature Wright peak flowmeters. Agreement between the calibration flow rate and meter reading was poorest at low flows and was worse for the miniature meter than the Wright peak flowmeter. They concluded that whereas reasonable comparison of measurements taken with different Wright peak flowmeters on the same patient may be made, they did not recommend comparing peak flows measured on different mini peak flow meters at flow rates less than about 400 L/min.

In the clinical use of peak flowmeters it is essential that the patient understands what is required of him and blows with his mouth correctly applied to the mouthpiece. Peak flow measurements with pursed lips may grossly overestimate the true measurement.

Dry Gas Meters

There are a number of these: the most common in

medical use is the Parkinson-Cowan meter which has the same basic design as those used throughout Britain in metering domestic gas. The description which follows would apply in general to all of these meters: in detail they vary considerably. There are three sections (see Fig. 7.18); the one at the top con-

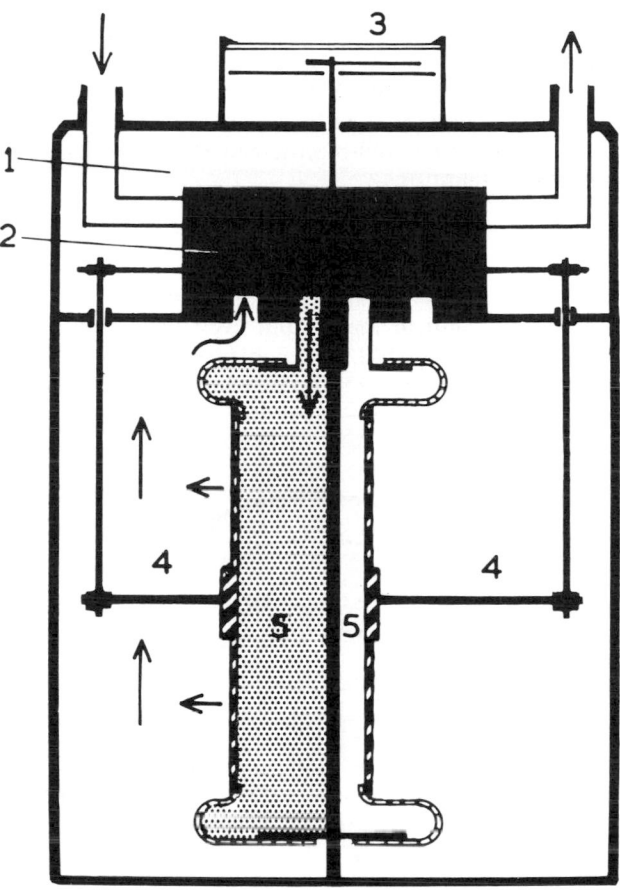

Fig. 7.18 Diagram of a dry gas meter: (1) valve section; (2) valve box; (3) display: dial and pointer; (4) measuring sections; (5) bellows.

tains the valve and display mechanisms; the two identical hermetically sealed sections below each contains bellows. Gas enters the bellows in the sealed section, or into the chamber outside the bellows. As the bellows fill so the gas in the surrounding chamber is forced out of the meter. When the bellows are full, gas enters the outer chamber and compresses the bellows, so that the gas contained is discharged to the exterior. A similar mechanism comes into operation in the other section a quarter of a cycle later.

The movements of the pair of bellows control the opening and closing of the valves across the ports into, and out of, each section. In addition the movement of the bellows is mechanically transmitted to the pointer which moves around the dial.

The arrangement of the valves is such that the pressure drop is kept at a minimum; nevertheless observation of the rotation of the pointer indicated that this is greater in some phases of the operation. In domestic meters the pressure drop is stated not to exceed 0.13 kPa at the maximum flow rate of 100 L/min. The arrangement also ensures that both bellows are not completely empty at the same moment.

Provided that the cumulative volume over the full cycle is collected, both adult and neonatal, minute volume ventilation can be accurately measured but leaks are more likely to cause serious errors at low flows. An accuracy of within 1% is claimed (Adams et al., 1967) when a well-maintained meter is used with suitable precautions.

Wet Gas Meters

The dry gas meter is capable of much greater accuracy than many clinical meters but even higher levels of accuracy are required, and achieved, in other fields. The wet gas meters (see Fig. 7.19), or gas clocks, are a

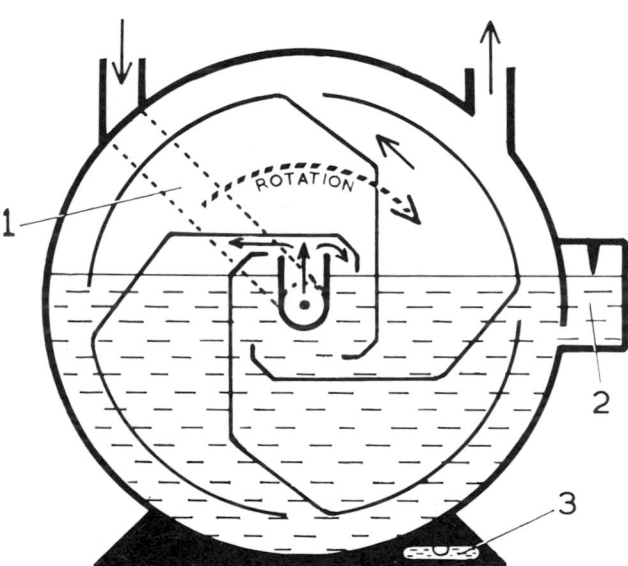

Fig. 7.19 Wet gas meter. Gas pathway shown by solid arrows; rotation by broken arrow. (1) entrance port to hollow spindle; (2) water level; (3) spirit level.

group of instruments whose accuracy may be as good as ±0.1%. Their limitation is that the maximum flow rate which may be passed is about 8 L/min. In order to visualize the mechanics imagine four identical chambers of known volume which rotate about a central axis. The gas enters through the hollow spindle and passes to each chamber in sequence thus maintaining the rotation of the spindle. As each chamber rotates the water causes the gas therein to be displaced peripherally through the outlet of the chamber situated on its circumference. The rotation of the spindle

is displayed on a calibrated dial. It is clear that both filling with water to a prescribed depth and precise levelling, are critical factors in determining the accuracy of this instrument. This is a precision instrument and it is extremely valuable in an anaesthetic laboratory in the calibration of other apparatus.

General Problems in Gas Volume Measurement

Cotes (1966) suggests maximum levels of additional resistance which can be tolerated in any apparatus for measuring ventilation. The pressure drop should not exceed 0.5 kPa at 85 L/min if ventilation is between 0–10 L/min and not over 0.25 kPa at 0–30 L/min. It is customary for this reason to use widebore tubing and connections but in the presence of back-pressure or of residual pressure these may be a further source of error because of the additional compressible volume and the compliance of the tubing.

A volume of one litre is compressed to approximately 999 ml by the application of 0.1 kPa pressure (Boyle's Law); so in large volume systems residual pressures should be kept at a minimum when accuracy is important. In a metre of distensible rubber tubing 10–40 ml are lost for each kPa applied pressure (Mushin et al., 1969). A further problem of additional compliance is that once filled it may discharge through pathways other than the measuring system.

(The Authors are pleased to thank Professors W. W. Mushin and W. W. Mapleson for many helpful discussions about this subject over several years.)

REFERENCES

Adams A.P., Vickers M.D.A., Munroe J.P. et al. (1967). Dry displacement gas meters. *Br. J. Anaesth.*, **39**, 174.

Biomedical Engineering (1969). Ultrasonic flowmeter **4**, 524.

Bird C.G. (1985). Translocation of flowmeter tubes. *Anaesthesia*, **40**, 1232.

British Standard 1042: Pt. i. (1964). *Methods for the Measurement of Fluid Flow in Pipes. Pt. 1; Orifice, Plates, Nozzles and Venturi Tubes.* London: British Standard Institution.

Clutton-Brock J. (1972). Static electricity and rotameters. *Br. J. Anaesth.*, **44**, 86.

Collins M.M., McDermott M., McDermott T.J. (1964). Bellows, spirometer and transistor timer for the measurement of forced expiratory volume and vital capacity. *J. Physiol.*, **172**, 39P.

Cooper E.A., Pask E.A. (1960). A bag for measuring respiratory volumes. *Lancet.* **i**, 369.

Cotes J.E. (1966). Respiratory Function Tests in Pneumoconiosis, p. 93, Geneva: International Labour Organization.

Cotes J.E. (1968). *Lung Function* 2nd edn., p. 23. Oxford: Blackwell Scientific.

Cox L.A., Almeida A.P., Robinson J.S. et al. (1974). An electronic respirometer. *Br. J. Anaesth.*, **46**, 302.

Drew C.D.M., Hughes D.T.D. (1969). Characteristics of the Vitalograph spirometer. *Thorax*, **24**, 703.

Fisher J., Shaw A. (1980). Calibration of some Wright peak flowmeters. *Br. J. Anaesth.*, **52**, 461.

Grenvik A., Hedstrand U., Sjogren H. (1966). Problems in pneumotachography. *Acta. Anaesthesiol. Scand.*, **10**, 147.

Hedenstierna G., Lundberg S., Rawlings D. et al. (1976). Evaluation of a new spirometer based on a fluidistor technique. *Acta Anaesthesiol. Scand.*, **20**, 7.

Hobbes A.F.T. (1967). A comparison of methods of calibrating the pneumotachograph. *Br. J. Anaesth.*, **39**, 899.

Kafer E.R. (1973). Errors in pneumotachography as a result of transducer design and function. *Anesthesiology*, **38**, 275.

Lunn J.N., Hillard E.K. (1970). The effect of repairs on the performance of the Wright respirometer. *Br. J. Anaesth.*, **42**, 1127.

McDowall D.G. (1964). Anaesthesia in a pressure chamber. *Anaesthesia*, **19**, 321.

Millar R.A., Marshall B.E. (1963). A respiration monitor for use during anaesthesia. *Br. J. Anaesth.*, **35**, 447.

Mushin W.W., Rendell-Baker L., Thompson P.W. et al. (1980). *Automatic Ventilation of the Lungs.* 3rd. edn. p. 43., Oxford: Blackwell Scientific.

Nunn J.F. (1956). A new method of spirometry applicable to routine anaesthesia. *Br. J. Anaesth.*, **28**, 440.

Nunn J.F., Ezi-Ashi T.I. (1962). The accuracy of the respirometer and ventigrator. *Br. J. Anaesth.*, **34**, 422.

Richardson W., Shaw A. (1986). Flowmeters: an old problem reappears. *Anaesthesia*, **41**, 675.

Smith W.D.A. (1964). The measurement of uptake of nitrous oxide by pneumotachography. I. Apparatus, methods and accuracy. *Br. J. Anaesth.*, **36**, 363.

Visick W.D., Fairley H.B., Kicket R.F. (1971). Evaluation of a new electronic spirometer. *Anesthesiology*, **34**, 475.

Wright B.M., McKerrow C.B. (1959). Maximum forced expiratory flowrate as a measure of ventilatory capacity. *Br. Med. J.*, **2**, 1041.

Wright B.M. (1978). A miniature Wright peak flowmeter. *Br. Med. J.*, **2**, 1627.

FURTHER READING

British Standard 1042 (1964). *Methods for the Measurement of Fluid Flow in Pipes.* Pt. I. London: British Standards Institution.

Hayward A.T.J. (1977). *Measuring the Repeatability of Flowmeters.* National Engineering Laboratory Report No. 636.

Ower E., Pankhurst R.C. (1966). *The Measurement of Air Flow.* Oxford: Pergamon Press.

8. Methods of Analysis in the Gas and Vapour Phase

N. J. H. Davies and
D. M. Denison

Principles of respired gas analysis
Individual methods of analysis
   Continuous gas analysis
   Discrete sample analysis

For practical purposes, classical methods of gas analysis by chemical absorbants have been superseded by physical instruments which allow continuous and rapid measurements. Their electrical outputs permit problems of linearity and gas specificity to be corrected, and facilitate data presentation. There are four main techniques of value in modern anaesthesia: mass spectrometry, infrared analysis, O_2 polarography and gas chromatography. Some guidelines on respired gas analysis in general will be discussed first, and then these physical methods will be considered in turn, with a brief description of other techniques.

PRINCIPLES OF RESPIRED GAS ANALYSIS

Most gases are odourless and invisible, and may be grossly contaminated, or badly mixed without this being apparent. There can be, for example, large concentration gradients within an anaesthetic or Douglas bag, and along the length or across the radius of anaesthetic hoses. Laminar flow will preserve these differences. In addition, when gas is supplied from pressurized sources or exhaled from a warm lung, there can be considerable temperature changes along the length of a delivery circuit or expiratory hose. These will lead to marked changes in vapour pressures. Similarly, analysers that have appreciable sampling rates disturb flow patterns at the sampling point. If sampling rates exceed respired flows, gas will be drawn in from undesired sites. Small inboard leaks near sampling points introduce profound though highly localized concentration errors. At different points in breathing circuits, absolute pressures vary and influence the measurements.

For all of these reasons, respired gas analysis is very dependent on the quality of sampling. Ideally, gas should be sampled at the lowest possible sample flow via a fine tube at right angles to the gas stream. This avoids ram jet effects where entry into the sampling tube is affected by the surrounding flow of respired gas. The orifice of the sampling tube should be in the axis along which the bulk of the gas stream flows. This is especially true at complex junctions such as respiratory valveboxes.

Most modern analysers depend on sequential amplification of small electrical signals, and often use digital circuits and logic boards to linearize curvilinear relationships. Devices may be linear when first used but can readily slip out of linearity unnoticed. Calibration circuits which insert standard currents or voltage do this downstream of the primary signal, and so provide no guarantee that the analyser is accurate or linear. The minimum test of reliability and accuracy is a three-point check of linearity which *spans* the range of use for each gas concerned. The strength of this lies in the centre point falling on the line generated by the other two. Its weakness lies in the reliability of the standard gas mixture.

Standard gas mixtures of analytic quality are expensive. It is often possible to begin with one or two pure gases or reliable mixtures, and dilute one with another serially, in a water-sealed spirometer, moving the bell between fixed points, drawing in the same volume of diluent each time. This will generate an exponential washout curve, with as many points as movements, which should be linear when plotted on semilogarithmic paper. Highly reliable gas mixing pumps are also available which can generate a great variety of calibration mixtures from a small set of cheap elemental gases.

Any gas analyser takes time to establish its signal. Part of this is the delay as the gas travels up the sampling tube and enters the analysing chamber. During this time the pressure, temperature, vapour content, and concentration gradient distribution of the sample may alter. Subsequently there is a sigmoid change in analyser output as the device senses any new material in the chamber. The first signal delay, the sample transit time, is often unimportant unless the output is married to some other real time variable, such as respired flow in breath-by-breath analysis. The second characteristic, the response time of the device, determines the fastest change in concentration it can see accurately. The 90% response time, the time needed to rise from the fifth to the ninety-fifth percentile of the signal, should be less than a fifth (or ideally one-tenth) of the respiratory cycle. This is critical in selecting analysers for studying high-frequency jet ventilation or respiration in infants.

Lastly, there are limitations to the interpretation of exhaled gas analysis. During inspiration the gas flowing down the bronchial tree slows down dramatically. Long before it reaches the alveoli it is essentially idle, and gas exchange occurs by the development of a diffusion gradient, which varies from alveolus to alveolus. On expiration, complex gas fronts, leaving 300 million alveoli nearly simultaneously, travel at different rates along paths of widely different lengths, to reach the mouth sequentially. The more diseased the lungs, the more gross are these differences and the more difficult it is to interpret this so-called alveolar plateau in an unequivocal way (Engel, 1985). Therefore measurements derived from singlebreath sampling or continuous waveforms have to be made with great caution. Rebreathing measurements reduce this source variability but hide true alveolar values. They are good for the estimation of: accessible alveolar volumes by insoluble gas dilution; effective pulmonary blood flow by the rate of soluble gas uptake; pulmonary capillary blood volume by carbon monoxide transfer; and mixed venous gas tensions from plateau or predicted asymptotic values.

INDIVIDUAL METHODS OF ANALYSIS

There are two levels at which gases may be analysed:

1. accurate continuous gas analysis
2. extremely accurate discrete sample analysis.

Continuous Gas Analysis

Mass Spectrometry

Modern respiratory mass spectrometers are capable of following rapidly changing concentrations of up to eight components of a gas mixture simultaneously while sampling at flows below 10 ml/min (Scheid, 1984). A pump sucks the sample along a fine capillary tube into the instrument where some diffuses across a molecular leak into a steel chamber maintained at a very low pressure (around 10^{-6} mmHg). In this chamber it is bombarded with electrons which ionize a representative portion of the gas. These ions are electrically accelerated into a device which separates them according to their mass/charge ratio, or, since the charge is generally the same for each ion, their molecular weight. This device can be one of two types. It may be a powerful permanent *magnetic* field, in which case ions of differing mass/charge ratios fall on dedicated collector plates for measurement. Alternatively it may be an array of four steel rods, a *quadrupole*, to which is applied a radio-frequency oscillating voltage. For any given voltage only ions of a particular mass/charge ratio can pass through the quadrupole and be measured by a common detector at the far end.

There are important differences between the two types of mass spectrometer. The collector plates of a magnetic instrument have to be moved physically to the correct position for a particular ion species and only four to six can be crammed into the small space. Each species is being collected continuously. A quadrupole instrument, by changing the voltage on the four rods, can look at up to eight gases sequentially using the same collector and electronic circuits that sample its output at the correct time. This sequencing is done very rapidly (every 2.5 ms) giving the illusion of truly continuous analysis. Because of this sharing of the detector, the quadrupole is less sensitive. Its big advantage however is versatility. The choice of which eight gases to analyse is made by the turn of a potentiometer. A quadrupole can also scan through its entire mass range and display a mass spectrum. This is useful when examining unknown gases.

The typical mass range of a quadrupole is 1–200 atomic mass units, rather less for a magnetic instrument, but even organic vapours that may be heavier than this will split up in the ionization chamber to produce measurable fragments below 200. If the mixture to be analysed contains two gases with the same mass, as for example CO_2 and N_2O, or CO and N_2, then such fragments may be used to distinguish one gas from the other. An alternative approach would be to use a stable isotope of one of the pair.

The response time to all gases is less than 0.1 s and only slightly slower for organic vapours. Water vapour however behaves oddly in a vacuum, tending to stick to the sides of any container which slows the response for this vapour only to several seconds. Automatic compensation can be applied for the presence of water vapour, and such a circuit will also allow for partial blockage of the sampling capillary and pressure swings at the patient end (Scheid et al., 1971). The response time and therefore the details of respiratory waveforms is well preserved even when sampling down capillary tubes as much as 30 m long (Davies and Denison, 1979). This makes it possible to use the instrument remotely and allows one relatively expensive spectrometer to be time-shared between many users, ITU beds or operating theatres (Severinghaus and Ozanne, 1978; Gothard et al, 1980).

Infrared Absorption
When infrared light (wavelength from 2.5 to 25 μm) falls on a molecule it may enhance its vibrational energy both in the stretching and bending of interatomic bonds, and also make the molecule rotate faster. This causes the infrared to be absorbed at wavelengths that are characteristic of the molecule concerned.

The analyser sucks gas through a sample chamber at around 200 ml/min, and the infrared absorption is compared with that of a reference chamber (Morgan, 1983). A mechanical 'chopper' blade switches the light between the two chambers at a frequency of 10 to 20 Hz. In modern instruments light-emitting diodes are cheap and reliable sources of infrared; solid-state devices with filters detect the radiation; the chopper blade is unnecessary and microprocessors can quickly compare absorption at several different wavelengths. These infrared analysers may be used to follow breath by breath changes in CO_2, N_2O, halothane, enflurane and isoflurane. Their response time varies for the different gases, being around 250 ms for CO_2 but as long as 750 ms for the volatile agents whose true end-tidal and inspired values will therefore only be identified at slow respiratory rates.

Polarography/Fuel Cell
Polarographic methods use the Clark electrode (Clark, 1956). Just as in blood gas analysers, oxygen diffuses across a membrane into an electrolyte between two polarized electrodes, the resulting current being related to P_{O_2}. The silver anode is gradually destroyed by the current. Such an analyser can be battery powered, but gets its robustness and electrode life-span from having a relatively thick membrane and a large volume of electrolyte. Both of these factors make the response time slow to check oxygen concentrations in breathing circuits and in oxygen tents.

A fuel cell is very similar to the Clark electrode, but the electrode metals are chosen so that the reduction of oxygen at the cathode (and hence the flow of current) will occur without the need for a polarizing voltage. The response time is slow for reasons mentioned above.

Ultraviolet Absorption
At these very short wavelengths (from 0.004 to 0.4 μm) the energy quanta absorbed by molecules is sufficient to disrupt them. Although many gases will absorb such radiation, including CO_2 and N_2, a clinical analyser has been developed only for halothane. Its principle is the same as that of infrared analysers. The response time is slow (over 1 s) although faster analysers have been described (Tatnall et al., 1978), and the ultraviolet light causes breakdown products of halothane that are toxic. Therefore the gas sample must not be returned to the breathing circuit unless passed through soda-lime first.

Paramagnetism
The presence of two unpaired electrons spinning in the same direction in the outer electron shell of the oxygen atom makes the molecules paramagnetic. They will behave like miniature magnets and try to align themselves with a magnetic field. In a paramagnetic oxygen analyser the stream of sample gas containing oxygen enhances a magnetic field in which a glass dumb-bell is suspended. The dumb-bell contains N_2, a gas with no intrinsic magnetic properties and which is repelled (rotated) by the field; the presence of oxygen causes the dumb-bell to rotate further. No other gases of clinical interest have this property.

The paramagnetic oxygen analysers are compact, relatively cheap devices and are unaffected by other common gases. The analytic chamber is rather large however and so the response time is slow (5–20 s). They have been largely replaced by polarographic or fuel cell analysers.

Thermal Conductivity
A katharometer takes advantage of the fact that some gases have a thermal conductivity very different to that of air. For example CO_2 is some 35% less, whereas helium is nearly six times greater. Thus as a gas stream is passed over a heated wire it will cool it to an extent which varies with gas composition, and as it cools its electrical resistance increases. This wire forms one element of the Wheatstone bridge circuit which senses these changes.

Such an analyser is sensitive to several gases including N_2O. Its response time is slow (5 s), unless operated at a low pressure (100 mmHg). It has been used for CO_2 but finds most use in the measurement of helium concentrations when making lung volume estimations.

Miscellaneous

A variety of other physical properties have been used in analysers that are of historic interest only. These include refractive index (Rayleigh refractometer), ultraviolet emission between high-voltage electrodes in a vacuum tube (for nitrogen), and absorption into silicone rubber (Drager Narkotest for halothane).

Discrete Sample Analysis

Gas Chromatography

A steel tube (the 'chromatographic column') about 2 m long and 3–5 mm in diameter is packed with diatomaceous earth particles coated with a non-volatile liquid (the 'stationary phase'), and placed in an oven whose temperature is carefully regulated. An inert carrier gas such as nitrogen or helium is passed continually through this tube at 30–50 ml/min and the effluent gas examined by any relatively non-specific gas detector such as a katharometer. When a small sample (1–10 ml) of an unknown test gas is injected into the carrier upstream of the column its component gases are absorbed by the stationary phase to various extents that depend in part on their volatility. The more volatile ones are swept on faster and reach the detector first. In this way all the components of the test gas are separated in time and arrive sequentially at the detector. The interval between the first component to arrive at the detector and the last might be some minutes and the output of the detector can be drawn on a slowly responding chart recorder. The concentration of any one gas will be proportional to the area under its peak, although measurement of peak heights is often sufficient (Wagner and Lopez, 1984).

The detector depends on the gases to be analysed, but three types are in common use. A katharometer is suitable for normal respired gases and for N_2O, but for some volatile agents a flame ionization detector is better. As its name implies, the gas is ionized by a flame in an electrical field and so increases the current flowing between the electrodes. The electron capture detector measures the reduction in current flowing between two electrodes, one of which is a beta particle (electron) emitter, when the intervening gas molecules are avid for electron capture and this detector is most sensitive to them, although its inherent nonlinearity makes it more difficult to use.

A gas chromatograph can only analyse discrete samples, and each sample will take several minutes to pass through the column. It is however extremely sensitive and accurate at the level of parts per million. It is particularly suited to the analysis of contaminants. By extracting gases out of solution by a Van Slyke technique or equilibration with an inert gas (Wagner et al., 1974) the method can be used to measure the concentration of all anaesthetic gases in blood at very low levels.

Miscellaneous

The traditional estimation of respired gas composition was with chemical analysers. In the Haldane apparatus (Haldane, 1920) and its modification by Lloyd (1958) a 10 ml gas sample is introduced into a graduated burette and its change in volume measured after passage through potassium hydroxide to absorb CO_2 and then pyrogallol to absorb O_2. The Scholander micro-method does the same in an apparatus which uses a micrometer screw to measure the volume changes. This needs a sample size of only 0.5 ml (Scholander and Roughton, 1943). The Van Slyke apparatus degasses a blood sample by applying a vacuum, and determines the O_2 and CO_2 contents of the extracted gas in a similar way to the Haldane apparatus, but measures changes in pressure after each absorption at a constant volume. These methods were a springboard for understanding physiology but are now only of historic interest.

REFERENCES

Clark L.C. (1956). Monitor and control of blood and tissue oxygen tensions. *Trans. Am. Soc. Artif. Internal Organs*, **2**, 41.

Davies N.J.H., Denison D.M. (1979). The uses of long sampling probes in respiratory mass spectrometry. *Respir. Physiol.*, **37**, 335.

Engel L.A. (1985). Intraregional gas mixing and distribution. In *Gas Mixing and Distribution in the Lung*, pp. 287–358. (Engel L.A., Paiva M., eds.). New York: Marcel Dekker.

Gothard J.W.W., Busst C.M., Branthwaite M.A. et al. (1980). Applications of respiratory mass spectrometry to intensive care. *Anaesthesia*. **35**, 890.

Haldane J.S. (1920). *Methods of Air Analysis*. (3rd edn.). London: Griffin.

Lloyd B.B. (1958). Developments of Haldane's gas analysis apparatus. *J. Physiol: (Lond.)*, **143**, 5.

Morgan P. (1983). Physical gas analysers. In *Measurement in Clinical Respiratory Physiology*, pp. 113–130. (Laszlo G., Sudlow M.F., eds.). London: Academic Press.

Scheid P. (1984). Mass spectrometers in respiratory physiology. In *Techniques in Respiratory Physiology*. P.402/1-P402/21. (Otis A.B., ed.) Shannon: Elsevier.

Scheid P., Slama H., Piiper J. (1971). Electronic compensation of the effects of water vapour in respiratory mass spectrometry. *J. Appl. Physiol.*, **30**, 258.

Scholander P.F., Roughton F.J.W. (1943). Microgasometric estimation of the blood gases. *J. Biol. Chem.*, **148**, 551.

Severinghaus J.W., Ozanne G. (1978). Multioperating room monitoring with one mass spectrometer. *Acta. Anaesthesiol. Scand. [Suppl.]*, **70**, 186.

Tatnall M.L., West P.G., Morris P. (1978). A rapid-response U.V. halothane meter. *Br. J. Anaesth.*, **50**, 617.

Wagner P.D., Lopez F.A. (1984). Gas chromatography techniques in respiratory physiology. In: *Techniques in Respiratory Physiology*. P.403/1–P.403/24 (Otis A.B. ed.) Shannon: Elsevier.

Wagner P.D., Naumann P.F., Laravuso R.B. (1974). Simultaneous measurement of eight foreign gases in blood by gas chromatography. *J. Appl. Physiol.*, **36**, 600.

9. Blood Gas Analysis and Oxygen Measurement

C. D. Hanning and M. E. Bone

The accurate determination of arterial blood gas status is an essential part of the management of many patients. The rapid advances in electrode and microprocessor technology have changed a research technique into a clinical, bed-side investigation in less than two decades. The history of these developments has been full recorded by two of the major participants, *Poul Astrup* and *John Severinghaus* (1987).

The miniaturization of electrodes has also made possible the *continuous* monitoring of arterial blood gases by intravascular and transcutaneous electrodes. The increased information on the transient, but clinically important changes in oxygenation and the immediacy with which it is available have been particularly helpful in the management of neonates.

The development of reliable methods of measurement of oxygen content and oxyhaemoglobin saturation (S_{O_2}) has been more recent but the pulse oximeter may well lead to a reorientation away from oxygen tension (P_{O_2}) and back to S_{O_2} as our principal clinical guide to oxygenation.

OXYGEN MEASUREMENT

Arterial oxygenation may be assessed by measuring oxygen tension (Pa_{O_2}), oxyhaemoglobin saturation or blood oxygen content. The relationship between these three factors is determined by the shape and position of the oxyhaemoglobin dissociation curve (Fig. 9.1).

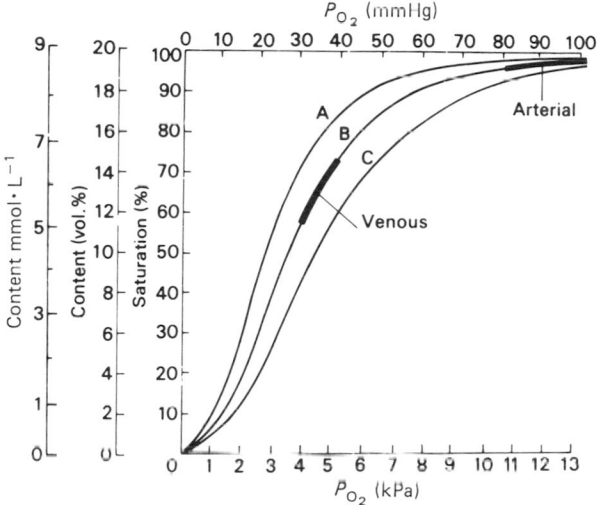

Fig. 9.1 Oxyhaemoglobin dissociation curves for (A) $P_{CO_2} = 2.7$ kPa, (B) $P_{CO_2} = 5.3$ kPa and (C) $P_{CO_2} = 8$ kPa. The normal arterial and mixed venous ranges are shown.

The shape of the curve has been defined mathematically by Severinghaus (1962). The formula is used for the calculation of S_{O_2} in many of the automatic blood gas analysers which only measure P_{O_2} and is reasonably accurate provided the P_{50} is normal (Chapter 41). Accurate work requires the separate measurement of P_{O_2} and S_{O_2}.

MEASUREMENT OF OXYGEN TENSION

In vitro—Bench Analysis

The Polarographic Electrode
The P_{O_2} electrode in common use is a polarographic cell in which the working electrode consumes oxygen.

The principle of polarography was developed in the 1920s (Clark et al., 1953) although the modern form of the oxygen electrode was not described until the 1950s (Clark, 1956). The electrochemical reduction of oxygen results in the production of an electrical current proportional to the oxygen tension and the applied voltage.

$$O_2 + 4e^- \rightarrow 2\,O^{--}$$

The simplest polarographic cell consists of a gold or platinum cathode and a silver/silver chloride anode immersed in the solution to be measured. Application of a polarizing DC voltage results in the reduction of oxygen at the cathode and a small current which can be read from a sensitive galvanometer. Increasing the applied voltage increases the current up to a plateau (Fig. 9.2) when the oxygen molecules cannot reach the

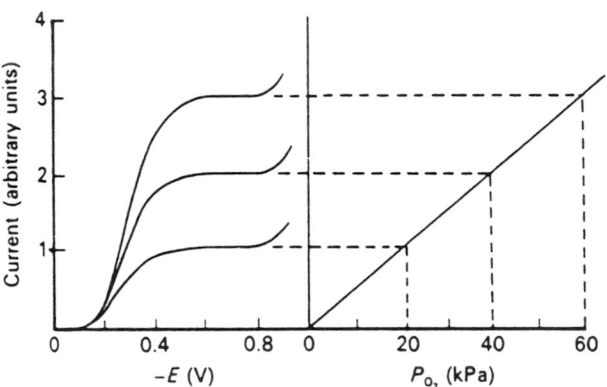

Fig. 9.2 The polarographic electrode shows changes in voltage with current at different oxygen tensions.

cathode fast enough. There is then little change of current with increasing voltage. The current at this plateau is determined by the rate of supply of oxygen to the cathode and thus to the concentration of the oxygen in solution. Henry's law states that the number of molecules in solution is proportional to the partial pressure. A series of voltage–current curves can be drawn (Fig. 9.2) where the height of the plateau is proportional to the partial pressure for oxygen.

A polarograph uses a fixed voltage selected so as to just correspond to the plateau of the voltage–current curve. Too high a voltage leads to rapid deposition of protein on the cathode with a consequent loss of accuracy and sensitivity. Covering just the cathode with a membrane in order to prolong its life increased the diffusion distance and reduced the response time. The practical difficulties of these electrodes restricted their use to the laboratory. Calibration of the polarograph was with solutions of known partial pressure of oxygen.

The Clark Electrode

Clark's great breakthrough was to cover both the cathode and the reference silver/silver chloride anode with a membrane to prevent protein deposition. This resulted in a usable electrode which was further improved by limiting the surface area of the cathode thus reducing its oxygen consumption and the problem of depletion of oxygen near the cathode. A further advance was the use of a pulse polarizing potential which also reduced the oxygen consumption.

A typical electrode (Fig. 9.3) consists of a fine (20 µm) platinum wire sealed into a glass rod ground

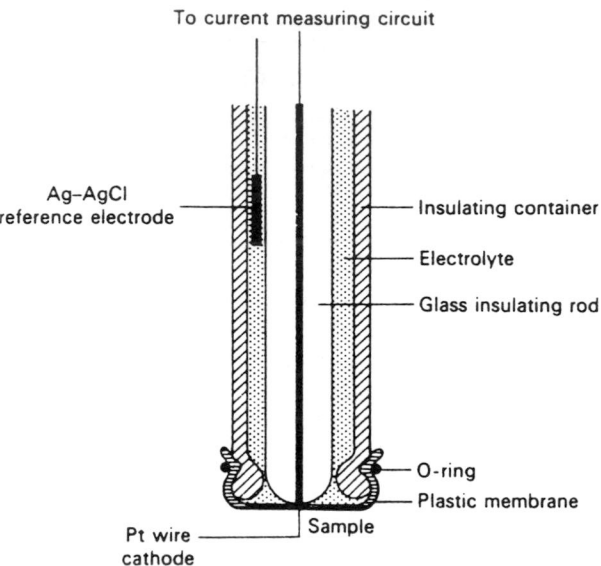

Fig. 9.3 A typical Clark oxygen electrode. (After Hahn, 1987).

so as to expose the wire. The silver/silver chloride reference electrode is sited immediately adjacent and both electrodes are covered by a thin film of buffered potassium hydroxide and enclosed in a thin polypropylene or Teflon membrane which is permeable to gases but not solvents. The choice of membrane determines the response of the electrode and is usually chosen to give a 95% response time of 40–60 s. The whole assembly is mounted in a cuvette and maintained at 37°C by a thermostatically controlled water bath.

A polarizing voltage of 0.6 V is applied which is high enough to ensure that the current of approximately 10^{-10} A.kPa^{-1} is proportional to the oxygen tension. Oxygen molecules are reduced at the cathode thus:

$$O_2 + 2H_2O + 2e^- \rightarrow H_2O_2 + 2OH^-$$
$$H_2O_2 + 2e^- \rightarrow 2OH^-$$

Four electrons flow for each molecule of oxygen reduced. The hydroxyl ions are buffered by the electrolyte layer.

Calibration. A two point calibration is required utilizing an oxygen free gas to set the zero point and a gas of known concentration to set the slope of the response. Most commercial analysers use gases of known composition which are automatically passed into the cuvette. A one point calibration is performed regularly and after each sample, and a two point calibration is performed several times daily. Good practice requires that at least daily calibration is performed with liquid standards (Minty, 1980). Ideally, these should be human blood equilibrated with gases of known composition in a tonometer (Bird and Henderson, 1971). However, this process is time consuming and modern commercial standards are satisfactory (Leary et al., 1980). Well maintained equipment should have a standard deviation of 0.15–0.3 kPa for samples with a P_{O_2} of 0–20 kPa and a planned quality control programme is essential if these standards are to be maintained, particularly for instruments not located in biochemical laboratories (Burnett et al., 1986).

Sources of Error with Clark-type Electrodes
Blood Gas Factor. A lower reading is generally obtained with blood samples than gases of identical P_{O_2} (Rhodes and Moser, 1966). This is thought to be related to the slower diffusion of oxygen in blood and depletion of oxygen at the cathode. The difference is usually less than 4% of the reading with modern electrodes and is internally corrected by the microprocessor.

Non-linearity. A minor degree of non-linearity is inherent in all electrodes due to oxygen depletion and loss of oxygen from the cuvette. Accurate measurements require that the calibrating gases have oxygen tensions that lie just above and below the tension to be measured.

Stability. Deposition of protein and lipid on the membrane or the formation of gas bubbles in the electrolyte will result in a slow drift in the calibration. This emphasizes the importance of regular cleaning of the electrode and rigorous quality control.

Interference. Nitrous oxide and halothane may also be reduced at the cathode and interfere with the analysis (Dent and Netter, 1976; Samra, 1983). This problem has been overcome in most modern analysers by a careful choice of membrane and polarizing voltages.

Hysteresis. Peroxide molecules from the first step in the reduction of oxygen can escape from the area of the cathode into the electrolyte thus reducing the indicated P_{O_2}. The ions may diffuse back if the subsequent sample has a lower P_{O_2} thereby increasing its apparent value. When samples of widely differing P_{O_2} are to be analysed it is wise to analyse each sample in duplicate and to rely on the second reading.

The Galvanic Cell
This cell differs from the Clark electrode in having a cathode of silver and an anode of lead. These metals are sufficiently electronegative with respect to each other that no polarizing voltage is required for the electrochemical reduction of oxygen. An electrolyte of molar potassium bicarbonate is used to minimize the effect of CO_2. Galvanic cells are mostly used in intravascular electrodes and in the measurement of oxygen content.

Blood Sampling Technique
Poor blood sampling technique is the commonest cause of error in blood gas analysis. The range of possible P_{O_2} values is so wide that such errors are difficult to detect.

Arterial blood is the best source, drawn either from a cannula or from direct arterial puncture. Venous blood from the dorsum of the hand is suitable for measurement of pH and P_{CO_2} provided that a brisk blood flow is induced by surface warming to about 45°C. Blood should be drawn without use of a tourniquet.

Capillary blood is also a satisfactory alternative for pH and P_{CO_2} in babies when drawn from a vasodilated earlobe or heel. The blood flow should be brisk and there should be no peripheral vasoconstriction (Gandy et al., 1964).

Anaerobic collection of the sample is most important. The syringe plunger should be freely moving so that there is less likelihood of aspirating air. Air bubbles, even of small size, have a significant effect on gas tensions (Biswas et al., 1982). Glass syringes have some advantages, in particular there is less loss of oxygen by diffusion (Scott et al., 1971). This is of less importance when the sampling to analysis time is short.

The sample should be heparinized to prevent it clotting in the analyser. A small quantity of heparin 1000 iu/ml should be drawn into the syringe and the walls wetted. All air bubbles should be carefully expelled and only sufficient heparin left to just fill the deadspace of the syringe. The syringe should be capped after the sample is drawn and then rotated to mix the heparin. Syringes designed for arterial sampling containing dry lithium heparin have been introduced. They eliminate some of the sampling errors but none succeed entirely (Hutchinson et al., 1986).

Heparin coated capillary tubes may be used for samples from babies. A 60 µl sample is drawn into the tube by capillary action and a small stainless steel bar inserted into the tube. The ends are sealed with plasticine and the sample mixed by moving the bar with a magnet.

Metabolism by leukocytes and loss of gases by diffusion results in a progressive reduction in P_{O_2} and pH with storage. This may be a particular problem in patients with a very elevated white blood cell count. Storage at 0°C in ice is usually satisfactory for up to three hours (Siggaard-Andersen, 1961).

TEMPERATURE CORRECTION

Blood gas analysers measure at 37°C and correction of the parameters is necessary if the patient's temperature differs by more than two degrees from the normal. Many automated blood gas analysers correct the values if given the patient's temperature. The calculations on which these corrections are made have been reviewed by Andritsch et al. (1981) and a comprehensive set of correction tables can be found in Nunn (1987) and other similar works.

In vivo Measurement of Oxygen Tension

Only a few years elapsed from Clark's original description of the oxygen electrode to the development of intravascular and transcutaneous applications. More recently the mass spectrometer has been applied to *in vivo* measurement of gas concentrations and the optical fluorescence techniques (optodes) have given a new lease of life to intravascular monitoring.

Intravascular Oxygen Electrodes

The Clark electrode is used most commonly although the galvanic type has also been utilized. The bipolar type with both cathode and anode mounted in a fine tube and covered by an oxygen permeable membrane has entirely supplanted the monopolar. A typical electrode is shown in Fig. 9.4. The catheter often has two

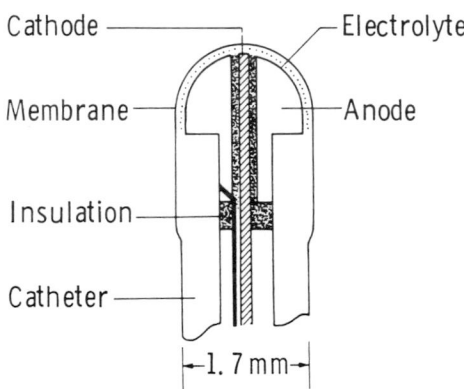

Fig. 9.4 A typical intravascular oxygen electrode. (After Putnam et al., 1984).

lumina, one for the electrode and the other for blood sampling. The catheters are generally small enough (0.4 mm diameter) to be passed through an 18G cannula and leave enough space for measurement of intravascular pressure and blood sampling.

The principle disadvantage of these electrodes is the drift in calibration that occurs due to protein deposition and deterioration of the electrode (Putnam et al., 1984). Regular recalibration is required by reference to bench blood gas analysis. The electrodes are also sensitive to temperature and to the blood flow past the

cathode. This latter effect is analogous to the blood gas factor in bench electrodes. Variations in blood flow at the electrode alter the delivery of oxygen to the cathode. The effect can be minimized at low flow rates by pulsing the polarizing voltage (Scott et al., 1983).

Nitrous oxide may falsely increase the reading if a silver cathode is used with a polarizing voltage in excess of 0.6 V (Evans and Cameron, 1978).

The 95% response is usually between 5–60 s. A fast response is generally associated with an increased sensitivity to changes in blood flow.

Mass Spectrometer

The mass spectrometer (Chapter 8) has the capacity to measure a number of gases simultaneously and requires only a very small sample. A perforated metal intravascular catheter, covered with a gas permeable membrane, is connected directly to the high vacuum inlet of the mass spectrometer and gas sampled at a rate of 5×10^{-6} ml/s (Wald et al., 1971). Calibration may be achieved by use of a known gas mixture or, preferably, by equilibrating the patient with an inert gas such as argon at a known concentration. The system is flow sensitive in the same manner as the Clark electrode and reducing the sensitivity usually increases the response time. The thickness of the membrane, the length and diameter of the sampling tube and the sampling rate all influence the 95% response time which varies from 3–50 s. Deposition of fibrin on the membrane will gradually increase the response time.

Gases can also be sampled from above the skin using a heated probe similar to that of the transcutaneous oxygen and carbon dioxide electrodes (*see below*) (Targett et al., 1984; Spencer et al., 1987). The complexity and cost of a mass spectrometer have restricted its use to research and there is little clinical experience.

Optodes

Oxygen has the property of quenching the fluorescence of certain dyes. Exposure of the dyes to light excites electrons to a higher energy state which then release photons when they return to their original state (fluorescence). Oxygen absorbs the energy from the excited electrons thus permitting them to return to their original state without emitting a photon (Fig. 9.5). The absorption of energy and thus the reduction in the light emitted is proportional to the P_{O_2}.

The probe consists of an optical fibre with a coating of dye at the tip covered by an oxygen permeable membrane. The dye is activated by a flash of light and the fluorescence measured by counting the photons emitted with a photomultiplier (Barker et al., 1987). The zero point is set during manufacture and a single calibration in room air is performed before insertion.

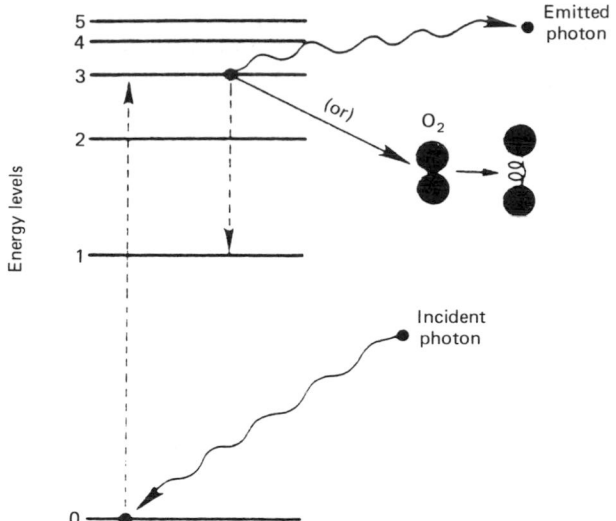

Fig. 9.5 Fluorescence quenching: an electron of the fluorescent dye is excited to a higher energy level by an incident photon. This excited electron can return to a lower energy level either by emitting a photon or by interacting with an oxygen molecule. (After Barker et al., 1987).

A thermocouple is included in the catheter to permit temperature correction.

Initial clinical results were most encouraging with good response time and stability although they may be sensitive to volatile anaesthetic agents (Peterson et al., 1984). Unlike the systems described above, the optodes do not 'consume' oxygen and are not sensitive to blood flow but are sensitive to fibrin deposition. Prolonged use leads to deterioration of the dye and a reduction in light intensity. Phosphorescent dyes are under investigation where the duration, rather than the intensity, of light emission is proportional to the oxygen tension. This property may offer improved stability.

Cardiopulmonary Bypass

The extracorporeal circulation is ideally suited to continuous blood gas monitoring since there is little re-striction on probe size and the patient is fully anticoagulated. Commercial systems are available where Clark type oxygen electrodes and pH and P_{CO_2} electrodes of similar dimensions to those in bench analysers are built into T connectors in the bypass circuit (Claremont and Pagdin, 1985). The sensors are separated from the blood by permeable membranes. Such systems appear to be both accurate and clinically useful and eliminate the need for temperature correction of blood gases.

Transcutaneous Oxygen Electrodes

Early workers attempted to measure the Pa_{O_2} by equilibrating a gas bubble applied to heated skin and measuring its oxygen concentration by chemical analysis. It was thus a logical use of the Clark electrode to apply it to the skin and to the surface of organs (Huch et al, 1972). However a number of factors control the skin surface P_{O_2} (Rithalia and Booth, 1985), usually known as the transcutaneous P_{O_2} (tcP_{O_2}) and confound the measurement of Pa_{O_2}.

Skin Surface P_{O_2}.

Oxygen reaches the skin surface by diffusion from the blood in the capillaries through the dermis which is 100–1400 μm thick and the avascular epidermis which is a similar thickness (Lubbers, 1981). Heating the skin increases capillary blood flow so that capillary P_{O_2} approaches that of the artery. However heat also increases the metabolic rate and thus the oxygen consumption of the dermis. The net effect is that the tcP_{O_2} increases with temperature up to a point where tissue damage occurs at approximately 44–46°C. The factors affecting tcP_{O_2} are summarized in Table 9.1.

A typical transcutaneous electrode is shown in Fig. 9.6. The cathode is mounted centrally and surrounded by a ring shaped anode. The electrolyte is contained by a gas permeable membrane. Heating elements and a thermistor are also built into the electrode housing which is fixed to the skin with a double sided adhesive disk. A control unit regulates the skin temperature and measures the power necessary to maintain that temperature. The power expended,

TABLE 9.1
FACTORS AFFECTING THE TRANSCUTANEOUS OXYGEN TENSION tcP_{O_2}

Oxygen delivery		Oxygen consumption		Oxygen diffusion	
Skin blood flow	• temperature • hypovolaemia • cardiac output • vasoactive drugs • hyperoxia	*Skin*	• temperature • trauma	*Skin thickness*	• age • site • oedema
Oxygen content	• arterial P_{O_2} • haemoglobin	*Electrode*	• cathode area • polarizing voltage	*Membrane*	• thickness • permeability

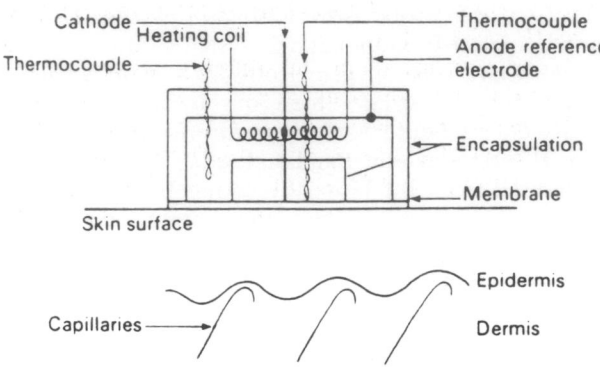

Fig. 9.6 A diagrammatic transcutaneous oxygen electrode. (After Hahn, 1987).

usually expressed in milliwatts, is related to skin blood flow and can be used as an index of perfusion.

Calibration is achieved *in vitro* by reference to gases of known composition. Two concentrations are required to set the slope and zero point. The response time is primarily related to the diffusion distance from capillary to skin rather than the electrode characteristics. Ninety per cent response times vary from 10–15 s in infants with thin skins to 45–60 s in adults. Drift in the calibration may be due both to the electrode and to the tissue (Severinghaus and Thunstrom, 1978). The electrode will deteriorate for the same reasons outlined for all Clark electrodes. Excessive heating leads to tissue damage and to an increased diffusion distance. Multiple micro-cathodes (3–25 μm diameter) are used in some systems to reduce the problem of oxygen depletion seen with large cathodes (4 mm diameter) which have a greater sensitivity.

An upward drift in the indicated tcP_{O_2} often suggests a small leak of air under the adhesive disk. It is important that the attachment of the electrode is checked frequently.

Relationship of Pa_{O_2} to tcP_{O_2}. The principal determinant of the relationship between Pa_{O_2} and tc$_{O_2}$ is the capillary blood flow and it is thus preferable to regard the tcP_{O_2} as a measure of skin oxygen delivery rather than Pa_{O_2} (Barker and Tremper, 1984). Any factor which induces cutaneous vasoconstriction such as hypotension, hypothermia, vasoactive drugs and high oxygen tensions will alter the relationship. The correlation is best in infants who are well perfused and when the electrode is heated to 44°C (Huch et al., 1974; Peabody et al., 1978). However, this temperature will result in tissue damage and the electrode site must be changed every few hours.

Clinical applications. Transcutaneous electrodes are widely used in neonatal practice and may be better than pulse oximetry at detecting hyperoxia although the longer response times are a disadvantage in detecting hypoxia. They are little used in adult practice to follow arterial oxygenation but have been used to

determine the viability of skin flaps (Achauer et al., 1980) and ischaemic limbs as an aid in choosing the level of amputation (Mustapha et al., 1983).

Conjunctival Oxygen Tension

The palpebral conjunctiva is a better site than skin for the indirect estimation of Pa_{O_2} since it does not have a keratinized layer, diffusion distances are much shorter (30 μm) and heating is unnecessary (Fatt and Deutsch, 1983). It is supplied by the carotid artery and may thus reflect cerebral oxygen delivery (Shoemaker and Lawner, 1983).

The sensor consists of a miniaturized Clark electrode mounted in an oval, ring shaped, ophthalmic former. One design consists of a gold ring cathode and a silver anode covered with a layer of silicon oxide. Another has a platinum cathode and a silver–silver chloride anode covered by a polyethylene membrane (Fig. 9.7). A thermistor is incorporated into the ring to measure conjunctival temperature (Fink et al., 1983).

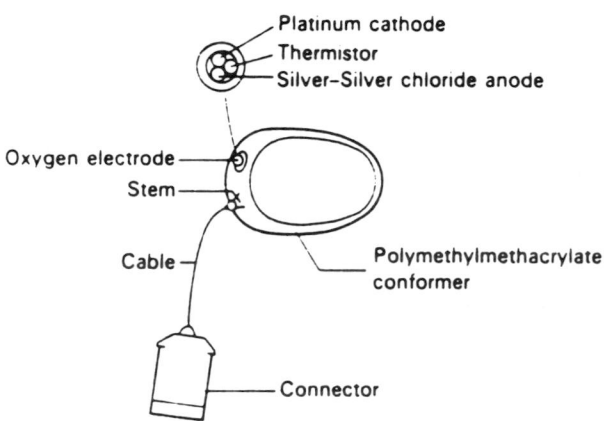

Fig. 9.7 A conjunctival oxygen sensor. (After Hahn, 1987).

The former is placed under the eye lids in the superior and inferior conjunctival fornices so that the electrode is held against the temporal palpebral conjunctiva by the action of the orbicularis muscle. Local anaesthesia is necessary in conscious subjects. Calibration is achieved before insertion by reference to gases of known composition. The response times are similar to the transcutaneous electrodes.

The correlation between the cjP_{O_2} and the Pa_{O_2} is generally better than between tcP_{O_2} and Pa_{O_2} except in the presence of hypothermia and hypotension when neither measurement correlates well (Fink et al., 1984). The sensor is well tolerated for up to 24 h. The preparation of the electrodes and their expense have precluded widespread use but they have proved useful in carotid artery surgery and other circumstances where cerebral oxygen delivery may be at risk.

OXYGEN CONTENT

Oxygen is held in the blood in physical solution and, more importantly bound to haemoglobin. The content is given by:

Oxygen content (ml/100 ml) =

$$\left(\frac{S_{O_2}}{100} \times Hb \times 1.34\right) + (0.025 \times P_{O_2})$$

Where S_{O_2} is the percentage oxygen saturation and Hb is the haemoglobin concentration (g/100 ml). The S_{O_2} can be measured directly or calculated from the P_{O_2} using the Severinghaus equations. The latter method is not recommended for accurate measurements. A number of analytical techniques have been described for direct measurement of oxygen content.

Van Slyke Analysis

The Van Slyke apparatus is the best of the techniques for chemical analysis of oxygen content and was developed to permit the analysis of small sample volumes (Van Slyke and Neill, 1924). Oxygen is driven from the sample by denaturing the haemoglobin with acid saponin. The oxygen and carbon dioxide are then absorbed sequentially by different reagents, and the volume of the evolved gases calculated from the reduction in pressure in the chamber. The technique calls for a precise, methodical approach and considerable skill is required for consistent results. Nevertheless, it remains the standard against which other methods are compared (Brix, 1981).

Galvanic Cell

A commercial apparatus has been described, the Lex–O_2–Con, which uses a galvanic cell (Adams and Cole, 1975). A small (20 μl) sample of blood is injected into a column and the oxygen eluted from the haemoglobin by displacement with carbon monoxide. The oxygen is carried by an oxygen-free carrier gas to a galvanic cell. The current produced by the cell is proportional to the number of oxygen molecules. The current is amplified and the oxygen content calculated and displayed. Calibration is achieved with samples of water equilibrated with room air.

The principle advantage over the Van Slyke technique is that less skill is required and multiple measurements can be made in a short time. The accuracy is slightly less than that attained by an expert with the Van Slyke apparatus (Dornbusch et al., 1983).

OXYHAEMOGLOBIN SATURATION; OXIMETRY

The principal alternative to the measurement of oxygen tension as a measure of oxygenation is oximetry, the measurement of the percentage saturation of haemoglobin with oxygen (S_{O_2}). The S_{O_2} is related to oxygen tension by the oxyhaemoglobin dissociation curve (Fig. 9.1 p. 119).

Oximetry relies upon the differing absorption of light at different wavelengths by the various states of haemoglobin. Oxyhaemoglobin and reduced haemoglobin differ at both the red and infrared portions of the spectrum (Fig. 9.8). The absorption is identical at

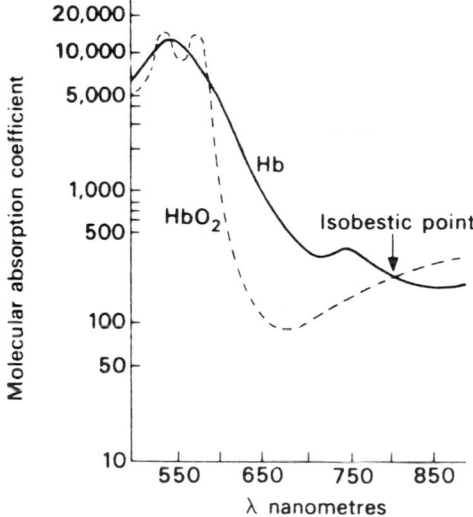

Fig. 9.8 The absorption spectra of oxygenated and reduced haemoglobin.

805 nm, the isobestic point. The principles of transmission of light through liquids are described by the Beer–Lambert law:

$$I = I_0 \, e^{-kCl}$$

Where I is the transmitted light, I_0 is the incident light, l is the path length, C is the concentration of the absorbant and k is the absorption coefficient of the substance at the wavelength used and is the base of the natural logarithm. This equation refers to the transmission of light through simple solutions and cannot be directly applied to *in vivo* transmission where light is also reflected and refracted from particles such as red blood cells and tissue interfaces.

The use of two wavelengths at different points on the absorption spectrum permits the measurement of the relative proportions of two compounds. In the case of oximetry, the ratio of the absorption at wavelengths in the red and infrared regions is proportional to the ratio between the concentrations of oxygenated and reduced haemoglobin. Further wavelengths can be added to permit calculation of the proportions of other haemoglobins such as carboxyhaemoglobin and methaemoglobin.

An alternative approach to the measurement of S_{O_2} has recently been proposed (Byrne and Clark, 1989). The S_{O_2} is related to the shift in the peak absorption between 400 and 450 nm. The position of the peak is determined from the light transmitted or reflected from the sample when illuminated by a scanning monochromator. The technique may have particular application in *in vivo* reflectance measurements.

Oximeters may be classified into transmission and reflectance instruments. The former can be divided into the cuvette types, where the absorption is measured *in vitro*, and *in vivo* methods, which includes pulse oximetry. The latter relies upon the reflection of light from blood and is restricted to *in vivo* measurements.

Transmission oximetry

In Vitro **Methods.** These instruments, commonly called *Co-oximeters*, are a direct application of spectrophotometry to oxyhaemoglobin saturation measurement (Brown, 1980). A sample of blood is introduced into a cuvette and haemolyzed, either by chemical means or freezing and thawing. The absorption of a number of different wavelengths of light is measured and the proportions of oxyhaemoglobin, reduced haemoglobin, carboxyhaemoglobin, methaemoglobin and total haemoglobin calculated. The instruments are calibrated by use of synthetic calibration standards or whole blood equilibrated with gases of known composition. These instruments are usually regarded as the gold standard of oxyhaemoglobin measurement. It is important to remember that they are calibrated for normal adult haemoblogin and may not give accurate results with other haemoglobin species unless recalibrated with the appropriate standards (Reichart, 1966; Dennis and Valeri, 1981).

In Vivo **Methods.** The transmission of light through tissues is complicated by a number of factors not found in the laboratory. Light is absorbed by tissues and pigments other than the arterial blood, particularly venous blood and is reflected from interfaces, particularly red blood cells. The length of the light path is an important factor in the Beer–Lambert law and thus any movement of the light source or detectors will introduce an error. The first attempts at *in vivo* oximetry were made by Kramer and Matthes in 1935 and subsequently developed by Goldie, Brinkman, Millikan and others predominantly in response to the need to investigate the effects of altitude on aviators (Severinghaus and Astrup, 1987). Light was passed through either the pinna of the ear or the web between thumb and first finger. Absorption by venous blood was eliminated by heating the tissues so as to 'arterialize' the tissue. The zero point was set by squeezing the tissue to render it 'bloodless' and the 100% saturation obtained by giving the subject 100% oxygen to breathe. Despite the inaccuracies inherent in the method much valuable work was achieved. The principle was further developed by Shaw who designed an instrument, subsequently marketed by Hewlett–Packard (Merrick and Hayes, 1976), which

used eight different wavelengths of light from a revolving filter disk transmitted to the ear through a fibreoptic cable. Calibration was achieved by inserting the earpiece into an 'artificial ear' contained within the instrument. This instrument was the first clinically usable oximeter, but the size of the probe restricted its use to adults over short time periods.

Pulse oximetry was described by Takuo Aoyagi in 1974 (Aoyagi et al., 1974). He realized that the transmission of light through tissues was not constant but varied with each pulse beat since blood flow is pulsatile in capillaries. The change in light absorbed from one time point to the next is due entirely to arterial blood. Thus the ratio of the change of absorption of red and infrared light is proportional to the ratio of oxyhaemoglobin to deoxyhaemoglobin, effectively 'subtracting' the contribution to light absorption of the tissues and venous blood (Fig. 9.9). The formula relating the changes is:

$$Sa_{O_2} = \frac{k_1 + k_2 \times \dfrac{\Delta R}{\Delta IR}}{k_3 + k_4 \times \dfrac{\Delta R}{\Delta IR}}$$

Where ΔR and ΔIR are the changes in red and infrared absorption respectively and k_1–k_4 are constants obtained empirically from measurements made on normal volunteers.

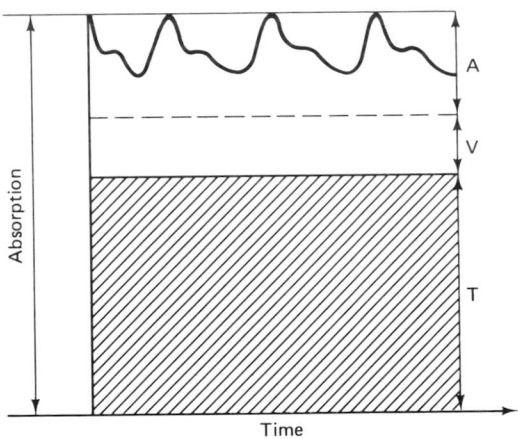

Fig. 9.9 Modulation of light absorbed by tissues by arterial pulsation. A, absorption by arterial blood; V, absorption by venous blood; T, absorption by other tissues.

The concept that all the change in light transmission is due to the capillary pulsation has been challenged by Kim and his colleagues (Kim et al., 1986). The observation that there is some pulsatility in venous blood may help to explain some of the minor inaccuracies noted when peripheral perfusion changes.

The advantages of pulse oximeters are that they are convenient to use and accurate (Hanning, 1985; New, 1985; Taylor and Whitwam, 1986). They require no calibration and the small size of the light emitting diodes used as the light sources permits probes small enough to be used on the smallest of premature infants. The principle disadvantages are that an adequate pulse wave must be detected for accurate measurements (Wilkins et al., 1989). Instruments which permit the display of a pulse waveform are therefore preferred. The use of only two wavelengths does not permit the instruments to differentiate oxy-haemoglobin from other species of haemoglobin, in particular carboxyhaemoglobin, and some dyes (Barker and Tremper, 1987; Scheller et al., 1986).

A large number of different instruments have become available in recent years. The differences between them lie in the computer programmes used to calculate the displayed Sa_{O_2}. A few instruments make multiple measurements throughout the pulse wave whereas some others take measurements at the peak and trough of the wave. A weighted average is then calculated and displayed. The system of weighting used by different manufacturers influences the ability of the instrument to detect a rapid change in oxygenation, reject movement artifact and to function when the arterial waveform is of low amplitude (Wilkins et al., 1989). Space does not permit a detailed assessment of every instrument but the limitations must be considered in choosing an instrument for a particular application.

The principle of pulse oximetry, at present, can only be reliably applied to transmission oximetry. The penetration of red and infrared light by tissues differs so that the path lengths are different if the emitters and sensor are adjacent to each other. It is anticipated that these problems will be overcome which will permit the use of pulse oximetry to measure foetal oxygenation by a probe placed on the scalp through the open cervix. Another, more feasible, application is the attachment of emitter and sensor to an oesophageal probe, directed at the pulmonary artery, for measurement of 'noninvasive' mixed venous oxygen saturation.

Reflectance Oximetry

A number of *in vitro* methods have been described in the past where light has been reflected from blood held in cuvettes (Cole and Hawkins, 1967). None of these techniques are in current use.

The main use of reflectance oximetry is in the measurement of mixed venous saturation ($S\bar{v}_{O_2}$) (Divertie and McMichan, 1984). A pulmonary artery catheter containing two fibre optic bundles is placed in the pulmonary artery. At least two wavelengths of light are transmitted along one bundle and reflected from the red blood cells down the other to the detector. A microprocessor calculates the $S\bar{v}_{O_2}$ and compensates for the effects of blood velocity. Calibration

is required for each catheter due to slight differences in manufacture (Gettinger et al., 1987). Some instruments may also be used for measurement of cardiac output by a dye dilution method.

Future developments may permit the light emitting diodes and the sensors to be placed at the tip of an intravascular catheter, eliminating the problems associated with fibre optic systems (Schmidt et al., 1986).

CARBON DIOXIDE MEASUREMENT

Carbon dioxide is carried in the blood in physical solution, as carbaminohaemoglobin and as bicarbonate. The three forms are in equilibrium and CO_2 content is usually expressed as CO_2 tension. P_{CO_2}, pH and bicarbonate are related by the Henderson–Hasselbalch equation (Chapter 0):

$$pH = pK + \log\frac{[\alpha P_{CO_2}]}{[HCO_3^-]}$$

The predictable relationship between pH and P_{CO_2} was the basis for the Astrup interpolation method (Astrup et al., 1960). The pH of a blood sample was measured and the blood then equilibrated with two gases of known CO_2 content and the pH measured for each gas. The values for the pH corresponding to the known P_{CO_2} values were plotted on the Siggaard-Andersen nomogram (1962) and a line drawn through them. The P_{CO_2} corresponding to the original pH value could then be read from this buffer line. The process was time consuming and inaccurate and has been superseded by the development of specific CO_2 electrodes.

In vitro Analysis

The Carbon Dioxide Electrode

The CO_2 electrode was first described by Stow (1957) and subsequently modified by Severinghaus and Bradley (1958) and is essentially a modified pH electrode (Chapter 10). A thin layer of sodium bicarbonate solution is held within a cellophane or nylon mesh over a pH electrode and contained by a membrane of silicone rubber or Teflon which is permeable to CO_2 but not hydrogen ions (Fig. 9.10). The pH sensitive glass electrode and the silver/silver chloride reference electrodes are contained within the membrane and are mounted in a water bath maintained at 37°C. The reaction can be summarized as:

$$CO_2 + H_2O \rightleftharpoons H_2CO_3 \rightleftharpoons H^+ + HCO_3^-$$

CO_2 molecules diffuse through the membrane until the electrolyte layer is in equilibrium with the gas or liquid in the cuvette. The measured pH can then be converted to the P_{CO_2} and displayed. The electrode is calibrated by reference to gases of known CO_2 concentration chosen to be above and below the expected range for the samples. Most automatic commercial

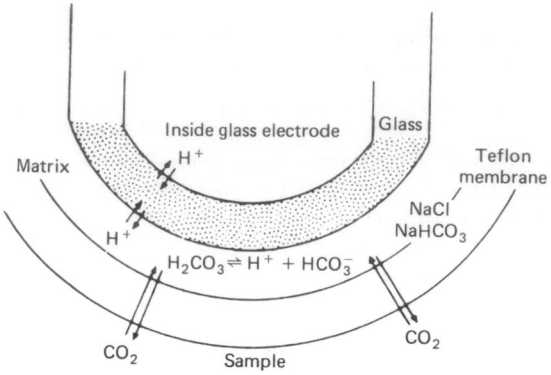

Fig. 9.10 A diagrammatic carbon dioxide electrode. (After Hahn, 1987).

instruments perform a two point calibration several times each day and a one point check before or after each determination.

The response time depends not only on the permeability of the membrane but also on the speed of reaction. A shorter response time can be obtained by adding carbonic anhydrase to the electrolyte layer. The response time can also be reduced by using a dilute solution of $NaHCO_3$ but at the expense of reducing the sensitivity measured as pH change for a given change in P_{CO_2}.

Carbon dioxide electrodes are generally accurate and stable (Severinghaus, 1962). CO_2 is not consumed, unlike an oxygen electrode, thus eliminating any blood gas effect. However a small hole in the membrane will give inaccurate results with liquids but not gases due to the loss of H^+ ions. The integrity of the membrane is usually checked electrically by measurement of its resistance. The accuracy should be ± 0.15 kPa which is considerably better than the Astrup interpolation method even in good hands.

In vivo Measurement

Intravascular Probes
Several workers have miniaturized the Stow–Severinghaus electrode to be inserted through an arterial cannula. The glass electrode is very fragile and electrode instability and drift have been recurrent problems. A palladium oxide electrode has been used in an attempt to overcome some of these problems.

Clinical experience has been limited although a commercial system has been described which combined CO_2 and oxygen electrodes in the same catheter (Parker et al., 1978).

Optodes. Optical sensors using the same principle as for the measurement of oxygen have been described for the measurement of pH and P_{CO_2} (Gehrich et al., 1986). A pH sensitive fluorescent dye is used to measure the pH of a layer of buffer separated from the

blood by a CO_2 permeable membrane. The dye emits light at two wavelengths depending upon the pH. The ratio between the light intensities of the two wavelengths is proportional to the pH and thus the P_{CO_2}.

Transcutaneous CO_2 Electrode
John Abernethy, a surgeon at St. Bartholomew's Hospital, demonstrated the release of carbon dioxide from the skin in 1793. More recently the CO_2 electrode has been developed to measure the transcutaneous P_{CO_2} (tcP_{CO_2}) as a means of estimating the Pa_{CO_2}. The modifications required are similar to those for the oxygen electrode. The glass electrode is covered by a permeable membrane which encloses the bicarbonate buffer. A heating element and thermistor maintain the skin temperature at 42–44°C and the electrode is secured to the skin by a double sided adhesive disk (Clutton-Brock and Rithalia, 1984).

The tcP_{CO_2} is a balance between cutaneous CO_2 production and its removal which is dependent on both blood flow and on the Pa_{CO_2}. Heating the skin increases metabolism and thus CO_2 production while also increasing its solubility and cutaneous blood flow. The tcP_{CO_2} is generally greater than Pa_{CO_2} (Severinghaus et al., 1978) and the relationship can be expressed as:

$$tcP_{CO_2} = 1.33 \times Pa_{CO_2} + 0.5 \text{ kPa}$$

tcP_{CO_2} increases still further with respect to Pa_{CO_2} when peripheral perfusion diminishes due to the reduction in CO_2 removal (Tremper et al., 1980). This effect is more prominent in adults than in infants (Versmold et al., 1981).

The response time is longer than for oxygen, the 63% response to a step change in Pa_{CO_2} taking 2–3 minutes at an electrode temperature of 43°C. Calibration is achieved *in vitro* by reference to gases of known composition. In common with transcutaneous oxygen measurement, the best results are obtained on sites where the skin is thin, such as the upper chest. Correlation coefficients between tcP_{CO_2} and Pa_{CO_2} vary between 0.79–0.98 in both infants and adults.

The electrodes have been extensively used in neonatal practice but have not been so widely used in adults. Combined oxygen and CO_2 electrodes have been devised (Wimberley et al., 1983; Mahutte et al., 1984). However the hydroxyl ions produced by the oxygen electrode can alter the pH of the electrolyte solution and affect the CO_2 electrode. An aluminium electrode is included which consumes the hydroxyl ions (Severinghaus, 1981). The main advantage is the reduction in the skin surface coverage and thus thermal damage compared with the use of separate sensors.

Non-invasive Mixed Venous P_{CO_2}
The principle of estimating the mixed venous P_{CO_2} ($P\bar{v}_{CO_2}$) by equilibrating a gas mixture by rebreathing

was elaborated by Campbell (Powles and Campbell, 1978). The Pa_{CO_2} is usually 0.8 kPa less than the $P\bar{v}_{CO_2}$ under normal circumstances. The technique was useful when infrared CO_2 analysers were more readily available than blood gas analysers. It has recently been automated (Leavell et al., 1986) and may be of value when repeated noninvasive estimates are required.

REFERENCES

General References

Astrup P., Severinghaus J.W. (1987). *The History of Blood Gases, Acids and Bases.* Munksgaard: Copenhagen.

Beetham R. (1982). A review of blood pH and blood gas analysis. *Ann. Clin. Biochem.*, **19**, 198.

Hahn C.E.W. (1987). Blood gas measurement. *Clin. Phys. Physiol. Meas.*, **8**, 3.

Nunn J.F. (1987). *Applied Respiratory Physiology.* 3rd edn. Butterworths: London.

Payne J.P., Severinghaus J.W. eds. (1986). *Pulse Oximetry.* Springer-Verlag: Berlin.

Seitz W.R. (1984). Chemical sensors based on fiber optics. *Anal. Chem.*, **56**, 16.

Spence A.A. ed. (1982). *Respiratory Monitoring in Intensive Care.* Churchill Livingstone, Edinburgh.

Tremper K.K., Barker S.J. eds. (1987). Advances in oxygen monitoring. *Int. Anesth. Clin.*, **25**, No 3.

Oxygen Tension

Achauer B.M., Black K.S., Lilke D.K. (1980). Transcutaneous P_{O_2} in flaps: a new method of survival prediction. *Plas. Reconst. Surg.*, **65**, 738.

Adams L., Cole P.V. (1975). A new method for the direct measurement of blood oxygen content. *Cardiovas. Res.*, **2**, 443.

Andritsch R.F., Muravchick S., Gold M.I. (1981). Temperature correction of arterial blood gas parameters. *Anesthesiology*, **55**, 311.

Barker S.J., Tremper K.K. (1984). Transcutaneous oxygen tension: a physiological variable for monitoring oxygenation. *J. Clin. Monitor*, **1**, 130.

Barker S.J., Tremper K.K., Hyatt J., et al. (1987). Continuous fibreoptic arterial oxygen tension measurements in dogs. *J. Clin. Monit.*, **3**, 48.

Bird B.D., Henderson F.A. (1971). The use of serum as a control in acid base determination. *Br. J. Anaes.*, **43**, 592.

Biswas K., Ramos J.M., Agroyannis B., et al. (1982). Blood gas analysis: Effect of air bubbles in syringe and delay in estimation. *Br. Med. J.*, **284**, 923.

Brix O. (1981). A modified Van Slyke apparatus. *J. Appl. Physiol.*, **50**, 1093.

Burnett D., Henfrey R.D., Woods T.F., et al. (1986). Regional quality assessment of pH and blood gas analysers. *Ann. Clin. Biochem.*, **23**, 26.

Claremont D.J., Pagdin T.M. (1985). Evaluation of a new reusable electrode for continuous monitoring of blood P_{O_2} during open heart surgery. *J. Med. Eng. Tech.*, **9**, 174.

Clark L.C., Wolf R., Granger D., et al. (1953). Continuous reading of blood oxygen tensions by polarography. *J. Appl. Physiol.*, **6**, 189.

Clark L.C. (1956). Monitor and control of blood and tissue oxygen tensions. *Trans. Am. Soc. Artif. Int. Organs*, **2**, 41.

Dent J.G. and Netter K.J. (1976). Errors in oxygen tension measurement caused by halothane. *Br. J. Anaes.*, **48**, 195.

Dornbusch E.A., Duke G., Collins J.E., et al. (1983). Blood oxygen contents: Van Slyke analyser *vs.* Lex-O_2-Con. *Heart Lung*, **12**, 522.

Evans M.C., Cameron I.R. (1978). Oxygen electrodes sensitive to nitrous oxide. *Lancet*, **2**, 137.

Fatt I., Deutsch T.A. (1983). The relation of conjunctival P_{O_2} to capillary bed P_{O_2}. *Crit. Care Med.*, **11**, 455.

Fink S.E., Ray W., McCartney S.F., et al. (1983). A new device for measuring conjunctival oxygen tension and its application to hyperoxic and hypoxic states. *Crit. Care Med.*, **11**, 224.

Fink S., Wayne W.C., McCartney S., et al. (1984). Oxygen transport and utilisation in hyperoxia and hypoxia: relation of conjunctival and cutaneous oxygen tensions to haemodynamic and oxygen transport variables. *Crit. Care Med.*, **12**, 943.

Gandy E., Grann L., Cunningham N., et al. (1964). The validity of pH and P_{CO_2} measurements in capillary samples in sick and healthy newborn infants. *Pediatrics*, **34**, 192.

Huch R., Lubbers D.W., Huch A. (1972). Quantitative continuous measurement of partial oxygen pressure on the skin of adults and new born babies. *Pflug. Arch.*, **337**, 185.

Huch R., Lubbers D.W., Huch A. (1974). Reliability of transcutaneous monitoring of arterial P_{O_2} in new born infants. *Arch. Dis. Child.*, **49**, 213.

Hutchinson A.S., Dryburgh F.J., Ralston S.H. (1986). Sampling errors in pH and blood gas analysis—an evaluation of three new arterial blood samplers. *Ann. Clin. Biochem.*, **23**, 329.

Leary E.T., Graham G., Kenny M.A. (1980). Commercially available blood gas quality controls compared with tonometered blood. *Clin. Chem.*, **26**, 1309.

Lubbers D.W. (1981). Theoretical basis of the transcutaneous blood gas measurements. *Crit. Care Med.*, **9**, 721.

Minty B.D. (1980). Problems of blood gas quality control. In *Quality Control in Clinical Laboratories.* Stevens J.F. (ed). *Ann. Clin. Biochem.*, **17**, 61.

Mustapha N.M., Redhead R.G., Jain S.K., et al. (1983). Transcutaneous partial oxygen pressure assessment of the ischemic lower limb. *Surg. Gynecol. Obstet.*, **156**, 582.

Peabody J.L., Gregory G.A., Willis M.M. (1978). Transcutaneous oxygen measurements in sick infants. *Am. Rev. Respir. Dis.*, **118**, 83.

Peterson J.I., Fitzgerald R.V., Buckhold D.K. (1984). Fibreoptic probe for *in vivo* measurement of oxygen partial pressure. *Ann. Chem.*, **56**, 62.

Putnam S.P., Rolfe P., Albery W.J. (1984). Electrochemical aspects of intravascular transducers. *J. Biomed. Eng.*, **6**, 22.

Rhodes P.G., Moser K.M. (1966). Sources of error in oxygen tension measurement. *J. Appl. Physiol.*, **21**, 729.

Rithalia S.V.S., Booth S. (1985). Factors influencing transcutaneous oxygen tension. *Intens. Care World*, **2**, 126.

Samra S.K. (1983). Halothane interference with transcutaneous oxygen monitoring: *in vivo* and *in vitro*. *Crit. Care Med.*, **11**, 612.

Scott I.L., Black A.M.S., Maynard P., et al. (1983). Pulsed polarography and intravascular oxygen electrodes. *Br. J. Anaes.*, **55**, 559.

Scott P.V., Horton J.N., Mapleson W.W. (1971). Leakage

of oxygen from blood and water samples stored in plastic and glass syringes. *Br. Med. J.*, **3**, 512.

Severinghaus J.W., Thunstrom A. (1978). Problems of calibration and stabilization of transcutaneous oxygen electrodes. *Acta. Anaes. Scand.*, **Suppl 68**, 68.

Shoemaker W.C., Lawner P.M. (1983). Method for continuous conjunctival oxygen monitoring during carotid artery surgery. *Crit. Care Med.*, **11**, 946.

Siggaard-Andersen O. (1961). Sampling and storage of blood for determination of acid base status. *Scand. J. Clin. Lab. Invest.*, **13**, 196.

Spencer J.A.D., Wolton R.S., Rolfe P., et al. (1987). Mass spectrometer system for continuous skin-surface and intravascular blood gas measurement of maternal-fetal respiration in labour. *J. Biomed. Eng.*, **9**, 161.

Targett R.C., Kocher O., Muramatsu K., et al. (1984). Skin gas tensions and resistances measured by mass spectrometry in adults. *J. Appl. Physiol.*, **56**, 1431.

Van Slyke D.D., Neill J.M. (1924). The determination of gases in blood and other solutions by vacuum extraction and manometric measurement. *J. Biol. Chem.*, **61**, 523.

Wald A., Hass W.K., Ransohoff J. (1971). Tutorial: experience with a mass spectrometer for blood gas analysis in humans. *J. Assoc. Advanc. Med. Instr.*, **5**, 325.

Oximetry

Aoyagi T., Kishi M., Yamaguchi K., et al. (1974). Improvement of an earpiece oximeter. In *Abstracts 13th Jap. Soc. Med. Elec. Biol. Eng.*, **90** (Jap).

Barker S.J., Tremper K.K. (1987). The effect of carbon monoxide inhalation on pulse oximetry and transcutaneous P_{O_2}. *Anesthesiology*, **66**, 677.

Brown L.J. (1980). A new instrument for the simultaneous measurement of total hemoglobin, % oxyhemoglobin, % carboxyhemoglobin, % methemoglobin and oxygen content of whole blood. *Trans. Biomed. Eng.*, **27**, 132.

Byrne P., Clark D. (1989). *Oximetry*. British Patent Application No. 8917187.0. Northern Regional Medical Physics Dept./NRDC.

Cole P.V., Hawkins L.H. (1967). The measurement of the oxygen content of whole blood. *Biochem. Eng.*, **2**, 56.

Dennis R.C., Valeri C.R. (1980). Measuring percent oxygen saturation of hemoglobin, percent carboxyhemoglobin and methemoglobin and concentrations of total hemoglobin and oxygen in blood of man, dog and baboon. *Clin. Chem.*, **26**, 1304.

Divertie M.B., McMichan J.C. (1984). Continuous monitoring of mixed venous oxygen saturation. *Chest*, **85**, 423.

Gettinger A., De Traglia M.C., Glass D. (1987). *In vivo* comparison of two mixed venous saturation catheters. *Anesthesiology*, **66**, 373.

Hanning C.D. (1985). Monitoring oxygen during anaesthesia. *Br. J. Anaes.*, **57**, 359.

Kim J.M., Arakawa K., Benson K., et al. (1986). Pulse oximetry and circulatory kinetics associated with pulse volume amplitude measured by photoelectric plethysmography. *Anesth. Analg.*, **65**, 1333.

Merrick E.B., Hayes T.J. (1976). Continuous noninvasive measurements of arterial blood oxygen levels. *Hewlett-Packard J.*, p2.

New W. (1985). Pulse oximetry. *J. Clin. Monit.*, **1**, 126.

Reichert W.J. (1966). The theory and construction of oximeters. In *Oxygen measurement in blood and tissues and their significance.*, eds Payne J.P., Hill D.W. Churchill: London.

Scheller M.S., Unger R.J., Kelner M.J. (1986). Effects of intravenously administered dyes on pulse oximetry readings. *Anesthesiology*, **65**, 530.

Schmitt J.M., Mihm F.G., Meindl J.D. (1986). New methods for whole blood oximetry. *Ann. Biomed. Eng.*, **14**, 35.

Severinghaus J.W., Astrup P. (1987). History of blood gas analysis. *Int. Anesth. Clin.*, **25**, 4.

Taylor M.B., Whitwam J.G. (1986). The current state of pulse oximetry. *Anaesthesia*, **41**, 943.

Wilkins C.J., Moores M., Hanning C.D. (1989). Comparison of pulse oximeters: Effects of vasoconstriction and venous engorgement. *Br. J. Anaes.* **62**, 439.

Carbon Dioxide

Astrup P., Anderson O.S., Jorgensen K., et al. (1960). The acid base metabolism: a new approach. *Lancet*, **i**, 1035.

Clutton-Brock T.H., Rithalia S.V.S. (1984). Transcutaneous CO_2 monitoring. *Br. J. Hosp. Med.*, March: 225.

Gehrich J.L., Lubbers, D.W., Opitz N., et al. (1986). Optical fluorescence and its application to an intravascular blood gas monitoring system. *IEEE Trans. Biomed. Eng.*, **BME33**, 117.

Leavell K., Finkelstein S.M., Warwick W.J., et al. (1986). Automated noninvasive determination of mixed venous P_{CO_2}. *Med. Instrumen.*, **20**, 248.

Mahutte C.K., Michiels T.M., Hassell K.T., et al. (1984). Evaluation of a single transcutaneous P_{O_2}–P_{CO_2} sensor in adult patients. *Crit. Care Med.*, **12**, 1063.

Parker D., Delpy D., Lewis M. (1978). Catheter tip electrode for continuous measurement of P_{O_2} and P_{CO_2}. *Med. Biol. Eng. Comput.*, **16**, 599.

Powles A.C.P., Campbell E.J.M. (1978). An improved rebreathing method for measuring mixed venous carbon dioxide tension and its clinical application. *J. Canad. Med. Assoc.*, **118**, 501.

Severinghaus J.W. (1962). Electrodes for blood and gas P_{CO_2} and blood pH. *Acta. Anaes. Scand.*, **Suppl 11**, 207.

Severinghaus J.W. (1981). A combined transcutaneous P_{O_2}–P_{CO_2} electrode with electrochemical HCO_3 stabilisation. *J. Appl. Physiol.*, **51**, 1027.

Severinghaus J.W., Bradley A.F. (1958). Electrodes for blood P_{O_2} and P_{CO_2} determination. *J. Appl. Physiol.*, **13**, 515.

Severinghaus J.W., Stafford M., Bradley A.F. (1978). Transcutaneous carbon dioxide electrode design, calibration and temperature gradient problems. *Acta. Anaes. Scand.*, **68**, 118.

Tremper K.K., Mentelos R.A., Shoemaker W.C. (1980). Effect of hypercarbia and shock on transcutaneous CO_2 and different electrode temperatures. *Crit. Care Med.*, **11**, 608.

Siggaard-Andersen O. (1962). The pH/log P_{CO_2} blood acid base nomogram revised. *Scand. J. Clin. Lab. Invest.*, **14**, 598.

Stow R.W., Baer R.F., Randall B. (1957). Rapid measurement of the tension of CO_2 in blood. *Arch. Phys. Med. Rehabil.*, **38**, 646.

Versmold H.T., Brunstler I., Enders A., et al. (1981). Transcutaneous P_{CO_2} monitoring of new born infants in shock at electrode temperature of 41°C–44°C. *Intens. Care Med.*, **7**, 251.

Wimberley P.D., Pedersen K.G., Thode J., et al. (1983). Transcutaneous and capillary P_{CO_2} and P_{O_2} measurements in healthy adults. *Clin. Chem.*, **29**, 1471.

10. The Determination of pH

M. K. Sykes

In 1923 Brønsted defined an acid as a molecule capable of donating an hydrogen ion, and a base as a molecule capable of accepting an hydrogen ion. The 'strength' of an acid or base may be related to the abundance of hydrogen or hydroxyl ions. This in turn depends on the concentration of the substance present in the aqueous solution and on the degree of dissociation. In practice the concentration of H^+ ions varies from 1 g/L for a molar solution of the strongest acids, to 10^{-14} g/L for the strongest alkalis. To cover this wide range of concentrations Sørensen (1909) proposed that a logarithmic scale should be used so that

$$pH = -\log_{10}[H^+]$$

where $[H^+]$ = the concentration of H^+ ions.

Water is unique in that it has equal proportions of H^+ and OH^- ions; the concentration of H^+ ions is therefore 10^{-7} g/L and the pH is 7.0. Since a base, even when it is fully dissociated, contains a smaller concentration of H^+ ions than water, its pH must be greater than 7.0. The converse applies to acids. The relationship of the concentration of H^+ ions to pH is shown more clearly in Table 10.1. It will be noted that a change in pH from 7.4 to 7.2 represents a greater change in hydrogen ion concentration than a change from pH 7.6 to 7.4.

TABLE 10.1
THE RELATION OF PH TO HYDROGEN ION CONCENTRATION

pH Scale	nmol/L	
7.0	100	
7.2	63	
7.4	40	i.e. ten-*fold* change in
7.6	25	concentration for 1 pH unit.
7.8	16	
8.0	10	

METHODS OF MEASUREMENT

Although most of the hydrogen ions in the body are within the cells it is not possible to make a direct measurement of intracellular pH. Measurements are therefore usually confined to extracellular fluids and blood. There are three methods in common use.

Indirect Measurements

In biological fluids pH can be calculated from P_{CO_2} and plasma bicarbonate by utilizing some form of the Henderson-Hasselbach equation:

$$pH = pK' + \log\frac{(HCO_3^-)}{0.004 \times P_{CO_2}}$$

It has now become apparent that a constant value of pK' of 6.10 can no longer be accepted since pK' varies with temperature, P_{CO_2} and the non-respiratory component of acid-base balance (Severinghaus et al., 1956; Siggaard-Andersen, 1962). Although the estimate of pH obtained by this method is satisfactory for most clinical purposes (Ludbrook, 1959) it is not adequate for accurate work.

Colorimetric Methods

The use of indicator dyes for measurement of pH was widespread before electrometric measurements were simplified but it is now less commonly used. For a rapid but very inaccurate estimation (± 1 pH unit) a 'universal' indicator may be used. This consists of a mixture of indicators which cover a wide pH range (e.g. BDH Universal indicator pH 4.1–11.0). A few drops of the indicator are added to the liquid under test and the colour compared with a chart which relates the colour to the pH. Greater accuracy (± 0.4 units) can be obtained by using this type of indicator in the form of test papers. More accurate measurements (± 0.3 pH units) can be obtained by using a simple comparator. This consists of a small stand backed by an illuminated ground glass screen. The solution under test is mixed with the appropriate concentration of indicator in a tube and the colour is then compared with the colour of the indicator in a number of other tubes containing buffers of known pH. Methods utilizing light absorption are difficult to apply to turbid solutions and many indicators undergo specific reactions with proteins. For these reasons indicator techniques are now rarely used for clinical estimations of the pH of plasma.

Electrometric Methods

Most measurements of pH are now made by means of pH-sensitive electrodes. The hydrogen electrode has always been the standard by which other methods are judged. Of all electrodes, its response to hydrogen ions is the most clearly understood. However, the technical difficulties associated with its use have precluded its employment in the clinical field. The quinhydrone electrode is simpler technically but lacks versatility. The glass electrode is extremely versatile, does not affect the solution to be measured and can be used with oxidizing or reducing solutions and with colloidal suspensions. It can be adapted for micro-measurements, and can be used for measurements in flow systems or even *in vivo*. It is therefore the electrode of choice for clinical work.

Measurement of pH with the Glass Electrode

When a metal is placed in a solution of one of its salts there is a tendency for the metal ions to go into solution thus leaving the metal with an excess negative charge. If two different metals and their salts are separated by a porous partition, as in the *Daniell* cell (Fig. 10.1) an electromotive force (EMF) is produced

taining a constant concentration it is possible to maintain a constant EMF. This is accomplished in both half-cells of the Weston standard cell (EMF 1.018 V at 20°C). When current flows, cadmium ions enter the solution from the cadmium amalgam (negative terminal) and mercurous ions leave the solution to form mercury at the positive terminal. However, the concentration of the solutions in the cell is accurately maintained since the solutions remain saturated with both sulphates (Fig. 10.2).

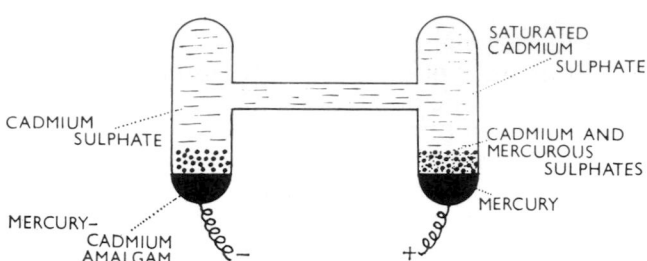

Fig. 10.2 The standard Weston cell.

In the measurement of pH, two half-cells are used (Figs. 10.3 and 10.4). One, the reference electrode, resembles half of the Weston cell but uses mercury and a saturated solution of mercurous chloride (Hg_2Cl_2) or calomel. This is connected to the solution under test by a salt bridge of saturated potassium chloride solution, the actual junction being formed at a porous plug or at the end of a capillary tube. The EMF produced by this cell remains constant as long as the temperature is kept constant.

The other half-cell is the glass electrode. This consists of a glass tube with a bulb of pH-sensitive glass sealed onto the end. The bulb contains an electrolyte, usually 0.1M HCl, into which a silver wire dips to effect an electrical connection. Again, the combination of a metal and its salt ensures a stable potential within the cell. The outside of the pH-sensitive glass makes direct contact with the test solution, the potential developed between the glass and test solution depending on the concentration of hydrogen ions in the solution. It is the variation in this potential which indicates the difference in pH between buffer and test solution.

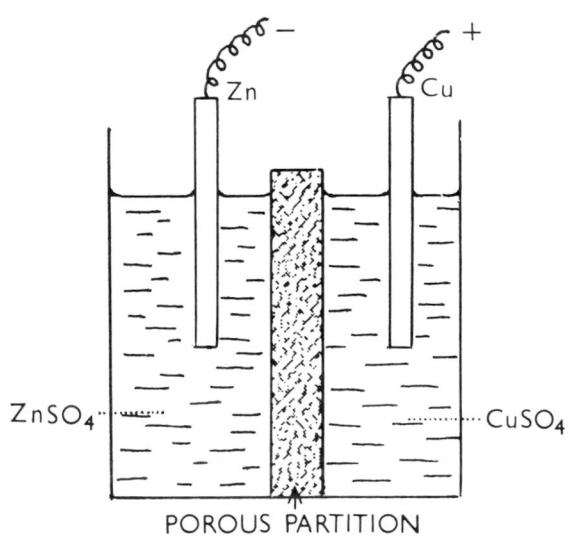

Fig. 10.1 The Daniell cell.

because there is a greater tendency for the zinc ions to go into solution than for copper ions to do so. The EMF of the whole cell may be regarded as the difference between the separate EMFs produced by the two half-cells.

The EMF of a cell depends not only on the nature of the solution but also on its concentration. By main-

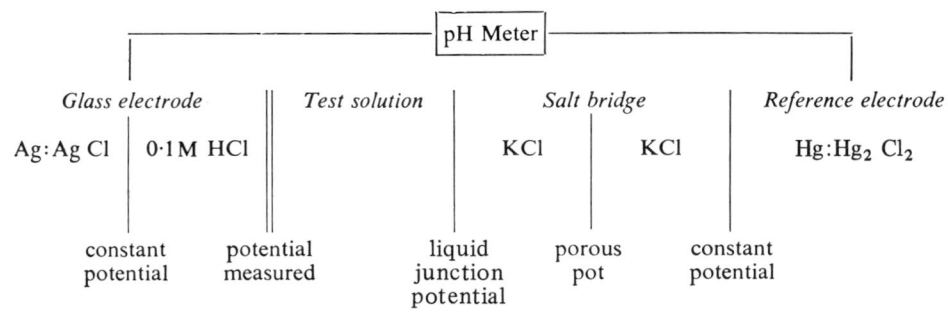

Fig. 10.3 The cell system used in the measurement of pH with the glass electrode.

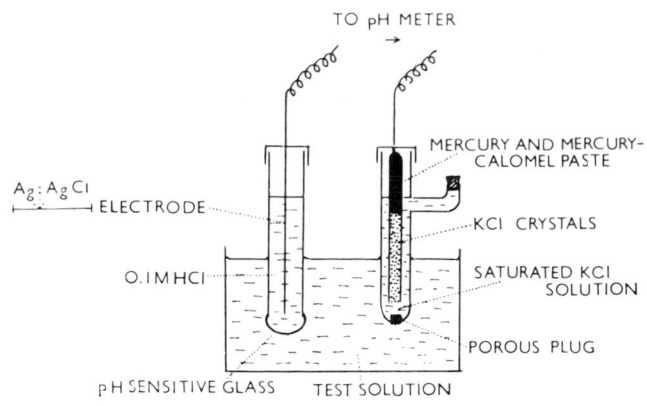

Fig. 10.4 The glass-calomel electrode system.

In addition to the three potentials already mentioned there is a fourth, the liquid junction potential, which is generated at the junction between the test solution and salt bridge. This kind of potential is always developed at the interface between two solutions of different compositions or strengths because of differences in ionic transport across the boundary layer. The magnitude of this potential depends on a number of factors, but in any individual electrode system the commonest cause of variation in the liquid junction potential is a variation in the geometry of the junction itself. For this reason electrode manufacturers take great care to design a liquid junction which can be accurately reproduced each time a measurement is made.

If a reproducible liquid junction potential can be achieved it becomes apparent that the only variable EMF in the system is that generated at the surface of the glass electrode. The total EMF of the system should therefore be governed solely by the temperature and the pH of the test solution. By applying thermodynamic principles it can be shown that the EMF of the cell should be approximately 61.5 mV per pH unit change at 37°C. Unfortunately this theoretical relationship does not apply in practice. There are three reasons for this. Firstly, the thermodynamic *activity* of a solution is not accurately related to the *concentration* of ions except in infinite dilution. This is because attractions arise between migrating anions and cations. Secondly, the exact magnitude of the liquid junction potential is not known. The liquid junction potential can be minimized by using concentrated solutions of potassium chloride (Semple, 1961), and it is possible to design electrode systems which do not rely on a liquid junction, but even so the accuracy of pH measurement can be no better than the accuracy of the convention used to estimate the activity of the chloride ion at the reference electrode. This limits the accuracy of 'true' pH determination to ± 0.02 units at the best (Semple, 1967). The third source of inaccuracy is the variability in the response of the glass electrode. The 'asymmetry potential' (the potential developed across the glass due to the difference in

hydrogen ion concentration on the two sides) decreases with time and after 6–12 months the electrode ceases to function effectively. In addition, the electrode is easily poisoned by protein deposition or other contaminants and may not be linear over all parts of the pH scale.

For these reasons it is necessary to refer the pH measurement to a conventional scale of pH which is, in turn, defined in terms of a number of buffer solutions. The pH electrode is therefore standardized against two known buffers so that the proportionality factor (mV per pH unit change) can be determined and all measurements are then compared with a known buffer so that the actual value of pH can be determined with reference to an agreed standard.

BUFFERS

Buffer solutions are solutions composed of a weak acid and its salt with a strong base, or a weak base and its salt with a strong acid. These dissociate to produce a constant concentration of hydrogen ions at any given temperature and show little variation in pH on the addition of small quantities of a strong acid or base. Unfortunately a number of different pH scales exist and one of the oldest, that of Sørenson, differs by 0.04 pH units from some of the scales used today. The choice of scales is now limited to the British Standards scale (BS) or that of the National Bureau of Standards (NBS) in the USA. While the NBS scale is based on the theoretically derived value of pH, the BS scale ignores this completely and defines the standard on the basis of a phthalate buffer; furthermore, none of the BS buffers are near the pH of blood. For these reasons most workers now prefer the NBS scale. (Report of *ad hoc* Committee on Methodology, 1966). However, as was pointed out previously such a theoretical scale is based on certain assumptions and even if these are correct there is still the unknown potential at the liquid junction. Not only is this junction variable in the individual cell, but it also varies with the design of the electrode and with the composition of the test solution (Siggaard-Andersen, 1961). It may therefore differ with buffer and blood (Kater et al., 1968). For these reasons measured blood pH probably does not bear a fixed relation to the hydrogen ion concentration of the sample.

In clinical practice two buffers are usually used to set up the electrode system. The primary standard for blood pH measurements is a mixture of KH_2PO_4 (0.0087 molal) and Na_2HPO_4 (0.0304 molal). This has a pH of 7.386 at 37°C. A second buffer is used to adjust the gain of the pH meter. A mixture of the same salts in 0.026 molal concentrations is usually used, the pH of this being 6.840 at 37°C (Bates, 1962).

Measurement of Potential

The EMF developed by a glass electrode assembly is

approximately 61.5 mV/pH unit at 37°C, but the internal resistance of the cell is high. Consequently, if the potential across the cell is measured when a current is flowing the reading obtained will be lower than the true EMF. It is, therefore, essential to measure the potential difference when little or no current is flowing. This can be achieved by using a measuring circuit with a very high impedance (about 10^{11} ohms).

As mentioned previously, the EMF of a glass electrode system varies somewhat from day-to-day. The fact is ignored in some commercial pH meters which assume a constant mV–pH unit ratio. The reading can be corrected by noting the pH difference between known buffers and then applying an appropriate correction factor. This process is facilitated by reading the output directly in millivolts. Modern accurate pH meters have a buffer adjustment control, which enables the user to align the buffer reading on the scale with the pH of a known buffer, and a span control which enables the user to adjust the sensitivity of the instrument so that it matches the difference in pH between two known buffers. The latter adjustment corrects for variations in electrode output.

In modern automated analysers the electrode output resulting from the injection of the two buffer solutions is stored in the memory of a microprocessor and subsequently used to correct the output from the test solution so that the correct pH is displayed digitally (Selman and Tait, 1976; Rubin et al., 1979).

Sources of Error in pH Measurement

Errors in pH measurement occur frequently despite the apparent simplicity of the technique. Anyone who wishes to convince himself of this fact should attempt to duplicate all blood pH measurements on two electrode systems. Even with meticulous care agreement to within 0.005 of a pH unit will be the exception rather than the rule! Indeed, the author has on a number of occasions noted errors of up to 0.3 pH units when the same blood sample has been measured on two electrode systems which were set up on the same pair of buffers and which gave almost identical readings on a third buffer. The only way to guard against such errors is to check the electrode system at least once a day. This can be accomplished either by comparing a pH reading of a *blood* sample with that determined on another electrode system, or by the use of a stabilized serum preparation (G. W. Burton—*see* Adams et al., 1967 and 1968). Other solutions for checking the accuracy of pH electrodes are now available commercially (Minty and Nunn, 1977).

Temperature Corrections

If the blood is sampled at one temperature, stored anaerobically and measured in an electrode system maintained at another temperature it is necessary to apply a correction factor to the observed reading,

there being a rise in pH as the temperature of the blood falls or vice versa. The reason for the change in pH is that the degree of ionization of the protein elements of blood is reduced as temperature falls. This releases more cations (Na^+ and K^+) for the carriage of CO_2 as HCO_3^- and the bicarbonate content of the plasma increases. P_{CO_2} therefore falls and pH rises (Brewin et al., 1955).

The factor commonly used to correct pH for temperature changes is that of Rosenthal (1948), namely pH rises 0.0147 of a pH unit for each °C fall in temperature. However, this factor is affected by the respiratory and, to a lesser extent, the non-respiratory state of the blood (Burton, 1965). Unfortunately, the significance of a pH measurement at low body temperatures is not clear and most units utilizing induced hypothermia assess the non-respiratory component at 37°C and only adjust the P_{O_2} and P_{CO_2} values to body temperature.

Blood Sampling and Storage

Blood samples may be venous, capillary or arterial. Venous samples taken from the median cubital vein are completely unreliable as the pH is influenced by the degree of stasis introduced by the tourniquet, the activity of the muscles, and the proportions of skin and muscle blood flow in the sample. Brooks and Wynn (1959) have shown that 'arterialized' venous blood obtained from the back of the hand without constriction and under certain specified conditions may provide a useful estimate in some cases. Astrup has proposed that capillary blood should be used. In the warm vasodilated ear of a patient at rest this may yield a reasonable comparison with arterial blood, but in babies and under certain conditions (Cooper and Smith, 1961) the relation to arterial blood pH is extremely variable.

Arterial samples are therefore used whenever possible. Arterial blood may be sampled by intermittent puncture with a 23 SWG needle or an indwelling plastic catheter. Catheters may be of the disposable type, which are inserted over a needle, or may be threaded over a flexible guide by the Seldinger (1953) technique. To minimize complications the catheter should be made of Teflon, should have parallel sides and should not be larger than 20 gauge (Davis and Stewart, 1980). Catheters should be flushed at frequent intervals with small quantities of heparinized saline (10 iu mL^{-1}) or connected to a device which ensures that a slow, continuous flush passes through the catheter.

If the blood sample is to be obtained by direct puncture the barrel of the syringe should be well lubricated with heparin (1000 iu mL^{-1}) by taking about 1 ml of heparin into the syringe, holding the syringe with its nozzle uppermost and then working the plunger up and down a few times. The syringe is then tapped to allow the air bubbles to rise to the surface of the heparin and any bubbles and excess heparin are expelled before attaching the syringe to the needle in the artery. A slight force must be applied to the plunger to overcome the friction present in plastic syringes but care must be taken not to apply excessive pressure for this may cause the syringe to leak or may even cause dissolved gas to come out of solution, so altering the pH.

After sampling, firm pressure must be applied to the artery. The required duration and extent of pressure cannot be predicted but should be related to the size of needle used and to such other factors as the arterial pressure, use of anticoagulants, etc. For direct puncture an occlusive pressure of 2–3 minutes duration followed by more gentle pressure for a further 2–3 minutes is usually adequate. However, the artery must always be observed for a further 5–10 minutes and it is a wise precaution always to apply a pressure dressing. Haematoma formation is very common (Gillies et al., 1979).

The syringe should be capped with a plastic or metal cap and then rotated between the palms to mix the sample. Mixing should be repeated before the pH is measured and the measurement should be completed as soon as possible after sampling. If immediate analysis is impossible the syringe should be stored in ice and water. Under these conditions the pH falls approximately 0.004 pH units per hour.

THE VALUE OF pH MEASUREMENTS

Measurements of the pH of blood reflect changes in the extracellular compartment of the body but this may bear little relation to changes in the intracellular compartment. Changes within the cells cannot be measured directly and little is known about the significance of intracellular changes in pH. However it is also important to realize that changes in the blood may not parallel changes in other body fluids. For example, an acute non-respiratory acidosis will cause a fall in blood pH but a rise in CSF pH.

From the Henderson-Hasselbach equation (p. 131) it may be seen that pH depends on the ratio between the quantities of base and acid present. Using the bicarbonate system as an example, the ratio of HCO_3^- to CO_2 is normally 20:1. Any increase in bicarbonate or decrease in CO_2 will therefore cause an alkalaemia and any reduction in bicarbonate or increase in CO_2 will cause an acidaemia (Report of *ad hoc* Committee on Acid-base Terminology, 1966). It is obvious therefore that the significance of acid-base changes cannot be decided on the basis of a measurement of pH alone. However, if one of the other two variables (i.e. HCO_3^- or P_{CO_2}) is measured then the full acid-base picture can be derived from the Henderson-Hasselbach equation or from one of the nomograms based on it (Siggaard-Andersen, 1971).

Changes in either the respiratory or non-respiratory components of acid-base balance are usually compensated by an alteration in the other component so that the pH is returned towards 7.4, but the rate at which this compensation occurs varies. For example, a change in the non-respiratory component usually induces a rapid but opposing change in the respiratory component so that pH is quickly returned towards normal levels. On the other hand the non-respiratory response to a respiratory change takes a matter of hours or days to develop: marked changes of pH may therefore result from acute changes of P_{CO_2}. In both situations the direction of the primary change is indicated by the direction of change in pH, for compensation is seldom complete. It is, however, unwise to base clinical judgements on such an assumption for two reasons. Firstly, there may be some complicating factor which causes an alteration in one of the components independently of the primary change. For example, a patient with respiratory failure may also have been treated with diuretics for heart failure. The pH, instead of being on the acid side of normal (indicating a primary respiratory disturbance) might then be above 7.4. This would wrongly suggest a primary non-respiratory alkalosis with compensating respiratory acidosis. The second reason for treating this assumption with caution is that there may be an alteration in the respiratory state due to the disturbance caused by blood sampling. For example, a patient in chronic respiratory failure with a high P_{CO_2} and compensatory increase in bicarbonate may develop a pH above 7.4 due to transient over-breathing at the moment of sampling. All pH values must therefore be considered in relation to the patient's history and present state. If this is done then pH may provide much useful clinical information. As an example one can consider again the patient with chronic obstructive airways disease who develops acute respiratory failure due to an infection. The P_{CO_2} will rise and cause a marked fall in pH. The bicarbonate will then rise gradually over the next one to two days until the pH is restored towards normal. If the patient has a high P_{CO_2} and a low pH on admission it suggests that the bicarbonate level is normal and that the patient is suffering from acute respiratory failure. If, however, the pH on admission is not low when the P_{CO_2} is high it suggests that the CO_2 retention has existed for some time and that the patient has a compensating non-respiratory alkalosis. The difference between these two situations may well affect the plan of treatment.

RECENT ADVANCES IN pH MEASUREMENT

The major advance has been the development of safe, rapid-response intravascular pH sensors. Although intravascular pH sensors have been available for over 20 years (Band and Semple, 1967), they have been difficult to produce, inconsistent in performance and have required the placement of a reference electrode to maintain an electrical connection with the subject.

Recently, a new type of electrode has been developed which does not create any electrical hazard for the patient, for it utilizes fibreoptics to detect the change of colour of a dye situated at the end of an intravascular catheter (Peterson et al., 1980). The catheter consists of two 0.15 mm diameter plastic optical fibres situated within a 0.30 mm ID cuprophan hollow dialysis tube which is covered for most of its length by a protective plastic sleeve. The tip of the dialysis tube is filled with microspheres of polyacrylamide to which is bound the pH-sensitive dye phenol red. The microspheres contain even smaller polystyrene spheres which provide very effective light scattering so that the light from a tungsten source, which is transmitted along one optical fibre, is then returned along the other fibre to the measuring instrument. The probe is calibrated by immersion in buffers at 37°C and can be passed through an 18 gauge needle. The probe is stable, has a 63% response time of 0.7 min and gives pH values which are within ± 0.02 pH unit within the pH range 7.0–7.4. However, it is subject to the usual problems of fibrin deposition on the probe. A similar probe which will pass through a 22 gauge needle has performed well in the experimental situation (Abraham et al., 1985).

Another recent development utilizes dyes in which there is a change in the intensity of fluorescence in response to changes in pH. Such dyes are weak electrolytes which can exist in both acid and base forms in solution, the proportion depending on the pH. The excitation spectrum of the acid and base forms of the dye differ, the former peaking at 410 nm whilst the latter peaks at 460 nm but both emit at a peak of 520 nm. Hence the ratio of the fluorescence intensity at 520 nm measured with 460 nm excitation to that measured with 410 nm excitation is a measure of the basic and acid forms of the dye. This ratio is relatively insensitive to changes in optical throughput.

By incorporating bicarbonate in the pH sensor the device can be made sensitive to P_{CO_2} (as in the Severinghaus CO_2 electrode). P_{O_2} can be measured with a similar device, the three sensors having been incorporated in a single catheter which will pass through a radial artery cannula (Gehrich et al., 1986).

CONCLUSIONS

Accurate pH measurements can only be achieved by meticulous attention to detail and repeated checking of the electrode system. One only has to compare pH determinations made by a number of different workers on the same system or by the same workers on different systems, to realize how wide can be the variation in results. However, if care is taken, reproducible results can be obtained and the measurement of blood pH can then provide an invaluable guide to the acid-base status of the patient.

REFERENCES

Abraham E., Markle D.R., Fink S., et al. (1985). Continuous measurement of intravascular pH with a fiberoptic sensor. *Anesth. Analg.*, **64**, 731.

Adams A.P., Morgan-Hughes J.O., Sykes M.K. (1967a).

pH and blood-gas analysis: methods of measurement and sources of error using electrode systems, Part 1. *Anaesthesia*, **22**, 575.

Adams A.P., Morgan-Hughes J.O., Sykes M.K. (1967b). pH and blood-gas analysis: methods of measurement and sources of error using electrode systems, Part 2. *Anaesthesia*, **23**, 47.

Band D.M., Semple S.J.G. (1967). Continuous measurement of blood pH with an indwelling arterial glass electrode. *J. Appl. Physiol.*, **22**, 854.

Bates R.G. (1962). Revised standard values for pH measurements from 0 to 95°C. *J. Res. Nat. Bur. Std. A.*, **66A**, 179.

Brewin E.G., Gould R.P., Nashat F.S. et al. (1955). An investigation of problems of acid-base equilibrium in hypothermia. *Guy's Hosp. Rep.*, **104**, 177.

Brønsted, J.N. (1923). Einige Bemerkungen uber den Begriff der Säuren und Basen. *Rev. trav. chim. Pays-Bas*, **42**, 718.

Brooks D., Wynn V. (1959). Use of venous blood for pH and carbon-dioxide studies. Especially in respiratory failure and during anaesthesia. *Lancet*, **1**, 227.

Burton, G.W. (1965). Effects of the acid-base state upon the temperature coefficient of pH of blood. *Br. J. Anaesth.*, **37**, 89.

Cooper E.A., Smith H. (1961). Indirect estimation of arterial P_{CO_2}. *Anaesthesia*, **16**, 445.

Davis F.M., Stewart J.M. (1980). Radial artery cannulation. A prospective study in patients undergoing cardiothoracic surgery. *Br. J. Anaesth.*, **52**, 41.

Gehrich J.L., Lubbers D.W., Opitz N., et al. (1986). Optical fluorescence and its application to an intravascular blood gas monitoring system. *IEEE. Trans. Biomed. Eng.*, **BME 33**, 117.

Gillies I.D.S., Morgan M., Sykes M.K., et al. (1979). The nature and incidence of complications of peripheral arterial puncture. *Anaesthesia*, **34**, 506.

Kater J.A.R., Leonard J.E., Matsuyama G. (1968). Junction potential variations in blood pH measurements. *Ann. N.Y. Acad. Sc.*, **148**, 54.

Ludbrook J. (1959). Estimation of P_{CO_2} by means of the Henderson-Hasselbach Equation. In *A Symposium on pH and Blood Gas Measurement*, p. 34. (Woolmer R.F. ed.). London: Churchill.

Minty B.D., Nunn J.F. (1977). Regional quality control survey of blood-gas analysis. *Ann. Clin. Biochem.*, **14**, 245.

Peterson J.I., Fitzgerald R.V., Buckhold D.K. (1980). Fibreoptic pH probe for physiological use. *Anal. Chem.*, **52**, 864.

Report of the *ad hoc* committee on acid-base terminology: current concepts of acid-base measurement (1966). *Ann. N.Y. Acad. Sci.*, **133**, 251.

Report of *ad hoc* committee on methodology: current concepts of acid-base measurement (1966). *Ann. N.Y. Acad. Sci.*, **133**, 259.

Rosenthal T.B. (1948). The effect of temperature on the pH of blood and plasma *in vitro*. *J. Biol. Chem.*, **173**, 25.

Rubin P., Bradbury S., Prowse, K. (1979). Comparative study of automatic blood-gas analysers and their use in analysing arterial and capillary samples. *Br. Med. J.*, **i**, 156.

Seldinger S.I. (1953). Catheter replacement of the needle in percutaneous arteriography. *Acta Radiol.* (Stockh), **39**, 368.

Selman B.J., Tait A.R. (1976). Towards blood-gas autoanalysis. An evaluation of the radiometer ABL1. *Br. J. Anaesth.*, **48**, 487.

Semple S. (1961). Observed pH differences of blood and

plasma with different bridge solutions. *J. Appl. Physiol.*, **16**, 576.

Semple S. (1967). Problems in measurement and interpretation of blood acid-base state. *Bio-med. Engng.*, **2**, 500.

Severinghaus J.W., Stupfel M., Bradley A.F. (1956). Variations of serum carbonic acid pK' with pH and temperature. *J. Appl. Physiol.*, **9**, 197.

Siggaard-Andersen O. (1961). Factors affecting the liquid-junction potential in electrometric blood pH measurement. *Scand. J. Clin. Lab. Invest.*, **13**, 205.

Siggaard-Andersen O. (1962). The first dissociation exponent of carbonic acid as a function of pH. *Scand. J. Clin. Lab. Invest.*, **14**, 587.

Siggaard-Andersen O. (1971). An acid-base chart for arterial blood with normal and pathophysiological reference areas. *Scand. J. Clin. Lab. Invest.*, **27**, 239.

Sørensen S.P.L. (1909). Etudes enzymatiques. Part 2. Sur la mésure et l'importance de la concentration des ions hydrogèns dans leurs reactions enzymatiques. *Comt. rend. trav. lab. Carlsberg*, **8**, 1.

Other Suggested Reading

Adams A.P., Hahn C.E.W. (1979). *Principles and practice of blood-gas analysis*. London: Franklin Scientific Projects.

Davenport H.W. (1969). *The ABC of Acid-base Chemistry*. 5th edn. Chicago: University of Chicago Press.

Flenley D.C. (1978). Interpretation of blood-gas and acid-base data. *Brit. J. Hosp. Med.*, **20**, 384.

Nunn J.F. (1962). Nomenclature and presentation of hydrogen ion regulation data. In *Modern Trends and Anaesthesia*, 2: Aspects of hydrogen ion regulation and biochemistry in anaesthesia. (Evans F.T., Gray T.C. eds.). London: Butterworths.

Siggaard-Andersen O. (1967) Therapeutic aspects of acid-base disorders. In *Modern Trends in Anaesthesia*, 3: Aspects of metabolism and pulmonary ventilation. (Evans F.T., Gray T.C. eds.). London: Butterworths.

Siggaard-Andersen O. (1974). *The acid-base status of the blood*, 4th edn. Copenhagen: Munksgaard.

11. Physical Basis of Radioisotopic Techniques

A. Hilson

Structure of atoms-isotopes
Half-life
Types of radioactive decay
  Spontaneous fission
  Alpha decay
  Beta decay
  Positron decay
  Electron capture
Detection of radioactivity
Uses of tracers
  Choice of tracers
  Comparison of activities
  Time-activity studies
  Profile studies
  Planar scintigraphy
  Tomographic scintigraphy
  Dynamic scintigraphy

This chapter describes the underlying basis of techniques in clinical use involving radioisotopes. These are the techniques of nuclear medicine, although inevitably there is an overlap with other specialities. The techniques which will be considered fall into three groups: *in vitro* methods (which overlap with pathology); therapeutic techniques using unsealed sources (which overlap with radiotherapy); and diagnostic imaging (which overlaps with radiology).

All of these fields rely on the use of radioactive materials as *tracers* which follow a pathway, metabolic or otherwise, which is shared by a stable compound. This is often, but not always, based on the use of radioactive atoms as tracers for stable isotopes of the same element.

STRUCTURE OF ATOMS–ISOTOPES

To understand the atomic basis of radioactivity, it is first necessary to consider the structure of the atom. Current thinking is based on the model proposed by Rutherford, and modified by Bohr. In this model, the atom consists of a nucleus, surrounded by electrons.

The *nucleus* of an atom consists of protons, which have a positive charge, and neutrons which have no charge. The number of protons in the nucleus of any atom is known as the atomic number (symbol Z), and this determines which element the atom represents. The number of neutrons (symbol N), added to the number of protons, Z, gives the atomic mass number (symbol A). Atoms sharing the same proton number (Z) are all atoms of the same substance, even if they have different mass numbers (A) and are referred to as *isotopes*. The term *nuclide* is used to refer to a specific nucleus, with a stated atomic number Z and mass number A. The notation used to specify a nuclide X, of mass number A, and atomic number Z, is

$$_{Z}^{A}X$$

Examples of specific nuclides are $_{1}^{1}H$, $_{6}^{12}C$, $_{8}^{16}O$ and $_{11}^{23}Na$, the common stable isotopes of hydrogen, carbon, oxygen, and sodium.

Although this is the correct formal notation, it is often replaced, for simplicity, by the chemical symbol or name of the element, together with the mass number A, as the value of Z is implied by the chemical symbol. In this notation the nuclides listed above would be written as 1-H or Hydrogen-1; 12-C or Carbon-12; 16-O or Oxygen-16; and 23-Na or Sodium-23.

The protons in the nucleus have a positive charge, and so tend to repel one another. On the other hand, all the nucleons, both protons and neutrons, are bound together by a stronger force, the nuclear force, which is of short range. There is a relationship between the number of neutrons and protons needed to form a stable nucleus. As the number of protons increases, so does the total electrostatic repulsive charge, and therefore the number of neutrons needed to stabilize them. For a stable nucleus, the number of neutrons needed is slightly larger than the number of protons. If the number of neutrons is larger or smaller than needed for stability, the nucleus will be unstable, and will undergo rearrangement to give a stable configuration. This process is known as *radioactive decay*. This may occur by the expulsion of a charged particle, or by the capture of an electron by the nucleus. The product of this process is by definition the nucleus of another nuclide. This may be stable, or may be unstable itself, undergoing further decay. Even if it is stable, the nucleus may be left with excess energy, in which case it is said to be 'excited'. In this case, the energy is given up as electromagnetic radiation (*a gamma-ray*) of characteristic energy. Occasionally this excited state may be stable for long enough to be identified separately, and it is then said to be *metastable*. This is denoted by adding the suffix 'm' to the designation of the nuclide (e.g. ^{99m}Tc).

HALF-LIFE

If a nuclide is unstable, and so undergoing radioactive decay (i.e. it is a *radionuclide*), the rate of decay is characteristic of that radionuclide. It is not affected by physical or chemical conditions. The time at which any given atom decays is random, but the probability of that decay is constant, regardless of the time which has elapsed. This probability may be expressed as the *decay constant*, or transformation constant, which has the unit of time^{-1} and is represented by the symbol λ. The same information may be expressed as the *half-life*, which is the time taken for half the atoms present to decay. The two are related by

$$T_{1/2} = \frac{0.693}{\lambda}$$

For instance, the rate of decay of ^{131}I may be expressed by stating that it has a decay constant of $\lambda = 0.086 \text{ d}^{-1}$, or that it has a half-life of $T_{1/2} = 8.06$ days.

It is possible to show that the number of atoms N at time t, after starting at time 0 with N_0 atoms is given by the relationship

$$N = N_0 \exp^{-\lambda t}$$

where λ is the decay constant. Using this relationship it is possible to correct for radioactive decay.

It is important to realize that we are dealing here with an exponential process, with a constant proportion of the remaining atoms decaying in each time interval. It follows that if the amount of radioactivity is plotted against time using log/linear axes (so-called semi-log paper), a straight line is obtained. Furthermore, it will take an infinitely long time for all the atoms to decay.

TYPES OF RADIOACTIVE DECAY

There are five types of radioactive decay. Two of these, spontaneous fission and alpha decay, are associated with change in the mass of the nucleus. In the other three there is a change in the charge of the nucleus, but not mass—these are electron decay, positron decay, and electron capture.

Spontaneous Fission

Spontaneous fission occurs only in the nuclei of the very heavy elements. An example is the spontaneous fission of (^{238}U) (Z = 92) into smaller nuclei, such as bromine (Z = 35) and lanthanum (Z = 57). Each of these daughter nuclides is unstable and undergoes further decay. This type of decay is of direct importance in reactor and weapon technology, but is of medical interest only in that it may represent a source of some radioisotopes.

Alpha Decay

Alpha decay is also only found in the decay scheme of the heavier elements, where the nucleus has an excess of both protons and neutrons over the stability ratio. The nucleus gives off an alpha particle, which is a helium nucleus consisting of two protons and two neutrons. This reduces the mass of the parent nucleus by four units and the charge by two units. The alpha-particle has a high energy of 3.7 MeV, and because of its relatively high mass and high charge it only has a short range in tissue (measured in microns) before interacting with another atom and releasing its energy, which is large because of the high kinetic energy. This release of energy, if it occurs in a cell, causes the high radiation damage typical of alpha emitters. This radiation damage makes alpha emitters unsuitable for diagnostic use in medicine (although there is a little interest in their possible therapeutic use).

Beta Decay

In beta decay (also known as electron decay) a neutron in the nucleus of the atom decays to a proton and an electron. The proton remains in the nucleus, and thus the charge increases by one unit, and therefore Z, so that the daughter nucleus is that of a different element. The electron is emitted from the nucleus, along with a particle known as an anti-neutrino. The energy released in the decay is shared between the electron and the anti-neutrino, and so the electrons have a range of energies.

An example of beta decay is the decay scheme of $^{90}_{38}Sr$ which decays with a half-life of 27.7 years to $^{90}_{39}Y$ with the emission of an electron of maximum energy of 0.54 MeV. The yttrium in turn decays with a half-life of 64 hours to $^{90}_{40}Zr$ with the emission of an electron of maximum energy 2.27 MeV. Note that all three nuclides have the same mass number, but that the atomic number Z increases with each decay. It is common for beta decay to occur in chains of sequential beta decays. Beta decay is found in nuclei which show an excess of neutrons, and is thus common in products of reactor irradiation where the radioactivity is produced by bombardment with neutrons.

The electron interacts with matter by colliding with orbital electrons (the volume of the nucleus being relatively minute). This may cause the target electron to move to a higher energy level (excitation), from which it will return with emission of characteristic X-rays (which depend on the energy level between the orbits), or it may displace it completely, causing ionization. It is this ionization which is responsible for radiation damage. Electrons having a low mass, travel only a relatively short distance in tissue (of the order of millimetres), but cause a considerable amount of ionization as a result of their charge.

Because of their short range, isotopes which undergo beta decay are not used in imaging aspects of Nuclear Medicine when there is any alternative, but are of importance in therapeutic aspects. For instance, ^{32}P, ^{131}I and ^{90}Y are all used therapeutically, the electrons being responsible for the therapeutic effect. However, ^{131}I, which also emits gamma rays, is only used for imaging when ^{123}I, which shares the same chemistry but is not a beta emitter, cannot be used.

Positron Decay

Positron decay is the converse of electron decay. The positron is a particle of the same mass as an electron, but of positive charge. Positrons are produced during the decay of nuclei which are relatively poor in neutrons, in which a proton changes to a neutron, with the emission of a positron and a neutrino. The nuclear charge, and therefore the atomic number Z, reduces by one unit, with no change in the mass number. An example is the decay of $^{18}_{9}F$ to $^{18}_{8}O$ with a half-life of 110 minutes, and the emission of a positron. Positron emitters all have short half-lives, and because they are poor in neutrons they must be produced by irradiation in reactors. They are usually produced by irradiation with particles such as protons in a cyclotron, which is a much more expensive method of production. Because the positron is of low mass and has a positive charge, it has a high probability of interaction with an electron (which is its anti-particle) in tissue.

This interaction of two oppositely charged particles causes the annihilation of both, their mass being converted into energy which is emitted as two gamma rays which have an energy of 511 keV each and which are emitted at 180 degrees to each other. It is this unusual annihilation radiation which makes positron-emitters of such interest, since the two photons can be recorded by opposed detectors and the position at which the annihilation occurred can be calculated. Since positrons only travel a short distance before annihilation, this point is effectively the location of the decaying atom. Tomography with positrons is therefore relatively simple.

Electron Capture

Electron capture is the other form of radioactive decay which may occur in a nucleus with a relative neutron deficit. Here one of the orbital electrons is captured by the nucleus, where it combines with a proton to form a neutron, with a decrease in atomic number but no change in mass number. The nucleus thus formed may be in an excited state, and will then give off its excess energy as a gamma ray of characteristic energy. Since gamma rays may be considered as 'pure energy', they have a relatively long range in tissue (typically of the order of several centimetres) and cause less ionization, and thus less radiation damage.

Isotopes which decay by electron capture are therefore the preferred ones for imaging procedures since they tend to emit mainly gamma rays which leave the patient (and can thus be detected) with relatively low radiation dose, as opposed to beta emission which does not travel far in tissue and is therefore difficult to detect whilst giving a relatively high radiation dose.

It must be realized that the above is a relatively simple account, and most radionuclides show complex decay schemes. For instance, ^{131}I decays by electron capture to ^{131}Xe, but there are three different energies of electron which may be emitted, and each produces a different excitation level of the resultant ^{131}Xe nucleus, which then de-excites with emission of gamma rays to one of five energies.

DETECTION OF RADIOACTIVITY

For all practical purposes, human beings are unable to detect ionizing radiation, and we are therefore forced to rely on indirect methods for its detection and measurement. This involves allowing the radiation to interact with matter, and then measuring the degree of interaction which has occurred. One of the simplest is the ability of radiation to produce ionization in photographic film, thus 'exposing' it. The amount of darkening is related to the amount of ionization and thus, approximately, to the amount of radiation. This is the basis of the familiar film badge dosimeter. It is also used as the basis of localization of specific molecules in molecular genetics, where a chromatography strip containing a radioactive compound of interest is placed over a sheet of film, and the film exposure indicates the location of the molecule of interest.

A second effect of beta and gamma radiation which has been known since the early part of the century is their ability to produce ionization in a substance such as a gas. If an electrical potential is applied across the gas, the ions produced will carry a current, which will be related to the degree of ionization. At its simplest, this is used in the Geiger counter where the pulses produced by the ionization are amplified and, typically, converted to sound. In this form the Geiger counter is a simple, robust, detector but it is only of real value as a detector of low levels of radiation, since the ionization detector cannot respond to high count rates (and indeed may positively mislead by 'paralysing' and suggesting that no radiation is present). Furthermore, the system provides no information as to the type or energy of the incident radiation.

A specialized type of ionization detector is the isotope calibrator, to be found in all Nuclear Medicine departments. This is an ionization chamber of relatively low sensitivity, but of high accuracy, in which relatively large amounts of activity may be placed. The current flowing (typically of the order of picoamps) is measured using an electrometer. This current is then proportional to the amount of activity in the chamber, the relationship being known for the isotope concerned.

The second major type of radiation detection is by scintillation detection. This relies on the fact that certain materials, when excited by radiation, de-excite by emitting energy in the UV and visible portions of the electromagnetic spectrum. These materials have the advantage that the amount of light emitted is proportional to the energy deposited in the detector, and thus to the energy of the radiation. Each interaction produces a flash of light and these pulses of light are amplified using one or more photomultiplier tubes. Scintillation detection is the most widely used method of radiation detection in Nuclear Medicine today. The system in most general use utilizes a crystal of sodium iodide, to which has been added 0.1%–0.5% of thallium to produce the NaI(Tl) detector. As this material is hygroscopic, it is enclosed in an aluminium 'can', with a transparent window to which the photomultiplier is attached. Crystals of NaI(Tl) are regularly manufactured up to 50 cm in diameter.

A scintillation detector sample counter consists of an NaI(Tl) crystal, often incorporating a well into which the sample is placed, a photomultiplier and electronics for counting that number of pulses, together with discriminant circuitry to ensure that only pulses of the appropriate energy are counted. Such a counter may also have a mechanism for changing the samples automatically, as well as built-in computing facilities.

The simplest detector used in clinical practice for *in vivo* work consists of an NaI(Tl) crystal and photo-multiplier assembly, surrounded by lead shielding except over one end of the crystal, forming a probe which may be used for counting the activity under it. Such a probe is used in renography, splenic sequestration and in thyroid uptake studies.

Following the development of the surface scintillation probe, which could not only be used to measure the uptake at one site but also to compare activities at different sites, it became apparent that it was logical to move the probe mechanically. This is the basis of the rectilinear scanner, in which the probe is moved to-and-fro across the patient and the distribution of activity is plotted as the degree of exposure of a photographic film. The probe is usually fitted with a collimator, consisting of a lead insert with tapered holes to restrict the volume from which activity is detected The rectilinear scanner has the advantage of high sensitivity and resolution, but is slow and bulky and takes what may be a relatively long time to cover the volume of interest. This may not matter overmuch for an organ such as the thyroid, but makes imaging of organs such as the liver very difficult.

An alternative approach is the use of a gamma-camera. Here a large diameter, thin NaI(Tl) crystal has multiple (usually between 37 and 91) photomultiplier tubes behind it, each seeing a portion of the crystal. By comparing the signals from all the tubes it is possible to reconstruct the position of the crystal at which the gamma ray hit it. Since the gamma-camera is usually fitted with a collimator which ensures that only gamma rays incident normal to the plane of the crystal can reach it, the distribution of scintillations in the crystal mirrors the distribution of activity in the patient. The gamma-camera has a lower sensitivity than the scanner, but can 'see' a larger area *at any one time* than the scanner and can also be used to detect changes in activity with time. Incidentally, it is this replacement of the rectilinear scanner by the gamma-camera which is one reason for the replacement of the term 'scan' by 'scintigram'. (The other is the use of 'scan' for other modalities, such as CT and ultrasound).

The other type of scintillation detector of routine value is the liquid scintillator. This is a complex of organic chemicals which gives off light in response to radiation. Liquid scintillation is used for measuring samples containing beta emitters, such as ^{14}C and ^{3}H, which are mixed with the scintillant, and the resultant light output measured by an external photomultiplier system. It is necessary to use this method as a result of the short range of electrons, which will only travel a few millimetres in liquid.

USES OF TRACERS

Having considered the basis of the methods by which tracers may be utilized, we can study the ways in which they are used. First we may consider the factors which lead to the choice of a specific tracer and then the method of application. The best classification of the latter is that of Rassow (1970). What is measured in a Nuclear Medicine study is a count rate which is hopefully proportional to a count rate or activity, A. At its simplest two activities, A_1 and A_2 are compared. At the most complex, the variations in A with space and time are measured. This may be expressed mathematically by saying that A is a function of the three spatial dimensions and time, i.e. $A = f(x,y,z,t)$. In any one study the variation of A with respect to one or more variables may be examined, ignoring the effects of the others. Using this approach, Nuclear Medicine studies may be grouped as follows:

1. Comparison of two activities
2. Time–activity studies $A = f(t)$
3. Profile studies $A = f(x)$
4. Planar scintigraphy $A = f(x,y)$
5. Tomographic scintigraphy $A = f(x,y,z)$
6. Dynamic scintigraphy $A = f(x,y,t)$

Choice of Tracers

Since the purpose of Nuclear Medicine studies is to examine physiological processes, it is necessary to have a tracer which follows the normal pathway of interest. This requires finding a suitable molecule, and labelling it with a appropriate radionuclide. Ideally, the radionuclide should have a half-life which is long enough not to be a problem during the study, but is as short as possible to reduce the radiation dose to the patient. In practical terms, the ideal radionuclide should have a half-life about twice the length of the procedure being undertaken, should be a gamma emitter, and should not affect the molecule in which it is inserted. This is not always possible. The most widely used radionuclide is technetium-99m (^{99m}Tc), which has a half life of six hours, multiple valency states, and can be obtained by elution of a chromatography column loaded with Molybdenum-99(^{99}Mo). Ammonium molybdate remains attached to the column, the daughter pertechnetate comes off the column when it is eluted with saline. However, many materials of biological interest cannot be labelled with technetium. These include many small biological molecules, and the only practical labels are radionuclides of low atomic number, which are often positron emitters of short half-life. Therefore these can only be used in the vicinity of the cyclotron in which they are prepared.

The trend in radiopharmacy is for initial studies to be performed with cyclotron-prepared tracers. Once the feasibility of the technique has been shown, the next step is often a tracer labelled with an 'intermediate' radionuclide, such as ^{131}I, ^{111}In, or ^{123}I. Eventually, a Technetium-labelled method is evolved.

Comparison of Activities

Three types of studies come into this category: methods using dilution analysis; methods using saturation analysis; and methods using transport analysis.

Dilution Analysis

If a known quantity of a labelled tracer is mixed with an unknown quantity of the unlabelled substance, and the mixture is sampled, then the amount by which the tracer is diluted depends only on the amount of unlabelled tracer present. The simplest study in which dilution analysis is used is the estimation of red blood cell volume using ^{51}Cr-labelled red blood cells. If 1 ml of labelled red blood cells of activity A_1 is injected intravenously, allowed to mix, and a 1 ml blood sample of activity A_2 and dilution D is obtained, then the volume of red blood cells in which the labelled tracer dose has been distributed is given by:

$$V = \frac{A_1 \times D}{A_2}$$

To obtain the blood volume, it is then only necessary to correct for the haematocrit. Similarly, the plasma volume can be estimated using labelled albumin.

Saturation Analysis

This is very similar to dilution analysis, in that a known quantity of labelled tracer is mixed with an unknown quantity of unlabelled substance. Following complete mixing, a portion of the mixture is then separated from other substances using a specific binding method. The quantity of radioactivity bound is then a function of the ratio between the amount of labelled and unlabelled compounds present. By using known quantities of the unlabelled compound, it is possible to derive a calibration curve expressing the ratio between the bound activity and the total amount of activity for different amounts of unlabelled compound, and to read off the concentration of any unknown sample from this curve. This is the basis of radioimmunoassay, in which the binding compound is an antibody, specific for the compound being measured.

Transport Analysis

Since the total amount of radioactivity (allowing for decay) administered to a patient is equal to the sum of the excreted and distributed activities, it is possible to make statements about the transport mechanism by measuring the activities administered and excreted. The best known example of this approach is the Schilling test, where the storage capacity is saturated with stable Vitamin B_{12}, and the urinary excretion of labelled B_{12} depends only on the patient's absorption ability.

Time-activity Studies

These are concerned with the changes of activity with time in a volume of the patient being studied. The volume may be an anatomical structure, such as a kidney, or an abstract space such as the volume of distribution of a tracer. One of the simplest of these studies is the use of ^{51}Cr labelled RBCs to study red blood cell survival. By taking serial blood samples over a period of days, it is possible to measure the rate of disappearance from the blood, and hence the mean red cell life. At the same time, it is also possible to measure the count rate over the spleen and liver using a surface probe, and so derive time-activity curves for these organs which show whether there is abnormal sequestration of RBCs in the spleen.

A more complex example is the measurement of cardiac output. If a probe is positioned over any vessel and a small amount of radioactivity injected as a bolus, the area under the curve produced by the detector depends on the cardiac output and the proportion of the cardiac output seen by the detector. If the tracer remains in the intravascular compartment, then this latter can be estimated as it is the proportion of the blood volume seen by the detector. This in turn can be calculated by dilution analysis if a blood sample is taken after equilibration and its activity compared with that injected. (For further details *see* Chapter 4).

A further example is the measurement of glomerular filtration rate. If a substance such as ^{51}Cr–EDTA is injected intravenously, the rate of disappearance from the blood depends on its rate of diffusion into the extravascular space and on the glomerular filtration rate. The first of these is relatively rapid, and if serial samples are taken between two and four hours after injection, the rate of decline of activity in the blood is an exponential determined by the GFR and the volume of distribution. Knowing the activity injected, by extrapolating the exponential back to the time of injection, the volume of distribution is given by dilution analysis, and hence the GFR may be calculated.

These are relatively simple examples of these techniques, and there has been a considerable effort devoted to the mathematical models involved in the analysis of activity–time problems, the field being known as tracer theory.

Profile Studies

If a detector is moved relative to a patient, it is possible to derive a profile showing the distribution of activity along a patient. This is not a technique of great value, but is used in some techniques of whole-body counting when the amount of radioactivity in the patient is small and a large detector must be used for sensitivity while attempting to localize the distribution of the activity.

Planar Scintigraphy

Scintigraphy is the general name for the technique of producing images showing the distribution of activity within a patient. This requires a detector with spatial resolution. As discussed above, this is usually a gamma-camera, but is still occasionally a rectilinear scanner. It is important to realize that a simple scintigram is built up over a period of time which is long compared with a radiograph, as a result of the relatively slow rate at which information is recorded.

Scintigraphy depends on the use of appropriate pharmaceuticals. A typical agent is the compound obtained by reacting technetium-99m with methylene diphosphonate in the presence of a reducing agent, the so-called Tc-MDP complex. This is taken up in bone in relation to the blood flow and also to the rate of bone turnover. (It is also excreted unchanged by the kidneys, probably by glomerular filtration.) If, therefore, a patient is imaged some four hours after the intravenous injection of the Tc-MDP complex, an image is obtained which shows the bones, with increased uptake at sites of increased bone turnover, such as fractures or metastases: this is the bone scintigram or bone scan. It is important to realize that the image obtained represents a functional distribution, not an anatomical one, and also that the pharmaceutical is distributed throughout the patient, not only to sites imaged. This is very different from the radiograph, which produces an image reflecting density or structural variation, and only involves irradiating the site imaged. For instance, the bone scintigram will show increased metabolic activity within 48 hours or less of a small stress fracture, reflecting the increased blood flow and bone turnover, whereas the radiograph may only become positive some weeks later when sclerotic healing bone is seen, by which time the scintigram has returned to normal.

Tomographic Scintigraphy

In the same way that computed transmission tomography is used to obtain images reflecting the three-dimensional distribution of structure, it is possible to obtain emission tomograms reflecting the distribution of function. There are two basic approaches. In Positron Emission Tomography (PET) advantage is taken of the annihilation radiation produced by positron emitters (*see* above) to reconstruct the volumetric distribution of the tracer. Early work with this method has led to the use of 18-fluoro-deoxy-glucose (FDG) as a tracer of brain metabolism, and thence to the use of changes in brain metabolism to differentiate between, for instance, Alzheimer-type dementia, multi-infarct dementia, Parkinsonian dementia and Huntington's chorea. Current fields of interest in PET work include the study of cerebral receptors and cardiac metabolism. PET is limited by the need for a cyclotron and specialized imaging devices (because of the short half-lives of positron-emitters), but is capable of studying major metabolic paths in the body.

A more generally available approach is Single Photon Emission Tomography (SPET). Here the isotopes are the more generally available ones, such as

^{123}I or ^{99m}Tc. Because only single photons are imaged, the mathematics is somewhat more complex, but it is possible to perform tomography by rotating a gamma-camera around the patient, and so no 'extra' equipment is needed. Pharmaceuticals optimized for SPET are now becoming available, such as ^{99m}Tc-HMPAO, which allows visualization of relative cerebral blood flow by any Nuclear Medicine department.

Dynamic Scintigraphy

In dynamic scintigraphy advantage is taken of the fact that a gamma-camera can be placed over an organ of interest and data recorded over a period of time which is relatively long, whilst the function of the organ is assessed as it handles the radiopharmaceutical. For instance, in dynamic renal scintigraphy the gamma-camera is positioned behind the patient, with the kidneys in the field of view, and a bolus injection of ^{99m}Tc-DTPA is given intravenously. This is handled purely by glomerular filtration. During the first passage of the activity through the kidney, however, the image obtained depends almost entirely on the blood flow. Images from 60–150 s show the distribution of functioning renal parenchyma, and later images show the renal outflow tract.

The technique may be further refined by the use of a small computer to allow quantitation of the data obtained. For instance, in renal scintigraphy it is possible to derive renal blood flow, divided function, glomerular filtration rate and response to diuretic as proof of obstruction, all from a single study.

It is this ability of scintigraphy to obtain information which allows the quantitation both of the spatial distribution of function and its variation with time which has been responsible for the spread of Nuclear Medicine and its methods.

A more sophisticated method is the use of gate-synchronized acquisition, in which a repetitive physiological function is recorded as a series of images spread over the cycle and triggered from the start of the cycle, such as gated cardiac imaging in which a quantitative image of the beating heart is built up using circuitry triggered by the QRS complex of the ECG. From such images it is possible to derive such parameters as the ejection fraction and dV/dT, and to study their change with intervention.

CONCLUSION

Radioisotope techniques in general and nuclear medicine in particular are evolving rapidly, and this review has deliberately not attempted to give details of any technique. Further details may be obtained from the reading list below, together with discussion with the hospital department of nuclear medicine where the majority of clinical studies will be undertaken.

FURTHER READING

Maisey M.N., Britton K.E., Gilday D.L. (eds.). (1983). *Clinical Nuclear Medicine*. London: Chapman and Hall.

Parker R.P., Smith P.H.S., Taylor D.M. (1984). *Basic Science of Nuclear Medicine*. 2nd edn. London: Churchill Livingstone.

Rassow G. (1970). *Basic Information on Routine Diagnosis in Nuclear Medicine*. Berlin: Siemens.

Journal of Nuclear Medicine, monthly. New York: Society of Nuclear Medicine.

Nuclear Medicine Communications, monthly. London: Chapman and Hall.

Seminars in Nuclear Medicine, quarterly. New York: Grune and Stratton.

12. Nuclear Magnetic Resonance Theory
D. G. Gadian

Outline of the basic principles
The basis of NMR spectroscopy
The basis of NMR imaging
   The relaxation times T_1 and T_2

Nuclear magnetic resonance (NMR) is finding increasing application in clinical practice and in biomedical research as a noninvasive method of obtaining human images and of studying tissue metabolism. In this chapter, an introduction is given to the principles underlying the use of NMR in biomedicine.

OUTLINE OF THE BASIC PRINCIPLES

NMR is a branch of spectroscopy, and in common with other spectroscopic techniques, it detects the interaction of radiation with matter. The technique relies on the fact that certain atomic nuclei, such as hydrogen, the proton, (^{1}H), carbon (^{13}C), phosphorus (^{31}P), and fluorine (^{19}F) have intrinsic magnetic properties. When a sample containing such nuclei is placed in a magnetic field, the nuclei (in analogy with compass needles) tend to align along the direction of the field. This magnetic interaction between the nuclei and the applied field can be detected by applying pulses of radiofrequency radiation to the sample and observing the frequencies at which radiation is absorbed and subsequently re-emitted. The frequencies of the various emitted signals are proportional to the field experienced by the nuclei. In NMR spectroscopy, these frequencies provide chemical information, whereas in imaging, they provide spatial information. Although there are several types of interrelationship between imaging and spectroscopy, it is most logical to discuss the two types of application separately.

It should be noted that of the nuclei mentioned above, all except for ^{13}C are 100% (or very close to 100%) naturally abundant, so that it is only in the case of ^{13}C (which has a natural abundance of about 1%) that the introduction of any labelling may be necessary.

THE BASIS OF NMR SPECTROSCOPY

Nuclei in different chemical environments give rise to signals of slightly different frequencies. This reflects the fact that the local field experienced by any nucleus differs slightly from the applied field, because of the secondary fields generated by the local electrons. This frequency separation, which forms the main basis of NMR spectroscopy, is commonly expressed in terms of the parameter known as the chemical shift. This is just one of the several parameters that characterize NMR signals (among the other are the relaxation times T_1 and T_2 which, as discussed later in this chapter, are of particular importance in imaging).

Figure 12.1 shows a ^{31}P spectrum obtained from the brain of an anaesthetized rat. The vertical axis represents signal amplitude, and the horizontal axis reflects signal frequency, expressed in terms of the chemical shift, which has dimensionless units of parts per million (ppm). Thus in the spectrum shown, the separation of 4.9 ppm between the phosphocreatine and inorganic phosphate signals means that at the

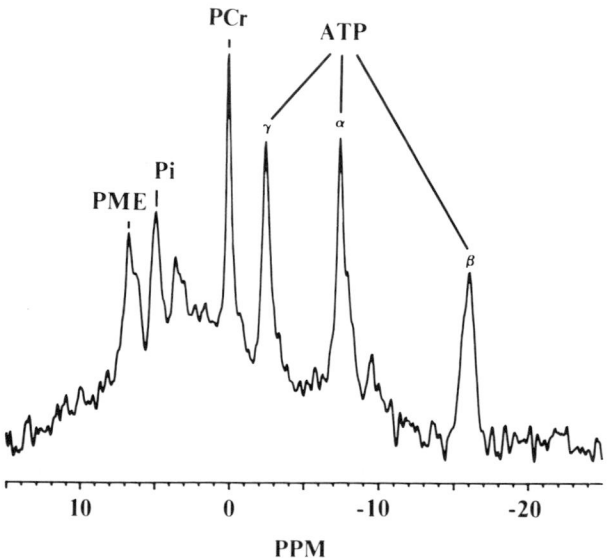

Fig. 12.1 ^{31}P NMR spectrum obtained from the brain of an anaesthetized rat, showing the characteristic signals from the β, α, and γ phosphates of ATP, phosphocreatine (PCr), inorganic phosphate (Pi), and phosphomonoesters (PME).

operating frequency of 146 MHz (which is determined by the strength of the magnetic field), these two signals are separated by about 700 Hz. The various signals can be assigned on the basis of their chemical shifts to the β, α, and γ phosphates of ATP, phosphocreatine (PCr), inorganic phosphate (P$_i$), and phosphomonoesters (PME). A particularly useful feature of ^{31}P spectra is that the chemical shift of the inorganic phosphate signal is sensitive to pH variations in the physiological range. This signal therefore provides a monitor of intracellular pH. The sensitivity to pH arises because the state of ionization of inorganic phosphate changes in the physiological pH range.

The concentrations of the various metabolites are, under certain conditions, proportional to the areas, or intensities of their respective signals. NMR spectroscopy therefore provides a noninvasive method of monitoring the metabolic state of tissues *in vivo*, and any changes that may occur in these metabolites (e.g. loss of high energy phosphates during exercise or ischaemia) can be followed noninvasively simply by monitoring how the signal areas vary with time.

NMR spectroscopy can be used in biomedical research to monitor metabolites in a wide variety of systems, including body fluids, cellular suspensions, isolated tissues, whole animals and humans. Such studies should lead to a better understanding of the metabolic and functional abnormalities that occur in disease, could assist in evaluating the efficacy of different therapies, and could aid diagnosis. The most commonly used nuclei are ^{31}P, ^{1}H, ^{13}C, and ^{19}F, and some of their applications can be found in the references given below.

It is important to consider the technical limitations of NMR spectroscopy, in particular the spatial resolution that will be available for human studies. The technique requires the use of high (and very homogeneous) fields (about 1.5 T or above) in order to obtain the requisite sensitivity and spectral resolution. However, even at these fields, the spatial resolution that can be achieved for detection of metabolites is very much poorer than for ^{1}H imaging. This is because the metabolites of interest are present at concentrations in the millimolar range (metabolites in the micromolar range produce insufficient signal), in contrast to water which has a concentration in soft tissue of about 40 M. The metabolites therefore generate relatively weak signals, and sufficiently high signal-to-noise ratios can only be achieved by increasing the size of the volume elements, typically to linear dimensions of 2 cm or above. The development of techniques for obtaining localized spectra is a very active area of research.

THE BASIS OF NMR IMAGING

Whereas NMR spectroscopy detects signals from a range of metabolites, NMR imaging is based primarily on the detection of ^{1}H signals from the water protons, with additional contributions from fats.

If the body were in a totally uniform magnetic field, then on application of the pulses of radiofrequency radiation that are used to generate the NMR signals, all of the water protons would give a signal of the same frequency, and no spatial information would be available. In imaging studies, well-defined magnetic field gradients are superimposed upon the applied magnetic field. As a result, different points in space can be identified with specific field values and hence with specific signal frequencies. Therefore the frequency distribution reflects the spatial distribution of the molecules, rather than their chemical features. By far the easiest molecule to image is water, because of the abundance of water molecules and because protons give stronger signals than other nuclei.

The generation of a cross-sectional image is achieved by computer analysis of data obtained with a range of different gradient conditions, in analogy with image reconstruction in X-ray scanning. One of the advantages of NMR is that the gradients can be applied equally easily along each axis, so that transverse, coronal, or sagittal images can all be obtained directly.

The Relaxation Times T_1 and T_2

The application of a radiofrequency pulse perturbs the magnetization away from its equilibrium orientation, which is along the direction of the applied field. The return back to equilibrium is termed relaxation, and is characterized by two relaxation times. The return along the direction of the magnetic field is known as spin-lattice or longitudinal relaxation and is characterized by the spin-lattice relaxation time T_1. The return of the magnetization in the plane perpendicular to the field is termed spin-spin or transverse relaxation and is characterized by the relaxation time T_2. In general, T_2 is significantly shorter than T_1.

In conventional NMR spectroscopy, T_1 and T_2 can be measured by the use of well-established sequences of radiofrequency pulses. These pulses are specified in terms of the angle through which they rotate the magnetization. Thus a $90°$ pulse tilts the magnetization through an angle of $90°$, whereas a $180°$ pulse rotates it through $180°$ so that the magnetization ends up opposite in direction to the applied field. As an example of the use of pulse sequences, T_1 can be measured using the 'inversion recovery' sequence $[180°-T-90°]$ and monitoring the signal intensity as a function of the delay time T. Pulse sequences of this type are incorporated into imaging studies in order to obtain images that are weighted according to T_1 or T_2 or some function of the two. In fact, most of the contrast between soft tissues is generated not so much by differences in water concentration (which vary over a relatively narrow range; from about 69% in skin to 83% in grey matter), but by the much larger differences in relaxation times. Thus soft tissue contrast is strongly dependent on the precise nature of the pulse sequence that is used, and appropriate choice of sequence depends on the clinical problem that is being addressed. Some pulse sequences are also sensitive to flow, and there is considerable interest in using such sequences not only to visualize blood vessels but also to measure flow velocity.

Fig. 12.2 illustrates the contrast and spatial resolu-

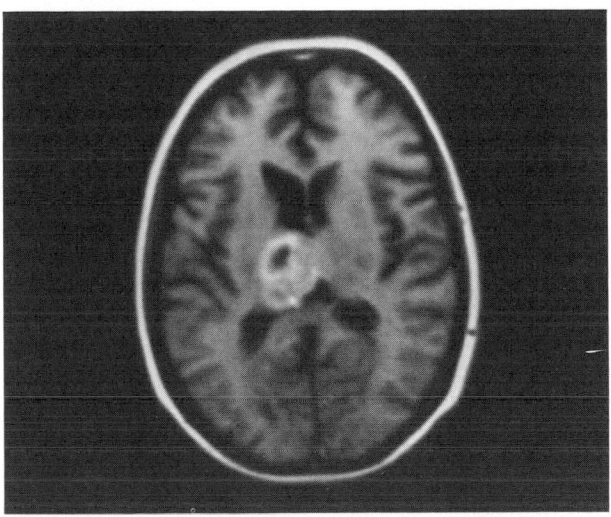

Fig. 12.2 T_1-weighted ^{1}H NMR image showing a glioma. This study involved the use of gadolinium-DPTA as a contrast agent. (Courtesy of Dr G. Bydder, Hammersmith Hospital)

tion that can be obtained with ^{1}H imaging at a relatively low (0.15 T) field strength, and indicates the obvious diagnostic usefulness of the technique. The wide range of clinical applications is indicated by the references given below.

FURTHER READING

Avison M.J., Hetherington H.P., Shulman R.G. (1986). Applications of NMR to studies of tissue metabolism. *Ann. Rev. Biophys. Biophys. Bioeng.* **15**, 377.

Gadian D.G. (1982). *Nuclear Magnetic Resonance and its Applications to Living Systems.* Oxford: Clarendon Press.

Morris P.G. (1986). *Nuclear Magnetic Resonance Imaging in Medicine and Biology.* Oxford: Clarendon Press.

Radda G.K., Taylor D.J. (1985). Application of nuclear magnetic resonance in pathology. In *Intern. Rev. Exp. Pathol.* **27** pp. 1–58. (Richter G.W., Epstein M.A., eds.) New York: Academic Press.

Stark D.D., Bradley W.G. (eds.) (1988). *Magnetic resonance imaging.* St Louis: The C.V. Mosby Co.

Steiner R.E. (1987). Nuclear magnetic resonance imaging. *Br. Med. J.* **294**, 1570.

Steiner R.E., Radda G.K. (eds.) (1984). Nuclear magnetic resonance and its clinical applications. *Br. Med. Bull.* **40**, 113.

Williams S.R., Gadian D.G. (1986). Tissue metabolism studied *in vivo* by nuclear magnetic resonance. *J. Exp. Physiol.* **71**, 335.

**PHYSIOLOGICAL BASIS OF THE
SCIENCE OF ANAESTHESIA**
A. CARDIOVASCULAR SYSTEM

13. Cardiac Performance
K. R. LaMantia, R. L. Hines and P. G. Barash

Despite the presence of severe cardiac dysfunction and its associated risk, an increasingly aged patient population is scheduled for major surgery. To deliver the most effective anesthetic care, minimize preoperative delays and optimize the probability of favorable outcomes, the anesthesiology consultant must integrate newer concepts of cardiovascular physiology into clinical practice.

Our scientific understanding of cardiac performance has progressed through two distinct phases (Strobeck and Sonnenblick, 1986). At first, the heart was thought of as a mechanical pump with its output related to the end-diastolic volume pressure required to eject a stroke volume. Starling synthesized these early concepts into the *Law of the Heart*, 'The law of the heart is therefore, the same as that of skeletal muscle namely that the mechanical energy set free on the passage from the resting to contracted state

depends on the area of chemically active surfaces, i.e., on the length of the muscle fibers' (Starling, 1915). This prophetic statement was not verified until techniques of skeletal muscle research were applied to the study of cardiac muscle physiology (second phase).

Terminology

Basic to our understanding of cardiac function is precise definition of terminology used to describe cardiac performance. *Ventricular performance* relates the ability of the heart to eject a volume of blood over the period of measurement which may be confined to a single heart beat (stroke volume) or averaged over a minute (cardiac output) (Braunwald, 1988). Frequently, comparisons are necessary between subjects. Therefore, measurements are adjusted for the size of the subject by indexing cardiac output to body surface area (BSA). *Work* is defined as the product of force and distance ($W = f \times d$). For the cardiovascular system, force is ventricular pressure and distance is the volume of blood moved. *Stroke work* is expressed as the product of ventricular pressure and stroke volume. *Contractility* refers to the specific property of cardiac muscle that reflects the level of activation of myofibril cross-bridge formation. While contractility remains a difficult quantity to assess clinically, it is important as it represents one of the four determinants of cardiac performance (heart rate, afterload, preload and contractility).

MYOCARDIAL MUSCLE MECHANICS

The study of isolated muscle preparations has greatly enhanced our understanding of cardiac function by enabling the investigator to examine the determinants of cardiac muscle function in isolation (Barash and Kopriva, 1984). These include:

1. Tension development
2. Rate of shortening or velocity
3. Instantaneous length
4. Time after onset of contraction.

Each of these variables can be understood by considering the isolated, papillary muscle preparation (Fig. 13.1). This preparation allows the investigator to place the resting muscle under a known amount of tension known as *preload*. Mechanically this is accomplished by adding weight to one end of the lever arm resulting in the stretching of the muscle fibers. The amount of preload added results in resting fiber length which increases with increasing preload.

The next step in an isolated muscle experiment is to place the *stop* on the muscle side of the lever arm. At this point, additional weight can be added to the stack, but will no longer stretch the preparation as the stop prevents the muscle from experiencing any further increases in preload. This additional load can only affect the muscle after the onset of active contraction and is termed *afterload*.

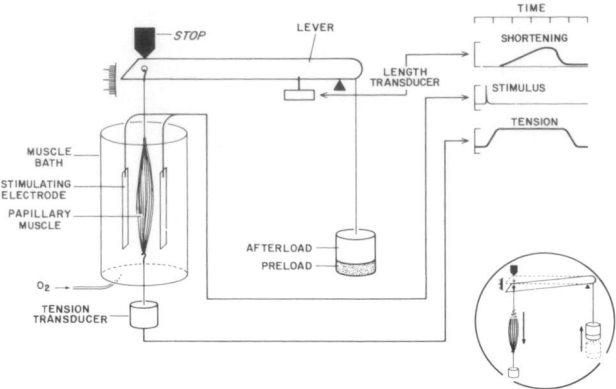

Fig. 13.1 A schematic diagram of an isolated papillary muscle preparation. The *stop* which is applied subsequent to preload stretching of the muscle, prevents the afterload weight from altering function until shortening of the muscle occurs. (Reproduced with permission from P.G. Barash, C.J. Kopriva 1984. *Manual of Cardiac Anesthesia*, New York: Churchill Livingstone.)

Phases of Contraction

Cardiac muscle contraction can be divided into three distinct phases: (*see* Fig. 13.2 A-C)

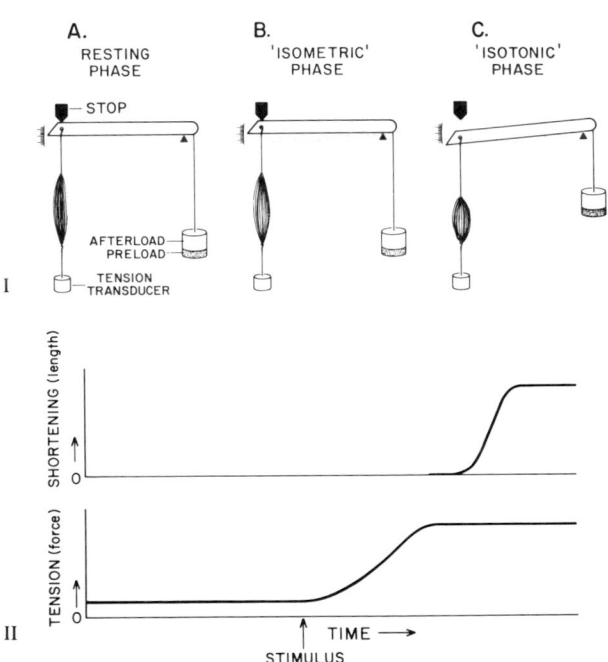

Fig. 13.2 (I) The three phases of muscle contraction: resting, isometric and isotonic are schematically shown for the isolated papillary muscle preparation. (II) The time course of muscle tension development and shortening for an isotonic contraction is depicted. Note that tension is maximally developed (isometric phase) before muscle shortening occurs (isotonic phase). (Reproduced with permission from P.G. Barash, C.J. Kopriva, 1984. *Manual of Cardiac Anesthesia*. New York: Churchill Livingstone.)

A) Resting Phase

Prior to electrical stimulation of the muscle, the strain gauge measures an amount of tension equal to the preload (Fig. 13.2A). At resting muscle length, the stiffness of the tissues is defined by the *length-resting tension relation*. This is analogous to the compliance characteristics of the intact ventricular chamber. In comparison to skeletal muscle, cardiac muscle is stiffer and elongates less for any increment of preload (Sonnenblick and Skelton, 1974).

B) Isometric Contraction Phase

During the *isometric* phase (constant length) tension is developed beyond the resting level without muscle shortening (Fig. 13.2B). Thus, no movement of the lever arm is detected during this phase. Tension (total tension) as measured by the strain gauge is the sum of active-tension and resting-tension (Fig. 13.3).

C) Isotonic Contraction Phase

During the *isotonic* (constant tension) contraction phase, muscle shortening occurs when sufficient tension develops to overcome the total load (Fig. 13.2C). This is defined as the sum of preload and afterload. When this level of tension is achieved, tension remains constant while shortening then proceeds.

Muscle Models

Models of cardiac muscle contraction are based on the behavior of isolated skeletal muscle preparations and help to form a unified view of muscle function (Parmley et al., 1967). Current models of cardiac muscle include a *contractile element* (CE), a *series elas-*

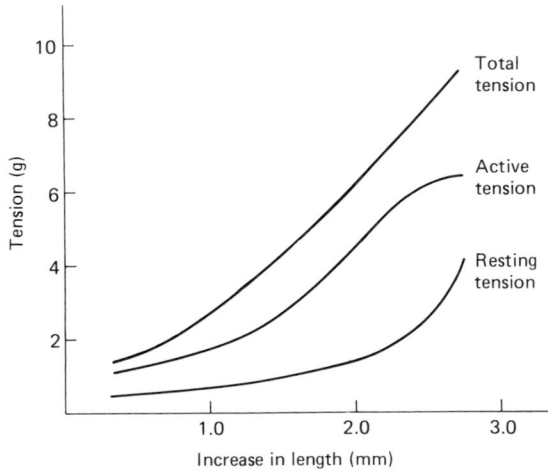

Fig. 13.3 Length-tension relation for an isolated papillary muscle preparation. Preload is defined by the resting tension measured by the strain gauge. As contraction begins tension (total tension) increases progressively. The difference between total tension and resting tension equals the tension generated by the muscle (active tension).

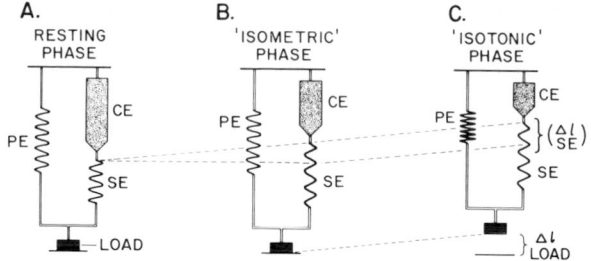

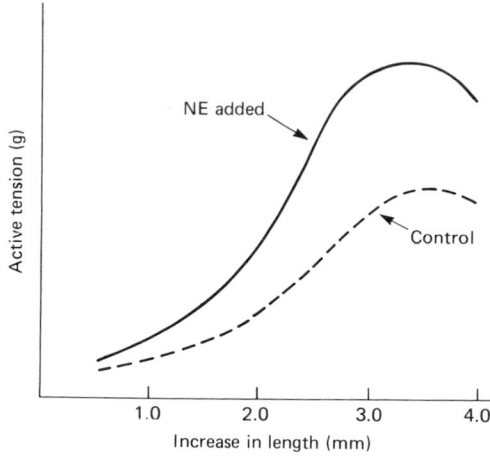

Fig. 13.4 Behaviour of a model of muscle function during the three phases of contraction: A. = resting phase, B. = isometric phase, C. = isotonic phase. The series elastic element (SE) elongates during isometric contraction at (B) as the contractile element (CE) shortens. The isotonic phase is characterized by shortening of the parallel elastic element (PE) with further elongation of the SE. Muscle length (l) decreases during the isotonic phase. (Reproduced with permission from P.G. Barash, C.J. Kopriva, 1984. *Manual of Cardiac Anesthesia*. New York: Churchill Livingstone.)

Fig. 13.5 Length-activity tension curves depicting an increase in slope with increasing contractility induced by the addition of norepinephrine (NE) to the muscle preparation.

tic element (SE) and a *parallel elastic element* (PE) (Fig. 13.4). CE represents the contracting portion of the muscle while the SE element represents a passive elastic component attached in series. By converting potential energy stored in chemical bonds to mechanical energy at the onset of contraction, the SE is stretched after the CE begins to shorten. During isotonic contraction the CE at first develops tension and stretches the SE with no overall shortening of the muscle during the isometric phase. When tension equals total load, shortening continues in the CE (no further change in the SE) resulting in muscle shortening. The PE element is postulated to account for such properties as stress relaxation which is muscle elongation during prolonged contraction.

Length-Tension Relations

By plotting the active tension versus the resting or preload length during an isometric contraction, the length-active tension curve is defined (Braunwald, 1988). The tension generated by an isometric contraction is dependent on two factors:

1. Resting length,
2. Contractility.

A change in the length-active tension relation secondary to augmentation of contractility as induced by noradrenaline (norepinephrine NE) is indicated by an increase in the slope of the length-tension plot (Fig. 13.5).

Isotonic contraction requires four variables to define mechanical function:

1. *Force* (tension)
2. *Velocity* of shortening (rate)
3. Instantaneous *length*
4. *Time* after activation.

For a particular muscle, increasing preload results in:

1. Increased resting tension
2. Increased initial velocity
3. Increased developed tension
4. Constant maximal velocity of shortening (V_{max})
5. Constant extent of shortening.

In the case of increasing afterload (constant preload) the following is observed:

1. Constant resting tension
2. Increased active tension
3. Decreased extent of shortening
4. Decreased V_{max}.

Overall, there is an inverse relationship between the velocity of shortening and the developed tension. An increase in contractility is detected by a shift in the length-tension or tension-velocity curves to the right (Fig. 13.6).

Force-Velocity-Length Relations as a Measure of Contractility

While no universally acceptable definition of contractility or inotropic state exists, it may be functionally defined as a unique relationship between force, velocity, and resting length that is time independent (Fig. 13.7). Each contractile state is graphically represented by a three dimensional surface defined by force, length, and velocity. Increases in contractility are denoted by shifts in the surface upward and to the right.

While isolated models of muscle contraction have been useful in defining muscle behavior independent of other structural and physiologic influences, ultimately these concepts must be tested in the intact heart both experimentally and clinically.

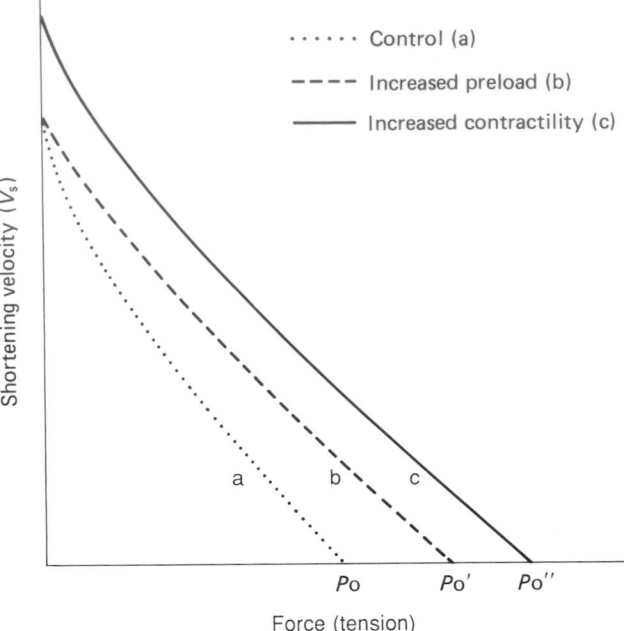

Fig. 13.6 Force (tension)-velocity curve showing the characteristic changes with increased preload or contractility. The Y-intercept represents V_{max} while the x-intercept (P_o is the maximum afterload against which the muscle preparation can shorten). An increase in contractility (c) is characterized by a shift to the right and an increase in V_{max}. Preload augmentation (b) results in only a shift to the right.

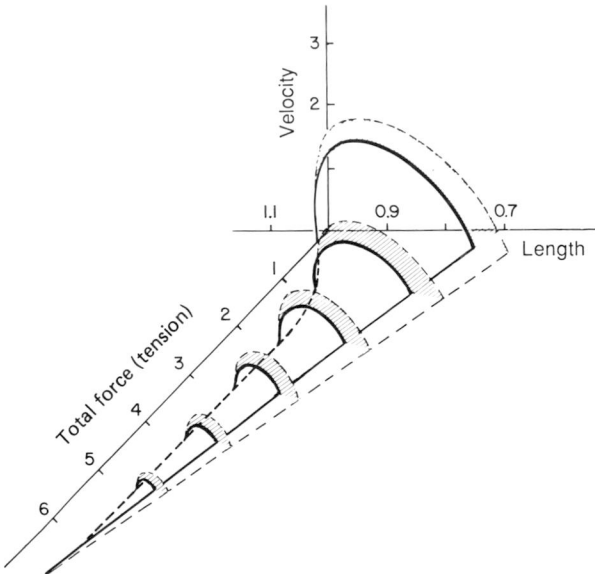

Fig. 13.7 Three-dimensional plot of tension, velocity and resting length of isolated muscle demonstrating characteristic shift of the surface upward and to the right with increased contractility. Each contractile state is defined by a three-dimensional surface. Solid curves define the baseline surface and cross-hatching indicates the shift with increased inotopy.

Cellular Basis of Cardiac Contraction

The ventricular myocardium is composed of cells arranged in a syncytium. Contained within the muscle cells are myofibrils traversing the length of the cell and composed of repeating units termed sarcomeres. Surrounding the myofibrils are numerous mitochondria in which adenosine triphosphate (ATP) is synthesized via oxidative phosphorylation. The sarcomere, the basic unit of contraction, is composed of an arrangement of filaments termed myofilaments (Fig. 13.8). Myofilaments consist of alternating thin filaments (actin), and thick filaments (myosin). The arrangement of filaments allows them to interdigitate and transform chemical energy (i.e., ATP) into mechanical work.

The anatomy of the sarcomere is important in understanding the contractile mechanism. Actin filaments are anchored at the Z line and adjacent Z lines comprize the I band. Myosin distribution is limited to the middle of the sarcomere (A-band) with actin being distributed peripherally on the sarcomere. The sarcolemma, the cell membrane penetrates the sarcoplasm to form a transverse or T-tubular system. T-tubules communicate with the sarcoplasmic reticulum and are responsible for the intracellular release and reuptake of calcium ions. Contraction is initiated by calcium release into the sarcoplasmic reticulum, with magnesium ATPase providing the energy for this transfer. As the action potential propagates, permeability of the sarcoplasmic reticulum is altered resulting in a release of calcium into the cytoplasm. This acute increase in calcium initiates the final phase of the contractile process.

During contraction, the actin and myosin filaments interdigitate resulting in a shortening of the sarcomere. As this shortening occurs, cross linkages are formed, broken and reformed between the actin and myosin filaments. The energy for this bond formation comes from the hydrolysis of the ATP by ATPase enzymes contained with the myosin filaments. The extent of muscle shortening is dependent upon the speed at which the actin-myosin cross linkages are formed and broken and on the number of bridges (calcium-actin-myosin) that are occupied at any one time.

FUNCTION OF THE INTACT VENTRICLE: THE HEART AS A PUMP

The concepts of loading and contractility are useful in developing a clearer understanding of the heart as a pump. The early appreciation of the necessity of merging the concepts of muscle performance and cardiac pump function are credited both to Otto Frank (1895) and to Ernest Starling (1914). Starling demonstrated the dependence of both stroke volume and cardiac output on venous return and ventricular end-diastolic volume. From experiments utilizing heart-lung preparations, concepts were synthesized into the Frank–Starling relation which relates filling pressure

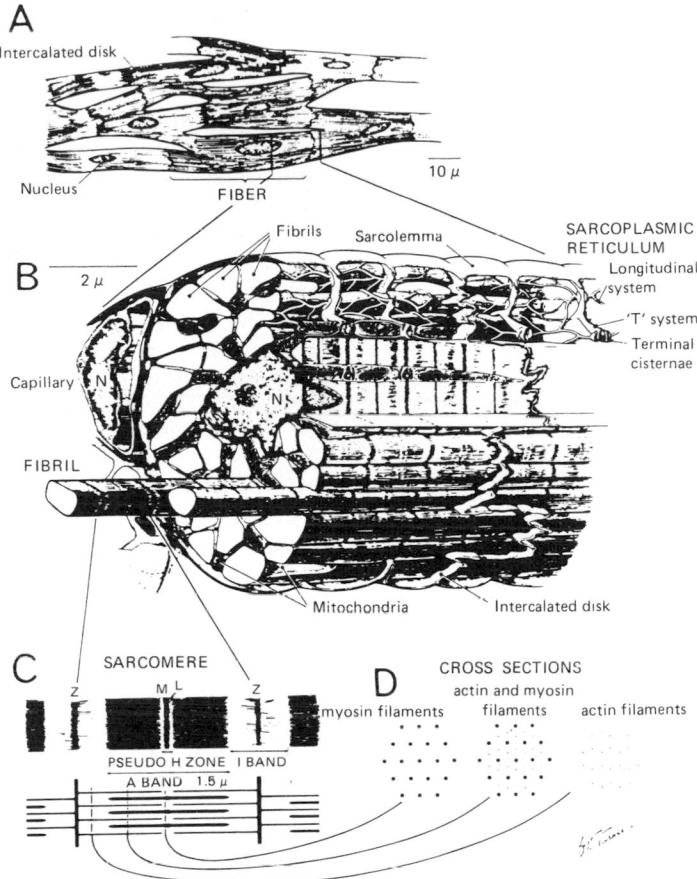

Fig. 13.8 Schematic of the anatomy of a cardiac muscle fiber. (A) Cardiac muscle fiber syncytium composed of numerous interconnected cardiac muscle cells. (B) Cardiac muscle fiber (cell) comprised of bundles of fibrils. Note the numerous mitochondria contained within the fibril bundle. (C) Sarcomere muscle unit defined by interdigitating myosin and actin filaments. (D) Cross-section of the sarcomere demonstrating the geometric arrangement of the myosin and actin filaments. (Reproduced with permission from E. Braunwald, S. Ross, E. Sonnenblick. (1988). *Mechanisms of Contraction of the Normal and Failing Heart*. Philadelphia: W.B. Saunders Co.)

or filling volume to the output of the heart (cardiac output or stroke volume). Starling also observed that the failing heart (decreased contractility) delivered a smaller stroke volume at normal filling pressures. Subsequent investigators including Sarnoff examined stroke work of the ventricle over a broad range of filling pressures and termed the resulting relation *Ventricular Function Curve* (VFC) (Fig. 13.9). Movement along an individual curve illustrates the operation of the Frank–Starling principle, while the shift to a different curve denotes altered contractility. The family of VFC corresponds to the length-tension relationship of isolated cardiac muscle.

Stroke volume and cardiac output vary inversely with outflow resistance (Fig. 13.10). This is analogous to the inverse relation between tension and velocity in

isolated cardiac muscle. Further, with decreasing levels of contractility stroke volume becomes more dependent upon outflow resistance.

Determinants of Pump Function

The determinants of cardiac performance, in the intact heart, include: preload, afterload, contractility, and heart rate. Although these variables are easily defined in isolated preparations, their application to the intact heart is more complex.

Preload

Preload is defined as the end-diastolic fiber length of the muscle prior to contraction. Since preload cannot

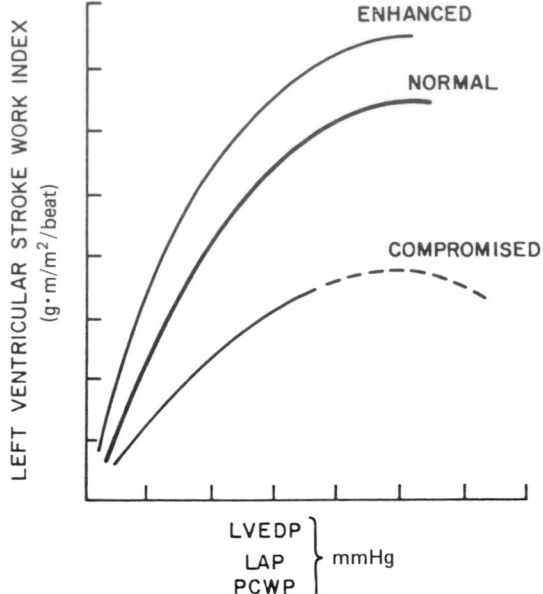

Fig. 13.9 Ventricular function curves demonstrating the effects of enhanced and compromised contractility on the normal curve (LVEDP = left ventricular end-diastolic pressure; LAP = mean left atrial pressure; PCWP = mean pulmonary capillary wedge pressure. (Reproduced with permission from P.G. Barash, C.J. Kopriva, 1984). Cardiac Pump Function and How. *Manual of Cardiac Anesthesia*. New York: Churchill Livingstone.)

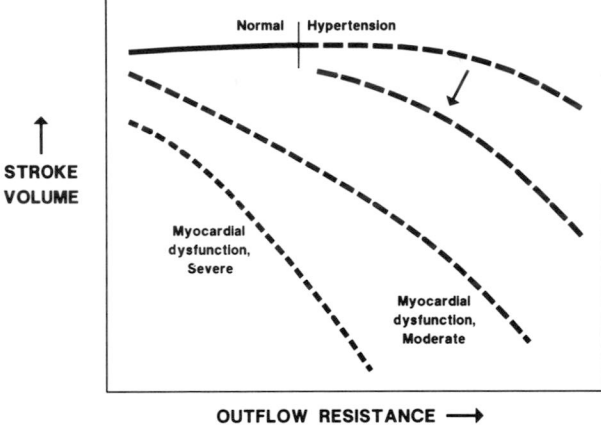

Fig. 13.10 The inverse relation between stroke volume and outflow resistance is demonstrated for hearts with normal and depressed function. (Reproduced with permission from J.N. Cohn, J.A. Francosa, 1977. *New Engl. J. Med.* **297**, 27.)

be directly measured in the intact heart it is clinically assessed by measurement of ventricular volume:

1. Indicator-dilution techniques
2. Contrast angiography
3. Echocardiography
4. Radionuclear angiography
5. Magnetic resonance imaging (MRI).

While each technique has its advantages, only radionuclear and indicator-dilution techniques are relatively free of geometric assumptions concerning the shape of the heart. Both contrast angiographic and echocardiographic techniques are based on formulae modeling the ventricle to an idealized geometric shape, such as an ellipsoid of rotation. In disease states such formulae may no longer be valid. Clinically, however, preoperative assessment of preload is most often based on pressure correlates of ventricular volumes. Unfortunately for the clinician, many variables confound the correlation of pressure with volume. The relationship between pressure and volume defines ventricular compliance.

$$\text{Compliance} = \frac{\text{Change in volume}}{\text{Change in pressure}} = \frac{\Delta V}{\Delta P}$$

In states where compliance is altered, for example, myocardial ischemia, filling pressures no longer correlate with ventricular end-diastolic volumes. In such circumstances reliance on measured intravascular pressures (e.g. central venous pressure, pulmonary capillary wedge pressure) to guide assessment of preload may lead to misinterpretation of data. Examples of factors that may interfere with the use of pressure measurements to assess preload are listed in Table 13.1.

TABLE 13.1
FACTORS ALTERING THE RELATION BETWEEN PRESSURE MEASUREMENTS AND VENTRICULAR PRELOAD

Site of pressure measurement	*Confounding factor*
Left ventricle	Left ventricular compliance
Left atrium	Above + mitral stenosis
Pulmonary capillary	Above + airway pressure
Pulmonary artery	Above + pulmonary vascular resistance
Right atrium	Above + right ventricular compliance tricuspid stenosis

Afterload

In the intact ventricle, afterload is defined as the tension operating on the muscle fibers to resist change, subsequent to the onset of contraction. Analogous to the isolated muscle preparation, afterload is functional only after the onset of contraction. Afterload is determined by factors related to the peripheral circulation and the ventricular chamber itself. The latter is predicted by the *law of La Place* which defines ventricular wall tension:

$$T = \frac{Pr}{2h}$$

Where P = chamber pressure
r = chamber radius
h = wall thickness

This assumes the ventricle to be a thick walled sphere,

which is not totally accurate, but is conceptually useful. For the normal heart, impedance to ejection is due mainly to systemic vascular resistance (SVR). Other commonly used terms to estimate afterload include left ventricular systolic pressure, and mean aortic pressure. Acute increases in afterload are associated with:

1. Increased end-diastolic and end-systolic volume
2. Decreased stroke volume
3. Increased ventricular radius and increased wall tension
4. Increased preload
5. Decreased velocity of shortening and extent of shortening.

Heart Rate

Cardiac output is dependent on both stroke volume and heart rate

$$CO = SV \times HR$$

With a fixed stroke volume, cardiac output is directly dependent on heart rate. This becomes an important consideration in disorders such as aortic stenosis, with relatively fixed stroke volume secondary to outflow tract obstruction. Increased heart rate is associated with demonstrable increases in contractility, the *Bowditch effect*. Availability of calcium ions, at the level of the contractile apparatus is at least partially responsible for this effect.

Contractility

Contractility, or the inotropic state, is a change in the force of contraction independent of loading conditions. A change in contractility can be demonstrated by comparing some measure of cardiac contractility which is independent of preload, afterload and heart rate. Clinically applicable methods of evaluating contractility must, therefore, be independent of other determinants of cardiac performance (*see* Clinical Evaluation of Pump Function).

THE CARDIAC CYCLE

An appreciation of normal cardiac events is essential to understand the various modalities to assess cardiac performance. Simultaneous measurement of electrical activity (ECG), intracardiac pressures, and chamber volumes yield the most comprehensive view of normal and abnormal cardiac performance (Fig. 13.11 A-B). This information is summarized by plotting a pressure-volume (*PV*) loop. The inscribed loop is analogous to length-tension curves from isolated muscle preparations and is composed of four phases (Fig. 13.12):

I (D-A)   Diastolic filling. Phase with two components (a) early to mid by passive filling, (b) atrial contraction. This phase begins mitral valve opening and is ter-

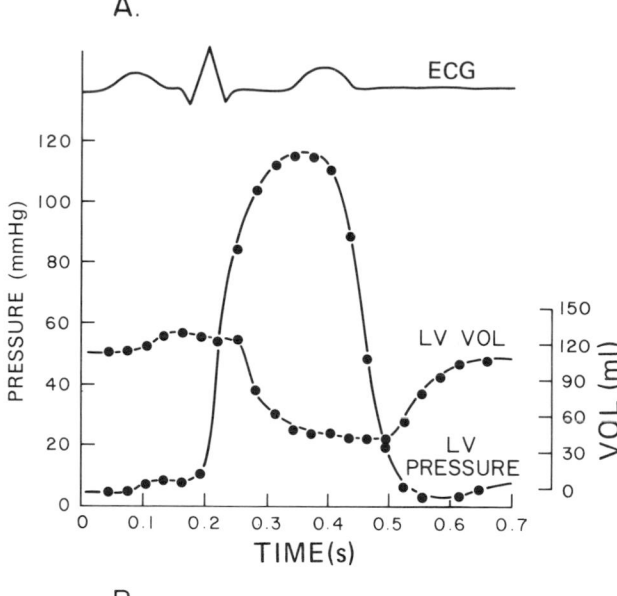

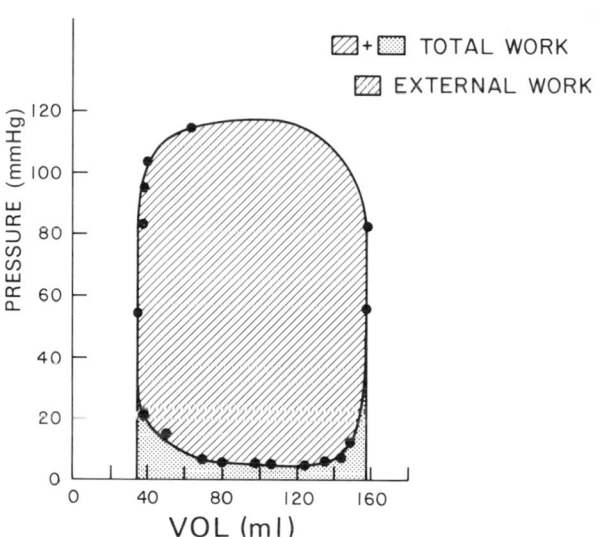

Fig. 13.11 A. Display of simultaneous left ventricular (LV) volume and pressure measurements along with the electrocardiogram (ECG). B. Simultaneous left ventricular pressure and volume determinations used to construct a *P-V* loop.

minated by mitral valve closure, ('a' = atrial component).

II (A-B)   Subsequent vertical limb indicating isovolumetric contraction. Isovolumetric contraction ends with the aortic valve opening.

III (B-C)   Upper horizontal limb representing systolic ejection. Systolic ejection is completed by aortic valve closure.

IV (C-D)   Isovolumetric relaxation. Ends with mitral valve opening when left atrial pressure exceeds LV pressure.

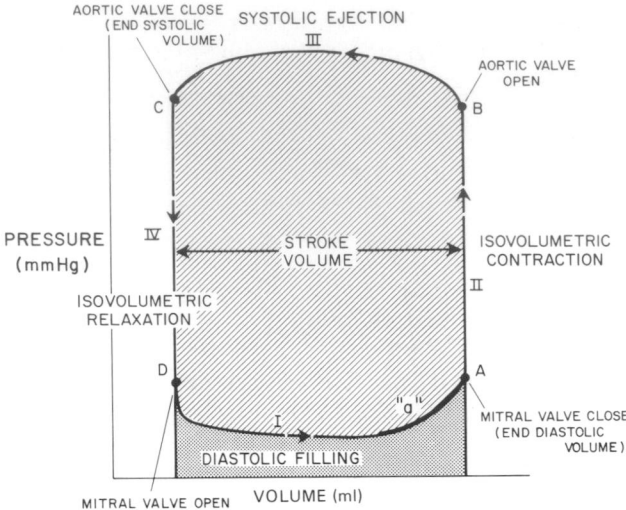

Fig. 13.12 The idealized pressure-volume loop obtained by simultaneous measurement of pressure and volume (*see* text for details). (Reproduced with permission from P.G. Barash, C.J. Kopriva 1984. *Manual of Cardiac Anesthesia.* New York: Churchill Livingstone.)

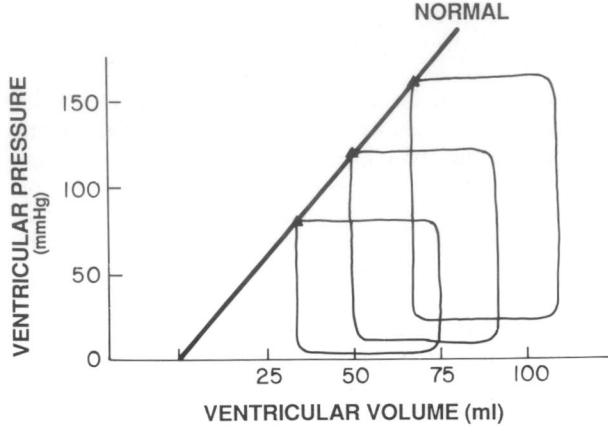

Fig. 13.13 Multiple pressure-volume loops are generated at varying conditions of preload and afterload to define the end systole pressure volume relation (ESPVR). The linear ESPVR is established by connecting the end systolic points on the various *PV* loops. The X-intercept is known as *V*d (dead volume) which is the minimal ventricular volume at which no pressure is generated by a contraction.

Transition points located between phases correspond to approximate valvular opening and closing. Isovolumetric periods refer to changes in pressure in the absence of volume changes (equivalent to isometric contraction). As work = pressure × volume, the area contained within the *P-V* loop defines the external work necessary for the heart to expel the stroke volume (ventricular stroke work). While the area between phase I and the X axis represents the work required by the right heart and left atrium to fill the left ventricle in diastole (internal work). The sum of these two components is the total work (Fig. 13.11B). This analysis can also be used to assess contractility in the clinical setting.

The End-Systolic Pressure Volume Relation

The slope of the line determined by connecting the transition points between phase III and IV (i.e., the end-systolic pressure volume relation) of multiple *P-V* loops generated at different loading conditions is an index of contractility (Fig. 13.13) (Sagawa, 1981). This concept was developed by Suga and Sagawa, during a series of experiments employing isolated perfused hearts (Suga et al., 1979). The end-systolic pressure volume relation (ESPVR) is analagous to the length-active tension curve generated for isolated cardiac muscle. Utility of the ESPVR is related to the following:

1. For two or more isovolumetric beats at varying afterloads, the end-systolic points define a linear relation with the equation: $Pes = Ees (Ves-V_d)$.

Where Pes and Ves are the end-systolic pressure and volume, respectively. Ees is the slope of the ESPVR line and V_d is the X intercept.

2. The slope (Ees) is a measure of the contractile state and this measure is largely load independent.
3. Ees increases with increasing contractility and decreases with compromized ventricular function (Fig. 13.14).
4. Ees can be calculated for ejecting beats, as well as isovolumetric beats, using the end-systolic pressure and volume.
5. The relation between ventricular pressure and volume defines *elastance*, which is the time vary-

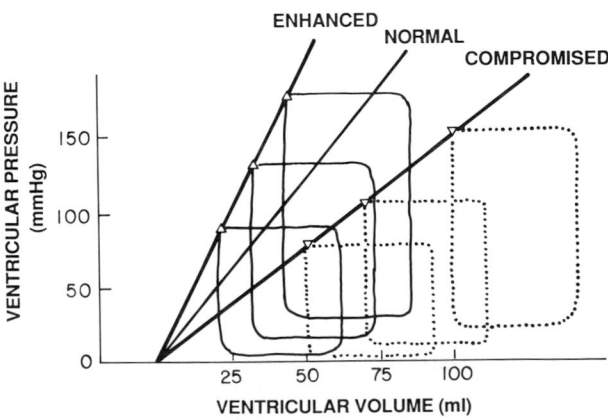

Fig. 13.14 Two series of pressure-volume loops demonstrating the change in slope of the linear ESPVR with enhanced (solid loops) or compromised (discontinuous loops) ventricular function. The line labelled normal defines the normal ESPVR for comparison.

ing property of the ventricle and causes it to return to the resting state after contraction.

The use of the ESPVR to assess contractility has several advantages over ventricular function curves: 1. Relative insensitivity to changes in afterload and preload during the measurement, 2. the independence of the ESPVR to compliance changes. However, clinical use of the ESPVR does face several clinical hurdles: 1. comparison of elastance (i.e., contractility) between patients requires normalization of volume data as end-systolic volume varies widely, 2. variation in ventricular wall thickness is considerable between patients especially in those with chronic pressure overload. Thicker walled ventricles generate higher pressure at a given volume independent of contractility. For this reason, in the setting of increased ventricular thickness, wall stress rather than pressure is utilized in ESPVR calculations. Wall stress is defined as force per cross-sectional area and is calculated by:

$$\text{Stress} = \frac{P_{\text{LV}} \times r}{2h}$$

P_{LV} = left ventricular pressure
r = radius of left ventricle
h = wall thickness

Use of the wall stress calculation is important in the presence of ventricular hypertrophy (e.g., aortic stenosis or hypertension).

In conclusion, while the concept of ESPVR is an important theoretical advance in quantitating contractility its application is not without problems. However, it remains the best of current measures of contractility available today.

Determinants of Cardiac Performance in the Intact Circulation

The determinants of performance in the intact circulation are the same as those in the isolated heart or muscle preparation:

1. Heart rate
2. Afterload
3. Preload
4. Contractility.

Ventricular Preload

Factors influencing the ventricular end-diastolic volume include:

Ventricular Diastolic Function. This is the relation between ventricular filling pressure and volume (Compliance = V/P), which is dependent on both active relaxation and passive stretch. Acute changes in left ventricular compliance are seen with myocardial ischemia, right ventricular dilatation, and states associated with increased pericardial pressure such as tamponade. Chronic changes in diastolic function are

seen secondary to left ventricular hypertrophy, and increased pericardial pressure (chronic constrictive pericarditis).

Venous Return. Dependent on blood volume, venous capacitance, intrathoracic pressure, the skeletal muscle pump and postural changes.

Atrial Contraction. Changes in the cardiac rhythm (e.g., nodal rhythm frequently observed during the use of halothane and anesthesia).

Left Ventricle—Right Ventricle Interaction. Traditionally, the right ventricle (RV) has been viewed as a conduit or reservoir for moving blood from the right side of the heart through the lungs into the left side (Starr et al., 1943). It was not until the work of Donald and Essex, that the importance of the right ventricle in influencing global cardiac performance was appreciated (Donald and Essex, 1954). The RV is an integral factor in determining left ventricular function. The RV is anatomically bonded to the LV by subepicardial muscle fibers that run from the free wall of the right ventricle to the anterior wall of the LV. The interventricular septum (IVS) is formed by subendocardial muscle bands from both ventricles. In addition, both ventricles are enclosed by the pericardium and are within the thoracic cavity.

Changes in pleural pressure, status of the pericardium (i.e., open or closed) and alteration in the geometry and location of the interventricular septum are all vital in maintaining normal left-right heart interactions. Jardin has demonstrated that alteration in right ventricular afterload (secondary to PEEP) can cause a *shift* of the interventricular septum, resulting in increasing right ventricular volumes and a secondary decrease in LV volumes (Jardin et al., 1981).

The interaction of the two ventricles results in alteration of both diastolic and systolic function of each. Several studies have demonstrated that increased distention of either ventricle results in altered distensibility of the other (Santamore et al., 1976).

Afterload

During anesthesia, afterload is dependent on the interplay of arterial pressure, ventricular chamber size and drug effects. The determinants of arterial pressure include:

1. Systemic vascular resistance (SVR)
2. Cardiac output.

Changes in the peripheral vasculature secondary to painful stimuli during *light* anesthesia may cause large increases in SVR resulting in decreased ventricular ejection and acutely increased filling pressures especially in the setting of decreased contractility. The use of inhalational anesthetic agents to decrease neurohumorally induced increases in PVR may be essential to augment cardiac performance. Manipulation of afterload with vasodilator therapy, may be essential in patients with decreased contractility (Tinker, 1979).

CLINICAL ASSESSMENT OF CARDIAC PERFORMANCE

Available diagnostic and monitoring modalities can be divided into methods to measure pressure, volume or flow. Since preload, afterload and heart rate seldom remain constant, measurement of contractility is difficult in the clinical setting. A more appropriate term is *pump function* which allows for changes in these important variables.

At the level of isolated cardiac muscle, contractility is a unique relation between force, length and velocity. As all clinical measures of contractility are based on properties of the intact heart, such assessments reflect cardiac function beyond muscle properties. With this limitation clinical indices of contractility may be divided into two general groups:

1. Isovolumetric phase,
2. Ejection phase.

Isovolumetric Phase Indices

Isovolumetric phase indices are derived from measurements made prior to ventricular ejection. Examples of such measurements include maximum velocity of shortening (V_{max}) and rate of change of left ventricular pressure development (dP/dt). Isovolumetric phase indices characteristically are sensitive to changes in contractility and relatively insensitive to changes in loading conditions (preload and afterload). These measurements are not useful in assessing absolute levels of contractility or in comparing individuals to a normal value, but are useful for comparing acute changes in contractility for a given patient.

dP/dt. The rate of pressure development is the counterpart of the maximum rate of force development in isometrically contracting isolated cardiac muscle. A variant of this index is dP/dt at 40 mmHg of DP (developed pressure) ($dP/dt|DP40$). This index partially corrects for preload variation of dP/dt. It does not correct for other weaknesses of this calculation which include variations based on increased ventricular wall thickness seen with chronic pressure overload.

V_{max}. This index is analogous to the theoretical maximum velocity of shortening of the ventricular contractile element under zero load. V_{max} is determined by plotting $dP/dt|P$ versus instantaneous wall stress. While this derived index is attractive as it controls for changes in wall thickness which influence dP/dt, it is difficult to obtain due to intersubject variation confining its use to research investigations.

Isovolumetric indices of contractility require invas-

ive pressure measurements employing high fidelity transducer tipped catheters placed in the left ventricle at cardiac catheterization. For this reason, such measurements are not likely to become part of the anesthetists clinical armamentarium.

Ejection Phase Indices

In contrast to the isovolumetric indices, these measurements are useful in assessing basal levels of contractility in patient groups (or individuals) over periods of time. Ejection phase indices include ejection fraction (EF), fractional shortening (FS), and mean velocity of shortening of the contractile element (V_{ce}). As all of these measurements are made during ventricular ejection, sensitivity to afterload is present. Ejection indices require imaging techniques including angiography, echocardiography, and radionuclear techniques. With the exception of echocardiography these modalities are infrequently seen in the operating room. Cardiac output determination is considered an ejection phase measurement and is sensitive to both afterload as well as preload.

Ejection fraction (EF) is the ratio of stroke volume to end-diastolic volume:

$$EF = \frac{SV}{EDV} = \frac{EDV-ESV}{EDV}$$

EDV = End–diastolic volume
ESV = End–systolic volume
SV = Stroke volume

Left ventricular ejection fraction (LVEF) above 55% is considered normal. Comparisons of LVEF should be made at similar afterloads. In the presence of mitral regurgitation, LVEF may be falsely increased as afterload is effectively *decreased* by valvular incompetence.

Fractional shortening (FS) is a correlate of ejection fraction in which distance change (echocardiographic) rather than volume change is measured. FS is a comparison between a dimensional change of the left ventricle during systole and its diastolic value:

$$FS = \frac{EDD-ESD}{EDD}$$

EDD = End-diastolic dimension
ESD = End-systolic dimension

The advantage of this index which is also affected by afterload, is that only a single echocardiographic imaging plane is required.

Mean and maximum circumferential fiber shortening (VcF) is a noninvasive index of contractility. Its measurement requires a combination of echocardiography, phonocardiography, ECG, and carotid pulse tracings.

$$\text{Mean V}_{CF} = \frac{EDD - ESD}{EDD \times ET}$$

EDD = End-diastolic diameter
ESD = End-systolic diameter
ET = Ejection time

V$_{CF}$ may be more sensitive to changes in contractility secondary to the inclusion of a time dimension. It is cumbersome to measure and is not likely to find widespread use in the preoperative setting except as a part of the preoperative cardiologic workup.

Methodology to Evaluate Cardiac Performance

Clinical Examination

Traditional examination of heart sounds, pulses and blood pressure provide important information on the adequacy of cardiac performance which is noninvasive and easily available to the anesthetist. These modalities should always be assessed to confirm data obtained from more sophisticated technology.

Echocardiography

The application of echocardiography to assess cardiac performance in the perioperative period has been the most significant improvement in ventricular function monitoring since the introduction of the pulmonary artery catheter. Echocardiography is rapidly becoming an important tool for the anesthesiologist due to its clinical utility and research potential.

Cardiac ultrasound is the noninvasive application of sound waves (1–10 MHz) to produce images of anatomical structures and measure blood velocity by the Doppler principle. Applications of both these ultrasonic techniques are valuable to cardiac performance. Motion mode (M mode) and two dimensional (2D) techniques can be utilized to measure ventricular volumes and derived indices of function such as ejection fraction and area change fraction (Thys, 1987). The ultrasonic transducer can be applied to the chest wall, epicardial surface or placed within the esophagus. This latter technique termed transesophageal echocardiography (TEE), has great applicability in the anesthetized patient.

Doppler echocardiography is the measurement of blood velocity utilizing ultrasound. This technique is based on the Doppler principle which relates the shift in sound frequency that occurs as red cells move in an ultrasonic beam to their velocity relative to the transducer. An example of the *Doppler effect* is the passage of a train sounding its whistle past a stationary observer. The pitch of the whistle increases as the train approaches and decreases as it fades into the distance. The velocity of the moving object (i.e., train) is proportional to the shift in sound frequency (*Doppler shift*) observed by the listener. Doppler systems quantitate the frequency changes and display blood velocity measurements digitally. Cardiac output monitors

based on this principle employ transducers monitored within esophageal stethoscopes for use during general anesthesia (Mark, 1986).

Pulmonary Artery Catheter

The balloon-tipped pulmonary artery flotation catheter (PAC) has been an important advance in assessing cardiac function. The PAC allows the clinician to measure intravascular pressures, volumes and cardiac output, saturation and RVEF.

Pulmonary capillary wedge pressure (PCWP) correlates with left atrial pressure (LAP) and indirectly with LV end-diastolic pressure (LVEDP) over a wide range of LVEDP (5–25 mmHg) (Walston and Lendall, 1973). In the absence of pulmonary artery hypertension, pulmonary artery end-diastolic pressure (PAEDP) can be used as an estimate of PCWP. The gradient between PAEDP and PCWP is 1–4 mmHg. The ability to rapidly obtain accurate measurements of cardiac output in patients and to repeat them as often as desired is a principal advantage of the pulmonary artery catheter. Thermodilution cardiac output is a variant of the indicator-dilution technique, with *cold* used as the trace indicator. Cooling of the blood is accomplished by injection of cold 5% dextrose (21° or 0°C) and the change in temperature at the downstream sampling site is inversely proportional to cardiac output.

Rapid response thermistors for pulmonary artery catheters facilitate the measurement of right ventricular ejection fraction (RVEF). The response time of such thermistors (50 ms) is rapid enough to record beat-to-beat temperature variation. Temperature fluctuation due to the injection of a known volume of cold solution is used to calculate the RVEF (normal = 40%) by the thermodilution principle (Kay et al., 1983).

Radionuclear Techniques

Radionuclear techniques can be classified into those methods which assess cardiac performance through the use of radioactive tracers that remain in the intravascular space, and those which visualize myocardial intracellular uptake of the tracer. The most frequently utilized radionuclear techniques are the first pass radionuclide angiography and equilibrium gated pool imaging. Both allow precise and accurate measurement of several parameters including: ventricular volume, ejection fraction, systolic ejection time, peak filling rate, and peak ejection rate.

The first pass technique utilizes a bolus of radioactive tracer, and is based upon the indicator-dilution theory. With this technique ejection fraction (EF) is usually calculated from the end-diastolic and end-systolic counts, which are proportional to relative volume (normal LVEF is 55–66% and RVEF is 50%). Ejection fraction and assessment of regional wall motion abnormalities determined by the first pass technique correlate well with values measured via contrast ventriculography.

The equilibrium gated pool technique utilizes labeled red cells (once equilibrium of the radiotracer with the intravascular pool has occurred) and analyses several hundred cardiac cycles with only a single bolus of radioactive tracer. This method provides a relatively stable pool of labelled cells for 6–8 hours. The patient's electrocardiogram is used as a physiologic gating signal and synchronization of counts during systole and diastole is achieved over 8–20 minute period. Measurement of ejection fraction (LVEF) by this method has a variability of 5% in patients with abnormal LVEF < 55% (Upton et al., 1980). An absolute change of 5% in patients with abnormal ventricular function or 10% in patients with normal ventricular function are the guidelines used for determining significant changes in LVEF in an individual patient. A major advantage of the equilibrium gated technique is that multiple studies can be performed from a single radionuclide injection.

Angiography

The invasive measurement of ventricular volumes by contrast angiography is the benchmark for noninvasive methods of assessment including echocardiography and radionuclide angiography (Braunwald, 1988). From single plane or biplane views of the opacified ventricle, volumes at end-systole and end-diastole are calculated from the geometric model of the left ventricle (Rackley, 1976). Volumes are compared to determine ejection fraction and stroke volume. Volume measurements may be combined with intraventricular pressure measurements to derive pressure volume relations such as the ESPVR (Ross, 1984).

Magnetic Resonance Imaging

Magnetic resonance imaging (MRI) has great potential in adding to the diagnostic armamentarium in assessing cardiac function (Pohost, 1987, Higgins, 1988). MRI depends on resonance of charged nuclei within a strong magnetic field when subjected to radiofrequency energy. Hydrogen is the nucleus most frequently used in the imaging process and its use has given rise to the name proton MRI. The image is created by detecting and quantitating the energy emitted during hydrogen resonance. This resonance is processed to create tomographic slices of anatomy by exploiting regional variation in proton density and relaxation times of nuclei undergoing excitation. Such regional variation produces a natural contrast between blood pool and cardiovascular structures with blood appearing black (low signal strength) on MRI scans. Contrast material is therefore, unnecessary. Additionally, a wide range of soft tissue MRI densities exist and are used to define anatomical structures. The ECG is used to gate image acquisition and can produce serial frames of moving anatomical structures in three dimensions (cine MRI). MRI produces information on both morphology and function. Ventricular volumes throughout the cardiac cycle are measured and can be used to determine ejection fraction. MRI calculation of the ejection fraction is similar to radionuclear techniques in that it is independent of geometry. Measurement of ventricular thickness and mass is possible along with wall stress calculations. The ultimate application of MRI in the study of cardiac performance awaits further study (Laschinger, 1987).

REFERENCES

Barash P.G., Kopriva C.J. (1984). Cardiac pump function and how to monitor it. In *Manual of Cardiac Anesthesia*. pp. 1–34, (Thomas S. ed.). Churchill Livingstone: New York.

Braunwald E. (1988). Assessment of cardiac function. In *Heart Disease*, pp. 449–470, (Braunwald E. ed.), Philadelphia: W.B. Saunders Co.

Braunwald E., Sonnenblick E.H., Ross J. (1988). Mechanisms of cardiac contraction and relaxation. In *Heart Disease*, pp. 383–425, (Braunwald E. ed.). Philadelphia: W.B. Saunders Co.

Donald D.E., Essex H.E. (1954). Pressure studies after inactivation of the major portion of the canine right ventricle. *Am. J. Physiol.*, **176**, 155.

Higgins C.S. (1988). New cardiac imaging modalities: magnetic resonance, fast computed tomography, positron emission tomography. In *Cardiology*, Chapter 43, pp. 1–24, (Parmley W.W., Chatterjee K. eds). Philadelphia: J.B. Lippincott, Co.

Jardin F., Farcot J.C., Boisante L., et al. (1981). Influence of positive end-expiratory pressure on left ventricular performance. *New Engl. J. Med.*, **304**, 387.

Kay H., Afshari M., Barash P. (1983). Measurement of ejection fraction by thermal dilution techniques. *J. Surg. Rev.*, **34**, 337.

Laschinger J.C., Vannier M.W., Gronemeyere S., et al. (1987). Three dimensional reconstruction of the heart using EKG triggered magnetic resonance images. *J. Med. Imaging.*, **1**, 228.

Mark J.B., Steinbrook R.A., Gugine L.D., et al. (1986). Continuous noninvasive monitoring of cardiac output with esophageal Doppler ultrasound during cardiac surgery. *Anesth. Analg.*, **65**, 1013.

Parmley W.W., Sonnenblick E.H. (1967). Series elasticity. In *Relation to Contractile Element Velocity and Proposed Muscle Models*. Circ. Res., **20**, 112.

Pohost G.M., Canby R.C. (1987). Nuclear magnetic resonance imaging: current applications and future prospects. *Circulation*, **75**, 88.

Rackley C.E. (1976). Quantitative evaluation of left ventricular function by radiographic techniques. *Circulation*, **54**, 862.

Ross J. Jr. (1979). Acute displacement of the diastolic pressure volume curve of the left ventricle: Role of the pericardium and right ventricle. *Circulation*, **59**, 32.

Ross J. (1984). Applications and limitations of end-systolic measures of ventricular performance. *Fed. Proc.*, **43**, 2418.

Sagawa K. (1981). The end-systolic pressure-volume relation of the ventricle: Definition, modifications and clinical use. *Circulation*, **63**, 1223.

Santamore W.P., Lynch Meier G. (1976). Myocardial interaction between the ventricles. *J. Appl. Physiol.*, **41**, 362.

Sonnenblick E.H., Skelton C.L. (1974). Reconsideration of the ultrastructural basis of the cardiac length tension relation. *Circ. Res.*, **35**, 517.

Starling E.H. (1915). *Linacre Lecture on the Law of the Heart.* London: Longmans, Green.

Starr I., Jeffers W.A., Meade R.H. (1943). The absence of conspicuous increments in venous pressure after severe damage to the right ventricle of the dog, with a discussion of the relation between clinical congestive failure and heart disease. *Am. Heart J.*, **3**, 291.

Strobeck J., Sonnenblick E.H. (1986). Myocardial contractile properties and ventricular function. In *The Heart and Cardiovascular System*. pp. 31–49. (Fozzard H.A. ed.), New York: Raven Press.

Suga H., Katabatake A., Sagawa K. (1979). End-systolic pressure determines stroke volume from a contractile state. *Circ. Res.*, **44**, 238.

Thys D.M., Hillel Z., Goldman M.E., et al. (1987). A comparison of hemodynamic indices derived by invasive monitoring and two dimension echocardiography. *Anesthesiology*, **67**, 630.

Tinker J. (1979). A pharmacological approach to the treatment of shock. *Br. J. Hosp. Med.*, **21**, 261.

Upton M.T., Rerych S.K., Newman G.E., et al. (1980). Detecting abnormalities in left ventricular function during exercise before angina and ST-segment depression. *Circulation*, **45**, 1301.

Walston A., Kendall M.E. (1973). Comparison of pulmonary wedge and left atrial pressure in man. *Am. Heart J.*, **86**, 159.

14. Control of the Systemic Circulation
J. A. Reitan and N. D. Kien

Mechanical factors
Central control
    Efferents from the central control systems
    Afferent segment of reflex arc
Humoral control
Local control
Regional circulations
    Coronary Circulation
    Renal circulation
    Splanchnic circulation
    Skin circulation
    Muscle circulation

The task of the cardiovascular system is to deliver oxygen and nutrients to the cells of the body and to pick up their waste for disposal. The overall index of this work has been judged historically by the measurement of the cardiac output. Whether this pump function is regulated by peripheral circulatory factors or by variables influencing the actual pumping capability of the heart is a general topic of discussion in cardiac physiology. Certainly under steady-state conditions, there is reasonable agreement that regulation of cardiac output may be viewed as a balance between venous return and the pumping ability of the heart. While about 85% of man's blood volume resides in the venous and pulmonary vasculature (Wiedeman, 1963), it ordinarily does not change rapidly enough (except in hemorrhage) to exert significant short-term control of cardiac output. Rather there is a blend of intrinsic cardiac adaptation to varying venous return (such as the Frank–Starling mechanism), extrinsic nervous control of heart rate and stroke volume, and slow changes in blood volume regulated mainly by the kidney.

MECHANICAL FACTORS

A vast majority of all local blood flow in the body is controlled by *in situ* metabolic variables and the sum of all blood flow is the cardiac output. When local flow increases, blood is transferred at an increased rate from the arterial to venous circulation. This increased venous volume begets an increased pressure in the capacitance veins. The driving pressure to fill the heart (the difference in pressure between the venous capacitance reservoir and the right atrium) rises and venous return to the heart is enhanced. The relationship between capacitance reservoir pressure and the filling pressure of the heart is shown in Fig. 14.1. In this diagram the venous reservoir is separated from

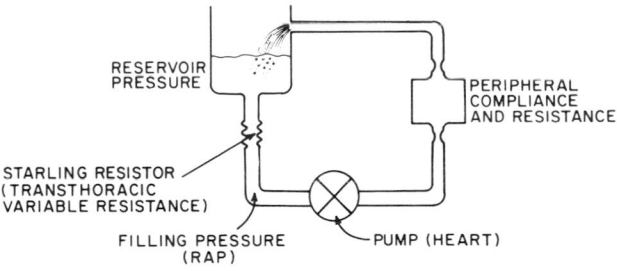

Fig. 14.1 A diagram of the circulation with the pulmonary circuit included as part of the heart. The driving pressure to fill the right heart is reservoir pressure minus right atrial pressure (RAP). The variable resistance between the venous reservoir and the heart is a limiting factor in venous return when RAP is low (*see text*).

the right atrium by a *Starling resistor* which *in vivo* relates to the propensity of the great veins to collapse upon entering the chest when right atrial pressure falls below atmospheric—a sort of transthoracic variable resistance. Under these conditions an effective stable resistance to flow exists from the venous capacitance reservoir to the right atrium. Flow to the right heart becomes constant because the driving pressure is simply the reservoir pressure minus atmospheric pressure (the value necessary for venous collapse at the point of entry of the great veins into the chest under these conditions). The cycle of mechanical control of the circulation is completed as the venous load to the heart is pumped effectively to the periphery and the sequence begins again.

The importance of this *in line* variable resistance in overall vascular flow control is controversial (Levy, 1979; Green, 1982), but it must be considered a significant cause for reduced cardiac output during positive pressure ventilation and anesthesia when the phasic rise in mean intrathoracic pressure tends to collapse the great veins.

The coupling between the peripheral circulation and the heart exists at the right atrium (Engler and Covell, 1987). The pressure in this chamber determines not only the gradient for blood return from the venous capacitance reservoir, but also loading for the heart. At any one moment it influences both the venous return and the pumping effectiveness of the heart.

Overall regulation of the cardiac pumping function should be considered in view of the preload, afterload, inotropy and heart rate (Braunwald, 1974). Because intrinsic cardiac factors affected by preload can account for an increased output of only three-*fold* under conditions of augmented venous return, extrinsic control mechanisms that modify afterload (blood pressure), inotropy (contractility) and heart rate must be activated to raise cardiac output to peak levels during exercise or sustained stress (Guyton, 1986). An example will explain this concept. If only the intrinsic mechanical cardiac factors were used during the initiation of high performance athletics, systemic flow would only double or triple before right atrial pressure would rise sufficiently to limit venous return to the heart. With the activation of extrinsic neurohumoral systems, inotropy and heart rate are increased as peripheral vascular resistance decreases. Pump efficiency improves and reduces right atrial pressure which, in turn, augments venous return. The cycle gains flow until the limits of both the internal and external factors are reached at a maximum of five to six-*fold* increase in cardiac output.

CENTRAL CONTROL

The central control mechanisms that modify the circulation have the ability to affect large parts of the system simultaneously. This is done by assimilation and integration of a constant barrage of afferent input from the periphery. The chemical transmitters in the brain include noradrenaline (norepinephrine), dopamine, adrenaline (epinephrine), 5-hydroxytryptamine (5-HT), acetylcholine and gamma-aminobutyric acid (GABA). The transmitters act on specific neurons to cause either excitation or inhibition. In the vasomotor center, release of noradrenaline generally has an adrenergic excitatory function while 5-HT produces a depressor action (Shepherd and Vanhoutte, 1979). A majority of the afferent fibers from the peripheral mechanoreceptors (those receptors that respond primarily to stretch) terminate in the solitary tract nucleus. This nucleus acts as a sort of clearing house for the considerable information relayed concerning pressure and volume in the central circulation. It, in turn, passes discrete impulses to the vasomotor center in the reticular formation and to the vagal nucleus (including the dorsal motor nucleus of the vagus and nucleus ambiguus) in the brain stem. The vagal nuclei control numerous peripheral vasculature functions through cholinergic innervation. The hypothalamus also has nerve tracts that interact with the solitary tract nucleus and the vasomotor center. These connections are thought to exert neuroendocrine control during emotional stress and to mediate the release of hormones such as vasopressin (anti-diuretic hormone). An excellent review of central neural control is available (Brody et al., 1986).

Efferents from the Central Control System

The efferent portion of the adrenergic nervous sequence is shown in Fig. 14.2. Afferent inputs into the solitary tract nucleus are integrated into the vasomotor center. The bulbospinal tract emerges as preganglionic neurons in the anterolateral columns of the spinal cord. Here the *pressor* transmitter, noradrenaline, and the *depressor* transmitter, 5-HT, may be found. Sympathetic ganglia as well as the adrenal medulla utilize acetylcholine as the transmitter, while at the target organs, noradrenaline is the effective neurotransmitter. Specific dopamine receptors apparently are scattered in the basal ganglia and in blood vessels—particularly in the renal and mesenteric vasculature. The cholinergic nervous sequence is shown in Fig. 14.3. From the solitary tract nucleus, connections to the vagal nuclei are made in the brain stem. Acetylcholine is the transmitter in the ganglia on the surface of the target organs. In general, the effect of vagal stimulation is dilatation in blood vessels, slowing of the heart and negative inotropy. GABA receptors, on the other hand, affect areas of the brain involving benzodiazepine binding sites.

Afferent Segment of Reflex Arc

The most common reflex modulation of activity in the vasomotor centers occurs with input from the afferent arc of the mechanoreceptors in the periphery. These

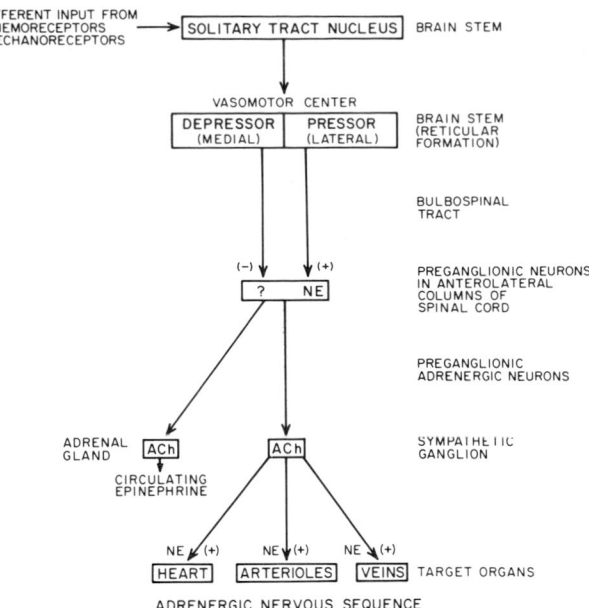

Fig. 14.2 The adrenergic nervous system sequence. On the right side anatomic locations are noted. Noradrenaline (NE) is the pressor neurotransmitter in the brain stem and 5-HT may be the chemical necessary for 'depressor' or inhibitory transmission. Acetylcholine (ACh) is the transmitter at the adrenergic ganglia and adrenal gland whereas NE is the chemical effector on the listed target organs. (+) designates stimulation or contraction and (−) suggests inhibition or dilatation. Both low and high pressure baroreceptors have input into the adrenergic system.

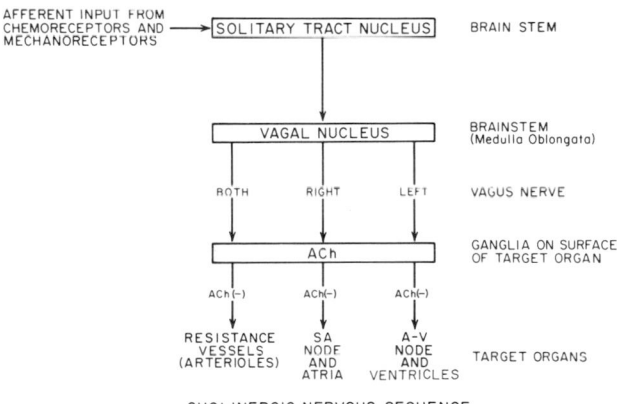

Fig. 14.3 The cholinergic nervous system showing anatomic locations in the right column. ACh is the neurotransmitter at both the ganglia and the target organs. The right vagus nerve has the predominant role in the atria and SA node while the left vagus influences the A-V node and the ventricles. The source of input is similar to that in the adrenergic system.

specific receptors include the high and low pressure systems.

Arterial Mechanoreceptors
The high pressure system, called the carotid sinus reflex, originates from mechanoreceptors located in the adventitia and media of the internal carotid artery near the bifurcation of the common carotid. These receptors are both rate and pressure dependent (Brown, 1980). Afferents from the receptors include both myelinated (fast conducting) and unmyelinated (slow conducting) fibers that form the carotid sinus nerve (Fig. 14.4). This nerve joins the glossopharyn-

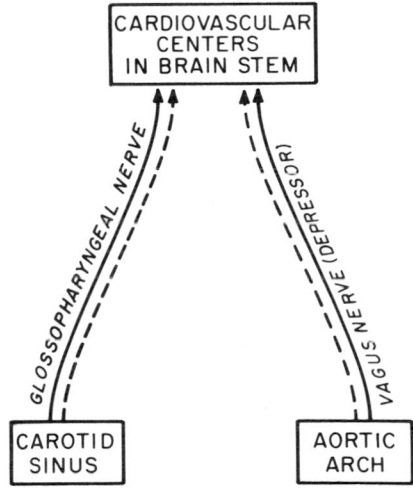

ARTERIAL MECHANORECEPTOR
SEQUENCE

Fig. 14.4 The high pressure baroreceptors circuit including sensors from the carotid sinus and arch of the aorta. Efferents from these specialized organs travel with the glossopharyngeal and vagus nerves as myelinated (solid line) and unmyelinated (dashed line) fibers.

geal for its cephalad projection. In the wall of the ascending aorta are similar receptors whose nerve fibres form the *depressor nerves* and join the vagus to reach the brain stem.

The high pressure mechanoreceptors have a set threshold: that is, below a given pressure there is no activity from these receptors. In normal man, there is evidence of activity beginning at about 65–70 torr (Pelletier et al., 1972). In hypertension this threshold is increased, depending upon the amount of blood pressure elevation present (Mancia et al., 1979). The exact mechanism whereby resetting occurs in either the subacute or chronic hypertensive patient, is unknown (Brown, 1980). In the normal individual, as the arterial blood pressure gradually increases, firing in the myelinated afferent fibers increases rapidly. Maximum output from the receptors occurs at about

180 torr. The aortic receptors have a slightly higher threshold, although their maximal firing range is similar to those receptors at the carotid sinus. There is also a difference between the thresholds of the unmyelinated and myelinated fibers from the high pressure mechanoreceptors. The myelinated nerves fire at a lower threshold and reach their maximal firing rate at a lower pressure than the slow unmyelinated nerves (Jones and Thoren, 1977). Thus, it would appear that the unmyelinated fibers tend to reinforce the fast-responding myelinated nerves and act as a recruitment phenomenon for grossly exaggerated arterial blood pressure.

When the high pressure mechanoreceptor nerves are attenuated with lower blood pressures, the *depressor* activity of the vagal center and vasomotor center is equally attenuated. Consequently, increased adrenergic activity to the heart and blood vessels occurs. Resistance vessels in the splanchnic, skin, renal and muscle beds are constricted and systemic vascular resistance is increased. The vast pool of blood from the splanchnic capacitance venous system is mobilized through contraction of these veins. Venous return to the heart increases. Heart rate and inotropy are augmented by an increase in cardiac sympathetic tone. The overall result is an increase in cardiac output and an attempt to maintain arterial blood pressure.

When blood pressure or heart rate acutely rises above a normal level for an individual, the reverse sequence occurs.

Cardiopulmonary Mechanoreceptors:

The low pressure baroreceptors or cardiopulmonary mechanoreceptors are located in the endocardium at the junction of the inferior and superior venae cavae with the right atrium and at the junction of the pulmonary veins and left atrium (Abboud et al., 1976). These receptors give rise to myelinated nerves that terminate in the cardiovascular centers of the brain including the solitary tract nucleus (Fig. 14.5). Unmyelinated nerve fibers arise from the scattered stretch receptors in all chambers of the heart. Both the unmyelinated and myelinated fibers from the cardiopulmonary mechanoreceptors join the vagus nerve. In addition there are discrete sympathetic afferents throughout the heart that connect to the spinal cord travelling along with efferent sympathetic nerves.

Following their activation from chamber distention, the traditionally ascribed function of the low pressure mechanoreceptors at the atriovenous junctions has been the increase in heart rate and decrease in sympathetic tone to the kidney. Later work with negative pressure devices in humans suggests that the arteriomechanoreceptors (high pressure system) regulate the heart rate and the splanchnic resistance vessels, whereas the cardiopulmonary receptors regulate predominantly muscle and skin resistance vessels (Abboud, 1979). In addition, activation of the cardiopulmonary mechanoreceptors produces a relative di-

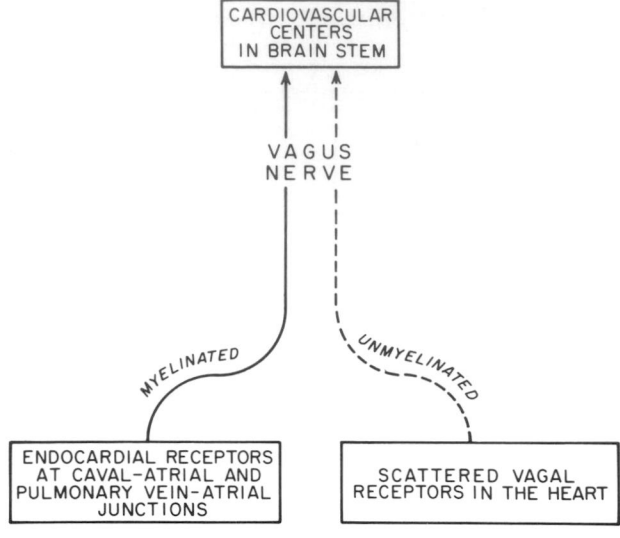

Fig. 14.5 The low pressure baroreceptor scheme. The vagus nerve transmits signals from both atrial border receptors (myelinated) and from sites throughout the endocardium (unmyelinated).

uresis, probably caused by suppression of the antidiuretic hormone from the posterior lobe of the pituitary (Linden, 1979).

The scattered vagal receptors in the heart are activated by increases in atrial or ventricular volume (Zucker, 1986). Upon stimulation they act similarly to the high pressure mechanoreceptors in that the depressor neurons of the vasomotor center and vagal nuclei are activated. This brings about an increase in vagal control of the cardiovascular system. Because of the decrease in heart rate, inotropy, and venous return caused by splanchnic pooling, cardiac output is diminished. Since these receptors are within the myocardium, they may act independently of the high pressure mechanoreceptors. For example, if a patient is in heart failure with a lowered systemic pressure and with distended atria, the two receptor systems would have opposing effects.

The Chemoreceptors

Two areas in man contain specialized cells that are oxygen, carbon dioxide, and hydrogen ion sensitive (Pelletier, 1972). These are the chemoreceptors of the carotid and aortic bodies. The carotid body is located near the bifurcation of the common carotid artery and has been studied in detail in both animal and man. The aortic chemoreceptor is located near the aortic component of the high pressure baroreceptors. The afferent nerves leaving the carotid body join with those from the carotid sinus to form the sinus nerve (Fig. 14.6). This, in turn, becomes part of the glosso-

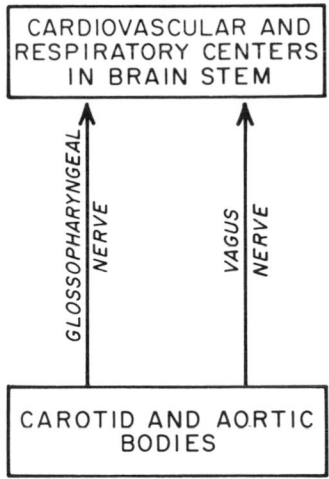

CHEMORECEPTOR
SEQUENCE

Fig. 14.6 A schematic drawing of chemoreceptor anatomy. From the carotid and aortic sensors information reaches the brain stem via cranial nerves IX and X.

pharyngeal on its cephalad course. The aortic body nerves join together with the nerves from the mechanoreceptors as part of the depressor nerve which subsequently joins the vagus. It is of interest that the receptor organs within the carotid and aortic bodies are amongst the most highly perfused areas in the body. They receive approximately 2000 ml/ (100 g·min). Apparently, this controlled hyperemia increases the sensitivity of the chemoreceptors to changes in proton, CO_2, and O_2 concentration in the blood. The threshold for chemoreceptor activity varies depending upon the stimulus. Increased firing by the afferent nerves in the carotid body does not occur until P_{O_2} falls below 80 torr in the normal individual. On the other hand P_{CO_2} values above 40 torr or a pH below 7.37 will initiate increasing activity proportional to the change in the stimuli (Pelletier, 1972). During respiratory acidosis wherein P_{CO_2} rises and pH falls, there is a marked increase in the activity of the chemoreceptor afferents.

Indirectly the chemoreceptors correlate with arterial blood pressure since acidemia and hypoxemia may be induced by hypotension. Stimulation of the chemoreceptors causes (1) an increase in minute volume mediated by the respiratory centers and an interaction with the cardiovascular centers of the brain stem which (2) increase cardiac vagal output and (3) increase sympathetic activity to the splanchnic venous pool and the arterial resistance beds of muscle, gut, and kidney. The overall result is an increase in ventilation, a decrease in heart rate and inotropy with a concomitant vasodilatation of the coronary arteries, and a support of blood pressure by increasing systemic vascular resistance and venous return. In the vaso-

motor center itself, there are chemoreceptors that activate when extreme acidosis or hypoxemia exists and the pressure is very low (30–40 torr). The output from the vasomotor center chemoreceptors under these extreme circumstances causes an unusually powerful stimulation in the sympathetic nervous system, as seen under agonal conditions (Sagawa et al., 1961).

HUMORAL CONTROL

Three blood borne vasoconstricting substances have significant control in maintaining cardiovascular stability. Circulating catecholamines, secreted from the adrenal medulla or from free nerve endings in the periphery, modify blood flow in many organs. Vasopressin, produced near and stored in the posterior hypophysis, is involved in long-term homeostasis by renal tubular control and possesses direct vasoactive qualities under some conditions. The renin-angiotensin-aldosterone pathway produces angiotensin II, a potent vasoconstrictor, and aldosterone for conservation of blood volume by sodium resorption in the kidney.

Adrenaline and *noradrenaline* are formed from tyrosine in adrenergic nerve endings and in the adrenal medulla. The sequence of

tyrosine → DOPA → dopamine → noradrenaline

is common to both locations, although little adrenaline is synthesized outside the adrenal gland. Adrenaline is produced from noradrenaline by the addition of a methyl group on the NH_2 moiety, accelerated by the enzyme ↑ phenylethanolamine-N-methyltransferase. Storage and release of noradrenaline is common to all adrenergic nerve terminals and involves repository vesicles and their release under calcium ion stimulation. Four times more adrenaline is stored in the adrenal medulla than noradrenaline and, as such, adrenaline is the primary circulating catecholamine effector. Upon release caused by stress such as hemorrhage, exercise, or emotion (fight and flight), adrenaline produces several circulatory modifications. β-adrenergic stimulation in the heart increases rate and inotropy while the coronary vasculature dilates. Splanchnic venous capacitance beds are constricted and most arteriole systems increase resistance. Muscle and some liver arterioles under β-adrenergic control dilate. Overall peripheral vascular resistance decreases with adrenaline release and cardiac output markedly increases. Mean blood pressure may rise slightly. The combination of α and β-adrenergic effects by adrenaline produces this mixture of responses. Circulating noradrenaline, on the other hand, causes predominantly α-adrenergic stimulation in the periphery and systemic vascular resistance and blood pressure rise concurrently. Little noradrenaline is released in the adrenal medulla so that most of it free in the blood comes from overflow at the adrenergic nerve endings.

Vasopressin is synthesized in neurons located in the

supraoptic and paraventricular nuclei. This polypeptide is transported by axons to the posterior pituitary gland and bound to other polypeptides for storage. Release of vasopressin (also called the anti-diuretic hormone or ADH) is triggered by several mechanisms. First, a small decrease in blood volume sensed by the low pressure mechanoreceptors induces an increase in ADH blood levels. Secondly, osmoreceptors in the hypothalamus and excessive blood levels of angiotensin II cause release of the hormone from storage. Finally, with the sudden loss of pressure occurring in hemorrhage or other forms of shock, arterial baroreceptors increase the rate of vasopressin secretion up to 40 times the normal. At these plasma levels, significant vasocontriction in the muscle, splanchnic and coronary vascular beds occurs by direct effect (Philbin, 1986). However, the main function of ADH is maintaining blood volume by selectively altering the permeability of the terminal portions of the renal tubule to water and urea. As the name implies, accelerated secretion of ADH leads to increased resorption of water and tends to restore blood volume. Suppression of the hormone by alcohol or nicotine may deplete the body of substantial vascular volume and reduce the effectiveness of reflex mechanisms in preserving homeostasis under stress.

The *renin-angiotensin-aldosterone* pathway is discussed as part of the renal circulation. In summary, angiotensin II enhances the response to circulating catecholamines and production of the neuroeffector substance in addition to its direct vasoconstricting action. The cardiovascular centers of the brain stem are stimulated as well by low concentrations of this hormone, and this latter function serves to create a basal tone within the adrenergic autonomic system. Finally, angiotensin II augments production of aldosterone in the adrenal cortex which increases reabsorption of the sodium ion in the distal renal tubule. All these factors tend to support a fundamental blood volume and pressure in man.

LOCAL CONTROL

Aproximately 75% of regulation in the systemic circulation comes from local factors in the microcirculation (Guyton, 1977). These include the effect of perivascular P_{O_2}, pH, P_{CO_2}, osmolality, the potassium, phosphate, magnesium, and lactate concentrations, the Bayliss myogenic response, and adenosine and prostaglandin production. Several review articles are available that investigate in depth and propose possible mechanisms of action for local vascular control (Dusting et al., 1979; Sparks and Belloni, 1978; Johnson and Henrich, 1975) and the mechanism for autoregulation in general (Johnson, 1986; Mellander, 1988). It would seem as though local processes controlling blood flow may differ in specific regions. Consequently, several vascular systems need to be reviewed and individual variation noted.

REGIONAL CIRCULATIONS

Coronary Circulation

Anatomy

The heart is perfused by the right and left coronary arteries which originate from the sinuses located at the root of the aorta above the anterior and left posterior coronary cusps of the aortic valve. The right coronary artery provides blood flow to the right atrium and ventricle. In 55% of hearts, the sinus node is perfused by the sinus node artery which originates from the right coronary artery and the blood supply to the atrioventricular node is provided by the posterior interventricular branch of the right coronary artery in 90% of hearts. The left coronary artery divides into the anterior interventricular and the circumflex arteries as it emerges from behind the pulmonary trunk. The anterior interventricular artery and its branches perfuse the anterior wall of the ventricle and most of the ventricular septum. The circumflex artery supplies blood flow to the left atrium, the posterior ventricular wall, and, in 45% of hearts, the sinus node. The circumflex artery also perfuses the anterior papillary muscle of the left ventricle, while the posterior papillary muscle receives blood supply from branches of both the right and left coronary arteries. There are also collateral and communicating vessels that channel between the right and left coronary arteries. These vessels have an important role in regulating blood flow distribution when myocardial ischemia occurs.

The venous drainage of the left coronary artery is carried by an elaborate system which empties predominantly into the coronary sinus via the great cardiac vein. The right coronary artery drains either into the coronary sinus or directly into the right atrium via smaller cardiac veins (Schlant and Silverman, 1986).

Control of Coronary Blood Flow

The main purpose of the coronary circulation is to provide adequate oxygen and nutrients to the contracting myocardium. Even at rest, the heart extracts most of the oxygen contained in its blood supply. As a result, when the myocardial oxygen consumption exceeds its normal range from 7.5–10.5 ml/(100 g·min) little or no oxygen can be made available from augmented extraction (Cohan and Gewertz, 1985). Instead, the increased oxygen delivery must be made with an increase in coronary blood flow. According to physical principles, coronary blood flow is dependent upon aortic pressure and coronary vascular resistance. Since coronary blood flow varies only slightly over a wide range of aortic pressure, and an increase in aortic pressure would produce an increased oxygen demand, the control of coronary blood flow must act predominantly through alterations in coronary vascular resistance. Thus, the coronary circulation autoregulates its blood flow by adjusting the vascular tone in response to the metabolic needs of the myocardium. The factors modulating the coronary auto-regulation are thought to be physical, metabolic and neurohumoral.

Physical Factor. The blood ejected from left ventricular contraction forces the cusps of the aortic valve to open which, in turn, intrude into the valsalva sinuses and impede blood flow to the coronary ostia. During diastole, the aortic pressure and the flow vortices formed at the aortic root following aortic valve closure are the major forces that drive blood into the coronary bed along with the reduction in intra–myocardial compression. Therefore, 80% of blood flow to the left ventricle occurs during this period. As the coronary vessels penetrate the ventricular wall to perfuse the endocardial layer, the vessels are compressed by extravascular forces that markedly inhibit blood flow. It is well known that there is a gradient of forces between the epicardial and endocardial layers during systole. This force gradient impedes endocardial blood flow and results in a gradient of blood flow distribution across the ventricular wall. In addition to the systolic compression, blood flow in the coronary vessels is impeded by shear forces caused by vessel bending which occurs during systolic contraction. During diastole, the endocardial vessels become dilated and the flow gradient is reversed in order to maintain a uniform blood distribution across the heart wall. In the event that the endocardial vessels become maximally dilated and the transmural distribution of coronary blood flow is no longer regulated, the endocardium is most vulnerable to ischemic damage. Therefore, the maldistribution of myocardial blood flow favoring the epicardial layer is often regarded as a sign of myocardial ischemia.

In contrast to the left ventricular blood flow, blood flow to the right ventricle occurs throughout the cardiac cycle with slightly higher flow during systole. This is possible due to a less significant compressive extravascular force because of the thinner wall and lower intracavitary pressure generated in the right ventricle. A comparison of phasic blood flow through the left and right coronary arteries in relation to aortic pressure is seen in Fig. 14.7.

The viscosity of blood is also a factor that can change the resistance to flow and thereby alter coronary blood flow, particularly in the presence of coronary disease. Similar to other vascular beds, the coronary vessels respond to an increase in perfusion pressure by stretching their vascular smooth muscle. This stretching triggers contraction which increases the compressing forces and, in turn, returns blood flow to control levels. Whether this myogenic reflex provides an important contribution to the autoregulation of coronary blood flow is not clear.

Metabolic Factor. This factor is believed to have the most important role in determining autoregulatory resistance of the coronary circulation. Fig. 14.8 shows

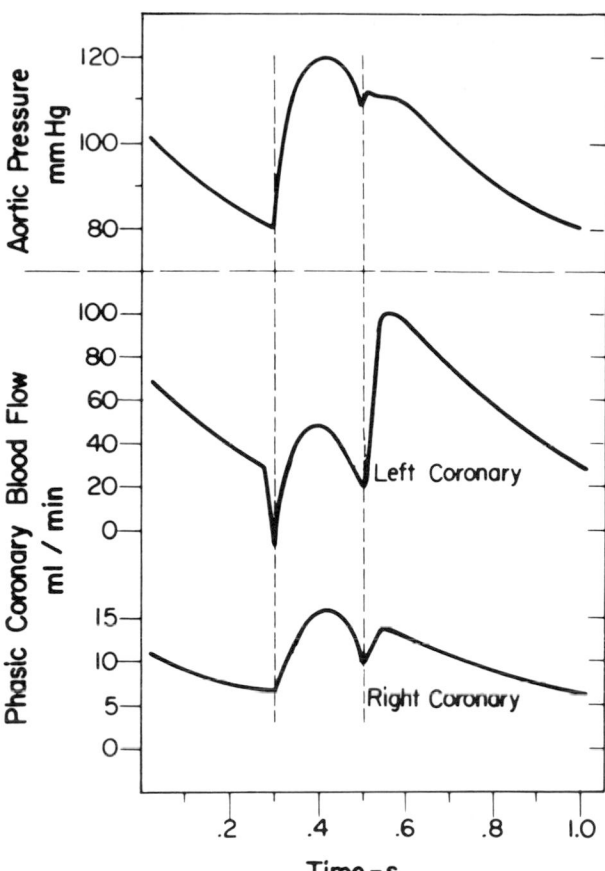

Fig. 14.7 Comparison of phasic blood flow in the left and right coronary arteries in relation to aortic pressure. The left coronary artery has a higher flow rate and greater fluctuation within one cardiac cycle. (From Berne and Levy, 1986 with permission).

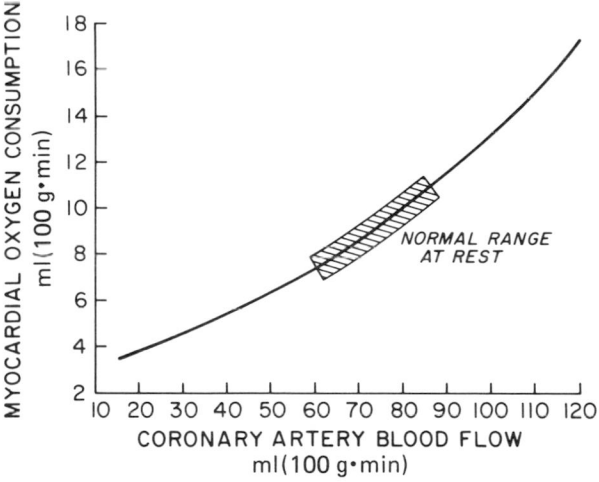

Fig. 14.8 A comparison of coronary artery blood flow and myocardial oxygen consumption. Mean resting flow and oxygen consumption are 70 ml/(100 g · min) and 9 ml/(100 g · min), respectively. The regression equation from the experimental data describes a nearly linear best fit line. (Canine data redrawn from Rubio, 1975 with permission).

a near linear relationship between coronary blood flow and myocardial oxygen consumption ($M\dot{V}O_2$). An increase in $M\dot{V}O_2$ causes a release of mediators that vasodilate the coronary vessels and result in a proportional increase in coronary blood flow. A number of agents are thought responsible for the communication link between coronary blood flow and $M\dot{V}O_2$.

Oxygen tension may regulate coronary blood flow by two mechanisms: first, by a direct transmural effect on the smooth muscle cells from the P_{O_2} level itself and secondly, through the effect of oxygen deficiency on the parenchymal cells of the vasculature which produce metabolites with vasodilatory properties. While oxygen may have some direct vasoactive control, it is doubtful that a significant amount of overall autoregulatory vasodilatation can be attributed to the reduced arteriolar P_{O_2} alone. Experimental work has shown that coronary vascular resistance correlates more closely with coronary venous P_{O_2}, than with arterial oxygen tension (Berne et al., 1957; Arnold et al., 1968). Thus, it appears that parenchymal cell metabolism is more reflected directly by venous P_{O_2} than intra-arterial P_{O_2}. Although hypoxia causes potent coronary vasodilatation, it is most likely that the vasodilatation is due to metabolites released from the hypoxic myocardium whether oxygen itself has a direct effect on local control of coronary vascular resistance is uncertain because of the experimental difficulty in separating the effects of oxygen from those of vasoactive metabolites (Dole, 1987).

Carbon dioxide and pH are reported to have some influence on the coronary blood flow. However, again it is difficult to distinguish their direct effects from other vasodilator mechanisms.

The prime vasoactive metabolite is thought to be adenosine, a potent coronary vasodilator found in the myocardium. Its concentration is related to changes in $M\dot{V}O_2$ and is measurable in the venous outflow from the heart. Adenosine is formed after dephosphorylation of AMP by a specific nucleotidase in the myocardial cell membrane. It has been suggested that with hypoxia there is a buildup of AMP, which produces more substrate for the reaction and subsequently more adenosine (Klocke, 1976). Adenosine can readily cross the myocardial cell membrane and act locally to induce relaxation of the vascular smooth muscle by activating the adenosine receptors in the coronary vessels. The involvement of adenosine in the regulation of coronary perfusion is illustrated in Fig. 14.9. The exact mechanism by which adenosine elicits vasodilatation is not known. However, it has been postulated that adenosine acts via cyclic AMP or via inhibition of calcium uptake (Berne and Rubio; Belardinelli, 1979, 1989).

Other vasoactive substances such as prostaglandins and kinins may also have a role in autoregulation. Experimental work has shown that a significant amount of coronary vasodilatation results from treatment with the arachidonic acid metabolite prostacyclin (Dusting et al., 1979). In isolated muscle studies this

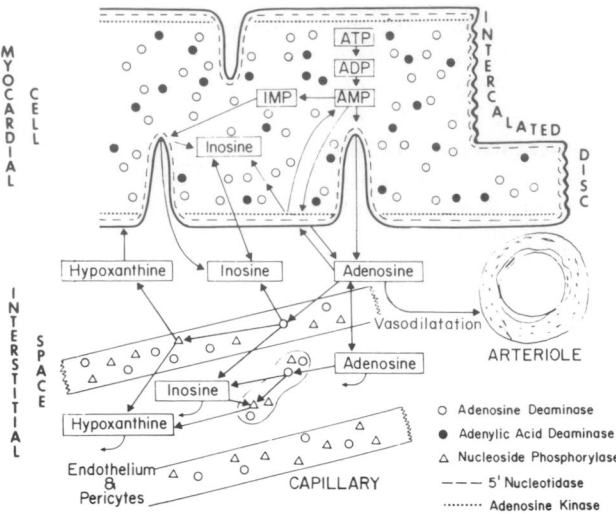

Fig. 14.9 Diagram depicting formation, site of action and degradation of adenosine. Adenosine is formed from the dephosphorylation of AMP, crosses the sarcolemma to induce vasodilatation and either is phosphorylated to AMP or is deaminated to inosine. The degradation of adenosine can occur in the myocardial cell, interstitial space or capillary bed. (From Rubio et al., 1972 with permission).

substance is found normally in small amounts in the vessel walls and its concentration increases with tissue bath hypoxia. Unfortunately, no definite study in intact animals has demonstrated a clear-cut cause effect relationship.

With autoregulation, the coronary vasculature reacts to varying perfusion pressures to maintain a constant blood flow. The solid line in Fig. 14.10 outlines the normal autoregulatory curve for coronary perfusion with the point of maximum vessel dilatation

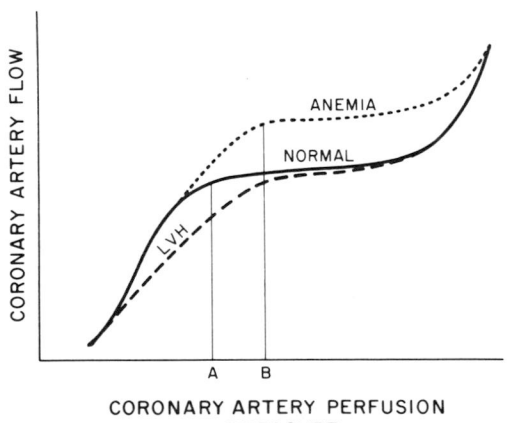

Fig. 14.10 Pressure-flow curves for myocardial perfusion. Autoregulation occurs during the horizontal slope of the lines, normally from pressures of 40-150 torr. Left ventricular hypertrophy (LVH) and anemia shift the curves and alter the zone of autoregulation. *See text*.

marked by the letter A. At pressures below maximum dilatation, flow is pressure dependent in a near linear fashion. The perfusion pressure is calculated as the difference between inflow (diastolic pressure) and outflow (right atrial pressure) of the coronary circulation. Studies have shown that the *downstream* outflow pressure may be considerably higher than previously conceived because of local tissue forces (Klocke et al., 1980). Consequently, the actual perfusion pressure may be significantly less than just the aortic diastolic pressure. This factor becomes important when cardiac muscle mass increases in excess to its nutrient vasculature as in left ventricular hypertrophy (LVH). The dashed line in Fig. 14.10 describes the shift to the right of the coronary autoregulatory curve with LVH and the point of maximum dilatation moves from A to B. This suggests that higher perfusion pressures are needed to maintain flow and prevent 'falling down the curve' below the point of maximum dilatation (B). Similarly, a higher flow is needed to meet myocardial demand in anemia because of the lowered oxygen carrying capacity of the blood. This adjustment elevates the autoregulatory curve as shown by the dotted line. Again, the point of maximum dilatation is shifted to the right (point B) and higher perfusion pressures are necessary to avoid hypoperfusion. Consequently, both of these conditions may lead to an increased likelihood of myocardial ischemia during hypotension.

Neurohumoral Factor. While metabolic activity may induce a five to six-*fold* change under stress in coronary artery resistance, neuroreflex stimulation accounts for changes of only 30–40% from resting control (Rubio and Berne, 1975). Sympathetic nervous activation results in initial vasoconstriction followed by vasodilatation (McRaven et al., 1971). This duality of effect is explained by investigation with both α and β-adrenergic antagonist drugs. After β blockade, sustained sympathetic nerve stimulation produces only vasoconstriction, and, after α-blockade, sympathetic stimulation results in vasodilatation (Vatner et al., 1970). Thus, it is apparent that both α and β receptors are present in the coronary vasculature. Recent studies have demonstrated the presence of both receptor subtypes in the large coronary arteries. It has been postulated that activation of the receptor subtypes modulates perfusion to different myocardial layers during exercise. Furthermore, there is evidence of direct vagal control of coronary resistance in that vagal stimulation in a β-blocked animal preparation produces vasodilation that may be blocked by atropine (Berne et al., 1965). However, the role of the parasympathetic nervous system in regulation of the coronary circulation circulation remains highly controversial (Young, 1987). A number of humoral agents have been reported to exert some influence on the coronary vascular resistance. The role of these substances in coronary regulation is not likely to be of great significance. However, their activities on the coronary vessel may provide some buffering effect, particularly in the presence of high sympathetic tone or severe hypotension. Among these agents, norepinephrine (noradrenaline), angiotensin II, vasopressin at high dose and thromboxane A_2 cause coronary vasoconstriction, whereas vasodilatation is observed with dopamine, thyroid hormone and prostaglandins (E_2, F and I_2). Recently, atrial natriuretic factor (ANF), a hormone-like substance found in atrial cells, has been thought to play a role in the regulation of blood volume. Whether ANF contributes to the coronary autoregulation awaits further elucidation.

Anesthetics and Coronary Circulation

Halothane, isoflurane and enflurane are known to relax vascular smooth muscle and decrease coronary vascular resistance. In addition to the direct coronary vasodilatation, coronary vascular resistance may be reduced by autoregulation in response to a decrease in systemic blood pressure. While autoregulation may be significantly attenuated during anesthesia, there is no evidence that it is completely blocked. Systemic vasodilatation unloads the congested heart and decreases myocardial oxygen consumption. This is particularly beneficial in the heart with significant coronary artery disease. Ironically, coronary artery dilatation may lead to *coronary steal*, a phenomenon in which blood flow is redistributed to benefit the normal myocardium at the expense of the ischemic bed. In animal studies, halothane maintains endocardial perfusion probably by a decrease in intramyocardial pressure. However, overall coronary blood flow decreases as a result of coronary vasoconstriction secondary to the decreased myocardial oxygen demand. The likelihood for coronary steal to occur without a net increase in coronary blood flow is minimal. Compared to halothane, isoflurane and enflurane are more potent coronary vasodilators, but whether they are associated with a coronary steal in the ischemic heart remains unclear and controversial (Buffington et al., 1987; Cason et al., 1987; Moore, 1989).

Recently, narcotics have become popular anesthetic agents in patients undergoing cardiac surgery. Despite the vasodilatory effect of opioids, cardiovascular stability appears to be well maintained during narcotic anesthesia. Since the cardiovascular responses to opioids are complex and vary from species to species, experimental evidence is incomplete and seems to justify continued investigation of these agents. On the other hand, nitrous oxide, alone or in addition to inhalational anesthetics, stimulates the sympathetic system, decreases coronary perfusion pressure and produces a myocardial depressant effect. Because of this, nitrous oxide may upset the myocardial oxygen balance and potentiate ischemic damage. Consequently, N_2O is seldom used in patients with significant ischemic heart disease.

In summary, regulation of coronary artery resistance is a complex mixture of systolic compression with myogenic mechanisms, predominant metabolic control related to oxygen demand, and neural feedback consisting of a moderate resting sympathetic vasoconstriction reflexly modulated by vagal vasodilatation. Figure 14.11 summarizes the factors influencing resistance to myocardial perfusion.

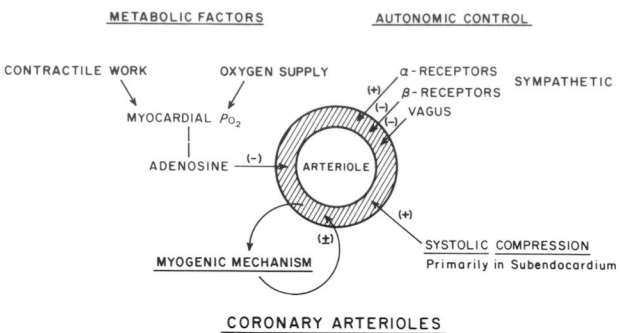

Fig. 14.11 Mechanisms by which coronary arteriole resistance is increased (+) or decreased (−). (Modified after Johnson, 1974.)

Renal Circulation

Total blood flow to the kidney equals approximately ¼ of the cardiac output. In the human kidney almost ¾ of the renal blood flow perfuses the cortex containing the glomeruli. The control of renal blood flow is regulated by three mechanisms:

1. Sympathetic innervation to the resistance vessels
2. Autoregulation
3. Endogenous hormonal systems including the circulating catecholamines and angiotensin II.

The sympathetic control is exerted mainly in the afferent arterioles of the glomeruli (Ljungqvist and Wagermark, 1970). Activation of the sympathetic system follows stimuli mediated through the brain stem centers (Fig. 14.12). These include afferents from the arterial and cardiopulmonary mechanoreceptors and indications of hypoxemia from arterial chemoreceptors. Muscle afferents may have an effect as well in reducing renal flow. Autoregulation in the kidney is remarkable in that blood flow remains relatively constant over a varying perfusion pressure from 80–250 torr. The mechanisms by which autoregulation occurs are not understood fully, but include the suggestion that the smooth muscle in the afferent arterioles to the glomeruli is pressure sensitive and a myogenic type of autoregulation exists similar to that present in the coronary circulation. Experimental work has shown that 'E' series prostaglandins exert a significant role in this vascular regulation, particularly by vasodilatation (Dusting et al., 1979).

Angiotensin II is the most active endogenous vasoconstrictor agent in the body and exerts a significant effect on renal vascular resistance. The sequence of its formation is shown in Fig. 14.13: an α_2-globulin

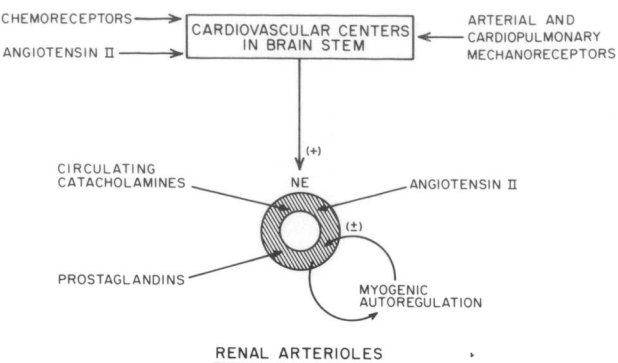

Fig. 14.12 A summary of factors influencing renal arterial flow. Mechanoreceptor, chemoreceptor, and angiotensin II input to the cardiovascular centers of the brain stem modulate sympathetic activity to the resistance arterioles. The neurotransmitter, NE, causes vasoconstriction (+) by activating the α-adrenoceptor. Circulating catecholamines and direct-acting angiotensin II influence renal flow similarly.

formed in the liver serves as a circulating substrate for the action of renin, a proteolytic enzyme. This enzyme is produced in the juxtaglomerular cells in the endothelium of the afferent arterioles to the glomeruli of the kidney. Production and release of the enzyme from these cells is dependent upon an increased activity in the renal adrenergic nerves, a decrease in perfusion distension of the afferent arterioles, or a fall in the amount of sodium delivered to the distal tubule (an

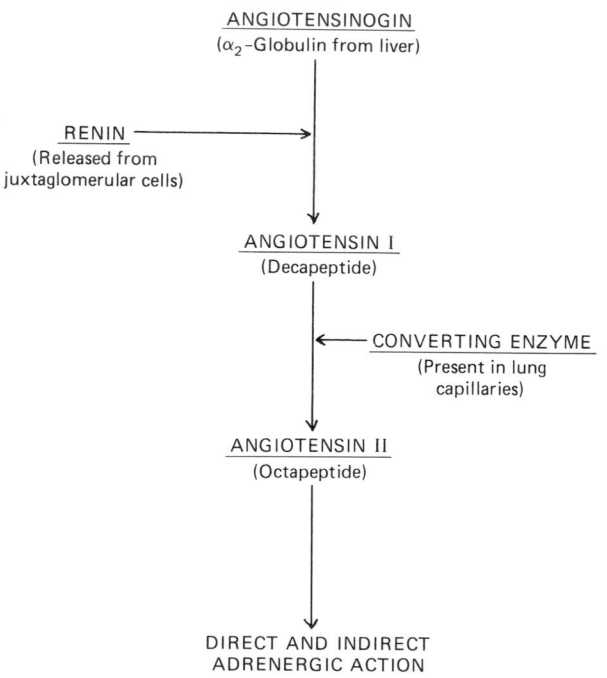

THE RENIN-ANGIOTENSIN SYSTEM

Fig. 14.13 *See text* for details.

area known as the macula densa). Of the three proposed mechanisms, arteriolar pressure decrease appears to be the most potent. Renin acts on the α_2 globulin to split off an inactive precursor, the decapeptide angiotensin I. The decapeptide is degraded further to an octapeptide by a specific converting enzyme found predominantly in the lung and kidney. This octapeptide is the active vasopressor angiotensin II.

Renin secretion is under the influence of two parallel feedback systems. First, angiotensin II produces a rise in blood pressure, which, in turn, slows down renin production. Additionally, angiotensin II stimulates production of aldosterone which increases sodium resorption and thereby attenuates renin release. It has been postulated that angiotensin II elevates the systemic blood pressure by actions on the vasomotor center in the brain, by potentiation of sympathetic ganglionic transmission, by enhancement of norepinephrine effects on α receptors, though direct constricting action on the smooth muscles of resistance vessels, and lastly, through augmented production of aldosterone and the resultant sodium retention (Reid et al., 1978). The last mechanism bears significantly on blood volume control in humans. A specific antagonist to angiotensin II activity known as saralasin, has been helpful in delineating the mechanisms of action of this potent vasopressor. Using this drug, investigators have shown that angiotensin II secretion is a major antagonist to sodium nitroprusside-induced hypotension (Delaney and Miller, 1980). Indeed, it may explain the tachyphylaxis and rebound phenomenon associated with the use of some hypotensive agents.

General anesthetics depress urine output with a concomitant fall in both free water and osmolar clearance (Deutsch, 1986). The mechanisms by which this restriction in output occurs include the effect of anesthesia on tubular transport and the result of vasopressin liberated by anesthesia. Undoubtedly, the major cause for lowered urine formation comes from a decreased glomerular filtration rate and renal blood flow. The reasons for the hemodynamic changes in the kidney under anesthesia are enigmatic, but, again, probably involve liberation of vasoactive substances such as vasopressin and angiotensin and a change in renal sympathetic tone. Regional block appears to preserve renal function unless blood pressure falls below the autoregulatory range (Hoffman, 1986).

Splanchnic Circulation

The splanchnic circulation is comprised of blood flow through the gastrointestinal tract, omentum, spleen, pancreas, gall bladder and liver. Blood from the extrahepatic splanchnic viscera reaches the liver via the portal vein. The liver is also supplied by the hepatic artery, a division of the coeliac artery. The hepatic artery provides about 30 40% of the total hepatic blood flow, while the portal vein contributes the rest

(Andreen and Irestedt, 1979). Splanchnic blood flow requires about 25% of the cardiac output in normal awake man and the splanchnic capacitance venous system serves as a large reservoir for about ⅓ the blood volume (Greenway and Lautt, 1986). Awake subjects, bled of 20% of their total blood volume, showed no change in splanchnic blood flow or resistance, even though almost 50% of the shed blood came from the splanchnic reservoir bed (Price et al., 1966).

Control of the splanchnic vessels is a combination of neuroreflex and hormonal factors (Fig. 14.14). Overall sympathetic vascular control comes by way of the splanchnic nerves from the coeliac and superior and inferior mesenteric ganglia. α-adrenergic stimulation causes an increase in splanchnic vascular resistance and a decrease in splanchnic blood flow. In addition, sympathetic stimulation of the venous capacitance system leads to a dramatic emptying of the 'splanchnic venous reservoir' and adds a significant amount of blood to the circulating volume. There do not appear to be cholinergic vasodilator nerves involved in the splanchnic circulation. Enterochromaffine cells under the control of the cardiovascular centers in the brain stem and circulating gastrointestinal hormones release 5-HT, which has a dilating effect on the splanchnic resistance vessels (Shepherd and Vanhoutte, 1979). The mechanoreceptor reflexes are closely involved in splanchnic arterial and venous vascular tone.

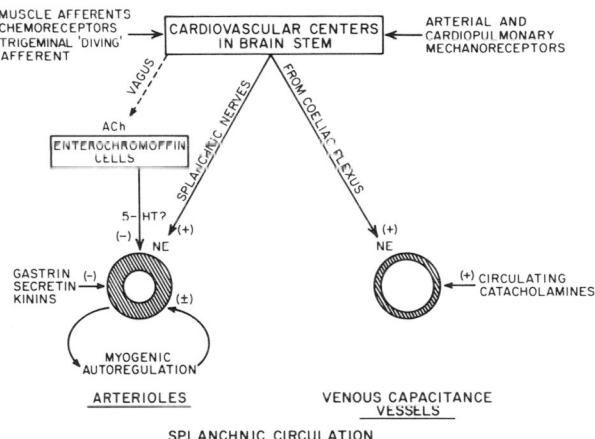

Fig. 14.14 A diagram of arterial and venous control in the splanchnic circulation. Cardiovascular centers in the brain stem regulate sympathetic outflow to the arterioles and veins while they, in turn, receive input from several sources. The contribution of the mechanoreceptors and chemoreceptors is described in the text. Muscle afferents from stretch receptors or free endings increase sympathetic outflow in order to attenuate splanchnic circulation during exercise. Similarly, sensory endings around the nose and eyes in the distribution of the trigeminal nerve elicit splanchnic, muscle, and renal vasoconstriction with bradycardia and apnoea. This is the so-called *diving reflex* and may influence blood flow and distribution in neonates when cold gases are blown across their faces.

In hemorrhage, initial vasoconstriction occurs through attenuation of the low pressure baroreceptor input to the cardiovascular centers of the brain. As blood loss increases, the carotid sinus and aortic mechanoreceptors assume the predominant role. Experimental evidence in man suggests that up to ⅓ the total blood volume adjustment to simulated hemorrhage is mediated through splanchnic baroreceptor pathways (Rowell et al., 1972). While chemoreceptors contribute centrally to the initial splanchnic vasoconstriction, the local effects of prolonged hypoxia and acidosis tend to override this with metabolic vasodilatation. Interestingly, in man, the sympathetic outflow to the splanchnic vessels appears to be directly proportional to the stress whether it be the result of hemorrhage, hyperthermia, or exercise.

A number of circulating hormones produce an effect on splanchnic vascular resistance. These include secretin, gastrin, and various kinins released by gastrointestinal mucosal glands. All of these substances cause a marked vasodilatation in the splanchnic resistance arterioles. Circulating catecholamines may have some small effect as well since the resistance vessels contain both α and β-adrenergic receptors (Price et al., 1967); yet, from studies in hypertensive patients, their role appears minor, at best, in the regulation of splanchnic arterial blood flow (Wilkins et al., 1951). However, the circulating catecholamines undoubtedly have significant influence on venoconstriction in the splanchnic bed and may be one of the ways in which the venous pool is expelled from the splanchnic area during blood loss (Greenway and Lautt, 1972).

With venoconstriction in the splanchnic capacitance circulation as a result of hemorrhage, there is an increased pressure gradient between the splanchnic pool and the depleted central venous volume. In effect, this hydrostatic mechanism accelerates the transfer of blood from the splanchnic area and hastens restoration of central circulating volume.

The effects of anesthesia on the splanchnic blood flow are varied and controversial (Gelman, 1986). Of the inhalation agents, halothane causes a dose dependent attenuation of portal blood flow in the monkey model, but the decrease in splanchnic circulation is proportional to the overall fall in observed cardiac output. Enflurane and isoflurane seem to support hepatic artery flow to a greater degree than halothane. Spinal and peridural block decrease splanchnic flow up to 25% during a T5 level block in man and this effect has been confirmed subsequently in a more detailed monkey preparation (Hoffman, 1986). Opioids—particularly morphine sulfate—cause changes in splanchnic blood flow. At low dose, morphine apparently lessens sympathetic tone and opens vascular beds while at higher doses it may increase catecholamine release and lead to splanchnic vasoconstriction.

Controlled ventilation with anesthesia causes a decrease in splanchnic flow during inspiration because of the compression of the liver by the diaphragm. This raises intrahepatic venous pressure and reduces the gradient between the hepatic and portal pressures. Additionally large tidal volumes and positive end-expiratory pressure elevate right atrial pressure and decrease venous return gradients into the right heart.

Skin Circulation

Skin blood flow is controlled by a complex assortment of mechanisms, both neural and regional in nature. The skin has the ability to increase blood flow far in excess of its nutritional needs. This potential for large increases in vascular conductance makes the cutaneous circulation an important regional flow area during changes in physical activity, environment and during anesthesia (Johnson, 1986).

Temperature sensors lie in the preoptic area of the anterior hypothalamus and may also occur in the deep vessels of the abdominal viscera and spinal cord (Shepherd and Vanhoutte, 1979). Heat to these areas causes vasodilatation and coolness results in cutaneous vasoconstriction. Both of these effects are neurally mediated through the cardiovascular center of the brain stem (Fig. 14.15) so that either a sympathetic pressor response occurs from cooled blood or a depressor action is initiated from heated blood perfusing the temperature receptors. The depressor action

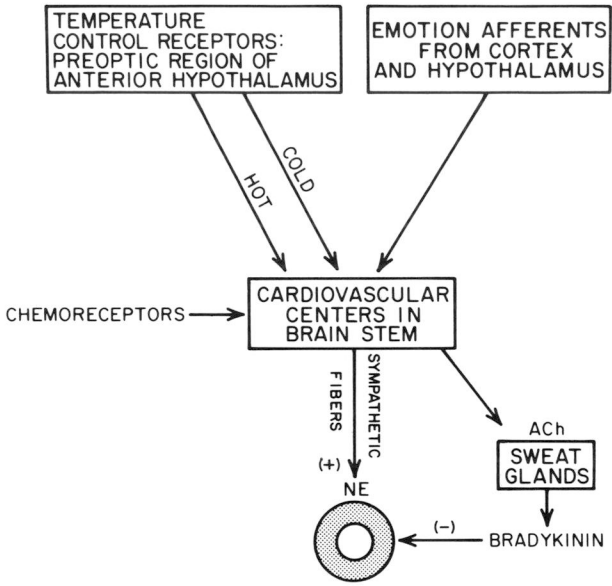

Fig. 14.15 A block diagram of control variables in regulation of skin blood flow. Temperature receptors in the hypothalamus respond to hot and cold by respectively decreasing or increasing the sympathetic stimulation to resistance arterioles and A-V shunts. Chemoreceptors and central afferents following emotional stress modulate the adrenergic tone as well. Sweating is associated with local bradykinin formation and vasodilatation (*see text*).

causes an inhibition of normal sympathetic vasoconstriction at the preganglionic neuron level (*see* Fig. 14.2). At normal temperature sympathetic tone to the cutaneous vascular bed is the primary modulating factor. While resting blood flow in the skin constitutes only about 4% of the total cardiac output (Mellander and Johansson, 1968), it has the potential to increase fifteen-*fold*, in part by the opening of arteriovenous anastomoses in the extremities, nose, ears and mouth. These shunts are under direct sympathetic vasoconstrictor influence and are normally closed. When they open following withdrawal of sympathetic input, as in hyperthermia, superficial venous flow is increased and body cooling is enhanced. Interestingly, the partial sympathoplegia related to some potent inhalation anesthetics may be one of the causes for dilated superficial veins when these agents are used (Eger et al., 1970). The same depression of resting sympathetic vasoconstriction in the skin by anesthesia may lead to accelerated body hypothermia as well.

Aortic and carotid chemoreceptor activity from acidemia, hypercarbia, or hypoxemia causes a decrease in sympathetic tone to cutaneous vessels with relative vasodilatation (Calvelo et al., 1970). This effect is opposite to the constrictive action of the chemoreceptors in the muscle, splanchnic, and renal circulation. Similarly, under sudden emotional stress, visceral resistance vessels constrict, but skin flow may increase by direct action (as with blushing) or indirectly as a result of sweating. On the other hand, sustained stress such as mental arithmetic causes increased cutaneous sympathetic activity and a decrease in skin blood flow (Delius et al., 1972).

The regional control of blood flow to the skin includes the cholinergic pathway to apocrine glands that triggers the release of bradykinin, a local vasodilator substance, to cause reactive hyperemia after skin compression. The only parasympathetic innervation to affect skin blood vessels reaches the sweat glands via the sudomotor nerve. When sweating is induced, an increased output of the enzyme kallikrein occurs. This enzyme, in turn, splits the polypeptide bradykinin from globulin in the perivascular interstitial fluids (Guyton, 1986). Bradykinin is a potent vasodilator and probably is the cause for increases in cutaneous blood flow whenever sweating takes place (Heistad and Abboud, 1974) and may also contribute to the reactive hyperemia in skin following prolonged occlusion of its blood-supply.

Muscle Circulation

Resting blood flow in human muscle ranges between 2–5 ml/(100 g·min). Yet the same muscle has the potential for a twenty to thirty-*fold* increase during exercise. Obviously, such wide variations in flow must have precise mechanisms for control in order to maintain cardiovascular homeostasis. Since skeletal muscle constitutes about 40% of body mass, blood flow changes to striated muscle can effect marked shifts in cardiac output and systemic vascular resistance. The determinants of skeletal muscle blood flow include a combination of neurogenic, autoregulatory, and local metabolic factors.

Sympathetic nerve stimulation causes vasoconstriction in the resistance vessels of skeletal muscle by excitation of α-adrenergic receptors (Fig. 14.16). The

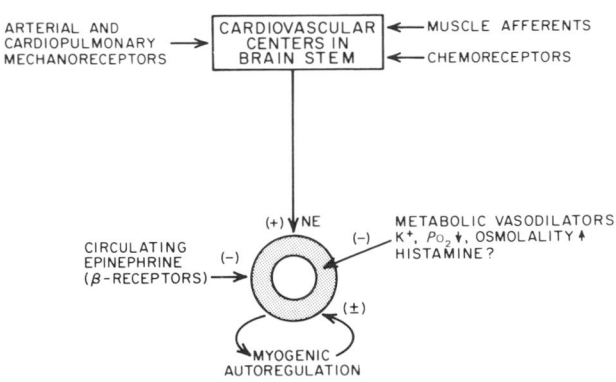

MUSCLE RESISTANCE ARTERIOLES

Fig. 14.16 A schema illustrating control of vascular resistance in muscle. Various mechanisms causing increased (+) or decreased (−) resistance are explained in the text. The effects of muscle compressive force on venous and arterial resistance are not included.

outflow tract originates in the vasomotor *pressor* center of the brain stem and is under constant degrees of attenuation from the *depressor* areas. While cessation of sympathetic input to skeletal muscle vascular resistance vessels will only double blood flow to the area, this control mechanism still permits important changes in total body vascular resistance because of the great bulk of skeletal muscle. The vascular smooth muscle cells in the resistance vessels respond to β-adrenergic stimulation with relaxation (Mellander and Johansson, 1968). Circulating adrenaline from adrenal stimulation acts upon the numerous receptors causing dilatation of the vessels. The potential for β-adrenergic control of muscle blood flow exceeds that of α-adrenergic because of the relatively greater number of β-adrenergic receptors in muscle resistance arterioles (Furchgott, 1970). Whether there are any significant cholinergic mechanisms for modifying vascular tone in the resistance vessels of striated muscle in man is unknown.

Reflex regulation of muscle blood flow is mediated through the high and low pressure mechanoreceptors, the chemoreceptors, and from somatic afferent stimuli in the muscle itself.

The carotid sinus and aortic mechanoreceptor activity is inverse to the α-adrenergic tone in muscle resistance vessels. With increased systemic pressure, additional baroreceptor nerve activity is generated. These signals augment the *depressor* modulation of sympathetic afferents to the resistance vessels. The result is a relative vasodilatation in the muscle bed (Bevegard and Shepherd, 1966).

The cardiopulmonary mechanoreceptors have a similar effect on muscle blood flow, that is, increased stretch in the receptors from dilatation of the heart chambers results in diminished α-adrenergic activity and relaxation in the resistance vessels.

The carotid and aortic chemoreceptors have some control over muscle blood flow in that animal studies have shown that hypoxemia and acidemia cause reflex vasoconstriction in the muscle beds (Pelletier, 1972). The exact contribution of the chemoreceptors is difficult to ascertain because the peripheral (local) response to the same stimulus is vasodilatation. In man there has been no isolated study of the effects of chemoreceptors on muscle vessels. It must be presumed that central acidosis or hypoxia contributes to increased α-adrenergic activity in these arterioles.

The striated muscles contain mechanoreceptors, thermoreceptors, and chemoreceptors that may trigger the afferent limb of a central pressor response (Mitchell, 1983). Varying stimuli from passive muscle stretch to severe exercise produce a graded effect response to the central vasomotor centers. The efferent limb of this reflex causes selective vasoconstriction. In active muscles local vasodilators overcome the α-adrenergic effect so that muscles that need blood flow receive it, and quiescent areas are relatively under perfused.

Indeed, the primary role of neurogenic control of muscle blood flow appears to be that of a buffer used in non-working muscle to offset the immense drain exercise hyperemia puts on the cardiac output. Combined with the splanchnic and renal circulation, the muscle resistance vessels, at rest, control the majority of total systemic vascular resistance. Much of this is under direct neurogenic influence. It has been suggested that the decrease seen in muscle blood flow during anesthesia by halogenated hydrocarbons is due to the release of vasopressin—a constricting substance—stimulated by the baroreflex response to relative hypotension (Hoffman, 1986).

Autoregulation in muscle resistance vessels may be attributed to myogenic or metabolic factors (Johnson, 1986: Borgstrom, 1987). The myogenic basis for control of constant flow under varying perfusion pressures is well-known and historically documented (Bayliss, 1902). It probably has a significant role in regulating blood flow in the resting muscle arterioles and during moderate changes in pressure gradients. Metabolic factors in the chemical milieu surrounding the arterioles tend to act in concert with the myogenic action in maintaining resting homeostasis. For example, a sudden decrease in perfusion pressure will cause a relative hypoxia in the perivascular fluid and the metabolic basis of vasodilatation now acts synergistically with myogenic autoregulation to maintain flow in spite of reduced pressure.

The substances involved in the metabolic basis of vascular control in the muscle are numerous. However, oxygen, potassium ions, and osmolality appear to have powerful effects on vascular tone in muscle (Sparks and Belloni, 1978).

The metabolic factors activated with muscle contraction have the potential to increase local blood flow nearly twenty-*fold*. The acute increase in venous blood osmolality at the initiation of muscle activity may have a primary role in the early vasodilatation while K^+ accumulation augments sustained resistance vessel relaxation (Scott et al., 1970). Certainly local hypoxemia is related closely to vascular dilatation in muscle vessels (Skinner and Powell, 1967). But whether it causes the effect by direct action or is only an indirect correlate still needs positive identification.

The total control of skeletal muscle vascular resistance involves a complex interaction among the neurogenic, autoregulatory and metabolic factors. From an anesthetic standpoint, the resting control by sympathetic innervation, vasopressin levels and autoregulatory mechanisms count significantly towards total systemic vascular resistance. The redistribution of cardiac output with hemorrhage, anesthetics, and mild hypothermia is influenced markedly by the striated muscle circulation.

CONCLUSION

Control of the systemic circulation relies on several interacting variables. The metabolic control of local blood flow depends on a stable perfusion pressure so that specific changes in resistance will provide for equally specific changes in flow. This constancy of blood pressure is maintained, to a large extent, through neurohumoral pathways superimposed on the intrinsic control mechanisms of the heart. The job of the cardiovascular system is to supply all tissue with appropriate amounts of blood. With the complex network of control mechanisms described in this chapter, the task is done remarkably well by consistently avoiding significant perturbations.

REFERENCES

Abboud F.M. (1979). Integration of reflex responses in the control of blood pressure and vascular resistance. *Am. J. Cardiol.*, **44**, 903.

Abboud F.M., Heistad D.D., Mark A.L., et al. (1976). Reflex control of the peripheral circulation. *Prog. Cardiovasc. Dis.*, **18**, 371.

Andreen M., Irestedt L. (1979). Effects of enflurane on splanchnic circulation. *Acta Anaesth. Scand. Suppl.*, **71**, 48.

Arnold G., Kosche F., Miessner E., et al. (1968). The importance of the perfusion pressure in the coronary arteries for the contractility and the oxygen consumption of the heart. *Pflügers Arch.*, **299**, 339.

Bayliss W.M. (1902). On the local reactions of the arterial wall to changes in internal pressure. *J. Physiol.* (London), **28**, 220.

Belardinelli L., Linden J., Berne R.M. (1989). The cardiac effects of adenosine. *Prog. Cardiovasc. Dis.*, **22**, 73.

Berne R.M., Blackmon J.R., Gardner T.H. (1957). Hypoxemia and coronary flow. *J. Clin. Invest.*, **36**, 1101.

Berne R.M., DeGeest H., Levy M.N. (1965). Influence of the cardiac nerves on coronary resistance. *Am. J. Physiol.*, **208**, 763.

Berne R.M., Rubio R. (1979). Coronary circulation. In *Handbook of Physiology, Sec. 2 The Cardiovascular System, and Vol. 1: The Heart*, Bethesda, Md., American Physiological Society.

Berne R.M., Levy M.N. (1986). *Cardiovascular Physiology*. 5th ed., St. Louis. CV Mosby Co.

Bevegard B.S., Shepherd J.T. (1966). Circulatory effects of stimulating the carotid arterial stretch receptors in man at rest and during exercise. *J. Clin. Invest.*, **45**, 132.

Borgstrom P., Gestrelius S. (1987). Integrated myogenic and metabolic control of vascular tone in skeletal muscle during autoregulation of blood flow. *Microvasc. Res.* **33**, 353.

Braunwald E. (1974). Regulation of the circulation. *N. Engl. J. Med.*, **290**, 1124.

Brody M.J., Alper R.H., O'Neill T.P., et al. (1986). Central neural control of the cardiovascular system. In *Handbook of Hypertension, Vol. 8: Pathophysiology of Hypertension—Regulatory Mechanisms*, (Zanchetti A., Tarazi R.C., eds.). Amsterdam: Elsevier Science Publishers.

Brown A.M. (1980). Receptors under pressure, an update on baroreceptors. *Circ. Res.*, **46**, 1.

Buffington C.W., Romson J.L., Levine A., et al. (1987). Isoflurane induces coronary steal in a canine model of chronic coronary occlusion. *Anesthesiology*, **66**, 280.

Calvelo M.G., Abboud F.M., Ballard D.R., et al. (1970). Reflex vascular responses to stimulation of chemoreceptors with nicotine and cyanide activation of adrenergic constriction in muscle and noncholinergic dilatation in dog's paw. *Circ. Res.*, **27**, 259.

Cason B.A., Verrier E.D., London M.J., et al. (1987). Effects of isoflurane and halothane on coronary vascular resistance and collateral myocardial blood flow: their capacity to induce coronary steal. *Anesthesiology*, **67**, 665.

Cohan G., Gewertz B.L. (1985). Measurement of myocardial oxygen consumption. *J. Surg. Res.*, **38**, 305.

Delaney T.J., Miller E.D. Jr. (1980). Rebound hypertension after sodium nitroprusside prevented by saralasin in rats. *Anesthesiology*, **52**, 154.

Delius W., Hongau A., Hogbarth K.E., et al. (1972). Maneuvers affecting sympathetic outflow in human skin nerves. *Acta Physiol. Scand.*, **84**, 177.

Deutsch S. (1986). Effects of anesthetics on renal circulation. In *Cardiovascular Actions of Anesthetics and Drugs Use in Anesthesia*, Basel, Karger.

Dole W.P. (1987). Autoregulation of the coronary circulation. *Prog. Cardiovasc. Dis.*, **29**, 293.

Dusting G.J., Moncada S., Vane J.R. (1979). Prostaglandins, their intermediates and precursors: cardiovascular roles in normal and abnormal circulatory systems. *Prog. Cardiovasc. Dis.*, **21**, 405.

Eger E.I., Smith N.T., Stoelting R.K. (1970). Cardiovascular effects of halothane in man. *Anesthesiology*, **32**, 396.

Engler R.L., Covell J.W. (1987). Influence of the venous system on ventricular/arterial coupling. In *Handbook of Hypertension, Vol. 8: Pathophysiology in Hypertension—Regulatory Mechanisms*, (Zanchetti A., Tarazi R.C., eds.). Amsterdam: Elsevier Science Publishers.

Furchgott R.F. (1970). Pharmacologic characteristics of adrenergic receptors. *Fed. Proc.*, **29**, 1352.

Gelman S. (1986). Effects of anesthetics on splanchnic circulation. In *Cardiovascular Actions of Anesthetics and Drugs Used in Anesthesia*, Basel, Karger.

Green J.F. (1982). *Fundamental Cardiovascular and Pulmonary Physiology*, Philadelphia: Lea and Febiger.

Greenway C.V., Lautt W.W. (1972). Effects of infusions of catecholamines, angiotensin, vasopressin and histamine on hepatic blood volume in the anesthetized cat. *Br. J. Pharmacol.*, **44**, 177.

Greenway C.V., Lautt W.W. (1986). Blood volume, the venous system, preload, and cardiac output. *Canad. J. Physiol. Pharmacol.*, **64**, 383.

Guyton A.C. (1977). An overall analysis of cardiovascular regulation. *Anesth. Analg.*, **56**, 761.

Guyton A.C. (1986). *A Textbook of Medical Physiology*. Philadelphia: W.B. Saunders Co.

Heistad D.D., Abboud F.M. (1974). Factors that influence blood flow in skeletal muscle and skin. *Anesthesiology*, **41**, 139.

Hoffman W.E. (1986). Influence of anesthetics on regional blood flow. In *Cardiovascular Actions of Anesthetics and Drugs Used in Anesthesia*, Basel, Karger.

Johnson J.M., Brengelmann G.L., Hales J.R.S., et al. (1986). Regulation of the cutaneous circulation. *Fed. Proc.*, **45**, 2841.

Johnson P.C. (1974). The microcirculation and local and humoral control of the circulation. In *Cardiovascular Physiology*, (Guyton, A.C., Jones C.E., eds.). London: Butterworths.

Johnson P.C., Henrich H.A. (1975). Metabolic myogenic factors in local regulation of the microcirculation. *Fed. Proc.*, **34**, 2020.

Johnson P.C. (1986). Autoregulation of blood flow. *Circ. Res.*, **59**, 483.

Jones J.V., Thoren P.N. (1977). Characteristics of aortic baroreceptors with non-medullated afferents arising from the aortic arch of rabbits with chronic renal vascular hypertension. *Acta Physiol. Scand.*, **101**, 286.

Klocke F.J. (1976). Coronary blood flow in man. *Prog. Cardiovasc. Dis.*, **19**, 117.

Klocke F.J., Ellis A.K., Orlick A.E. (1980). Sympathetic influences on coronary perfusion and evolving concepts of driving pressure, resistance, and transmural flow regulation. *Anesthesiology*, **52**, 1.

Levy M.N. (1979). The cardiac and vascular factors that determine systemic blood flow. *Circ. Res.*, **44**, 739.

Linden R.J. (1979). Atrial reflexes and renal function. *Am. J. Cardiol.*, **44**, 879.

Ljungqvist A., Wagermark J. (1970). The adrenergic innervation of intrarenal glomerular and extra-glomerular circulatory routes. *Nephron*, **7**, 218.

Mancia G., Ferrari A., Gregorini L., et al. (1979). Control of blood pressure by carotid sinus baroreceptors in human beings. *Am. J. Cardiol.*, **44**, 895.

McRaven D.R., Mark A.L., Abboud F.M., et al. (1971). Responses of coronary vessels to adrenergic stimuli. *J. Clin. Invest.*, **50**, 773.

Mellander S. (1988). Myogenic mechanisms of local vascular control. *Acta Physiol. Scand.*, **571**, 25.

Mellander S., Johansson B. (1968). Control of resistance, exchange, and capacitance functions in the peripheral circulation. *Pharmacol. Rev.*, **20**, 117.

Mitchell J.H., Kaufman M.P., Iwamoto G.A. (1983). The exercise pressor reflex: its cardiovascular effects, afferent mechanisms and central pathways. *Ann. Rev. Physiol.*, **45**, 229.

Moore P.G., Kien N.D., Reitan J.A., et al. (1989). Lack of coronary steal with isoflurane anesthesia. *Anesthesiology*, **71**, A1156.

Pelletier C.L. (1972). Circulatory responses to graded stimulation of the carotid chemoreceptors in the dog. *Circ. Res.*, **31**, 431.

Pelletier C.L., Clement D.L., Shepherd J.T. (1972). Comparison of afferent activity of canine aortic and sinus nerves. *Circ. Res.*, **31**, 557.

Philbin D.M. (1986). Cardiovascular effects of neurohumoral substances released during anesthesia. In *Cardiovascular Actions of Anesthetics and Drugs Used in Anesthesia*, Basel, Karger.

Price H.L., Deutsch S., Marshall B.E., et al. (1966). Hemodynamic and metabolic effects of hemorrhage in man, with particular reference to splanchnic circulation. *Circ. Res.*, **18**, 469.

Price H.L., Cooperman L.H., Warden J.C. (1967). Control of splanchnic circulation in man: role of beta-adrenergic receptors. *Circ. Res.*, **21**, 333.

Reid I.A., Morris B.J., Ganong W.F. (1978). The renin-angiotensin system. *Ann. Rev. Physiol.*, **40**, 377.

Rowell L.B., Detry J.M.R., Blackmon J.R., et al. (1972). Importance of the splanchnic vascular bed in human blood pressure regulation. *J. Appl. Physiol.*, **32**, 213.

Rubio R., Berne R.M. (1975). Regulation of coronary blood flow. *Prog. Cardiovasc. Dis.*, **18**, 105.

Rubio R., Wiedmeier V.T., Berne R.M. (1972). Nucleoside phosphorylase localization and role in the myocardial distribution of purines. *Am. J. Physiol.*, **222**, 550.

Sagawa K., Taylor A.E., Guyton A.C. (1961). Dynamic performance and stability of cerebral ischemic pressor response. *Am. J. Physiol.*, **201**, 1164.

Schlant R.C., Silverman M.E. (1986). Anatomy of the heart. In *The Heart*, (Hurst J.W. ed.), New York: McGraw-Hill Book Co.

Scott J.B., Rudko M., Radawski D. (1970). Role of osmolality, K^+, H^+, Mg^{++} and O_2 in local blood flow regulation. *Am. J. Physiol.*, **218**, 338.

Shepherd J.T., Vanhoutte P.M. (1979). *The Human Cardiovascular System, Facts and Concepts*. New York: Raven Press.

Skinner N.S. Jr., Powell W.J. Jr. (1967). Action of oxygen and potassium on vascular resistance in dog skeletal muscle. *Am. J. Physiol.*, **212**, 533.

Sparks H.V., Belloni F.L. (1978). The peripheral circulation: local regulation. *Ann. Rev. Physiol.*, **40**, 67.

Vatner S.F., Franklin D., Van Citters R.L., et al. (1970). Effects of carotid sinus nerve stimulation on the coronary circulation of the conscious dog. *Circ. Res.*, **27**, 11.

Wiedeman M.P. (1963). Dimensions of blood vessels from distributing artery to collecting vein. *Circ. Res.*, **12**, 375.

Wilkins R.W., Culbertson J.W., Ingelfinger F.J. (1951). The effect of splanchnic sympathectomy in hypertensive patients upon estimated hepatic blood flow in the upright as contrasted with the horizontal position. *J. Clin. Invest.*, **30**, 312.

Young M.A., Knight D.R., Vatner S.F. (1987). Autonomic control of large coronary arteries and resistance vessels. *Prog. Cardiovasc. Dis.*, **30**, 211.

Zucker I.H. (1986). Left ventricular receptors: physiological controllers or pathological curiosities? *Basic Res. Cardiol.*, **81**, 539.

15. Coronary Circulation

G. Koski and E. Lowenstein

Since William Harvey's demonstration that the heart receives its nutrient blood supply from the coronary arteries, generations of cardiovascular physiologists have endeavoured to understand the many factors involved in regulation of this highly specialized circulation. All higher forms of life depend, on a moment-to-moment basis, upon the functional integrity of the coronary circulation. If the supply of nutrients and oxygen to the heart is inadequate to meet its metabolic demand, the resulting decline in myocardial function may lead to cardiovascular collapse. Recognition of this fact and the widespread occurrence of coronary vascular disease in man, emphasize the importance of an understanding of coronary physiology and myocardial metabolism.

To appreciate fully the complexity of the coronary circulation, one must understand not only the unique anatomical and physical determinants of flow in the coronary vascular bed, but also the metabolic, humoral and nervous mechanisms involved in the regulation of coronary vascular tone. Our intent is to provide an overview of the coronary circulation, emphasizing those points that may provide clinically useful insights into coronary physiology for physicians involved in acute cardiovascular management of patients with or without coronary artery disease. For more detailed consideration of these subjects, the reader is referred to the comprehensive works by Berne and Rubio (1979) and Olsson and Bugni (1986). These articles critically evaluate methods which have been used to obtain the data on which current understanding of the coronary circulation is based. They are therefore most valuable to those wishing to explore this complex field in great depth. It is important to recognize that much of this information has been obtained from laboratory studies of experimental animals and *in vitro* preparations. While species differences and pathophysiological processes undoubtedly limit the general applicability of these experimental studies to the clinical setting, these data provide the scientific foundation for understanding the physiology of the coronary circulation.

MYOCARDIAL METABOLISM AND CORONARY BLOOD FLOW

Determinants of Myocardial Oxygen Demand

During rhythmic cardiac contraction and relaxation, the metabolic machinery of the heart must be supplied with energy for supporting both contractile function and maintenance of cellular integrity, as outlined in Table 15.1. Generation of this energy requires almost exclusively oxidative metabolism of substrates to generate high energy phosphate compounds which are fuel for the ion-pumps and metabolic processes underlying myocardial function. Modern techniques have shown that the pool of high energy phosphates in myocardial muscle is subject to significant depletion and regeneration during a single cardiac cycle. Compared with skeletal muscle, the heart has limited capacity for anaerobic metabolism or accumulation of an *oxygen debt*. Consequently, energy supply must match demand on a beat-to-beat basis if normal function is to be maintained. Together, the various components of myocardial metabolism consume 6–10 ml O_2 per 100 g of myocardial tissue per minute in the normal human at rest. This increases dramatically during strenuous exercise and during heart failure, as detailed in Table 15.2.

Myocardial Oxygen Delivery

Because the heart extracts a great fraction of the available oxygen from coronary blood even at rest, in-

TABLE 15.1

DETERMINANTS OF MYOCARDIAL METABOLIC REQUIREMENTS IN THE NORMAL BEATING HEART AT
REST

Parameter	Contributing Factors	*Contribution to Total M_{VO_2}
Basal metabolism	Cellular integrity, protein synthesis, ion gradients, substrate metabolism	25–35%
Wall tension	Cavitary pressure, wall thickness	30%
External work	Stroke volume, arterial pressure	10–15%
Activation of contraction	Transport of activator calcium	10–15%
Electrical excitation	Propagation of action potentials	1%
Fiber shortening	Physical shortening of myocardial sarcomeres	?

Note

*The total contribution of each parameter over time will vary as a function of heart rate. Adapted from
Gibbs and Chapman (1979).

TABLE 15.2

MYOCARDIAL OXYGEN CONSUMPTION AND CARDIOVASCULAR PARAMETERS MEASURED IN A NORMAL
SUBJECT, AN ATHLETE, AND IN HEART FAILURE

	Normal Subject		Athlete		Heart Failure
	At Rest	Heavy Exercise	At Rest	Heavy Exercise	At Rest
Cardiac output, L/min	4.9	22.0	5.0	36.0	4.5
Heart rate, beat/min	70	200	50	200	90
Stroke volume, ml	70	110	100	180	50
End-diastolic volume, ml	130	130	220	200	300
LV heart weight, g	200	200	330	330	410
Mean blood pressure, mmHg	100	110	100	120	90
Peak systolic blood pressure, mmHg	120	180	120	180	110
LV stroke work, kg m/(100 g·min)	2.2	10.9	2.2	17.4	1.8
LV developed tension, g/cm²	190	290	190	290	120
LV oxygen consumption, ml/(100 g·min)	9	28.7	7.3	28.7	10.7
Total LV oxygen consumption, ml/min	18.0	57.4	24.0	94.7	43.9
LV total mechanical efficiency	11.9	18.4	14.6	29.4	8.2
LV active mechanical efficiency	17.8	20.6	24.8	32.9	11.4

Note

Data used in constructing this table came from a wide variety of sources, with particularly heavy reliance
on Astrand and Rodahl (1970) and Levine and Wagman (1962). Calculations were made on the basis that
the LV (left ventricle) approximates to a sphere. With a known end-diastolic volume the inner radius, a,
was calculated. Midwall stress was taken to be 190 g/cm², and this information together with the peak
intraventricular pressure, P, allowed the outer radius, b, to be calculated and also determined ventricular
weight. The same procedure was used for all the different physiological conditions. Hypertrophy was
assumed to keep peak wall stress approximately constant. (Adapted from Gibbs and Chapman (1979) and
reproduced with permission from the American Physiological Society).

creased extraction cannot contribute importantly to
increased oxygen supply. The only ways to meet increased demand are to increase the efficiency of oxygen utilization by the tissue or to increase oxygen
delivery to the tissue. Although the heart has some

capacity to improve its mechanical efficiency during
exercise, by far the most important contribution
towards satisfying increased oxygen demand comes
from increasing coronary arterial supply. To a greater
extent than other vascular beds, the coronary circula-

tion at rest is constricted (Hoffman, 1984), providing it with a remarkable capacity to increase flow by decreasing coronary vascular tone. Accordingly, coronary blood flow is precisely regulated, largely through vasodilatation by mechanisms that have not been fully characterized, to maintain the balance between myocardial oxygen supply and demand.

Myocardial Oxygen Balance

Under normal physiological conditions, *coronary blood flow is directly and very tightly correlated with myocardial oxygen consumption* (Fig. 15.1). The mechanistic implications of this dramatic correlation are subject to various interpretations, according to whether or not the coupling is dependent upon oxygen *per se*, as discussed by Olsson et al. (1986). From a practical point of view, this coupling means that increased myocardial energy metabolism will, if physically possible, be accompanied by increased coronary blood flow. It also implies that *luxury perfusion* in excess of demand is not a normal physiological occurrence. Any condition that impairs the ability of coronary blood flow to increase adequately in response to

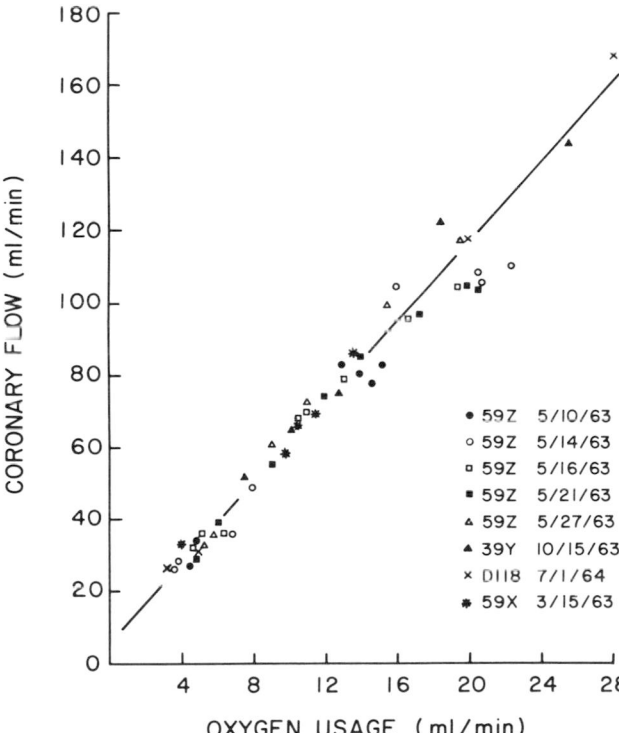

Fig. 15.1 Relationship between coronary blood flow and myocardial oxygen consumption in conscious dogs. Each dog is represented by a separate symbol. A tight correlation between the two variables is evident over a 7-fold physiological range. (Reproduced by permission of the American Heart Association, Inc. Khouri et al., (1965). Effect of exercise on cardiac output, left coronary flow and myocardial metabolism in the unanesthetized dog. *Circ. Res.*, **17**, 427.)

increased demand, or interferes with the normal distribution of blood flow to an area of increased demand, may result in the rapid onset of myocardial oxygen imbalance and dysfunction. Our goal in the remainder of this chapter is to analyze the anatomical, physical and biochemical factors involved in the regulation of coronary blood flow and the precise matching of myocardial oxygen supply and demand.

ANATOMICAL FEATURES OF THE CORONARY CIRCULATION

Gross Anatomy

The general features of the gross anatomy of the coronary vasculature are easily appreciated in Figs. 15.2 and 15.3. Two major arteries, the right and left coronary arteries, arise from the coronary ostia in the sinuses of Valsalva near the aortic valve. The ostia are generally located above the free margins of the valve leaflets. The valve leaflets do not directly impede coronary blood flow, even during systole. The main coronary arteries run along their respective atrioventricular grooves, where they bifurcate repeatedly to form an extensive network coursing over the epicardial surface around the cardiac chambers.

In general, the branches arising from the left coronary artery supply the major portion of the left ventricle, the anterior portion of the right ventricle and the interventricular septum, while the right coronary distribution includes the remainder of the right ventricle and the posterior portion of the left ventricle through its posterior interventricular branch. Extensive anastomoses are commonly present between the branches of the right and left coronary systems. The term *dominant* is conferred upon that coronary artery which gives rise to the posterior interventricular artery supplying the posterior surface of the left ventricle and the atrioventricular conduction system. The right coronary artery is dominant in about 90% of normal human hearts.

These large epicardial coronary arteries, which are commonly affected by atherosclerotic processes in ischemic heart disease, are also those most readily accessible to study, both in laboratory and clinical settings. Consequently, much of our current understanding of the coronary circulation has been based on studies of these superficial vessels. Unfortunately, any description of coronary physiology based primarily on studies of epicardial vessels is grossly inadequate, because most of the coronary vascular bed lies within the muscular myocardial wall.

The intramyocardial vessels receive flow from the epicardial arteries through branches arising at near right angles and plunging deep into the muscle (Fig. 15.4). Further divisions occur within the muscle to generate an elaborate network of small arteries and arterioles, from which the myocardial capillary beds are supplied. Of special interest are the two types of branches arising from the epicardial vessels. One class

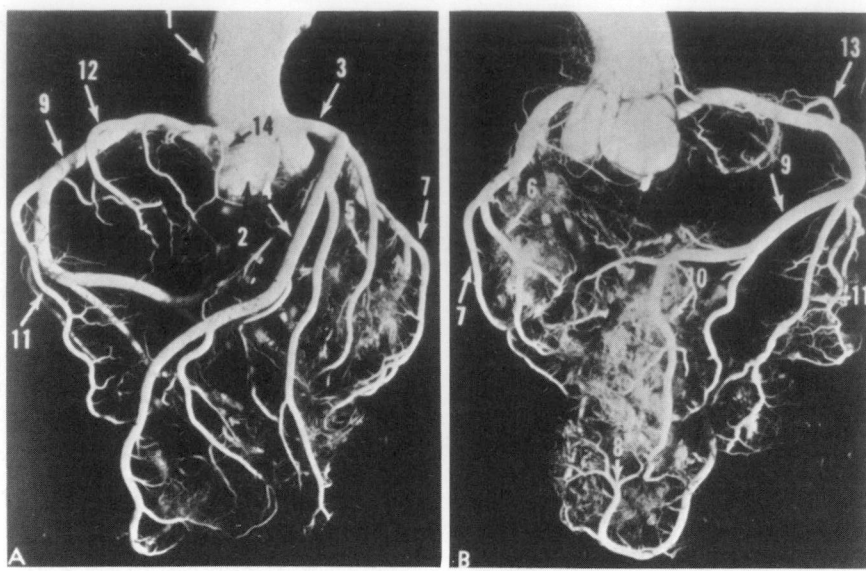

Fig. 15.2 Plastic cast of coronary arteries of human heart in which myocardial walls have been digested in concentrated hydrochloric acid solution. A: view from anterior surface of heart. B: view from posterior surface of heart. 1, Aorta; 2, aortic valves; 3, main coronary artery; 4, left anterior descending branch; 5, left diagonal branch; 6, left circumflex branch; 7, left marginal branch; 8, posterior ascending branch; 9, right coronary artery; 10, posterior descending branch; 11, right marginal branch; 12, right arterior branch; 13, main atrial branch; 14, third coronary artery. Observe the junction of two main coronary arteries (3 and 9) with aorta lies above cusp of aortic valves. Notice that anterior descending branch (4) curves about apex to ascend and give rise to a posterior ascending branch (8). In this particular heart, right coronary artery (9) gives rise to posterior descending branch (10); i.e. right coronary artery is dominant. (Reproduced with permission from Baroldi and Scomazzoni, 1967.)

of vessels arborize in the subepicardial region whereas the second class of vessels penetrates into the sub-endocardial region before forming a dense plexus of vessels (Fig. 15.5). Differential regulation of the tone in these two types of major branches from the epicardial vessels provides a mechanism for altering the distribution of flow to the subepicardial and subendocardial regions of the myocardium (Feigl, 1987).

Microvascular Coronary Anatomy

At the microscopic level, the coronary vasculature is truly extraordinary. Each arteriole gives rise to a dense network of capillaries which run in long parallel bundles, with few interconnections, entirely encompassing each muscle fiber (Fig. 15.6). The capillaries themselves are very long, ranging from 300–1200 μm in length, and the intercapillary distances are quite small 16–19 μm (Fig. 15.7). Venules, which are three to four times more numerous than arterioles, exit the capillary bed and coalesce to form veins that leave the myocardium along the course of the arteries. While some veins, notably the Thebesian veins, empty directly into the ventricular cavities or the right atrium, most join to form a confluence at the coronary sinus

emptying into the right atrium. All vessels providing the coronary arterial supply and the myocardial capillaries contain smooth muscle cells or non-endothelial cells with contractile elements which are subject to contraction thereby reducing the caliber of the vessels. It is likely that such constriction accounts for much of the high basal tone of the coronary bed and plays an important role in regulation of coronary blood flow distribution.

Collateral Coronary Circulation

Although early anatomical studies suggested that coronary arteries are end arteries, more recent evidence clearly demonstrates the existence of extensive inter and intracoronary anastomoses at all levels of the coronary circulation except the capillaries, even in the normal myocardium (Schaper, 1971). In normal human hearts, these vessels are quite small but they enlarge considerably and take on important functional roles in the presence of significant atherosclerotic stenoses ($>80\%$) (Fig. 15.8). In other species, notably the dog, collaterals are more prominent under normal conditions, contributing to interspecies discrepancies in some experimental studies.

The stimulus for development of collateral vessels

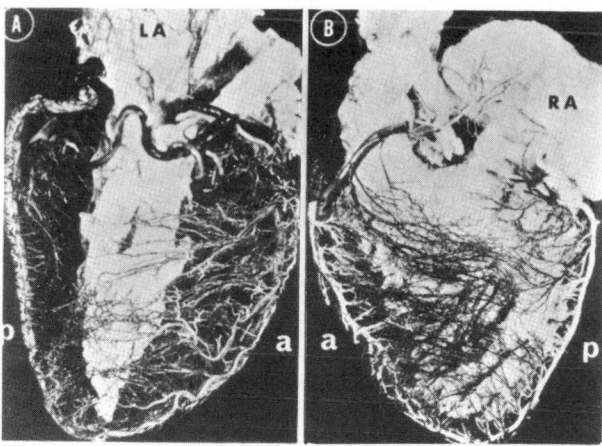

Fig. 15.3 Preponderance of left anterior descending coronary artery in human interventricular septum. Vessels cast in dark plastic are the arteries. A: heart is viewed from right side, with left ventricular chambers cased in white. LA, left atrium. B: heart is viewed from left side, with case of right ventricle in background. RA, right atrium. Cast of left anterior descending coronary artery is to the right in A and to the left in B. a, Anterior; p, posterior. Note large number of arterial branches that supply the septal wall. Artery opposite to left anterior descending artery that also supplies the septum corresponds to posterior descending coronary artery. (Reproduced with permission from James, 1971.)

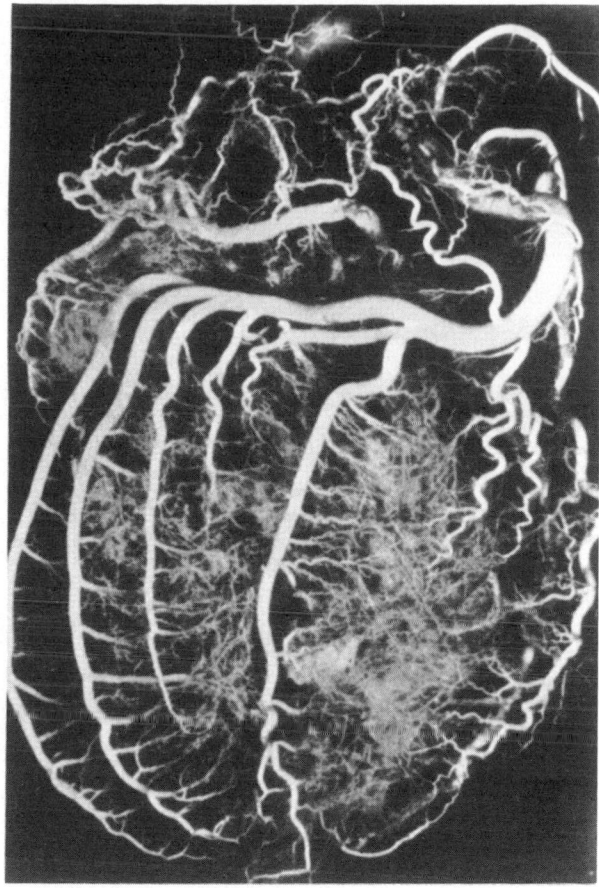

Fig. 15.4 Perpendicular penetration of intramural coronary arteries into left ventricular wall. Posterior view of human heart. Main arterial branch is circumflex artery. (Reproduced with permission from Baroldi and Scomazzoni, 1967.)

appears to be chronic tissue hypoxia (Schaper, 1971), but significant collateral flow to an ischemic region of myocardium can be demonstrated within an hour of an acute coronary arterial occlusion (Marcus et al. 1976). Once functional, collateral vessels are subject to the same physical determinants of flow as other coronary vessels, but they are apparently insensitive to vasoactive drugs and neurohumoral agents (Wiggers and Green, 1936). Thus, they function primarily as passive conduits, their flow being determined by extrinsic factors regulating circulation to the vascular beds served by the vessels from which the collaterals arise.

Functional Implications of the Coronary Anatomy

Unlike other organs, the heart is unique in that it generates the pressure for its own perfusion. Like other muscle vascular beds, vessels within the muscle are necessarily subject to varying tissue pressures and geometric configurations during muscle contraction. However, no other muscle vascular bed has to meet the large, sustained metabolic demand for flow placed on the coronary circulation by the heart.

This unique anatomic and physiologic arrangement has important functional implications. First, and perhaps most importantly, *the coronary vessels are exposed to continuously varying intramyocardial pressure during the cardiac cycle* (Sabiston and Gregg, 1957). This tissue pressure, which constitutes a major impediment to coronary blood flow (Downey and Kirk, 1974), differs regionally between the right and left cardiac chambers, atrial and ventricular muscle, and from the epicardial to the endocardial surface of the heart.

Secondly, the coronary vessels are not only contractile, but also elastic and compressible. Consequently, contraction of the spiral bands of muscle comprising the ventricular chambers of the heart subjects the perpendicularly penetrating intramyocardial branches of the coronary arteries to lateral shearing forces which may completely obstruct flow in certain regions during systole (Downey and Kirk, 1975). At the same time, the smaller intramyocardial vessels, including the capillaries running parallel to the muscle fibers, are compressed, thereby pumping blood further downstream into the venous system. In fact, coronary venous flow occurs almost exclusively during systole. Clearly, flow to various regions of the heart varies during the cardiac cycle, but these variations are only in part due to changes in systemic hemodynamic determinants.

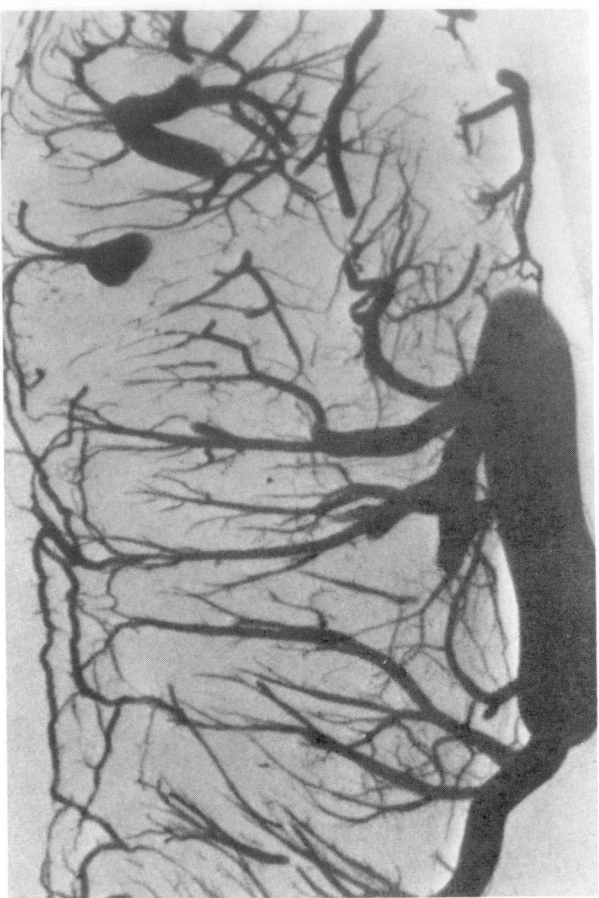

Fig. 15.5 Subendocardial plexus of anastomotic arterial vessels in human myocardium. This specimen was obtained by sectioning perpendicularly to ventricular wall. Right, epicardial surface of heart. Note almost perpendicular penetration of intramural branches, some of which give rise to branches that terminate in subendocardial network (Reproduced with permission from W.F.M. Fulton, (1965). *The Coronary Arteries: Arteriography Microanatomy and Pathogenesis of Obliterature Coronary Artery Disease.* Courtesy of Charles C. Thomas, Publisher, Springfield, Illinois.)

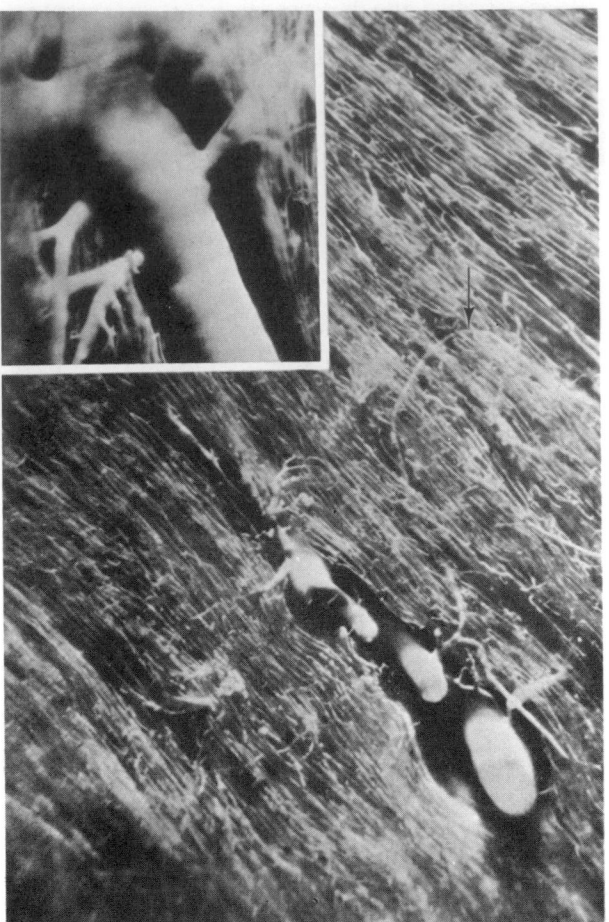

Fig. 15.6 Subepicardial vasculature. Section parallel to epicardium, 1 mm deep. Scale divisions 10 and 100 µm. A 60 µm arteriole, accompanied by two venules, gives rise to three 10 µm arterioles, two short and one long (at arrow). The insert (same scale) shows a 160 µm vein giving rise to small venules and branching rapidly into the parallel capillaries. (Reproduced with permission from Bassingthwaighte et al., 1974.)

The density of capillaries in the myocardium reflects the high metabolic demand of the heart. The absolute requirement for a continuous supply of energy and oxygen to each muscle fiber and the great length of the capillaries supplying them pose an interesting physiological problem. The arterioles from which these capillaries arise must be able to determine the quantity of blood flow needed downstream to ensure that an adequate supply of nutrients is delivered to the most distal muscle fibers supplied by that bed. Each arteriole must be able to sense changes in metabolic demands of the muscle bed in order to increase supply appropriately. This *feedback* could easily be provided through a counter-current mechanism similar to that found in the kidney, where afferent and efferent vessels lie in close apposition. However,

this anatomical arrangement is not present in the heart, and would perhaps be detrimental because it would permit diffusional shunting of oxygen and nutrients. Such shunting is present but limited in the coronary circulation (Feigl and Roth, 1981). Other factors must therefore be involved.

Recently, Segal and Duling (1987) have shown that intercellular communication, possibly electrical coupling through gap junctions, may play an important role in regulation of vascular resistance. They found that ionophoretic application of acetylcholine to intact arteriolar segments induced vasodilatation that rapidly propagated *bidirectionally*. Even in the absence of flow secondary to occlusion of the vessel proximal to the site of acetycholine application, vasodilatation was observed in the upstream segment. Such electrotonic coupling may be present in the

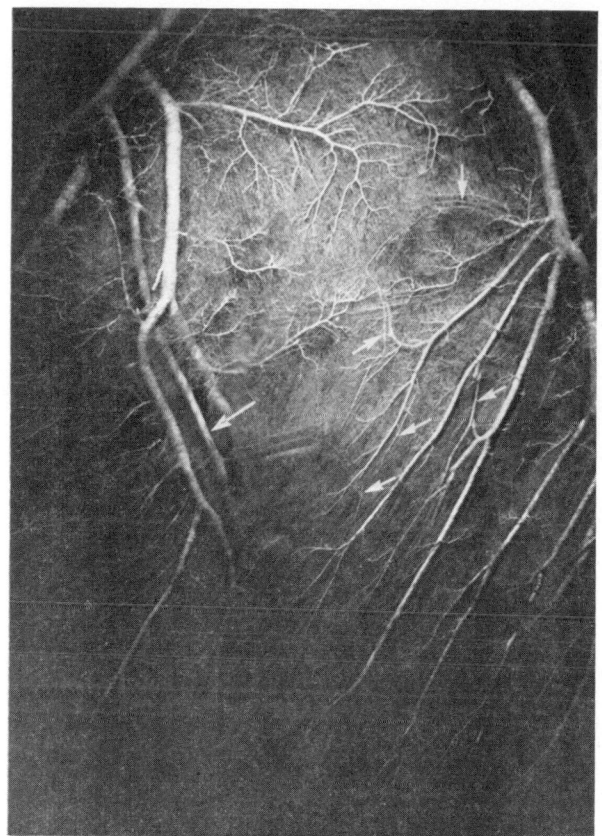

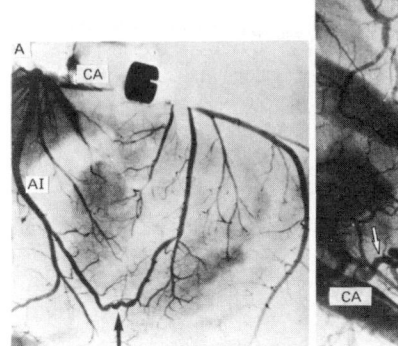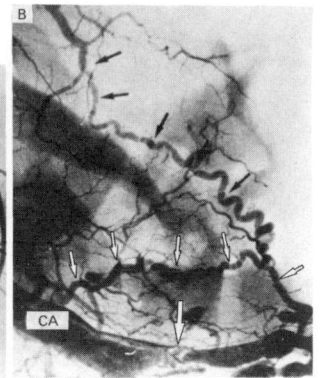

Fig. 15.8 Collateral coronary blood vessels in dog and human. A: arteriogram of anterior view of a dog heart 8 week after placement of an Ameroid constrictor on the left circumflex coronary artery, AICA. CA. Arrow points to a large collateral vessel connecting the AI with the CA. B: collateral vessels, small white arrows, originating from right coronary artery in a human heart with a calcified occlusion of left circumflex coronary artery, CA, marked by large white arrow. Black arrows point at tortuous collateral vessels originating from sinus node artery. Note that both sets of collaterals join and form a single large collateral, arrowhead, which empties into CA distal to point of occlusion. (Reproduced with permission from Schaper, 1971.)

Fig. 15.7 Vasculature of the left ventricular epicardium filled with Microfil. Scale divisions are 1 mm. The top is toward the base of the heart. The capillaries form dense parallel networks in the middle upper region running 30 to the right of the ventricular axis and in the lower half running 30 to the left. Most of the larger vessels are veins. The arrow tips mark arterioles. (Reproduced with permission from Bassingthwaighte et al., 1974.)

coronary bed and could be a mechanism for dilatation of arterioles upstream from a vascular bed requiring additional blood flow. This may be a fruitful area for future investigation of coronary vascular regulation.

Because of technical difficulties associated with accurately measuring intramyocardial pressures and flows, it has been very difficult to fully characterize the relationships between them. To further complicate matters, the pressures generated by and within the muscular walls of the cardiac chambers are strongly influenced by extracardiac factors, including the independently varying resistances and capacitance of the systemic and pulmonary vascular beds. The interdependence of myocardial function and coronary perfusion requires an elaborate control system for integrated regulation of myocardial performance, coronary blood flow and systemic hemodynamics. Interference with the normal function of this control system by pathologic processes or pharmacologic agents may be expected to destabilize the system. This

situation is frequently encountered clinically, particularly during anesthesia.

In view of these complexities, it is difficult to develop simple hydraulic or electrical models to characterize the dynamics of flow in the coronary circulation. The mechanisms underlying these regulatory process are unknown, but are the subject of intense investigation and will be addressed later in this chapter.

PHYSICS OF FLOW IN THE CORONARY CIRCULATION

Physical Determinants of Coronary Blood Flow

Two factors governing coronary blood flow are purely physical: the coronary driving pressure and the intramural myocardial pressure. In addition, coronary vascular myocytes contract in response to stretching, a physical stimulus dependent upon pressure. This response is the basis for myogenic autoregulation of coronary artery blood flow (Fig. 15.9). As mentioned earlier, these physical factors vary continuously throughout the cardiac cycle, accounting for the specific characteristics of the phasic coronary flow waveforms in various regions of the heart.

Coronary driving pressure is identical with instantaneous aortic blood pressure except in the presence of coronary stenosis. It is opposed by the myocardial tissue pressure, which occurs as a result of cardiac

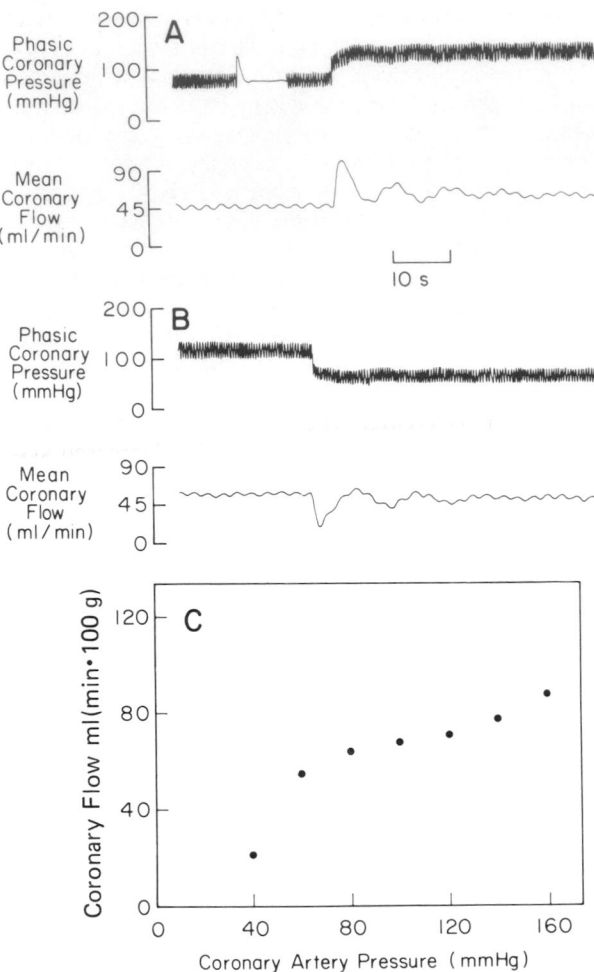

Fig. 15.9 Demonstration of dynamic and static coronary autoregulatory flow responses to a step increase (A) and a step decrease (B) in coronary perfusion pressure of 50 mmHg. Note that the dynamic flow responses consist of a series of damped oscillations that ultimately reach a new steady-state level only slightly different from that prior to the change in perfusion pressure. C: Steady-state coronary flow rate is relatively independent of perfusion pressure over the autoregulatory range, which in this example extends between roughly 60 and 120 mmHg. Redrawn from original records kindly furnished by Dr. William P. Dole, University of Iowa. (Reproduced with permission from Olsson R., Bugni W. (1986). Coronary circulation. In *The Heart and Cardiovascular System*. Chapter 48, pp 987–1037. New York, Raven Press.)

contraction. Direct compression and transmitted cavitary pressure together compose myocardial tissue pressure, which constitutes the major impediment to coronary flow (Downey and Kirk, 1974). As both the driving pressure and the opposing downstream pressures are continuously varying, and because of the presence of a significant intracoronary capacitance, simple calculation of *coronary vascular resistance* from pressure-flow relationships, though often performed and reported, is inappropriate and its limitations must be recognized.

When myocardial tissue pressure surrounding the coronary vessel exceeds coronary venous pressure, it will represent outflow pressure for blood flow. This is consistent with a *vascular waterfall*, first described in the lung, when the alveolar pressure exceeded the left atrial pressure (Fig. 15.10). Evidence that tissue pres-

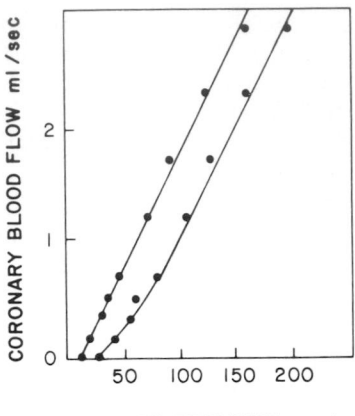

Fig. 15.10 Coronary pressure-flow curves from an open-chest anesthetized dog, illustrating the kind of evidence used to support the vascular waterfall hypothesis. The curve at left is from an arrested heart; that on the right from a beating heart. In both, pharmacological vasodilatation abolished autoregulatory tone. Note that in the absence of systolic extravascular compression, flow is linearly pressure-dependent and ceases at a pressure distinctly higher than zero. In the beating heart, flow is linearly dependent on perfusion pressure if this pressure is higher than ventricular systolic pressure, but alinear if pressure is lower than systolic ventricular pressure. The nonlinear portion of the curve is interpreted as evidence that flow ceases in vessels whose distending pressure is less than local intramyocardial tissue pressure. (Reproduced by permission of the American Heart Association, Inc. Downey J.M., Kirk E.S. (1975). Inhibition of coronary blood flow by a vascular waterfall mechanism. *Circ. Res.*, **36**, 75.)

sure is the limiting value was obtained in hearts in which the coronary circulation was maximally dilated by adenosine (Downey and Kirk, 1975). In that case, the pressure flow curve was shifted towards a higher pressure in beating, as opposed to asystolic hearts. When perfusion pressure exceeded left ventricular cavity pressure, the pressure-flow curve was parallel to that of the non-beating heart. Below this pressure, the pressure-flow lines converged. The inflection point was equal to the highest systolic pressure, whereas the intercept on the pressure axis was the lowest diastolic pressure.

Recognition that these pressures both exceed coronary sinus or right atrial pressures has prompted most investigators to use ventricular diastolic pressure (rather than right atrial pressure) as the outflow pressure when calculating coronary perfusion pressure to the left ventricle, however inappropriate such a calculation may be. Though it does not incorporate a direct measure of myocardial tissue pressure, it is probably closer to the correct outflow pressure in most circumstances.

Pressure-Flow Relationships in the Coronary Circulation

Left ventricular epicardial coronary artery flow is predominantly diastolic. Coronary flow rate increases rapidly early in diastole, and decreases linearly as diastolic pressure falls and left ventricular intracavitary pressure rises (Fig. 15.11). Atrial contraction is associated with a momentary decrease in coronary flow (the *atrial cove*), whether or not sinus rhythm is present. This is thought to be due to compression of intramural ventricular blood vessels due to the increase of ventricular cavity pressure. Epicardial coronary flow decreases at onset of ventricular systole, and may actually reverse. Expression of blood from intramural blood vessels by ventricular contraction is responsible for the reverse flow component. Normally, right epicardial coronary flow is similar during systole and diastole because the compressive forces generated by the right ventricle remain lower than the aortic driving pressure. However, with the appearance of right ventricular hypertension, the characteristics of right epicardial coronary flow progressively resemble that of the left coronary system, and systolic coronary flow becomes less prominent. Similarly, systolic left coronary artery flow becomes proportionally greater when left ventricular hypotension occurs (Fig. 15.12), reflecting the decreased sys-

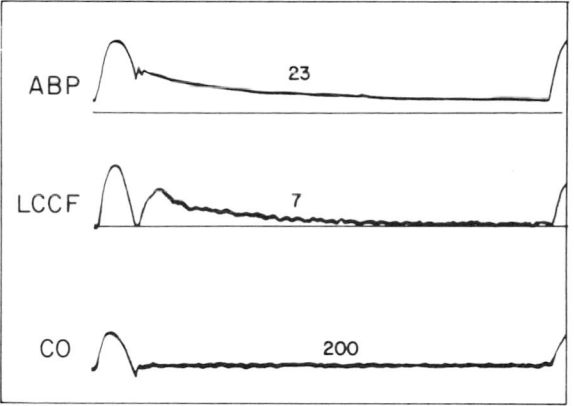

Fig. 15.12 Phasic flow pattern in the left circumflex coronary artery in a dog during profound hypotension. Symbols are the same as in Fig. 11. In the later states of cardiovascular decompensation following hemorrhage, systolic coronary flow constitutes a large fraction of stroke coronary flow. (Reproduced with permission from Granata et al., 1969.)

tolic left ventricular compressive forces and diastolic driving pressures. In summary, the epicardial coronary blood flow in the absence of coronary stenosis is largely dependent upon principles of hydraulic physics. Determinants of flow change throughout the cardiac cycle, and are in turn dependent upon the hemodynamic conditions generated by the ventricle.

Whether epicardial blood flow represents simultaneous intramyocardial blood flow is an important question which is difficult to evaluate due to technical problems associated with measurement of instantaneous intramyocardial blood flow. Flow velocity profiles of septal (intramyocardial) and small epicardial coronary arteries reveal differences between them and those registered in large epicardial arteries (Chilian and Marcus, 1982). For instance, early systolic backflow is consistently present in the former but not in the latter. Thus, it is likely that epicardial flow recordings only qualitatively reflect instantaneous

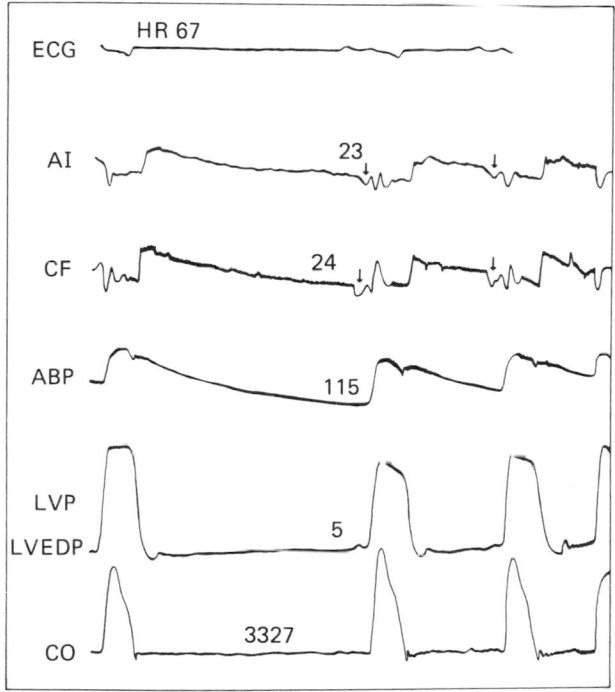

Fig. 15.11 Examples of phasic flow patterns in left epicardial coronary branches in a dog resting quietly some weeks after thoracotomy for instrumentation. From above downward, curves are electrocardiograms (ECG), flow in the anterior descending (AI) and circumflex (CF) branches of the left coronary artery, aortic root (ABP) and left ventricular cavitary (LVP) pressures, and cardiac output (CO). Numbers indicate mean heart rate (HR), blood flow rates (ml/min), and pressures (mmHg). Note the similarity of the flow patterns in the coronary branches, the atrial coves (arrows) in the coronary flow curves, and the pronounced sinus arrhythmia typical of this experimental preparation. (Reproduced by permission of the American Heart Association, Inc. P.H.B., Gregg D.E. (1968). Coronary hemodynamic effects of increasing ventricular rate in the unanesthetized dog. *Circ. Res.*, **22**, 753.)

intramyocardial capillary blood flow. The extent to which this is true has been the subject of a great deal of as yet unresolved controversy during the past decade.

Coronary Vascular Autoregulation

Autoregulation is a major principle governing coronary blood flow. In brief, blood flow remains approximately constant within the autoregulatory range, which is normally between approximately 50–150 mmHg (*see* Fig. 15.9). There is a small flow increase over this range, probably due to increased myocardial oxygen demand as wall tension increases. Above and below this range, however, epicardial blood flow is linearly related to pressure. Thus, within the autoregulatory range, resistance decreases as pressure decreases. Most of the modulation of resistance normally occurs in the small coronary blood vessels rather than the large conductance vessels. An exception is variant angina and coronary vasospasm, in which reversible contraction of smooth muscle in large coronary arteries limits coronary flow.

Until recently, it was thought that only after the vessels had reached the limits of vasodilatation would flow become linearly related to pressure. However, recent information indicates that even in the presence of severe ischemia, further dilatation may be induced by adenosine (Most et al., 1985).

Flow in the Presence of a Coronary Constriction

Fig. 15.13 illustrates the situation when there is a constriction in a coronary artery. Initially, the small vessel resistance ($R_{v\,small}$) decreases enabling flow to increase. After $R_{v\,small}$ is as low as it can become, blood flow will be determined by the physical laws governing flow through a narrowed tube rather than physiologic mechanisms regulating blood flow to the myocardium. Steady linear flow across a constriction is proportional to the square root of the pressure difference. Thus, a four-*fold* drop in inflow (aortic) pressure will produce a halving of coronary blood flow. Likewise, a doubling of inflow pressure will be associated with only a 25% increase of flow.

The consequences of these physical principles are that flow across a constriction will be decreased only to a minor degree at a constant pressure until the cross sectional area is reduced by 80–90%. Then a precipitous decline will occur with only a small further increment of narrowing. This mathematical analysis assumes a single, rigid, uniform narrowing with essentially no length to it, and laminar flow. None of these conditions is met in man with coronary disease. Atherosclerotic plaques have length, are usually sequential, virtually always eccentric, and often contain both rigid and compliant elements. Turbulent flow is thus inevitable. Feldman et al. (1979) examined the effect of stenosis length and sequential narrowings on

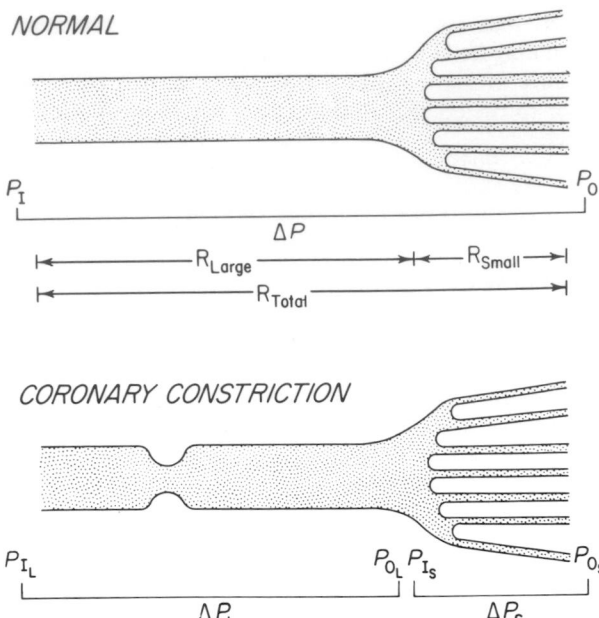

Fig. 15.13 Diagram of a normal coronary vascular unit and one supplied by a constricted coronary artery. Total resistance (R) is the sum of the resistance of the large (R_{Large}) extramyocardial and small (R_{Small}) intramyocardial blood vessels. In the normal unit, autoregulation is important in determining blood flow. The pressure (P) is the difference between the inflow pressure (P_I) and outflow pressure (P_O). In the presence of a severe coronary constriction, there may be a pressure gradient across the narrowing (P_{I_L}—P_{O_L}). Therefore, the small vessel bed is not exposed to P_{I_L}, and P_{O_L} represents the inflow pressure to the small vessel bed (P_{I_S}). When the small vessel bed is dilated completely, as when the myocardium is ischemic, the pressure-flow characteristics of the constriction limit the blood flow available to the small vessel bed. (Reproduced with permission from Lowenstein et al., 1982.)

canine coronary blood flow. They demonstrated that, for instance, a 60% stenosis 15 mm long caused the same flow limitation as a 90% stenosis 1 mm long. Sequential stenoses have similar effects. Obviously, a given degree of stenosis in a small vessel will present a greater impediment to flow than a comparable degree of stenosis in a large vessel.

Paradoxically, decreased resistance or pressure distal to the stenosis may be associated with increased stenosis resistance and decreased flow across a *severe, compliant* stenosis (Fig. 15.14). Both intracoronary isoproterenol and nitroglycerine decreased regional coronary blood flow through such a stenosis (Santamore and Walinsky, 1980). Increased outflow pressure was associated with increased canine circumflex coronary blood flow in a compliant, but not a rigid, stenosis (Schwartz, 1983). These observations are consistent with passive collapse and distension of the stenotic segment.

Most coronary stenoses in man involve both diseased and relatively normal sections of the vessel wall.

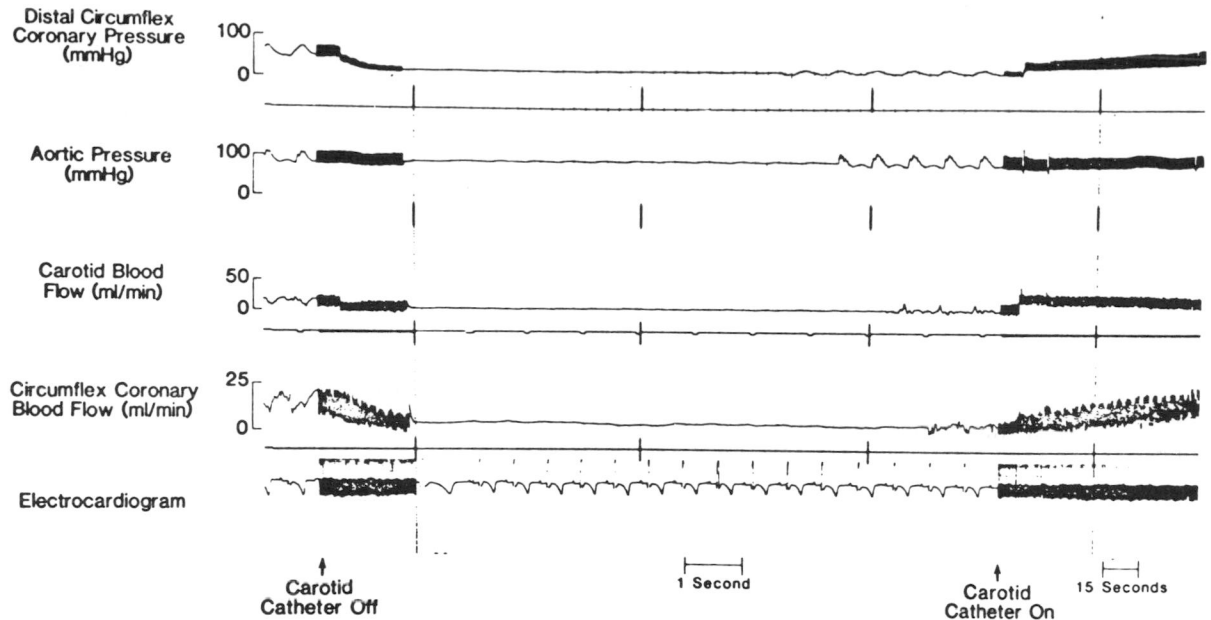

Fig. 15.14 Effect of lowering or raising pressure distal to compliant severe coronary stenosis. Lowering distal circumflex coronary pressure by closing carotid-to-coronary catheter caused marked decrease in flow pressure by reopening carotid-to-coronary catheter results in increased circumflex CBF. Carotid blood flow = flow through carotid to coronary catheter. (Reproduced with permission from Schwartz, 1983.)

In physical terms, these translate into rigid and flexible elements. The latter may have normal, or even hypersensitive, contractile properties, as well as being compliant. Thus, stenosis diameter and resistance may vary both actively and passively, causing a continuously changing set of resistances which blood must traverse to reach the capillary beds supplying regional myocardium.

METABOLIC REGULATION OF CORONARY BLOOD FLOW

Metabolic Mediators of Coronary Vasodilatation

The specific mediators involved in metabolic regulation of coronary blood flow are unknown, despite intense investigation. It has generally been assumed that such mediators would be generated by myocardial cells as a function of their metabolic activity. Criteria for such mediators have been proposed by Berne (1980). They must be vasodilators, produced and released endogenously in sufficient quantity to account for the observed vasodilatation, and must have access to the resistance vessels of the coronary circulation under physiological conditions. Furthermore, there should be a close relationship between the concentration of mediator and observed vascular tone over the entire physiologic range, and the effects of the endogenous mediator should mimic those of the same substance administered exogenously. Agents that potentiate or attenuate the vascular response to the mediator should have similar effects whether the mediator is released endogenously or administered exogenously. Finally, release of the proposed mediator and coronary blood flow should exhibit a cause and effect relationship under all physiological and pathophysiological conditions.

Several possible mediators have been studied (*see* Table 15.3), but none has been shown to meet all of the criteria outlined above. Perhaps the best case can be made for adenosine, but it seems unlikely that this is the only mediator involved in metabolic regulation of coronary flow. It is more likely that several mediators are involved, each exerting its own influence and modulating the actions of other mediators.

Notably absent from the list of widely studied candidates is nitric oxide, recently identified as endothelial-derived relaxing factor (EDRF), an important local vasodilator derived from endothelial cells in other vascular beds (Moncada et al, 1987), and the substance responsible for the vasodilating effects of sodium nitroprusside and organic nitrates. Further study of endogenous nitric oxide and other endothelial-derived relaxing factors in regulation of the coronary circulation is warranted.

Reactive Hyperemia

When flow to a region of myocardium is interrupted for a period of several seconds and then restored, flow to the ischemic region increases dramatically and then slowly returns to normal. This phenomenon, known as reactive hyperemia, has been a valuable experimental tool for studying local metabolic regulation of

TABLE 15.3

POTENTIAL MEDIATORS FOR LOCAL METABOLIC REGULATION OF CORONARY BLOOD FLOW

Mediator	Pro	Con	References
Acetate	Only glycolytic intermediate known to dilate coronary vessels	High concentrations required unlikely to be achieved *in vivo*	Molnar et al. (1962)
Adenosine	Meets nearly every established criterion for local metabolic mediator	Experimentally altered adenosine levels not always correlated with local changes in resistance; interstitial concentrations unmeasured	Berne (1980); Gewirtz et al. (1983)
CO_2/H^+	Continuously produced at rate coupled to oxidative metabolism; hyper and hypocapnia respectively constrict and dilate coronary vessels	No evidence relating endogenous $[CO_2]$ with coronary vascular resistance	Feigl (1983)
K^+	Coronary plasma $[K^+]$ correlated with initial metabolic rate and coronary resistance changes accompanying a step increase in HR	Persistant decrease in coronary resistance accompanied by falling level of $[K^+]$	Murray et al. (1979)
Nitric oxide (EDRF)	Recently identified as endothelial-derived relaxing factor; hypoxic coronary vasodilatation is endothelium dependent; coronary vessels very sensitive to enogenous generators of nitric oxide (nitroglycerine, sodium nitropusside)	Little direct evidence available from studies of coronary vessels *per se*	Busse et al. (1983) Holtz et al. (1984)
Oxygen	Hypoxia vasodilates, hyperoxia vasoconstricts coronary vessels	Unlikely that P_{O_2} in vicinity of resistance arterioles falls low enough to cause vasodilatation under physiological conditions	Gellai et al. (1973)
Prostaglandins	Extremely potent coronary vasodilators produced endogenously	No known mechanism for metabolic coupling; synthesis inhibitors have little effect on coronary vascular vasomotion	Hintz et al. (1977) Holtz et al. (1984)

coronary blood flow. Although the underlying mechanisms of reactive hyperemia are unknown, they are generally presumed to be the same as those which subserve local metabolic regulation of flow under normal conditions. This assumption, which is implicit in such studies, may not be justified, because it represents an extreme case unlikely to be encountered physiologically, except in the presence of reversible vasospasm. For a more detailed discussion of this phenomenon, the reader is referred to Olsson et al. (1986).

NEUROHUMORAL AND PHARMACOLOGIC REGULATION OF THE CORONARY CIRCULATION

Neurohumoral Influences on Coronary Blood Flow and its Distribution

In addition to myogenic and metabolic regulation, the coronary vasculature is subject to direct and indirect neural and humoral effects. The heart is richly innervated by sympathetic and parasympathetic autonomic fibers which course along the branches of the arterial tree to the arteriolar level, each arteriole receiving its own neural input (Abraham, 1969). The coronary vessels are also known to contain both α and β adrenergic receptors, as well as receptors for several other humoral mediators including vasopressin, histamine, angiotensin, prostanoids and serotonin. Assessment of the direct effects on the coronary circulation on the activation of specific classes of receptors has been difficult. Most studies have focused on their systemic hemodynamic actions. However, coronary vascular smooth muscle does not seem to differ greatly from that found in other vascular beds so the direct effects of agonists for these receptors on the coronary vessels are probably similar. The major cardiovascular effects of these agents are summarized in Table 15.4. Resultant changes in coronary blood flow will depend upon interactions among the multiple variables involved in determining myocardial oxygen consumption and delivery, and systemic hemodynamics.

The use of selective receptor-antagonists has facilitated understanding of the pharmacology of the coronary circulation. In general, one may conclude

TABLE 15.4
RECEPTOR-MEDIATED CARDIOVASCULAR RESPONSES THAT INFLUENCE CORONARY BLOOD FLOW

Receptor	Subtype	Principal Action(s) of Agonist
Adrenergic		
Alpha	1	Vasoconstriction, (+)Inotropy
	2	Vasoconstriction, Vasodilatation
Beta	1	(+)Inotropy, (+)Chronotropy
	2	(+)Chronotropy, Vasodilatation
Cholerinergic		
Nicotine	Neuronal	Vasoconstriction 2° to catecholamine release
	Neuromuscular	Increase preload and resistance 2° to muscular contraction
Muscarinic	M_1	Vasodilatation
	M_2	(−)Inotropy
Histamine	H_1	Vasoconstriction, (+)Inotropy?
	H_2	Vasodilatation, (+)Inotropy
Glucagon	No	(+)Inotropy
Angiotensin	No	Vasoconstriction
Vasopressin	Yes	Vasoconstriction
Adenosine	Yes	Vasodilatation
Prostaglandins	Yes	
PGE		Vasodilatation, (+)Inotropy?
prostacyclin		Vasodilatation
thromboxane		Vasoconstriction

Note
All agents have been shown to alter coronary blood flow but some of these effects may be secondary to changes in myocardial oxygen consumption or systemic hemodynamic variables. Antagonists may be expected to have opposite effects in the presence of agonists. Data used to compile this table were summarized from multiple sources including Berne and Rubio (1979); Olsson and Bugni (1986); Gilman et al. (1985) and Antonaccio (1985).

that α receptors mediate coronary vasoconstriction and β receptors mediate vasodilatation. In the latter case, the effect appears to be due to both a direct action on the vascular smooth muscle, as well as to increased myocardial oxygen demand and the coupled production of local vasodilators. Recent studies suggest a direct role for both $β_1$ and $β_2$ receptors in dilatation of large epicardial coronary arteries (Vatner et al., 1986) with $β_1$ receptors predominating, but the properties of small resistance vessels are less well characterized. Direct sympathetic activation may be expected to produce initial vasoconstriction, particularly in the presence of β receptor blockade (Guidicelli et al., 1980). Epinephrine (adrenaline) or norepinephrine (noradrenaline) released into the circulation during a sympathetic response may produce either vasoconstriction (α receptor-mediated) or vasodilatation (β receptor-mediated) depending upon the responsiveness of the receptors to agonists. Similarly, exogeneously administered sympathomimetic drugs will also have coronary vascular effects that may be quite variable, depending upon the existing tone of the coronary vessels and the metabolic and physical factors concurrently affecting flow (Johanssen et al., 1982).

Vasodilators and Coronary Steal

The effects of direct-acting vasodilators on the coronary circulation are much the same as their effects on the systemic resistance vessels. This becomes a very important consideration because of the role of basal coronary tone in regulating the regional distribution of coronary flow. For instance, during exercise, increased tone (i.e. resistance) in epicardial vessels in response to sympathetic activation helps to preserve perfusion of subendocardial regions (Feigl, 1987). Direct-acting vasodilators may interfere with these regulatory mechanisms, resulting in maldistribution of flow and possibly myocardial oxygen imbalance. This condition is most likely to occur when a critical stenosis occurs in an artery supplying both a normal and a collateral-dependent zone of myocardium (Gross and Warltier, 1981). In this situation, the vascular bed of the collateral dependent zone would be maximally dilated by local factors, whereas the normal bed would exhibit characteristically high vascular tone. Vasodilatation of the normal bed would provide a low resistance pathway for coronary blood flow away from the collaterally supplied vessels, thereby *stealing* flow from the post-stenotic collateral-dependent bed (Fig. 15.15). This phenomenon may account for ischemia induced by sodium nitroprusside, hydralazine, dipyridamole and some inhalation anesthetics with pronounced vasodilating properties.

Many other substances undoubtedly effect the coronary circulation, either directly or indirectly, and these effects should be considered when multiple pharmacological interventions are anticipated, as is usually the case in anesthesia.

REGULATION OF CBF DURING ANESTHESIA

Effect of Anesthetics on the Coronary Circulation

Inhalation anesthetics appear to impair regulation of coronary blood flow. The principal evidence for this is an increase in coronary venous oxygenation consistent with flow in excess of metabolic demand. Narcotics, in contrast, appear to leave coronary regulation intact. A decrease in myocardial oxygen extraction would intuitively appear to offer the advantage to the myocardium of an increased oxygen reserve. However, under specific anatomical circumstances as discussed previously, in which regional myocardial blood flow is dependent upon collateral blood vessels, inappropriate coronary vasodilatation may be associated with a coexistence of regional luxury perfusion and regional myocardial ischemia (Fig. 15.15). Impairment of coronary autoregulation is most pronounced during isoflurane inhalation and least during halothane. Enflurane appears to be intermediate in this respect (Fig. 15.16). Because this is an

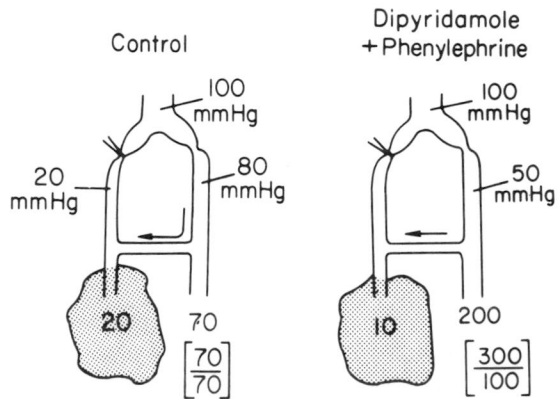

Fig. 15.15 Schematic diagram of the coronary circulation showing proposed mechanism for a vasodilator-induced coronary steal. The coronary artery divides into two branches, one completely occluded, and the other stenosed but providing collaterals to the first. In the control situation on the left, distal pressure is low in the occluded arterial bed and there is a small gradient in mean pressure across the stenosis. Flow in the ischemic region (dotted area) is 20 ml/(100 g · min) and is determined by the collateral driving pressure, or the difference between distal pressures in the bed supplying collaterals (80 mmHg) and the ischemic bed (20 mmHg). Flow in the distribution of the stenotic vessel is normal at 70 ml/(100 g · min) and is evenly distributed between subendocardium (lower value in bracket) and subepicardium (upper value). During dipyridamole administration, with blood pressure maintained constant by phenylephrine, flow increases in the nonischemic bed to 200 ml/(100 g · min), but becomes maldistributed between subendocardium and subepicardium. In addition, pressure distal to the stenosis falls to 50 mmHg causing a reduction in collateral driving pressure. As a result, flow to the ischemic region decreased to 10 ml/(100 g · min) interpreted as a coronary steal. (Reproduced by permission of the American Heart Association, Inc. Becker L.C. (1978). Conditions for vasodilator-induced coronary steal in experimental myocardial ischemia. *Circulation*, **57**, 1103.)

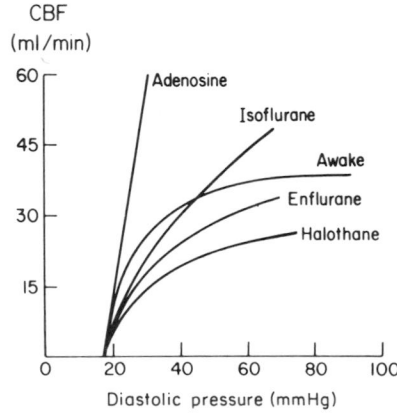

Fig. 15.16 Diastolic pressure—coronary blood flow relations in the awake and anesthetized dog. Halothane, enflurane, and isoflurane are effective vasodilators, though none impairs autoregulation comparably to adenosine. Isoflurane is more potent than either halothane or enflurane. (Reproduced with permission from Sybert et al., 1983.)

area of current controversy that may have important clinical implications, we will review the pertinent data in detail.

The most convincing human data demonstrating coronary steal by anesthetics were presented by Reiz et al. (1983). Unpremedicated vascular surgical patients with coronary artery disease (CAD) received 1 MAC isoflurane. Five out of ten patients studied developed ECG signs of ischemia in association with a reduced systemic arterial and calculated coronary perfusion pressure, unchanged coronary sinus blood flow and decreased myocardial oxygen extraction. Electrocardiographic ST segment changes compatible with ischemia and increased coronary sinus oxygenation persisted in three out of five patients despite restoration of hemodynamics to preanesthetic levels by pharmacologic intervention and atrial pacing, suggesting persistent coronary vasodilatation. This phenomenon has not been demonstrated during similar studies of halothane by Reiz et al. (1982). Similarly, Moffitt and associates demonstrated myocardial lactate production in 3 out of eleven patients in whom isoflurane was administered to an end point of arterial pressure reduced by 30%. They did not observe lactate production in similar studies using enflurane/oxygen anesthesia (Moffitt et al., 1984). Only one out of twelve patients receiving halothane/oxygen demonstrated lactate production, this during sternotomy (Moffitt et al., 1982).

There is an indication that the coronary vasodilatation induced by isoflurane may be dose dependent. O'Young et al. (1987) noted no abnormality of myocardial oxygenation when 0.5% isoflurane was administered to treat hypertension during high-dose synthetic narcotic anesthesia. Confirmatory evidence for the role of redistribution of coronary blood flow during isoflurane anesthesia has recently been obtained in animal models. Buffington et al. (1987) performed experiments in dogs four weeks after gradual occlusion of the anterior interventricular (AI) artery and consequent collateralization of the AI territory. In this preparation, administration of 1% isoflurane shifted blood flow from collateral-dependent to normal myocardium, despite constant heart rate, blood pressure, and total coronary blood flow. The maldistribution primarily affected the subendocardial zone (Fig. 15.17), and was associated with impairment of contraction in the area of the myocardium perfused by collaterals.

Priebe (personal communication, 1987) has recently conducted crossover experiments in dogs with acutely narrowed AI arteries. At the same perfusion pressure,

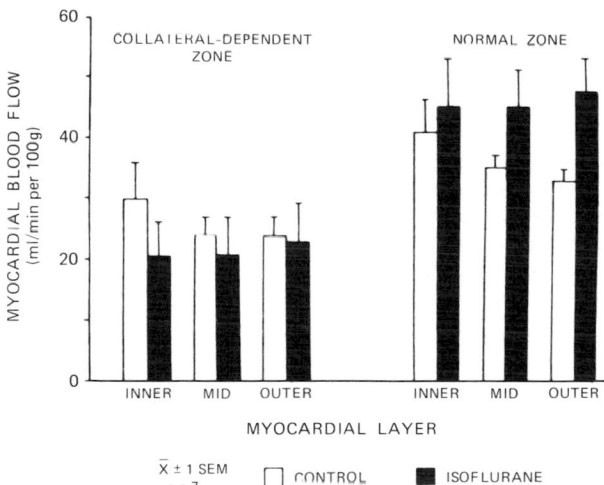

Fig. 15.17 Effect of isoflurane upon distribution of coronary blood flow in a canine model of chronic coronary occlusion. Isoflurane (1%) caused a redistribution of coronary blood flow away from collateral-dependent myocardium and away from the inner layers of the heart. (Reproduced with permission from Buffington et al., 1985.)

heart rate, and left ventricular end-diastolic filling pressure, coronary blood flow in the region supplied by the stenosed artery was higher, and shortening was greater during halothane than during isoflurane anesthesia. In contrast, flow to the area supplied by the nonstenosed coronary artery was higher during isoflurane anesthesia, and contraction was normal during both anesthetics. Using quantitative angiography, Sill et al. (1987) have demonstrated that distal coronary arterioles constitute the site of isoflurane-induced coronary vasodilatation. These are the same vessels thought to be responsible for physiological regulation of coronary blood flow and its distribution.

Importantly, data documenting a difference in myocardial infarction rate among patients receiving different anesthetics is lacking. This may be because adequately designed clinical studies have not been performed, because other pharmacologic properties of anesthetics are more important in the generation of myocardial infarction, because differences in skill of anesthetic and surgical postoperative care providers overwhelm intrinsic differences of the drugs, or other as yet unidentified factors. It is also possible that no such difference exists.

Effects of Laryngoscopy and Endotracheal Intubation

Evidence is mounting that laryngoscopy and tracheal intubation are associated with enhanced coronary vasomotion. Figure 15.18 demonstrates decreased coronary sinus blood flow and ejection fraction, with abnormal wall motion, concurrent with laryngoscopy and intubation, preceding detectable hemodynamic changes. In a series of thirty patients demonstrating myocardial ischemia during laryngoscopy, coronary sinus blood flow was transiently decreased by approximately one quarter. This was not true in other patients who did not demonstrate ischemia (Reiz et al., 1985). Bellows et al. (1984) demonstrated abnormal anterior left ventricular wall motion in 8 out of 24 patients with AI artery disease during laryngoscopy and tracheal intubation. Only three experienced adverse changes in hemodynamic variables. Kleinman et al. (1986) observed development of heterogeneous myocardial perfusion in 45% of patients undergoing endotracheal intubation under either halothane or narcotic anesthesia. All of the above data are compatible with coronary vasospasm.

Changes in Coronary Blood Flow Secondary to Systemic Hemodynamics During Anesthesia

Although autoregulation may be impaired, it nevertheless remains a principal determinant of coronary blood flow during all anesthetics. Thus, within limits, coronary blood flow usually remains appropriate despite anesthesia associated with 20–30% decreases in arterial blood pressure.

Most information regarding coronary blood flow

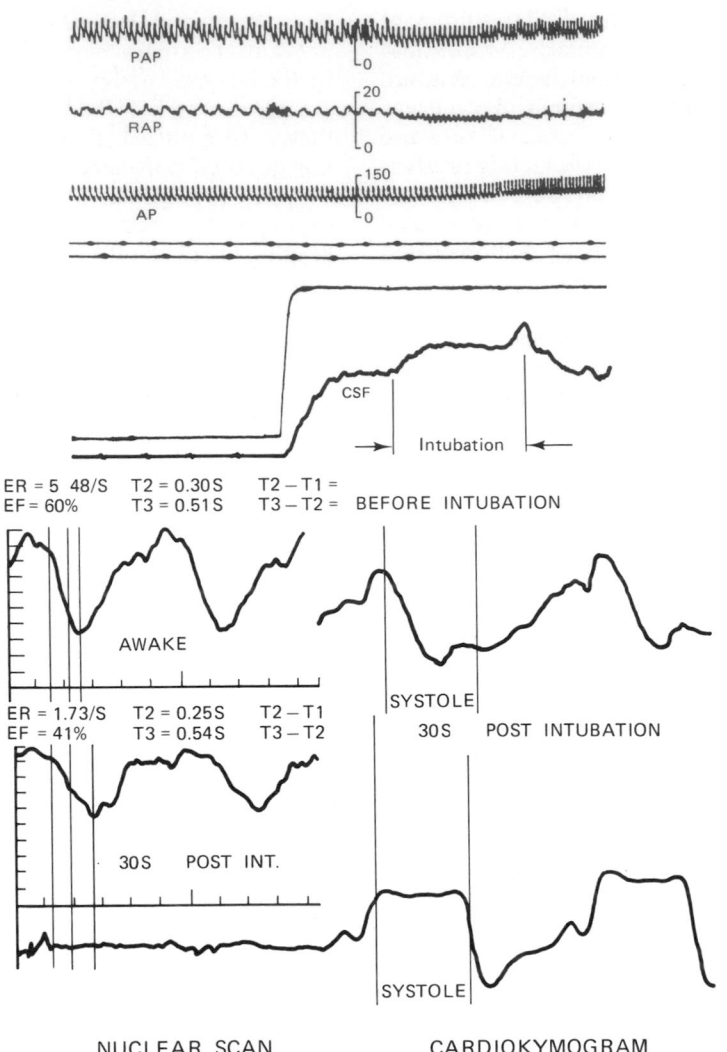

Fig. 15.18 Effects of laryngoscopy and intubation on hemodynamics and coronary blood flow (upper panel), scintigraphically-
determined ejection fraction (lower left), and the cardiokymogram,
which reflects anterior left ventricular wall motion (lower right) in
one anesthetized patient with coronary artery disease. The upward
shift of the mixed blood indicator resistance denotes a decrease in
left ventricular coronary blood flow (CSF) which precedes changes
in arterial pressure (AP), pulmonary artery pressure (PAP), right
atrial pressure (RAP) was removed, despite the increased heart rate
at this time. The associated ischemia is demonstrated by outward
anterior wall motion and decreased ejection rate and ejection fraction. It is likely that the decreased coronary blood flow is due to
vasospasm. (Reproduced with permission from Reiz et al. (1985).
Acta Anaesth. Scand., **29**, 106.)

and hemodynamics in humans is indirect, and necessarily obtained from studies of patients with CAD
undergoing anesthesia. Instead of a measurement of
coronary blood flow, an index of ischemia (such as
ECG change, ventricular wall motion abnormality, or
increase in ventricular filling pressure with abnormal
wave form) is employed. Clearly, this approach has
major limitations. From the low incidence of recognized ischemia and myocardial infarction in patients

without heart disease despite major abnormalities in
all hemodynamic variables, we can infer, however,
that coronary flow meets metabolic demands during
anesthesia, much as it does in the unanesthetized
state.

Systemic hemodynamics remain perhaps the most
important determinants of coronary blood flow under
anesthesia both in normal patients and in those with
coronary artery disease. Hypotension (Mauney et al.,

1970) and tachycardia (Slogoff and Keats, 1985) have been related to perioperative myocardial infarction. Relief of myocardial ischemia is routinely observed when adverse hemodynamics are relieved, both in experimental models of myocardial ischemia (Bland and Lowenstein, 1976) and in patients with CAD (Hess et al., 1983; Roizen et al., 1981). However, the precise drug or combination of drugs (both anesthetics and adjuvants) which are most advantageous have not been determined. For instance Hess and associates demonstrated that isoflurane is better than halothane for normalizing PCWP during hypertension, Roizen et al. showed that both halothane and enflurane were equally effective. Moreover, Roizen showed a decreased systemic vascular resistance with halothane, whereas Hess and his colleagues did not. It is likely that similar contradictory findings would be observed were the coronary blood flow to be measured during similar circumstances. This emphasizes the need for direct measurements, not only for greater understanding but also for optimum patient care.

REFERENCES

Abraham A. (1969). *Microscopic Innervation of the Heart and Blood Vessels in Vertebrates Including Man.* New York: Pergamon Press.

Antonaccio M.J. (1984). *Cardiovascular Pharmacology.* New York: Raven Press.

Astrand P.O., Rodahl K. (1970). *Textbook of Work Physiology.* pp. 115–178. New York: McGraw-Hill.

Baroldi G., Scomazzoni G. (1967). *Coronary Circulation in the Normal and the Pathologic Heart.* Washington, D.C.: Office of the Surgeon General, Department of the Army.

Bassingthwaighte J.B., Yipintsoi T., Harvey P.B. (1974). Microvasculature of the dog left ventricular myocardium. *Microvasc. Res.,* **7**, 229.

Becker L.C. (1978). Conditions for vasodilator-induced coronary steal in experimental myocardial ischemia. *Circulation,* **57**, 1103.

Bellows W.H., Bode R.H. Jr., Levy J., et al. (1984). Non-invasive detection of peri-induction ischemic ventricular dysfunction by cardiokymography in man: preliminary experience. *Anesthesiology,* **60**, 155.

Berne R.M. (1980). The role of adenosine in the regulation of coronary blood flow. *Circ. Res.,* **47**, 807.

Berne R., Rubio R. (1979). Coronary Circulation, In *Handbook of Physiology, Section 2, Volume 1, The Cardiovascular System,* pp. 873–952, (Berne R. et al., eds.) Bethesda, MD.: American Physiological Society.

Blaise G., Sill J.C., Nugent M., et al. (1987). Isoflurane causes endothelium-dependent inhibition of contractile responses of canine coronary arteries. *Anesthesiology,* **66**, 513.

Bland J.H.L., Lowenstein E. (1976) Halothane-induced decrease in experimental myocardial ischemia in the non-failing canine heart. *Anesthesiology,* **45**, 287.

Buffington C.W., Romson J.L., Duttlinger N.C. (1985). Does isoflurane cause coronary steal? *Anesthesiology,* **63**, A9.

Buffington C.W., Romson J.E., Levine A., et al. (1987). Isoflurane induces coronary steal in a canine model of chronic coronary occlusion. *Anesthesiology,* **66**, 280.

Busse R., Pohl V., Kellner C., et al. (1983). Endothelial cells are involved in the vasodilatory response to hypoxia. *Pflugers Arch.,* **397**, 78.

Chilian W.M., Marcus M.L. (1982). Phasic coronary blood flow velocity in intramural and epicardial coronary arteries. *Circ. Res.,* **50**, 775.

Downey J.M., Kirk E.S. (1974). Distribution of the coronary blood flow across the canine heart wall during systole. *Circ. Res.,* **34**, 251.

Downey J.M., Kirk E.S. (1975). Inhibition of coronary blood flow by a vascular waterfall mechanism. *Circ. Res.,* **36**, 753.

Feigl E.O. (1983). Coronary physiology. *Physiol. Rev.,* **63**, 1.

Feigl E.O. (1987). The paradox of adrenergic coronary vasoconstriction. *Circulation,* **76**, 737.

Feigl E.O., Roth A.C. (1981). Diffusional shunting in the canine myocardium. *Circ. Res.,* **48**, 470.

Feldman R.L., Nichols W.W., Pepine C.J., et al. (1979). The coronary hemodynamics of left main and branch coronary stenoses. *J. Thorac. Cardiovasc. Surg.,* **77**, 377.

Fulton W.F.M. (1965). *The Coronary Arteries: Arteriography, Microanatomy and Pathogenesis of Obliterative Coronary Artery Disease,* Springfield, Ill.: Thomas.

Gellai M., Norton J.M., Detar R. (1973). Evidence for direct control of coronary vascular tone by oxygen. *Circ. Res.,* **32**, 279.

Gewirtz H., Brantigan D.L., Olsson R.A., et al. (1983). Role of adenosine in the maintainance of coronary vasodilation distal to a severe coronary artery stenosis: Observations in conscious domestic swine. *Circ. Res.,* **53**, 42.

Gibbs C.L., Chapman J.B. (1979). Cardiac Energetics. In *Handbook of Physiology, Section 2, Volume 1, The Cardiovascular System,* pp. 775–804. (Berne R.M. et al. eds.) Bethesda, MD.: American Physiological Society.

Gilman A.G., Goodman L.S., Rall T.W., et al. (1985). The *Pharmacological Basis of Therapeutics,* 7th ed., New York: Macmillan.

Granata L., Huvos A., Pasque A., et al. (1969). Left coronary hemodynamics during hemorrhagic hypotension and shock. *Am. J. Physiol.,* **261**, 1583.

Gross C.J., Warltier D.C. (1981). Coronary steal in four models of single or multiple vessel obstruction in dogs. *Am. J. Cardiol.,* **48**, 84.

Guidicelli J., Berdeaux A., Tato F., et al. (1980). Left stellate stimulation: Regional myocardial flows and ischemic injury in dogs. *Am. J. Physiol.,* **239**, H359.

Hess W., Arnold B., Schulte-Sasse V., et al. (1983). Comparison of isoflurane and halothane when used to control intraoperative hypertension in patients undergoing coronary artery bypass surgery. *Anesth. Analg.,* **62**, 15.

Hintze T.H., Kaley G. (1977). Prostaglandins and the control of blood flow in the canine myocardium. *Circ. Res.,* **40**, 313.

Hoffman J.I.E. (1984). Maximal coronary flow and the concept of coronary vascular reserve. *Circulation,* **70**, 153.

Holtz J., Forstermann V., Pohl V., et al. (1984). Flow-dependent endothelium mediated dilation of epicardial coronary arteries in conscious dogs: Effect of cyclo-oxygenase inhibition. *J. Cardiovasc. Pharmacol.,* **6**, 1161.

Johanssen V.J., Mark A.L., Marcus M.L. (1982). Responsiveness to cardiac sympathetic nerve stimulation during maximal coronary dilation produced by adenosine. *Circ. Res.,* **50**, 510.

Khouri E.M., Gregg D.E., Rayford C.R. (1965). Effect of exercise on cardiac output, left coronary flow and myocardial metabolism in the unanesthetized dog. *Circ. Res.*, **17**, 427.

Kleinman F., Henkin R.E., Glisson S.N., et al. (1986). Qualitative evaluation of coronary flow during anesthetic induction using Thallium-201 perfusion scans. *Anesthesiology*, **64**, 157.

Klocke F.J. (1976). Coronary blood flow in man. *Prog. Cardiovasc. Dis.*, **19**, 117.

Levine H.J., Wagman R.J. (1962). Energetics of the human heart. *Am. J. Cardiol.*, **9**, 372.

Lowenstein E., Hill R.D., Rajasopalan B., et al. (1982). Winnie the Pooh revisited, or, the more recent adventures of piglet. *Anesthesiology*, **56**, 81.

Marcus M.L., Kerber R.E., Ehrhardt J., et al. (1976). Effects of time on volume and distribution of coronary collateral flow. *Am. J. Physiol.*, **230**, 279.

Mauney F.M. Jr., Ebert P.A., Sabiston D.C. Jr. (1970). Postoperative myocardial infarction: A study of predisposing factors, diagnosis and mortality in a high risk group of surgical patients. *Ann. Surg.*, **172**, 497.

Moffitt E.A., Sethna D.H., Bassell J.A., et al. (1982). Myocardial metabolism and hemodynamic responses to halothane or morphine anesthesia for coronary artery surgery. *Anesth. Analg.*, **61**, 979.

Moffitt E.A., Imrie D.D., Scovil J.E., et al. (1984). Myocardial metabolism and hemodynamic responses with enflurane anesthesia for coronary artery surgery. *Can. Anaesth. Soc. J.*, **31**, 604.

Moffitt E.A., Barker R.A., Glenn J.J., et al. (1986). Myocardial metabolism and hemodynamic responses with isoflurane anesthesia for coronary artery surgery. *Anesth. Analg.*, **65**, 53.

Molnar J.I., Scott J.B., Frolich E.D., et al. (1962). Local effects of various anions and H^+ on dog limb and coronary vascular resistances. *Am. J. Physiol.*, **203**, 125.

Moncada S., Herman A.G., Vanhouette P. (1987). Endothelium-derived relaxing factor is identified as nitric oxide. *Trends Pharmacological Sci.*, **8**, 365.

Most A.S., Williams D.O., Gewirtz H. (1985). Elevated coronary vascular resistance in the presence of reduced resting blood flow distal to a severe coronary stenosis. *Cardiovasc. Res.*, **19**, 599.

Murray P.A., Belloni F.L., Sparks H.V. (1979). The role of potassium in the metabolism control of coronary vascular resistance of the dog. *Circ. Res.*, **44**, 767.

Olsson R., Bugni W. (1986). Coronary circulation. In *The Heart and Cardiovascular System*, Chapter 48, pp. 987–1037. (Fozzard H.A. et al. eds.) New York: Raven Press.

O'Young J., Mastrocostopoulos G., Hilgenberg A., et al. (1987). Myocardial circulation and metabolic effects of isoflurane and sufentanil during coronary artery surgery. *Anesthesiology*, **66**, 653.

Pitt B., Gregg D.E. (1968). Coronary hemodynamic effects of increasing ventricular rate in the unanesthetized dog. *Circ. Res.*, **22**, 753.

Reiz S., Balfours E., Gustavsson B., et al. (1982). Effects of halothane on coronary hemodynamics and myocardial metabolism in patients with ischemic heart disease and heart failure. *Acta. Anesth. Scand.*, **26**, 133.

Reiz S., Balfour E., Sorensen M.B., et al. (1983). Isoflurane—a powerful coronary vasodilator in patients with coronary artery disease. *Anesthesiology*, **59**, 91.

Reiz S., Ryduall A., Haggmark S. (1985). Coronary hemodynamic effects of surgery during enflurane-nitrous oxide anesthesia in patients with ischemic heart disease. *Acta. Anaesth. Scand.*, **29**, 106.

Roizen M., Hamilton W.K., Solm Y.J. (1981). Treatment of stress-induced increases in pulmonary capillary wedge pressure using volatile anesthetics. *Anesthesiology*, **55**, 446.

Sabiston D.C. Jr., Gregg D.E. (1957). Effect of cardiac contraction on coronary blood flow. *Circulation*, **15**, 14.

Santamore W., Walinsky P. (1980). Altered coronary flow responses to vasoactive drugs in the presence of coronary arterial stenosis in the dog. *Am. J. Cardiol.*, **45**, 276.

Schaper W. (1971). *The Collateral Circulation of the Heart*, Amsterdam: North Holland.

Schwartz J.S. (1983). Effect of distal coronary pressure on rigid and compliant coronary stenoses. *Am. J. Physiol.*, **245**, H1054-H1060.

Segal S.S., Duling B.R. (1987). Flow-control among microvessels coordinated by intracellular conduction. *Science*, **234**, 868.

Sill J.C., Bove A.A., Nugent M., et al. (1987). Effects of isoflurane on coronary arteries and coronary arterioles in the intact dog. *Anesthesiology*, **66**, 273.

Slogoff S., Keats A.S. (1985). Does perioperative ischemia lead to post-operative myocardial infarction? *Anesthesiology*, **62**, 107.

Sybert P.E., Hickey R.F., Hoar P.F., et al. (1983). Effects of volatile anesthetics on the regulation of coronary blood flow. *Anesthesiology*, **59**, A24.

Vatner D.E., Knight D.R., Homey C.J. et al. (1986). Subtypes of β-adrenergic receptors in bovine coronary arteries. *Circ. Res.*, **59**, 463.

Wiggers C.J., Green H.D. (1936). The ineffectiveness of drugs upon collateral flow after experimental coronary occlusion in dogs. *Am. Heart J.*, **11**, 527.

16. The Pulmonary Circulation
J. M. Leigh

Volatile anaesthetic agents gain access to the circulating blood through the media of the respiratory gases, the alveoli and the pulmonary capillary blood flow. The anaesthetist relies upon this, sometimes for induction but mostly for the maintainance of anaesthesia in the modern 'anaesthetic sequence'. At the same time he fulfils his responsibilites to the patient by ensuring gaseous homeostasis via the same route. For these reasons the pulmonary circulation is an important area for his interest.

The existence of the pulmonary circulation was an essential feature of William Harvey's postulations on the unidirectional circulation of the blood (1628). In 1669 Richard Lower in *Tractatus de Corde* described how venous blood became arterialized in traversing the lungs and that the absorption of a vital chemical from the air was involved. In 1868 Adolph Fick at a meeting of the Physical-Medical Association of Wurzburg theorized on the determination of stroke volume, based upon the exchange of the respiratory gases and their arterio-venous content difference. The figure which he arrived at was 77 ml per beat and thus a cardiac output or pulmonary blood flow of 4.9 litres per minute.

GENERAL FEATURES OF THE PULMONARY CIRCULATION

The pulmonary circulation is unique among the regional circulations in that it is in series rather than in parallel. The right ventricular output passes through one capillary bed but the left ventricular output becomes subdivided to pass through several capillary networks which are in parallel with each other. It is also unique in that it has its own heart pump, the right ventricle.

The pulmonary vessels can be seen on a plain chest film and are responsible for most of the markings in the lung fields. Under conditions of a very high pulmonary blood flow these markings are more pronounced. The opposite, i.e., a paucity of markings, is seen where there is a low pulmonary blood flow.

The pulmonary circuit is a low resistance and therefore a low pressure system in contrast to the systemic circulation, which has a resistance about ten times as high. The systemic circuit has a higher systolic pressure than the pulmonary circuit, that is 120 mmHg compared to 20 mmHg systolic. The mean capillary pressure in the systemic circulation is about 20 mmHg whereas in the pulmonary circulation it is about 10 mmHg and is pulsatile. The systemic circulation contains twice as much blood as the pulmonary. The pulmonary capillary blood volume is about 60–100 ml and the capillary transit time varies from about 1 second down to about 0.4 seconds depending upon cardiac output.

The cardiac output subserves the demands of the systemic organs and is regulated by the venous return volume and the Starling mechanism. Since the pulmonary circuit is in series, the flow through it is modified at the same time. As, in an average size adult, the cardiac output in health can vary from about 3 litres per minute during sleep to 25 litres or more per minute during exercise, the pulmonary circuit must cope with these flows firstly without disturbing its function and secondly without overloading its heart pump. The resistance in the system is kept down under conditions of high flow due to its high compliance. The latter results from the distensibility of the large vessels, by dilatation of already opened capillaries and by recruitment of hitherto unopened capillaries.

The function of the pulmonary circulation is the exchange of respiratory gases according to their tension gradient with the alveolar gas. In this way something like 360 litres of oxygen are exchanged for 288 litres of carbon dioxide in a single day. The pulmonary capillaries and their accompanying 350 000 000 alveoli provide a gas exchange surface of some 70 square metres, that is about 40 times the body surface area. The capillary blood volume is spread out in this area as if in a sheet about 4 micrometres thick.

It is important that intracapillary blood pressure does not exceed the oncotic pressure of the plasma proteins lest transudation of plasma and pulmonary oedema ensue. The mean capillary blood pressure in the pulmonary circuit is of the order of 10 mmHg and is much lower than the plasma colloid oncotic pressure of about 25 mmHg. This gradient between intrapulmonary capillary pressure and the oncotic pressure is highly important in keeping the lung dry for proper function.

The demonstration of arterio-venous anastomoses within the lungs has been achieved by a variety of workers but not always confirmed by others (Liebow, 1962; Tobin, 1966.) It would be surprising if they did not exist since A-V anastomoses are an important feature of other circulations. Their possible role in the lung could be to by-pass a high flow load away from the capillaries, i.e., to relieve what would otherwise be an excessive pressure load on them.

The low resistance characteristics of the pulmonary circuit are reflected in the structure of its different elements. The right ventricle is one third the thickness of the left ventricle, reflecting its lower work load. The main pulmonary arteries are elastic conducting vessels only about twice as thick as the venae cavae and one third the thickness of the aorta. The muscular pulmonary arteries range from 100–1000 micrometres in diameter and are characterized by circularly oriented smooth muscle between two elastic laminae. In the systemic arteries muscularization occurs at a much larger diameter. Pulmonary arterioles are vessels of less than 100 micrometres diameter, the walls consist of a single elastic lamina and an endothelial lining. There is no muscular media except at the origin from the parent artery. The pulmonary capillaries are about 4 micrometres in diameter. The walls or septa between alveoli consist of capillary endothelium and alveolar epithelium.

The nutrient flow to the pulmonary structures themselves is via the bronchial arteries. While some venous drainage enters the systemic venous system via the pleurohilar veins the majority drains into the pulmonary veins and therefore constitute shunt. The bronchial flow is approximately 50 ml/min.

Pulmonary Lymph Flow. Interstitial water from the lung drains like any other structure via the lymphatics. The flow normally amounts to approximately 500 ml per day. There is experimental evidence to suggest that it might increase up to 28 times in disease. The formation of lung water is discussed in detail by Harris and Heath (1986) and Nunn (1987).

Vasomotor Control in the Pulmonary Circulation

Experimental stimulation and pharmacologic challenges are capable of demonstrating vasomotor reactions in the pulmonary circuit. The presence of pulmonary vasomotor nerves is undisputed but their importance under physiological conditions is difficult to assess. This is especially so since all the distributional characteristics of the pulmonary bed are present in the denervated lung of the adrenalectomized animal and also in the completely isolated but perfused lung. The particular features of interest are: *the autoregulation of flow at alveolar level by oxygen tension and the passive hydrostatic effects of gravity on pulmonary flow.*

The Effect of Oxygen

In 1946 Von Euler and Liljestrand demonstrated that alveolar hypoxia caused a rise in pulmonary artery pressure in the cat. This response to hypoxia is enhanced by extra-cellular acidosis and by hypercapnia. The characteristic response of muscular pulmonary arteries to alveolar hypoxia is thus to *constrict*. This is important at the local level since the mechanism will divert perfusion to better ventilated alveoli without a rise in main pulmonary artery pressure. However, when alveolar hypoxia is generalized and continuous as it is in the permanent inhabitants of the high altitude situation, these whether animals or man, suffer a state of chronic pulmonary hypertension with hypertrophy of the muscular pulmonary arteries and the right ventricle, a state which is amenable to reversal by oxygen therapy or return to low altitude. The arterial constriction associated with alveolar hypoxia raises two questions. Firstly, as the arteries are proximal to the capillaries, how can they 'sense' the change in oxygen tension? And secondly, how is it that hypoxia which is a dilator of systemic arteries causes constriction of pulmonary arteries?

Firstly, it is apparent from the thin walls of the small arteries and veins that they could participate in gas exchange. That alveolar gas does indeed penetrate into quite large arteries has been demonstrated in the most elegant manner by Sobol and his colleagues (1963) Fig. 16.1.

If a breath of hydrogen is taken, it is absorbed into the blood stream and travels round the circulation producing an acute change in potential as it passes. This can be sensed by a platinum tipped hydrogen sensitive electrode. In this particular experiment a double lumen catheter with a hydrogen electrode at its tip and another one 4 cm proximally was passed through the right heart to a wedged position in the pulmonary artery. The hydrogen electrode at the tip is giving the output 'PC' and the one 4 cm proximally the output PA, confirmed by the pressure tracings in the top right hand corner of Fig. 16.1. A third hydrogen electrode was placed in the brachial artery-BA. The time lines are one second apart. At the arrow a breath of hydrogen was taken. Not only did the inhaled hydrogen appear at the wedged position within 2 seconds, but it also appeared virtually at the same time at the pulmonary artery electrode. The fact that the BA electrode does not register a change in potential for a further 5 seconds shows that there is not sufficient time for the hydrogen to have recirculated. The findings demonstrate that the gas has rapidly penetrated pulmonary arteries of 1.5–3.0 mm in diameter. Since such arteries do contain smooth muscle this is strong evidence that they are directly accessible to alveolar gas and could therefore influence the distribution of blood according to the composition of that gas.

Having demonstrated that the alveolar gases diffuse into vessels which influence distribution it is necessary to consider the problem of the arterial muscle which constricts in the face of hypoxia.

Lundholm and Mohm-Lundholm (1963) believe that the contractile process of systemic vascular smooth muscle depends upon the continuing production of high energy compounds. Evidence points to a direct relationship between oxygen availability and

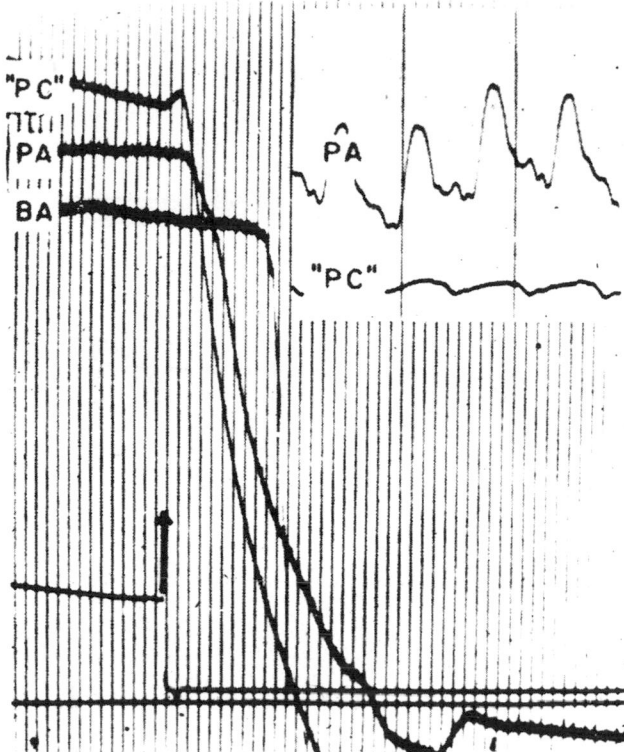

Fig. 16.1 A double lumen catheter was wedged in the pulmonary artery. The pressure tracings (inset) confirm that the tip was wedged 'PC' and the second lumen, 4 cm proximally, was in the pulmonary artery PA. Each lumen was also equipped with a platinum tipped hydrogen sensitive electrode. The potential measured at these is shown in the main part of the Fig. 'PC' and PA respectively. A third hydrogen electrode was placed in the brachial artery-BA. The time lines are one second apart. At the arrow a breath of hydrogen was taken in. A sudden change in potential at both the 'PC' and PA electrodes occurred virtually simultaneously two seconds later while the change in potential at the BA electrode did not occur for a further five seconds. The findings demonstrate that the gas has rapidly penetrated pulmonary arteries of 1.5–3.0 mm diameter. (Reproduced with permission from Sobol et al., 1963).

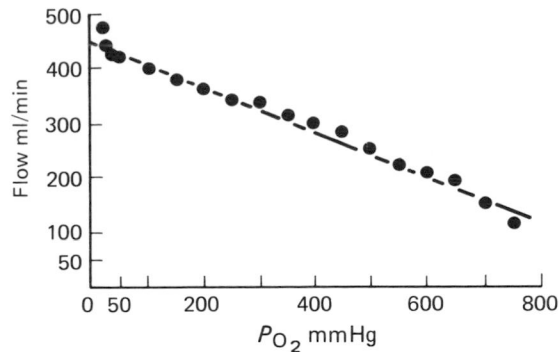

Fig. 16.2 The negative correlation between the flow permitted by the isolated lamb ductus arteriosus (ordinate) and the oxygen tension of the perfusate (abscissa). (Reproduced with permission from Assali et al., 1963).

the contractile strength of systemic vascular smooth muscle. This is very well demonstrated by the ductus arteriosus in which tonic contraction in the face of an increased oxygen tension is an essential feature of the transition from fetal to neonatal existence. Figure 16.2 is from the work of Assali and his colleagues (1963) and shows the flow permitted by the isolated ductus when the oxygen tension of the perfusate was varied over the range shown. Measurements *in vivo* on the fetal lamb when ventilated with different mixtures have also demonstrated this effect (Born et al., 1956).

By contrast hypoxia has the opposite effect on the pulmonary artery (Fig. 16.3). The tracing is from a cat anaesthetized and ventilated with a double lumen tube in place. The lungs were denervated and the total pul-

monary blood flow was controlled. The lower trace shows the flow in the left pulmonary artery obtained by an electro-magnetic flowmeter and the upper trace shows ventilation pressure. When the ventilation of the left lung was discontinued (Figs. 16.3(A) and (B)), the left pulmonary artery flow fell as a result of hypoxic vasoconstriction. In Fig. 16.3(B) the ventilation of the lung was recommenced at the arrow. Some hyperinflations were given to achieve re-expansion and the flowrate immediately rose.

When Lloyd (1967) investigated the contractile properties of isolated strips of pulmonary artery, he found that the responses to changes in oxygen tension were the reverse of those *in vivo*. This showed that the muscle itself responds like any other vascular smooth muscle. The pressor response to alveolar hypoxia therefore involves an activating mechanism present in the lung which overrides the tendency for the muscle itself to relax consequent upon oxygen deprivation. The available evidence points to this being a humoral response.

The search for a chemical mediator consisted of two basic steps. Firstly, the postulation and demonstration that a given substance was a pulmonary vasoconstrictor and secondly, that treatment with a substance which is a blocking agent of the first attenuated or abolished the pressor response to hypoxia. Early work by Barer (1966) suggested that noradrenaline was involved, while Hauge (1968) and Hauge and Melmon (1968) were able to demonstrate that histamine had the appropriate actions on the pulmonary vasculature, i.e., its pressor action was reversed by antihistamines and restored after the exhibition of semi-carbazide which is a specific antihistaminase. Histamine is manufactured in the mast cells of the vessel walls and accumulates in non-mast cell stores in the endothelial cells.

At subcellular level calcium ion flux is demonstrably important. Recently Burghuber (1987) has demonstrated that the calcium blocking drug nifedipine attenuates acute hypoxic pulmonary vasocon-

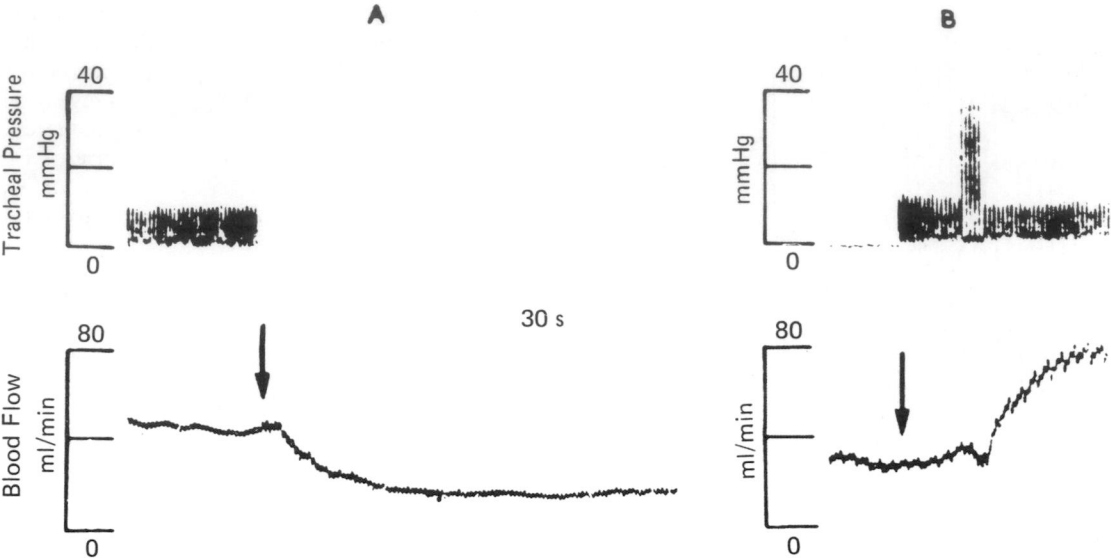

Fig. 16.3 Tracings from a cat anesthetized with a double lumen tube in place. Upper trace airway pressure. Lower trace left pulmonary artery flow. In A, at the arrow, ventilation of the left lung ceased and pulmonary blood flow fell away as a result of hypoxic vaso-constriction. In B, at the arrow, ventilation of the left lung was recommenced. Some hyper-inflations were given to achieve re-expansion and the flow rate immediately rose. (Reproduced with permission from Barer, 1966).

striction in patients with chronic obstructive pulmonary disease.

It is now well known that the endothelial cells of the lung capillaries not only provide an inert surface for gas exchange but are also significantly involved in the removal, production or modification of other bio-active materials as well as those mentioned above.

The endothelial cells have invaginations of the cell membrane, the pinocytotic vesicles, which are thought to be involved in the transcapillary movement of lipid-insoluble macromolecules. These vesicles are the site of the biotransformation of the 'autocoids' angiotensin I, bradykinin, noradrenaline, 5-HT and the site of production of the arachidonic acid metabolites known collectively as the eicosanoid substances—prostaglandins, prostacyclins, thromboxanes and leukotrienes (Bakhle and Ferreira, 1985).

Substances, such as angiotensin I and bradykinin are transformed on the surface of the endothelial cell by converting enzymes, producing activation to angiotensin II in the case of the former, and the in-active peptide in the case of the latter. Noradrenaline and 5-HT are actively taken up and degraded by monoamine oxidase.

During profound metabolic responses, i.e., allergic and anaphylactoid reactions, these substances, especially histamine, reach a critical level and 'over-flow' into the capillary lumen.

Pulmonary Oxygen Toxicity

The pathogenesis of this condition is poorly under-stood. Airway irritation occurs in normal men after 12 hours of 100% oxygen at 1 ATA. In conscious dogs consolidation of lung tissue and death occur within approximately 30–80 hours. The rate of development and degree of lung damage are proportional to the inhaled oxygen tension and the duration of exposure. The picture is one of damage to the alveolar-capillary membrane similar to that seen in toxic pneumonitis with oedema, haemorrhage and cellular infiltration, mediated by the autocoids mentioned earlier.

The Effect of Gravity

Because the pulmonary circulation is a low pressure system, the pulmonary blood flow is subject to hydro-static effects due to gravity. These effects may be illus-trated by a four zone model (Hughes et al., 1968). For full discussion of the effects of gravity on pulmonary blood flow, see Chapter 22, *Ventilation/perfusion re-lationships*.

Ventilation/Perfusion Relationships

Of special importance to proper lung function is the relationship or matching between ventilation (V) and perfusion (Q). Figure 16.4 is a model which explains the matching of ventilation and perfusion. This model permits there being two conditions of the alveoli, i.e., open (the two on the right) and closed (the one on the left), and two kinds of capillary similarly open and closed. There are thus three kinds of relationship established. On the left there is perfusion without ventilation causing a right to left shunt of venous blood and on the right is the reciprocal situation, i.e.,

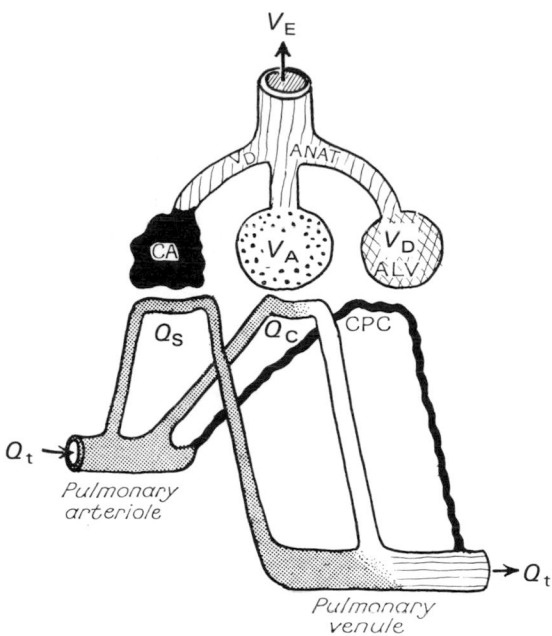

Fig. 16.4 Model to explain the possible relationships (matching) between ventilation and perfusion. The model states that matching can be explained 'as if' there were two kinds of alveoli and two kinds of pulmonary capillary, i.e., open and closed. There are thus three possibilities: perfusion without ventilation, on the left: ventilation without perfusion, on the right: the ideal situation is shown in the centre. CA = closed alveolus. CPC = closed pulmonary capillary. Q_t = cardiac output. Q_s = shunted blood flow. Q_c = ideal pulmonary capillary blood flow. $(Q_t = Q_s + Q_c)$. V_E = ventilatory volume measured during expiration. $V_{D\,ALV}$ = alveolar dead space ventilation. $V_{D\,ANAT}$ = obligatory 'wasted' anatomical dead space ventilation. $(V_{D\,ALV} + V_{D\,ANAT}$ = physiological dead space ventilation). V_A = ideal alveolar ventilation. $(V_E = V_A + V_{D\,ANAT} + V_{D\,ALV}.)$

ventilation without perfusion, resulting in alveolar dead space. Only in the centre is the situation ideal i.e., an open capillary in contact with an open alveolus, so that gaseous equilibrium can occur. The vertical hatching in the bronchial tree represents the anatomical dead space ventilation. The latter plus the cross-hatched area is the total physiological dead space. The venous admixture effect of the shunt past the closed alveolus is represented by the change in shading in the right hand side of the venule. This model is a useful one because the volumes represented by all these shaded areas can be quantitated if suitable measurements are taken (see appendix to this chapter). However, it must be remembered that there are 350 000 000 alveoli and therefore there are possibly 350 000 000 variants of the interrelationships.

The Effects of Alterations in V/Q on the Uptake of Anaesthetic Agents

The effect of alterations in shunt and dead space on

the uptake of anaesthetics have been elaborated by Saidman and Eger (1967) utilizing a simple V/Q model. In Fig. 16.5(A), the ventilation and perfusion are ideally matched. Inhalation of a highly soluble gas and a slightly soluble gas is being considered. In order to achieve an alveolar partial pressure of 10 mmHg a very much higher inspired tension of the highly soluble gas, i.e., 50 mmHg, has to be given than the insoluble gas, i.e., 12 mmHg. Because there is no V/Q abnormality, the effluent pulmonary venous blood has a partial pressure equal to that in the alveoli, and the end-tidal tension (mixed alveolar tension), which in this model is the average tension in the two alveoli, is also equal to that in the alveoli and in the pulmonary venous blood.

Figure 16.5(B) shows the effect of a shunt on the highly soluble agent. The shunt is shown in this case as the result of the blockage of the alveolus on the left. Alveolar ventilation is assumed to be the same and therefore the alveolus on the right becomes doubly ventilated, which effectively doubles the partial pressure of the highly soluble agent. The partial pressure in the effluent blood from this alveolus is thus 20 mmHg. However, the shunted blood from the non-ventilated alveolus has a zero partial pressure, and therefore the effect on the effluent pulmonary venous blood is that the partial pressure in this two unit model is the average of the two i.e., 10 mmHg, which is no different from that in the ideal arrangement in Fig. 16.5(A). On the other hand, the end-tidal tension is 20 mmHg, i.e., double.

Figure 16.5(C) shows the effect of a shunt on the slightly soluble gas. The arrangement is as previously, i.e., with the left hand airway blocked off and the alveolar ventilation doubled to the right hand unit.

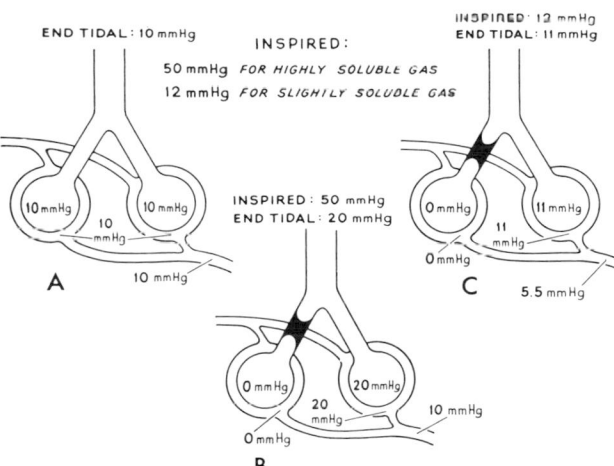

Fig. 16.5 The effect of a large shunt (venous admixture) on the uptake of anaesthetic agents (for full description see text). A. The normal lung with a normal end-tidal anaesthetic partial pressure equal in both lungs and in the arterial blood. B. Highly soluble gas. C. Slightly soluble gas. (Reproduced with permission from Saidman and Eger, 1967).

This has a very small effect on the alveolar partial pressure of the insoluble agent because the inspired to end-tidal gradient was very small in the first place. There is only a rise of 1 mmHg in this partial pressure, which is also reflected in the end-tidal partial pressure; however, the effect in the blood phase is much more significant. The partial pressure in the blood from the ventilated alveolus becomes halved, as it was with the soluble agent, but the effluent pulmonary venous blood partial pressure is very much lower than in the ideal situation i.e., 5.5, as opposed to 10 mmHg. Thus a shunt has a greater effect on an insoluble agent. In practice, induction with a soluble anaesthetic agent would not be faster than with an insoluble one, rather more normal anaesthetic time course would ensue with a soluble anaesthetic than with an insoluble anaesthetic and the inspired concentration would have to be raised less with the soluble agent to achieve a normal rate of induction.

Figure 16.6 shows the effect when alveoli are ventil-

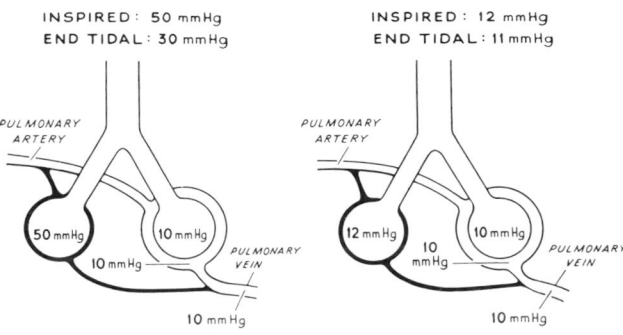

Fig. 16.6 The effect of a large dead space on the uptake of anaesthetic agents (for full description *see* text. (Reproduced with permission from Saidman and Eger, 1957).

ated but not perfused, i.e., there is an increase in dead space. The same two agents are being considered. The alveolus on the left has no perfusion so in neither case is the effluent pulmonary venous blood partial pressure affected—both are 10 mmHg. However, the non-perfused alveoli undergo no exchange with the blood and thus the anaesthetic agent partial pressure in them is in equilibrium with the inspired. The end-tidal partial pressure in the two unit model is the average of the two alveolar partial pressures and is very much higher in the case of the highly soluble agent (on the left) than in the ideal situation shown earlier, i.e., 30 mmHg instead of 10 mmHg. The effect on the insoluble agent (on the right) is minimal. This would mean that with a soluble agent the patient would not be as deeply anaesthetized as the end-tidal partial pressure would suggest, if indeed it was measured.

The choice of the two unit model of course greatly exaggerates these effects. While they are of theoretical

interest they are probably seldom of major clinical significance.

The Effects of V/Q Abnormalities on Oxygen and Carbon Dioxide Homeostasis

Shunting: The result of pulmonary shunting is that the pulmonary venous effluent blood has a lower arterial oxygen content than that of the end-pulmonary capillary blood. The ratio of shunt flow to cardiac output, the Q_s/Q_t ratio, can be derived from an application of the Fick principle. An indirect estimate of the shunt flow may also be obtained from the alveolar to arterial oxygen tension gradient (A–a$_{O_2}$ gradient), i.e., the gradient between the oxygen tension in the ideal capillary or ideal alveolus and that in the pulmonary venous blood. The relationship between A–a oxygen gradient and the oxygen content difference, which is of course the clinically important quantity, is non-linear because of the shape of the oxygen dissociation curve, thus when considering alveolar to arterial oxygen tension gradients at least one of the figures must be quantitated.

Hypoxaemia in Anaesthesia. An increase in alveolar to arterial oxygen tension gradient under conditions of a constant inspired oxygen tension has been shown to occur after premedication and after the induction of anaesthesia itself, especially when IPPV is employed, with prolongation into the postoperative period if surgery is lengthy. The effect is increased with age as there is a negative correlation between age and arterial oxygen tension.

The increase in A–a$_{O_2}$ gradient is not associated with alveolar hypoventilation as the arterial P_{CO_2} is not raised. Although it was first considered to be associated with atelectasis this has not been demonstrated by X-ray studies; also since the lesion is amenable to oxygen administration, frank atelectasis is an unlikely explanation. There remain two possible explanations:

Firstly if there is a fall in cardiac output at a constant oxygen consumption, it is obvious that as output falls mixed venous oxygen content falls and therefore the venous admixture effect of a constant shunt will be a greater depression of arterial oxygen tension at a given alveolar oxygen tension. However, it is possible that shunt values do not remain constant during changes in cardiac output. Sykes and his co-workers (1970) showed that in the high output state produced by over-transfusion in dogs there is an increase in Q_s/Q_t ratio. At the other end of the scale, work carried out by the author and M. F. Tyrrell, in which dogs had their cardiac outputs lowered, showed that Q_s/Q_t ratio decreases with cardiac output, an effect which tends to offset the effect of progressive venous desaturation until very low levels are reached (Fig. 16.7). Each line represents the regression line for a group of dogs, Q_s/Q_t ratio is on the ordinate. In the GBA group the blood pressure and cardiac output were lowered

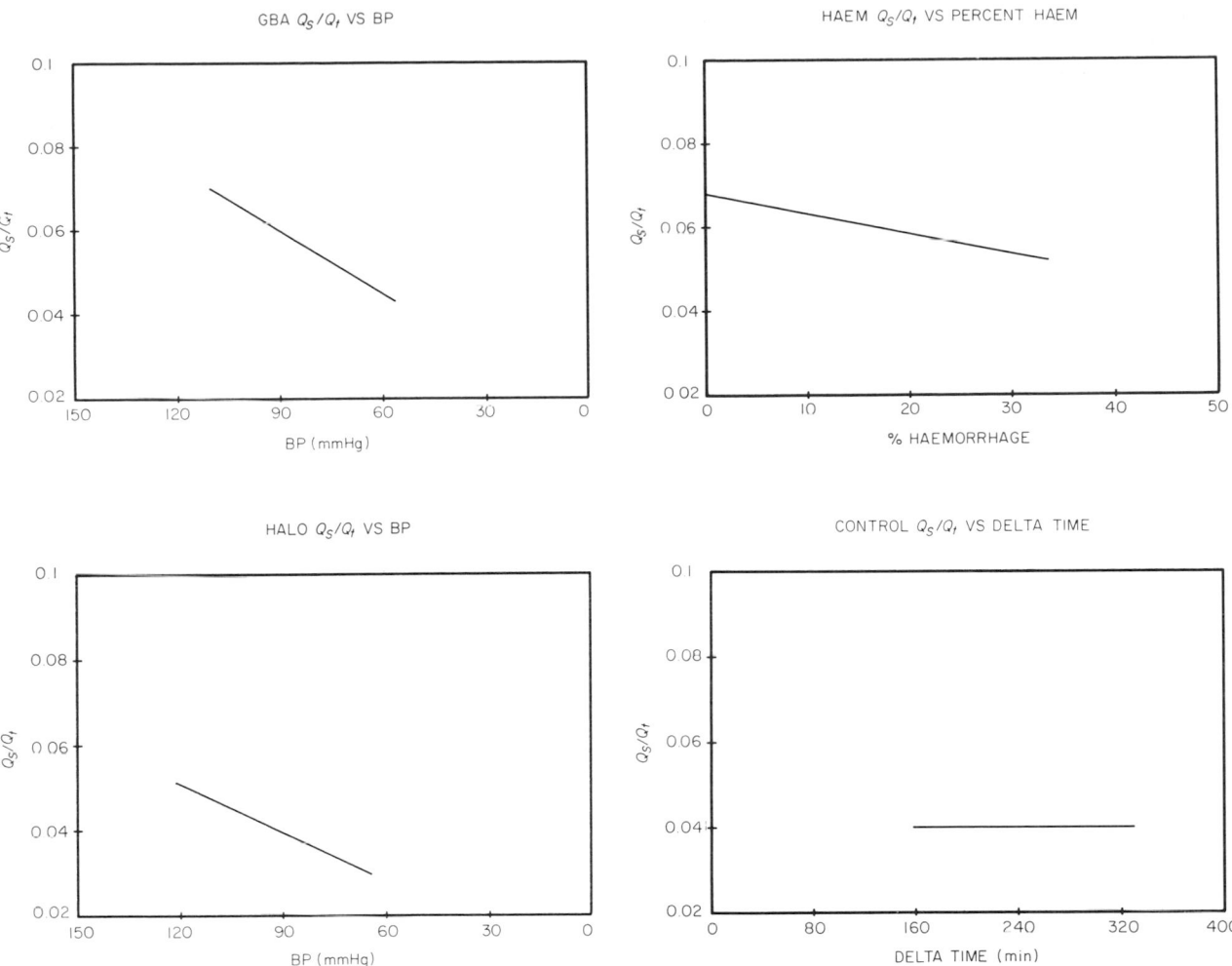

Fig. 16.7 Regression of Q_s/Q_t—shunt ratio—(ordinate) in anaesthetized ventilated dogs. GBA 11 dogs—blood pressure and cardiac output lowered with pentolinium (abscissa—mean arterial blood pressure mmHg). HALO 5 dogs—blood pressure and cardiac output lowered with halothane (abscissa—mean arterial blood pressure. HAEM 6 dogs—blood pressure and cardiac output lowered by haemorrhage (abscissa—percentage of estimated blood volume removed). CONTROL 6 dogs—anaesthesia (abscissa—time in minutes). This work demonstrated that Q_s/Q_t decreases when blood pressure and cardiac output are lowered by pentolinium tartrate, halothane and haemorrhage when compared with the effect of the passage of time alone.

with pentolinium tartrate, and the shunt ratio decreased as the blood pressure fell, as shown. In the HALO group, blood pressure and cardiac output were lowered with halothane and Q_s/Q_t ratio also decreased. In the HAEM group the effect of haemorrhage and a fall in cardiac output on Q_s/Q_t is shown; once more there is a decrease. The control group is plotted against time and there was very little change in Q_s/Q_t ratio.

The *second* and probable cause is maldistribution of ventilation and perfusion. In this respect there could be two possible mechanisms for the increase in shunting:

1. Decreased aeration due to the effect of small airways closure during expiration.

2. An increase in shunting through non-aerated areas resulting from a disorder of the hypoxic pressor response.

Evidence has accumulated to substantiate (1.) above particularly after abdominal surgery (Spence and Alexander, 1972; Alexander et al., 1972). The arguments are as follows: FRC is reduced after surgery and more so after upper abdominal surgery; the net increase in transpulmonary pressure as a result of the causal process brings the airways closing point (CP) closer to the end-tidal position (ETP). Alexander and his colleagues (1972) reported significant negative correlation between the index (ETP—CP) and the A–a$_{O_2}$ gradient. Davis and Spence (1972) showed that the situation is worse in the elderly and that these also obtain least benefit from an increase in inspired oxygen concentration. These facts further substantiate the above explanation since it is well known that closing volume becomes closer to end-tidal volume with increasing age.

There is also evidence that the second hypothetical mechanism, i.e., a disorder of the hypoxic pulmonary pressor response, may also contribute to the hypoxaemia. Sykes and his colleagues (1973) demonstrated the abolition of this response in the isolated perfused cat lung during the administration of 1–1.5% halothane, 0.5–0.75% trichlorethylene, 2–4% ether and 74% nitrous oxide. While these findings cannot neccessarily be extrapolated to the human situation, they provide presumptive evidence of a contributory role of clinical anaesthetics, at least in early postoperative hypoxaemia.

Instances of gross shunting associated with anaesthesia are seen, for example with the use of an endobronchial blocker, although hypoxic vasoconstriction would tend to offset this. The worst form is seen in the chemical pneumonitis associated with acid aspiration, where shunting through areas of oedematous nonventilated lung occurs, and these can be seen on a plain chest X-ray.

Dead Space: Changes in dead space during anaesthesia are associated with changes in cardiac output and the consequent passive changes in capillary perfusion. These may be seen particularly during haemorrhage and induced hypotension. Figure 16.8 shows the changes in dead space ratio (V_D/V_E) in the studies mentioned earlier. The values are on the ordinate and are of total functional dead space, i.e., including anatomical and apparatus dead space which are of course

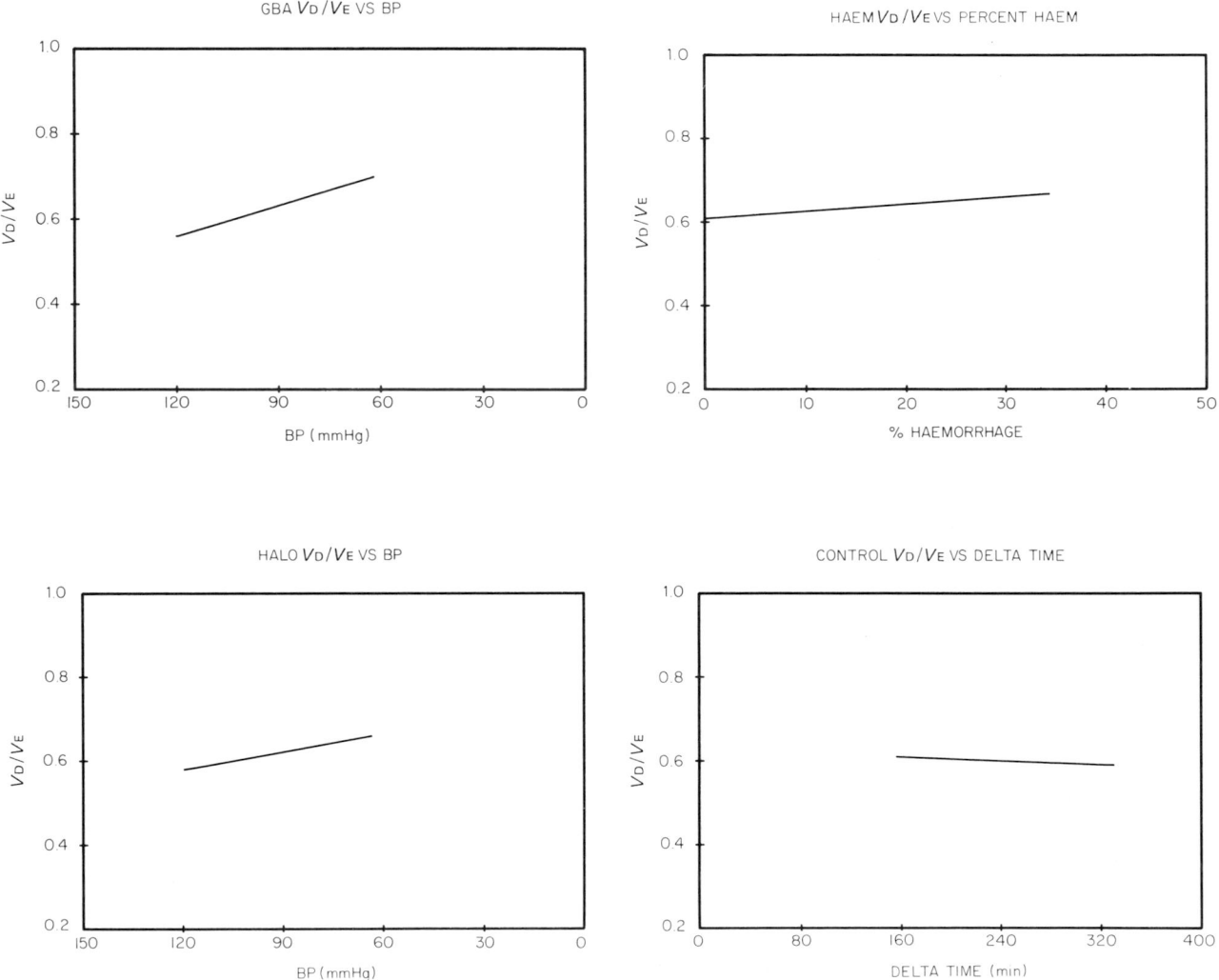

Fig. 16.8 Regression of V_D/V_E—physiological dead space ratio—(ordinate) in the same groups of dogs as are shown in Fig. 16.7. The values on the ordinate are of *total functional* physiological dead space, i.e., including apparatus dead space which was of course unchanged in each individual animal. This work demonstrates that V_D/V_E increases when blood pressure and cardiac output are lowered by pentolinium tartrate, halothane and haemorrhage when compared with the effects of the passage of time alone.

unchanged in each animal. It can be seen that the dead space ratio increased in association with the fall in blood pressure and cardiac output produced by ganglion blockade, by halothane and by haemorrhage in contrast with the control group.

Assessment of the changes in alveolar dead space alone can be achieved by measurement of the arterial to end-tidal carbon dioxide gradient. Figure 16.9 is from a clinical study by the author and P. W. R. Smethurst. The record was made during a faciomaxillary procedure on a male patient aged 45 years. Hypotension was induced by means of a trimetaphan infusion, during controlled ventilation with nitrous oxide/oxygen and trichlorethylene. The upper tracing is of blood pressure from 0–200 mmHg and the lower is end-tidal carbon dioxide concentration from 0–10%. The changes in blood pressure are quite clearly seen to be accompanied by parallel changes in end-tidal carbon dioxide concentration. The arterial to end-tidal gradients at the two times of sampling were 1.25 and 0.72 kPa respectively, giving alveolar dead space ratios of 24% during the hypotension and 13.5% at the higher blood pressure.

The Effects of Drugs on the Pulmonary Circulation

Finally, it is appropriate to ask whether individual para-anaesthetic drugs or anaesthetic agents themselves exert any specific and significant effects on the pulmonary circulation of intact animals or man. There is litle work on this because firstly, before any phenomenon can be demonstrated to have an active vasomotor effect on the pulmonary circulation it must be proved to act independently of changes in the systemic circulation and of changes in respiration. Ideally flow and respiratory tract pressure should be constant when drugs are assessed. Having achieved this, if possible, measurements of changes in vascular tone require that the pressure drop across the pulmonary circuit be measured. Pulmonary arterial pressure is of course easy to obtain by cathcterization, i.e., persuading the catheter to traverse the tricuspid and pulmonary valves. This is relatively easy as the catheter travels with the blood stream. However, the distal part of the circuit cannot be approached with such ease. Left heart catheterization is carried out against the blood stream and it is virtually impossible to persuade the tip of a catheter through the mitral valve. There are several manoeuvres for obtaining access to the left atrium—sometimes it can be entered through a patent foramen ovale from the right atrium; alternatively the atrial septum can be deliberately breached by a trans-septal puncture from the right atrium; when it is absolutely necessary more heroic procedures can be adopted; for example, puncture at the sternal notch and successive puncture of aorta, pulmonary artery and then left atrium; percutaneous puncture of the left ventricle and then a transmitral approach; an endobronchial approach; or finally a percutaneous approach from the rear. Of course, none of these can be justified, for the purposes of research in the human subject. Recourse is usually made to a wedged pulmonary artery catheter. It is considered that as no flow past the wedged catheter can occur, the

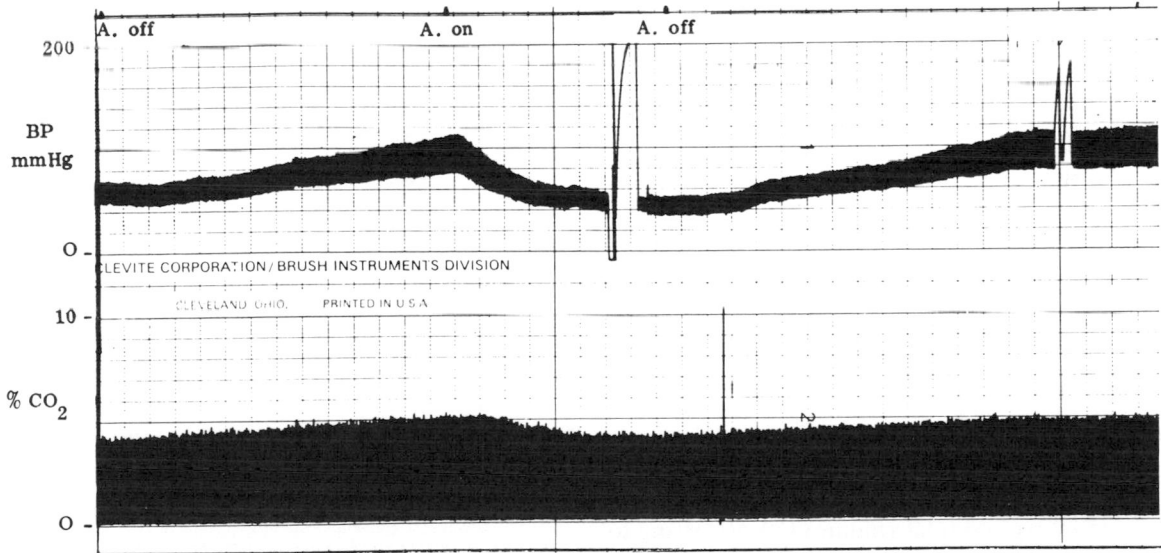

Fig. 16.9 Record of intra-arterial blood pressure (upper trace) and end-tidal carbon-dioxide (lower trace) during induced hypotension by trimetaphan (arfonad) in a male patient aged 45 during controlled ventilation with nitrous oxide/oxygen and trichlorethylene. 'A off' and 'A on' denote stopping and starting the arfonad infusion. The two interruptions in the arterial tracing represent times when arterial blood was sampled. The time scale is one minute per division. Blood pressure changes are clearly paralleled by changes in the end-tidal carbon dioxide concentration. The a-ETpP$_{CO_2}$ gradients at times of sampling were 9.0 and 5.4 mmHg respectively; the ratios of $V_{D\,ALV}/V_E$ were 24% during the hypotension and 13.5% at the higher blood pressure.

static column of blood ahead of the catheter is in continuity with the left atrium and therefore accurately reflects the left atrial pressure. However, this technique is very liable to artefacts and some workers prefer to use the left ventricular end-diastolic pressure.

Since the pressure gradient across the pulmonary circuit is very small, any errors in measurement will grossly effect the calculated derived resistance. High fidelity measurements and careful technique are thus required. Both the controlled conditions required and the measurements indicated are virtually impossible to achieve, especially during clinical anaesthesia itself. Although drugs can be shown to effect the pulmonary artery calibre, it seems certain that these are overriden by the systemic effects of cardiac output, or by the effects of P_{O_2} on pulmonary vascular tone.

Summary

As the pulmonary circuit is in series, the flow through it is governed by events in the systemic circulation. Its function is gaseous exchange and the low resistance in the circuit is subservient to this function. Regional flow is affected by the passive hydrostatic effects due to gravity, and by the active, probably humorally mediated, effects of the intra-alveolar oxygen tension, although excessive oxygen is toxic to the alveolar capillary membrane.

When perfusion is wasted there is a shunt effect which can be evaluated by the alveolar to arterial oxygen tension gradient, and when perfusion is reduced there is a dead space effect which can be evaluated by the arterial to end-tidal carbon dioxide gradient. As far as the state of anaesthesia is concerned, there is a partially explained increase in alveolar to arterial O_2 gradient in association with that state. Changes in dead space are associated with the low cardiac output state of induced hypotension. Specific effects of individual agents on the pulmonary circulation are difficult to measure and probably masked under clinical conditions by systemic events.

APPENDIX

Solution of the Ventilation/Perfusion Model

Ventilation

Solution of the ventilation compartments of the model usually consists of deriving the ratio of each subdivision to expired tidal volume (V_E). Referring to Fig. 16.4,

$$V_{D\,ALV} + V_{D\,ANAT} = V_{D\,PHYS}$$
$$\text{and, } V_{D\,PHYS} + V_A = V_E$$

The full interrelationship between these quantities may be expressed with reference to the gas R line in an O_2/CO_2 diagram (Fig. 16.10).

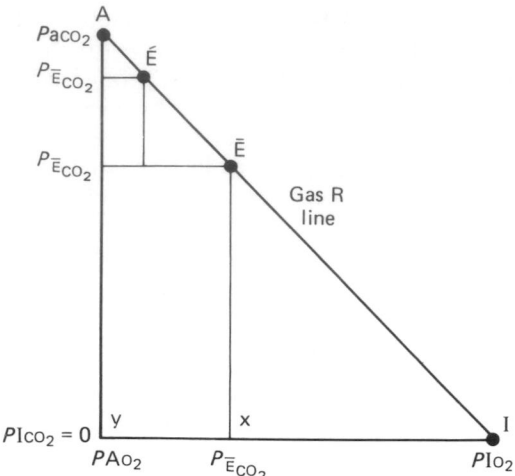

Fig. 16.10 Geometric interrelationship of the respiratory gases in the O_2-CO_2 diagram (Abscissa = P_{O_2} ordinate = P_{CO_2}).
A = ideal alveolar gas. É = end-tidal gas. Ē = mixed expired gas. I = inspired gas. $Pa_{CO_2} = P_{A_{CO_2}}$. AI is the gas R line. For further explanations *see* text.

In this diagram AI is the gas R line and,

$$A\bar{E} \propto V_{D\,PHYS}$$
$$A\acute{E} \propto V_{D\,ALV}$$
$$\acute{E}\bar{E} \propto V_{D\,ANAT}$$
$$\bar{E}I \propto V_A$$
$$\text{and, } AI \propto V_E$$

As can be seem, the co-ordinates of these defined points make up a series of similar triangles. Since, in similar triangles, the ratios of any pair of similar sides are equal, derivation of the various equations is easy (Leigh and Tyrrell). Thus:

$$\frac{V_D}{V_E} = \frac{A\bar{E}}{AI} = \frac{Pa_{CO_2} - P\bar{E}_{CO_2}}{Pa_{CO_2}} \quad \text{(Bohr equation)}$$

$$\frac{V_{D\,ALV}}{V_E} = \frac{A\acute{E}}{AI} = \frac{Pa_{CO_2} - P\acute{E}_{CO_2}}{Pa_{CO_2}}$$

$$\frac{V_{D\,ANAT}}{V_E} = \frac{\acute{E}\bar{E}}{AI} = \frac{P\acute{E}_{CO_2} - P\bar{E}_{CO_2}}{Pa_{CO_2}}$$

$$\frac{V_A}{V_E} = \frac{\bar{E}I}{AI} = \frac{P\bar{E}_{CO_2}}{Pa_{CO_2}} \quad \text{(Farhi equation)}$$

The following measurements are required:

Pa_{CO_2}, using a direct-reading electrode or interpolation from pH.

$P\bar{E}_{CO_2}$, measured on expired gas (collected classically through a one-way valve into a Douglas bag) with a direct reading electrode, Haldane apparatus or infrared CO_2 analyser.

$P\acute{E}_{CO_2}$, measured during tidal expiration using the writeout from an infrared CO_2 analyser for accuracy.

To convert percentage CO_2 to tension multiply by (barometric pressure $-47)/100$.

Finally if V_E is measured, then the ventilation model can be fully quantitated.

High frequency ventilation: The interpretation of the mechanics of high frequency ventilation in terms of the ventilation model seems at first to be difficult. However, if the arterial CO_2 level can be measured and CO_2 production obtained by collection of expired gas, then the model can be solved to determine the effective alveolar ventilation using the classical alveolar air equation

$$F_{A_{CO_2}} = F_{I_{CO_2}} + \frac{\dot{V}_{CO_2}}{\dot{V}_A}$$

Ideal Alveolar Oxygen Tension

The ideal alveolar oxygen tension ($P_{A_{O_2}}$) is the key figure in the ventilation/perfusion model as it is assumed to exist both in the V_A compartment and the Q_C compartment. The equation for its calculation may be easily obtained from Fig. 16.10.

$$\frac{Iy}{Ix} = \frac{AI}{\bar{E}I}$$

$$\frac{P_{I_{O_2}} - P_{A_{O_2}}}{P_{I_{O_2}} - P_{\bar{E}_{O_2}}} = \frac{P_{a_{CO_2}}}{P_{\bar{E}_{CO_2}}}$$

$$\therefore \quad P_{A_{O_2}} = P_{I_{O_2}} - P_{a_{CO_2}} \left(\frac{P_{I_{O_2}} - P_{\bar{E}_{O_2}}}{P_{\bar{E}_{CO_2}}} \right)$$

(Nunn equation)

In addition to the measurements mentioned above the following are required: $P_{I_{O_2}}$ and $P_{\bar{E}_{O_2}}$; these can be measured directly by polarographic electrode, or by Haldane apparatus or paramagnetic oxygen analyser. Both the latter give $O_2\%$ which requires conversion to tension.

Perfusion

Quantitating the perfusion part of the model involves solution of the *shunt equation*, which may be derived as follows:

Referring to Fig. 16.4, $Qt = Qc + Qs$,

and, since $\qquad Qc = Qt - Qs$

$\therefore \qquad\qquad Qt = (Qt - Qs) + Qs$

The oxygen flow through these compartments is:

$$Qt \cdot Ca_{O_2} = (Qt - Qs)C\acute{c}_{O_2} + Qs \cdot C\bar{v}_{O_2}$$

(where C = content; $\acute{c}$ = end-pulmonary capillary; $\bar{v}$ = mixed venous)

$\therefore \quad Qt \cdot Ca_{O_2} = Qt \cdot C\acute{c}_{O_2} - Qs \cdot C\acute{c}_{O_2} + Qs \cdot C\bar{v}_{O_2}$

$\therefore \quad Qt(Ca_{O_2} - C\acute{c}_{O_2}) = Qs(C\bar{v}_{O_2} - C\acute{c}_{O_2})$

$$\therefore \quad \frac{Qs}{Qt} = \frac{Ca_{O_2} - C\acute{c}_{O_2}}{C\bar{v}_{O_2} - C\acute{c}_{O_2}}$$

which may be rewritten:

$$\frac{Qs}{Qt} = \frac{C\acute{c}_{O_2} - Ca_{O_2}}{C\acute{c}_{O_2} - C\bar{v}_{O_2}}$$

Ca_{O_2} is measured on arterial blood; $C\bar{v}_{O_2}$ is strictly only measurable on blood obtained from the pulmonary artery. These content measurements in ml $O_2/100$ ml blood can be made by chemical and volumetric methods (e.g. on a Van Slyke's apparatus), by gas chromatography, by derivation from saturation measurements (oximetry) or from P_{O_2} (polarography). Both the latter have to be converted to content assuming a normal saturation curve.

End-pulmonary capillary blood cannot, of course, be sampled but the basic assumption of the model is that this blood is in equilibrium with ideal alveolar gas. The ideal alveolar oxygen tension ($P_{A_{O_2}}$) is therefore calculated from the Nunn equation and thence $C\acute{c}_{O_2}$ assuming a normal saturation curve. Finally, the Qs/Qt ratio can be obtained and the normal value is less than 0.04 (4%). If the cardiac output is also measured, Qs can be fully quantitated.

REFERENCES

Alexander J.I., Horton P.W., Miller W.T., et al. (1972). The effect of upper abdominal surgery on the relationships of airway closing point to end tidal position. *Clin. Sci.*, **43**, 137.

Assali N.S., Morris J.A., Smith R.W., et al. (1963). Studies on ductus arteriosus circulation. *Circ. Res.*, **13**, 478.

Bakhle Y.S., Ferreira S.H. (1985). Lung metabolism of cicosanoids: prostaglandins, prostacyclin, thromboxane and leukotrienes. *Handb. Physiol. Section 3*, **1**, 365.

Barer, G. (1966). Reactivity of vessels of collapsed and ventilated lungs to drugs and hypoxia. *Circ. Res.*, **18**, 366.

Born G.V.R., Dawes G.S., Mott J.C., et al. (1956). The constriction of the ductus arteriosus caused by oxygen and by asphyxia in newborn lambs. *J. Physiol.*, **132**, 304.

Burghuber O.C. (1987). Nifedipine attenuates acute hypoxic pulmonary vasoconstriction in patients with chronic obstructive pulmonary disease. *Respir.*, **52**, 86.

Davis A.G., Spence A.A. (1972). Postoperative hypoxaemia and age. *Anesthesiology*, **37**, 663.

Fick A. (1870). Uber die Messung des Blutquantums in den Herzventrikeln. *Sitsungsb. der phys-med Ges. zu Wurzburg.* **XIV**, XVI.

Harris P., Heath D. (1986). *The Human Pulmonary Circulation*. London: Churchill Livingstone.

Harvey W. (1628) *Exercitatio de Motu Cordis et Sanguinis.* Trans. K.J. Franklin (1957). Springfield, Illinois: Thomas.

Hauge A. (1968). Role of histamine in hypoxic pulmonary hypertension in the rat: I. blockade or potentiation of endogenous amines, kinins and ATP. *Circ. Res.*, **22**, 371.

Hauge A., Melmon K.L. (1968). Role of histamine in hypoxic pulmonary hypertension in the rat: II. depletion of histamine, serotonin and catecholamines. *Circ. Res.*, **22**, 385.

Hughes J.M.B., Glazier J.B., Maloney J.E., et al. (1968). Effect of lung volume on the distribution of pulmonary blood flow in man. *Resp. Physiol.*, **4**, 58.

Leigh J.M., Tyrell M.F. Unpublished observations.

Leigh J.M., Smethurst P.W.R. Unpublished observations.

Liebow A.A. (1962). Recent advances in pulmonary anatomy. In: *Pulmonary Structure and Function.* p. 2. London: J.A. Churchill.

Lloyd T.C. (1967). Influence of P_{O_2} and pH on resting and active tensions of pulmonary arterial strips. *J. Appl. Physiol.*, **22**, 1101.

Lower R. (1669). *Tractatus de Corde.* Trans. K.J. Franklin in R.T. Gunther's *Early Science in Oxford* (1932). Vol. IX. Oxford: Oxford University Press.

Lundholm L., Mohme-Lundholm E. (1963). Dissociation of contraction and stimulation of lactic acid production in experiments on smooth muscle under anaerobic condition. *Acta Physiol. Scand.*, **57**, 111.

Nunn J.F. (1987). *Applied Respiratory Physiology.* London: Butterworths.

Saidman L.J., Eger E.I. (1967). The influence of ventilation/ perfusion abnormalities upon the uptake of inhalation anaesthetics. In: *Clinical Anaesthesia. Lung Disease.* p. 79. Oxford: Blackwell.

Sobol B.J., Bottex G., Emirgil C., et al. (1963). Gaseous diffusion from alveoli to pulmonary vessels of considerable size. *Circ. Res.*, **13**, 71.

Spence A.A., Alexander J.I. (1972). Mechanisms of postoperative hypoxaemia. *Proc. Roy. Soc. Med.*, **65**, 12.

Sykes M.K., Adams A.P., Finlay W.E.I., et al. (1970). The cardiorespiratory effects of haemorrhage and overtransfusion in dogs. *Brit. J. Anaesth.*, **42**, 573.

Sykes M.K., Davies D.M., Chakrabarti M.K., et al. (1973). The effect of inhalational anaesthetic agents on the pulmonary vasculature of the isolated perfused cat lung. *Brit. J. Anaesth.*, **45**, 114.

Tobin C.E. (1966). Arteriovenous shunts in the peripheral pulmonary circulation in the human lung. *Thorax*, **21**, 197.

Von Euler U.S., Liljestrand G. (1946). Observations of the pulmonary artery blood pressure in the cat. *Acta Physiol. Scand.*, **12**, 301.

17. Fluid Dynamics of the Cerebral Circulation

P. J. A. Lesser and J. Gareth Jones

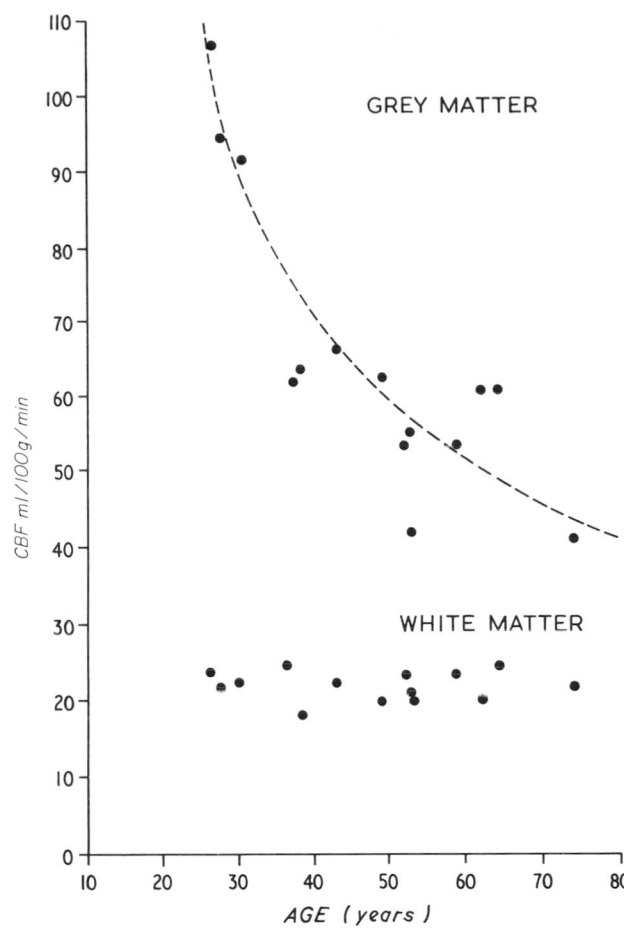

Fig. 17.1 Regional cerebral blood flow (rCBF) decreases with age in grey tissue while remaining constant in white tissue. (Modified from Frackowiak et al., 1980.)

CEREBRAL BLOOD FLOW AND METABOLISM OF THE BRAIN

It is an extraordinary fact that resting normal young adults have an almost identical mean cerebral blood flow (CBF) of 50 ml/100 g of brain/min. Although the mean CBF shows a decrease with age of the order of 0.5% per year, it is otherwise independent of gender, race, country, climate, or of the method used to measure CBF. It must be noted that this mean value lumps together the quite different blood flows in grey and white cerebral tissue of about 70 and 20 ml/(100 g · min) respectively. The oxygen consumption of grey tissue is about 6 ml/(100 g · min) and white tissue about 2 ml/(100 g · min). Blood flow shows an age related reduction in grey, but remains constant in white tissue (Fig. 17.1). This chapter is concerned with the factors that maintain such a constant CBF, the anaesthetic factors which may influence CBF and the measurement of CBF in man and experimental animals.

In most organs there is a tight coupling between metabolic demand and blood flow. This is certainly true for different parts of the brain where there is a close dependency of regional CBF (rCBF) on the regional metabolic rate (rCMR). One example of this close link between flow and metabolism is the effect of spontaneous movement of one arm which immediately enhances the rCBF in the contralateral Rolandic region. The development of positron emission tomography (PET) produced further evidence of the normally close coupling of flow/metabolism showing that mental activity caused an increase in both rCBF and rCMR, there being marked differences between the right and left hemispheres. This close coupling of flow/metabolism may be disrupted by a number of factors such as head injury and epilepsy. Volatile anaesthetics, particularly halothane, produce a fall in rCMR, but a considerable rise in rCBF. Tumours are hyperaemic, but their flow is not coupled to metabolism.

FLUID MECHANICS

Cerebral Arterial System

The pattern branching of small intracerebral vessels avoids the transmission of high arterial pressure onto the capillary bed. A topological approach is used to analyse the complex branching geometry and haemodynamics in pial branches (30–320 μm in diameter) of the middle cerebral arteries (Hudetz et al., 1987). This shows that the greatest resistance occurs in proximal vessels greater than 100 μm in diameter. Resistance (R) is calculated using the Poiseuille equation:

$$R \propto \frac{\eta l}{\pi d^4}$$

where n = viscosity of blood, l = length and d = the diameter of the vessel. This expression shows how quite small changes in diameter of small vessels produce vast changes in resistance and emphasizes how factors which change the tone of vascular smooth muscle can readily alter rCBF.

The concept of Poiseuille flow is not applicable at very low rates of shear in microvessels whose diameters are similar to those of red cells or under low flow conditions during incomplete occlusions. Traditional studies with the cone and plate viscometer assume that the relative viscosity of blood may increase by as much as a hundredfold at these very low shear rates. However in the microcirculation, red cells migrate from the wall where the shear rate is maximal, towards the centre of the vessel where the shear rate is zero. This gives a reduction rather than a large increase of relative viscosity for blood flowing in the microcirculation. This is called the Fahraeus-Lindqvist effect, but as the capillary radius falls towards that of the red cell, there is an abrupt rise in relative viscosity.

There is an optimum haematocrit of 0.42 which is associated with an optimum cerebral oxygen delivery (Hudetz et al., 1987). A change in haematocrit from this optimum value causes a change in CBF due to autoregulation. However, if the vessels are already fully dilated in hypoperfused tissue, there is a *reduction* in oxygen delivery if haematocrit is reduced (Gaehtgens and Marx, 1987).

Venous System

Most of the adult intracranial blood volume of 200 ml is contained in the venous sinuses and pial veins. With an increase in intracranial pressure (ICP), the thin walled venous system is compressed and the cerebral blood volume (CBV) and the cerebrospinal fluid (CSF) volume are both reduced. Measurement of ICP is nowadays an important part of the monitoring of the brain. When 1 ml of saline is injected and the change in ICP is measured, the compliance of the intracranial contents can be derived from:

$$\text{Compliance} = \frac{\text{increase in volume}}{\text{increase in ICP}} = \frac{\Delta V}{\Delta P}$$

An instructive hydraulic model of the intracranial venous system employs the Starling resistor. This is a collapsible tube surrounded by a fluid filled rigid container in which the pressure external to the tube can be made to exceed the tube luminal pressure at the outflow end. With a brisk flow through the tube, a slow infusion of fluid into the chamber produces a nonlinear increase of chamber pressure which causes an abrupt fall of tube flow as the downstream end of the tube collapses. Injection into the chamber then further compresses the Starling resistor with continued reduction in flow.

This system models the intracranial pressure response to an ever increasing intracranial tissue volume and causes progressive collapse of a hierarchy of compressible structures. Thus the compression of the cerebral veins by progressive cerebral oedema depends on (1) venous volume, (2) systemic arterial pressure, (3) CSF volume and (4) sagittal sinus pressure, all of which are probed by measurements of intracranial compliance.

The mechanics of autoregulation can be modelled by two resistances in series, with a capacitance element added (Fig. 17.2). The autonomic nervous system regulates the large extraparenchymal vessels in series with the small intraparenchymal vessels, which are regulated by intrinsic metabolic or myogenic mechanisms. Effects on one element may be masked by compensatory changes in the other.

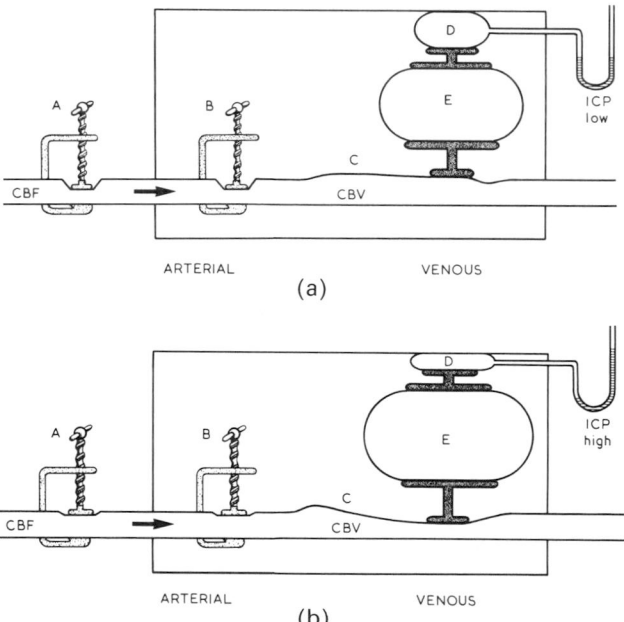

Fig. 17.2 (a) Normal cerebral state. (b) Brain swelling and arterial vasodilatation; decreased CBF, CBV, increased ICP. A = large extracerebral; B = small intracerebral resistance vessels; C = capacitance vessels (Starling resistor); D = displaceable skull contents (cerebrospinal fluid, brain water); E = non-displaceable skull contents (brain, meninges). These variables may be manipulated independently.

Fluid Balance in the Microcirculation

In vascular beds other than those in the brain, the capillary endothelium presents a semipermeable barrier of varying degrees of leakiness to hydrophilic macromolecules such as albumin (mol.wt. 65 000 daltons). In contrast, the endothelium of the cerebral vessels is remarkably non-leaky, even to very small molecules (e.g., mannitol, mol.wt. 180 daltons) because of the high resistance tight junctions between endothelial cells. Solutes with high lipid solubility can penetrate the barrier and non-lipid soluble molecules may enter and leave the interstitial space of the brain via a number of active transport systems.

The unique properties of the vascular junctions are due to factors secreted by the brain itself. If normal, leaky capillaries from the gut are implanted into the brain they will develop the same impermeable blood barrier as the normal cerebral vessels. Note that the blood brain barrier and the blood-cerebrospinal fluid barrier are two independent barriers, the former having a surface area 5000 times greater than the latter.

The barrier properties are remarkably resistant to the effects of cerebral ischaemia; days or weeks may elapse after cerebrovascular occlusion before the barrier breaks down. This explains why mannitol can be used to reduce cerebral oedema for a considerable time after the initiation of brain injury (Cook et al., 1989).

REGULATION OF CBF

Cerebral blood flow is regulated to satisfy the metabolic requirements of brain tissue under a range of physiological circumstances. This process of *autoregulation* may be disturbed by pathological or non-physiological events such as brain injury, changes in blood gas tensions or the administration of anaesthetic drugs. When some regions of brain have pathologically non-reactive vasculature, the *steal phenomenon* is found. Reactive vasculature dilates to take flow preferentially away from the pathological area. Conversely in inverse steal, the reactive brain is vasoconstricted, diverting flow to the diseased area.

Autonomic Influences

The autonomic nervous system regulates the calibre of the carotid, vertebral and basilar arteries and major trunks of the middle and anterior cerebral arteries. In contrast, changes in the calibre of smaller intracerebral vessels depend on the metabolism of surrounding tissue. The net effect of a catecholamine is the summation of direct α and β receptor stimulation plus sympathetic perivascular innervation. For example, if a catecholamine is injected intravenously, it does not cross the blood brain barrier, and does not affect small resistance vessels (Tuor and McCulloch, 1986). Nevertheless, there are also β mediated effects on metabolism and thus indirectly on flow.

Receptors

β_1 receptors are relaxant and α_2 constrictors. A large number of neurotransmitters affect the cerebral vasculature. Their effects may be direct and non-synaptic. Intact endothelium is necessary for bradykinin and acetylcholine to produce vasodilatation (Verrechia et al., 1986).

The cervical sympathetic ganglia (Sadoshima et al., 1986), are involved in autoregulation. Sympathetic stimulation constricts cerebral vessels (Alafaci et al., 1986) and shifts the pressure autoregulation curve to the right (Lacombe et al., 1986). This protects the brain and blood brain barrier against a cerebral perfusion pressure (CPP) above the normal upper limit of autoregulation by decreasing high blood flows (Lacombe et al., 1986). Here CPP is defined as the difference between mean arterial pressure (MAP) and either the jugular venous or intracranial pressure (JVP or ICP), whichever is the greater. This is usually abbreviated to CPP = MAP—ICP. All pressures including MAP should be measured at the head rather than the heart level. In haemorrhagic hypotension, the sympathetic tone mediated by α_2 receptors produces vasoconstriction and reduces CBF inappropriately. This is particularly significant in head injured hypovolaemic patients suffering pain, who will have both a low CPP and sympathetically mediated cerebral vasoconstriction combining to impair blood flow.

Pressure Autoregulation

CBF is usually independent of CPP between 60–130 mmHg MAP in normal man (McDowall, 1985). A series of autoregulation curves are shown in Fig. 17.3 in normotensive and hypertensive subjects. Different regions of the brain have different ranges of autoregulation (Sadoshima et al., 1986; Burke et al., 1987). Those with the narrowest range being regions which are vulnerable to haemorrhage (Burke et al., 1987). Cortical grey matter is particularly vulnerable as the pial resistance vessels are furthest upstream and thus the microvascular pressure is higher. The vessels in the spinal cord have a similar autoregulation and CO_2 reactivity to those in the brain (Porter et al., 1985).

It is interesting to note that symptoms of brain hypoperfusion in awake subjects appear at MAPs of about 60% of the lower limit of autoregulation (Strandgaard, 1976).

Chronic hypertension resets the autoregulation curve to the right (Fig. 17.3). Treatment in some cases eventually returns the curve to the left, though some individuals will not reset their curve (Strandgaard, 1976). Autoregulation is not an instantaneous process and may take several minutes to have effect. There have been cases reported of a rapid reduction of blood pressure to 'normal' levels in less than 2 h, resulting in the death of hypertensive patients. Long-term antihypertensive treatment does not decrease CBF (Ram et

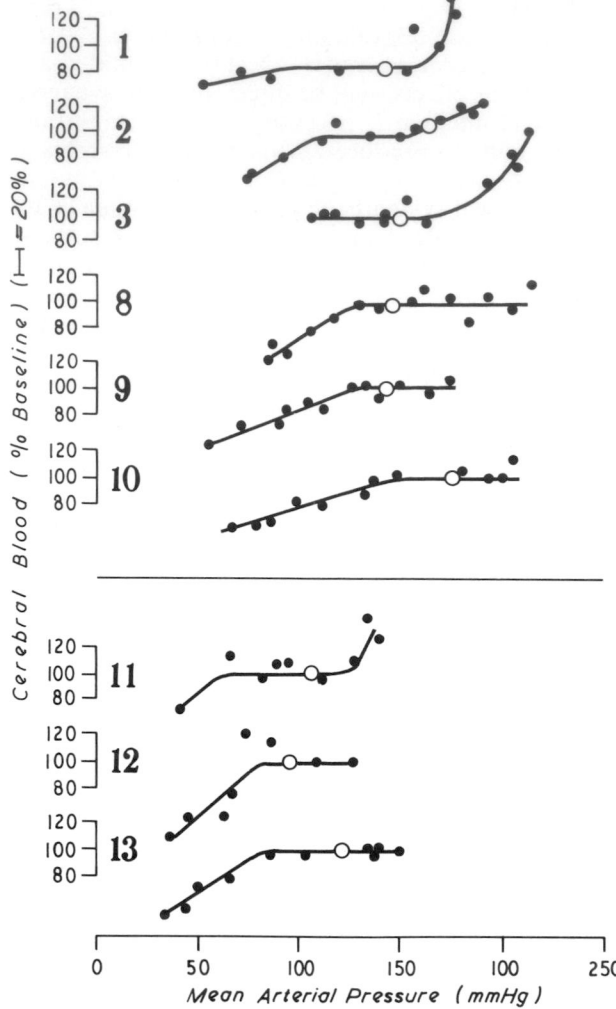

Fig. 17.3 Autoregulation curves. Hypertensive patients above the horizontal line and normotensive patients below. These curves illustrate the shift to the right with chronic hypertension. The dissimilarity to the common idealized curve is evident. Open circles represent an estimate of habitual MAP. (Modified from Strandgaard et al., 1973.)

al., 1987) and can actually increase it due to decreasing cerebrovascular resistance (Meyer et al., 1985).

Plateau waves seen on the ICP trace, lasting many minutes, can be precipitated by a fall in CPP, for example by elevating the head of the bed. Plateau waves are a result of at least partially intact autoregulation compensating for the decreased CPP by vasodilatation. This increases ICP and decreases CPP further in a positive feedback loop until brainstem ischaemia produces a rise in MAP, or MAP is raised therapeutically to abort the plateau wave (Rosner and Becker, 1984).

Local Factors Affecting Flow

Carbon dioxide and oxygen tensions, metabolism, the pH of extracellular fluid (ECF), temperature, haematocrit and viscosity have all been shown to affect CBF. These can be viewed as different facets of metabolic equilibrium. Non-physiological intervention affects the balance. For example, an increase in inspired CO_2 concentration will release ECF pH and P_{CO_2} from the constraints of substrate supply and lactate production.

Carbon Dioxide

CBF is proportional to arterial and venous P_{CO_2} (Wilson et al., 1985) subject to the upper limit of maximal vasodilatation and the lower limit of vasoconstriction beyond which tissue hypoxia would result. Although the relationship between CBF and P_{CO_2} is said to be linear, a logarithmic curve produces a better fit. The effects of CO_2 on vessel calibre are mediated locally rather than by the brainstem (Wilson et al., 1985). The effect of CO_2 on the cerebrovascular circulation is transient and blood flow returns to pre-existing levels within a few hours mediated by the pH of ECF. Some concepts of the management of head injured patients assume that the benefits of ICP reduction by hyperventilation are maintained for a prolonged period. It is apparent that *some individuals have a very transient response*, lasting less than 90 min, while others have a longer lasting response. The distinction must be made between ventilation for the purpose of avoiding hypoxaemia and hyperventilation for the primary purpose of brain shrinkage, which may well be temporary in effect and be accompanied by an opposite effect on cerebral fluid dynamics at the termination of hyperventilation. This is not to say that hyperventilation is undesirable, but that its limitations must be realized.

Oxygen

Cerebral blood flow is inversely proportional to oxygen concentration (Ca_{O_2}, as is apparent in Fig. 17.4a. By modifying this data to take the sigmoid dissociation curve into account and taking the reciprocal, the more familiar relationship between Pa_{O_2} and CBF is seen, as in Fig. 17.4b and Ca_{O_2} is the main factor (Brown et al., 1985). Hypoxic vasodilatation overrides hypocapnic vasoconstriction (Hansen et al., 1986). Haematocrit affects viscosity and Ca_{O_2} and although a change in haematocrit produces a proportional change in CBF, it is difficult to isolate the influences of haematocrit, viscosity and Ca_{O_2} on autoregulation. A change in CBF due to an alteration of haematocrit is likely to be mediated predominantly (56–100%) by the change in vascular resistance to maintain a constant oxygen delivery and minimally by rheological factors (Hudak et al., 1986). Thus autoregulation by C_{O_2} is the main factor (Brown et al., 1985).

Metabolism

There is a close correlation between glucose utiliza-

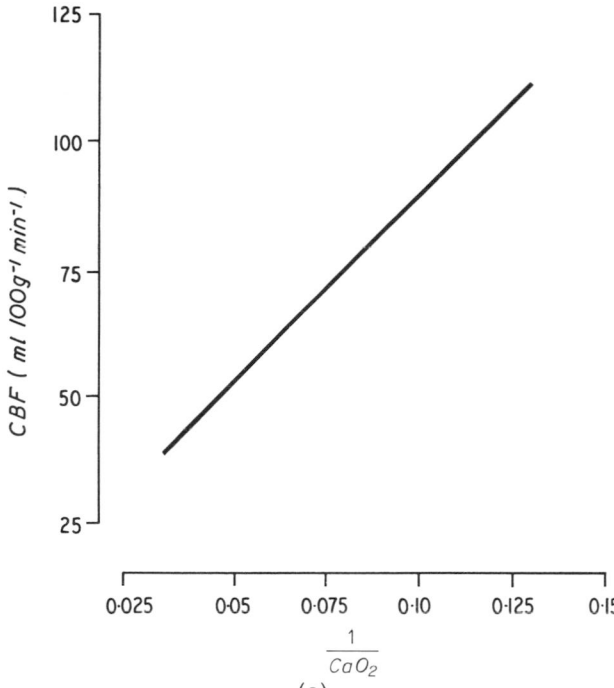

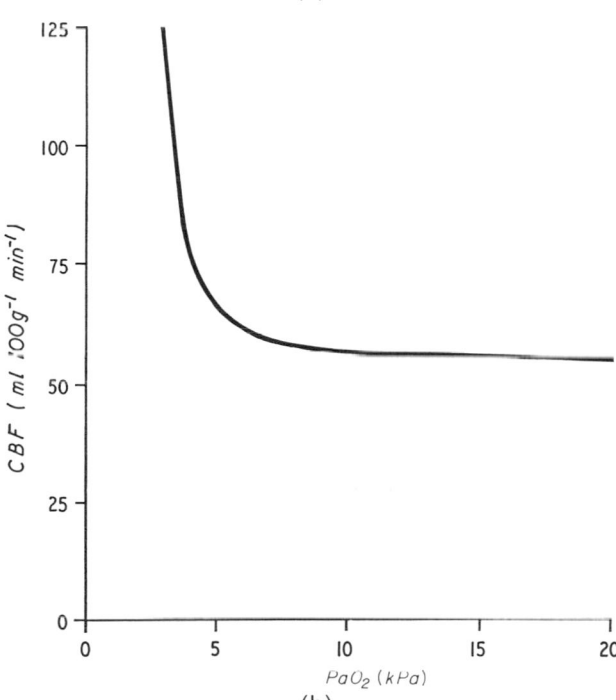

Fig. 17.4 (a) CBF is inversely proportional to Ca_{O_2}. (Data from Brown et al., 1985, Fig. 2.) (b) Replotting the straight line in (a) by applying a sigmoid O_2 dissociation curve and taking the reciprocal, produces the more familiar asymptotic curve of Pa_{O_2} vs CBF which disguises the dependence of CBF on Ca_{O_2}.

tion and local CBF (Gaehtgens and Marx, 1987). Tissue alkalosis may increase glycolytic rate and thus increase lactate even in the absence of ischaemia.

The above variables probably all act locally (Wilson et al., 1985; Brown et al., 1985), through a common pathway involving ECF, pH and ATP.

CEREBRAL ISCHAEMIA

Ischaemia describes a continuum between normal cell function and cell death. There are thresholds of flow assuming normally oxygenated blood below which cellular processes are no longer able to continue.

Electrical activity of the brain diminishes when rCBF is reduced below 20 ml/(100 g · min), membrane failure and cell death occurring when rCBF reaches 10 ml/(100 g · min). Values of rCBF which fall for minutes or hours into the range of 10–20 ml/(100 g · min) are associated with reversible neurological deficits. These thresholds are not uniform throughout the brain (Symon, 1985), though possibly, in terms of supply and demand, they may be more homogenous. The cortex in particular requires a high flow. Generally, thresholds may be considered to be as in Table 17.1.

TABLE 17.1
RELATIONSHIP BETWEEN CEREBRAL BLOOD FLOW ACTIVITY
AND ION HOMEOSTATIS

	CBF ml/(100 g · min)
Change in electrical activity	20–23
Loss of electrical activity and oedema formation	12–17
Loss of ionic homeostasis with initial maintenance of energy (ATP) stores	8–10
Ultimately cell death Recovery is inversely related to duration	<8

(From Symon, 1985; Olsen, 1986)

Ionic homeostasis is lost if flows fall below 10 ml/(100 g · min), though at this flow ATP levels are close to normal and some energy is still available for ion pumping. Flow thresholds for disruption of K^+ and Ca^{2+} are not simultaneous. First extracellular K^+ (K^+e) rises, then as the process of ionic disruption continues, extracellular Ca^{2+} ($Ca^{2+}e$ falls. Homeostasis fails due to overload of the clearance mechanisms and falling ATP levels. Cell death is mediated by high intracellular Ca^{2+} stimulating phospholipase A2. This is modified by Ca^{2+} influx being decreased by a low $Ca^{2+}e$. Ca^{2+} channel blockers have been used successfully in animals and humans to reduce brain injury, but their place is uncertain (Symon, 1985). It has now become clear that the response of cerebral neurons to *acute short-term ischaemia* is too complex to be described by simple threshold concepts. Using PET scans in patients with chronic occlusive cerebrovascular disease (Powers et al., 1985) an rCBF of 19 ml/(100 g · min) is adequate to maintain normal cerebral function and a rCBF of 15 ml/(100 g·min) is adequate for tissue viability. However, these are amalgamated values for grey and white tissue and the minimum grey flow is certainly higher than 15 ml/(100 g·min). Values of rCMRO$_2$ as low as 1.3 ml/(100 g·min) were sufficient to sustain cerebral function, whereas values of rCMRO$_2$ less than 1.3 ml/(100 g·min) implied irreversible infarction. The ratio of CBF to CMRO$_2$ in normal subjects and those with transient cerebral ischaemia was 16, in patients with reversible ischaemic neurological defects 11, and in infarction was 27, a considerable increase of the normally high ratio of perfusion to metabolism.

Autoregulation is lost in ischaemic brains (Muizelaar et al., 1986) and metabolism/flow coupling is lost after severe head injury (Cold, 1986), the loss of coupling has been related to poorer outcome. CMRO$_2$ is not reduced in hypotension producing mild ischaemia (Strandgaard, 1976).

The question of increasing the tolerance of brain cells to reduced perfusion has been the subject of intensive study. The effect of *hypothermia* in reducing cerebral metabolism and thus the tolerance to reduced perfusion is now well established. The effects of various *anaesthetics*, particularly barbiturates, in increasing tolerance to ischaemia has been more controversial. Michenfelder and Theye, (1975) have made the important distinction between the basal metabolism of neuronal cells and the metabolism for specialized neuronal function. Hypothermia reduces the metabolism of both components, whereas anaesthetics reduce only that for specialized function leaving basal metabolism unchanged. Thus the effects of hypothermia and general anaesthesia could not be equated. Nevertheless there is now evidence that sodium thiopentone therapy, in selected high risk patients undergoing cardiopulmonary bypass, will improve the outcome in terms of neurological benefit (Nussmeier et al., 1986). Barbiturates and probably propofol reduce neurological damage in vascular occlusion (Maekawa et al., 1986) presumably by a metabolic effect, whereas volatiles increase infarct size (Maekawa et al., 1986) presumably due to steal (McDowall, 1985). Isoflurane induced hypotension has been reported to maintain a normal EEG down to flows just above 8 ml/(100 g·min) (Gibson et al., 1986).

Hyperglycaemia exacerbates neuronal injury in reversible brain ischaemia (Ginsberg et al., 1987; McDowall, 1985) because of the increased osmotic load due to anaerobic metabolism being facilitated. This produces more small molecular weight metabolites as well as causing acidosis. Preoperative fasting is thus beneficial in this respect. Conversely, hyperglycaemia is actually beneficial in thrombotic infarction and reduces infarct size (Ginsberg et al., 1987). Cimetidine blocks H2 mediated hypoxic vasodilatation and may be harmful (Clozel et al., 1985). Other mechanisms relevant to this problem of brain protection are beyond the brief for this chapter.

Mitochondria require 0.13–0.27 kPa of O$_2$ pressure. Some neurons exist in an environment of only 0.3 kPa O$_2$ pressure. Krogh in 1919 elaborated a cylindrical model of the territory around a capillary and the O$_2$ pressures available at a distance from the vessel. This has been modified, but the concept is still valid. The proportion of capillaries perfused in a vascular bed varies, rising from 50% at normoxia to 90% at an F_{IO_2} of 6% (Francois-Dainville et al., 1986). This increases blood flow and decreases the diffusion distance to any cell.

Some parts of the brain can function normally with a flow of 10–15 ml/(100 g·min), whereas boundary zones, i.e., the areas supplied by vessels at the edges of the territories of the main cerebral arteries, are particularly vulnerable to ischaemia (McDowall, 1985). The presence of arterial disease, the distance of a cell from an open capillary as well as the desaturation of the capillary blood are all influences which emphasize that local ischaemia may occur in the presence of apparently adequate global flow.

DRUG EFFECTS

Anaesthetic agents generally decrease cerebral metabolism and thus flow, though gaseous agents and ketamine have particular vasodilating effects which increase CBF thus compromising ICP.

Intravenous Agents

Thiopentone can reduce flow and metabolism to the absolute normothermic minimum during N$_2$O/halothane anaesthesia (Astrup et al., 1984). Care must be taken to maintain MAP, in order to optimize CBF and promote inverse steal.

Etomidate produces a dose dependent fall in CBF, CMRO$_2$, ICP, and EEG activity with a minimal fall in MAP, thus maintaining CPP, and CO$_2$ reactivity (Cold et al., 1986). An infusion of 60 μg/(kg·min), which is approximately four times the minimum infusion rate (MIR), produces metabolic supression comparable to barbiturates (Ginsberg et al., 1987). Unfortunately, its use by infusion is now prevented by an association with marked increases in mortality related to corticosteroid depletion. Recovery times were in any case undesirably long.

Propofol similarly appears to have a beneficial effect on ICP by reducing brain metabolism.

Ketamine is unusual as it increases CBF independently of metabolism, due to a cholinergic mechanism which is blocked by hyoscine (Reicher et al., 1987). There is thus a secondary increase in ICP which contraindicates its use in the cerebrally compromised patients. Midazolam and diazepam decrease CBF and CMRO$_2$ (Hoffman et al., 1986).

Muscle relaxants have no effect on CBF or cerebral metabolism (Rosa et al., 1986a, b), though there are theoretical considerations of histamine release and laudanosine excitation (Rosa et al., 1986a).

Gaseous Agents

Nitrous oxide increases cerebral metabolism and blood flow which complicates interpretation of studies which use N_2O concurrently with volatile agents (Hoffman et al., 1986; Manohar, 1985) (Fig. 17.5).

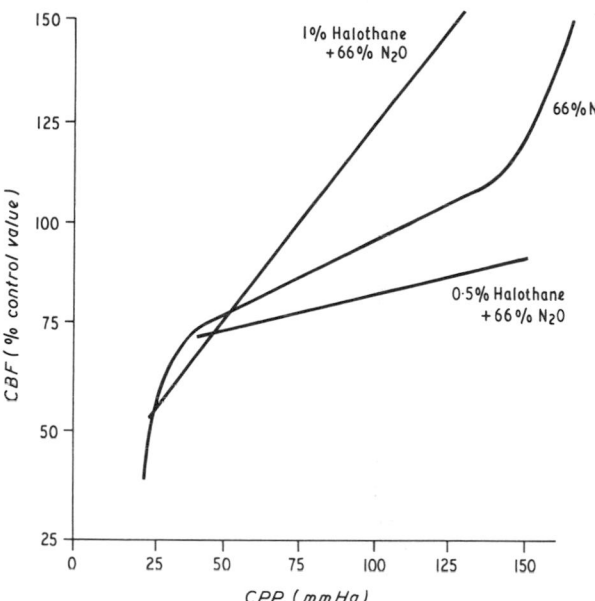

Fig. 17.5 The effect of nitrous oxide and halothane on autoregulation. Low concentrations of halothane reduce metabolism and thus flow. At higher concentrations the direct vasodilator action predominates. (Data from Morita et al., 1977.)

Volatile agents affect ICP, CBF, metabolism and autoregulation. The effects on CBF are a summation of flow/metabolism coupling, a direct effect of unknown mechanisms and the effects of other agents (Drummond et al., 1986). The smooth muscle relaxation and thus vasodilatation induced by halothane is mediated by cAMP and not affected by β blockade (Nikki et al., 1987). If metabolism is already maximally depressed, only this direct dilating effect, which is the same for halothane and isoflurane (Drummond et al., 1986) will be evident, thus diminishing the relative advantage of isoflurane in low metabolism states.

Autoregulation is abolished by 1 MAC of halothane or enflurane though a return to 0.5 MAC partially restores it (Miletich et al., 1976). Less than 0.5 MAC of halothane or enflurane does not affect autoregulation, whereas isoflurane up to 1 MAC, does not affect autoregulation although loss of autoregulation after cessation of 1.4 MAC anaesthesia persists for some time. Hypocarbia has a beneficial effect on autoregulation impaired by halothane (Miletich et al., 1976) (Fig. 17.6). Carbon dioxide reactivity is greater with isoflurane than halothane, which it is in turn greater than N_2O alone, so the consequences of

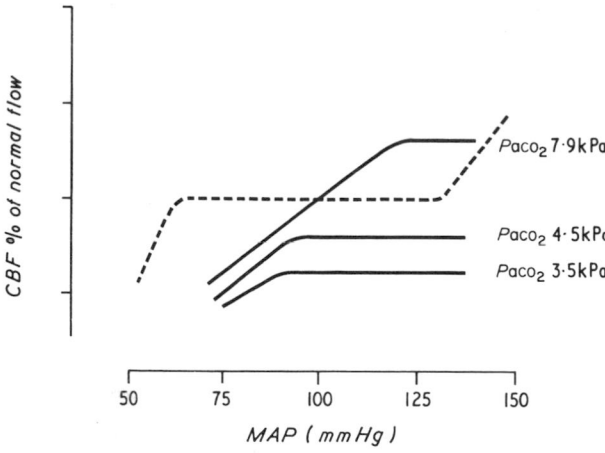

Fig. 17.6 Schematic representation of the changes in autoregulation caused by manipulating Pa_{CO_2} during 0.5 MAC halothane anaesthesia. Note the increase both in the minimal MAP at which autoregulation occurs as well as the actual flow when Pa_{CO_2} is raised. (Data from Miletich et al., 1976.)

hypercapnia are more pronounced with isoflurane than halothane (Eintrei et al., 1985). Anaesthesia with 1 MAC of halothane increases CBF at all levels of CO_2, including hypocapnia (Scheller et al., 1986). Halothane anaesthesia increases CO_2 reactivity as MAP falls which may be related to vessel wall tone (Lifson et al., 1985).

TABLE 17.2
CHANGE IN CBF WITH A TOTAL OF 1.5 MAC OF 70 PER CENT N_2O AND VOLATILE AGENT

Volatile	*Multiples of control values of CBF*
Halothane	2.66
Enflurane	1.35
Isoflurane	1.0

(From Eintrei et al., 1985)

The increased flow induced by halothane falls with time (Nikki et al., 1987). On 1% halothane, it takes more than 2.5 h to approach control levels (Albrecht et al., 1983).

Isoflurane is a vasoconstrictor below 0.95%. It does not change CMR glucose (CMRg) at up to 2 MAC (Maekawa et al., 1986), but decreases $CMRO_2$/flow coupling and $CMRO_2$. $CBF/CMRO_2$ is influenced favourably during isoflurane induced hypotension down to MAP 51 mmHg in humans (Newman et al., 1986). At similar pressures in dogs, cerebral energy state is maintained at normal levels (Newberg et al., 1984).

Enflurane alone at up to 1.5 MAC has no effect on

CBF, but addition of 50% N_2O produces a large increase (Manohar and Parks, 1984). Enflurane has an epileptogenic property, with spike activity or burst supression induced on the EEG by inspired concentrations above 2–3%. At 3.5 MAC, inspired $CMRO_2$ is lowered and CBF increased with no evidence of anaerobic metabolism (Seo et al., 1984).

Sevoflurane decreases CBF and $CMRO_2$, but O_2 flux decreases almost as much (Manohar, 1986).

Opioids

Direct effects of moderate doses of opioid are negligible, but an increase in CO_2 levels from opioid administration can produce significant secondary effect. Morphine in very large doses increases the proportion of cardiac output that goes to the brain (Law et al., 1985). Alfentanil does not affect autoregulation or CO_2 response (McPherson et al., 1985). Naloxone increases CBV (Sandor et al., 1986).

Hypotensive Agents

Sodium nitroprusside (SNP) has a direct vascular action and produces a higher rCBF than trimetaphan (TMP) which can mean a higher ICP with SNP. SNP produces the most homogenous brain surface oxygenation (Maekawa et al., 1979) and electrical activity is maintained to a lower MAP with SNP than TMP (Prior, 1985) (Fig. 17.7). SNP opens the blood

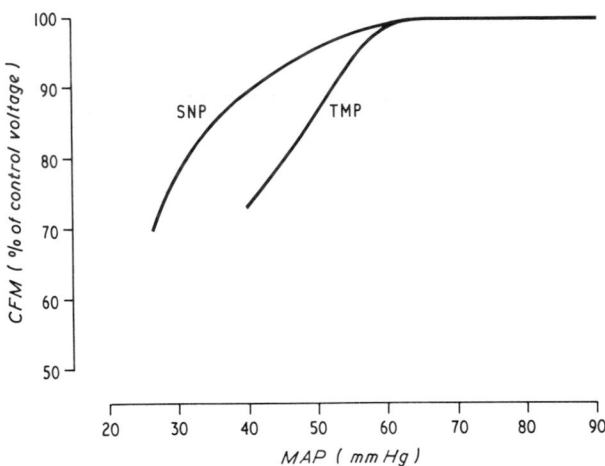

Fig. 17.7 Electrical activity is maintained better at low flows with SNP compared to TMP. (Simplified Prior, 1985.)

brain barrier more than TMP (Ishikawa et al., 1983). Haemorrhage as a means of induced hypotension is very undesirable.

Fluids

Mannitol decreases ICP, with longer effect if given after frusemide. A single bolus of 1.5 g/kg has a measurable effect for up to 24 h (Jafar et al., 1986). In clinical practice 0.5 g/kg is more appropriate. The mechanism may be a combination of brain water reduction and decreased blood viscosity improving O_2 flux (Mendelow et al., 1985), causing reflex vasoconstriction (Muizelaar et al., 1986). It is most likely to be of benefit in patients with focal injuries or high ICP or CPP below the limit of autoregulation.

METHODS FOR MEASURING CEREBRAL BLOOD FLOW IN MAN

A large number of different methods has been described and most of these are listed in Table 17.3.

TABLE 17.3
METHODS FOR MEASURING CBF

1.	Kety-Schmidt	Sequential cerebral venous sampling N_2O, ^{133}Xe, ^{85}Kr
2.	Mallett and Veal	External isotope detection, ^{133}Xe
3.	Positron emission tomography	On-site cyclotron
4.	Single photon emission computerized tomography (SPET)	New radionuclides
5.	Plethysmography	Neonates
6.	Infrared	Neonates (transmission) Adults (reflection)
7.	Hydrogen clearance	Animal studies
8.	Umbelliferone	Animal studies
9.	Microspheres	Animal studies
10.	Doppler methods	Non-invasive

Kety-Schmidt Method—Global Cerebral Blood Flow

The gold standard for measuring cerebral blood flow is based on the Kety-Schmidt method described in 1948 (Kety and Schmidt, 1948). This technique was based on the known solubility of N_2O in brain tissue and on measurements of nitrous oxide in arterial and cerebral venous blood during a 10 min period breathing a mixture containing the gas. The mean CBF in the original study was 56 ml/(100 g·min), but Lassen and his colleagues concluded that the short duration of the study and extra cerebral contamination gave a 10% error and a true CBF of 51 ml/(100 g·min) was found using ^{85}Kr instead of N_2O. Lassen and Monk, (1955) and Lassen et al., (1960) found values slightly less than 50 ml/(100 g·min) and similar results were found with ^{133}Xe.

This method measures global CBF, without discriminating between grey and white brain substance and is insensitive to regional changes in cerebral blood flow.

Regional Cerebral Blood Flow

A major advance in methodology for demonstrating regional differences in CBF was made by Mallett and Veal (1965) who used $^{133}Xenon$ administered by inhalation and external scintillation detectors. Other workers have administered ^{133}Xe (or other radio-molecules) by intracarotid injection. This method can be used to differentiate between grey and white flow by analysis of the washout curves. Some of the problems with ^{133}Xe include its low solubility in blood and tissue with limited absorption from the lung, its varying partition coefficient in normal and abnormal brain and its 81 keV photon making energy discrimination of scattered radiation a problem.

Nevertheless, most of the information on CBF in man in health and disease has, until recently, been obtained with the ^{133}Xe method because of its simplicity and portability.

Positron Emission Tomography (PET)

At the opposite extreme of technical complexity is *Positron Emission Tomography* (*PET*) which requires an on site cyclotron to produce the short lived radionuclides as well as a complex detecting and computing system. This method is based on the Kety-Schmidt principle and examines the regional CBF in terms of uptake pattern of positron emitting tracers such as $C^{15}O_2$, $H_2^{15}O$, ^{77}Kr or C labelled alcohol. In addition to CBF, it measures oxygen extraction rate and glucose consumption and can produce a unique metabolic map of physiological and disease processes in tomographic slices of the brain. The method is sufficiently sensitive to be able to detect regional changes in CBF and metabolism produced by subtle changes in modalities of sensory information.

Brooks et al. (1986) have used ^{11}C-methyl albumin microspheres and PET to measure rCBF and compared these results with the more standard $C^{15}O_2$ technique. The results correlate within 10%.

Nuclear Magnetic Resonance

This can give superior images to conventional computerized radiographic tomography and also gives information about biochemical changes in tissue *in vivo*. It is not yet possible to combine these techniques to give information about regional differences in biochemical activity in discrete regions.

Single Photon Emission Computerized Tomography (SPECT or SPET)

This provides an alternative method for measuring regional cerebral blood flow that can be carried out at a small fraction of the cost of PET. SPET equipment is available in many departments in the UK and is based on recording single photons emitted from radionuclides using a rotating gamma camera detector system. However, until recently the main problem was the lack of adequate radiopharmaceuticals. The solution to this problem was the development of a demethylated derivative of propylene amine oxime (CERETEC) which entered the brain very rapidly in proportion to rCBF and leaves the brain very slowly at less than 1% per hour.

Plethysmography

The neonate, because of its expansible skull, allows the use of a plethysmographic technique. A mercury in rubber strain gauge is placed around the fronto-occipital head circumference of the sleeping infant and the jugular veins are compressed. The change in circumference during 10 heart beats is recorded (Cowan et al., 1983). The method is unsuitable for routine measurements.

Infrared Spectrophotometry

Cerebral oxygenation and haemodynamics may be quantified using near infrared spectrophotometry using laser diodes transmitting in the range 700–1300 nm. In the neonate, transmission through the whole brain may be measured whereas, in the adult, reflection from brain tissue is employed. With this approach, on line measurements can be made of oxygenated and reduced haemoglobin, cerebral blood volume, mixed venous saturation, cerebral blood flow and oxidized cytochrome, (Fox et al., 1985).

TECHNIQUES USED IN LABORATORY STUDIES

Hydrogen Clearance

This technique uses platinum electrodes implanted within the surface of the brain. The advantages of the method are the focal nature of the recording, ability to repeat the measurements, and the simple electronic equipment. However, a craniotomy is needed and there may be wide differences in the values derived, depending on the size of the electrode. This may represent real differences in regional CBF in that the smaller the electrode the greater the variability in the derived CBF (Young, 1980).

Umbelliferone

Umbelliferone (7-hydroxycoumarin) is a fat soluble, pH sensitive fluorescent indicator with both molecular and ionic fluorophors. Because of this, it is freely diffusible across the blood brain barrier and can be used to measure equivalent intracellular pH and CBF (Anderson et al., 1987). Measuring the fluorescence from a small area of brain surface shows a different response to inhaled CO_2 compared to larger regions studied with ^{133}Xe or ^{85}Kr in cats and rabbits. This suggests that the method minimizes the contribution from larger vessels.

Labelled Microspheres

The technique employs labelled particles, 15 μm in diameter, which behave rheologically like red cells (Heymann et al., 1977). Such microspheres are virtually 100% extracted from arterial blood by the microvasculature in one passage of the circulation and remain trapped. Their relative distribution indicates the regional distribution of flow. Studies can be carried out by injecting aliquots of microspheres labelled with different radionuclides. Between each injection various physiological manoeuvres are performed, which may change regional distribution of flow. Most of the studies have entailed postmortem examination of organs, but Brooks et al. (1986) recently described this technique in man.

Doppler Flow Velocity

Doppler flow velocity methods have been described for non-invasive measurements of total CBF. However, no quantitative measure of CBF can be obtained and a change in calibre of a vessel will change velocity without there being a change in flow. Nevertheless, the technique is useful in newborn infants (Greisen et al., 1984) and in the determination of flows in individual arteries (Kirith, 1986).

CONCLUSION

The consequences of changes in cerebral blood flow, volume and pressure as a result of anaesthetic manipulations must be considered in the normal course of anaesthesia. The relevance of such understanding transcends neuro-anaesthesia to affect our practice in our daily work particularly in acutely ill patients in intensive care. This chapter is an outline of the salient features of cerebral haemodynamics. A more comprehensive review may be found in (Wood, 1987 and Michenfelder, 1988).

REFERENCES

Alafaci C., Cowen T., Crockhard H.A., et al. (1986). Perivascular nerve types supplying cerebral blood vessels of the gerbil. *Acta Physiol. Scand. Suppl.*, **552**, 9.

Albrecht R.F., Miletich D.J., Madala L.R. (1983). Normalisation of CBF during prolonged halothane anesthesia. *Anesthesiology*, **58**, 26.

Anderson R.E., Sundt T.M., Yaksh T.L. (1987). rCBF and focal cortical perfusion: a comparative study of 133Xe, 85Kr and umbelliferone as diffusible indicators. *J. Cereb. Blood Flow Metab.*, **7**, 207.

Astrup J., Rosenørn J., Cold G.E., et al. (1984). Minimum CBF and metabolism during craniotomy. Effect of thiopental loading. *Acta Anaesthesiol. Scand.*, **28**, 478.

Brooks D.J., Frackowiak R.S.J., Lammertsma A.A. (1986). A comparison between rCBF measurements obtained in human subjects using 11C methalbumin microspheres, the $C^{15}O_2$ steady state method and PET. *Acta Neurol. Scand.*, **73**, 415.

Brown M.M., Wade J.P.H., Marshall J. (1985). Fundamental importance of arterial O_2 content in the regulation of CBF in man. *Brain*, **108** (Ptl), 81.

Burke A.M., Greenberg J.H., Sladky J. (1987). Regional variation in cerebral perfusion during acute hypertension. *Neurology*, **37**, 94.

Clozel J.P., Amend P., Saunier C., et al. (1985). Cimetidine inhibits the hypoxia induced increase in CBF in dogs. *Crit. Care Med.*, **13**, 976.

Cold G.E. (1986). The relationship between $CMRO_2$ and CBF in the acute phase of head injury. *Acta Anaesthesiol. Scand.*, **30**, 453.

Cold G.E., Eskesen V., Eriksen H., et al. (1986). Changes in $CMRO_2$, EEG and concentration of etomidate in serum and brain tissue during craniotomy with cont. etomidate suppl. to N_2O and fentanyl. *Acta Anaesthesiol. Scand.*, **30**, 159.

Cook P.R., Myers D., Barker M., et al. (1989). Blood-brain barrier to pertechnetate following drug-induced hypotension. *Br. J. Anaesth.* **62**, 402.

Cowan F., Erikson M., Thoresen M. (1983). An evaluation of the plethysmographic method of measuring cranial blood flow in the newborn infant. *J. Physiol.*, **335**, 41.

Drummond J.C., Todd M.M., Scheller M.S., et al. (1986). A comparison of the direct cerebral vasodilating potencies of halothane and isoflurane in the New Zealand white rabbit. *Anesthesiology*, **65 (5)**, 462.

Eintrei C., Leszniewski W., Carlsson D. (1985). Local application of 133Xe for measurement of rCBF during halothane, enflurane and isoflurane anesthesia in humans. *Anesthesiology*, **63 (4)**, 391.

Fox E., Jobis-Vandervliet F.F., Mitnick M.H. (1985). Monitoring cerebral oxygen sufficiency in anaesthesia and surgery. *Adv. Exp. Med. Biol.*, **191**, 849.

Frackowiak R.S.J., Gian-Luigi L., Jones T., et al. (1980). Quantitative measurement of rCBF and O_2 metabolism in man using $^{15}O_2$ and Positron emission tomography: theory, procedure and normal values. *J. Comput. Assist. Tomogr.*, **4**, 727.

Francois-Dainville E., Buchweitz E., Weiss H.R. (1986). Effect of hypoxia on percent of arteriolar and capillary beds perfused in the rat brain. *J. Appl. Physiol.*, **60**, 280.

Gaehtgens P., Marx P. (1987). Hemorheological aspects of the pathophysiology of cerebral ischaemia. *J. Cereb. Blood Flow Metab.*, **7**, 259.

Gibson B.E., McMichan J.C., Cucciara R.F. (1986). Lack of correlation between transconjunctival O_2 and CBF during carotid artery occlusion. *Anesthesiology*, **64**, 277.

Ginsberg M.D., Prado R., Dietrich W.D., et al. (1987). Hyperglycaemia reduces the extent of cerebral infarction in rats. *Stroke*, **18**, 570.

Greisen G., Johansen K., Ellisen P.H. (1984). CBF in the newborn infant. Comparison of doppler ultrasound and 133 Xe clearance. *J. Pediatr.*, **104**, 411.

Hansen N.B., Nowicki P.T., Miller R.R., et al. (1986). Alterations in CBF and O_2 consumption during prolonged hypocarbia. *Pediatr. Res.*, **20**, 147.

Heymann M.A., Payne B.D., Hofman J.I.E., et al. (1977). Blood flow measurements with radionuclide-labelled particles. *Prog. Cardiovasc. Res.*, **20**, 55.

Hoffman W.E., Miletich D.J., Albrecht R.F. (1986). The effects of midazolam on CBF and O_2 consumption and its interaction with nitrous oxide. *Anesth. Analg.*, **65 (7)**, 729.

Hudak M.L., Koehler R.C., Rosenberg A.A., et al. (1986). Effect of hematocrit on CBF. *Am. J. Physiol.*, **25 (1pt.2)**, H63.

Hudetz A.G., Conger K.A., Halsey J.G., et al. (1987). Pressure distribution in the pial arterial system of rats based on morphometric data and mathematical models. *J. Cereb. Blood Flow Metab.*, **7**, 342.

Ishikawa T., Funatsu N., Okamoto K., et al. (1983). Blood brain barrier function following drug-induced hypotension in the dog. *Anesthesiology*, **59**, 526.

Jafar J.J., Johns L.M., Mullan S.F. (1986). The effect of mannitol on CBF. *J. Neurosurg.*, **64**, 754.

Kety S.S., Schmidt C.F. (1948). The N_2O method for the quantitative determination of CBF in man: theory, procedure and normal values. *J. Clin. Invest.*, **27**, 476.

Kirith A.M. (1986). Transcranial measurement of blood velocities in the basal cerebral arteries using pulsed Doppler ultrasound velocity as an index of flow. *Ultrasound Med. Biol.*, **12**, 15.

Krogh A. (1919). The number and distribution of capillaries in muscle, with calculations of the O_2 pressure head necessary for supplying the tissue. *J. Physiol.*, **52**, 391.

Lacombe P., Miller M.C., Seylaz J. (1986). Variability of the sympathetic influence on CBF as related to different physiological situations. *Acta Physiol. Scand.*, **Suppl. 552**, 58.

Lassen N.A., Monk O. (1955). The CBF in man determined by the use of radioactive Krypton. *Acta Physiol. Scand.*, **33**, 30.

Lassen N.A., Feinberg I., Lane M.H. (1960). Bilateral studies of cerebral oxygen uptake in young and aged normal subjects and in patients with organic dementia. *J. Clin. Invest.*, **39**, 491.

Law W.R., Ritzmann R.F., Lee J.M., et al. (1985). The effects of acute and chronic morphine on regional distribution of cardiac output in brain. *Experientia*, **15**, **41**, 78.

Lifson J.D., Rubenstein E.H., Scremin O.U., et al. (1985). Cerebrovascular reactivity to CO_2: modulation by arterial pressure. *Experientia*, **15**, **41**, 467.

Maekawa T., McDowall D.G., Okuda Y. (1979). Brain surface O_2 tension and cerebral cortical blood flow during haemorrhagic and drug induced hypotension in the cat. *Anesthesiology*, **51**, 313.

Maekawa T., Tommasino C., Shapiro H.M., et al. (1986). Local CBF and glucose utilization during isoflurane anesthesia in the rat. *Anesthesiology*, **65**, 144.

Mallet B.L., Veal N. (1965). Measurement of regional cerebral clearance rates in man using Xe 133 inhalation and extracranial recording. *Clin. Science*, **29**, 179.

Manohar M. (1985). Impact of 70% N_2O administration on regional distribution of brain blood flow in unmedicated healthy swine. *J. Cardiovasc. Pharmacol.*, **7**, 463.

Manohar M., Parks C.M. (1984). Porcine brain and myocardial perfusion during enflurane anesthesia without and with N_2O. *J. Cardiovasc. Pharmacol.*, **6**, 1092.

Manohar M. (1986). rCBF and cerebral cortical O_2 consumption during sevoflurane anesthesia in healthy isocapnic swine. *J. Cardiovasc. Pharmacol.*, **8**, 1268.

McDowall D.G. (1985). Induced hypotension and brain ischaemia. *Br. J. Anaesth.*, **57**, 110.

McPherson R.W., Krempasan Ka E., Eimerl D. (1985). Effects of alfentanil on cerebral vascular reactivity in dogs. *Br. J. Anaesth.*, **57**, 1232.

Mendelow A.D., Teasdale G.M., Russell T., et al. (1985). Effect of mannitol on CBF and CPP in human head injury. *J. Neurosurg.*, **63**, 43.

Meyer J.S., Rogers R.L., Mortel K.F. (1985). Prospective analysis of long term control of mild hypertension on CBF. *Stroke*, **16**, 985.

Michenfelder J.D. (1988). *Anesthesia and the Brain* New York: Churchill Livingstone.

Michenfelder J.D., Theye R.A. (1975). The influence of anesthesia and ischaemia on the cerebral energy state. In *Cerebral Vascular Diseases*, pp. 243–250. (Whisnat J.P., Sandok B.A., eds.) New York: Grune and Stratton.

Miletich D.J., Ivankovich A.D., Albrecht R.M. (1976). Absence of autoregulation of CBF during halothane and enflurane anesthesia. *Anesth. Analg.*, **55**, 100.

Morita H., Nemoto E.M., Blayaert A.L. (1977). Brain blood flow autoregulation and metabolism during halothane anaesthesia in monkeys. *Am. J. Physiol.*, **233**, H670.

Muizelaar J.P., Wei E.P., Kontos H.A., et al. (1986). CBF is regulated by changes in blood pressure and in blood viscosity alike. *Stroke*, **17**, 44.

Newberg L.A., Milde J.H., Michenselder J.D. (1984). Systemic and cerebral effects of isoflurane induced hypotension in dogs. *Anesthesiology*, **60**, 541.

Newman B., Gelb A.W., Lam A.M. (1986). The effect of isoflurane induced hypotension on CBF and $CMRO_2$ in humans. *Anesthesiology*, **64 (3)**, 307.

Nikki P.H., Nemoto E.M., Blayaert A.L., et al. (1987). Absence of beta adrenergic receptor involvement in cerebrovascular dilation by halothane in monkeys. *Anesth. Analg.*, **66**, 39.

Nussmeier N.A., Ralund C., Slogoff S. (1986). Neuropsychiatric complications after cardiopulmonary bypass: cerebral protection by a barbiturate. *Anesthesiology*, **64**, 165.

Olsen T.S. (1986). rCBF after occlusion of the middle cerebral artery. *Acta Neurol. Scand.*, **73**, 321.

Porter S.S., Albin M.S., Watson W.A., et al. (1985). Spinal cord and CBF responses to subarachnoid injection of local anesthetics with and without epinephrine. *Acta Anaesthiol. Scand.*, **29**, 330.

Powers W.J., Grubb R.L., Darriet D., et al. (1985). CBF and $CMRO_2$ requirements for cerebral function and viability in humans. *J. Cereb. Blood Flow Metab.*, **5**, 600.

Prior P.F. (1985). EEG monitoring and evoked potentials in brain ischaemia. *Br. J. Anaesth.*, **57**, 63.

Ram C.V.S., Meese R., Kaplan N.M., et al. (1987). Antihypertensive therapy in the elderly. Effects on BP and CBF. *Am. J. Med.*, **82**, 53.

Reicher D., Bhalla P., Rubinstein E.H. (1987). Cholinergic cerebral vasodilator effect of ketamine in rabbits. *Stroke*, **18**, 445.

Rosa G., Orfei P., Sanfilippo M., et al. (1986a). The effects of atracurium besylate (Tracrium) on ICP and CPP. *Anesth. Analg.*, **65**, 381.

Rosa G., Sanfilippo M., Vilardi V., et al. (1986b). Effects of vecuronium bromide on ICP and CPP. A preliminary report. *Br. J. Anaesth.*, **58**, 437.

Rosner M.J., Becker D.P. (1984). Origin and evolution of plateau waves. Experimental observations and a theoretical model. *J. Neurosurg.*, **60**, 312.

Sadoshima S., Fujii K., Yao H., et al. (1986). Regional CBF autoregulation in normotensive and spontaneously hypertensive rats. Effects of sympathetic denervation. *Stroke*, **17**, 981.

Sandor P., Put J.C.-V., de Jong W., et al. (1986). Continuous measurement of cerebral blood volume in rats with the photo-electric technique: effect of morphine and naloxone. *Life Sci.*, **39**, 1657.

Scheller M.S., Todd N.M., Drummond J.C. (1986). Isoflurane, halothane and rCBF at various levels of Pa_{CO_2} in rabbits. *Anesthesiology*, **74**, 598.

Seo K., Maekawa T., Takeshita H., et al. (1984). Cerebral energy state and glycolytic metabolism during enflurane anaesthesia in the rat. *Acta Anaesthsiol. Scand.*, **28**, 215.

Strandgaard S. (1976). Autoregulation of CBF in hypertensives. The modifying influence of prolonged treatment on the tolerance to acute drug induced hypotension. *Circulation*, **53**, 720.

Strandgaard S., Olesen J., Skinhoj E., et al. (1973). Autoregulation of brain circulation in severe arterial hypertension. *Br. Med. J.*, **1**, 507.

Symon L. (1985). Flow thresholds in brain ischaemia and the effects of drugs. *Br. J. Anaesth.*, **57**, 34.

Tuor U.I., McCulloch J. (1986). Regional cerebral perfu-

sion during hypertension depends on the hypertensive agent. *Neurosci. Lett.*, **63**, 253.

Verrechia C., Hamel E., Edvinsson L., et al. (1986). Role of the endothelium in the pial artery responses to several vasoactive peptides. *Acta Physiol. Scand.*, **Suppl. 552**, 33.

Wilson D.A., Traystman R.J., Rapela C.E. (1985). Transient analysis of the canine cerebrovascular response to CO_2. *Circ. Res.*, **56**, 596.

Wood J.H. (1987). *Cerebral Blood Flow, Physiologic and Clinical Aspects*. New York: McGraw-Hill Company.

Young W.H. (1980). Clearance measurement of blood flow. A review of technique and polarographic principles. *Stroke*, **11**, 552.

18. Pathophysiology, Monitoring, Outcome Prediction and Therapy of Shock States

W. C. Shoemaker and H. B. Kram

Shock is a syndrome that is recognized by subjective symptoms and signs and managed by anecdotal approaches based on these subjective signs and symptoms. Although most patients eventually get all the therapy they need, it is not necessarily at the right time, in the right amount, or in the right order.

Common misconceptions of the nature of shock have led to ineffective therapy. The concept of shock as hypotension, low flow, and high resistance arose from early studies of hemorrhage and cardiogenic shock (Wiggers and Shoemaker, 1940; Cournand et al., 1943). However, patients with hypovolemia or myocardial infarction are not representative of most clinical shock states*. Second, shock is often regarded as a single physiologic picture rather than a wide variety of life-threatening circulatory syndromes whose physiologic patterns evolve in time. A third misconception is that the goal of therapy is to restore blood pressure (BP) and cardiac output values to their normal range. However, normal or high cardiac output values do not indicate that further volume therapy is not needed and that only vasopressors are required to maintain pressure. These simplistic notions based on subjective and arbitrary definitions lead to suboptimal therapy (Shoemaker et al., 1988).

CONVENTIONAL ETIOLOGIC APPROACH TO SHOCK

Traditionally, the etiologic approach to shock includes hemorrhagic, cardiogenic, traumatic, septic, and rarely, neurogenic shock syndromes. Each of these categories are described by signs and symptoms, laboratory findings, and primary pathophysiologic derangement; therapeutic principles readily follow from these (Table 18.1). Each cause of shock is assumed to have a characteristic clinical and laboratory pattern

*(Clowes and Del Guercio, 1960; Heilbrunn and Allbritten, 1960; Del Guercio et al., 1964; Wilson et al., 1965; Shoemaker et al., 1967; Siegel et al., 1971; Shoemaker et al., 1973; Bland et al., 1985; Bland and Shoemaker, 1985a; Shoemaker et al., 1988.)

TABLE 18.1
APPROACH TO VARIOUS ETIOLOGIC TYPES OF SHOCK

Hemorrhagic	Cardiogenic	Traumatic	Septic
Signs and Symptoms			
Pallor, fainting	Pallor, fainting	History of injury	Fever, chills
Skin clammy, cold	Skin clammy, cold	Physical evidence of injury, fractures	Skin warm
Tachycardia	Arrhythmias		Tachycardia
Oliguria	Oliguria	Oliguria	Oliguria
Collapse	Collapse	Tachycardia	Altered mental status
		Collapse	Collapse
Laboratory			
↓ Hct, Hgb	↓ Cardiac enzymes ECG	X-rays, CT scan, Angiograms for organ and vascular injury	Positive smears and cultures
Pathophysiology			
↓ Blood volume	↓ Cardiac output	Direct injury to organs and tissue	↓ Peripheral resistance
Therapy			
1. Fluids	1. Antiarrhythmics	1. Repairs injuries	1. Antibiotics
2. Blood	2. Vasopressors	2. Fluids	2. Fluids
3. Control bleeding	3. Vasodilators	3. Blood	3. Drain abscesses

and that therapeutic principles are apparent. This etiologic approach is straightforward, unambiguous, easily understood, and widely accepted. Unfortunately, this approach is a simplistic answer to a complex problem. Each etiologic event does not begin and end with a single physiologic alteration that can be treated by correcting the primary cause. The primary event produces complex and potentially lethal interactions. For example, in hemorrhage, reduced blood volume decreases flow and oxygen transport; in cardiogenic shock, the reduced flow decreases BP and oxygen transport; in traumatic and septic shock, flow increases but these increases may not be sufficient for the concomitantly increased metabolism. Irrespective of the initiating event, circulatory compensations and their decompensations stimulated by the primary event produce the shock syndrome. Changes in volume, flow, and oxygen transport lead to the characteristic patterns of survival or to death. The real problem with this simplistic unidimensional approach is that it leads to simplistic unidimensional therapy. Therapy must be directed to all components of the disturbed circulation, not just the primary initiating event; an automobile wreck produced by a tyre blowout is not corrected by the tyre's replacement.

The conventional approach also involves a search for specific defects, their documentation, and correction. This one at a time search for defects followed by their normalization leads to fragmented, episodic, incoherent patient care. An appropriate alternative is to base therapy on the pattern of survivors and on underlying circulatory mechanisms that determine survival. If the pathophysiology is not understood and monitoring is not appropriate, death will be attributed to the patient's disease rather than to the inappropriate therapy.

Traditional Approach to Monitoring

Routine monitoring consists of repeated measurements of the superficial manifestations of shock, such as the vital signs, hematocrit (Hct), and urine output. In a series of critically ill postoperative survivors and nonsurvivors commonly monitored variables [mean arterial pressure (MAP), heart rate (HR), central venous pressure (CVP), pulmonary artery wedge pressures (WP), and cardiac output] were returned to the normal range in 76% of nonsurvivors, who nevertheless still went on to die; by comparison, 75% of the survivors also had two or more values in the normal range (Table 18.2). Clearly, the wrong variables were measured and normal ranges for these conventional variables were the wrong therapeutic goals (Bland et al., 1978).

Invasive Circulatory Monitoring

Invasive hemodynamic and oxygen transport variables may be repeatedly monitored with systemic arterial and pulmonary arterial catheters to provide frequent measurements of arterial and venous pressures in the systemic and pulmonary circulations, cardiac output, arterial and mixed venous gases and saturations, core temperature, hemoglobin (Hb), and Hct (Shoemaker et al., 1973, 1985a, 1987; Bland et al., 1985, 1985a). From these measurements, a variety of hemodynamic values may be derived including cardiac index, CI), the systemic and pulmonary vascular

TABLE 18.2

NUMBER AND PERCENT OF PATIENTS WITH TWO OR MORE VALUES IN THE NORMAL RANGE

	Nonsurvivors		Survivors	
	Number	%	Number	%
Mean arterial pressure	29	78	68	89
Heart rate	30	81	66	87
Central venous pressure	35	95	72	95
Pulmonary wedge pressure	11	30	21	28
Cardiac index	35	95	64	84
Mean of these variables		76		75

resistance index (SVRI and PVRI, respectively), the left and right ventricular stroke work index (LVSWI and RVSWI, respectively) and left and right cardiac work (LCW and RCW, respectively). When arterial and mixed venous gases are measured simultaneously with cardiac output, oxygen transport and metabolism may be evaluated; oxygen delivery ($\dot{D}o_2$) which is the product of CI and arterial O_2 content (Cao_2), oxygen consumption ($\dot{V}o_2$), the product of CI and arterio-venous O_2 content difference ($C(a\text{-}v)o_2$), oxygen extraction $C(a\text{-}\bar{v})o_2/Cao_2$ pulmonary venous admixture or shunting ($\dot{Q}sp/\dot{Q}t$), and the alveolar-arterial oxygen gradient [$P(A\text{-}a)o_2$]. Flow and volume-related variables are indexed according to body surface area (Table 18.3).

PATHOPHYSIOLOGY OF SHOCK

The natural physiologic history of clinical shock syndromes produced by hemorrhage, accidental and surgical trauma, sepsis, cardiogenic problems as single etiologies, and various combinations of these etiologies was described by sequential hemodynamic and oxygen transport changes observed during periods remote from therapy, i.e., before therapy was begun or after the immediate direct effects of therapy were over. Hemodynamic and oxygen transport patterns characterize the physiologic natural history of various etiologic shock syndromes (Shoemaker et al., 1967, 1973, 1985a, 1987; Bland et al., 1985, 1985a).

Dimensions of Circulatory Function

Circulatory function is often expressed in terms of cardiac hemodynamics, including intravascular pressures, flow, LVSW, dP/dt, etc. However, these cardiac functions are only one aspect of circulatory function. Circulatory dynamics include the fundamental dimensions that physically characterize fluid systems: pressure, volume, flow, and function; the latter is best characterized by the $\dot{V}o_2$, which represents the sum of all oxidative metabolic processes.

Figure 18.1 schematically represents the normal state of these four dimensions, each assigned a value of 100%, and represented as a square. Shock syn-

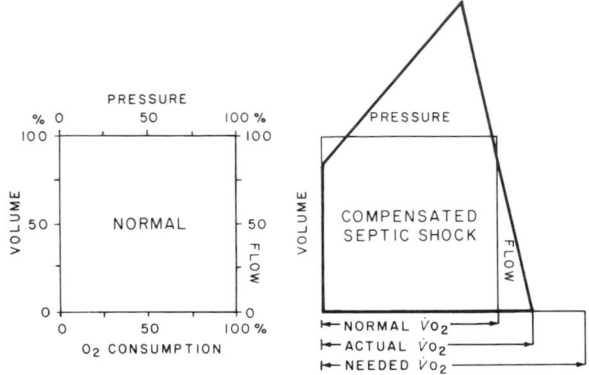

Fig. 18.1A Normal circulatory dimensions representing pressure, volume, flow, and function ($\dot{V}o_2$). The dimensions are drawn to a scale in which the normal values are shown as 100% and changes of each dimension above or below the normal expressed as percentage changes of that scale. B. Average values of patients with compensated septic shock showing 20% reduction in volume and 30% drop in pressure, but 75% increase in flow and 20% increase in $\dot{V}o_2$. Although the observed $\dot{V}o_2$ values are greater than normal, they are considerably less than needed.

dromes can be portrayed as changes in each of these dimensions. The average changes in these dimensions observed in a large series of patients with compensated septic shock are shown in Fig. 18.1. The normal values shown by the fine lines of the square may be compared to the thick lines representing decreased MAP and blood volume due to dehydration and fever, as well as increased flow and $\dot{V}o_2$. The lower horizontal dimensions, representing $\dot{V}o_2$, shows the normal value, the observed value, and the $\dot{V}o_2$ values that are required by patients with increased metabolism. Figure 18.2 illustrates circulatory dimensions in hemorrhagic, cardiogenic, traumatic, and septic shock. The initial primary changes of each dimension for each etiologic type of shock are shown in the second column; the decompensated state in the third column; and the terminal state, which is often very similar in each etiologic type of shock, is shown on the extreme right. The figure illustrates differences in the

TABLE 18.3

CARDIORESPIRATORY VARIABLES; ABBREVIATIONS, UNITS, CALCULATIONS, NORMAL VALUES, PREFERRED VALUES, AND PREDICTIVE CAPACITY

Variables	Abbreviations	Units	Measurements or calculations	Normal values	Preferred values	%
Volume-related						
Mean arterial pressure	MAP	mmHg	Direct measurement	82–102	>84	76
Central venous pressure	CVP	cm H_2O	Direct measurement	1–9	<5	62
Central blood volume	CBV	ml/m²	CBV = MTT × CI × 16.7	660–1000	>925	61
Stroke index	SI	ml/m²	SI = CI/HR	30–50	>48	67
Hemoglobin	Hgb	g/dl	Direct measurement	12–16	>12	66
Mean pulmonary artery pressure	MPAP	mmHg	Direct measurement	11–15	<19	68
Wedge pressure	WP	mmHg	Direct measurement	0–12	>9.5	70
Blood volume	BV	ml/m²	BV = PV/(1 − Hct)* × surface area	Men 2.74	>3.0	76
				Women 2.37	>2.7	
Red cell mass	RCM	L/m²	RCM = BV − PV	Men 1.1	>1.1	85
				Women 0.95	>0.95	
Flow-related						
Cardiac index	CI	L/(min·m²)	Direct measurement	2.8–3.6	>4.5	70
Left vent stroke work index	LVSWI	g·m/m²	LVSWI = SI × MAP × 0.0144	44–68	>55	74
Left cardiac work index	LCWI	kg·m/m²	LCWI = CI × MAP × 0.0144	3–4.6	>5	76
Right vent stroke work index	RVSWI	g·m/m²	RVSWI = SI × MAP × 0.0144	4–8	>13	70
Right cardiac work index	RCWI	kg·m/m²	RCWI = CI × MPAP × 0.0144	0.4–0.6	>1.1	69
Stress-related						
Systemic vasc resist	SVR	dyn·s·cm⁻⁵·m²	SVR = 79.92 (MAP-CVP)†/CI	1760–2600	>1450	62
Pulmonary vasc resist	PVR	dyn·s·cm⁻⁵·m²	PVR = 79.92 (MPAP-WP)†/CI	45–225	<226	77
Heart rate	HR	beat/min	Direct measurement	72–88	>100	60
Rectal temperature	temp	°F	Direct measurement	97.8–98.6	>100.4	64
Oxygen-related						
Hemoglobin saturation	Sao_2	%	Direct measurement	95–99	>95	67
Arterial CO_2 tension	$Paco_2$	torr	Direct measurement	36–44	>30	69
Arterial pH	pH	. . .	Direct measurement	7.36–7.44	>7.47	74
Mixed venous O_2 tension	$P\bar{v}O_2$	torr	Direct measurement	33–53	>36	68
Arterial-mixed venous O_2 content difference	$C(a-\bar{v})O_2$	ml/dl	$C(a-\bar{v})O_2 = Cao_2 − C\bar{v}o_2$	4–5.5	<3.5	68
O_2 delivery	$\dot{D}o_2$	ml/(min·m²)	$\dot{D}o_2 = Cao_2 × CI × 10$	520–720	>550	76
O_2 consumption	$\dot{V}o_2$	ml/(min·m²)	$\dot{V}o_2 = C(a-\bar{v})o_2 × CI × 10$	100–180	>167	69
O_2 extraction rate	O_2 ext	%	O_2 ext $= (Cao_2 − C\bar{v}o_2)/Cao_2$	22–30	<31	69

Note

vasc resist = vascular resistance.

*Hematocrit: (Hct) value corrected for packing fraction and large vessel hematocrit to total body hematocrit ratio.

†Venous pressures expressed in mm Hg.

primary changes of each etiology and their subsequent pattern of changes. It illustrates the interactions of circulatory dimensions of each primary etiologic event and the body's principal compensatory responses, increased flow and $\dot{D}o_2$. Decompensation and the terminal state, which result from inadequate CI and $\dot{D}o_2$, lead to inadequate $\dot{V}o_2$, Shoemaker et al., 1979, 1988; Bland et al., 1978, 1985, 1985a, 1985b.

In hemorrhage, volume is primarily reduced, while the other three dimensions are secondarily affected but to a lesser extent. After volume therapy restores blood volume to normal or slightly above, pressure is restored to the normal range, but compensations produce considerably greater than normal flow and $\dot{V}o_2$; their continued fall in the terminal state leads to death.

In cardiogenic shock the primary problem is reduced flow, which secondarily affects pressure and $\dot{V}o_2$; some degree of hypovolemia may be present because of dehydration from inadequate fluid intake and diuretic therapy. Vasopressors and fluids may augment compensations and restore pressure and flow; $\dot{V}o_2$ may increase to restore oxygen debt produced by the previous low flow state.

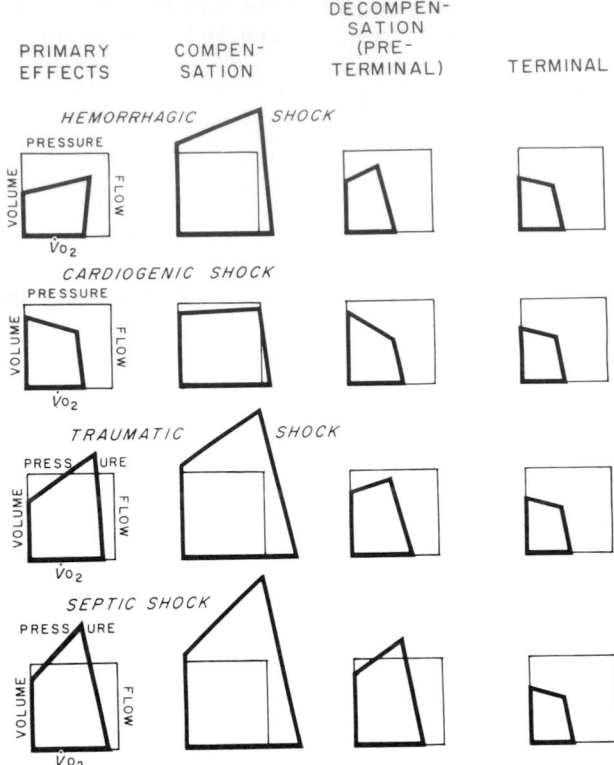

Fig. 18.2 Circulatory dimensions of patients with hemorrhagic, cardiogenic, traumatic, and septic shock. The primary effects of each etiologic type, their compensatory responses, their decompensations, and their terminal state are shown.

With trauma, the blood volume, pressure, and $\dot{V}o_2$ fall; flow may also fall, especially with associated hemorrhage, but there is often an early compensatory flow increase. In the compensated state, flow and $\dot{V}o_2$ are markedly increased. With decompensation and the terminal state, all four dimensions decrease.

With sepsis, the pressure and $\dot{V}o_2$ initially decrease; dehydration with decreased blood volume is often present. With therapy and compensations, there are marked flow and $\dot{V}o_2$ increases, the latter from increased metabolic demands. With decompensation and in the terminal state, these dimensions decrease markedly.

Survivor and Nonsurvivor Hemodynamic and Oxygen Transport Patterns after Surgical Trauma

The surgical operation provides a unique opportunity to analyse a specific type of shock, because physiologic measurements may be obtained in a pre-illness control period, during the hemodynamic crisis, and throughout the subsequent periods leading to recovery or death. In this regard, surgical shock may serve as a model for other shock syndromes. Despite the wide varieties of surgical diseases and surgical operations, rather consistent hemodynamic and oxygen transport patterns characterize the effects of surgical trauma (Bland et al., 1985; Shoemaker et al., 1973, 1985a, 1987; Bland and Shoemaker, 1985a). However, various preoperative conditions including age, sepsis, trauma, stress, cirrhosis, and cardiac failure affect these patterns (Bland and Shoemaker, 1985b).

Comparison of physiologic patterns of survivors to those who died provides insight into the nature and biological importance of these cardiorespiratory compensatory responses. Departure from the normal range may indicate compensatory responses, unrecognized complications, new physiologic processes, decompensations, or cardiorespiratory deterioration of the patient. Although carcinomatosis, transfusion reactions, pulmonary emboli, or other catastrophic events may be lethal, the great majority of nonsurvivors die of complications that may be directly or indirectly attributed to inadequate circulatory compensations or overwhelming surgical trauma.

Critically Ill Patients with Normal Preoperative Hemodynamics

Cardiorespiratory patterns were observed in high risk patients who preoperatively had normal cardiac output and no evidence of associated conditions that would affect baseline hemodynamic values (Figs. 18.3 and 18.4). Intraoperatively, CI, $\dot{D}o_2$ and $\dot{V}o_2$ fell in both survivors and nonsurvivors, but this fall was greater in the latter. Postoperatively, in those who died, these variables returned to or toward preoperative control values. In survivors, the $\dot{D}o_2$, $\dot{V}o_2$, and oxygen extraction steadily increased above control values during the first 12-24 postoperative hours. Thus, the cardiorespiratory responses of nonsurvivors were similar but less pronounced than those of the survivors; the nonsurvivors pattern was characterized by early compensatory stress responses which failed to achieve the magnitude of the survivors' responses. Later, the nonsurvivors were often unable to maintain normal, much less elevated, cardiac function despite elevated venous filling pressures; their $\dot{D}o_2$ and $\dot{V}o_2$ values remained below those of survivors, while oxygen extraction rose in partial compensation until they developed lethal complications. Despite normal blood gases, nonsurvivors' $\dot{Q}sp/\dot{Q}t$ and $P(\text{A-a})o_2$ rose intraoperatively and remained at high levels postoperatively (Bland et al., 1985).

Patients with Preoperative Low Flow

Patients with low preoperative cardiac output who were elderly, in cardiac failure, or in hemorrhagic shock had similar but less intense postoperative stress responses. That is, ventricular function started from lower control values and was minimally augmented postoperatively. In the postoperative period, the sur-

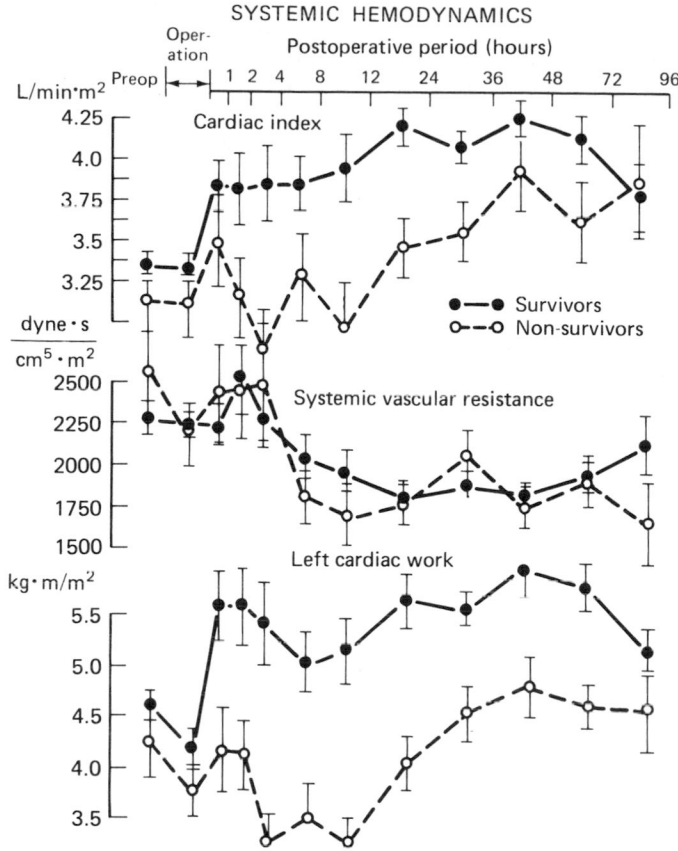

Fig. 18.3 Temporal patterns of systemic hemodynamic variables, cardiac index, systemic vascular resistance index, and left cardiac work index. Dots represent mean values; vertical bars represent SEM in the preoperative control period, intraoperative period, and at various time intervals in the postoperative period. (Reproduced with permission from Bland et al., 1985).

vivors' CI, $\dot{D}o_2$, and $\dot{V}o_2$ values increased from their low preoperative baseline values. The nonsurvivors had lower postoperative CI, $\dot{D}o_2$, and $\dot{V}o_2$ values despite high WP; i.e., they have less compensatory flow responses than did the survivors. The nonsurvivors also had significantly greater increases in PVR and $\dot{Q}sp/\dot{Q}t$ (Bland and Shoemaker, 1985a).

Patients with High Preoperative Cardiac Output

Septic patients, patients severely stressed by major preoperative trauma, and patients with advanced cirrhosis usually have high CI values indicative of the compensatory circulatory stress response. In the immediate postoperative period (first 72 h), the mean CI, $\dot{D}o_2$ and $\dot{V}o_2$ values increased above their preoperative baseline; this increase was greater in the survivors than in the nonsurvivors, while the WP, PVR and $\dot{Q}sp/\dot{Q}t$ were higher in the nonsurvivors. Both groups maintained intravascular pressures and other nonflow-related variables within relatively normal ranges (Bland and Shoemaker, 1985a).

Significance of Hemodynamic and Oxygen Transport Patterns

The basic underlying pathophysiologic problems of accidental and surgical trauma is that inadequate flow and oxygen transport values lead to tissue hypoxia and cumulative oxygen debts. The type of surgical operation is unimportant, but the duration of shock, extent of tissue hypoxia, the preoperative status, associated medical illness, and the capacity to compensate with increased CI, $\dot{D}o_2$ and $\dot{V}o_2$ are major determinants of outcome. The common physiologic problem is early reduced or inadequate $\dot{V}o_2$ that often occurs during or before the initial hypotensive crisis, produces tissue hypoxia, limits body metabolism, produces organ failure, and compromises survival. Limited $\dot{V}o_2$ may be produced by: (1) low cardiac output from hemorrhage or other causes of hypovolemia; (2) maldistribution of flow, particularly at the microcirculatory level from uneven vasoconstriction, neurohormonal mechanisms, and various mediator-induced responses; and (3) increased metabolic need (demand) that exceeds the basic transport function of the circulation (supply). The disparity between the supply and demand of oxygen may occur along with that of other nutrients.

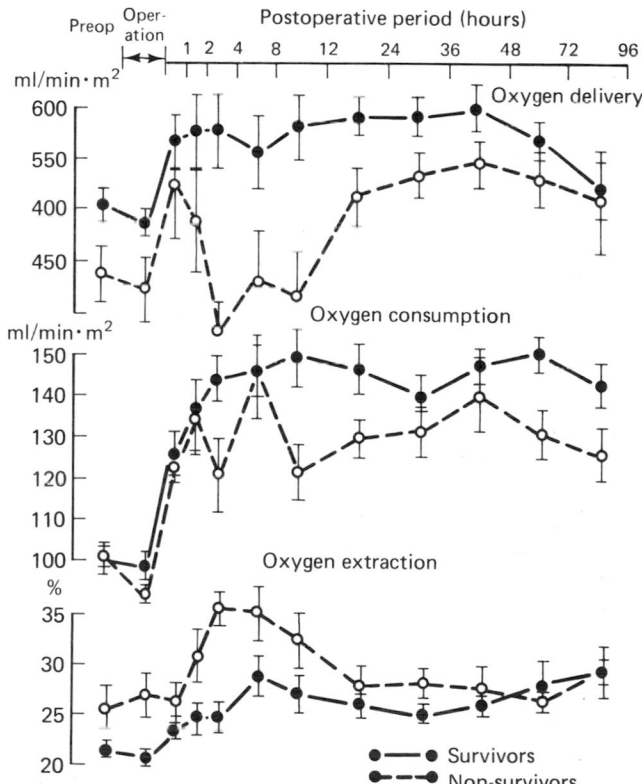

Fig. 18.4 Temporal patterns of oxygen transport variables, oxygen delivery index, oxygen consumption index, and oxygen extraction for survivors and nonsurvivors. See Fig. 18.3 for explanation. (Reproduced with permission from Bland et al., 1985).

This analysis may be seen on the background of circulatory physiology: (1) the transport of blood constituents, especially oxygen, is the major circulatory function; (2) oxygen has the highest extraction ratio and is the most flow-dependent blood constituent; (3) since oxygen cannot be stored, the rate at which oxygen is transported across the alveolar-capillary membrane in steady-state conditions is equivalent to the rate of oxygen consumed; (4) the overall circulatory function may be evaluated in terms of the $\dot{D}o_2$, while the $\dot{V}o_2$ reflects the sum of all oxidative metabolic reactions and is a measure of the body's overall metabolism; (5) $\dot{V}o_2$ may be rate-limited by reduced supply ($\dot{D}o_2$) or flow maldistributions produced by accidental trauma, surgical operations, anesthetic agents, sepsis, postoperative states, endocrine and metabolic disorders, and other forms of acute illness; (6) the sequential pattern of circulatory changes after various conditions may define the primary problem and the compensatory responses; and (7) the pattern of oxygen transport ($\dot{D}o_2$ and $\dot{V}o_2$) is strongly related to survival or death. Reduced or inadequate $\dot{V}o_2$ is greater and more prolonged in patients who die than in those who survive. Inadequate $\dot{V}o_2$ is the major pathogenic mechanism in the development of shock syndrome as well as a major determinant of outcome. Thus, $\dot{D}o_2$ and $\dot{V}o_2$ provide the best measure of the functional adequacy of both circulation and metabolism.

Therapeutic Goals

Therapeutic goals for high-risk postoperative patients were defined by the values of patients who have survived life-threatening critical illnesses as: (1) CI 50% greater than normal ($4.5\,L \cdot min^{-1} \cdot m^{-2}$); (2) $\dot{D}o_2$ slightly greater than normal ($>600\,ml \cdot min^{-1} \cdot m^{-2}$); (3) $\dot{V}o_2$ about 30% greater than normal ($>60\,ml \cdot min^{-1} \cdot m^{-2}$); and (4) blood volume 500 ml in excess of the norm, i.e., $3.2\,L/m^2$ for males, $2.8\,L/m^2$ for females (Shoemaker et al., 1973a, 1985a; Bland and Shoemaker, 1985a). These increments are needed to supply the increased metabolism associated with wound healing, fever, and the need for tissue repair. Severely traumatized, septic, and burn patients require even higher values (Bland et al., 1985; Shoemaker et al., 1985a; Bland and Shoemaker, 1985a); elderly patients may not have the reserve capacity to respond the way young previously healthy patients do.

Peripheral Perfusion Defect of Shock

Pulmonary blood flow maldistribution is the basic physiologic defect of acute pulmonary failure (Riley and Cournand, 1951; Comroe et al., 1962). Similarly, there is evidence for maldistribution of systemic blood flow in shock states. Direct microscopic observations have shown wide variations in microcirculatory flow with dilated metarteriolar capillary networks next to vasoconstricted networks. The tissue supplied by free-flowing microcirculation may be adequately nourished, while cells surrounding vasocontricted networks will be hypoxic (Shoemaker et al., 1976, 1976a).

Clinical Evaluation of Blood Volume and Fluid Status

The first primary goal in the treatment of hemorrhagic, traumatic, and septic shock is to restore blood volume, but criteria for this goal are not well defined. Based on experimental and clinical studies after sudden acute hemorrhage, tachycardia with reduced MAP, CVP, WP, urine output, and Hct values are often used. Unfortunately, these variables do not reflect the blood volume status in the subsequent course of these patients in the ICU. Moreover, in critically ill postoperative patients, these commonly used clinical criteria were unreliable compared with careful measurements of blood volume (Shippy et al., 1984).

Failure to differentiate between the status of total body water, interstitial water, and plasma volume is a common misconception. For example, the patients with peripheral edema may be hypovolemic even though there is excess total body water; these patients have maldistribution of their extracellular water with contracted plasma volume but expanded interstitial water. Indeed, this is the most common situation in the surgical or trauma patient thought to be adequately resuscitated (Shoemaker et al., 1973). The goal is to improve circulatory function by restoring plasma volume, despite the expanded interstitium (second space), and fluid escape into the third space (bowel lumen, peritoneal fluid, and pleural effusion, etc.).

Since the most important correctable clinical problem in acute circulatory shock is to restore blood volume, a reliable assessment of volume is essential. Measurement of plasma volume by ^{125}I-labeled albumin or red cell mass by ^{55}Cr-labeled red cells, is time-consuming, expensive, and usually used only in research centers. The CVP and WP were thought to have the needed accuracy and have largely replaced blood volume measurements. Low CVP and WP reflect low blood volume during acute hypovolemia; high venous pressures are associated with both acute blood volume overload in the initial resuscitation or in the immediate postoperative period and cardiac failure at any time. However, venous pressures are unreliable indicators of blood volume in ICU patients (Shippy et al., 1984); compliance changes in venous wall-tension occur with the changing neural and neurohormonal patterns over time in ICU patients. Venous pressures accommodate to either high or low blood volumes with values of about 10–15 mmHg. CVP and WP, which measure venous pressures not blood volume, are useful to prevent acute volume overload during rapid fluid restoration and fluid challenges. With rapid volume loading, the CVP and WP reflect the capacity of the vascular system to accept more volume without producing pulmonary edema. Notwithstanding, peripheral and pulmonary edema may result from massive crystalloid infusions that expand the interstitial space without fully restoring plasma volume or exceeding *safe* venous pressures.

Daily weight and fluid balance measurement are used to monitor fluid management; both measure changes in body water, not blood volume. Body composition studies are the definitive means to measure the distribution of body water between the plasma, interstitium, and intracellular compartments.

PREDICTION OF OUTCOME

Relative Importance of Hemodynamic and Oxygen Transport Variables

Traditionally monitored variables are useful descriptors of end stage circulatory failure, but they are not sensitive or accurate for early warning of impending circulatory problems in acutely ill surgical patients. However, the biologic importance of each cardio-respiratory variable may be assessed by its ability to predict outcome. The relationship of a given variable to survival or death is also the best criterion of its usefulness in making therapeutic decisions. The capability for each hemodynamic and oxygen transport variable to predict outcome varies from stage to stage as the patient's shock syndromes evolve, indicating that the predictors are stage-specific. For example, MAP is a poor predictor in the early stages, but a good late predictor. However, in the late stage, most variables predict outcome well, but at this time, clinical judgment is good and the clinical usefulness of predictions is minimal (Shoemaker and Czer, 1979). Rigor mortis may be the best indicator of all, but it occurs too late to be useful for therapeutic decisions.

Outcome Prediction

A simplified predictor was developed based on the survival rates of critically ill patients whose values for each variable fell within each of ten equally spaced divisions of the total range of values; the average score of each variable's prediction was computed to give an overall predictive index at successive times post-operatively (Shoemaker et al., 1985a; Bland and Shoemaker, 1985b). For example, Fig. 18.5 illustrates the survival rates of patients whose left ventricular stroke work index values ranged from 15–90 g·m/m² in the first 8 hours postoperatively in our initial retrospective postoperative series. Survival rates increased progressively from the low end of the spectrum until a plateau was reached; the height of the plateau reflects the predictive capacity of the variable and the width of this plateau defines the optimal values. Figure 18.6 illustrates $\dot{D}o_2$ and $\dot{V}o_2$ values in the same series; the wide, high plateau for $\dot{D}o_2$ indicates this variable is an excellent predictor; optimal values for survival were

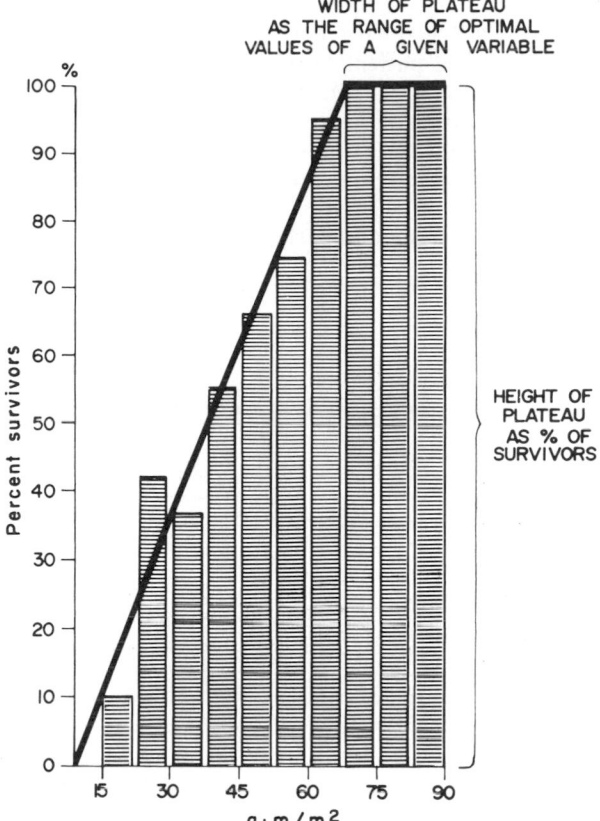

Fig. 18.5 Distribution of observed values for left ventricular stroke work in the first 8 hours postoperatively in our first series. The survival rates were calculated for the patients whose values fell into each of the ten divisions from the lowest to the highest value. Note the plateau at the top; the height of this plateau reflects how good the variable is as a predictor. The width reflects the values that are associated with good outcome. (Reproduced with permission from Shoemaker et al., 1983).

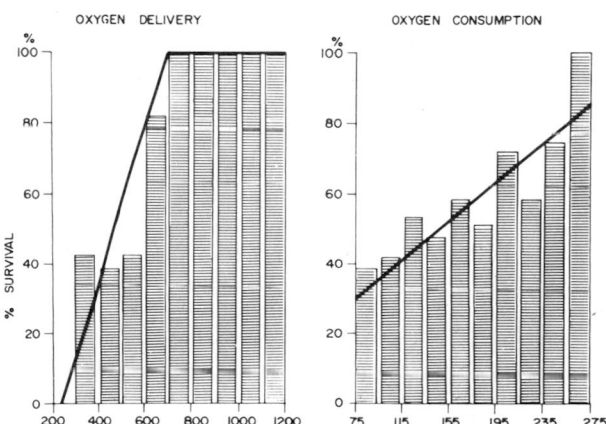

Fig. 18.6 Distribution of values for oxygen delivery (left) and oxygen consumption (right) in the same series. (Reproduced with permission from Shoemaker et al., 1983).

over 600 ml·min⁻¹·m⁻². The $\dot{V}_{O_2}$ pattern shows increasing survival with increasing $\dot{V}_{O_2}$ values. Figure 18.7 illustrates patient survival rates for HR were approximately 50% throughout the observed range, indicating poor prognostic capability. PVR values did not have a high plateau indicating that it was a poor predictor of survival, but the decrease to 0% survival above values of 500 dyn·s·cm⁵·m⁻² indicates that this variable was a good early predictor of death. This

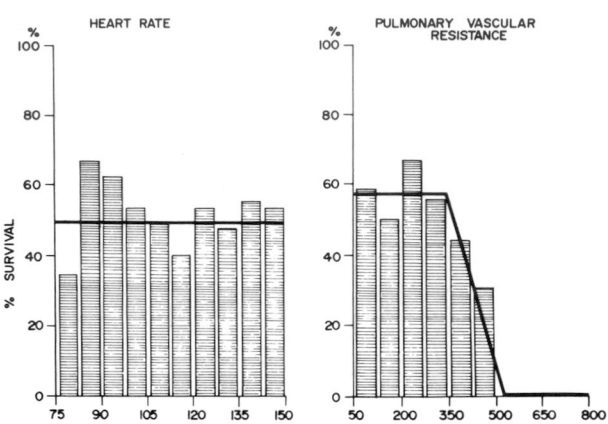

Fig. 18.7 Distribution of values for heart rate (left) and pulmonary vascular resistance index (right) in the same series. (Reproduced with permission from Shoemaker et al., 1983).

system of predictors was also tested in a prospective trial of a fresh series of patients and found to be 94% correct. Figure 18.8 shows significant separation between survivors and nonsurvivors beginning about 4 hours postoperatively (Bland et al., 1985b). The advantage of these predictors is that they objectively analyse the complex physiologic problems with no preconceptions and a minimum number of assumptions. The criteria are empirically and heuristically determined solely by the observed values of critically ill surgical patients who survived as compared with the values of those who subsequently died (Bland et al., 1985; Hankeln et al., 1987; Shoemaker et al., 1982, 1985a).

THERAPY

Physiologic compensatory responses maintain overall circulatory function and integrity after trauma, hemorrhage, sepsis, and other forms of stress. Fatal complications occur when these responses fail to compensate adequately. For example, increased cardiac output may compensate for reduced hematocrit, reduced P_{O_2}, or adequate tissue oxygenation. Since this compensatory flow increase has survival value, therapy should augment cardiac output rather than return it to the normal range. The use of propanolol or other β-blockers to reduce HR or to return high

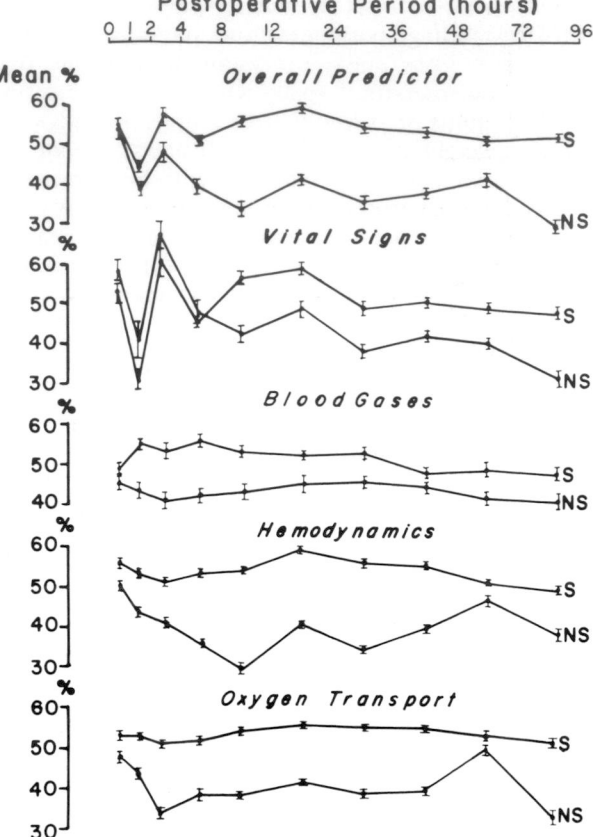

Fig. 18.8 Upper section: overall predictor for survivors (S) and nonsurvivors (NS) at each time interval postoperatively. Second Section: Predictions calculated from the vital signs variables for S and NS. Third Section: Predictions calculated from the blood gas variables for S and NS. Fourth Section: Predictions calculated from the hemodynamic variables for S and NS. Lowest Section: Predictions calculated from the oxygen transport variables for S and NS. Dots represent mean values, vertical bars SEM. (Reproduced with permission from Bland and Shoemaker, 1985b).

cardiac output values to the normal range in patients with traumatic or septic shock may result in precipitous circulatory and metabolic deterioration. The understanding of cardiorespiratory responses to stress in mechanistic terms is essential since the maintenance and augmentation of these compensatory responses is needed for survival.

Therapeutic Plan Using a Branched-Chain Decision Tree

Strategies for achieving therapeutic goals were determined empirically by evaluating the relative effectiveness of each therapy. Decision rules, priorities and a branch-chain decision tree were developed from the survivor and nonsurvivor patterns as well as patients' responses to specific therapeutic interventions (Fig. 18.9). Vigorous volume loading without exceed-

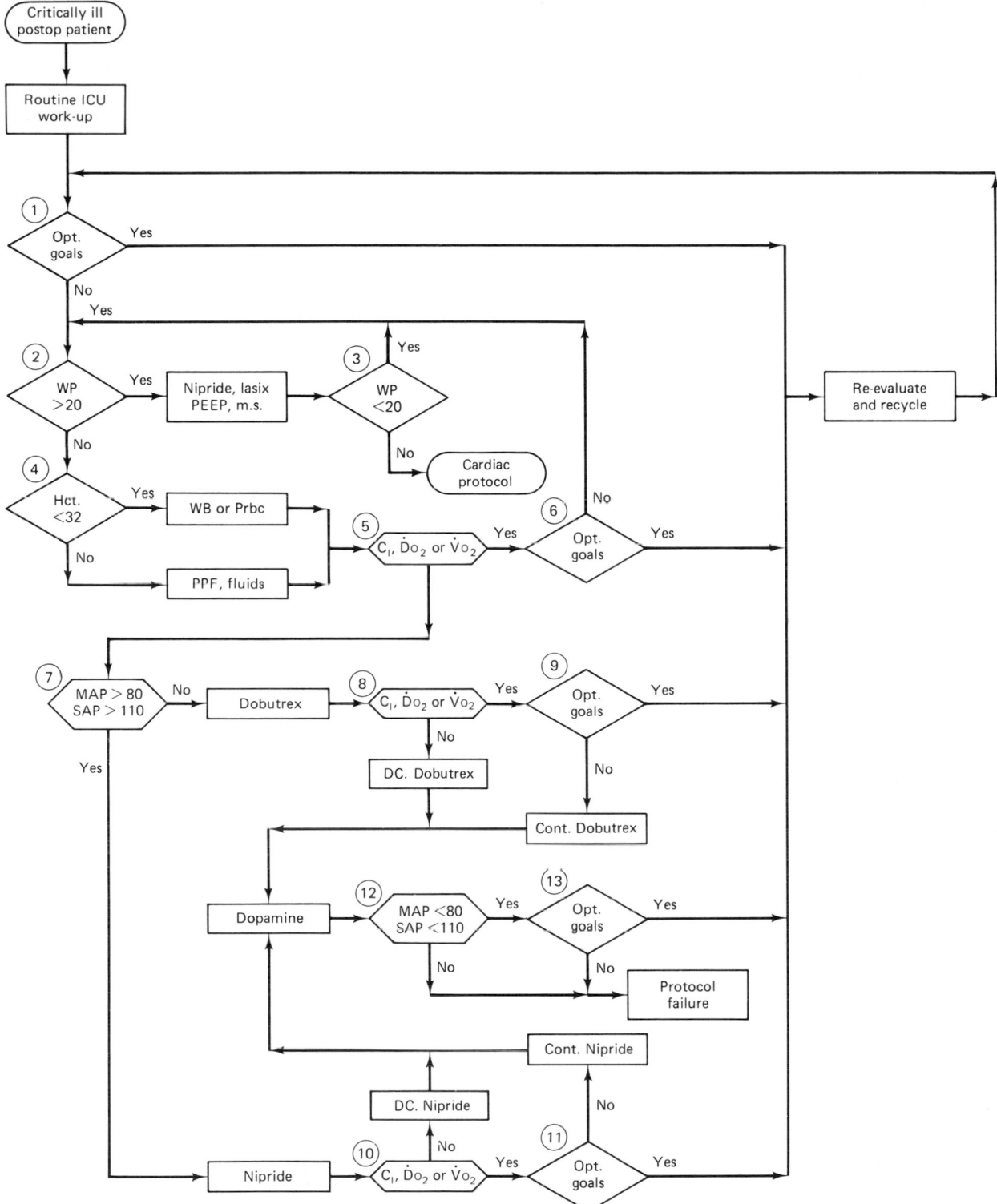

Fig. 18.9 Branch-chain decision tree for postoperative ICU patients. Preliminary evaluation of high-risk critically ill patients by routine ICU work-up that includes arterial blood gases, chest X-ray, routine blood chemistries, ECG, and coagulation studies. These tests should be either performed or in process and the observed defects corrected. *Step 1*. Measure CI, $\dot{D}_{O_2}$, $\dot{V}_{O_2}$ and blood volume (BV) to determine if the patient has reached the optimal goals. If CI < 4.5 L/min $\cdot$ m², $D_{O_2} < 600$ ml/(min $\cdot$ m²), $\dot{V}_{O_2} < 170$ ml/min $\cdot$ m², or BV < 3 L/m² for men or 2.7 L/m² for women, proceed to step 2, but if the goals are reached, the objective of the algorithm has been achieved; re-evaluate and recycle at intervals to maintain these goals. *Step 2*. Take pulmonary artery wedge pressure (WP). If > 20 mmHg, proceed to step 3; if < 20, proceed to step 4. *Step 3*. If WP > 20, give furosemide iv at increasing dose levels (20, 40, 80, 160 mg) if there is

continued on page 226

continued from page 225

clinical or X-ray evidence of salt and water overload or clinical findings of pulmonary congestion. If not, consider vaso-dilators, nitroprusside or nitroglycerin if MAP > 80 and systolic pressure > 110 mmHg. Recycle to titrate the dose as needed to reduce WP < 15 mmHg but maintain MAP > 80 mmHg. If unsuccessful, place on cardiac protocol. *Step 4*. If Hct < 32%, give 1 unit of whole blood (WB) or 2 units of packed red blood cells (Prbc)). If Hct > 32%, give a fluid load (volume challenge) consisting of one of the following (depending on clinical indications of plasma volume deficit or hydration): 500 ml of 5% PPF; 500 ml of 5% albumin; 50 ml of 25% albumin (25 g); 500 ml of 6% hydroxyethyl starch; 500 ml of 6% dextran-60; or 1000 ml of D5RL. *Step 5*. If the blood or fluid load improved any of the optimal therapeutic goals defined in step 1, proceed to step 6; if none is improved, proceed to step 7. *Step 6*. If goals are not reached, recycle steps 2 through 6 until these goals are met or WP > 20 mmHg. *Step 7*. If MAP > 80 or systolic arterial pressure (SAP) < 110 mmHg, give dobutamine by constant iv infusion in increasing doses to increase CI, $\dot{D}o_2$ and $\dot{V}o_2$. *Step 8*. Titrate dobutamine beginning with 2 µg/(min·kg) and gradually increase doses up to 10 µg/(min·kg) provided there is im-provement in CI, $\dot{D}o_2$, or $\dot{V}o_2$ without further lowering of arterial pressure until goals are met. *Step 9*. If goals are reached, re-evaluate and recycle. If goals are not reached or it becomes evident that higher doses of the drug are not more effect-ive or that they produce hypotension and tachycardia, continue dobutamine at its most effective dose range. *Step 10*. If MAP > 80 mmHg and SAP > 110 mmHg, give sodium nitroprusside or nitroglycerin in gradually increasing doses pro-vided there is improvement in CI, $\dot{D}o_2$ or $\dot{V}o_2$. *Step 11*. If there is no improvement in CI, $\dot{D}o_2$, or $\dot{V}o_2$ with the vasodilator, or if hypotension (MAP < 80 mmHg, SAP < 110 mmHg) ensues, discontinue the vasodilator. If there is improvement in CI, $\dot{D}o_2$ or $\dot{V}o_2$ titrate the vasodilator to its maximum effect consistent with satisfactory arterial pressures. *Step 12*. If opti-mal goals are reached, re-evaluate and recycle at intervals. If these goals are not reached and MAP < 80 mmHg, and SAP < 110, give vasopressors, dopamine or if ineffective, norepinephrine. *Step 13*. Titrate doses of vasopressor in the lowest doses possible to maintain arterial pressures, MAP > 80, SAP > 110. If the goals and pressures cannot be main-tained, the patient is considered to be a protocol failure. (Reproduced with permission from Shoemaker et al., 1983).

ing WP values greater than 18–20 mmHg is the first and most important therapy. Packed red cells or whole blood is given when the Hct is below 34%. Therapeutic goals may be easier to achieve with col-loids that expand the plasma volume without over-expansion of the interstitial water (Appel et al., 1981; Hauser et al., 1980; Shoemaker et al., 1973, 1977). It should not be assumed that plasma volume has been restored in patients with pitting edema who have received large volumes of crystalloids, because expanded interstitial water frequently occurs in the presence of hypovolemia. Concentrated (25%) albu-min, which expands plasma volume by shifting inter-stitial water back into the plasma volume may be given in these conditions (Appel and Shoemaker, 1981; Hauser et al., 1980).

After the maximum effect of fluids has been obtained, an inotropic agent such as dobutamine is started at about 2 µg·kg^{-1}·min^{-1} and titrated to achieve the desired CI, $\dot{D}o_2$ and $\dot{V}o_2$. If the patient has normal or high MAP with SVR, vasodilation with labetalol, nitroglycerine, or nitroprusside is con-sidered; the optimal dose is obtained by titration to achieve improved cardiac index without producing hypotension. If fluids, inotropic agents, and vasodila-tors fail to achieve optimal goals, vasopressors such as dopamine are then given in the lowest dose needed to maintain MAP above 80 mmHg and systolic arterial pressure (SAP) above 110 mmHg. Vasopressors are given last because they limit optimal fluid administra-tion by increasing venous pressures, pulmonary venous shunt, and lactic acidemia.

Goals and Strategies in Various Types of Shock

The therapeutic strategy is to open up unevenly vaso-

constricted microcirculatory networks. This may be done by increasing volume and flow with fluids, inotropic agents and vasodilators to force open the constricted circuits. Volume is given until optimal goals are achieved or WP is 18–20 mmHg. In this approach WP is not used as a measure of blood volume, because it clearly does not reflect blood volume (Shippy et al., 1984). Rather, WP is used as an upper limit for volume therapy in order to avoid pul-monary edema. In postinjury stress, cirrhosis, trau-matic shock or septic shock, the $\dot{V}o_2$ requirements cannot be measured directly because the $\dot{V}o_2$ even though high, may be limited by flow. Moreover, the widely varying increases in metabolism require a wide range of increased circulatory function to supply these increased needs. The answer to this dilemma is an operational definition of goals: continue to give each therapy as long as it improves CI, $\dot{D}o_2$ and $\dot{V}o_2$, unless limited by WP (in the fluid therapy), tachycar-dia > 130 (in inotropic agents), and hypotension < 80 MAP or < 110 SAP (for vasodilators). After adequate fluids and inotropic stimulation, vasopressors may be used to maintain sufficient MAP to provide for coron-ary and cerebral perfusion.

Therapeutic Goals and Strategies of Elderly and Cardiac Patients

Cardiac patients with otherwise healthy bodies have different physiologic problems than do patients with normal hearts but multiple organ failures. The heart may be the weak link in the former, but circulatory transport functions often limit survival in the latter. An appropriate strategy in cardiac patients may be to reduce cardiac work with vasodilators rather than to stimulate the heart with inotropic agents or overload it with salt and water. Unfortunately, critically ill patients do not always divide themselves neatly into cardiac and noncardiac categories.

The elderly patient and the cardiac patient also may have life-threatening multiple organ failures. Under these conditions, rigid interpretation with the decision tree is not appropriate. Volume therapy with concentrated albumin may be given in preference to sodium-rich solutions. Inotropic agents such as dobutamine may be tried in the lowest effective dose, while isoproterenol and vasopressors that increase cardiac work more than they increase myocardial blood flow should be avoided; vasodilators, particularly after plasma volume has been adequately restored by volume loading, may be effective. The hemodynamic effectiveness of each agent given separately should be established before combinations of agents are used. The most important principles in these complex clinical conditions are to: (1) document baseline hemodynamic and oxygen transport variables; (2) measure changes with each agent; and (3) titrate the dose to achieve values as close to optimal as possible.

Therapeutic Goals and Strategy in Surgical Patients Who Preoperatively have High Cardiac Output and $\dot{V}o_2$

In preoperative patients with severe trauma, stress, sepsis and hypercatabolic states, increased $\dot{V}o_2$ indicates increased metabolic requirements. Even though the $\dot{V}o_2$ is increased the patient's metabolic needs have not necessarily been met. Since therapeutic goals cannot be measured under conditions of increased metabolism, the adequacy of therapy cannot be determined directly. However, tissue oxygen demand may be indirectly evaluated empirically by a trial of therapy. If the therapy increases cardiac output and $\dot{V}o_2$, it may be assumed that therapy opened up additional microcirculatory channels that perfused relatively hypoxic tissues which, being hypoxic, extracted additional oxygen. Since tissues cannot take up more oxygen than they use, the increased $\dot{V}o_2$ after fluid challenge indicates that an oxygen debt had been present and that this debt was at least partially satisfied.

Prospective Clinical Trials of this Approach

A therapeutic plan which used the empirically defined median values of the survivors as a first approximation to therapeutic goals was tested prospectively in two clinical trials of high risk, high mortality patients; the control group had normal values as their therapeutic goals, while the protocol group had the supranormal median values of the survivors as their therapeutic goals (Shoemaker et al., 1982a, 1983, 1988). There were marked reductions in morbidity and mortality in the protocol patients. In a subsequent, three-leg trial, begun preoperatively and strictly randomized using sealed envelopes, CVP cath-

eters with normal values as goals, pulmonary artery catheters with normal values as goals, and pulmonary artery catheters with optimal values as goals of therapy were compared (Shoemaker et al., 1988). The results showed no statistically significant difference between the mortality of patients managed with CVP catheters (23%) and those with pulmonary artery catheter with normal values as therapeutic goals (33%). However, the pulmonary artery catheter with optimal goals led to significantly reduced (4%) mortality. Similarly, the number of complications, hospital days, ICU days, and ventilator days were reduced.

Fluid Therapy

Comparison of crystalloids and colloids in prospectively randomized studies in critically ill postoperative patients were reported by Skillman et al., 1975 and Boutrous et al., 1979, in burn patients by Jelenko et al., 1979, and in emergency hypotensive shock and trauma patients by Shoemaker et al., 1981; Rackow et al., 1982, 1983 and Modig, 1983. These studies showed statistically significant physiological and clinical advantages in colloid administration.

Physiologic criteria for fluid therapy are the most important questions. If the immediate, direct effects of sodium (increased blood pressure and urine output) are used as the criteria of efficacy, then sodium-rich solutions are most likely to be judged efficacious. However, if cardiac output, blood volume, $\dot{D}o_2$ and $\dot{V}o_2$ are the appropriate outcome measures, then colloids and blood are the most effective agents (Shoemaker and Monson, 1973a; Shoemaker et al., 1973, 1977; Hauser et al., 1980). The efficacy of alternative fluid therapies is best evaluated by physiologic responses that are related to survival, rather than commonly monitored variables that are routinely used because of their convenience.

The high risk critically ill postoperative patient requiring fluid resuscitation should have a pulmonary artery catheter to define physiologic problems and to titrate fluid therapy to the optimal goals defined by the pattern of the survivors of life-threatening operations. Achievement of these physiologic goals is of crucial importance; changes in the variables related to the bulk transport and utilization of oxygen provide the most sensitive and specific criteria of circulatory performance after various therapeutic/interventions.

The relative effectiveness of alternative therapies may be compared by hemodynamic and oxygen transport responses which use the patient as his own control (Shoemaker and Monson, 1973a; Shoemaker et al., 1977; Hauser et al., 1980). Figure 18.10 illustrates an example of resuscitation from burn shock from a series of burn patients who were given various colloids and lactated Ringer's solution alternately during the period of their critical illness (Shoemaker et al., 1977). Increases in CI, $\dot{D}o_2$ and $\dot{V}o_2$ were significantly greater after colloids than twice or four times the

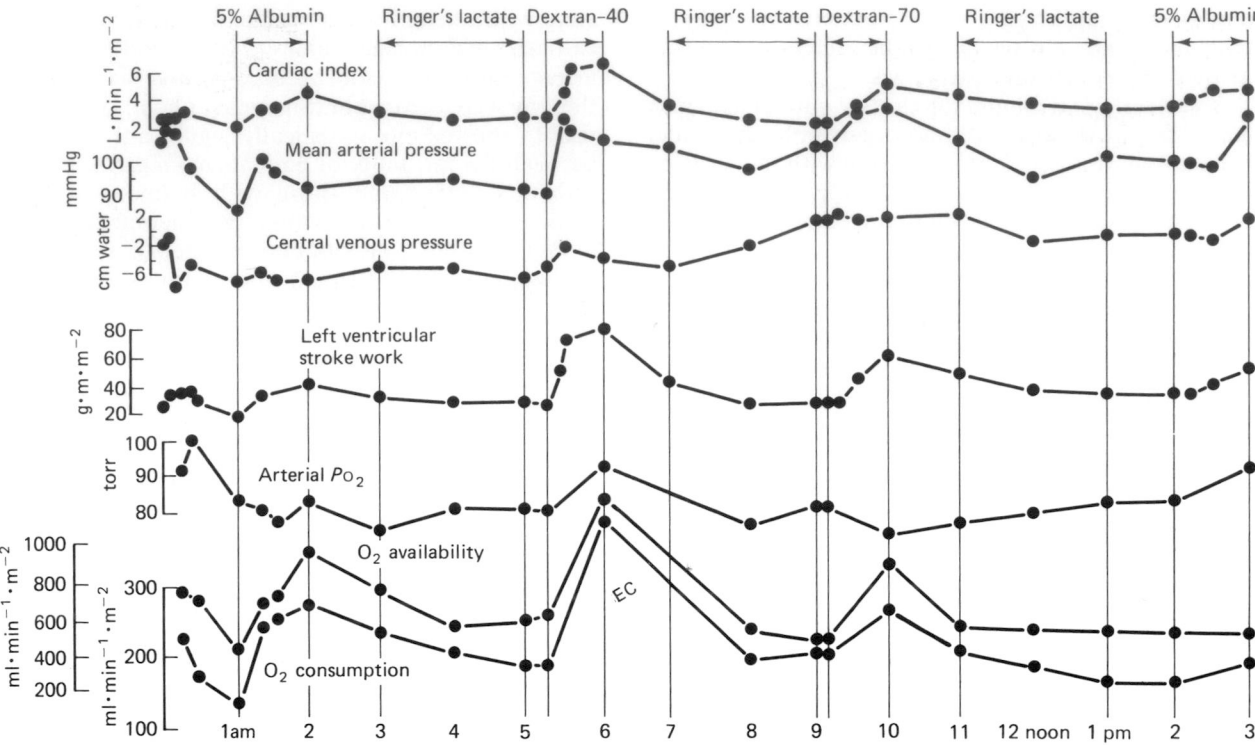

Fig. 18.10 Cardiorespiratory values during resuscitation of a patient with severe burns. (Reproduced with permission from Shoemaker et al., 1977).

volume of the crystalloids (Shoemaker et al., 1973, 1977; Hauser et al., 1980).

Hauser et al., 1980 compared the changes after 1 L of lactated Ringer's solution with those of 25 g of 25% albumin (100 ml) given in random order to a prospective series of critically ill surgical patients with early lung shock (Fig. 18.11). Albumin increased plasma volume 465 ± 47 (SE) ml by shifting over 350 ml of water from the interstitial water to the intravascular water. Simultaneously, albumin increased CI, MAP, left ventricular stroke work, $\dot{D}o_2$ and $\dot{V}o_2$; lung function variables were not worsened but in many instances actually improved. By contrast, 1 L of Ringer's lactate expanded plasma volume only 194 ± 18 ml at its maximum which was at the end of infusion, i.e., over 80% of the infused crystalloid almost immediately equilibrated or *leaked* into the interstitial water and the small proportion of fluid remaining in the plasma, then decreased exponentially. After Ringer's lactate administration, $\dot{V}o_2$ decreased despite the slightly increased $\dot{D}o_2$ and the pulmonary shunt worsened. The hemodynamic responses to the administered fluid were directly proportional to volume expansion. Thus, colloids improve hemodynamics and oxygen transport by plasma expansion, while crystalloids principally expand interstitial volume; when tolerated, they may restore plasma volume if massive amounts are given (Hauser et al., 1980).

Recently our series was expanded to include 400

fluid therapy interventions in 211 patients with early adult respiratory distress syndrome (ARDS) occurring postoperatively and in sepsis (Appel and Shoemaker, 1981; Shoemaker and Appel, 1985). Figures 12–14 illustrate the flow and oxygen transport variables in: (1) patients during ARDS, (2) these same patients not during ARDS, i.e., before or after the episode of ARDS, and (3) a concurrent group of critically ill patients who did not develop ARDS. These data show significant increases in oxygen transport and delivery after colloid infusion but no significant changes after infusion of Ringer's lactate except increased arterial pressure (Table 18.4); there was a similar lack of changes when the data were stratified into groups with high, normal, and low initial cardiac index values. Circulatory effects of colloids were similar in patients with and without ARDS. However, these therapeutic studies were made in the first day or two after onset of ARDS. By contrast, there were no significant differences in cardiac output after infusion of colloids, whole blood, or crystalloids in patients in the preterminal stage of ARDS defined as the last 24–48 hours of life (Shoemaker and Appel, 1985). Thus, clinical manifestations of the capillary leak syndrome develop after the clinical appearance of ARDS; the capillary leak appears to be the result, not the pathogenic cause of ARDS. Colloids may improve those physiologic variables that determine survival after ARDS until there is evidence that they significantly increase pulmonary shunting.

Inotropic Support

After the maximum effect of fluid therapy has been attained, inotropic agents may be used to improve cardiac output and flow-related variables. Norepinephrine (noradrenaline), epinephrine (adrenaline)

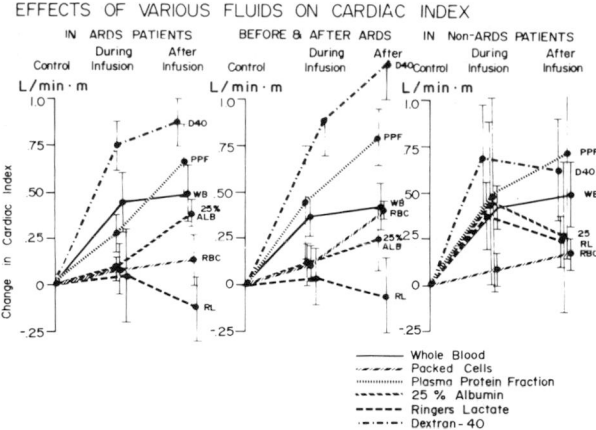

EFFECTS OF VARIOUS FLUIDS ON CARDIAC INDEX

Fig. 18.12 Cardiac index responses to various agents are shown in patients with ARDS during the episode of respiratory distress (left section), patients with ARDS not during the episode of respiratory distress (center section), and patients without ARDS (right section). The data represents changes in CI + SEM during and after the administration of each agent. (Reproduced with permission from Appel and Shoemaker, 1981).

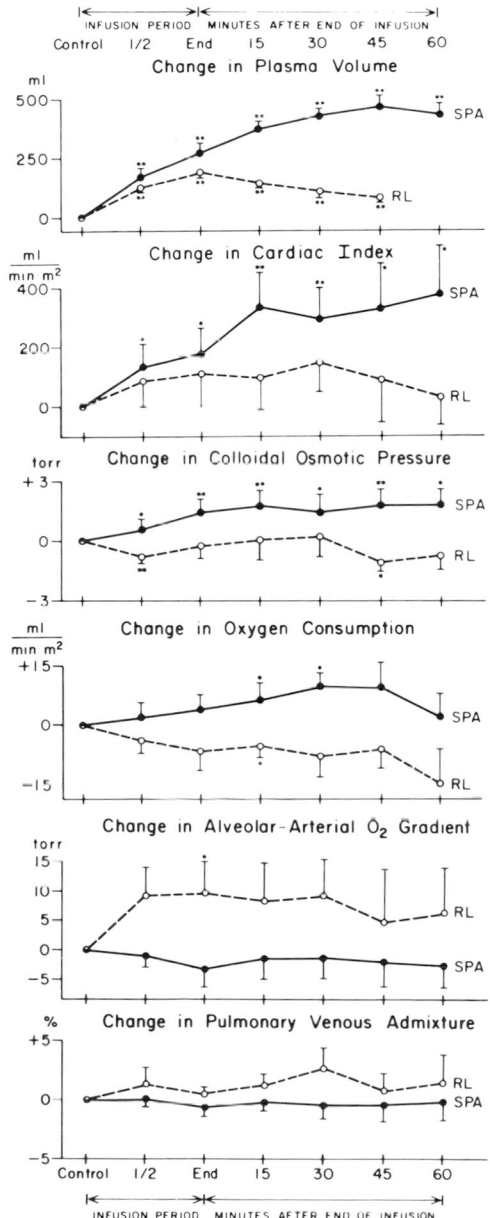

Fig. 18.11 Changes in plasma volume, cardiac index (CI), colloid osmotic pressure, $\dot{V}o_2$, $P(\text{A-a})o_2$ and $\dot{Q}sp/\dot{Q}t$ are compared after intervention with 1000 ml of lactated Ringer's solution (RL) and 100 ml of 25% albumin (SAP) in a crossover study. Note the greater increase in plasma volume, CI, colloid osmotic pressure, and $\dot{V}o_2$ after SPA. $P(\text{A-a})o_2$ as well as $\dot{Q}sp/\dot{Q}t$ were unaffected by SPA, whereas after infusion of RL, $P(\text{A-a})o_2$ increased. *P <0.05. (Reproduced with permission from Hauser et al., 1980).

and dopamine have α adrenergic effects that increase the MAP and SVR as well as β_1 effects that increase cardiac output. Dobutamine has both β_1 cardiotonic action as well as β_2 effects that dilate previously vasoconstricted metarteriolar-capillary networks; it must only be given after hypovolemia has been corrected by adequate fluid therapy. The net effect of dobutamine is to improve both cardiac output and tissue perfusion; the latter is indicated by improved $\dot{D}o_2$ and $\dot{V}o_2$ (Shoemaker et al., 1986). In prospective clinical trials, dobutamine has greater inotropic effects than dopamine at the same dosage; dopamine has greater vasopressor effect, but it produces hypoxemia from increased pulmonary shunting (Shoemaker et al., 1988).

Vasodilator Therapy

Vasodilators are frequently used in the presence of hypertension or increased SVRI. Nitroprusside and nitroglycerine are α-blocking agents that often increase cardiac output and decrease MAP and SVR. Labetalol is a selective α_1 blocking agent with nonspecific β_1 blocking action (MacCarthy et al., 1983; Morel et al., 1984). It may, therefore, be given in combination with dobutamine to override the negative inotropic effects of labetalol. Labetalol with or without dobutamine inproves both flow and tissue perfusion as reflected by increased $\dot{D}o_2$ and $\dot{V}o_2$ (Harrier and Shoemaker, in press).

All vasodilators should be given only after hypovolemia has been corrected with adequate fluid therapy, as vasodilation in the hypovolemic state will produce severe hypotension.

TABLE 18.4

CARDIORESPIRATORY RESPONSES TO FLUID THERAPY

Variable	Units	Lactated Ringer's Solution (N = 19)			Albumin 5% (N = 39)		
		Control	Mid-point (500 ml)	After infusion (1000 ml)	Control	Mid-point (250 ml)	After infusion (500 ml)
Mean arterial pressure	mmHg	90 ± 16*	95 ± 18	99 ± 16**	85 ± 20	90 ± 19**	89 ± 22**
Cardiac index	L/(min·m²)	3.97 ± .94	419 ± .85	4.22 ± 1.16	3.04 ± .99	3.57 ± 1.1**	3.68 ± 1.1*
CVP	cm H₂O	6.1 ± 5.2	7.3 ± 4.3	8.2 ± 5	4.7 ± 5.9	6.4 ± 6.6	7.5 ± 7.3**
Heart rate	beat/min	108 ± 29	108 ± 27	110 ± 24	103 ± 28	103 ± 19	103 ± 26
Mean pulmonary arterial pressure	mmHg	15.2 ± 6.5	17.3 ± 10.9	17.1 ± 6.1	16.5 ± 7.1	18.2 ± 6.3	20.2 ± 7**
Pulmonary wedge pressure	mmHg	8.5 ± 2.6	9.9 ± 3.3	9.7 ± 2.7	7.5 ± 6.1	9.0 ± 4.9	11.1 ± 6.5*
Systemic vasc. resistance	dyn·s· cm⁻⁵·m²	1647 ± 397	1589 ± 410	1458 ± 343	2307 ± 941	1969 ± 959**	1912 ± 808*
Pulmonary vasc. resistance	dyn·s· cm⁻⁵·m²	163 ± 76	167 ± 56	157 ± 117	246 ± 133	211 ± 90**	216 ± 111**
Left cardiac work	kg·m/m²	4.9 ± 1.7	5.3 ± 2.2	5.4 ± 1.8	3.5 ± 1.5	4.3 ± 1.5**	4.5 ± 1.8**
Right cardiac work	kg·m/m²	0.84 ± .41	0.96 ± .45	1.05 ± .45	0.69 ± .43	0.91 ± .37**	1.0 ± .45**
Hematocrit	%	30.2 ± 6.1	28.7 ± 6.5	29.2 ± 6.2	34.7 ± 4.7	33.2 ± 4	31.3 ± 4.1*
O₂ delivery	ml/(min·m²)	565 ± 176	580 ± 204	585 ± 208	458 ± 164	504 ± 149**	512 ± 157**
O₂ consumption	ml/(min·m²)	145 ± 31	149 ± 23	146 ± 34	128 ± 36	131 ± 33	129 ± 31
O₂ extraction	%	24 ± 3	24 ± 5	27 ± 8	29 ± 8	28 ± 4	29 ± 9

Note
 * Mean ± SD
 ** $P < 0.5$

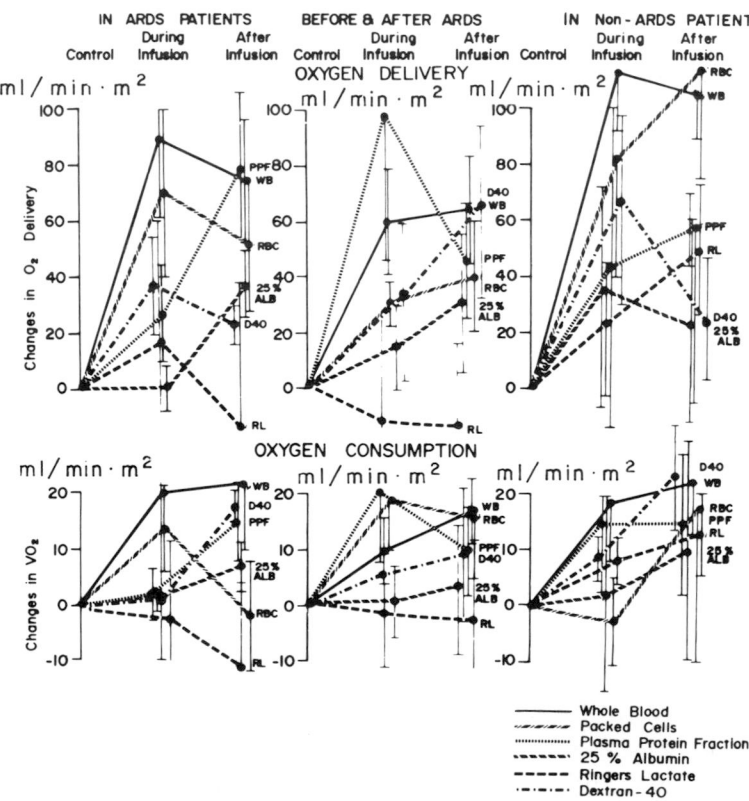

Fig. 18.13 Changes in $\dot{D}o_2$ and $\dot{V}o_2$ during and after adminstration of various agents are shown, as described in Fig. 18.12. (Reproduced with permission from Appel and Shoemaker, 1981).

CHANGE IN BLOOD VOLUME PLOTTED AGAINST
CHANGE IN CARDIAC INDEX AFTER VARIOUS FLUIDS

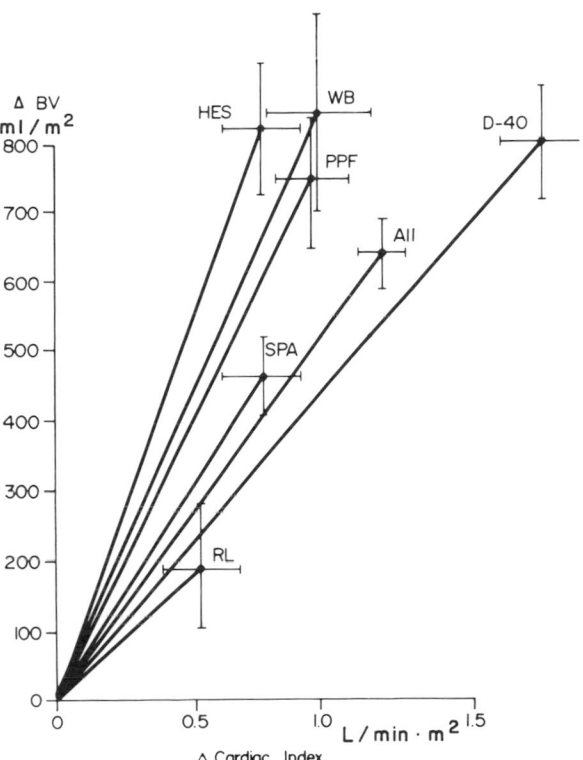

Fig. 18.14 Changes in blood volume index expressed as mean (dot) ISEM (vertical bars) plotted against changes in cardiac index mean (dot) ISEM (horizontal bars) for various fluids: WB 500 ml whole blood; HES 500 ml 6% hydroxy starch, PPF 500 ml plasma protein fraction; D-40, 500 ml 10% dextran-40; SPA 100 ml 25% (salt pool) albumen; RL 1000 ml Ringers-lactate. (Reproduced with permission from Shippy et al., 1984).

Other Factors

This approach directed towards fluid and pharmacologic management of shock obviously will not correct diagnostic errors, anatomical problems, misadventures at the time of surgery, transfusion reactions, idiosyncratic drug reactions, iatrogenic ineptitudes, or the lack of the patient's motivation to live. Furthermore, even if physiologic variables are optimized, the patient's cardiac and pulmonary reserve capacities may not be adequate for overwhelming trauma.

SUMMARY

In essence, most postoperative deaths are due to identifiable, predictable, and preventable physiologic problems. Second, therapy of the critically ill should be defined by physiologic criteria of survivors of life-threatening disorders. Third, administration of therapy should be monitored prophylactically to obtain optimal physiologic goals rather than giving

therapy to attain normal values after the deficiency has occurred. Fourth, the use of a branch-chain decision tree helps to achieve expeditiously these therapeutic goals by providing a coherent organized patient management plan that maintains prophylactically the optimal hemodynamic state and prevents tissue hypoxia from blood volume, hemodynamic, and oxygen transport deficits. Finally, therapy to optimize the important variables should be given as soon as possible after the onset of accidental trauma as well as before, during, and immediately after surgery in the high-risk patient.

REFERENCES

Appel P.L., Shoemaker W.C. (1981). Fluid therapy in adult respiratory failure. *Crit. Care Med.*, **9**, 862.

Bland R.D., Shoemaker W.C., Shabot M.M. (1978). Physiologic monitoring goals for the critically ill patient. *Surg. Gynecol. Obstet.*, **147**, 833.

Bland R.D., Shoemaker W.C., Abraham E., et al. (1985). Hemodynamic and oxygen transport patterns in surviving and nonsurviving postoperative patients. *Crit. Care Med.*, **13**, 85.

Bland R.D., Shoemaker W.C. (1985a). Common physiologic patterns in general surgical patients. Hemodynamic and oxygen transport changes during and after operation in patients with and without associated medical problems. *Surg. Clin. North. Am.*, **65**, 793.

Bland R.D., Shoemaker W.C. (1985b). Probability of survival as a prognostic and severity of illness score in critically ill surgical patients. *Crit. Care Med.*, **13**, 91.

Boutrous A.R., Ruess R., Olson L., et al. (1979). Comparison of hemodynamic, pulmonary and renal effects of use of three types of fluids following major surgical procedures on the abdominal aorta. *Crit. Care Med.*, **7**, 9.

Clowes G.H.A. Jr., Del Guercio L.R.M. (1960). Circulatory response to trauma of surgical operations. *Metab.*, **9**, 67.

Comroe J., Foster R.E., DuBois A.B., et al. (1962). *The Lung: Clinical Physiology and Pulmonary Function Tests.* 2nd edn. Chicago: Year Book Medical Publishers.

Cournand A., Riley R.L., Bradley S.E., et al. (1943). Studies of the circulation in clinical shock. *Surg.*, **13**, 964.

Del Guercio L.R.M., Commarswamy R.F., Feins N.R., et al. (1964). Pulmonary arteriovenous admixture and the hyperdynamic state in surgery for portal hypertension. *Surg.*, **56**, 57.

Hankeln K., Senker R., Schwarten J.M., et al. (1987). Evaluation of prognostic indices based on hemodynamic and oxygen transport variables in shock patients with adult respiratory distress syndrome. *Crit. Care Med.*, **15**, 1.

Harrier H.D., Shoemaker W.C., Appel P.L., et al. (In Press). Use of labetalol in critical surgical illness. *Crit. Care Med.*

Haupt M.T., Rackow E.C. (1982). Colloids osmotic pressure and fluid resuscitation with hetastarch, albumin, and saline solutions. *Crit. Care Med.*, **10**, 159.

Hauser C.J., Shoemaker W.C., Turpin I., et al. (1980). Hemodynamic and oxygen transport responses to body water shifts produced by colloids and crystalloids in critically ill patients. *Surg. Gynecol. Obstet.*, **150**, 811.

Heilbrunn A., Allbritten F.F., (1960). Cardiac output during and following surgical operation. *Ann. Surg.*, **152**, 197.

Jelenko C., Williams J.B., Wheeler M.L. et al., (1979).

Studies in shock and resuscitation. I: Use of a hypertonic, albumin-containing, fluid demand regimen in resuscitation: A physiologically appropriate method. *Crit. Care Med.*, **7**, 157.

MacCarthy E.P., Bloomfield S.S. (1983). Labetalol: a review of its pharmacology, pharmacokinetics, clinical uses and adverse effects. *Pharm.*, **3**, 193.

Modig J., (1983). Advantages of dextran–70 over Ringer's acetate solution in shock treatment and in prevention of adult respiratory distress syndrome: A randomized study in man after traumatic-hemorrhage shock. *Resuscitation.*, **10**, 219.

Morel D.R., Forster A., Suter P.M. (1984). Evaluation of i.v. labetalol for treatment of post-traumatic hyperdynamic state. *Intens. Care Med.*, **10**, 133.

Nolan L.S., Shoemaker W.C. (1982). Transcutaneous O_2 and CO_2 monitoring of high risk surgical patient during the perioperative period. *Crit. Care Med.*, **10**, 762.

Rackow E.C., Falk J.L., Fein I.A., et al. (1983). Fluid resuscitation in circulatory shock. *Crit. Care Med.*, **11**, 839.

Riley R.L., Cournand A. (1951). Analysis of factors affecting partial pressures of oxygen and carbon dioxide in gas and blood of lungs: Theory. *J. Appl. Physiol.*, **4**, 77.

Shoemaker W.C. (1987). Relation of oxygen transport patterns to the pathophysiology and therapy of shock stress. *Intens. Care Med.*, **13**, 230.

Shoemaker W.C., Appel P.L. (1985). Pathophysiology of adult respiratory distress syndrome after sepsis and surgical operations. *Crit. Care Med.*, **13**, 166.

Shoemaker W.C., Appel P.L., Bland R., et al. (1982). Clinical trial of an algorithm for outcome prediction in acute circulatory failure. *Crit. Care Med.*, **10**, 390.

Shoemaker W.C., Appel P., Bland R. (1983). Use of physiologic monitoring to predict outcome and to assist in clinical decision in critically ill postoperative patients. *Am. J. Surg.*, **146**, 43.

Shoemaker W.C., Appel P.L., Kram H.B. (1986). Hemodynamic and oxygen transport effects of dobutamine in critically ill general surgical patients. *Crit. Care Med.*, **14**, 1032.

Shoemaker W.C., Appel P.J., Kram H.B., et al. (1988). Hemodynamic management of high risk surgical patients using central venous and pulmonary artery catheterization: A prospective randomized study of 88 patients.

Shoemaker W.C., Appel P.L., Kram H.B., et al. (1989). Comparison of dobutamine and dopamine in prospective randomized clinical trials. *Chest*.

Shoemaker W.C., Appel P.L., Waxman K., et al. (1982a). Clinical trial of survivors' cardiorespiratory patterns as therapeutic goals in critically ill postoperative patients. *Crit. Care Med.*, **10**, 398.

Shoemaker W.C., Bland R.D., Appel P.L. (1985a). Therapy of critically ill postoperative patients based on outcome prediction and prospective clinical trials. *Surg. Clin. North Am.*, **65**, 811.

Shoemaker W.C., Bryan-Brown C.W., Makabali G., et al. (1976). Method for estimating nutritional and non-nutritional blood flow and O_2 transport in critical illness. *Crit. Care Med.*, **4**, 117.

Shoemaker W.C., Bryan-Brown C.W., Quigley L., et al. (1973). Body fluid shifts in depletion and post stress states and their correlation with adequate nutrition. *Surg. Gynecol. Obstet.*, **136**, 371.

Shoemaker W.C., Czer L.S.C. (1979). Evaluation of the biologic importance of various hemodynamic and oxygen transport variables. *Crit. Care. Med.*, **7**, 424.

Shoemaker W.C., Czer L.S.C., Change P., et al. (1979). Cardiorespiratory monitoring in postoperative patients: I. Prediction of outcome and severity of illness. *Crit. Care Med.*, **7**, 237.

Shoemaker W.C., Launder W.J., Costagna J., et al. (1976a). Method for estimation of the perfusion defect in shock. *J. Surg. Res.*, **20**, 77.

Shoemaker W.C., Matsuda T., State D. (1977). Relative hemodynamic effectiveness of whole blood and plasma expanders in burned patients. *Surg. Gynecol. Obstet.*, **144**, 909.

Shoemaker W.C., Monson D.O. (1973a). Effect of whole blood and plasma expanders on volume-flow relationships in critically ill patients. *Surg. Gynecol. Obstet.*, **137**, 453.

Shoemaker W.C., Montgomery E.S., Kaplan E., et al. (1973b). Physiologic patterns in surviving and nonsurviving shock patients. *Arch. Surg.*, **106**, 630.

Shoemaker W.C., Printen K.J., Amato J.J., et al. (1967). Hemodynamic patterns after acute anesthetized and unanesthetized trauma. *Arch. Surg.*, **95**, 492.

Shoemaker W.C., Schluchter M., Hopkins J.A., et al. (1981). Comparison of the relative effectiveness of colloids and crystalloids in emergency resuscitation. *Am. J. Surg.*, **142**, 73.

Shippy C.R., Appel P.L., Shoemaker W.C. (1984). Reliability of clinical monitoring to assess blood volume in critically ill patients. *Crit. Care Med.*, **12**, 107.

Siegel J., Goldwyn P.M., Friedman H.P. (1971). Pattern and process in the evolution of human septic shock. *Surg.*, **70**, 232.

Skillman J.J., Restall D.S., Salzman W.E. (1975). Randomized trial of albumin *vs* electrolyte solutions during aortic operations. *Surg.*, **78**, 291.

Wiggers C.J. (1940). *Physiology of Shock*. New York: Commonwealth Fund.

Wilson R.F., Thal A.P., Kinding P.H., et al. (1965). Hemodynamic measurements in shock. *Arch. Surg.*, **91**, 124.

19. Electrocardiography: Normal and Abnormal Cardiac Electrophysiology

J. L. Atlee

Normal Cardiac Electrophysiology
  Cardiac action potential
  Resting membrane potential (RMP)
  Depolarization
  Threshold potential
  Refractoriness
  Slow inward current
  Repolarization
  Spontaneous phase 4 (Diastolic)
    depolarization
  Electrical activity of sinus node and AV node
    cells
Abnormal Cardiac Electrophysiology
  Loss of membrane potential
  Depressed fast response
  Conduction of the depressed fast response
  Refractoriness in depressed fibers
  Abnormal automaticity
  Triggered activity
  Early afterdepolarizations
  Re-entry of excitation
  Incomplete repolarization, depressed fast
    response, premature action potentials
  Slow response
  Re-entry with an anatomical obstacle
  Reflection
  Leading circle concept for re-entry
  Slow conduction and re-entry caused by the
    anisotropic structure of cardiac muscle
  Summation and inhibition

The electrocardiogram (ECG) is a graphic recording of the changing potential of an electrical field generated by a group of myocardial cells. It is useful as an aid to diagnosis for anatomic, pathophysiologic, and drug-induced disturbances affecting the heart. In the operating theatre, the ECG is most often used for the detection of cardiac arrhythmias. Cardiac arrhythmias result from disturbances that adversely affect normal electrical properties of the heart, or that initiate abnormal ones.

An arrhythmia is any abnormality in the rate, regularity, or site of origin of the cardiac impulse. It can also be a disturbance in the conduction of that impulse, such that the normal sequence of activation of the atria and ventricles is altered (Cranefield et al., 1973). Arrhythmias continue to be thought of as disturbances of impulse initiation, impulse propagation, or both (Hoffman and Cranefield, 1964). Such disturbances may result from mild impairment of normal cardiac electrical properties, or more serious alterations that can induce abnormal forms of cardiac electrical activity. An understanding of normal and abnormal cardiac electrophysiologic mechanisms is essential for correct diagnosis and proper management of cardiac arrhythmias.

Arrhythmias are not only of passing interest to anesthetists. Cardiac arrhythmias: (1) occur in 60% or more of anesthetized patients (Atlee, 1990); (2) are often the initial sign of some physiologic or pharmacologic derangement; (3) may be the cause of profound circulatory insufficiency, upset a favorable myocardial oxygen balance, or predispose to lethal arrhythmias.

The following discussion considers those aspects of normal and abnormal cardiac electrophysiology pertinent to an understanding of the proposed mechanisms for and the ECG diagnosis of cardiac arrhythmias.

NORMAL CARDIAC ELECTROPHYSIOLOGY

Cardiac Action Potential

The normal, regular beating of the heart is accompanied by cyclic changes in the transmembrane potential (TMP) of cardiac cells. These changes are the basis for the cardiac action potential (AP). The use of intracellular, microelectrode recording techniques has allowed TMP changes with the AP to be measured directly, and AP's have been shown to vary in amplitude and with time as the impulse travels through the heart (Hoffman and Cranefield, 1960). The microelectrode technique involves passing a glass capillary tube with a tip diameter of about 0.1 μm through the cell membrane. As the microelectrode passes from the outside to the inside of the cell membrane, it records a negative potential in resting fibers (Fig. 19.1). Microelectrode studies are usually made on isolated bundles of cardiac fibers mounted in a tissue bath superfused with physiologic solutions. Action potentials may be stimulated in such preparations by the direct application of a brief pulse of current to the fiber surface.

Resting Membrane Potential (RMP)

The level of RMP is largely determined by the concentration gradient for potassium ions (K^+) across the cell membrane. At rest, the cell membrane is relatively permeable to K^+, but relatively impermeable to calcium (Ca^{2+}), sodium (Na^+), and chloride (Cl^-) ions. The outward movement of K^+ is not accompanied by a comparable movement of anions, since the latter are mostly large polyvalent ions such as proteins. Consequently, a net negative charge builds up within the cell (Fig. 19.2).

Potassium continues to leave the cell until forces driving it down its concentration gradient are balanced by negative intracellular charges that attract

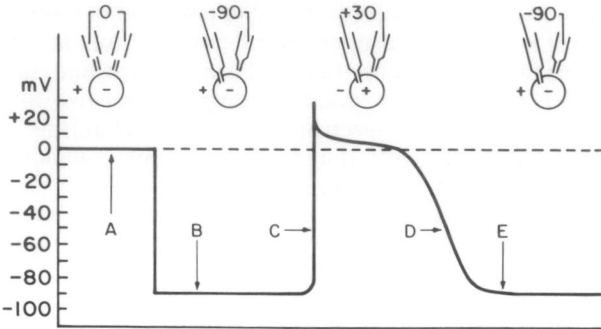

Fig. 19.1 The resting membrane and action potential (AP) of a cardiac cell. The upper row of diagrams show a cell and two microelectrodes. In A, both electrodes are extracellular, and there is no potential difference between them. B shows the tip of one microelectrode inside the cell. The potential diference between the inside and outside of the cell, the resting membrane potential, which in this example is −90 mV, is now recorded. In C, the upstroke of the AP is seen. The AP occurs when the cell is excited. At the peak of the upstroke the inside of this cell is 30 mV positive with respect to the outside. D represents the final phase of repolarization, which returns the membrane potential to its resting level, shown at E. (Reproduced with permission from Cranefield, 1975).

K$^+$ back into the cell. The sum of the electrical and chemical forces which determine the net flow of K$^+$ is called the *electrochemical potential gradient*. This gradient is zero when the two forces are equal and opposite. The potential at which this occurs is the K$^+$

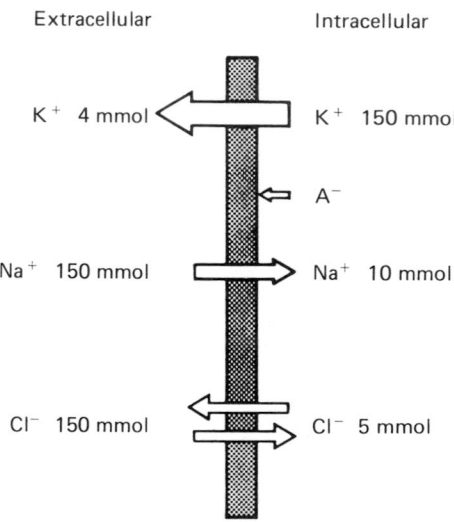

Fig. 19.2 Distribution of ions contributing to the resting membrane potential. Typical concentration of ions inside and outside the cell are shown. At rest the membrane is highly permeable to K$^+$, but impermeable to large anions (A$^-$). The permeability to Na$^+$ and Cl$^-$ are relatively low. The distribution of Cl$^-$ is most probably determined by the average value of the membrane potential. (Reproduced with permission from Gadsby and Wit, 1987).

electrochemical equilibrium potential—E_K. The value for E_K is given by the Nernst equation:

$$E_K = \frac{RT}{zF} \ln \frac{[K^+]_o}{[K^+]_i}$$

where R is the gas constant, T is the absolute temperature, z is the valence of the ionic species involved, F is the Faraday number, and $[K^+]_o$ and $[K^+]_i$ *are the extracellular and intracellular concentrations of K^+* respectively. For a Purkinje fiber at 36°C for which $[K^+]_o$ is 4 mmol/L and $[K^+]_i$ is 150 mmol/L, E_K would be:

$$E_K = \frac{RT}{F} \ln \frac{4}{150}$$

$$= 26.6 \ln \frac{4}{150}$$

$$= 61.4 \log \frac{4}{150}$$

$$= -96.6 \, mV$$

Examining the above, we can see that E_K will change by 61.4 mV following a ten-*fold* change in either $[K^+]_o$ or $[K^+]_i$. If the cell membrane were exclusively permeable to K$^+$, its RMP would change with variations in $[K^+]_o$ and $[K^+]_i$ as predicted by the Nernst equation. The RMP of atrial and ventricular muscle, and Purkinje fibers are in close agreement with values predicted by the Nernst equation for extracellular K$^+$ levels greater than 10 mmol/L. At lower values for $[K^+]_o$, the values for RMP are less negative than predicted by the Nernst equation and this discrepancy increases as $[K^+]_o$ is lowered further. The reason for this is that there is a small net inward movement of Na$^+$, which increases as $[K^+]_o$ is lowered. The depolarization consequent to the inward movement of Na$^+$ is negligibly small when $[K^+]_o$ is high (membrane K$^+$ conductance also high), but it becomes significantly greater as $[K^+]_o$ and consequently K$^+$ conductance, falls. The contribution of the small inward movement of Na$^+$ to the RMP as the result of reduced $[K^+]_o$ can be incorporated into a modification of the Nernst equation (Goldman, 1943; Hodgkin and Katz, 1949) termed the 'constant field' equation for RMP for cells permeable to both Na$^+$ and K$^+$:

$$E_M = \frac{RT}{F} \ln \frac{[K^+]_o + P_{Na}/P_K[Na^+]_o}{[K^+]_i + P_{Na}P_K[Na^+]_i}$$

where P_{Na} and P_K are the permeability coefficients of the cell membrane to Na$^+$ and K$^+$, respectively. However, E_M is approximate to the equilbrium potential for potassium, E_K, only when $[K^+]_o$ is much greater than 1.5 mmol/L (Gadsby and Wit, 1987). At $[K^+]_o$ of 1.5 mmol/L, E_M will be about 18 mV less negative than E_K.

So far, we have talked only in terms of the relative permeability of the membrane to Na$^+$ and K$^+$, not the absolute magnitude of their permeability coefficients. As the 'constant field' equation shows, the RMP is sensitive to the ratio of the permeabilities of the ions involved, but not to the individual permeability values themselves. Even if the Na^+ permeability were to be quite substantial, the RMP would still be determined predominantly by the K^+ concentration gradient as long as the membrane retained a much higher permeability to K^+ than to Na^+. The membrane channels through which K^+ ions move to generate the K^+ currents that determine the RMP are capable of inward-going rectification; that is, large *inward* K^+ currents can be passed when the difference between the membrane potential and E_k is large and negative, but only very small *outward* K^+ currents can be passed when the driving force is large and positive.

Calcium (ionized) contributes little to the RMP. However, changes in Ca^{2+} can affect membrane permeability to other ions. An increase in $[Ca^{2+}]_i$, for example, increases K^+ conductance. $[Ca^{2+}]_i$ is affected by several mechanisms, including uptake by the sarcoplasmic reticulum. Additionally, there appears to be Ca^{2+}/Na^+ exchange across the cell membrane. This exchange depends in part on the maintenance of the Na^+ concentration gradient by the Ca^{2+}/Na^+ exchange pump (*see* repolarization). Normally, one intracellular Ca^{2+} is exchanged for two or three extracellular Na^+. However, with some pathologic conditions and in the presence of certain drugs (e.g., digitalis), extracellular Ca^{2+} may be exchanged for intracellular Na^+. Cells that gain Na^+ tend also to gain Ca^{2+}, with a consequent loss in membrane potential. Indeed, loss of membrane potential may be a ubiquitous cause for clinical rhythm and conduction disturbances.

Depolarization

The electrical impulse that travels through the heart to initiate mechanical systole is termed the *propagated action potential*. With the arrival of the propagated AP, each cell transiently depolarizes. That is, the inside of the cell becomes positive. The cell then gradually returns to its initial, negative level of membrane potential. The latter process is termed repolarization. The cardiac AP has five distinct phases in atrial and ventricular muscle, and Purkinje fibers: (1) *phase 0*—initial, rapid depolarization; (2) *phase 1*—early rapid repolarization; (3) *phase 2*—plateau; (4) *phase 3*—final rapid repolarization; (5) *phase 4*—resting membrane potential or electrical diastole (Fig. 19.3). However, phases 1 and 2 are not so distinct in cells of the sinus and atrioventricular nodes. (Fig. 19.4).

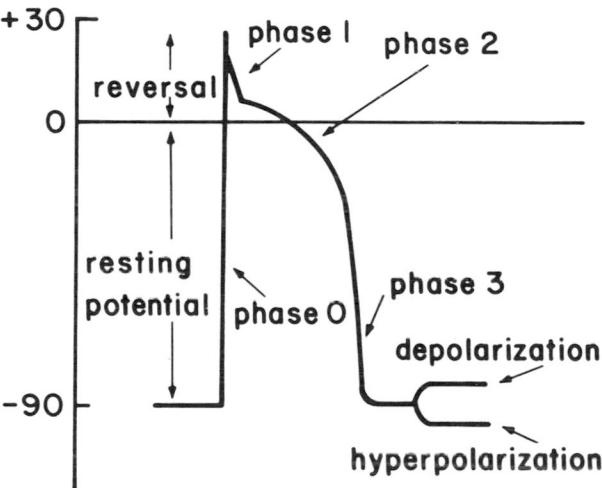

Fig. 19.3 Schematic of the action potential (AP) of a Purkinje fiber. When the fiber is quiescent the inside of the cell is −90 mV negative with respect to the outside which is the resting potential. At the peak of the upstroke of the AP, the interior of the cell becomes about 30 mV positive with respect to the outside so that there is a reversal or overshoot. The upstroke is also referred to as *phase 0*, and early rapid repolarization is *phase 1*. The plateau or period of persisting depolarization is *phase 2*, and final rapid repolarization is *phase 3*. A change in membrane potential away from the resting potential towards zero is depolarization. A change in the membrane potential that makes the inside of the cell more negative is a *hyperpolarization*. (Reproduced with permission from Cranefield, 1975).

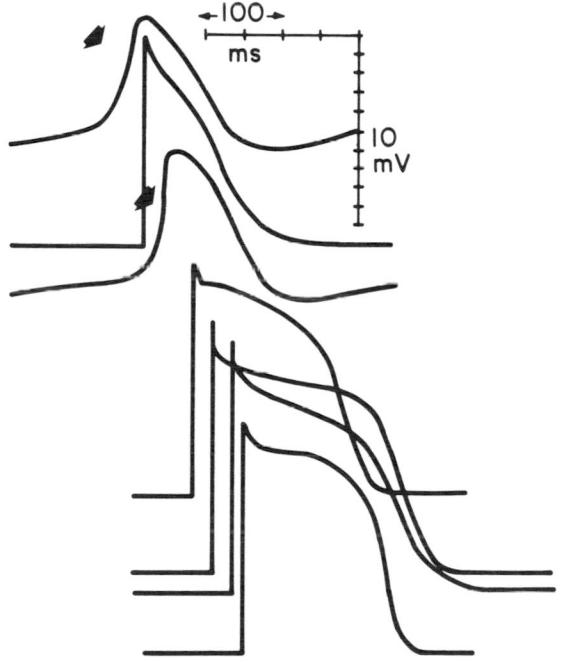

Fig. 19.4 Comparison of sinus node and AV nodal action potentials (AP), which are indicated by arrows with AP's of working myocardium and Purkinje fibers. Schematics of AP's recorded from the following sites, from top to bottom: sinus node, atrium, AV node, bundle of His, Purkinje fiber in a false tendon, terminal Purkinje fiber, and ventricular muscle fiber. Note that the upstroke velocity and amplitude of sinus and AV nodal AP's are both smaller than those of the AP's of the other cells. (Reproduced with permission from Hoffman and Cranefield, 1960).

Following an appropriate stimulus to a myocardial cell, the AP is initiated by a transient and marked increase in the cell membrane permeability to Na^+. The maximal rate at which depolarization occurs during phase 0 ($\dot{v}_{max}$, phase 0) is a measure of the rapidity of Na^+ entry via its ion-specific channel, and a major determinant of conduction velocity for the propagated AP (Weidmann, 1955). The changes in membrane permeability to Na^+ result from the opening and closing of cell membrane channels through which Na^+ can easily pass. It is generally believed that movement of gates control the opening and closing of ion-specific channels. The latter can exist in at least three conformations—*rest*, *activated* and *inactivated*. One gate, corresponding to the activation variable 'm' in the Hodgkin–Katz analysis (1949) of Na^+ currents in the membranes of squid giant axons, moves rapidly to open the channel when the membrane is depolarized by an applied stimulus or propagated AP. The other gate, corresponding to the inactivation variable

'h' in the Hodgkin–Katz analysis (1949), moves more slowly on depolarization, and its function is to close the channel. This *gated system model* (Hodgkin and Huxley, 1952) is depicted schematically in Fig. 19.5 for both the fast (Na^+) and slow (mainly Ca^{2+}) channels of a fiber with a normal RMP of -90 mV, the same fiber with its RMP reduced to -60 mV (inactivating the Na^+ channel), and the response of the fiber with a reduced RMP to catecholamines. Both the steady-state distribution of the gates within the specific ion-channel population and the speed with which they move into and out of position depend on the level of membrane potential. Consequently, *time-dependent* and *voltage-dependent* are adjectives used to describe membrane ion-conductance.

Threshold Potential

Rapid depolarization with the onset of the AP is caused by the inward movement of Na^+ ions flowing

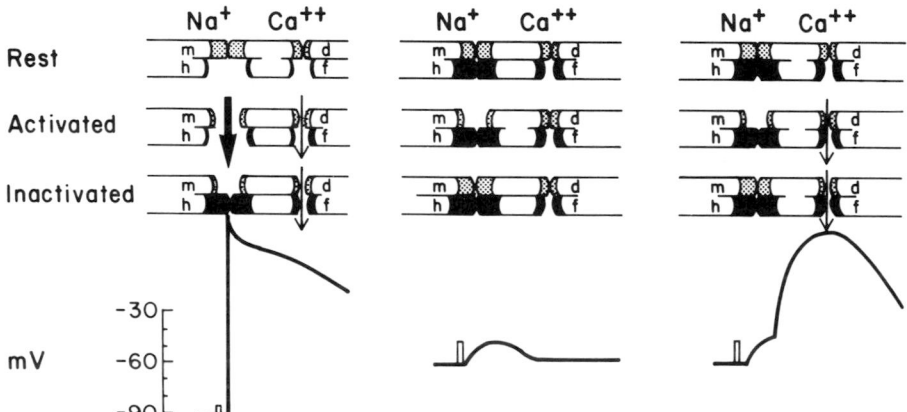

Fig. 19.5 Gated system model. Schematic representation of the membrane channels for Na^+ (fast channel) and Ca^{2+} (slow channel). Current movements are shown at resting membrane potential (Rest), following activation (Activated), and inactivation (Inactivated). The left panel depicts the membrane channels (top) and action potential (bottom) for a normal fiber with a resting membrane potential -90 mV. The middle panel depicts the same for a fiber with its membrane potential reduced to -60 mV (depressed fiber). The right panel depicts the response of the depressed fiber to catecholamines. The activation gates of the fast and slow channels are m and d, respectively. The corresponding inactivation gates are h and f, respectively. Left, the m and d gates are closed during the resting state; the h and f gates are open. With stimulation, the m gates (Na^+ channel) open for a brief time. The open m and h gates allow current to flow. This depolarizes the cell (phase 0). The h gates then close while the m gates remain open, inactivating Na^+ conductance. When the upstroke of the action potential exceeds the threshold for the slow (Ca^{2+}) channel, the d gates open, thereby permitting ingress of Ca^{2+}, which contributes to phase 2 (plateau) of the action potential. The f gates close more slowly during inactivation than do the h gates. Although the slow channel remains open longer than does the fast channel, less total current (smaller arrow) flows. Middle, reduction of the resting membrane potential to -60 mV inactivates the fast channel, because the h gates remain closed. Even though the m gates may open with activation, the majority of the inactivation gates remain closed so that the amount of Na^+ current is too small to elicit an action potential. The f gates (Ca^{2+}) are only partially closed, but the upstroke of the action potential does not exceed threshold for activation of the slow channel. Right, when the fiber is excited after the addition of catecholamines, the d gates open and permit flow of Ca^{2+}. This causes a slow-response type action potential. (Reproduced with permission from Wit and Bigger, 1975).

down their electrochemical potential gradient (Draper and Weidmann, 1951). For the Na^+ channel to open effectively, a critical portion of the cell membrane must be depolarized to a level of membrane potential termed threshold potential (TP). TP is -60 to $-70\,mV$ (Cranefield, 1975) in atrial and ventricular muscle and Purkinje fibers (Fig. 19.6). Experimen-

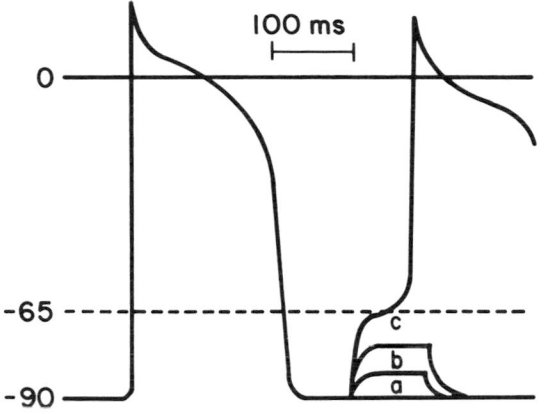

Fig. 19.6 Threshold potential. The AP shown at the left arises from a resting potential of $-90\,mV$; this occurs when the fiber is excited by a propagated AP or by any stimulus that rapidly lowers the membrane potential to below the threshold level of $-65\,mV$. At the right, the effects of two subthreshold stimuli and a third threshold stimulus are shown. The subthreshold stimuli (a and b) do not lower the membrane potential to threshold, and therefore an AP is not elicited. A threshold stimulus (c) reduces the membrane potential just to the threshold level from which an AP then arises. (Reproduced with permission from Hoffman and Cranefield, 1960).

tally, TP is determined by applying current through intra or extracellular electrodes. In situ, local current preceding the propagated AP wavefront bring quiescent cardiac fibers to TP. At TP, sufficient Na^+ channels are opened to initiate a regenerative Na^+ current.

By *regenerative* Na^+ *current* is meant that the movement of a little Na^+ causes an even greater number of Na^+ channels to open, thereby increasing the magnitude of the Na^+ current. The speed of regenerative depolarization, measured by the AP upstroke velocity ($\dot{v}_{max}$, phase 0), is about $500\,V/s$ in Purkinje fibers, about $200\,V/s$ in ventricular muscle, and $100–200\,V/s$ in atrial muscle (Hoffman and Cranefield, 1960). Na^+ dependent AP with characteristic rapid upstroke velocities are termed *fast responses*. AP's arising in fast response fibers (atrial and ventricular muscle, Purkinje fibers) with a reduced level of resting membrane potential (*see* Fig. 19.5) are termed *depressed fast responses* (*discussed later*).

Fast responses propagate rapidly through the heart. Conduction velocities in atrial and ventricular muscle range from $0.3–0.4\,m/s$, and in Purkinje fibers from $2–3\,m/s$ (Sperelakis, 1979). In contrast, conduction

through the AV and SA nodes—*slow response fibers* discussed later—is much slower ($0.1\,m/s$ and $<0.05\,m/s$, respectively). In cells with similar membrane capacitance and axial resistance properties, the speed of AP propagation is largely determined by the magnitude of the Na^+ inward current. This is because the local circuit currents that flow through the cells just ahead of the propagated AP wavefront are large with the fast upstroke of the fast response as compared to the depressed fast response or slow response. These larger local circuit currents can bring the membrane potential of quiescent fibers to threshold sooner than can small currents. While local circuit currents also flow across cell membranes just behind the propagated AP wavefront, they are unable to excite cells behind the propagating AP because they are refractory immediately following excitation.

Refractoriness

Prolonged refractoriness following excitation results from the long duration of the AP and the voltage dependence of the gating of Na^+ channels (Gadsby et al., 1987). Following phase 0 of the fast response AP, there is a period of from one hundred to several hundred milliseconds during which there is no regenerative response to a second stimulus. This is called the *absolute refractory period* (Fig. 19.7). The absolute refractory period usually lasts beyond the AP plateau (phase 2), during which time the Na^+ chan-

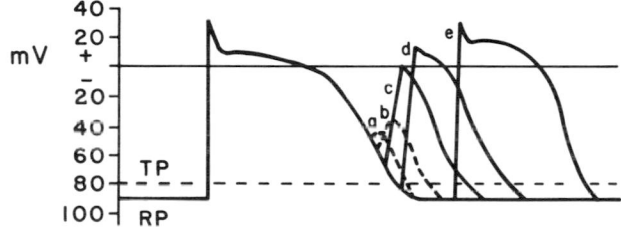

Fig. 19.7 Diagrammatic representation of a normal action potential (AP) and of responses elicited by stimuli applied at various stages of repolarization, where TP represents threshold potential and RP, resting potential. The amplitude and upstroke velocity of the responses elicited during repolarization are related to the level of the membrane potential from which they arise. The earliest response (a) defines the end of the absolute refractory period. Responses (a) and (b) arise from such low levels of membrane potential that they are too small to propagate (graded or local responses). Response (c) represents the earliest propagated AP, but it propagates slowly because of its low upstroke velocity and low amplitude. Response (d) is elicited just before complete repolarization, and its rate of rise and amplitude are greater than those of (c) because it arises from a higher membrane potential. It still propagates more slowly than normal, however, response e is elicited after complete repolarization and, therefore, has a normal rate of depolarization and amplitude, as well as rapid propagation. (Reproduced with permission from Singer and Ten Eick, 1969).

nels are inactivated by persistent depolarization. During phase 3, there is a progressive removal of inactivation so that an increasing number of Na^+ channels are available for subsequent activation. As a result, it is possible to induce only small inward Na^+ currents by applying a stimulus early during phase 3, but larger currents are obtained as the cell becomes more fully repolarized. Inward Na^+ currents excited when some Na^+ channels are inactivated provide *graded* responses (Fig. 19.7), and the time period during which graded responses are obtained is termed the *relative refractory period*. AP initiated during the relative refractory period have a slow rate of rise and lower amplitude which causes them to propagate slowly. Such AP may be the cause for conduction delay, decrement, and block. They can also be responsible for re-entrant excitation. Finally, concerning AP initiated during the relative refractory period, the voltage-dependence of the AP on level of membrane potential during removal of inactivation (Weidmann, 1955) is termed *membrane responsiveness* (Fig. 19.8).

Slow Inward Current

The fast, Na^+ inward current, largely responsible for the upstroke of the AP in fast response fibers, is followed by a relatively slow, inward current carried mainly by Ca^{2+}. This current is termed the *slow-inward current* (Reuter, 1967; Cranefield, 1975). It flows through the so-called *slow channel* (Reuter, 1973), which similar to the Na^+ channel, exhibits time

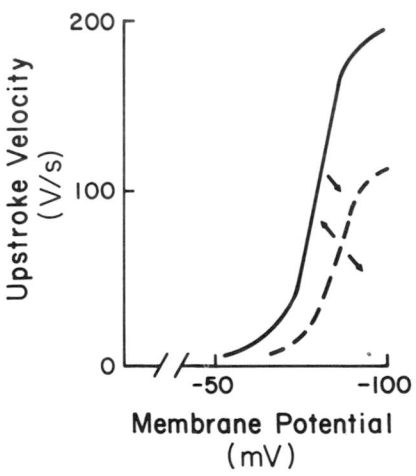

Fig. 19.8 Membrane responsiveness. The maximal upstroke velocity of the action potential (ordinate) is related to the level of membrane potential (abscissa) at the time of excitation. An hypothetical *normal* curve is depicted by the solid line; *reduced responsiveness* in a partially depolarized fiber by the dashed line. For the curve of reduced responsiveness, a shift upward and to the left (arrows) indicates *increased responsiveness*. For either curve, a shift downward and to the right (arrow) indicates *decreased responsiveness*.

and voltage-dependent conductance. The threshold potential for activation of the slow-inward current is -30 to -40 mV (Cranefield, 1975). Current flows through both the fast Na^+ and slow Ca^{2+} channels toward the latter part of the AP upstroke. Since the Ca^{2+} current is smaller than the Na^+ current, it contributes little to the AP until the Na^+ current is largely inactivated following the initial upstroke. The Ca^{2+} current contributes mainly to the plateau (phase 2) of the AP. An increase in extracellular Ca^{2+} shifts the plateau in a depolarizing (more positive direction); a decrease in extracellular Ca^{2+}, *vice versa*.

Repolarization

Following phase 0 of the AP in Purkinje fibers and some atrial and ventricular muscle fibers, there is rapid transient repolarization (*see* Fig. 19.3). This initial rapid repolarization is due partly to inactivation of the Na^+ inward current during phase 0 and to activation of a transient outward current carried by K^+, with possibly a small component carried by Cl^- (Kenyon and Gibbons, 1977). During phase 1, the membrane potential returns to near 0 mV as the result of a relative increase in intracellular negative charges. The plateau (phase 2) maintains this level of membrane potential.

During the plateau, the membrane conductance falls to low values for nearly all ions. In spite of its large electrochemical gradient, membrane conductance for K^+ is reduced due to *inward-going rectification* of a K^+ background current (I_{K_1}). This means that the channel passes outward current in response to positive potential changes less easily than it passes inward current in response to negative potential changes. Consequently, K^+ enters the cell more easily than it can exit, and few K^+ ions leave the cell. Sodium conductance is low because the Na^+ channel has been inactivated. Minor ionic movements occurring during phase 2 include electromagnetic, ATP-dependent, Na^+/K^+ exchange (normally, three Na^+ are pumped out in exchange for two K^+) and a small influx of Cl^-. The slow-inward current has a long time constant for inactivation. Consequently, it turns off slowly during the plateau. The slow-inward current balances net outward currents produced by the influx of Cl^- and exchange of Na^+ for K^+. Electrophysiologically, the plateau delays repolarization and restoration of excitability following excitation.

Repolarization during phase 3 (final rapid repolarization) is primarily the result of an outward current carried by K^+ (I_{K_2}). This current is due to *reversal of inward-going rectification* of I_{K_1}. Repolarization during phase 3 is also the result of time-dependent inactivation of the slow-inward current. As the new membrane current becomes more outward biased, the membrane potential shifts in a more negative direction. The latter causes an increase in K^+ conductance so that repolarization self-perpetuates in a regenerative manner, similar to initial fast depolarization.

Spontaneous Phase 4 (Diastolic) Depolarization

The membrane potential of working atrial and ventricular muscle fibers normally remains constant throughout diastole. In specialized fibers of the atria (including, muscle of tricuspid and mitral valves, along the inferior sulcus terminalis), the distal AV node, and in Purkinje fibers the membrane potential does not remain constant throughout diastole. Rather, it steadily declines to less negative values. If a propagating AP does not depolarize the cell before it reaches threshold potential, a spontaneous action potential may arise from that cell. When spontaneous, phase 4 depolarization leads to the initiation of AP, *automaticity* exists.

Normally, the rate of phase 4 depolarization in the sinus node exceeds that of other potential (latent) pacemaker sites. This is termed *sinus dominance*. Sinus dominance is due to the mechanism of *overdrive suppression*. Overdrive suppression is mediated by enhanced activity of the Na^+/K^+ exchange pump. When latent pacemakers are driven faster than their intrinsic rate, the enhanced outward current generated by the Na^+/K^+ pump suppresses automaticity at these sites (Vassale, 1970). When the dominant pacemaker is removed, overdrive suppression is responsible for a period of quiescence which lasts until the Na^+/K^+ pump current becomes small enough to allow the latent pacemaker cells to spontaneously depolarize to threshold. Spontaneous phase 4 depolarization which occurs in the sinus node and latent pacemaker cells is termed *normal automaticity*. Normal automaticity is differentiated from *abnormal automaticity* (discussed later). The ionic basis for phase 4 depolarization differs in slow response (sinus node) and fast response (Purkinje cells) fibers (Noble, 1985; Zipes, 1984). Irrespective of fiber type, for phase 4 depolarization to occur, there must be a net gain in intracellular positive charges.

In the *sinus node*, phase 4 depolarization occurs due to: (1) inactivation of a time-dependent K^+ current (I_{k_1}); (2) activation of an inward pacemaker current carried predominantly by Na^+; and (3) progressive activation of the slow-inward current carried mainly by Ca^{2+} (Brown and Noble, 1974; Noma and Irisawa, 1974). The resulting decrease in outward flux of K^+, and increased inward flux of Na^+ and Ca^{2+}, gradually depolarize the cell to a level of membrane potential at which the slow-inward current is fully activated. The latter is responsible for the upstroke of the sinus node AP.

Early studies suggested that phase 4 depolarization in *Purkinje fibers* was achieved by a decrease in the outward K^+ current (I_{K_1}), while a relatively constant, inwardly-directed, background current carried by Na^+ gradually depolarized the membrane to threshold potential for activation of the fast-inward current (Vassale, 1966; Noble and Tsien, 1968). More recent evidence is interpreted as suggesting that the normal pacemaker current is an inward current carried mainly by Na^+ that gradually increases with time,

thereby bringing the membrane to threshold potential (Di Francesco, 1981).

Electrical Activity of Sinus Node and AV Node Cells

The electrical activity of cells found in the sinus and AV nodes (slow response fibers) is quite different from that of working myocardial and Purkinje fibers (fast response fibers). By virtue of their unusual electrophysiologic characteristics, nodal cells are often involved in the initiation and maintenance of cardiac arrhythmias. Because of the above, normal electrical properties of these cells are considered separately.

The *resting potential* of sinus and AV node cells is about 20 mV less negative (-60 to -70 mV) than fast response fibers (Fig. 19.4). The measured intracellular concentration of K^+ (and consequently level of E_k) in sinus node cells appears to be similar to that of cardiac cells with much higher (more negative) resting potentials (Grant and Strauss, 1982). Consequently, it is likely that the lower resting membrane potential results from a higher ratio of the Na^+ to K^+ permeability coefficients (Gatsby et al., 1987). This could be due to an unusually high resting membrane permeability to Na^+, or a low permeability to K^+.

The *upstroke of the AP*, (phase 0) has a lower rate of rise (1–15 V/s) in sinus and AV nodal cells than in fast response cells (100–700 V/s). The *amplitude of the AP* is also much lower in sinus and AV nodal cells (60–80 versus 110–120 mV). The slower AP upstroke and reduced amplitude reflect the smaller amount of inward current that is responsible for phase 0 in nodal compared to fast-response cells. The current that flows through the slow channel (the slow-inward current, I_{si}) is carried mainly by Ca^{2+}. AP's of cells with their upstroke dependent on I_{si} are termed *slow-responses* to distinguish them from AP's dependent on the fast-inward current, i.e., *fast-responses* (Cranefield, 1975). Slow-responses conduct quite slowly (< 0.05–0.1 m/s).

Following phase 0, the slow-inward current contributes to depolarization throughout the *plateau*. The plateau is poorly defined in nodal cells (*see* Fig. 19.4). Activation of a time and voltage-dependent, outward K^+ current, coupled with inactivation of the slow-inward current, are the most important currents involved in *repolarization*.

The slow-inward channel conductance is also much slower to reactivate following membrane repolarization than the fast-inward channel conductance (Cranefield, 1975; Gatsby et al., 1987). Despite full repolarization, sufficient inactivation of slow channel conductance may persist so that the cells remain absolutely refractory to applied stimuli (Merideth, et al., 1968). *Reactivation* in slow-response fibers gradually occurs throughout diastole. Premature impulses initiated early in diastole have slow upstrokes and reduced amplitudes, and they conduct slowly. Impulses initiated later have faster upstrokes and higher amplitudes, and conduct more rapidly (Mendez and

Moe, 1966). The above behavior reflects the long time course for reactivation of slow-inward channels.

Differences in the proposed ionic mechanism for *spontaneous, diastolic (phase 4) depolarization* in the sinus node compared to Purkinje cells were discussed above. AV nodal cells can also exhibit spontaneous phase 4 depolarization, especially when disconnected from the surrounding atrial myocardium (Mendez et al., 1966).

ABNORMAL CARDIAC ELECTROPHYSIOLOGY

Loss of Membrane Potential

Many abnormalities of cardiac muscle and specialized conducting fibers that result in cardiac arrhythmias, especially myocardial ischemia and infarction, tend to depolarize the cell membrane, that is the membrane potential becomes less negative, equivalent to a *loss of membrane potential* (LMP). There are four ways to produce LMP: (1) an increase in extracellular K^+; (2) a decrease in intracellular K^+; (3) increased membrane permeability to Na^+; (4) decreased membrane permeability to K^+. Any one of these changes would by itself cause the membrane potential to decline; but more than one are likely to occur simultaneously in diseased cells.

A disease process or drug (e.g., digitalis) that affects the Na^+/K^+ exchange pump would produce LMP in the affected cells, probably as the net result of both an increase in extracellular K^+ and a decrease in intracellular K^+. The normal loss of cellular K^+ with replacement by Na^+ that occurs with excitation would not be repaired by the Na^+/K^+ exchange pump. Consequently, there would be a continuous net loss of K^+ from the cells. Since diffusion of ions from the extracellular spaces is somewhat restricted and slow, K^+ lost from cells tends to accumulate outside the cell. Therefore, both an increase in $[K^+]_o$ and decrease in $[K^+]_i$ simultaneously contribute to LMP.

Just as changes in $[K^+]_o$ and $[K^+]_i$ contribute to LMP, it is likely that complementary changes in membrane permeability to Na^+ (P_{Na}) and K^+ (P_K) also combine to produce LMP (Gatsby et al., 1987). A pathologic condition which produces an increase in the 'leakiness' of cell membranes to Na^+ would increase the ratio P_{Na}/P_K (from the Goldman, Hodgkin, Katz constant field equation p. 234) and lead to LMP. Since the LMP might occur in the absence of any significant change in $[K^+]_o$ or $[K^+]_i$, the K^+ equilibrium potential ($E_K = -96.6\,mV$) would remain unchanged. However, the outward driving force for K^+ (membrane potential, E_K) is now greater than normal (a less negative membrane potential is further from E_K). Additionally, as a result of inward-going rectification, the K^+ conductance and K^+ permeability coefficient (P_K), would be smaller than normal. Thus, LMP associated with the hypothetical increased 'leakiness' to Na^+ would result from increased P_{Na}/P_K due to an increase in P_{Na} and decrease in P_K.

Finally, a disease process might conceivably lead to a reduction in P_K. This might be a consequence of alterations in the cell membrane composition due to disordered protein or lipid metabolism. As a result, the ratio P_{Na}/P_K would increase leading to LMP, even though there was no increase in P_{Na}. While a specific disorder that reduces P_K has yet to be described, this situation has been modeled experimentally (Isenberg, 1976).

Depressed Fast Response

Loss of membrane potential prevents attainment of the large negative intracellular potentials required to reopen all the Na^+ (fast) channels following cardiac excitation. LMP from -70 to $-60\,mV$ inactivates about one-half, and to $-50\,mV$ all of the Na^+ channels. The smaller number of available Na^+ channels reduces the magnitude of the fast-inward current during depolarization. As a result, the AP upstroke velocity and amplitude are reduced (Fig. 19.9). AP's with their upstroke characteristics dependent on the magnitude of Na^+ inward current flowing through partially inactivated channels are termed *depressed fast responses* (Wit et al., 1974).

Conduction of the Depressed Fast Response

With steady state Na^+ channel inactivation and LMP, conduction velocity in depressed Purkinje

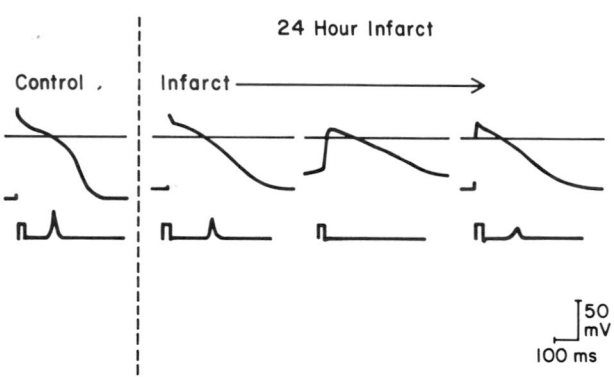

Fig. 19.9 Changes in action potentials (AP) recorded from Purkinje fibers as a result of infarction in the canine heart. The bottom trace in each panel (recorded with a faster sweep) shows the differentiated upstroke of the AP preceded by a differentiated calibration signal (200 V/s slope). The left (control) panel shows the AP recorded from a Purkinje fiber in a noninfarcted region; it has a normal maximum diastolic or resting potential and a rapid upstroke. The right panel shows AP's recorded from three different Purkinje fibers on the endocardial surface of the infarct. Note that maximum diastolic potential, action potential amplitude, and upstroke velocity ($\dot{v}_{max}$ were all diminished in the infarcted as compared to the control region. Depression of the resting potential and AP in the middle infarct panel is particularly severe. (Reproduced with permission from Friedman, Stewart, Fenoglio, et al., 1973).

fibers may be reduced from the normal of 2–3 m/s to less than 0.5 m/s. With more complete Na^+ channel inactivation AP upstroke velocity and amplitude becomes entirely dependent on the slow-inward current. The result is an even further slowing of conduction (<0.1 m/s) or conduction block. Varying degrees of depression of the fast response create areas that conduct slowly, and areas of unidirectional or complete conduction block (Fig. 19.10). Such uneven changes in conduction favor the development of re-entry (discussed later).

Refractoriness in Depressed Fibers

As discussed above, the relative refractory period of fast response fibers lasts until repolarization is complete. AP's elicited before full repolarization have a reduced upstroke velocity and amplitude due to partial inactivation of the Na^+ channel and its current (*see* Fig. 19.7). AP's elicited within a few milliseconds of full repolarization, however, have a normal upstroke velocity and amplitude. The rate of removal of inactivation of the Na^+ current is highly dependent on the steady level of membrane potential. Recovery occurs rapidly (<20 ms) at -90 mV, but takes 100 ms or more at -60 mV (Gettes and Reuter, 1974). Thus, in addition to slowed conduction consequent to LMP

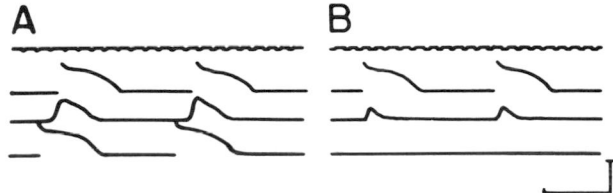

A   **B**

Fig. 19.10 Unidirectional conduction block in a bundle of canine Purkinje fibres. The top line shows time marks at 100 ms intervals. The three traces beneath show action potentials (AP) recorded from three different cells along the length of a bundle of Purkinje fibres. The AP's on the upper trace were recorded from the near end of the bundle, those on the middle trace were recorded from the center, and those on the bottom trace were recorded from the far end of the bundle. The cells in the center segment of the bundle were depolarized by perfusion with high $[K^+]_o$ solution, and the AP's recorded there have slow upstrokes and low amplitudes. Panel A shows records obtained by stimulating the bundle at the far end. The impulse was first recorded in the cell at the far end of the bundle (bottom trace), and then it conducted through the center segment (middle trace) to finally excite the cells at the near end of the bundle (top trace). Panel B shows records obtained when the near end of the bundle was stimulated instead. The cell monitored by the top trace was excited, since this was near the region of stimulation. Conduction block, however, occurred in the depressed area (middle trace). Consequently, the far end of the bundle (bottom trace) was not activated. (Reproduced with permission from Cranefield et al., 1973).

and the depressed fast response, prolonged refractoriness in depressed fibers may also lead to slowed conduction of premature impulses and the enhanced likelihood of sustained re-entry.

Finally, large alterations in refractory period duration can be brought about by changes in action potential duration (APD) in fast response fibers (Gadsby et al., 1987). In such cells, removal of Na^+ channel inactivation is complete soon following repolarization. Shortening the APD, as with increased heart rate, vagal stimulation (atrial fibers only), or immediately following the onset of ischemia (Downar et al., 1977), is accompanied by a corresponding shortening of the effective and relative refractory periods (Hoffman et al., 1960). In areas that are chronically ischemic, the APD is likely to be markedly prolonged (Lazzara, et al., 1974). Changes in APD and refractoriness, can markedly affect the conduction of both normal and premature impulses and thereby cause arrhythmias.

Abnormal Automaticity

While pacemaker activity is not generally a property of working myocardial fibers, myocardial ischemia may induce automaticity in such fibers. Based on the rate response to catecholamines for pacemaker fibers exhibiting normal automaticity, it is unlikely that heart rates much greater than 200 beats/minute are due to enhanced normal automaticity (Cranefield, 1975; Hoffman and Rosen, 1981). Working atrial and ventricular fibers do not normally show spontaneous diastolic depolarization or initiate the same, even when not excited by propagated AP's for long periods of time. When the resting membrane potential of working atrial and ventricular muscle fibers is reduced to around -60 mV by experimental methods or disease, spontaneous diastolic depolarization may occur and cause self-sustained impulse initiation (Surawicz and Imanishi, 1976; Katzung and Morgenstern, 1977). This is called *abnormal automaticity*. As shown in Fig. 19.11, Purkinje fibers, which exhibit normal automaticity at a normal level of membrane potential, also exhibit abnormal automaticity when the membrane potential is reduced to a lower level. However, if a low level of membrane potential were the only criterion for abnormal automaticity, sinus node automaticity would have to be considered abnormal. Hence, an important distinction between normal and abnormal automaticity is that the latter only occurs in a fiber with its membrane potential substantially reduced from the normal level (Hoffman et al., 1981).

At the low level of membrane potential at which abnormal automaticity occurs, it is likely that at least some of the ionic currents responsible for spontaneous depolarization are not the same ones responsible for normal automaticity. A likely candidate for automaticity at resting membrane potentials of around -50 mV is a deactivation of the K^+ outward current (I_{K_2}) attributed to reversal of inward-going

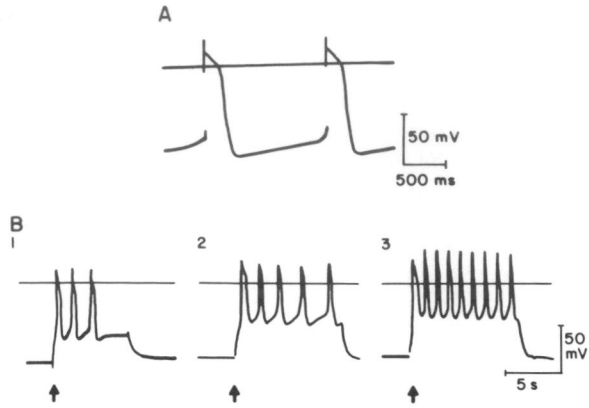

Fig. 19.11 Normal and abnormal automaticity in a canine Purkinje fiber. A shows normal automaticity in a Purkinje fiber with a maximum diastolic potential of -85 mV. B shows abnormal automaticity that can occur when membrane potential is decreased. In panel 1 (left), the fiber is depolarized (at the arrow) from a resting potential of -60 mV to -45 mV by injecting a long-lasting current pulse through a microelectrode. This causes three non-driven AP's. In panel 2 a larger amplitude current pulse reduces the membrane potential to -40 mV. This causes sustained rhythmic activity. In panel 3 a still larger current pulse at the arrow reduces membrane potential to -30 mV. Sustained rhythmic activity now occurs at a higher rate. (Reproduced with permission from Wit and Friedman, 1975).

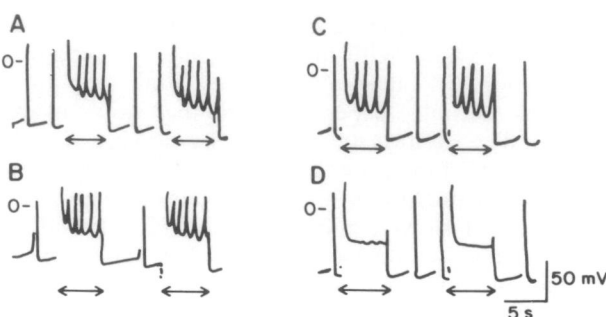

Fig. 19.12 Abnormal automaticity in canine Purkinje fibres with low levels of membrane potential. Depolarizing current pulses were delivered across a single sucrose gap at the times indicated by the intervals between arrowheads. A, control. Depolarization reduced the membrane potential from -85 to between -50 and -55 mV. This induced abnormal automaticity at a more rapid rate than that associated with normal automaticity in the first, second, seventh and eighth cycles. B, superfusion with lidocaine (3 mg/l) slowed the spontaneous discharge rate and reduced the amplitude of action potentials associated with normal automaticity, but had no effect on abnormal automaticity. C, return to control after 30 minutes of washout. D, superfusion with verapamil (3×10^{-6} M) suppressed abnormal automaticity associated with a reduced level of membrane potential, but had no effect on normal automaticity. (Reproduced with permission from Elharrar and Zipes, 1980).

rectification of I_{K_1} (Noble and Tsien, 1968). As discussed above, I_{K_2} under normal conditions functions to bring about repolarization following the upstroke of the AP.

Since the depolarizing ionic currents responsible for abnormal automaticity are not likely the same ones responsible for normal automaticity in Purkinje fibers, the two types of automaticity may respond differently to antiarrhythmic drugs (Fig. 19.12). Moreover, because of the low level of membrane potential from which AP's arise, the upstrokes of AP's caused by abnormal automaticity are dependent on the slow-inward current. The causes for the loss of membrane potential required to initiate abnormal automaticity are the same ones discussed above with the depressed fast response.

Abnormal automaticity occurs in Purkinje fibers that survive on the subendocardial surface of canine infarcts, and are possibly the cause of ventricular tachycardia in this model (Friedman et al., 1973, Lazzara et al., 1973). Moreover, preparations of diseased atrial and ventricular myocardium from human hearts show abnormal automaticity at membrane potentials in the range of -50 to -60 mV (Carmeleit, 1980; Dangman and Hoffman, 1983).

An abnormal automatic focus should emerge and cause an arrhythmia when the sinus rate is slower than that of the abnormal automatic focus, as discussed earlier for pacemakers exhibiting normal automati-

city. But unlike normal automatic pacemaker foci, abnormally automatic pacemakers cannot be overdrive suppressed (Carmeleit, 1980, Dangman and Hoffman, 1983). Consequently, even transient sinus pauses may permit an abnormally automatic focus to capture the heart for one or more beats. An ectopic focus exhibiting normal automaticity would probably remain quiescent during short and transient sinus pauses because of overdrive suppression.

Triggered Activity

Triggered activity or automaticity is sustained impulse generation that is critically dependent on prior impulses (Automatic or propagated AP's) for its initiation (Cranefield, 1977; Hoffman et al., 1981). In contrast, automatic pacemaker activity is initiated spontaneously and is not critically dependent on prior impulses. Triggered activity or automaticity arises from early or late afterdepolarizations. An afterdepolarization is a second subthreshold depolarization that occurs either during repolarization—*early afterdepolarization*, or following repolarization—*late* or *delayed afterdepolarization*.

Early Afterdepolarizations

Early afterdepolarizations usually occur during repolarization of an AP initiated from a high level (greater than -75 mV) of membrane potential

(Fig. 19.13). As shown in Fig. 19.13, early afterdepolarizations can lead to second upstrokes or sustained rhythmic activity (Wit et al., 1980). The membrane potential during the early afterdepolarization reaches threshold for activation of the slow-inward current, and a second AP occurs prior to complete repolarization. The second AP may or may not be followed by additional AP's, all occurring at a low level of membrane potential. Sustained rhythmic activity, so initiated, may continue at the low level of membrane potential, or it may terminate when the increase in membrane potential associated with repolarization of the first AP returns the membrane potential to its initial high level (Panel B, Fig. 19.13).

Concerning triggered activity arising from early afterdepolarizations, there are some conceptual difficulties (Cranefield, 1977). According to the definition of triggered activity (*see* previous section), there is no

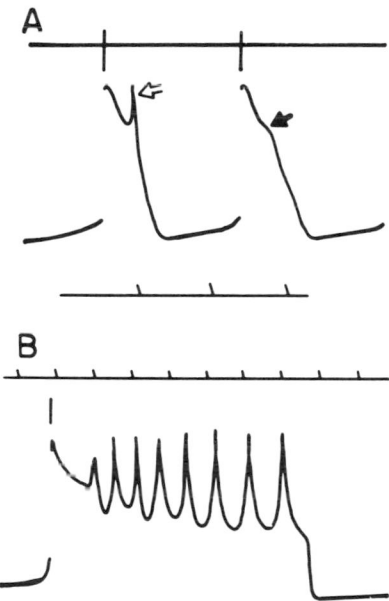

Fig. 19.13 Early after depolarization, second upstrokes, and sustained rhythmic activity in canine cardiac Purkinje fibres exposed to 4 mmol/L K$^+$-containing Tyrode's solution. The two spontaneous action potentials (AP) in Panel A show, respectively, a second upstroke arising from an early afterdepolarization (left-hand AP) and an early afterdepolarization or 'hump' during the repolarization phase (right-hand AP). These AP's were recorded while the fiber was recovering from a brief exposure to norepinephrine. Panel B shows a spontaneous AP recorded in another preparation shortly after replacing the bicarbonate/carbon dioxide buffering system with HEPES buffer (N-2-hydroxy-ethylpiperazine-N'-2-ethanesulfonic acid). The second upstroke is followed by a 'burst' of rhythmic activity arising from a low level of membrane potential. The maximum diastolic potential was −84 mV in Panel A and −87 mV in Panel B. The second upstroke in Panel A and the later slow responses in Panel B peaked near 0 mV. Time marks occur at 1 s intervals. (Reproduced with permission from Wit et al., 1980).

problem in characterizing the second AP upstroke as triggered. But if a series of AP's arise from a low level of membrane potential before the cell repolarizes to a high level of membrane potential, are these AP's triggered or do they occur because of an abnormal automatic mechanism? Perhaps only the first (i.e., early afterdepolarization) AP is triggered, and all remaining AP's from the low level of membrane potential are automatic. This consideration has led some authorities to more recently term sustained rhythmic activity following early afterdepolarizations triggered automaticity. As opposed to triggered activity, the term recommended for sustained rhythmic activity following late (delayed) afterdepolarizations (Wit and Rosen, 1986).

Early afterdepolarizations may be caused by the reversal of inward-going rectification for I_{K_1} (*discussed above*), as well as a steady-state inward current carried by Na$^+$ (noninactivated Na$^+$ channels) and the slow-inward current (Wit and Rosen, 1984). The second upstroke and any subsequent AP's that rise from low levels of membrane potential are presumably slow responses. Early afterdepolarizations have been produced *in vitro* by a variety of experimental interventions, including altering ionic concentrations in the superfusate and exposing the preparation to neurohumors and drugs (Cranefield, 1975). Early afterdepolarizations may also be caused *in vitro* by factors that are present in the *in situ* heart under some pathologic conditions (Wit et al., 1984). Among these are hypoxia, hypercarbia and catecholamines. Since any of these may be present in an ischemic or infarcted region of the heart, it is possible that triggering could be the cause for some arrhythmias associated with myocardial ischemia and infarction.

A late or *delayed afterdepolarization* is a transient depolarization that occurs after final repolarization of an AP, and that is induced by that AP (Fig. 19.14). Delayed afterpotentials occur under conditions in which there is a large increase in intracellular Ca^{2+} (Wit et al., 1984). Possible mechanisms by which an increase in [Ca^{2+}]$_i$ may cause delayed afterdepolarizations are discussed elsewhere (Kass et al., 1978a; 1978b). As illustrated in Fig. 19.15, one of the widely recognized causes for delayed afterdepolarizations is digitalis toxicity (Ferrier, 1977). Other causes include catecholamines and certain conditions affecting the heart as with atrial fibers from diseased hearts, Purkinje fibers surviving myocardial infarction and myocardial hypertrophy (Wit et al., 1984). Triggered activity caused by digitalis or catecholamines often terminated spontaneously, even in the presence of maintained levels of these drugs. Finally, triggered arrhythmias may be terminated at critical times by premature stimuli or overdrive stimulation (Wit et al., 1984).

Re-entry of Excitation

Normally, the propagating impulse dies out after sequential activation of the atria and ventricles. This

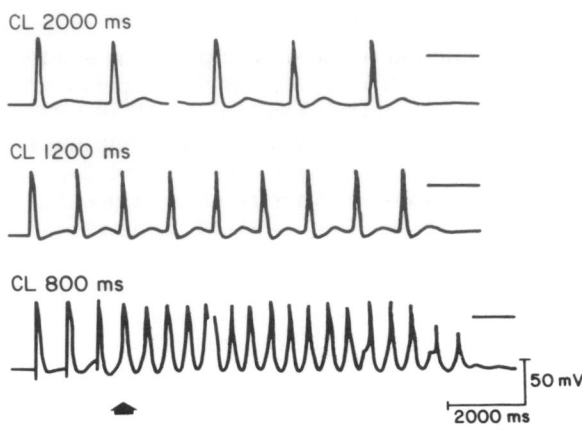

CL 2000 ms

CL 1200 ms

CL 800 ms

50 mV

2000 ms

Fig. 19.14 Triggered activity in an atrial fiber from the left atrium of a cat with hypertrophic cardiomyopathy. The preparation was superfused with 1.0 µg/ml of norepinephrine in Tyrode's solution. The resting potential of this fiber was −50 mV, and the action potential (AP) was characterized by a slow upstroke. The 0 reference is indicated by the horizontal line to the right of each tracing. Top panel, AP's and delayed afterdepolarizations recorded when the fiber was stimulated at a cycle length (CL) of 2000 ms. The first two AP were recorded just after stimulation began, and the three to the right, 10 seconds later. Middle panel, AP's and delayed afterdepolarizations recorded at stimulated CL of 1200 ms. Lower panel, when the fiber was stimulated at a CL of 800 ms, triggered activity began at the arrow. This panel shows the first five triggered impulses, although these continued for several minutes (during the break in the record). The last 12 impulses during triggered activity are shown in the right half of the panel. (Reproduced with permission from Wit et al., 1979).

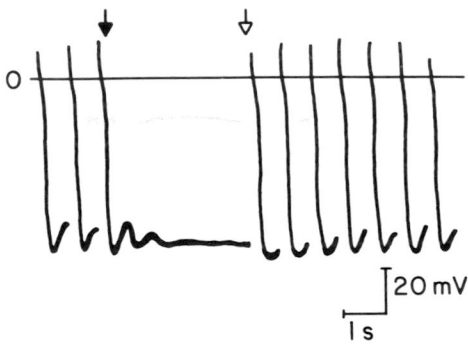

0

20 mV

1 s

Fig. 19.15 Delayed afterpolarizations caused by digitalis in a canine Purkinje fiber. The fiber was exposed to a toxic concentration of ouabain prior to obtaining this record. At the left, the 3 action potentials (AP) shown were stimulated at a cycle length of 700 ms. The stimulus was then turned off (black arrow). The last stimulated AP is followed by 2 subthreshold delayed afterdepolarizations. After a period of quiescence, stimulation was again began at the second (white) arrow. Delayed afterdepolarizations increase in amplitude after each stimulated AP. Each AP is actually being stimulated at the peak of the previous delayed afterdepolarization. (Reproduced with permission from Rosen et al., 1973).

occurs because this impulse is surrounded by tissue made refractory by recent excitation. Under certain conditions, however, the propagating impulse may not die out following complete activation of the heart. Rather it persists to re-excite the atria or ventricles after the end of the refractory period, a process termed re-entry of excitation.

Hoffman and Rosen (1981) have subdivided this mechanism into two sub-categories, *random* and *ordered re-entry*. The principal distinction between the two is that with the former, impulse propagation occurs over re-entrant pathways that continuously change their size and location with time—as with atrial fibrillation. With ordered re-entry, there is a relatively fixed re-entrant pathway—as with AV nodal re-entrant tachycardia. The basic requirements for both random and ordered re-entry are similar: the propagating impulse must block somewhere in the re-entrant circuit, and the block must be transient or unidirectional (Fig. 19.16). The zone where the block occurs enables an excitable pathway to persist for re-excitation by the re-entrant impulse. Additionally, the wave length of the re-entrant impulse (conduction velocity × refractory period) must be shorter than that of the length of the circuit so that the circuit has sufficient time to regain excitability (Mines, 1914). The consequence of this latter requirement is that re-entry of excitation may be promoted by slowing conduction velocity, shortening the refractory period, or both.

There can be a number of causes for slowed conduction and block that are required for re-entry. Conduction velocity in cardiac fibers is dependent on certain features of the transmembrane AP (particularly, those that affect upstroke velocity and amplitude), passive membrane electrical or 'cable' properties, and the microanatomical features of cardiac fibers (Wit et al., 1984). While different groups of investigators determining mechanisms for re-entrant arrhythmias have focused on one or another of these causes, and attempted to attribute all or most re-entry to a single cause, it is likely that one or more mechanisms for re-entry may be operational singly or in combination (Wit et al., 1984). Some of these are discussed below, but this list is not all inclusive. The cause of slowed conduction and block may vary with the specific arrhythmia and cardiac disease process, and are discussed below.

Incomplete Repolarization, Depressed Fast Response, Premature Action Potentials

Premature activation of the heart, whether by discharge from an automatic focus or external stimulation, can induce re-entry because impulses conduct slowly in regions of the heart that are not completely repolarized (some Na^+ channels remain inactivacted). Re-entry may also occur in cells with persistent low levels of membrane potential and consequent depressed fast responses (DFR). Among the factors that could be responsible for DFR's are excess digitalis, high extracellular K$^+$, and myocardial ischemia and infarction. Depending on the amount of Na$^+$ channel inactivation, DFR fibers could be the site for slowing or of blocking conduction.

Slow response

The slow-inward current, under certain conditions, may underlie the genesis of re-entrant arrhythmias

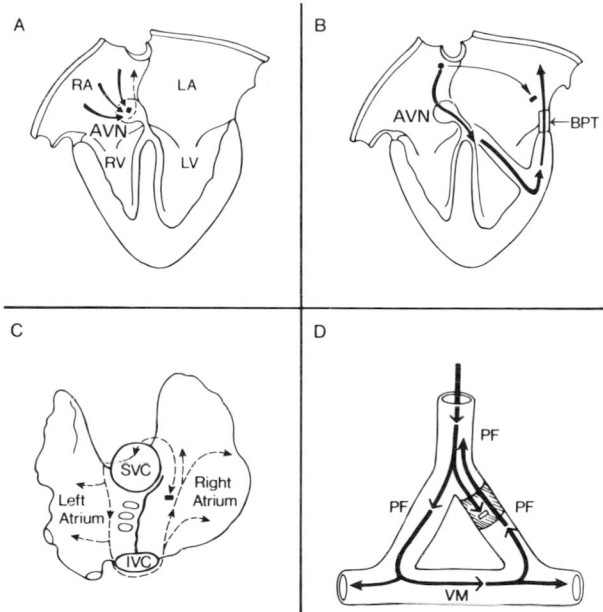

Fig. 19.16 Re-entry in different regions of the heart. In each panel, the arrows show the pattern of impulse conduction. Double parallel lines indicate sites of unidirectional block. Panel A shows how re-entry occurs in the AV node (AVN) when an impulse from the atria blocks in part of the node, but conducts slowly through remaining portions and back to re-excite the atria. Panel B shows re-entry utilizing an AV bypass tract (BPT). The impulse from the atria blocks at the atrial margin of the bypass tract but conducts in an anterograde direction through the normal AV conducting system. Retrograde conduction to the atrium is through the bypass tract. Panel C shows a mechanism proposed by Lewis (1925) for atrial re-entry around the superior and inferior venae cavae (SVC and IVC). Re-entry is initiated by rapid stimulation, which causes transient block in conduction in the direction from the superior to inferior vena cava. Conduction occurs around the cavae in the other direction, however. Conduction in one direction continues after rapid stimulation is stopped. Panel D shows re-entry in a loop comprised of Purkinje fiber bundles (PF) and ventricular muscle (VM). A depressed zone with unidirectional block of conduction (anterograde conduction) is indicated by the stippled zone. Conduction proceeds normally in the other bundle to excite VM in both directions. Conduction proceeds from VM to excite the distal PF beyond the depressed zone. If this zone has recovered sufficiently, conduction may proceed back to the proximal PF (retrograde conduction) to re-excite the fiber. (Reproduced with permission from Wit and Rosen, 1981).

(Cranefield, 1975). Propagated AP's that are dependent on conduction of the slow response include those in the SA and AV nodes and in fast response fibers with their membrane potential reduced to -50 mV (all Na$^+$ channels inactivated). Transient or unidirectional block of conduction may occur with propagated slow responses. As a result, arrhythmias may be due to SA or AV nodal re-entry (Fig. 19.17), or re-entry involving atrial, ventricular or Purkinje fibers when their membrane potentials are reduced sufficiently to activate the slow inward current.

Re-entry with an Anatomical Obstacle

Re-entrant excitation as the result of slowed conduction and block of conduction may also occur in large, anatomically distinct circuits. These may be loops formed by branching Purkinje fibers, bundles of surviving muscle fibres in healed infarcts, or fiberoptic regions of the atria or ventricles. Anatomically, distinct circuits are also involved in re-entry involving

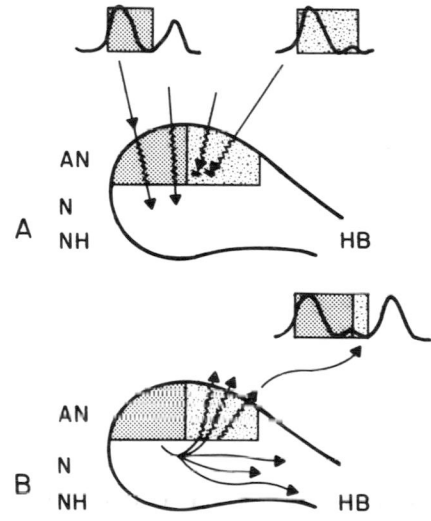

Fig. 19.17 Re-entry of an atrial impulse in the AV node. Panels A and B show diagrammatic representation of the AV node with the upper (AN), middle (N), and lower (NH) node indicated; HB indicates the His bundle. In A, action potentials (AP) recorded from two regions in the upper node are illustrated at the top: the AP at the left has a shorter refractory period than that shown at the right, as indicated by the shaded area. Therefore, when a premature atrial impulse enters the AV node (arrows), it may be able to propagate through part of the upper node with the shorter refractory period. However, it blocks in the region with the longer refractory period. This is also shown in the AP recordings at the top. Panel B shows a possible continuation of these events: the propagating impulse (indicated by the arrows) can return to excite the area of the node in which antegrade conduction block has occurred and thereby re-enter the atrium; AP's recorded from the return nodal pathway are shown above. The impulses can also conduct into the His bundle. (Reproduced with permission from Wit, Rosen and Hoffman, 1974).

the bundle branches or accessory AV conducting pathways.

Reflection

Re-entry can occur in contiguous pathways (Fig. 19.18) based on observations that such pathways can undergo functional longitudinal dissociation (Schmitt and Erlanger, 1929; Scherf, 1947). Re-entry of this type is also termed *reflection* (Cranefield et al, 1973), and occurs in unbranched bundles of depressed Purkinje fibers (incomplete activation of fast response). Reflection can also be caused by electrotonic transmission across a blocked segment (inexcitable gap) in a single fiber (Fig. 19.19).

Leading Circle Concept for Re-entry

Studies by Allessie and colleagues (1977) demonstrate a mechanism for re-entry that does not require an anatomical substrate or functionally depressed segment. The initiation of re-entry is made possible by the different refractory periods of atrial fibers in close proximity to one another. A premature impulse

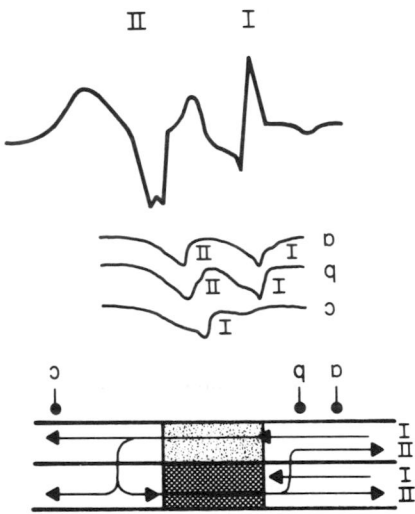

Fig. 19.18 Re-entry in contiguous pathways—reflection. Re-entry can occur in a single bundle of muscle or Purkinje fibers. The diagram depicts two adjacent fibers in a bundle; the entire shaded area is depressed, but depression in the darker area of the upper fiber is so severe that unidirectional conduction block occurs there. The arrows indicate the sequence of activation in the bundle; arrows labeled I show the impulse entering the bundle, and the arrows labeled II show the re-entrant impulse returning to re-excite the left end of the bundle. Action potentials (AP) recorded from sites a, b, and c in the lower fiber are shown below: AP's I were recorded as the impulse conducted from left to right, and AP's labeled II were recorded as the impulse returned to its origin. The bottom trace shows how such events would appear on the electrocardiogram. (Reproduced with permission from Wit and Bigger, 1975).

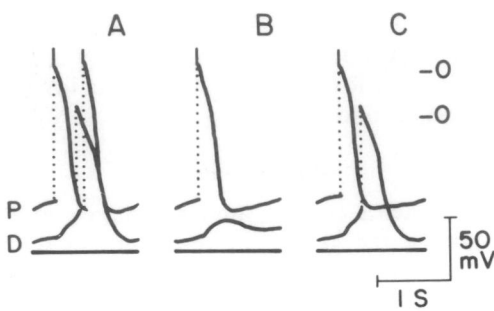

Fig. 19.19 Reflection caused by electrotonic transmission across an inexcitable gap. Transmembrane potentials were recorded from a bundle of Purkinje fibers. P shows recordings from the proximal side of an inexcitable region several mm wide; D shows transmembrane potentials recorded distal to the inexcitable region. In panel A, the first action potential (AP) in the P trace was stimulated and propagated up to the inexcitable region. Excitation occurred distal to the inexcitable region (D) because of electrotonic current flow. The delay before the distal region was excited was long enough to allow the proximal area to recover excitability and permitted a reflected AP to occur (second AP in trace P). In panel B, electrotonic current flow was not sufficient to excite the fiber distal to the inexcitable region. In panel C, the distal segment was activated too quickly and reflection did not occur because the proximal region had not yet recovered excitability. (Reproduced with permission from Antzelevitch et al., 1980).

initiates sustained activity blocks in fibers with long refractory periods and conducts in those with shorter refractory periods. The impulse eventually returns to the initial point of block after recovery of excitability there (Fig. 19.20), and the impulse may continue to circulate. Conduction through the re-entrant circuit is slowed because impulses are propagating in partially refractory tissue. The circumference of the pathway may be quite small (6–8 mm). Impulses spread centripetally from the circumference of the circulating wave front towards the centre. The upstroke velocities and amplitude of these AP's gradually decrease as the centre is approached. Cells in the centre show only local responses because they are kept refractory by the circulating impulse.

Slow Conduction and Re-entry Caused by the Anisotropic Structure of Cardiac Muscle

The anatomic and physical properties of cardiac muscle vary according to the direction in the cardiac syncytium in which they are measured (Clerc, 1976). More recently, Spach and his colleagues (1981, 1982a, 1982b) have shown that anisotropy can be a cause for re-entry in normal atrial and ventricular muscle. Briefly, their data show that impulse conduction velocity perpendicular to the long axis of myocardial fibers can be very slow, even when resting potentials are normal. Such slow conduction can facilitate the occurrence of re-entry.

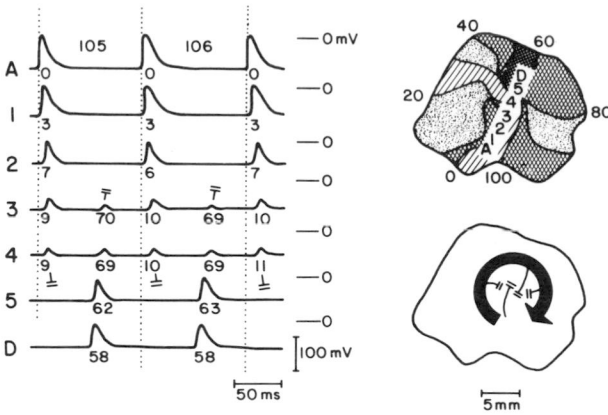

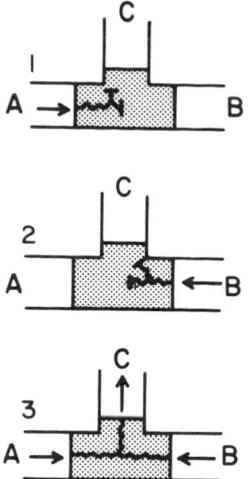

Fig. 19.20 Re-entry in isolated left-atrial myocardium by the leading circle mechanism. At the right, above, is the map of the activation pattern of the atrium during circus movement. The impulse continuously rotates in a clockwise direction; each number and different shading indicates the time in milliseconds during which a given region is activated. Activation proceeds from 0-100 ms; that is, 1 complete revolution takes 100 ms. At the left, the membrane potentials of 7 fibers (marked A, D and 1 through 5) located on a straight line through the center of the circus movement are shown (the locations from which these AP's were recorded are indicated on the map at the upper right). These records show that the fibers in the central point of the circuit (fibers 3 and 4) show double responses of subnormal amplitude during circus movement. These responses result from conduction of the impulse from the circulating wave toward the center. At the lower right, the activation pattern during circus movement is given schematically. It shows the circuit with the converging wavelets in the center. (Reproduced with permission from Allessie et al., 1977).

Fig. 19.21 Summation and inhibition in a branching Purkinje fiber with a depressed zone (stippled). Stimulation at either normal end, A (as in panel 1) or B (as in panel 2), results in a small depolarization, incapable of propagation, in the depressed segment. However, if A and B are stimulated simultaneously (as in panel 3), the resulting depolarizations *summate* in the depressed segment, thereby providing a sufficient response for activity to propagate to C and excite distal, normal tissue. The schematic (panel 3) also illustrates *inhibition*. Under conditions permitting the impulse to propagate successfully from branch B to C, the simultaneous presence of a depressed fast response (activated slow response) in branch A could block the spread of excitation from B to C and prevent the emergence of a re-entrant impulse in branch C. (Reproduced with permission from Hoffman and Rosen, 1981).

Summation and Inhibition

Studies on isolated and depressed mammalian Purkinje fiber preparations demonstrate two additional properties namely, *summation* and *inhibition* that make matters more complicated in attempting to provide simple and uniformly applicable rules to describe re-entrant excitation (Cranefield and Hoffman, 1971; Hoffman et al, 1981). Summation and inhibition can be considered in relation to Fig. 19.21, which depicts a branching Purkinje fiber with a central depressed zone. The likelihood of either summation or inhibition in such a fiber is critically dependent on the timing of impulses propagating toward the depressed segment.

REFERENCES

Allessie M.A., Bonke F.M., Schopman F.J.G. (1977). Circus movement in rabbit atrial muscle as a mechanism of tachycardia. III. The 'leading circle' concept: A new model of circle movement in cardiac tissue without the involvement of an anatomical obstacle. *Circ. Res.*, **41**, 9.

Antzelevitch C., Jalife J., Moe G.K. (1980). Characteristics of reflection as a mechanism of re-entrant arrhythmias and its relation to parasystole. *Circulation*, **61**, 182.

Atlee J.L. (1990). *Perioperative Cardiac Dysrhythmias: Mechanisms, Recognition, Management*. 2nd edn., 450 pp Chicago: Year Book Medical Publishers.

Atlee J.L. (1985b). Anaesthesia and cardiac electrophysiology. *Eur. J. Anaesth.*, **3**, 215.

Brown H.F., Nobel S.J. (1974). Effects of adrenaline on membrane current underlying pacemaker activity in frog atrial muscle. *J. Physiol.*, **238**, 51P.

Carmeleit E. (1980). The slow-inward current: Non-voltage-clamp studies. In *The Slow Inward Current and Cardiac Arrhythmias* pp. 97–10. (Zipes D.P., Bailey J.C., Elharrar V., eds.) The Hague: Martinus-Nijhoff.

Clerc L. (1976). Directional differences of impulse spread in trabecular muscle from mammalian heart. *J. Physiol.*, **255**, 335.

Cranefield P.F. (1975). *The Conduction of the Cardiac Impulse*. p. 404. Mt. Kisco, New York: Futura.

Cranefield P.F., Hoffman B.F. (1971). Conduction of the cardiac impulse. II. Summation and inhibition. *Circ. Res.*, **28**, 220.

Cranefield P.F., Wit A.L., Hoffman B.F. (1973). The genesis of cardiac arrhythmias. *Circulation*, **47**, 190.

Cranefield P.F. (1977). Action potentials, afterpotentials and arrhythmias. *Circ. Res.*, **41**, 415.

Dangman K.H., Hoffman B.F. (1983). Studies on overdrive

stimulation of canine Purkinje fibers: Maximum diastolic potential as a determinant of the response. *J. Am. Coll. Cardiol.*, **2**, 1183.

Di Francesco D. (1981). A new interpretation of the pace-maker current i_{K2} in Purkinje fibers. *J. Physiol.*, **314**, 359.

Downar E., Janse M.J., Durrer D. (1977). The effect of acute coronary artery occlusion on subepicardial transmembrane potentials in the intact porcine heart. *Circulation*, **56**, 217.

Draper M.H., Weidmann S. (1951). Cardiac resting and action potentials recorded with an intracellular electrode. *J. Physiol.*, **115**, 74.

Elharrar V., Zipes D.P. (1980). Voltage modulation of automaticity in cardiac Purkinje fibers. in *The Slow Inward Current and Cardiac Arrhythmias* pp. 357–373. (Zipes D.P., Bailey J.C., Elharrar V., eds.) The Hague: Martinus-Nijhoff.

Ferrier G.R. (1977). Digitalis arrhythmias. Role of oscillatory afterpotentials. *Prog. Cardiovasc. Dis.*, **19**, 459.

Friedman P.L., Stewart J.R., Fenoglio J.J., et al. (1973). Spontaneous and induced cardiac arrhythmias in subendocardial Purkinje fibers surviving extensive myocardial infarction in dogs. *Circ. Res.*, **33**, 612.

Gadsby D.C., Wit A.L. (1987). Normal and abnormal electrical activity in cardiac cells. In. *Cardiac Arrhthmias*. 2nd edn., p. 53–80. (Mandel W.J., ed.) Philadelphia: J.B. Lippincott.

Gettes L.S., Reuter H. (1974). Slow recovery from inactivation of inward current in mammalian myocardial fibers. *J. Physiol.*, **240**, 703.

Goldman D.E. (1943). Potential, impedance and rectification in membranes. *J. Gen. Physiol.*, **27**, 37.

Grant A.O., Strauss H.C. (1982) Intracellular potassium activity in rabbit sinoatrial node. Evaluation during spontaneous activity and arrest. *Circ. Res.*, **51**, 271.

Hodgkin A.L., Katz B. (1949). The effect of sodium ions on the electrical activity of the giant axon of the squid. *J. Physiol.*, **108**, 37.

Hodgkin A.L., Huxley A.F. (1952). A quantitative description of membrane current and its application to conduction and excitation in nerve. *J. Physiol.*, **117**, 500.

Hoffman B.F., Cranefield P.F. (1960) *Electrophysiology of the Heart*. 323 pp. New York: McGraw-Hill.

Hoffman B.F., Cranefield P.A. (1964) Physiologic basis of cardiac arrhythmias. *Am. J. Med.*, **37**, 670.

Hoffman B.F., Rosen M.R. (1981). Cellular mechanisms for cardiac arrhythmias. *Circ. Res.*, **49**, 1.

Imanishi S., Surawicz B. (1976). Automatic activity in depolarized guinea pig ventricular myocardium. Characteristics and mechanisms. *Circ. Res.*, **39**, 751.

Isenberg G. (1976). Cardiac Purkinje fibers: caesium as a tool to block inward rectifying potassium currents. *Pflugers Arch.*, **365**, 99.

Kass R.S., Tsien R.W., Weingart R. (1978a). Ionic basis of transient inward current induced by strophanthidin in cardiac Purkinje fibers. *J. Physiol.*, **281**, 209.

Kass R.S., Lederer W.J., Tsien R.W., et al. (1978b). Role of calcium ions in transient inward currents and aftercontractions induced by strophanthidin in cardiac Purkinje fibers. *J. Physiol.*, **281**, 187.

Katzung B.G., Morgenstern J.A. (1977). Effects of extracellular potassium on ventricular automaticity and evidence for a pacemaker current in mammalian ventricular myocardium. *Circ. Res.*, **40**, 105.

Kenyon J.L., Gibbons W.R. (1977). Effects of low-chloride solutions on action potentials of sheep cardiac Purkinje fibers. *J. Gen. Physiol.*, **70**, 635.

Lazzara R., El-Sherif N., Scherlag B.J. (1973). Electrophysiological properties of canine Purkinje cells in one-day-old myocardial infarction. *Circ. Res.*, **33**, 722.

Lazzara R., El-Sherif N., Scherlag B.J. (1974). Early and late effects of coronary artery occlusion on canine Purkinje fibers. *Circ. Res.*, **35**, 391.

Lewis T. (1925). *The Mechanism and Graphic Registration of the Heart Beat*. p. 529. London: Shaw.

Mendez C., Moe G.K. (1966). Some characteristics of transmembrane potentials of AV nodal cells during propagation of premature beats. *Circ. Res.*, **19**, 993.

Merideth J., Mendez C., Mueller W.J., et al. (1968). Electrical excitability of atrioventricular nodal cells. *Circ. Res.*, **23**, 69.

Mines G.R. (1914). On circulatory excitations in heart muscle and their possible relation to tachycardia and fibrillation. *Trans. R. Soc. Can. Sur.*, **9, Sect IV 8**, 43.

Noble D., Tsien R.W. (1968). The kinetics and rectifier properties of the slow potassium current in cardiac Purkinje fibers. *J. Physiol.*, **195**, 185.

Noble D. (1985). Ionic Bases of Rhythmic Activity in the Heart. In *Cardiac Electrophysiology and Arrhythmias*, pp. 3–11. (Zipes D.P., and Jalife J. eds.) Orlando, F.L.: Grune and Stratton.

Noma A., Irisawa H. (1974). Electrogenic sodium pump in rabbit sinoatrial node cell. *Pflugers Arch.*, **351**, 177.

Reuter H. (1967). The dependence of slow inward current in Purkinje fibers on the extracelular calcium concentration. *J. Physiol.*, **192**, 479.

Reuter H. (1973). Divalent cations as charge carriers in excitable membranes. In Progress in Biophysics and Molecular Biology, pp. 1–43. (Butler J.A.V. and Noble D., eds.) New York: Pergamon Press.

Rosen M.R., Gelband H., Merker C., et al. (1973). Mechanisms of digitalis toxicity. Effects of ouabain on phase four of canine Purkinje fiber transmembrane potentials. *Circulation*, **47**, 681.

Scherf D. (1947). Studies on auricular tachycardia caused by aconitine administration. *Proc. Soc. Exp. Biol. Med.*, **64**, 233.

Schmitt F.O., Erlanger J. (1929). Directional differences in the conduction of the impulse through heart muscle and their possible relation to extrasystolic and fibrillary contractions. *Am. J. Physiol.*, **87**, 326.

Singer D.H., Ten Eick R.E. (1969). Pharmacology of cardiac arrhythmias. *Progr. Cardiovasc. Dis.*, **11**, 488.

Spach M.S., Miller W.T., Geselowitz, D.B., et al. (1981). The discontinuous nature of propagation in normal canine cardiac muscle: Evidence for recurrent discontinuities of intracellular resistance that affect the membrane currents. *Circ. Res.*, **48**, 39.

Spach M.S., Miller W.T., Dolber P.C. (1982a). The functional role of structural complexities in the propagation of depolarization in the atrium of the dog: Cardiac conduction disturbances due to discontinuities of effective axial resistivity. *Circ. Res.*, **50**, 75.

Spach M.S., Kootsey J.M., Sloan J.D. (1982b). Active modulation of electrical coupling between cardiac cells of the dog: A mechanism for transient and steady state variations in conduction velocity. *Circ. Res.*, **51**, 347.

Sperelakis N. (1979). Origin of the Cardiac Resting Potential. In *Handbook of Physiology. Section 2. The Cardiovascular System. Vol I. The Heart*. pp. 187–267. Bethesda, Md: The American Physiological Society.

Surawicz B., Imanishi S. (1976). Automatic activity in depolarized guinea pig ventricular myocardium. Characteristics and mechanism. *Circ. Res.*, **39**, 751.

Vassale M. (1966). Analysis of cardiac pacemaker potential using a 'voltage clamp' technique. *Am. J. Physiol.*, **210**, 1335.

Vassale M. (1970). Electrogenic suppression of automaticity in sheep and dog Purkinje fibers. *Circ. Res.*, **27**, 361.

Weidmann S. (1955). The effect of the cardiac action potential on the rapid availability of the sodium-carrying system. *J. Physiol.*, **127**, 213.

Wit A.L. (1984) Cellular electrophysiologic mechanisms of cardiac arrhythmias. *Ann. N.Y. Acad. Sci.*, **432**, 1.

Wit A.L., Bigger J.T. (1975). Possible electrophysiology mechanisms for lethal arrhythmia accompanying myocardial ischemia and infarction. *Circulation (Suppl)*, **51** and **52**, 96.

Wit A.L., Boyden P.A., Gadsby D.C., et al. (1979). Triggered activity as a cause of atrial arrhythmias. In *Cardiac Arrhythmias: Electrophysiology, Diagnosis and Management*. pp. 14–31. (Narula O.S., ed.) Baltimore: Williams and Wilkins.

Wit A.L., Cranefield P.F., Gadsby D.C. (1980). Triggered activity. In *The Slow Inward Current and Cardiac Arrhythmias*. pp. 437–454. (Zipes D.P., Bailey J.C., Elharrar V., eds.) The Hague: Martinus-Nijhoff.

Wit A.L., Friedman P.F. (1975). Basis for ventricular arrhythmias accompanying myocardial infarction: Alterations in electrical activity of ventricular muscle and Purkinje fibers after coronary artery occlusion. *Arch. Intern. Med.*, **135**, 459.

Wit A.L., Rosen M.R. (1981). Cellular electrophysiology of cardiac arrhythmias. II. Arrhythmias caused by abnormal impulse conduction. *Mod. Conc. Cardiovasc. Dis.*, **50**, 7.

Wit A.L., Rosen M.R. (1984). Cellular electrophysiology of cardiac arrhythmias. In *Tachycardias: Mechanisms, Diagnosis, Treatment*. pp. 1–27. (Josephson M.E., Wellens H.J.J., eds.) Philadelphia: Lea and Febiger.

Wit A.L., Rosen M.R. (1986). Afterdepolarizations and triggered activity. In *The Heart and Cardiovascular System*, pp. 1449–1490. (Fozzard H.A., Haber E., Jennings R.B., et al., eds.) New York: Raven Press.

Wit A.L., Rosen M.R., Hoffman B.F. (1974). Electrophysiology and pharmacology of cardiac arrhythmias. II. Relationship of normal and abnormal electrical activity of cardiac fibers to the genesis of arrhythmias. A. Automaticity. *Am. Heart J.*, **88**, 515.

Zipes D.P. (1984) Genesis of Cardiac Arrhythmias: Electrophysiological Considerations. In *Heart Disease*, 2nd edn., pp. 605–647. (Braunward E., ed.) Philadelphia, W.B. Saunders.

B. RESPIRATION

20. Control of Breathing
D. Trenchard and W. Kox

Ventilatory 'drives'
The respiratory centre and rhythm generation
Optimization of breathing patterns
  Primary optimization
  Secondary optimization
  Tertiary optimization
  Protective mechanism

It is generally accepted that the principal function of breathing is to maintain adequate levels of O_2 and CO_2 within the body. In this way sufficient O_2 can be provided to meet a wide range of metabolic requirements, while removal of CO_2 generated by this metabolism ensures maintenance of a near constant, species-specific optimum value of intracellular pH (Reeves and Rahn, 1981). A simple analysis of how the control of breathing is able to affect the wide-ranging adjustments involved in such a system indicates that at least four functional components should be considered:

1. A mechanism(s) providing a 'drive' to breathe
2. A mechanism(s) for generating breathing in response to this 'drive'
3. Mechanisms for the optimization of breathing patterns
4. Protective mechanisms to prevent damage to the respiratory system.

This chapter can only give an outline of the respiratory control system. For more detailed coverage and extensive reference lists, the reader is referred to the latest relevant volumes of the Handbook of Physiology (Cherniack and Widdicombe, 1986).

VENTILATORY 'DRIVES'

For many years it was thought that a basic rhythmic pattern of breathing was automatically generated in a respiratory centre situated in the brain-stem (ponto-medullary region of the CNS) influenced by the direct action of CO_2 upon it. Two experiments in particular in recent years have changed this to a concept that the basic rhythm is not automatically generated, but depends critically on afferent information. Thus, in unanaesthetized dogs, Sullivan et al. (1978) studied the effects on breathing of successively suppressing the major sources of respiratory afferent information (wakefulness, vagal activity, peripheral and central chemoreceptors). Suppression and/or abolition of each afferent pathway in turn, led to progressive slowing of the frequency of breathing with little or no reduction in tidal volume, until finally the dogs were breathing as slowly as one breath per minute. A similar conclusion that afferent information was essential for the maintenance of rhythmic breathing was reached by See et al. (1983) in studies on cats in which central chemoreceptors had been abolished. Additional elimination of peripheral chemoreceptors and vagal afferents caused respiratory arrest, although breathing could still be elicited in response to a thermoregulatory afferent input from the hypothalamus.

These two studies—and many more—suggest the presence of at least five 'drives' that can generate breathing, of which two are dominant under normal circumstances, Fig. 20.1. Firstly, a major 'drive' arising from central chemoreceptors (CC) defined principally in cats, as two areas on the ventrolateral surface of the medulla at a depth of approximately 100–200 μm. Most evidence suggests CC respond directly to changes in the extracellular pH of their environment, which in turn can be affected by both metabolic and respiratory acid-base changes in arterial blood. The manner in which CC transmit their information to the rhythm-generating mechanism is as yet not fully understood, although the receptive mechanism itself appears to be cholinergic.

The second major 'drive' arises from a requirement for thermoregulation, derived from central thermoreceptors. Most mammals use breathing for thermoregulatory purposes by evaporative heat loss from the upper airways. This is normally achieved by increasing the frequency of breathing ($100–400$ min^{-1}) while reducing tidal volume to values close to, or below anatomical dead space. A large minute ventilation (for thermoregulation) can thus be achieved without increasing alveolar ventilation (for gas exchange). In the absence of a requirement for gas exchange, the thermoregulatory 'drive' can still produce sufficient 'drive' to maintain breathing (See et al., 1983).

The third 'drive' arises from peripheral chemoreceptors (PC), principally the carotid, but possibly also the aortic chemoreceptors in some species. These PC are sensitive to oxygen levels within the blood, but there is little or no effect at normal levels: the ventilatory change induced by the hypoxic 'drive' from PC only becomes clear cut at Pa_{O_2} values less than 60 mmHg. There is some controversy about the PC response to Pa_{O_2} (or [H^+]). Animal studies with and without PC indicate that under normal circumstances the 'drive' from PC related to Pa_{CO_2} contributes up to 30% of the total 'drive' to breathing, particularly when assessed as a Pa_{CO_2}/ventilatory response curve. On the other hand, animal studies eliminating central chemoreceptor function have demonstrated that although PC can still respond to hypoxic stimuli, there is a total absence of any ventilatory response to an increased CO_2/H^+ stimulus. The interpretation of such studies is still confused since either it means that

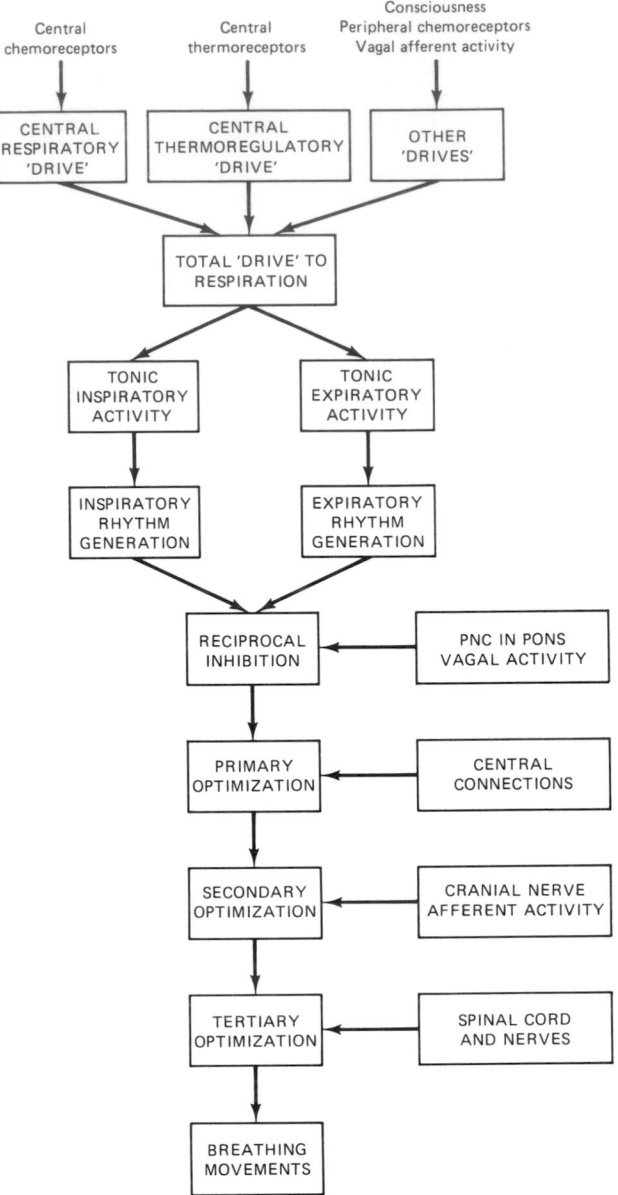

Fig. 20.1 Functional organization of the control of breathing.

PC have no CO_2/H^+ sensitivity or that the 'drive' from PC can only exert an effect in the presence of a 'drive' from CC. Part of this confusion may have arisen from the fact that the role of activity from PC appears to be two-*fold*, each acting at a different site. As just described, the PC input contributes to the total 'drive' to breathing, but additionally it has an optimizing role at a subsequent stage in the production of respiratory activity. The conflicting results could simply be a consequence of different experimental conditions or species differentially affecting these two roles.

The fourth 'drive' to breathing is indicated by the

reduction in ventilation produced by vagotomy (Sullivan et al., 1978). Although this is usually attributed to either the loss of mechanosensitive information from vagal lung receptors or to the loss of aortic chemoreceptor information, recent studies have demonstrated CO_2/H^+ sensitivities from two vagal lung receptors—pulmonary stretch receptors in dogs (Coleridge and Coleridge, in Cherniack and Widdicombe, 1986), and J receptors in rabbits (Trenchard, 1986). Further studies are needed to determine if chemoreceptor 'drives' for breathing can be attributed to either or both of these vagal receptors. The role of this vagal input parallels that from PC in having a two-*fold* function, contributing to the initial drive to breathing and subsequent optimization of the respiratory activity.

The fifth 'drive' relates to the presence of consciousness. Sullivan et al. (1978) clearly demonstrated that a significant proportion of the total 'drive' was lost when their dogs went from a state of quietly resting to slow-wave sleep. Although this observation has been known for many years, it is only now that attempts are being made to quantify it; it is still not known how much relates to the increased metabolism accompanying consciousness and how much to consciousness itself.

With the possible exception of the last one, all the former 'drives' can be considered as metabolic and hence are under involuntary (automatic) control. There is a final 'drive' that also relates to consciousness, concerning voluntary control. Thus (in Man at least) it is possible to alter the pattern of breathing at will, hyperventilating or breath-holding for example. Although this voluntary 'drive' to breathe cannot be considered as part of the normal 'drive', its life-saving value can be demonstrated in patients suffering from Ondine's Curse Syndrome for example, where there is complete loss of involuntary rhythmic breathing: respiration can be maintained by this voluntary 'drive' pathway activated by auditory or visual commands. This 'drive' related to voluntary control does not act centrally, and will subsequently be discussed in relation to interactions at spinal level.

THE RESPIRATORY CENTRE AND RHYTHM GENERATION

In unanaesthetized animals, respiratory related activity can be recorded in neurones of the CNS extending from mid-brain to the first few cervical segments, but there is a much higher probability of finding it in certain circumscribed areas. On the other hand, in deeply-anaesthetized animals such respiratory-related activity can only be recorded from these three circumscribed areas. Successive ablations of parts of the CNS have also shown that these three areas appear to be essential for retaining a basic respiratory rhythmicity. Two of these bilaterally-paired areas are to be found in the medulla—a dorsal respiratory group (DRG) and a ventral respiratory group (VRG)

while the third is found in the pons (PNC). Most, but not all, investigators accept that the generation of respiratory rhythm is related to the neuronal interconnection between these groups, with the two medullary groups generating inspiratory and expiratory activities that project to respiratory muscle neurones, while the third group in the pons is more concerned with phase-switching. Unfortunately there is little agreement as yet on how this is achieved or how it relates to these three regions. Current concepts—which to some extent have almost turned full circle to concepts held early this century—suggest that there are two half-centres (one for inspiration and one for expiration) each able to generate a rhythm in its own right, in addition to reciprocal inhibition between them. During quiet breathing when no expiratory muscle activity is present, rhythmic inspirations can occur, interspersed by periods of no inspiratory activity (expiration), generated solely within the inspiratory half-centre. Generation of expiratory activity is not therefore a prerequisite for rhythmic breathing, but if present, as ventilation is stimulated, rhythmic expirations would be produced in a parallel fashion in the expiratory half-centre and the two outputs synchronized by the reciprocal inhibition.

What can be termed a 'crude' primary pattern of a breath is therefore determined in this pontomedullary respiratory centre in that the magnitude is determined by the 'drives' and the durations of inspiration and expiration by the respective phase-switching mechanisms. (It should be noted that although the respiratory centre is usually thought of as controlling diaphragmatic, intercostal and abdominal muscles, parts of the respiratory centre project to other muscles associated with respiration—alae nasi, pharyngeal, laryngeal, tongue and accessory muscles for example. There is considerable interaction in the respiratory centre nuclei involved in all these pathways, so that the total breathing pattern can be synchronized.)

In a variety of studies in anaesthetized animals where the phase-switching mechanisms were eliminated (destruction of PNC in pons combined with vagotomy) apneustic breathing was produced, consisting of extremely prolonged inspirations due to a tonic level of inspiratory activity. The magnitude of these apneustic breaths are very dependent on Pa_{CO_2}/H^+, and in current concepts this is consistent with an origin as the 'drive' from central (and peripheral) chemoreceptors. The PNC therefore appears to be an essential part of the respiratory centre by its phase-terminating action in the generation of rhythmic compared with apneustic breathing, although the same function can also be performed by vagal mechanosensitive afferent information from pulmonary stretch receptors in the lung. It is of interest that studies in anaesthetized cats with apneustic breathing (due to PNC lesions combined with vagotomy) have revealed that if the same cats are allowed to recover consciousness then a relatively normal pattern of breathing develops. This could be attributable in part to a restoration of central thermoregulatory control (and hence the 'drive') associated with recovery of consciousness: alternatively it could suggest the existence of at least one more phase-switching mechanism, as yet poorly understood, but whose function depends on the presence of consciousness (St. John et al., 1972).

Thus the current overall concept of how the basic rhythmic breathing is produced is that it is not automatically generated within neural networks of the brain stem, but depends critically on sufficient afferent information from chemical (and/or thermoregulatory if appropriate) 'drives' to activate these neural networks. Thus, when sufficient chemical 'drive' is present to produce a requirement for ventilation, it will generate a single breath. If one breath is sufficient to annul the 'drive', then periodic breathing is produced—periods of a few breaths alternating with prolonged expiratory apneas while the 'drive' is building up again. On the other hand, if the whole system is delicately balanced, a continuous and regular rhythm could easily be established, as normally occurs.

OPTIMIZATION OF BREATHING PATTERN

Optimization should be considered in three ways. Firstly that the pattern of breathing is optimal in terms of energy expenditure in its primary role of responding to the 'drive' that generates it, usually the chemical 'drive'. Secondly, while responding to the primary 'drive' the pattern of breathing can be modified to provide an optimal compromise between this and other functions of breathing, thermoregulation or speech for example. Thirdly, there is optimization of respiratory control by integration with other control systems: perhaps the best example of this is the matching of ventilation with lung perfusion.

For most of this century, it has been known that the spontaneous pattern of breathing adopted under a wide variety of conditions in practically all the mammalian species studied, is the most optimal in terms of energy cost for the differing requirements of those species. It is still not known to what extent this is an active process—implying the presence of as yet undiscovered receptors and control systems. Alternatively it could have happened passively by evolutionary processes over many thousand of years.

As described previously a 'crude' primary breath is generated in the ponto-medullary respiratory centre, whose magnitude is determined by the 'drives' and the durations of inspiration and expiration by the respective rhythm generating mechanisms and reciprocal inhibitions. Optimization of the breathing pattern also occurs in this region by integration and interaction with other control systems (primary optimization) and also by modifications as a consequence of afferent inputs to this area via peripheral nerves (secondary optimization). These sub-divisions do not necessarily indicate an anatomical or sequential separation; they are merely used as a functional separation, since the actual sites or networks and the mechanism involved are still not fully understood.

Primary Optimization

Overall integration of the respiratory and cardiovascular control systems is the most obvious example that occurs in this region, leading to an optimization of the pattern of breathing in relation to the pulmonary circulation. Other examples include optimization in relation to centres in the cortex, thalamus and hypothalamus. Both consciousness and thermoregulation have previously been considered as contributing to the total 'drive' to respiration, but it is probable that they also contribute to a modification of the breathing pattern once it has been generated. Much current research is centred on the various factors determining the increased breathing accompanying the onset of exercise. One of these factors is believed to be a 'feed-forward', whereby the higher centres from where the output drive to the exercising muscles is derived, also sends parallel inputs to the respiratory (and cardiovascular) control systems: each system is therefore optimized in relation to the increased demands of exercise simultaneous with its commencement.

Secondary Optimization

As opposed to the primary optimization which is concerned with connections to other centres within the CNS, secondary optimization is based on feed-back information from distinct receptors external to the CNS, mediated by cranial nerves. The location of this secondary optimization in the ponto-medullary region of the CNS becomes obvious when the evolutionary origin of the respiratory system is considered. In lower vertebrates who used gills for this purpose, practically all the afferent information as well as the motor neurone output to respiratory-related musculature was derived from the cranial segments of this region. With the change from gills to lung breathing, the same cartilage, muscles and innervation of these segments were incorporated into the new system, but because of various anatomical changes the nerves often follow quite tortuous paths, although still projecting to and from the same area of the CNS. It is not surprising therefore that this site is the region of most of the secondary optimization of the 'crude' breath. Thus activity from peripheral chemoreceptors will tend to enhance inspiratory activity in both magnitude and duration if its arrival coincides with this phase of the generated breath, but decrease expiratory duration if its arrival coincides with the expiratory phase. Increased mechanosensitive vagal activity from pulmonary stretch receptors in the lung has the complementary action of decreasing inspiration and enhancing expiration. Such afferent information therefore serves the purpose of modifying a breath generated primarily by central chemoreceptors adjacent to the respiratory centre, in relation to up-to-date information from 'distance' receptors.

It is also in the respiratory centre that interactions occur between the various sensory and motor nuclei of other muscles associated with breathing, so that synchrony can occur. For example, it would be no use in having only minimal abduction of the vocal cords, or closure of the alae nasi in certain species, if a very large inspiration was about to be produced. There is also a time synchrony between motor outputs so that for example the glottis and larynx are dilated fractionally in advance of an inspiration commencing, a synchrony that appears to fall down during a hiccup.

Tertiary Optimization

A tertiary level of optimization of the pattern of breathing occurs at the spinal level in the appropriate phrenic, intercostal and abdominal nuclei. A major part of this optimization/integration is related to the proprioceptive information from the respective muscles, particularly in relation to their postural function. For example, if an animal is bending sideways so that one half of the chest wall is stretched and the other side compressed, there is adjustment of the respiratory-related output to the two sides. It is also at these spinal levels that integration occurs with activity in the direct voluntary pathways from the cortex. This becomes of major importance in Man, for apart from the voluntary control of the pattern of breathing, including its inhibition in a breath-hold, it is at this point that the delicate control of breathing (particularly expiration), required for the production of speech occurs.

Protective Mechanisms

While not contributing directly to the generation of breathing pattern, activation of protective mechanisms can completely override normal breathing. Impaction of a single, relatively small foreign body at the site of a single cough receptor in the larynx for example, is sufficient to produce a spasm of coughing involving the whole body, and producing a severe disturbance to ventilation.

A detailed description of all the receptive and reflexive processes involved in these protective mechanisms is beyond the scope of this chapter but for more information the reader is referred to the chapters by Widdicombe, and by Coleridge and Coleridge in Cherniack and Widdicombe 1986.

REFERENCES

Cherniack N.S., Widdicombe J.G. eds. (1986). *Handbook of Physiology, Section 3: The Respiratory System. Volume II: Control of Breathing*. Bethesda: Am. Physiol. Soc.

Reeves R.B., Rahn H. (1981). Patterns in vertebrate acid-base regulation. In *Evolution of respiratory processes*. (Wood S.C., Lenfant C. ed.) Dekker.

See W.R., Folgering H., Schlaefke M.E. (1983). Further studies of the central chemosensitive drive and the respiratory drive in hyperthermia. In *Central Neurone Environment and the control systems of breathing and circulation*. (Schlaefke M.E., Koepchen H.P., See W.R. ed.) Springer-Verlag.

St. John W.M., Glasser R.L., King R.A. (1971). Rhythmic respiration in awake, vagotomized cats with chronic pneumotaxic area lesions. *Resp. Physiol.*, **15**, 233.

Sullivan C.E., Kozar L.F., Murphy E., et al. (1978). Primary role in respiratory afferents in sustaining breathing rhythm. *J. Appl. Physiol.*, **45**, 11.

Trenchard D. (1986). CO_2/H^+ receptors in the lungs of anaesthetized rabbits *Resp. Physiol.*, **63**, 241.

21. Respiratory Mechanics
M. K. Sykes

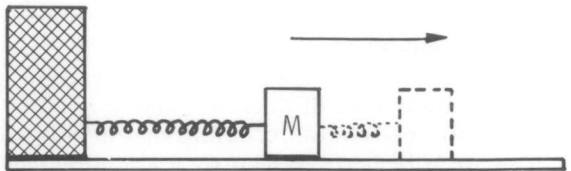

Fig. 21.1 Model to illustrate forces opposing movement of the respiratory system. The mass (M) is connected to a stationary object by a spring. Movement of the mass in the direction of the arrow is opposed by the elastic recoil of the spring, by the frictional resistance between the mass and the surface and by the inertive forces resulting from the acceleration of the mass.

This chapter is concerned with the factors which determine the resting lung volume, the changes in lung volume resulting from respiratory muscle activity or artificial ventilation, and the regional distribution of ventilation within the lung.

Throughout this analysis it is necessary to differentiate clearly between the static and dynamic properties of the respiratory system. The difference between these properties is best illustrated by a simple model consisting of a mass attached by a spring to a solid block (Fig. 21.1). To move the mass against the action of the spring it is necessary to apply a force. The movement of the mass generates three types of opposing force.

Firstly, the spring will be stretched, so generating an elastic recoil. The force generated by the spring will depend on the 'stiffness' of the spring and will increase progressively with the degree of stretch of the spring. The recoil force tending to return the mass to its resting position will thus be related solely to the position of the mass and will not be affected by the rate at which the mass is moving.

The second force opposing the movement of the mass is the frictional resistance between the mass and the surface on which it rests. This force is affected not only by the magnitude of the frictional resistance but also by the velocity of movement.

The third force to be considered is that resulting from the inertia of the block. This depends on the mass of the block and on the rate of change of velocity (or acceleration) of the block.

In the respiratory system the pressure (p) required to move gas into the lungs is opposed by the elastic recoil (the balance of forces between the lung and chest wall), the viscous resistance due to the movement of gases down the airways and to the deformation of tissues, together with the inertive component resulting from the acceleration of both gas and tissues. Since elastic recoil (E) is proportional to volume (V), resistance (R) is proportional to flow ($\dot{V}$) and inertia (I) is proportional to acceleration ($\ddot{V}$)

$$p = E \cdot V + R \cdot \dot{V} + I \cdot \ddot{V}$$

At normal breathing frequencies inertia is small; discussion will therefore be concentrated on the factors governing the elastic recoil pressure and the resistance.

Compliance

In the respiratory system the elastic properties of the lungs, chest wall or total respiratory system are usually defined by the static compliance.

$$\text{Compliance} \ (\text{L/cmH}_2\text{O}) = \frac{\text{change in volume (L)}}{\text{change in pressure (cmH}_2\text{O})}$$

The change in volume is easily measured by a spirometer or body plethysmograph (*see* p. 266). However, measurement of the appropriate pressure difference is more difficult. For lung compliance the pressure difference is from the alveolus to the pleural space; for chest wall compliance from pleural space to atmosphere; whilst total thoracic compliance is calculated from the sum of these pressure differences. At the end of expiration, pleural pressure is approximately 5 cmH$_2$O (0.5 kPa) less than alveolar (i.e. atmospheric) pressure, so that the transpulmonary pressure difference is $+5\,cmH_2O$ ($+0.5\,kPa$). At the end of inspiration pleural pressure falls to $-10\,cmH_2O$ ($-1.0\,kPa$) so that the transpulmonary pressure difference becomes $+10\,cmH_2O$ ($+1.0\,kPa$). If the change in the transpulmonary pressure of $5\,cmH_2O$ produces a volume change of $0.5\,L$, lung compliance $= 0.5\,L/5\,cmH_2O = 0.1\,L/cmH_2O$. ($0.5\,kPa$ produces a volume change of $0.5\,L$: lung compliance $= 1\,L/kPa$)

Unfortunately, it is usually impossible to measure pleural pressure directly: however, in the erect posture reasonable estimates of pleural pressure can be obtained by measuring the pressure in a lax, thin-walled balloon placed in the lower oesophagus. By relating this pressure to the pressure outside the thorax it is possible to derive the pressure difference which affects the volume of the thorax; this enables chest wall compliance to be calculated.

Obviously, the difference in pressure must be measured at a time when there is no respiratory muscle activity for this will affect the position of the chest wall. Although it is possible to make measurements of chest wall compliance in subjects who have been trained to relax their respiratory muscles, more satisfactory measurements are obtained when the respiratory muscles are paralysed. Under these circumstances the pressure difference between the alveoli and the atmosphere (i.e. the inflation pressure) can be related to the volume change to enable total thoracic compliance to be calculated.

Resistance

The second factor opposing respiratory movement, the non-elastic resistance, has two components, the resistance to gas flow along the airways and the viscous resistance resulting from the deformation of the tissues. Both of these are related to the rate of change of volume or flow rate. The viscous resistance of the tissues is usually between 20–40% of total resistance in normal subjects and is not commonly affected by disease processes. It will therefore not be considered further (Marshall and Dubois, 1956a, b). The frictional resistance to gas flow is defined by the instantaneous gas flow rate and the pressure difference between the mouth and alveoli:

$$\frac{\text{airway resistance}}{(cmH_2O/(L/s))} = \frac{\text{pressure difference } (cmH_2O)}{\text{flow rate } (L/s)}$$

(for SI units: cmH_2O becomes kPa)

Flow rate and mouth pressure can be measured directly but alveolar pressure has to be derived by an indirect method (p. 262; pp. 264–7).

The definition of airway resistance assumes that gas flow through the airways is laminar and obeys Poiseuille's law and that the diameter (and hence, resistance) of the airways does not change with the change in lung volume. As will be seen later neither of these assumptions is strictly true, but the definition provides a useful basis for an understanding of respiratory mechanics.

STATIC PROPERTIES

Lungs. The retractive forces which tend to cause collapse of the lung are the elasticity of the lung parenchyma and the liquid-gas interface in the alveolus. In the normal lung the surface tension forces generated at this interface are minimised by the presence of a complex lipo-protein known as surfactant: as a result the contribution of each component to the total retractive force is approximately the same.

When the lungs are removed from the thorax they contract to a volume which is well below the residual volume (i.e. the volume reached after a maximal expiration with the chest intact). A transpulmonary pressure gradient of $2–3\,cmH_2O$ ($0.2–0.3\,kPa$) must therefore exist at the residual volume to maintain the lungs at this degree of expansion. To expand the lungs to the normal resting expiratory position (functional residual capacity or FRC) this gradient must be increased (Figs. 21.2 and 21.3). Over most of the range

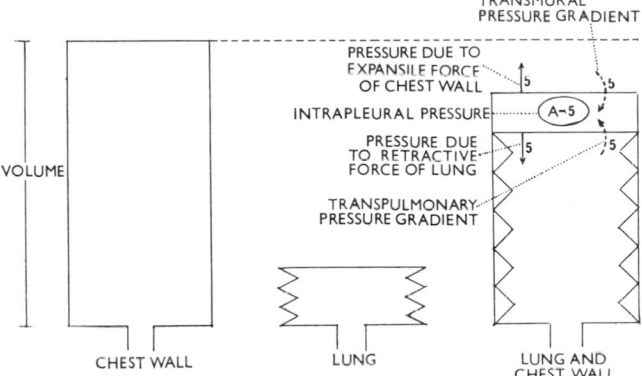

Fig. 21.2 Pressure gradients across lung and chest wall at the resting expiratory position (FRC). The resting position of the isolated lung and chest wall are also shown. Pressures in cmH_2O. A = atmospheric pressure, so that $A - 5 = 5\,cmH_2O$ below atmospheric pressure.

of lung expansion encountered in the intact chest the volume increment which results from unit pressure change across the lung (i.e. the compliance) is constant and equal to about $0.2\,L/cmH_2O$ ($2\,L/kPa$). However, at the upper limit of chest expansion smaller volume changes result from given increments of pressure. This reduction in lung compliance governs the upper limit of the vital capacity in the normal person.

Airways. The distal airways form an integral part of the lung structure and expand, both in length and diameter, in proportion to the rest of the lung parenchyma.

Chest Wall. The mobile portions of the chest wall are

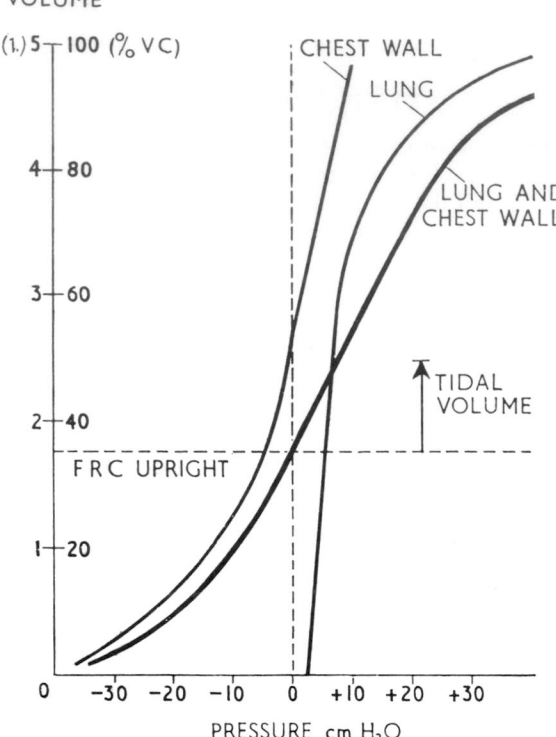

VOLUME

Fig. 21.3 Pressure-volume diagram of lungs, chest wall and lung-chest wall combination in erect position. A transpulmonary pressure gradient of 5 cmH$_2$O is required to inflate the lung to the resting expiratory level (FRC). This is balanced by an equal and opposite pressure gradient across the chest wall. The transthoracic pressure gradient at this point is zero. As the chest is expanded the transpulmonary and transthoracic gradients increase whilst the gradient across the chest wall decreases towards zero, reaches zero at its own resting expiratory position and then increases. (10 cmH$_2$O is approx. 1 kPa)

the rib cage and diaphragm. Throughout most of the range of chest movement in the upright position the compliance of the chest wall is constant and approximately equal to that of the lungs, i.e. 0.2 L/cmH$_2$O (2 L/kPa). However, below the normal end-expiratory position the pressure volume plot becomes curved, smaller changes in volume resulting from unit changes of pressure. It is this factor which largely governs the volume of air left in the lungs of a normal patient after a maximal expiration.

In the mid-range of lung inflation the pressure/ volume relationships of the lung and chest wall are reasonably linear and of approximately equal magnitude. To expand the thorax by 0.2 L it is necessary to apply a pressure gradient of 1 cmH$_2$O (0.1 kPa) across the lung and 1 cmH$_2$O (0.1 kPa) across the chest wall. The compliance of the thorax is therefore

$$\frac{0.2}{1+1} = 0.1 \text{ L/cmH}_2\text{O} \quad \text{i.e.} \quad \frac{1}{C_T} = \frac{1}{C_{CW}} + \frac{1}{C_L}$$

where C_T = total thoracic compliance
C_{CW} = chest wall compliance
C_L = lung compliance

As already mentioned the pressure/volume relationships of lung and chest wall are not linear at the extremes of lung volume. This leads to non-linearity in the pressure/volume plot for the complete thorax (*see* Fig. 21.3). This is usually only of clinical importance when lung compliance is grossly reduced by disease. However, it does lead to difficulties when comparing compliance values obtained by different authors. For example, the value obtained at a pressure of 30 cmH$_2$O will be less than one obtained at 10 or 5 cmH$_2$O.

Factors Determining the Normal Resting Expiratory Position of the Thorax

Upright. From Fig. 21.3 it can be seen that at the normal resting expiratory position there is a transpulmonary pressure difference of 5 cmH$_2$O tending to hold the lung inflated. If the respiratory muscles are relaxed this must be balanced by an equal and opposite pressure difference across the chest wall. Since the chest wall compliance is 0.2 L/cmH$_2$O, it can be calculated that the chest wall must be 0.2 × 5 = 1.0 L below its own resting position when it is pulled inwards by the lungs. This is equivalent to a change of position from 55 to 35% of the vital capacity (VC). At the resting position, therefore, the intrapleural pressure is 5 cmH$_2$O below atmospheric pressure and there are opposing pressure differences of 5 cmH$_2$O maintaining the balance between the retractive force of the lung and the expansile force of the chest wall.

Since the resting expiratory position is determined by the point at which the opposing pressure gradients across the lungs and chest wall are in balance, it follows that any alteration in compliance of either lungs or chest wall will alter the resting expiratory position. Thus as lung compliance is reduced, for example by atelectasis, the pressure gradient required to maintain a given lung volume will be increased. The point of balance will therefore only be achieved at a lower lung volume: this will predispose to further atelectasis. On the other hand, if lung compliance is increased, as in emphysema or old age, the lung retractive force will be decreased and the resting expiratory level will be greater than normal.

Supine. In the upright position the chest is relatively little affected by the weight of the abdominal contents or chest wall. However, as the subject changes to a more recumbent position the effects of gravity on the abdomen and chest wall become more important.

The major effects are due to the pressure exerted by the abdominal contents on the diaphragm. At the end of expiration there is negligible electrical activity in the muscle of the diaphragm and its position is determined by the pressure gradient between the abdominal and pleural cavities. Mechanically, the abdomen behaves like a bag containing fluid and, in the upright position, there is a gradient of pressure from the top to the bottom of the abdomen. The level at which this pressure equals atmospheric depends on the equilibrium between the elastic forces of the abdominal wall and thorax, and the gravitational force of the abdominal contents. At the resting end-expiratory position in the standing posture the zero point lies about 4 cm below the dome of the diaphragm, thus maintaining the sub-atmospheric intrapleural pressure. When the subject is supine the zero level corresponds with the ventral wall of the abdomen. The weight of the abdominal contents thus supplements the retractive force of the lung and the diaphragm rises into the chest. The final point of balance is then determined by the elasticity of the diaphragm itself. In the prone position the zero pressure point corresponds with the dorsal abdominal wall whilst in the lateral position it is mid-way between the two sides. These changes in the gravitational effects of the abdominal contents are chiefly responsible for the alterations in functional residual capacity with posture (Figs. 21.3, 21.4 and 21.5). Further changes may be introduced by alterations in intra-abdominal pressure due to air, fluid, tumour or external pressure.

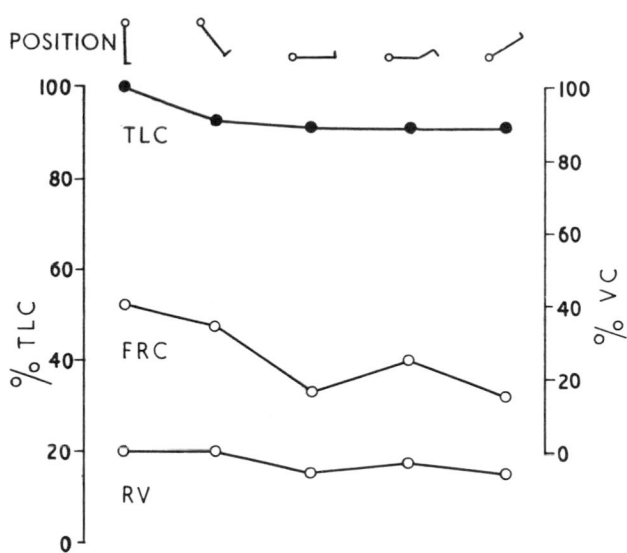

Fig. 21.5 Alterations in total lung capacity (TLC), vital capacity (VC), functional residual capacity (FRC) and residual volume (RV) with posture. Data from Agostoni and Mead (1964).

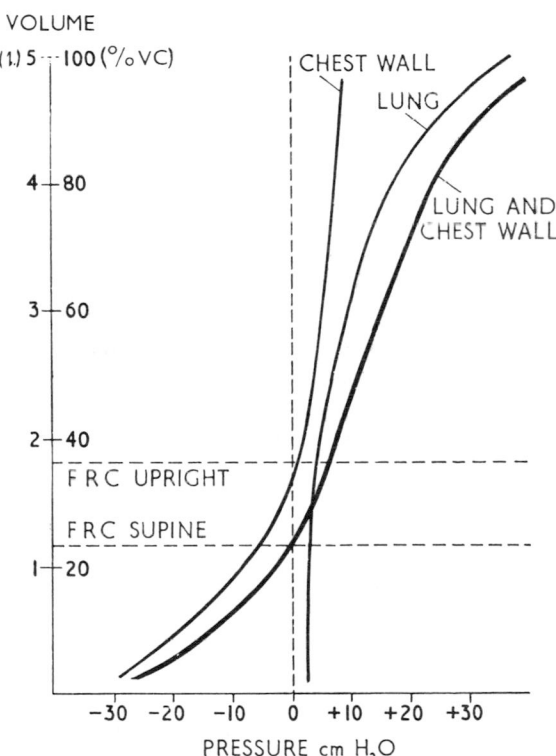

Fig. 21.4 Pressure-volume diagram of lungs, chest wall and lung-chest wall combination in supine position. The weight of the abdominal contents causes a shift of the chest wall pressure-volume plot and a reduction in FRC. (10 cmH$_2$O is approx. 1 kPa)

Differences in Pressure During Inflation of the Lungs

Since the full significance of a pressure/volume diagram is often difficult to comprehend a further diagram (Fig. 21.6) has been included to illustrate the changes in pressure gradient during inflation of the lungs.

Figure 21.6d illustrates the resting expiratory position of the lung-chest wall combination. To hold the lung expanded at this volume a pressure difference of 5 cmH$_2$O across the lung is required. The retractive force generated by the lung is balanced by the expansile force generated by the elasticity of the chest wall when this is below its own normal resting level. The pressure difference across the chest wall is therefore 5 cmH$_2$O and the intrapleural pressure is 5 cmH$_2$O below atmospheric pressure. If the compliance of the chest wall is 0.1 L/cmH$_2$O (as it may be in the supine position) the thoracic cage will occupy a position which is 500 ml below its own natural position.

When inspiration occurs the inspiratory muscles exert a force on the chest wall which then expands. After 250 ml of air have been drawn into the lungs (Fig. 21.6c) the transpulmonary pressure difference must have increased by 250/100 = 2.5 cmH$_2$O. The total pressure difference therefore equals 7.5 cmH$_2$O and the intrapleural pressure must be 7.5 cmH$_2$O below atmospheric. Since the chest wall is now only 250 ml below its own resting volume the pressure difference across the chest wall must be reduced to 2.5 cmH$_2$O. The inspiratory muscles must therefore be exerting a force equivalent to a pressure gradient of 7.5 − 2.5 = 5 cmH$_2$O.

When 500 ml of air has been drawn into the chest

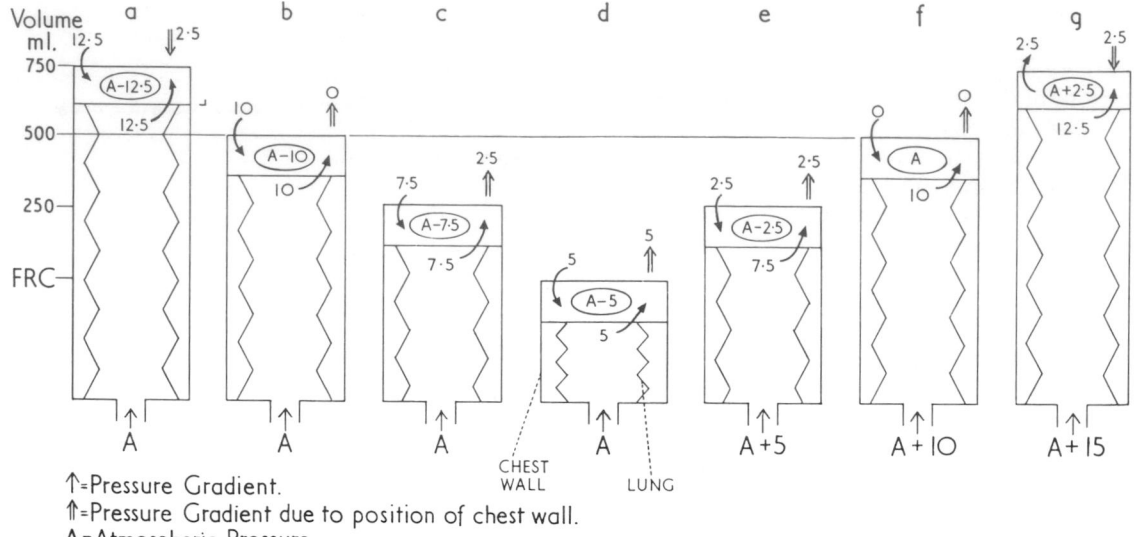

↑=Pressure Gradient.
⇑=Pressure Gradient due to position of chest wall.
A=Atmospheric Pressure.

Fig. 21.6 Pressure gradients during expansion of the thorax with spontaneous ventilation (a, b and c), at FRC (d) and during IPPV (e, f and g). Lung compliance and chest wall compliance assumed to equal 0.1 L cmH₂O. (10 cmH₂O is approx. 1 kPa).

(Fig. 21.6b) the transpulmonary pressure difference must be $5 + 500/100 = 10 \, cmH_2O$. At this degree of expansion the chest wall is at its normal resting position. All the inspiratory muscle force (equivalent to $10 \, cmH_2O$) must therefore be exerted against the lung. When the chest is inflated to volumes above this level, however, the inflating force must distend both lung and chest wall. For example, at a tidal volume of 750 ml (Fig. 21.6a) the transpulmonary gradient is $5 + 750/100 = 12.5 \, cmH_2O$ and the pressure difference across the chest wall is $-250/100 = -2.5 \, cmH_2O$. The force produced by the inspiratory muscles must therefore be equivalent to a total pressure difference of $15 \, cmH_2O$.

Similar considerations apply to the use of positive pressure ventilation (Figs. 21.6e, f and g). However, since the pressure inside the alveoli now becomes positive with respect to atmospheric, the intrapleural pressure becomes less negative with inspiration, then equals atmospheric and finally becomes positive with respect to atmospheric.

Airway Closure

So far it has been assumed that the intrapleural pressure is the same throughout the pleural cavity. However, it is now known that there is a gradient of pressure from the top to the bottom of the pleural space (Daly and Bondurant, 1963). This fact is of great importance for it not only determines the variation in alveolar size from the top to the bottom of the lung (Glazier et al., 1966) but also affects the regional distribution of ventilation and blood flow (Milic-Emili et al., 1966; Kaneko et al., 1966). Of greater importance to the anaesthetist is the recognition that this

gradient of pleural pressure may lead to airway closure and alveolar collapse in the dependent zones of the lung (Rehder et al., 1977a).

The cause of the gradient is still not clear (Agostoni, 1977). Originally it was postulated that the lung behaved as a bag with semi-fluid contents. The effect of gravity would have caused the lung to bulge outwards at the bottom and inwards at the top thus creating a greater subatmospheric pressure in the upper parts of the pleural space than in the dependent parts. Since the density of the lung is about a quarter of that of water the difference in pressure between the top and bottom of the pleural space of a lung 30 cm high would have been $30/4 = 7.5 \, cmH_2O$. (0.75 kPa). This agreed with observed values. However, it is now believed that the gradient of pressure is created by regional differences in the geometry of the lungs and chest wall which are produced by the effects of gravity on these structures. Whatever the cause, pleural pressure appears to be less subatmospheric in the dependent zones of the lung when the patient breathes spontaneously in the supine, lateral, prone or head-down position.

Reference to the pressure-volume curve of the lung shown in Fig. 21.7 illustrates the effects of this difference in pleural pressure on regional lung volume and ventilation. At FRC the alveoli and airways in the non-dependent zones of the lung will be exposed to a transpulmonary pressure difference of $+10 \, cmH_2O$ (1 kPa) and so will be expanded to about 70% of the volume they would occupy when the lung is fully expanded to the total lung capacity (TLC); alveoli and airways in the dependent zones will be exposed to a transpulmonary pressure difference of only $2.5 \, cmH_2O$ (0.25 kPa) and so will have a smaller rest-

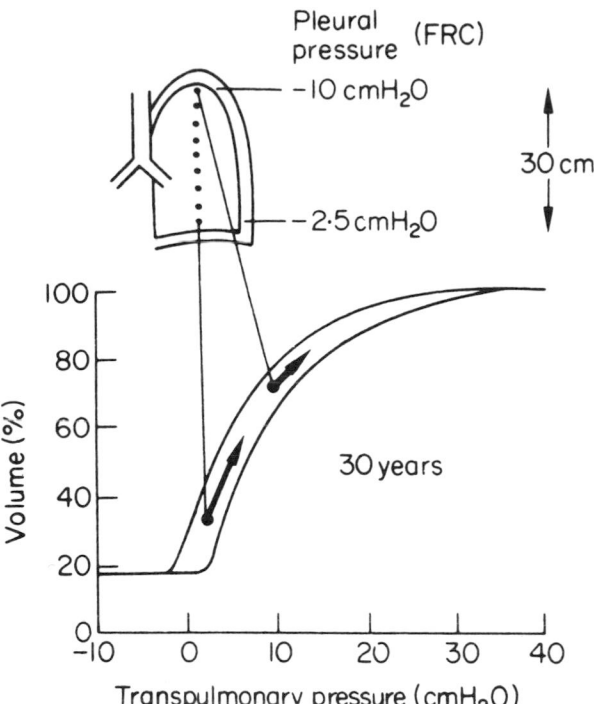

Fig. 21.7 Pressure-volume diagram of the lung to illustrate how regional differences in transpulmonary pressure influence regional lung volume and regional distribution of ventilation during spontaneous respiration. (10 cmH$_2$O is approx. 1 kPa).

ing volume. During inspiration the pleural pressure in both zones becomes more subatmospheric. Because of their position on the steep part of the pressure-volume curve the dependent alveoli will receive more ventilation than those in the non-dependent zones. This mechanism explains why ventilation tends to be greater in the dependent lung zones in the erect position and in the dependent lung in the lateral position when the patient breathes spontaneously from FRC.

When the patient breathes out towards residual volume the pleural pressures become less subatmospheric. Eventually a point will be reached at which the pleural pressure over the dependent lung zones approaches, or even exceeds atmospheric. There will be no distending pressure across the walls of the smaller airways and they will close. When the patient inspires from this lung volume gas will initially be directed towards the upper alveoli but when the dependent airways open the greater part of the ventilation will once again be directed to the dependent zones. The presence of airway closure in the dependent zones of the lung may thus modify the normal pattern of distribution of ventilation.

It has already been pointed out that the subatmospheric pleural pressure is generated by the elastic recoil of the lung. The elastic recoil of the lung is at a maximum in young adults and gradually decreases with increasing age. This produces two effects: it in-

creases FRC and decreases the pressure difference tending to hold the airways open. As a result airways close at progressively higher lung volumes as the patient ages (Leblanc et al., 1970). Since the lung volume at which airways close (the 'closing volume') increases more rapidly with age than FRC, a point is reached at which closing volume exceeds FRC. This usually occurs at about the age of 65 years in the erect patient with normal lungs. Since FRC is reduced in the supine position pleural pressure becomes less subatmospheric. Although the difference in pleural pressure between the dependent and non-dependent parts of the lung is reduced (because the antero-posterior diameter of the chest is less than its height in the erect posture), most patients over the age of 45 years may be expected to have closed airways in this position. A further reduction in FRC occurs in the head down position thus causing airway closure to occur in the tidal volume range at an even earlier age (Craig et al., 1971a).

Elastic recoil is also low in young children and increases progressively throughout childhood. As a result closing volume often exceeds FRC in supine children under the age of six years (Mansell et al., 1972). Closing volume may also be increased in a number of pathological conditions which either narrow the small airways or make pleural pressure or the interstitial pressure surrounding the airways more positive. Thus closing volume is higher in smokers and chronic bronchitics than in normals. An acute increase in closing volume can also be produced by the rapid intravenous infusion of 2 L of crystalloid solution (Muir et al., 1975).

The change in the relationship between closing volume and FRC suggests that patients may be divided into three broad categories. First, those with a closing volume below the FRC; these would not be expected to show any abnormality of gas exchange. A second group would include those whose airways were all open in the inspiratory position but who developed dependent zone airway closure during expiration. These patients would tend to have regional underventilation in dependent lung zones and so might have a small reduction in arterial P_{O_2}. The third group would have closed airways in dependent zones throughout the respiratory cycle and would therefore be expected to develop atelectasis and an intrapulmonary shunt (Craig et al., 1971b). Some support for these views is provided by the correlation between arterial P_{O_2} values and the relationships between closing volume and FRC from infancy to old age (Mansell et al., 1972). Thus, arterial P_{O_2} is about 70 mmHg at 1 week, 85 mmHg from 1–10 months, 90 mmHg at 4–8 years, 97 mmHg from 12–20 years and then declines to 80 mmHg at the age of 60 years. However, there are several factors which may modify the deleterious effects of airway closure on gas exchange. Probably the most important factor is that there are collateral channels between contiguous alveoli, alveolar ducts and terminal bronchioles. Collateral ventilation appears to be greatest in the very young and the very old and may prevent atelectasis in zones where airway closure occurs (Menkes and Traystman, 1977). A second factor is that blood flow in zones supplied by closed airways may be reduced by a parallel reduction in the diameter of extra-alveolar vessels and by hypoxic pulmonary vasoconstriction. Thirdly, there is little absolute proof that complete airway closure actually occurs (Rehder et al., 1977a).

Effect of Anaesthesia on Airway Closure

Bergman (1963) and later Laws (1968) demonstrated that the induction of anaesthesia was associated with a reduction in FRC. However, the magnitude of this change is variable. Don et al., (1970) originally claimed that the reduction in FRC was greater in short, fat patients than in their leaner colleagues. This observation correlated well with the greater reduction in lung compliance on induction of anaesthesia observed by Gold and Helrich (1965a). However, Hewlett et al., (1974a, b) have failed to substantiate this correlation. In their studies the reduction in FRC appeared to be somewhat greater in elderly patients but the scatter was wide. For many years it was believed that the reduction in FRC due to the assumption of the supine posture and induction of anaesthesia caused an increase in the number of closed airways and so accounted for the increase in alveolar-arterial P_{O_2} difference observed during surgery (Hickey et al., 1973; Weenig et al., 1974). This argument was based on the supposition that the lung volume at which airway closure occurred remained constant (Fig. 21.8). However, Westbrook et al., (1973) have clearly demonstrated that the reduction in FRC is associated with an increase in lung elastic recoil pressure. This must have caused pleural pressure to become more subatmospheric and so should have increased the distending pressure across the airways. The concept of an unchanged closing volume after induction of anaesthesia was subsequently challenged by Juno et al., (1978) who demonstrated that closing volume decreases *more* than FRC in those patients whose closing volume exceeded the FRC in the awake state. Thus anaesthesia should have increased the arterial P_{O_2}.

Effect of Anaesthesia on Gas Exchange

The concept that the increase in alveolar-arterial P_{O_2} difference during anaesthesia is due to an altered relationship between FRC and closing volume is now being questioned (Rehder et al., 1977a; Jones, 1987). It appears that anaesthesia with volatile agents, with or without muscle paralysis, may reduce FRC by producing an increase in thoraco-abdominal blood volume with a variable effect on the rib cage and diaphragm resulting from reduced ventilatory muscle tone. In contrast, anaesthesia with methohexitone or ketamine may preserve chest wall muscle tone and so may reduce the effects of the changes in blood volume on FRC.

Recent studies using CT scanning have shown that the dependent lung zones tend to collapse within a few minutes of induction of anaesthesia and that this collapse persists into the postoperative period. The collapse occurs with both spontaneous and controlled ventilation, though the shunt tends to be greater during muscle paralysis. The collapsed areas can often be re-expanded by rotating the patient so that these zones are placed in a non-dependent position. The collapsed areas can also be re-expanded by the application of PEEP, though the increase in shunt may not be completely reversed (Brismar et al., 1985; Hedenstierna et al., 1986; Tokics et al., 1987).

Although the dependent zone collapse explains the observed increase in shunt it is still not clear whether the collapse results from the decrease in FRC or whether the collapse is due to some other mechanism, the reduction in FRC then following as a consequence of the collapse.

Effect of Chest Wall Mechanics on Distribution of Ventilation in the Anaesthetized-Paralysed State

In the supine position the abdominal contents exert a lateral pressure which tends to push the diaphragm up into the chest. During spontaneous ventilation in the conscious state this pressure is opposed by the diaphragm, the dependent areas moving more than the anterior portions of the muscle. When anaesthesia with spontaneous respiration is established the diaphragm moves up into the chest (as would be expected from the reduction in FRC) but the largest excursion is still in the dependent portion of the muscle. How-

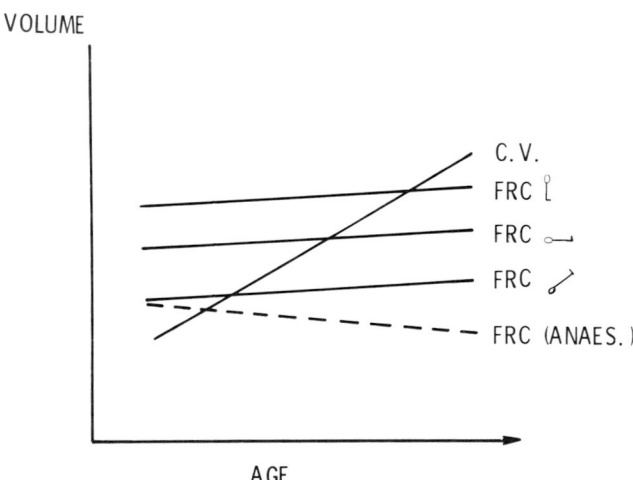

Fig. 21.8 Relation of closing volume (CV) and functional residual capacity (FRC) to age. The increase in FRC with age is much less than the increase in CV. FRC is lower in the supine (⌣) or head down (↗) position than in the erect position (P). It is further reduced by anaesthesia FRC (ANAES).

ever, when muscle paralysis is induced the amplitude of movement is reduced in the dependent zone and increased in the non-dependent zone. Similar changes occur in the lateral position (Froese and Bryan, 1974). These changes indicate that the hydrostatic pressure generated by the abdominal contents has a major influence on regional distribution in the supine position. By using large tidal volumes the ventilation can be rendered more uniform. This effect is probably due to the fact that the non-dependent alveoli are expanded onto the more horizontal portion of the pressure-volume curve at the height of inspiration: this forces more ventilation into the more compliant alveoli in the lower part of the lungs. However, this simplified description is modified by a number of other factors. Readers wishing to study the subject further should study the series of papers from the workers at the Mayo clinic (Landmark et al., 1977; Rehder et al., 1977b).

DYNAMIC PROPERTIES

Airway Resistance

Resistance to airflow normally accounts for 60–70% of the total non-elastic resistance of the lungs. It depends on the characteristics of the airway and the rate and pattern of airflow. There are three main patterns of airflow.

Laminar flow occurs when the gas passes down parallel-sided tubes at less than a certain critical velocity. With laminar flow the pressure drop down the tube is proportional to the flow rate and may be calculated from the equation derived by Poiseuille:

$$P = \frac{\dot{V} \times 8\, l \times \mu}{\pi r^4 \times 980}\ (\text{cgs})$$

$$P = \frac{\dot{V} \times 8\, l \times \mu}{\pi r^4} \times 10^{-3}\ (\text{SI})$$

where P = pressure drop (cgs) cmH$_2$O (SI) Pa
$\dot{V}$ = volume flow rate   cm^3/s   m^{3}s^{-1}
l = length of tube   cm   m
r = radius of tube   cm   m
μ = viscosity   poise   Pa · s

When flow exceeds the critical velocity it becomes turbulent. The flow at which this occurs may be calculated by determining Reynold's number (Re) from the equation:

$$Re = \frac{2\sigma \dot{V}}{\pi r \mu}$$

where σ is the density of the gas.

Turbulent flow occurs when Re exceeds 2000. However this type of calculation can only be applied to smooth tubes with parallel sides. Small variations in the diameter of the lumen or branching often cause turbulence in airways at much lower flow rates than would be expected from theoretical calculations.

The significant feature of turbulent flow is that the pressure drop along the airway is no longer *directly proportional to flow rate* but is proportional to the *square of flow rate* according to the equation:

$$P = \frac{\dot{V}^2 f l}{4\pi^2 r^5}$$

where f is a friction factor which depends on the roughness of the tube wall and on Reynold's number.

A third type of flow (*orifice* flow) occurs at constrictions such as the larynx. In these situations the pressure drop is also proportional to the square of flow rate but density replaces viscosity as the important factor in the numerator. This explains why a low density gas such as helium diminishes the resistance in severe obstructions to the upper airway.

At FRC the total resistance of the airways is normally 0.5–2 cmH$_2$O/L/s, i.e. 0.05–0.2 kPa·L^{-1}·s. However, since the airways expand and contract in parallel with the lungs and since resistance is greatly affected by both the radius and length of the airways, airway resistance changes with lung volume. This relationship is hyperbolic (i.e. airway resistance is very sensitive to small changes in lung volume below FRC) (Fig. 21.9a): however, if the reciprocal of resistance

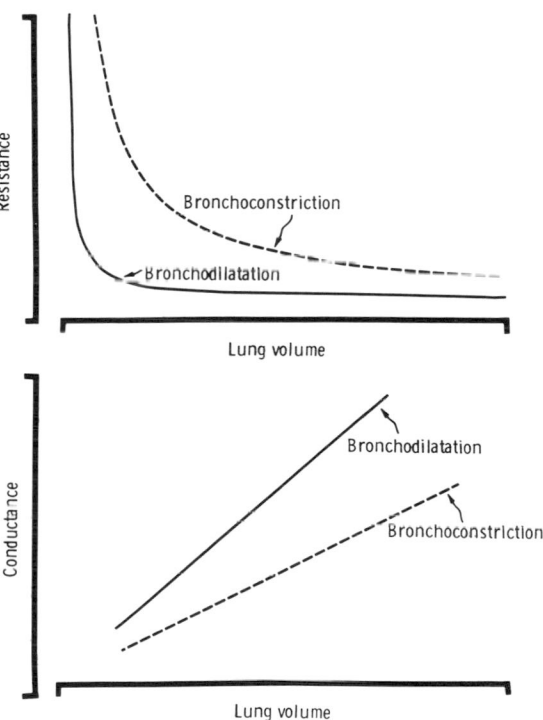

Fig 21.9 (a) Hyperbolic relationship between airways resistance and lung volume. (b) Relationship between conductance (reciprocal of resistance) and lung volume. The slope of this line is specific conductance, a measure which is independent of lung volume. Changes in airways calibre can be measured by determining specific conductance at a number of lung volumes and then comparing the slopes.

(conductance) is plotted against lung volume a straight line results (Fig. 21.9b). The slope of this line is known as specific conductance. Changes in the slope of this line provide a useful means of measuring changes in the calibre of the airways without having to know absolute values of lung volume (Lehane et al., 1980).

About half of the total airway resistance is situated in the naso-pharynx and larynx and about half in the trachea and smaller airways. Surprisingly, the very small airways (less than 2 mm in diameter) only contribute about 0.5 cmH$_2$O/L/s (0.05 kPa $\cdot$ L^{-1} $\cdot$ s) to the total airway resistance. This is because the total cross-sectional area of the terminal airways is much larger than the cross-sectional area of the trachea or medium-sized bronchi so that the velocity of airflow is greatly reduced. Thus, the early pathological changes of smoking and bronchitis, which affect these airways, do not affect airway resistance and are best detected by the measurement of frequency-dependence of compliance.

To sum up: The pressure gradients developed during inflation and deflation of the thorax overcome two types of resistance—elastic and non-elastic. The pressure gradient required to overcome the elastic resistance is proportional to the change in lung volume and may be plotted if the compliance and change in volume are known (Fig. 21.10). The remainder of the pressure gradient overcomes non-elastic resistance. The energy used in overcoming non-elastic resistance is roughly proportional to flow rate during most of the respiratory cycle.

Dynamic Compliance: Time Constants

Static compliance is normally measured during a breath-hold so that complete equilibrium is achieved between alveolar pressure and mouth pressure: this ensures that all the alveoli are filled to a volume which is determined by their regional compliance. However, in clinical practice more information can be gained by measuring compliance during respiration at normal breathing frequencies (Fig. 21.10). This yields a value termed dynamic compliance. If airway resistance is low, so that all the alveoli have reached full pressure equilibrium with the applied pressure at the end of inspiration, dynamic compliance should approximate to static compliance. In patients with lung disease (in which there are regional variations in compliance and airway resistance) alveolar filling may not be completed within the inspiration period so that dynamic compliance may be much less than static compliance. This discrepancy is increased as respiratory frequency is increased so leading to the phenomenon of frequency-dependent compliance (Otis et al., 1956).

The factors affecting the rate of alveolar filling are best understood by considering the pattern of filling in response to the application of a step increase pressure at the mouth. At the moment that this pressure is applied the pressure gradient down the airways is

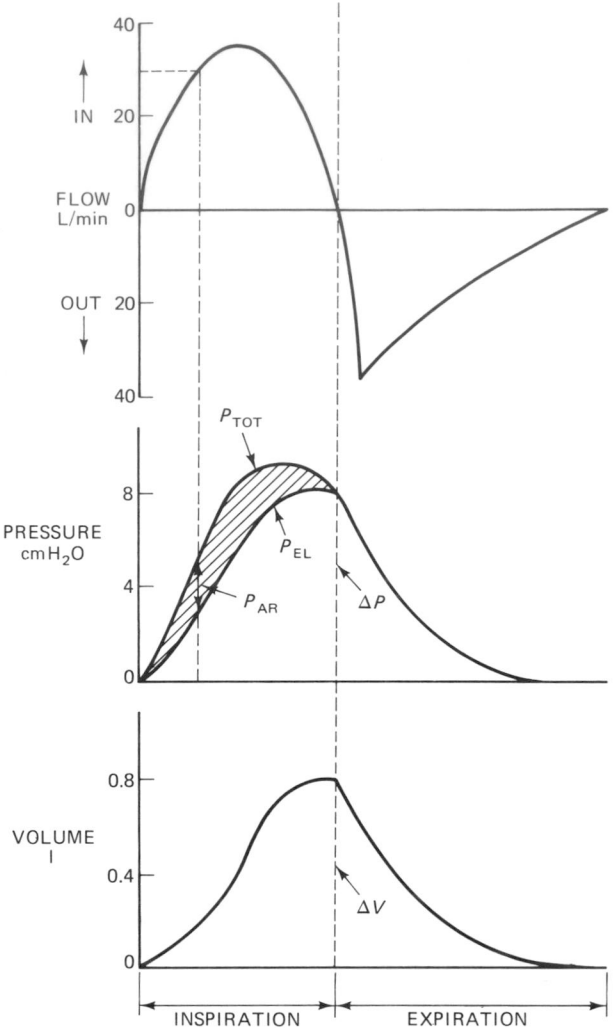

Fig. 21.10 Inspiratory and expiratory flow rate, transpulmonary pressure and volume in lung during one respiratory cycle. Dynamic compliance is measured by relating ΔV to ΔP at the point of inspiratory-expiratory flow reversal since airway resistance is zero when flow is zero and all the pressure gradient is exerted against the elastic component. The line (P_{EL}) shows the proportion of the total inflation pressure (P_{TOT}) which overcomes the elastic recoil during inflation. The remainder of the pressure gradient (shaded) shows the pressure which overcomes the non-elastic component (P_{AR}). By relating the latter to the flowrate non-elastic resistance is measured.

maximal. Flow is therefore also at a maximum (Fig. 21.11). As gas flows into the alveoli the alveolar pressure increases, so decreasing the pressure difference down the airways. This results in an exponential decrease in flow rate. The time taken for a given volume of air to flow down an airway will obviously vary with the pressure difference across the airway and with the airway resistance. If all the alveoli had the same compliance filling would therefore be completed most quickly in the alveoli which were supplied by airways with the lowest resistance. However, alveoli with a high compliance will accommodate a

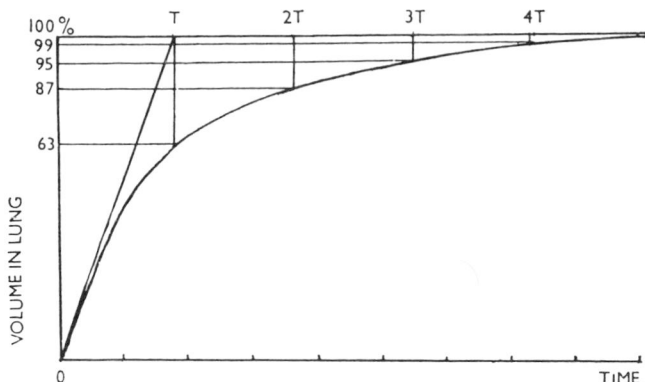

Fig. 21.11 Exponential pattern of filling of lung in response to constant applied pressure. The slight change in airway resistance during inspiration is ignored.

greater volume of gas than low compliance alveoli when exposed to the same applied pressure. Thus, if the airway resistance of all the airways was similar, areas of lung with a high compliance would take longer to fill than areas with a low compliance. Both airway resistance and compliance therefore affect the rate at which final equilibrium between alveolar pressure and mouth pressure is attained. Since the pattern of filling is approximately exponential, the rate of filling can be defined by the time constant (T) which can be calculated from the product of airway resistance (R) and compliance (C). Thus for the whole lung:

$$T = C \times R$$
$$= 0.1 \, \text{L/cmH}_2\text{O} \times 2 \, \text{cmH}_2\text{O/L/s}$$
$$= 0.2 \, \text{s}$$

From the characteristics of an exponential change one can conclude that the lung should achieve 95% of its final volume at $3T = 0.6 \, \text{s}$. Variations in regional time constants caused by lung disease will thus lead to incomplete filling of some alveolar units at normal breathing frequencies and to a difference between static and dynamic compliance. This difference will be minimised by prolonging the duration of inspiration and expiration.

THE MEASUREMENT OF THE MECHANICAL PROPERTIES OF THE LUNGS AND CHEST WALL

Before making any measurements of compliance the volume history of the lungs is standardized by asking the subject to make several maximal inspirations before making the relevant pressure and volume measurements at different lung volumes.

Static Compliance

In the patient who can breathe spontaneously static lung compliance is determined by recording the mouth to oesophageal pressure gradient while the patient holds his breath after inspiring a measured volume of gas from a spirometer. The measurement is repeated at a number of different volumes and the compliance is calculated from the slope of the pressure/volume plot so obtained. During the period of breath-holding the pressure gradient falls due to stress relaxation and to the displacement of blood from the lungs. The readings of pressure are accordingly taken after several seconds or when there is a satisfactory plateau. At this point airflow is zero so that mouth pressure may be taken to be equal to alveolar pressure.

Total thoracic compliance is more difficult to measure since it is difficult to eliminate inspiratory muscle tone in the conscious patient. Measurements have been made in trained subjects by recording the static pressures at the mouth after the subject has inspired various volumes from a spirometer and then relaxed against a shutter with an open glottis. However, the validity of the method is doubtful.

In the apnoeic or paralysed patient respiratory muscle tone is abolished. The measurement of lung, chest wall and total thoracic compliance is therefore easily achieved by measuring the appropriate pressure gradient when the lungs have been inflated to known volumes by the application of positive pressure to the mouth or subatmospheric pressure to the outside of the chest (tank ventilator). The lungs can either be inflated by pressure from a reservoir bag and the inflation pressure and expired volume recorded, or else a known volume of air can be insufflated from a large syringe and the pressure recorded after a fixed interval.

In the intensive care unit abnormalities of the pressure-volume curve may provide useful diagnostic information. Figure 21.12 shows an inflation-deflation curve obtained in an apnoeic patient by recording the airway pressure during the injection and withdrawal of 200 ml aliquots of O_2. It is apparent that in the patient with adult respiratory distress syndrome the initial inflation of the lung can only be achieved by

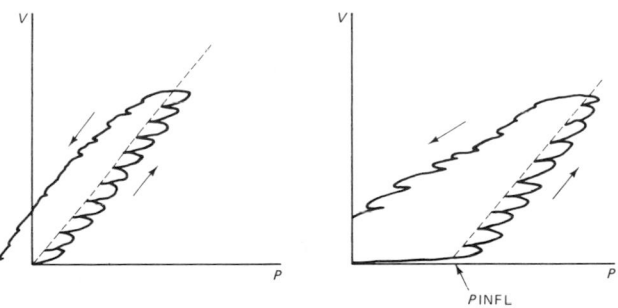

Fig. 21.12 Pressure-volume curves recorded by injecting aliquots of gas into the lungs from a syringe. *Left*: normal lungs. *Right*: Early adult respiratory distress syndrome. Pinfl is the inflection point where collapsed alveoli are re-expanded. The slope of the dotted lines represents the inspiratory static compliance.

applying a high airway pressure. A point is then reached at which each inflation results in a smaller increase in pressure, the slope of the P/V curve being similar to that of a normal lung, though at a higher transpulmonary pressure. The deflation limb shows that the lung remains at a higher lung volume for a given transpulmonary pressure (i.e. there is marked hysteresis). This type of curve is seen in the surfactant-deficient lung of the neonatal respiratory distress syndrome and in the early stages of the adult respiratory distress syndrome. It is believed that the inflection point represents the point at which collapsed alveoli re-open and it has therefore been suggested that optimal gas exchange may be obtained by setting the level of positive end-expiratory pressure to equal the pressure at the inflection point (Matamis et al., 1984). Whilst the syringe technique yields useful information the interpretation must take account of the O_2 consumption occurring during the manoeuvre (Gattinoni et al., 1987).

Dynamic Compliance

The dynamic compliance of the lungs is obtained by recording pressure, flow and volume traces during spontaneous ventilation (*see* Fig. 21.10). Flow is recorded by a pneumotachograph and the volume measured by integration of the flow rate or by a recording spirometer.

Compliance is measured by relating the inspired volume to the transpulmonary pressure gradient at the point of zero air flow at the height of inspiration. Since the intraoesophageal pressure is subject to interference from cardiac pulsations compliance is usually calculated over 6–10 cycles and the mean taken. During anaesthesia with controlled ventilation dynamic compliance can be measured by interposing an end-inspiratory pause of $>20\%$ of the inspiratory time (Fig. 21.13). During this zero flow interval the pressure at the mouth equilibrates with the alveolar pressure and so may be related to volume to give total thoracic compliance.

Dynamic compliance can also be obtained from a series of pressure-volume loops recorded on an oscilloscope or X-Y recorder (Fig. 21.14) or by a subtraction technique utilizing pressure flow-loops (Fig. 21.15).

Non-elastic Resistance

Since the dimensions of the airway vary with lung volume and since the proportions of turbulent and laminar flow vary with flow rate it is not possible to quote a value for non-elastic resistance which is applicable throughout the full range of lung volume. However, in most patients, non-elastic resistance is reasonably linear at flow rates up to $1.0\,L/s$ and therefore resistance values are usually quoted in $cmH_2O/L/s$ ($kPa/L^{-1}s$) as measured at a flow rate of $0.5\,L/s$.

When making this measurement the first require-

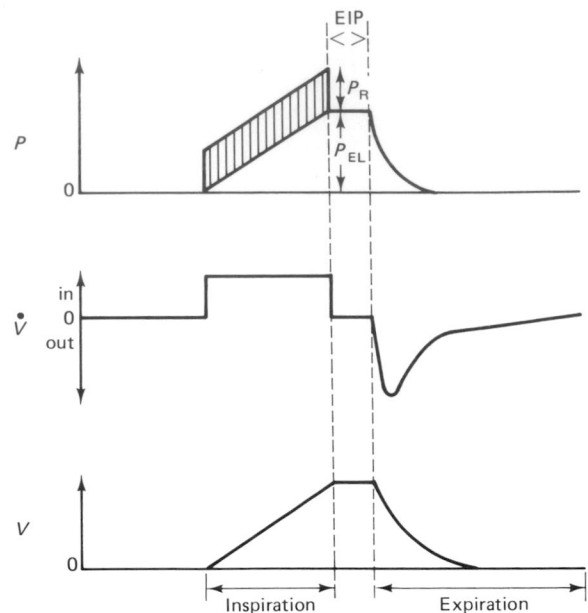

Fig. 21.13 Pressure (P), flow ($\dot V$) and volume (V) traces during constant flow ventilation of the lungs with an end-inspiratory pause (EIP). P_R, pressure difference between mouth and alveoli due to airway resistance. P_{EL}, elastic recoil pressure.

ment is to separate the pressure gradient exerted against elastic recoil from the total pressure gradient measured. This may be done in a number of ways.

Constant Flow Technique. One method which may be used during anaesthesia is to utilize a constant-flow ventilator with an end-inspiratory pause (*see* Fig. 21.13). The increase in pressure at the onset of

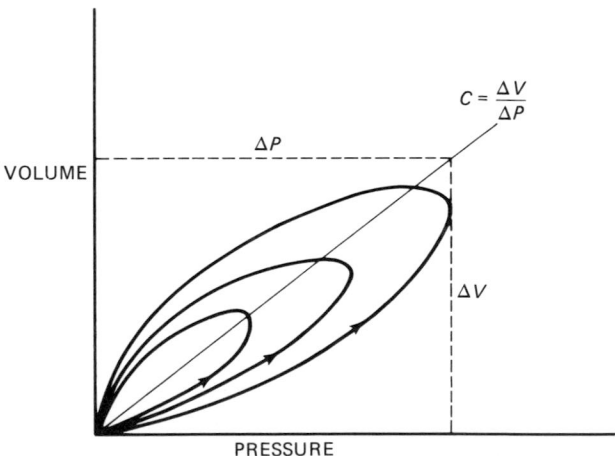

Fig. 21.14 Pressure-volume loops recorded during successive inspirations at increasing volumes. Compliance is calculated from the slope of the line joining the points of maximum volume. The deviation of the loop from the compliance line is due to the extra pressure required to overcome airway resistance during inspiration and expiration.

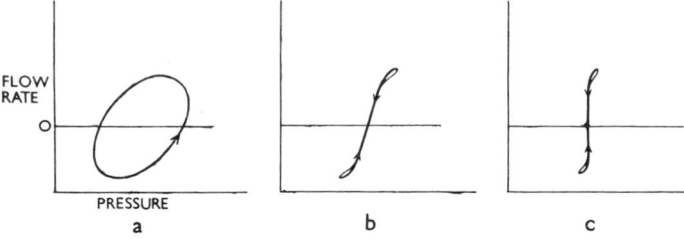

Fig. 21.15 Measurement of mechanics by subtraction method using pressure-flow loops. (a) Pressure-flow loop. (b) The same after the subtraction of increasing proportions of the volume signal from the pressure signal on the X-axis. When the loop becomes flattened to a straight line the only pressure signal displayed on the X-axis is that due to non-elastic resistance. Resistance can therefore be calculated from the relationship between pressure and flow. (c) A signal proportional to flow rate is now subtracted from the X-axis until the line becomes vertical, indicating that there is now no pressure signal on the X-axis. The reading on the potentiometer controlling the proportion of the volume signal subtracted in (b) can be calibrated to give a direct reading of compliance and the reading on the potentiometer controlling the proportion of the flow signal subtracted in (c) can be calibrated to give a direct reading of resistance (Reproduced with permission from Miller and Simmons, 1960).

flow or the decrease in pressure at the cessation of flow can then be related to the flow rate to give a measure of airway resistance (Don and Robson, 1965).

Subtraction Technique. A more sophisticated technique utilizes recordings of pressure, flow and volume during spontaneous or controlled ventilation (*see* Fig. 21.10). Compliance is first calculated from the relation of volume and pressure at the point of zero air flow at the height of inspiration. A suitable point during inspiration is then selected (e.g. when flow rate equals 0.5 L/s) and the pressure gradient overcoming elastic recoil is calculated from the volume inspired and the compliance. By subtracting this pressure gradient from the total pressure at this point the pressure gradient overcoming non-elastic resistance can be calculated. This is then related to the air flow to give non-elastic resistance. The resistance value obtained depends on the gradient which is recorded. If the transpulmonary gradient is used the resistance measured will be airway resistance plus lung tissue resistance. If the transthoracic pressure gradient is recorded chest wall tissue resistance will be included.

The subtraction of elastic pressure from the total pressure gradient can also be accomplished electrically. A signal proportional to flow is displayed on the Y-axis of an oscilloscope and the total pressure gradient is displayed on the X-axis. A pressure-flow loop results (*see* Fig. 21.15). A signal proportional to volume is now subtracted from the pressure signal on the X-axis. The proportion of the volume signal which

is subtracted is then increased: this causes the pressure-flow loop to narrow until it finally becomes a straight line. At this point the only pressure signal left on the X-axis is that exerted against the non-elastic resistance so that the slope of the pressure-flow plot indicates the non-elastic resistance. By calibrating the potentiometers used in this device and carrying the subtraction technique one stage further it is possible to obtain direct readings of compliance and non-elastic resistance (Miller and Simmons, 1960).

Interrupter Technique. Another method of determining non-elastic resistance utilizes a shutter which rapidly interrupts the air flow at the mouth for periods of 0.1 s during spontaneous breathing. When this technique was originally proposed it was assumed that at the moment of interruption the airflow would be reduced to zero so that mouth pressure would equal alveolar pressure. By recording the flow rates and pressures before and after the interruption it was thought that a pressure-flow plot could be constructed which would yield a value for airway resistance. It is now known that the technique yields a value closer to total non-elastic resistance since a true equilibrium between mouth and alveolar pressure cannot be achieved when the lung is moving.

Passive Expiration Technique. When the chest is artificially inflated and then allowed to deflate passively it does so in an approximately exponential fashion (Bergman, 1969). If the time constant (T) of this curve is derived (*see* Fig. 21.11) and the static compliance (C) calculated from the initial inflation pressure and volume expired, resistance (R) can be calculated from the equation:

$$T = C \times R \quad \text{or} \quad R = \frac{T}{C}$$

Plethysmographic Technique. This is now the standard by which all the other methods are judged since it can provide a measure of thoracic gas volume; this enables specific conductance to be calculated. The subject sits in an airtight box of 600–700 L capacity, supports the cheeks with the hands and pants rapidly through a pneumotachograph which is calibrated to measure air flow in and out of the lungs. The panting maneouvre is used to minimize changes in the temperature and composition of the gas passing through the pneumotachograph during the measurements and to minimize the resistance of the glottis. Airway pressure can be measured close to the mouth and the airway can be occluded by a remotely controlled shutter.

There are basically two types of plethysmograph. In the volume-displacement type (Fig. 21.16a) the subject breathes air from the outside of the box and the volume changes of the thorax are recorded by a small spirometer or a pneumotachograph connected to the inside of the box (Mead, 1960). However, for measurements of airway resistance it is more practical

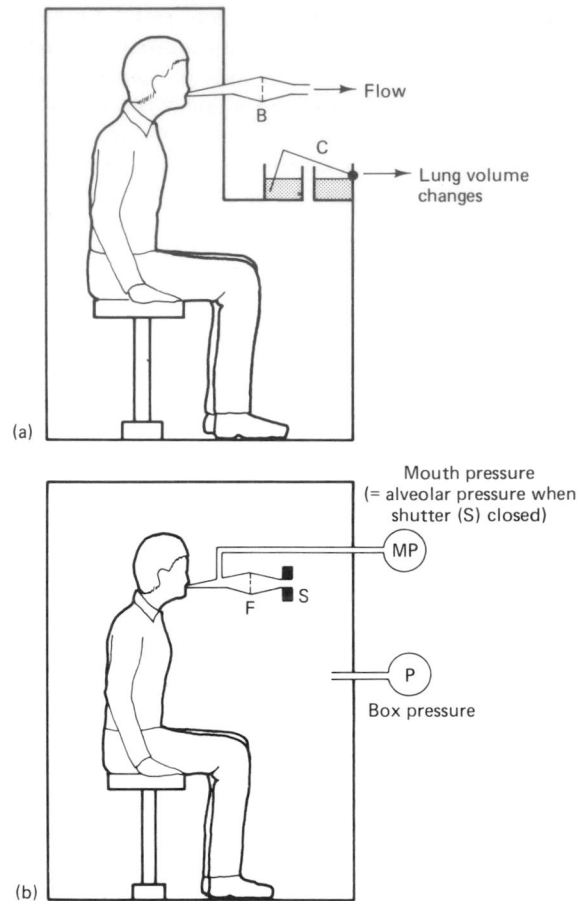

(a)

(b)

Fig. 21.16 (a) Constant-pressure body plethysmograph. Flow is measured by the pneumotachograph (B) and the change in volume by a small wedge spirometer (C). (b) Constant-volume body plethysmograph. The change in volume is obtained by measuring the change in pressure with the transducer (P). This is calibrated against a sinusoidal pump connected to the interior of the box. The second transducer (MP) measures mouth pressure, or alveolar pressure at the points of flow reversal when shutter (S) is closed. Flow is measured by the pneumotachograph (F).

to use the constant volume plethysmograph (Fig. 21.16b) in which the subject breathes air from within the box (DuBois et al., 1956a). When the subject breathes the volume of gas in the lung changes, not only because of the transfer of gas through the airways but also because there is a change in pressure in the alveoli due to the resistance of the airways. Since, the gas in the lungs has a constant temperature and humidity the change in volume is inversely proportional to the change in alveolar pressure. Furthermore, as the total volume of gas in the box and the patient is constant, any change in gas volume within the lungs will be reflected by a change in pressure within the box. Since the change in pressure within the box is very small (± 0.1 cmH$_2$O) it is necessary to use a very sensitive transducer with a high frequency re-

sponse. To measure airway resistance the subject first breathes through the pneumotachograph with the shutter open to establish the relationship between airflow and the pressure inside the box (P_{box}). This is recorded on an oscilloscope or X—Y recorder. The shutter is then closed whilst the subject continues to make breathing efforts and the relationship between mouth pressure and P_{box} is recorded. When the shutter is closed the pressure at the mouth equals alveolar pressure. Since the relationship of both alveolar pressure (P_{alv}) and airflow ($\dot{V}$) to P_{box} is now known, airway resistance (R) may be calculated:

$$R = \frac{P_{alv}}{\dot{V}} = \frac{P_{alv}/P_{box}}{\dot{V}/P_{box}}$$

To measure total thoracic gas volume (V) similar manoeuvres are employed, but in this case it is necessary to calibrate the change in box pressure in terms of volume (DuBois et al., 1956b). This is done by recording the change in P_{box} when known volumes of air are pumped in and out of the box whilst the subject is connected to the closed shutter. The volume of gas in the alveoli and airways can then be derived from the equation:

$$V = (BP - WVP) \cdot \frac{\Delta V}{\Delta P}$$

where (BP $-$ WVP) = barometric pressure $-$ water vapour pressure and ΔV and ΔP are the change in thoracic volume and change in mouth pressure during airway occlusion. The lung volume at which the panting maneouvre is performed can be related to the total lung capacity or residual volume by asking the subject to make a maximal inspiration or expiration and recording the change in volume with a pneumotachograph.

Forced Oscillation Technique. This is a useful non-invasive technique which may be used in conscious or anaesthetized subjects but requires a great deal of expertize to obtain reliable results (Lehane et al., 1979, 1980). The method is based on an electrical analogue of the respiratory system which assumes that the total impedance to an oscillating flow at the mouth is the sum of components due to compliance, resistance and inertance (DuBois et al., 1956c).

Because compliance is related to volume (the integral of flow) and inertia is related to acceleration (the differential of flow) the impedance values are opposite in sign, compliance contributing most of the impedance at low frequencies and inertia contributing most at high frequencies. At the resonant frequency of the respiratory system these two components exactly cancel each other out so that the difference in pressure at the mouth in response to the sinusoidal oscillation of flow is entirely due to the resistance of the airways and lung and chest wall tissue.

The flow oscillations (which have a volume of about ± 40 ml in an adult) are produced by a sine wave pump or loudspeaker and the resulting pressure and flow at the mouth are measured by a pressure transducer and a pneumotachograph and displayed on the X and Y axes of an oscilloscope. The frequency of oscillation is then adjusted until the pressure-flow loop approximates to a straight line (i.e. the phase difference between the pressure and flow is at a minimum, and resistance is then calculated from the peak-to-peak differences in pressure and flow (Fig. 21.17) (Fisher et al., 1968)). Various modifications of this technique have since been described (Goldman et al., 1970; Michaelson et al., 1975: Landser et al., 1976).

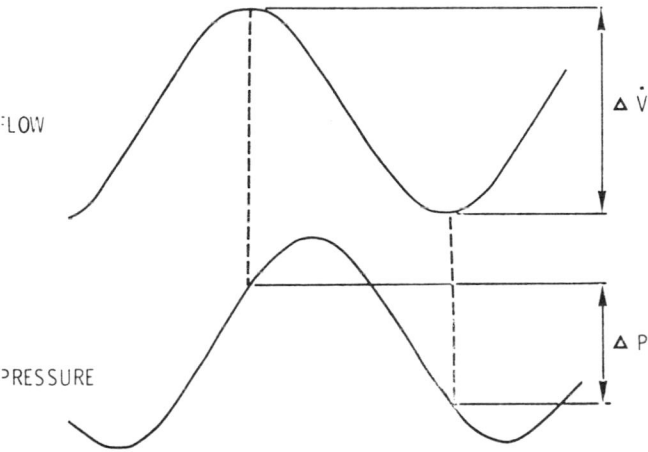

Fig. 21.17 Oscillation technique for measuring pulmonary resistance. The difference in pressure between the positive and negative peaks of flow is related to the peak flow rate.

Clinical Methods of Detecting Changes in Airway Resistance

Changes in airway resistance may be detected by measuring the air flow rate during a maximal inspiration or expiration. Since a maximal inspiratory effort is more difficult to achieve than a maximal expiration, the latter is most commonly used.

Peak Expiratory Flow Rate. Measurements made at the beginning of a maximal expiration (when the airways are maximally dilated) are very dependent on the patient's expiratory muscle power and are therefore less sensitive indices of airway obstruction than those obtained in the normal tidal volume range. Peak expiratory flow rate can be calculated from the slope of an expired volume/time plot recorded by a rapidly-responding spirometer or can be measured by a peak flow meter or peak flow gauge (Wright and McKerrow, 1959; Wright, 1974). The normal value is in the range 400–600 L/min for an average healthy adult.

Forced Expiratory Volume. The volume of air expired during 0.75 or 1.0 s ($FEV_{0.75}$ or FEV_1) is measured with a spirometer having minimal inertia. This measurement is best related to the forced vital capacity (FVC), more than 80% of the forced vital capacity being expired in 1.0 s if the airway resistance is normal.

Mid-Expiratory Flow Rate. Expiratory flow rate is usually very high at the commencement of expiration (when the bronchi are maximally dilated) and very slow at the end of expiration. A measurement of flow rate which ignores the first and last quarters of the expiration is therefore often used. Since this measurement covers the normal tidal volume range it is closely related to the actual changes in airway resistance experienced by the patient.

Constant Flow Techniques. These are illustrated by the method described by Don et al. (1965). Air is forced into the lungs at a constant, known rate for 0.75–1.0 s and the pressure at the mouth is recorded. The increase in pressure at the mouth when flow commences yields a value for airway resistance whilst the difference between the pressure before and after the lung inflation, together with the volume of gas insufflated into the lung, yields the static compliance (Fig. 21.13).

Exponential Methods. During anaesthesia similar measurements can be made by inflating the lung artificially and then allowing it to deflate naturally. It is found that the pattern of flow is roughly exponential. By utilizing the known properties of an exponential curve one can calculate various indices of airway resistance (Bergman, 1969).

FACTORS AFFECTING COMPLIANCE

The force required to extend a piece of elastic 10 cm long by 1 cm will be much greater than that required to extend a piece of similar elastic 100 cm long by the same amount. In other words the measure of elasticity used (in this case increase in length per unit of force) must be related to the initial length. In the same way compliance depends not only on the elasticity of the lung tissue but also on the initial volume of the lung before it is stretched. It is therefore necessary to determine whether an alteration in compliance represents a change in the elasticity of the lung tissue itself or whether it is due to a change in initial lung volume. Since lung compliance is related most closely to functional residual capacity (Marshall, 1957):

$$C_l (\text{L/cmH}_2\text{O}) = 0.05 \times \text{FRC (L)}$$

it has been proposed that the best method of eliminating the effects of a change in lung volume is to determine the specific compliance:

$$\text{Specific compliance} = \frac{C_L (\text{L/cmH}_2\text{O})}{\text{FRC (L)}} \text{ or } \frac{C_L (\text{LkPa}^{-1})}{\text{FRC (L)}}$$

The normal value is 0.05 L/cmH$_2$O/L, i.e. 0.5 LkPa^{-1}L, and the range is 0.038–0.070 L/cmH$_2$O/L, i.e. 0.38–0.70 LkPa^{-1}L.

This measure provides a useful method of comparing compliance in patients of different age and size. For example, although the compliance of the lungs of new-born babies of 3.5 kg body weight is approximately 5 ml/cmH$_2$O, this does not compare on a weight basis with adult values of compliance. However, the FRC of new-born infants is about 2½ times smaller than would be expected from adult values scaled down according to body weight. When specific compliance is calculated with an FRC value of 95 ml the result is 0.053 (L/cmH$_2$O)/L FRC, which is in agreement with the adult figures.

Age. Comparisons of compliance at different ages are rendered difficult by variations in the relationship of lung size to body size and by differences in the method of study. In general, the recoil pressure at 60% of the TLC increases from 4 cmH$_2$O at the age of 8 years to a maximum of 8 cmH$_2$O at the age of 14 years. Thereafter, it progressively declines to a value of 4 cmH$_2$O at the age of 60 years. Chest wall compliance is high in neonates and infants but the changes in later childhood have not been documented. A progressive increase in stiffness of the chest wall occurs in adult life.

Pathological Changes. The elastic recoil pressure of the lung is reduced in emphysema and asthma and lung volumes are generally increased (Gibson and Pride, 1976). The loss of functioning lung units produced by atelectasis, consolidation or lung resection results in a reduction in lung compliance. A variety of conditions associated with widespread alveolar fibrosis produce a reduction in TLC and compliance—the so called restrictive defect. Part of the reduction in compliance is due to a reduction in the number of functioning lung units but there also appears to be an increase in the 'stiffness' of the ventilated portions of lung. Pulmonary congestion or oedema may decrease the number of functioning lung units whilst the absence of surfactant in the respiratory distress syndrome of the newborn may greatly increase the static recoil pressure of the lung. Reductions in total thoracic compliance may also be seen when there is pleural thickening, pneumothorax or pleural fluid or when there is a reduction in chest wall compliance due to kyphoscoliosis, scleroderma or obesity.

Another important consideration in interpreting changes in compliance is the volume history of the lungs. Thus, if a lung is inflated with equal increments of volume and then deflated in a similar manner it is found that the pressure gradient generated by a given lung volume is less during deflation than inflation. This phenomenon is termed hysteresis or stress-relaxation and is attributed to the recruitment of additional alveoli during the expansion of the lung. Similarly it has been observed that compliance increases after hyperinflation of the lung and then gradually decreases when the original tidal volume is resumed.

Anaesthesia

Changes in total thoracic compliance associated with anaesthesia may be produced by changes in posture, by the effects of anaesthetic drugs, and by muscle paralysis and the use of intermittent positive pressure ventilation.

Posture. (Table 21.1). The effect of posture on FRC and the consequent reduction in compliance has already been mentioned. Lim and Luft (1959), for example, found that FRC decreased from about 3.7 to 2.5 L on changing from the erect standing to the supine position whilst lung compliance fell from 0.19

TABLE 21.1
FALL IN TOTAL THORACIC COMPLIANCE WITH POSTURE
(VALUES EXPRESSED AS % OF SUPINE CONTROL)
(Data of Safar and Aguto–Escarraga, 1959)

Supine control	100
Lithotomy	102
Head up 20°	118
Head down 20°	82
Gall-bladder support	91
Prone	78
Prone and jack-knife	75
Prone and head down	64
Lateral	94
Kidney support	83

to 0.14 L/cmH$_2$O. Attinger et al., (1956) found that lung compliance fell from 0.19 L/cmH$_2$O sitting to 0·14 L/cmH$_2$O supine and 0.15 L/cmH$_2$O prone. Lynch et al., (1959) found a decrease in static total thoracic compliance in the supine position and a further decrease in the prone position. These changes were particularly marked in patients with severe scoliosis.

Posner et al., (1965) also found a decrease in lung compliance in the prone position whilst Potgieter (1959) demonstrated a reduction in compliance in the dependent lung in the lateral nephrectomy position.

The effects of external pressure due to surgeons, retractors, packs and tight bandages must also be considered (Safar and Aguto-Escarraga, 1959). For example, Drummond and Martin (1978) showed that total thoracic compliance was increased by changing from the supine to the lithotomy position but was then markedly reduced when gas was insufflated into the peritoneum prior to laparoscopy. The reduction in chest wall compliance due to the increase in abdominal pressure resulted in a 19% decrease in FRC.

Finally it must be remembered that gravitational effects may be magnified by the presence of obesity.

Naimark and Cherniack (1960), for example, showed in the very obese that chest wall compliance was a third of normal and that the excess weight on the chest wall caused a marked reduction in total thoracic compliance in the supine position.

Anaesthetic Agents and Artificial Ventilation. Although there are many reports of compliance changes associated with anaesthesia the results must be interpreted with great caution. For example, oesophageal pressure measurements in the supine position are affected by the type of balloon used, the position in the oesophagus, the size of the heart and possible effects of the anaesthetic on oesophageal tone. Furthermore the pressure-volume curve is non-linear so that the values obtained depend on the lung volume at the time of measurement and on the volume history of the lung. Most investigators have found that lung compliance is decreased during anaesthesia (Rehder et al., 1975). For example, Westbrook et al., (1973) found that lung compliance fell from a mean of 0.204 L/cmH$_2$O awake to 0.143 L/cmH$_2$O during thiopentone-pethidine anaesthesia with spontaneous ventilation and 0.140 L/cmH$_2$O (1.40 L/kPa) when the volunteers were anaesthetized and paralysed, whilst Rehder et al. (1974) found a similar reduction in supine subjects given isoflurane and suxamethonium. The reduction in lung compliance is associated with a reduction in total thoracic compliance, values during anaesthesia ranging from about 0.04–0.08 L/cmH$_2$O (Rehder et al., 1975). However, it is not yet clear whether the primary cause of the change in total thoracic compliance is an alteration in lung compliance or an alteration in the mechanics of the chest wall (Westbrook et al., 1973). Possible causes of a reduction in lung compliance are a direct effect of anaesthetic drugs on the lung, airway closure or atelectasis, changes in intrathoracic blood volume, altered surfactant activity, altered intrapulmonary gas distribution and the accumulation of interstitial fluid. Changes in chest wall mechanics could be produced by altered muscle tone, an alteration in the shape of the chest or altered intrapulmonary gas distribution (Grimby et al., 1975; Rehder et al., 1977b; Jones et al., 1979).

Duration of Anaesthesia. The dependence of compliance on the volume history of the lungs has already been emphasized. It was the observations of Mead and Collier (1959) in dogs and Ferris and Pollard (1960) in humans which showed that shallow tidal volumes decreased compliance and that these changes could be reversed by maximal inflations. This is a manifestation of the stress-relaxation or hysteresis noted by Bernstein (1957) and Butler (1957). Egbert et al. (1963) studied changes in total thoracic compliance during anaesthesia and noted that this rose from a mean of 35.6 to 42.8 ml/cmH$_2$O after a series of deep breaths and then fell within 5–10 min to a mean of 36.1 ml/cmH$_2$O. In this, and a number of other studies on the changes in alveolar-arterial oxygen tension

differences with time, Bendixen and his colleagues stressed that the changes in compliance were closely related to the volume history of the lungs (Egbert et al., 1963). It was suggested that the tidal volume necessary to prevent progressive falls in compliance was about 7 ml/kg body weight in patients with normal lungs: at a respiratory frequency of 20/min this produced a mean arterial P_{CO_2} of 27 mmHg. To overcome the problem of decreasing compliance in patients respiring at lower tidal volumes it was suggested that deep breaths should be given every 5–10 min. A number of subsequent studies have thrown some doubt on the general applicability of these conclusions. Thus Fletcher and Barber (1966) found no change in dynamic lung compliance during spontaneous breathing in normal subjects and Panday and Nunn (1968) found no change in alveolar-arterial oxygen tension difference under similar conditions during anaesthesia. Colgan and Whang (1968) were also unable to find any fall in lung compliance or increase in intrapulmonary shunting with nembutal, methoxyflurane and halothane anaesthesia in dogs and humans. During controlled ventilation Judd and King (1967) found that if the lungs were hyperinflated and the tidal volume then maintained at normal levels by mechanical ventilation, the most rapid fall in compliance occurred during the first minute after the hyperinflation. After 15 min the lung compliance was decreased by 29% compared with the value obtained just after hyperinflation but thereafter they could detect no change even if the ventilation was continued for up to 3 hours. These findings are supported by the absence of change of alveolar-arterial oxygen tension differences noted by Askrog et al. (1964) and Lumley et al. (1969). Since there are a number of differences in the premedication, anaesthesia and type of ventilation used in these studies it would seem wise to use the maximum tidal ventilation compatible with a normal arterial P_{CO_2} and to utilize every opportunity to re-expand the lungs. This is particularly important after the patient has been in a position which reduces FRC: it should also be carried out after coughing, intubation and the aspiration of secretions.

FACTORS AFFECTING AIRWAY RESISTANCE

The diameter of the airways depends on body size, on the pressure gradients holding them open, on the thickness of the bronchial mucosa and on the degree of bronchomotor tone.

Body size. Above a functional residual capacity of 2.5 L, body size does not appear to affect airway resistance, the normal value being 0.5–2.0 cmH$_2$O/L/s, i.e. 0.05–0.2 kPaL^{-1}s at 0.5 L/s flow rate. Below an FRC of 2.5 L airway resistance increases as body size falls (Helliesen et al., 1958, Cook et al., 1958). In neonates the average resistance is 0.03 cmH$_2$O/(ml·s) (0.003 kPa/(ml·s)).

Pressure Gradients. In the thorax, the trachea and main bronchi are exposed to the gradient of pressure between the atmosphere and the intrapleural space. The airways within the lung are exposed to a similar gradient of pressure due to the elasticity of lung tissue. An increase in this gradient during inspiration therefore widens the airways whilst the converse occurs during expiration. Similarly any factor which alters the elastic recoil pressure of the lung will alter the diameter of the airways. At any given lung volume the airways will thus tend to be narrower in patients with emphysema.

Bronchial Mucosa. Small changes in the calibre of the smaller airways lead to marked changes in resistance. The presence of secretions or an increase in thickness of the mucosa are thus very common causes of an increased airway resistance. Little is known about the changes in the thickness of the bronchial mucosa resulting from physiological or pathological stimuli but it is probable that such variations play an important part in the changes of airway resistance due to posture or alterations in pulmonary blood volume. Certainly in patients with severe pulmonary oedema the mucosa is often extremely congested and oedematous and on occasions the author has noted almost complete occlusion of the main bronchi on bronchoscopic examination.

Bronchial Muscle Tone. Bronchial muscle tone is under the control of the autonomic system: bronchi are constricted by parasympathetic activity and dilated by sympathetic stimulation. Drugs produce similar effects. Thus isoprenaline, adrenaline, atropine and ganglion blocking drugs such as hexamethonium produce bronchodilatation whilst histamine, acetylcholine and irritant gases cause bronchoconstriction and an increase in airways resistance. An increase in smooth muscle contraction is probably the predominant cause of the increased airway resistance in asthma where resistance may increase to 20–50 cmH$_2$O/L/s, i.e. (2–5 kPaL^{-1}s).

In addition to the causes already mentioned it must be remembered that increases in airway resistance will occur when there are localized obstructions to air flow (foreign body, tumour, extrinsic pressure), and that bypassing the upper airways by a tracheostomy may lower the total airway resistance.

Anaesthesia

The factors which are most likely to affect airway resistance during anaesthesia are airway obstruction or the use of artificial airways, a reduction in lung volume due to posture or anaesthesia, changes in the alveolar gas tensions and drugs used in premedication and anaesthesia.

The Airway. In the normal patient 20–30% of the airway resistance is incurred above the cricoid cartilage.

Obstruction at the larynx or above may greatly increase airway resistance which may not be alleviated by the passage of an airway. Thus, Gold and Helrich (1965b) found that the induction of anaesthesia with thiopentone, nitrous oxide and either halothane or methoxyflurane resulted in an average increase in resistance of 123% over control values. When an oropharyngeal airway was inserted the resistance was 55% above control values, whilst the insertion of an oral endotracheal tube reduced the resistance to 18% below the control values. Wu et al. (1956) also noted that airway resistance could usually be kept within normal limits by the passage of an endotracheal tube.

Lung Volume. The average reduction in FRC resulting from the induction of anaesthesia is about 500 ml. However, the patient will already have suffered a decrease in FRC of up to 1 L on becoming supine and this change may have been accentuated by a head down tilt or external pressure on the chest. As a result, the expiratory reserve volume is greatly reduced and airway resistance increased. Such changes are frequently observed in the very obese.

Alveolar Gas Tensions. In man, hypocapnia has been shown to cause bronchoconstriction by a central effect mediated by the vagus. Hypercapnia tends to widen airways (Don et al., 1965). Changes in alveolar oxygen tension seem to produce variable effects on airway resistance.

Drugs. Of the drugs used in premedication only atropine produces a marked reduction in airway resistance. Morphine tends to increase airway resistance, whilst pethidine and the barbiturates produce little change. Airway resistance values during anaesthesia range from 5–9 cmH$_2$O/(L·s) (0.5–0.9 kPa/(L·s) and are obviously influenced by the variations in upper airway resistance resulting from the position of the tongue and the use of artificial airways or endotracheal tubes. The volatile anaesthetics are generally considered to produce bronchodilatation (Aviado, 1975). Both halothane and enflurane produce marked reductions in respiratory resistance though there are several case reports of bronchospasm during the use of these agents (Lehane et al., 1980). The only relaxant shown to alter airway resistance is d-tubocurarine. This increased airway resistance slightly in 7 out of 23 patients studied by Westgate et al. (1962).

CONCLUSIONS

It will be apparent that the changes in the mechanics of breathing associated with anaesthesia can be due to a multiplicity of causes. The variations encountered between normal patients are large and the variations due to pathological changes are sometimes great enough seriously to impair ventilation. However, respiratory failure rarely arises from a low compliance alone: it is nearly always due to a combination of low compliance with a high airway resistance and to the retention of secretions and central respiratory depression from drugs or toxaemia. Whatever the cause it is obvious that the most important factor in the prevention of respiratory failure is the maintenance of optimal mechanical function of the lungs. This can be accomplished by removal of secretions, re-expansion of all areas of atelectasis and bronchodilatation. Although detailed measurements of respiratory mechanics are seldom made in clinical practice a great deal can be learned from such simple tests as the vital capacity and forced expiratory volume. The application of these tests and the interpretation of the pressures and volumes measured during mechanical ventilation, are within the province of every anaesthetist and should be closely integrated into clinical practice.

REFERENCES

Agostoni E., Mead J. (1964). Statics of the respiratory system. *Handbook of Physiology: Respiration*, **1**, 387.

Agostoni E. (1977). Transpulmonary pressure. In *Regional Differences in the Lung*. (West, J.B., ed.). London: Academic Press.

Askrog V.F., Pender J.W., Smith T.C., et al. (1964). Changes in respiratory dead space during halothane, cyclopropane and nitrous oxide anesthesia. *Anesthesiology*, **25**, 342.

Attinger E.O., Monroe R.G., Segal M.S. (1956). The mechanics of breathing in different body positions. 1. In normal subjects. *J. Clin. Invest.*, **35**, 904.

Aviado D.M. (1975). Regulation of bronchomotor tone during anesthesia. *Anesthesiology*, **42**, 68.

Bergman N.A. (1963). Distribution of inspired gas during anesthesia and artificial ventilation. *J. Appl. Physiol.*, **18**, 1085.

Bergman N.A. (1969). Properties of passive exhalations in anesthetized subjects. *Anesthesiology*, **30**, 378.

Bernstein L. (1957). The elastic pressure-volume curves of the lungs and thorax of the living rabbit. *J. Physiol.*, **138**, 473.

Brismar B., Hedenstierna G., Lundquist H., et al. (1985). Pulmonary densities during anesthesia with muscular relaxation—a proposal of atelectasis. *Anesthesiology*, **62**, 422.

Butler J. (1957). The adaptation of the relaxed lungs and chest walls to changes in volume. *Clin. Sci.*, **16**, 421.

Colgan F.J., Whang T.B. (1968). Anesthesia and atelectasis. *Anesthesiology*, **29**, 917.

Cook C.D., Helliesen P.J., Agathon S. (1958). Relation between mechanics of respiration, lung size and body size from birth to young adulthood. *J. Appl. Physiol.*, **13**, 349.

Craig D.B., Wahba W.M., Don H.F. (1971a). Airway closure and lung volumes in surgical positions. *Canad. Anaes. Soc. J.*, **18**, 92.

Craig D.B., Wahba W.M., Don H.F., et al. (1971b). Closing volume and its relationship to gas exchange in seated and supine positions. *J. Appl. Physiol.*, **31**, 717.

Daly W.J., Bondurant S. (1963). Direct measurement of respiratory pleural pressure changes in normal man. *J. Appl. Physiol.*, **18**, 513.

Don H.F., Robson I.G. (1965). The mechanics of the respiratory system during anesthesia. *Anesthesiology*, **26**, 168.

Don H.F., Wahba W.M., Cuadrada L. and Kelkar K.

(1970). The effects of anesthesia and 100% oxygen on the functional residual capacity of the lungs. *Anesthesiology*, **32**, 521.

Drummond G.B., Martin L.V.H. (1978). Pressure-volume relationships in the lung during laparoscopy. *Br. J. Anaesth.*, **50**, 261.

DuBois A.B., Botelho S.Y., Comroe J.H. (1956a). A new method for measuring airway resistance in man using a body plethysmograph: values in normal subjects and in patients with respiratory disease. *J. Clin. Invest.*, **15**, 327.

DuBois A.B., Botelho S.Y., Bedell G.N., et al. (1956b). A rapid plethysmographic method for measuring thoracic gas volume: a comparison with a nitrogen washout method for measuring functional residual capacity in normal subjects. *J. Clin. Invest.*, **15**, 322.

DuBois A.B., Brody A.W., Lewis D.H., et al. (1956c). Oscillation mechanics of the lungs and chest in man. *J. Appl. Physiol.*, **8**, 587.

Egbert L.D., Laver M.B., Bendixen H.H. (1963). Intermittent deep breaths and compliance during anesthesia in man. *Anesthesiology*, **24**, 57.

Ferris B.G. Jr., Pollard D.S. (1960). Effect of deep and quiet breathing on pulmonary compliance in man. *J. Clin. Invest.*, **39**, 143.

Fisher A.B., DuBois A.B., Hyde R.W. (1968). Evaluation of the forced oscillation technique for the determination of resistance to breathing. *J. Clin. Invest.*, **47**, 2045.

Fletcher G., Barber J.L. (1966). Lung mechanics and physiologic shunt during spontaneous breathing in normal subjects. *Anesthesiology*, **27**, 638.

Froese A.B., Bryan A.C. (1974). Effects of anesthesia and paralysis on diaphragmatic mechanics in man. *Anesthesiology*, **41**, 242.

Gattinoni L., Mascheroni D., Basilico E., et al. (1987). Volume/pressure curve of total respiratory system in paralysed patients: artefacts and correction factors. *Intensive Care Med.*, **13**, 19.

Gibson G.J., Pride N.B. (1976). Lung distensibility. *Brit. J. Dis. Chest*, **70**, 143.

Glazier J.B., Hughes J.M.B., Maloney J.E., et al. (1966). Decreasing alveolar size from apex to base in the upright lung. *Lancet*, **2**, 203.

Gold M.I., Helrich M. (1965a). Pulmonary compliance during anesthesia. *Anesthesiology*, **26**, 281.

Gold M.I., Helrich M. (1965b). Mechanics of breathing during anesthesia: 2. The influence of airway adequacy. *Anesthesiology*, **26**, 751.

Goldman M., Knudson R.J., Mead J., et al. (1970). A simplified measurement of respiratory resistance by forced oscillation. *J. Appl. Physiol.*, **28**, 113.

Grimby G., Hedenstierna G., Lofstrom B. (1975). Chest wall mechanics during artificial ventilation. *J. Appl. Physiol.*, **38**, 576.

Hedenstierna G., Tokics L., Strandberg A., et al. (1986). Correlation of gas exchange impairment to development of atelectasis during anaesthesia and muscle paralysis. *Acta Anaesthesiol. Scand.*, **30**, 183.

Helliesen P.J., Cook C.D., Friedlander L., et al. (1958). Studies of respiratory physiology in children. 1: Mechanics of respiration and lung volumes in 85 normal children 5 to 17 years of age. *Pediatrics*, **22**, 80.

Hewlett A.M., Hulands G.H., Nunn J.F., et al. (1974a). Functional residual capacity during anaesthesia. II. Spontaneous respiration. *Br. J. Anaesth.*, **46**, 486.

Hewlett A.M., Hulands G.H., Nunn J.F., et al. (1974b).

Functional residual capacity during anaesthesia. III. Artificial ventilation. *Br. J. Anaesth.*, **46**, 495.

Hickey R.F., Visick W.D., Fairley H.B., et al. (1973). Effects of halothane anesthesia on functional residual capacity and alveolar—arterial oxygen tension difference. *Anesthesiology*, **38**, 20.

Jones J.G. (1987). Anaesthesia and atelectasis: the role of V_{TAB} and the chest wall. *Br. J. Anaesth.*, Editorial, **59**, 949.

Jones J.G., Faithfull D., Jordan C., et al. (1979). Rib cage movement during halothane anaesthesia in man. *Br. J. Anaesth.*, **51**, 399.

Judd B.C., King B.D. (1967). Human lung compliance during prolonged positive pressure ventilation. *Anesthesiology*, **28**, 257.

Juno P., Marsh H.M., Knopp T.J., et al. (1978). Closing capacity in awake and anesthetized-paralyzed man. *J. Appl. Physiol.*, **44**, 238.

Kaneko K., Milic-Emili J., Dolovich M.B., et al. (1966). Regional distribution of ventilation and perfusion as a function of body position. *J. Appl. Physiol.*, **21**, 767.

Landmark S.J., Knopp T.J., Rehder K., et al. (1977). Regional pulmonary perfusion and $\dot{V}/\dot{Q}$ in awake and anesthetized-paralyzed man. *J. Appl. Physiol.*, **43**, 993.

Landser F.J., Nagels J., Clement J., et al. (1976). Errors in the measurement of total respiratory resistance and reactance by forced oscillations. *Resp. Physiol.*, **28**, 289.

Laws A.K. (1968). The effects of induction of anaesthesia and muscle paralysis on functional residual capacity of the lungs. *Canad. Anaes. Soc. J.*, **15**, 325.

Leblanc P., Ruff F., Milic-Emili J. (1970). Effects of age and body position on airway closure in man. *J. Appl. Physiol.*, **28**, 448.

Lehane J.R., Jordan C., Jones J.G. (1979). Measurement of airways resistance during anaesthesia. *Br. J. Anaesth.*, **51**, 65P.

Lehane J.R., Jordan C., Jones J.G. (1980). Influence of halothane and enflurane on respiratory airflow resistance and specific conductance in anaesthetized man. *Br. J. Anaesth.*, **52**, 773.

Lim T.P.K., Luft U.C. (1959). Alterations in lung compliance and functional residual capacity with posture. *J. Appl. Physiol.*, **14**, 164.

Lumley J., Morgan M., Sykes M.K. (1969). Changes in arterial oxygenation and physiological dead space under anaesthesia. *Br. J. Anaesth.*, **41**, 279.

Lynch S., Brand L., Levy A. (1959). Changes in lung-thorax compliance during orthopedic surgery. *Anesthesiology*, **20**, 278.

Mansell A.,Bryan A.C., Levison H. (1972). Airway closure in children. *J. Appl. Physiol.*, **33**, 711.

Marshall R. (1957). The physical properties of the lungs in relation to the subdivisions of lung volume. *Clin. Sci.*, **16**, 507.

Marshall R., Dubois A.B. (1956a). The measurement of the viscous resistance of the lung tissues in normal man. *Clin. Sci.*, **15**, 161.

Marshall R., Dubois A.B. (1956b). The viscous resistance of lung tissue in patients with pulmonary disease. *Clin. Sci.*, **15**, 473.

Matamis D., Lemaire F., Harf A., et al. (1984). Total respiratory pressure-volume curves in the adult respiratory distress syndrome. *Chest*, **86**, 58.

Mead J. (1960). Volume displacement body plethysmograph for respiratory measurements in human subjects. *J. Appl. Physiol.*, **15**, 736.

Mead J., Collier C. (1959). Relation of volume history of

lungs to respiratory mechanics in anesthetized dogs. *J. Appl. Physiol.*, **14**, 669.

Menkes H.A., Traystman R.J. (1977). Collateral ventilation. *Amer. Rev. Resp. Dis.*, **116**, 287.

Michaelson E.D., Grassman E.D., Peters W.R. (1975). Pulmonary mechanics by spectral analysis of forced random noise. *J. Clin. Invest.*, **56**, 1210.

Milic-Emili J., Henderson J.A.M., Dolovich M.B., et al. (1966). Regional distribution of inspired gas in the lung. *J. Appl. Physiol.*, **21**, 749.

Miller J.H., Simmons D.H. (1960). Rapid determination dynamic pulmonary compliance and resistance. *J. Appl. Physiol.*, **15**, 967.

Muir A.L., Flenley D.C., Kirby B.J., et al. (1975). Cardiorespiratory effects of rapid saline infusion in normal man. *J. Appl. Physiol.*, **38**, 786.

Naimark A., Cherniack R.M. (1960). Compliance of the respiratory system and its components in health and obesity. *J. Appl. Physiol.*, **15**, 377.

Otis A.B., McKerrow C.B., Bartlett R.A., et al. (1956). Mechanical factors in distribution of pulmonary ventilation. *J. Appl. Physiol.*, **8**, 427.

Panday J., Nunn J.F. (1968). Failure to demonstrate progressive falls of arterial P_{O_2} during anaesthesia. *Anesthesia*, **23**, 38.

Posner A., Brody D., Ravin M. (1965). Effect of prone position with constant volume ventilation on Pa_{O_2} in man. *Anesth. Analg. Curr. Res.*, **44**, 435.

Potgieter S.V. (1959). Atelectasis: Its evolution during upper urinary tract surgery. *Br. J. Anaesth.*, **31**, 472.

Rehder K., Mallow J.E., Fibuch E.E., et al. (1974). Effects of anesthesia and muscle paralysis on respiratory mechanics in normal man. *Anesthesiology*, **41**, 477.

Rehder K., Marsh H.M., Rodarte J.R., et al. (1977a). Airway closure. *Anesthesiology*, **47**, 40.

Rehder K., Sessler A.D., Marsh H.M. (1975). General anesthesia and the lung. *Am. Rev. Resp. Dis.*, **112**, 541.

Rehder K., Sessler A.D., Rodarte J.R. (1977b). Regional intrapulmonary gas distribution in awake and anesthetized-paralyzed man. *J. Appl. Physiol.*, **42**, 391.

Safar P., Aguto-Escarraga L. (1959). Compliance in apneic anesthetized adults. *Anesthesiology*, **20**, 283.

Tokics L., Hedenstierna G., Strandberg A., et al. (1987). Lung collapse and gas exchange during general anesthesia: effects of spontaneous breathing, muscle paralysis, and positive end-expiratory pressure. *Anesthesiology*, **66**, 157.

Weenig C.S., Pietak S., Hickey R.F., et al. (1974). Relationship of pre-operative closing volume to functional residual capacity and alveolar-arterial oxygen difference during anesthesia with controlled ventilation. *Anesthesiology*, **41**, 3.

Westbrook P.R., Stubbs S.E., Sessler A.D., et al. (1973). Effects of anesthesia and muscle paralysis on respiratory mechanics in normal man. *J. Appl. Physiol.*, **34**, 81.

Westgate H.D., Gordon J.R., Van Bergen F.H. (1962). Changes in airway resistance following intravenously administered d-tubocurarine. *Anesthesiology*, **23**, 65.

Wright B.M. (1974). Peak-flow meter and peak-flow gauge. *Lancet*, **2**, 1151.

Wright B.M., McKerrow C.B. (1959). Maximum forced expiratory flow rate as a measure of ventilatory capacity with a description of a new portable instrument for measuring it. *Br. Med. J.*, **2**, 1041.

Wu N., Miller W.F., Luhn N.R. (1956). Studies of breathing in anesthesia. *Anesthesiology*, **17**, 696.

22. Ventilation-Perfusion Relationships
John B. West

The prime function of the lung is to exchange gas between the inspired air and the venous blood. It is clear at the outset therefore that if a given part of the lung receives either no inspired gas or no mixed venous blood, gas exchange cannot occur there at all. It is also true that if the amounts of ventilation and blood flow are poorly matched in the different regions, gas exchange becomes inefficient. The serious effects of mismatch of ventilation and blood flow have only been fully appreciated in the last few years, and it is now recognized that the commonest cause of hypoxemia and hypercarbia in lung disease is uneven ventilation and blood flow.

ALVEOLAR VENTILATION

Not all the gas which is inspired reaches the alveoli where gas exchange occurs. For example, if the tidal volume is 500 ml, only some 350 ml gets to the alveoli because approximately 150 ml remains in the bronchi and is exhaled with the next breath. Since the bronchi are not provided with pulmonary capillaries, gas exchange cannot occur within them and they constitute a *dead space*. The volume of fresh gas entering the alveoli per minute is known as the alveolar ventilation. The normal value is in the region of 5 litres per minute.

The alveolar gas is in a constant state of agitation because of molecular diffusion and, as a result, the whole volume is available for gas exchange at any time. Indeed, it is now believed that the gas only reaches the alveoli because of the rapid diffusion process within the airways. This is because ordinary bulk flow (like water flowing down a river) only carries the inspired molecules to the terminal or respiratory bronchioles. The rest of the distance to the alveoli is then accomplished by random diffusion. For this reason, large particles such as dust or aerosol droplets which diffuse very slowly often fail to penetrate to the alveoli and are deposited in the small airways.

Distribution of Ventilation

It is now known that during spontaneous respiration, the dependent regions of the lung are better ventilated than the upper zones. This is true whether the subject is seated upright, or is lying in the supine, prone, or lateral positions.

By contrast, if the subject breathes at an abnormally low lung volume, the distribution of ventilation is reversed; that is, the superior regions of the lung ventilate well, but the dependent zones are poorly ventilated or indeed no fresh gas may reach them at all. This reversed pattern of ventilation is also seen in older persons at normal lung volumes and also in some patients with chronic obstructive lung disease.

The difference in distribution is shown clearly when a normal subject breathes in slowly in steps from residual volume. At first, all the inspired gas enters the upper zones and the lower regions do not ventilate at all. However, after a certain lung volume has been passed, the lower regions receive most of the gas and this pattern is maintained up to maximal volumes.

Cause of the Distribution of Ventilation

The pressure in the intrapleural space is normally negative (less than atmospheric) in order to keep the lung expanded. However, recent measurements show that the pleural pressure is less negative at the base of the upright lung than it is at the top. This is not particularly surprising because the lung has weight and in order to support it, the pressure below it must be greater than the pressure above.

It is possible to explain the normal distribution of ventilation on the basis of these regional differences in pleural pressure. Fig. 22.1(A) shows that at normal lung volumes, because the expanding pressure at the base of the lung is smaller than that at the apex, the resting volume of the alveoli at the base is small. Furthermore, because of the curved shape of the pressure-volume curve of the lung, a small decrease in pleural pressure during inspiration will cause a larger increase in volume of the basal alveoli than at the apex. For both these reasons the basal regions are normally better ventilated than those at the apex.

Fig. 22.1(B) shows that the situation is changed dramatically at very low lung volumes. At residual volume, for example, the pleural pressure at the base of the upright lung actually exceeds atmospheric pressure. Thus this lung is not being expanded but is being compressed under these conditions. For this reason a small decrease in pleural pressure will result in good ventilation of the lung apex but no ventilation of the base. Only when the pleural pressure at the base of the lung goes below atmospheric pressure does the base of the lung begin to ventilate.

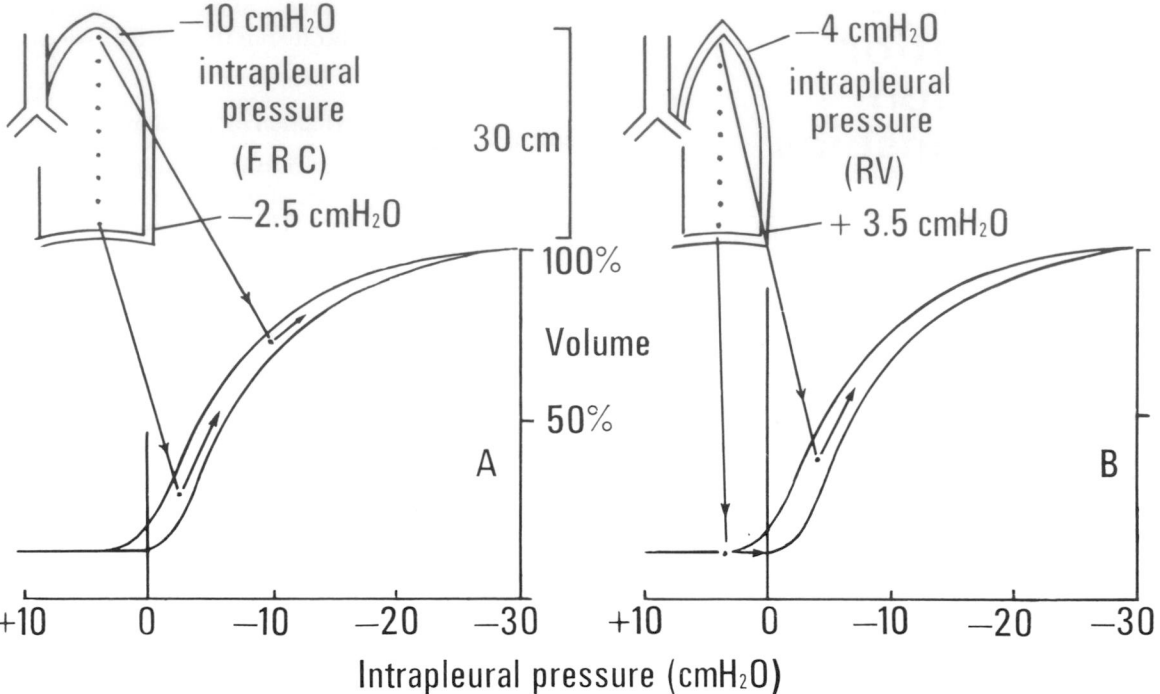

Fig. 22.1 Diagram to explain the distribution of ventilation in the normal upright lung. (A) shows that at normal lung volumes, the base is better ventilated than the apex because the basal alveoli have a smaller resting volume and a larger increase in volume than those at the apex. (B) shows that at residual volume, the basal alveoli do not receive any gas during a small inspiration and that only the apex is ventilated.

This explanation of the uneven distribution of ventilation is an oversimplification. For example, it assumes that the relationship between lung volume and transpulmonary pressure is the same irrespective of how the lung is distorted and this is not so. However, a more detailed analysis of this complex problem is not warranted here.

Regional Differences in Alveolar Size

Figure 22.1 implies differences in the resting volume of the alveoli between the apex and base of the lung. Figure 22.2 shows the results of direct histological measurements of the relative size of the alveoli down the lung of a dog in the upright (head up) position. These measurements were made after fixing the lungs *in situ* by freezing the anesthetized animal. Note that the alveoli at the apex are about four times larger by volume than those at the base. Furthermore, most of the change in volume occurs over the upper regions of the lung. Presumably a similar pattern occurs in man.

These striking differences in alveolar size and the pattern of ventilation associated with them have important implications in various clinical situations. For example, the small alveoli at the base are relatively unstable and tend to collapse. Since these regions are the best perfused, the impairment of gas exchange may then be severe. The reduced ventilation of the dependent regions at low lung volumes is important in obesity which causes a low lung volume, or following

abdominal surgery when the diaphragm may be elevated. These dangers are particularly important in patients with chronic bronchitis and emphysema where even at normal lung volumes the bases are often poorly ventilated.

PULMONARY BLOOD FLOW

Since the total output of the right heart goes through the lungs, the pulmonary blood flow is equal to the cardiac output, that is some five or six litres per minute. However, the actual volume of blood in the capillaries is probably less than 100 ml. This small figure contrasts with the volume of gas in the alveoli which is two to three litres. However, it is of interest that in spite of the very different volumes of blood and gas undergoing gas exchange in the alveoli at any moment, the volume of fresh gas entering the alveoli per minute, that is the alveolar ventilation, and the volume of blood flow are both approximately the same. Thus the normal ratio of alveolar ventilation to pulmonary blood flow is approximately one.

Distribution of Pulmonary Blood Flow

In the normal upright lung, blood flow per unit volume decreases rapidly from bottom to top, reaching very low values at the apex (Fig. 22.3). This pattern is affected by change of posture and exercise. When the subject lies supine, the apical and basal

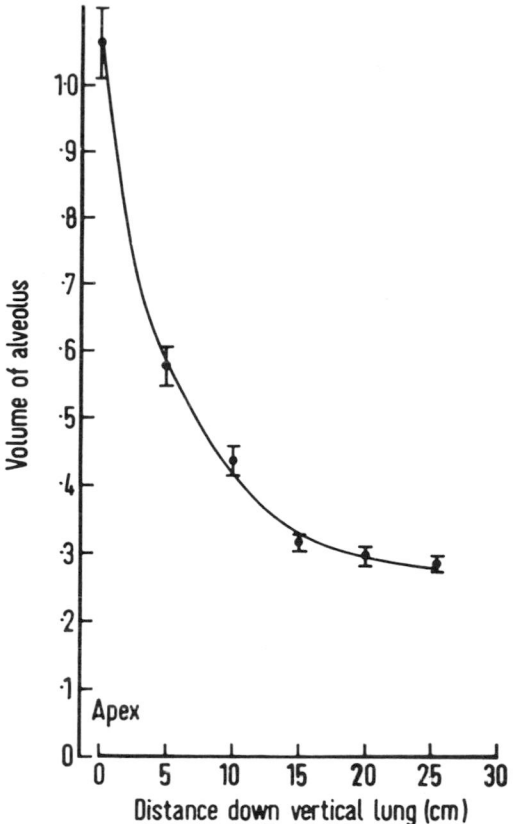

Fig. 22.2 Differences in alveolar size down the lungs of upright (head up) dogs. Note that the alveoli at the base are about four times smaller by volume than those at the apex.

blood flows become the same, but the posterior (dependent) part of the lung has a higher blood flow than the anterior region. In the lateral position, the dependent regions again are best perfused. On exercise in the upright position, both apical and basal blood flows increase so that the proportion of the total flow going to the apex rises.

Changes in lung volume affect the distribution of blood flow just as they do the distribution of ventilation. At low lung volumes, a zone of decreased blood flow is seen at the bottom of the lung, and indeed at residual volume this area of increased vascular resistance spreads up the lung until the apical blood flow actually exceeds basal flow.

Cause of the Distribution of Blood Flow

The uneven distribution of blood flow is caused by the hydrostatic pressure differences within the lungs. The pulmonary circulation is unique in that air and blood are separated by a very thin delicate membrane over a vertical distance of some 30 centimetres and consequently the hydrostatic effect of this large column of blood determines the calibre of the small vessels.

Figure 22.4 shows the importance of the relative magnitudes of the pulmonary arterial, alveolar, and venous pressures. There may be a *zone 1* at the top of the lung where pulmonary arterial pressure is less than alveolar pressure (normally atmospheric). The reason why the pulmonary arterial pressure is low here is the hydrostatic gradient within the pulmonary arterial tree. If arterial pressure is less than alveolar, this part of the lung is unperfused because the delicate pulmonary capillaries are directly exposed to alveolar pressure and collapse when the pressure outside them

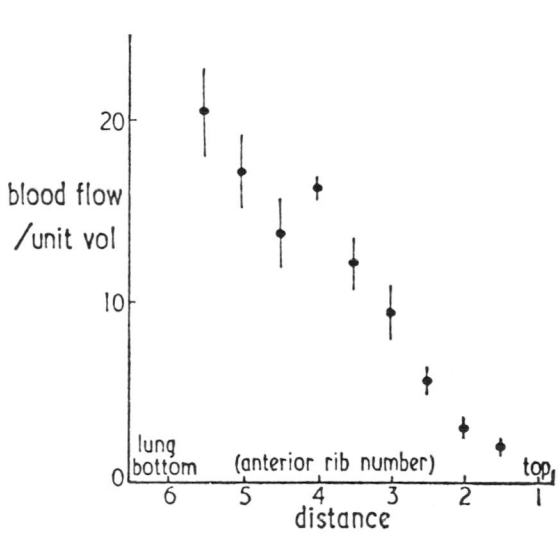

Fig. 22.3 Distribution of blood flow in the normal upright lung as measured with radioactive carbon dioxide. Note that blood flow decreases rapidly from bottom to top reaching very low values at the apex.

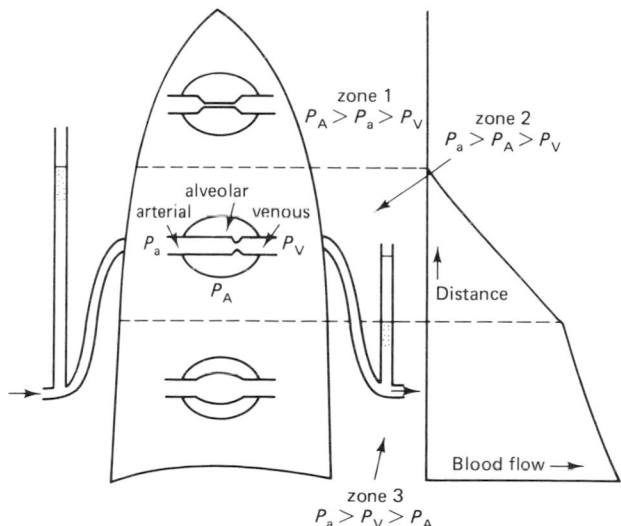

Fig. 22.4 Diagram to explain the distribution of blood flow according to the relative magnitude of the pulmonary arterial, alveolar and venous pressures. *See* text for details.

exceeds the pressure inside. Indeed, histological examination of lung rapidly frozen under these conditions shows collapsed bloodless capillaries. It should be emphasized that in the normal lung, the pulmonary arterial pressure is just sufficient to raise blood to the top. However, if the arterial pressure is reduced as in haemorrhage, oligemic shock, or exposure to acceleration, or if the alveolar pressure is raised as in positive pressure ventilation, then an unperfused zone may be present. This constitutes an alveolar dead space and is useless for gas exchange.

Further down the lung in *zone 2*, pulmonary arterial pressure exceeds alveolar pressure and alveolar exceeds venous pressure. Here it has been shown that blood flow depends on the difference between arterial and alveolar pressure. This is known as the vascular waterfall or Starling resistor effect and is caused by collapse of part of the thin walled capillaries. Consequently, since arterial pressure increases down the zone but alveolar pressure is constant, blood flow increases down the zone.

In *zone 3*, venous pressure exceeds alveolar pressure, the collapsible vessels are held open, and flow is determined in the ordinary way by the arterial-venous pressure difference. The reason why blood flow increases in this zone is that the pressure inside the vessels is increasing whereas the pressure outside is constant and therefore the calibre of the vessels gets larger. It has been shown in quick frozen lungs that the diameter of the pulmonary capillaries increases down this zone.

The cause of the zone of reduced blood flow at the base of the normal lung at low lung volumes can probably be ascribed to the extra-alveolar pulmonary blood vessels. These are held open by radial traction of the surrounding parenchyma much as the bronchi are. Consequently, at the base of the lung where the parenchyma is poorly expanded (*see* Fig. 22.2), the larger blood vessels have a small calibre and thus cause an area of increased vascular resistance. It is also possible that folds develop in the capillaries and increase their vascular resistance when the lung is poorly inflated.

Ventilation-Perfusion Ratio

Because blood flow increases more rapidly than ventilation from the top to the bottom of the upright lung, the ventilation perfusion ratio has a high value at the apex and a low value at the base of the lung. The key importance of this ratio is more easily understood if we consider a simple model of the lung (Fig. 22.5). In this model powdered dye is poured in (analogous to the addition of oxygen by ventilation), and the dye is removed by a flow of water corresponding to the blood flow. What determines the concentration of dye in the alveolar compartment (and thus the effluent blood) under steady state conditions? Intuitively it can be seen that both the rate at which the dye is poured in, and the rate at which the water is pumped through

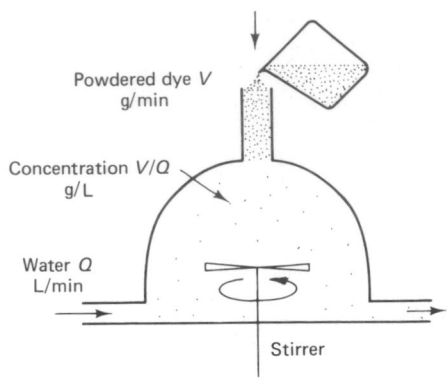

Fig. 22.5 Diagram to explain how the ventilation-perfusion ratio determines the concentration of gas in any lung region. In this analogy, dye is poured into a vessel through which water is pumped. *See* text for details.

the model determine the concentration of dye. In fact, if the dye is poured in at the rate of V grams per minute, and water is pumped through at the rate of Q litres per minute, the concentration of dye under steady state conditions is given by V/Q grams per litre. In exactly the same way the concentration (or partial pressure) of oxygen in the alveolar gas is given by the ratio of ventilation to blood flow. This ratio also determines the concentrations of carbon dioxide and nitrogen or any other gas under steady state conditions.

Regional Differences in Gas Exchange

Since the ventilation-perfusion ratio decreases down the upright lung and because this ratio determines the gas exchange which occurs in any region, it follows that regional differences in gas exchange must occur. Figure 22.6 shows that the alveolar oxygen tension is calculated to change by more than 40 mmHg between the apex and the base of the upright lung. The partial pressure is high at the top of the lung because the ventilation-perfusion ratio is high there, and therefore the amount of oxygen being added by ventilation is large by comparison with the amount which is being removed by the blood flow. Again the carbon dioxide tension varies by more than 10 mmHg. In this case, the high ventilation-perfusion ratio means that a relatively large amount of carbon dioxide is removed compared with the small amount coming in via the blood flow.

Appreciable differences in the gas contents of the blood draining from different regions of the lung can also be seen. Note that the apex contributes relatively little to oxygen uptake because of its low blood flow, though on exercise when the proportion of blood flow to the apex increases, it carries more of the load.

Overall Gas Exchange

Although these differences in ventilation-perfusion

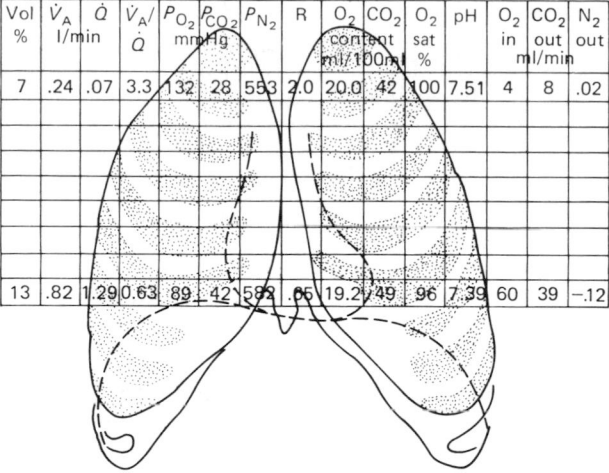

Vol %	$\dot{V}_A$ l/min	$\dot{Q}$	$\dot{V}_A/\dot{Q}$	P_{O_2} mmHg	P_{CO_2}	P_{N_2}	R	O_2 content ml/100ml	CO_2	O_2 sat %	pH	O_2 in ml/min	CO_2 out	N_2 out
7	.24	.07	3.3	132	28	553	2.0	20.0	42	100	7.51	4	8	.02
13	.82	1.29	0.63	89	42	582	.66	19.2	49	96	7.39	60	39	−.12

Fig. 22.6 Regional differences in gas exchange down the normal upright lung resulting from the differences in the ventilation-perfusion ratio. The lung is divided into nine imaginary slices but only the values for the top and bottom regions are shown.

ratio cause large changes in regional gas exchange, their effects on overall gas exchange can be of much greater physiological and clinical importance. It can be shown that a lung with uneven ventilation and blood flow is less efficient at transferring gas either from air to blood or *vice versa*, than an homogeneous lung. The reason for this impairment of gas exchange in the normal lung can be seen by referring to Fig. 22.6. This shows that the base of the lung is much more important than the apex in determining the arterial blood composition because it contributes most of the blood. However, the base has a low oxygen partial pressure (because of its low ventilation-perfusion ratio). Thus inevitably the arterial oxygen partial pressure is depressed because it is loaded with less well oxygenated blood. For the same reason, the carbon dioxide partial pressure in the blood is elevated. It is as if the presence of uneven ventilation-perfusion ratios sets up a barrier between the gas and the blood with the result that the arterial oxygen partial pressure is depressed, and the carbon dioxide partial pressure is raised.

There is an additional reason why the arterial oxygen partial pressure is reduced by ventilation-perfusion ratio inequality. While the oxygen content of blood draining from alveoli with a low ventilation-perfusion ratio is always abnormally low, alveoli with a high ventilation-perfusion ratio are not able to oxygenate their blood much more than normal alveoli. This is because the blood is normally almost fully saturated with oxygen owing to the shape of the oxygen dissociation curve. This additional reason does not apply to carbon dioxide.

In the normal lung, the effects of uneven ventilation-perfusion ratios on overall gas exchange are trivial; the arterial oxygen partial pressure is reduced by a few mmHg and the carbon dioxide partial pressure is raised by less than 1 mmHg. Both these liabilities can be met by the lung increasing its total ventilation and thus its overall ventilation-perfusion ratio. Indeed, the level of overall ventilation is normally set by the respiratory centre via the arterial carbon dioxide partial pressure. Thus, if uneven ventilation-perfusion ratios elevate the arterial carbon dioxide partial pressure, this is brought back by the increased respiratory drive and the consequently higher overall ventilation.

In the diseased lung, the effects of ventilation-perfusion ratio inequality on gas transfer may be very severe because the degree of uneven ventilation and blood flow is far greater than in the normal lung. The arterial oxygen partial pressure may be depressed by 50 or more mmHg and in practice no amount of increased ventilation can return it to its normal level. The carbon dioxide partial pressure, however, is often brought down by an increase in total ventilation though sometimes this is not possible and hypercarbia develops.

VENTILATION-PERFUSION INEQUALITY

Unfortunately, in the abnormal lung, it is not usually possible to map out the distribution of ventilation and blood flow as can be done in the normal lung using radioactive gas techniques (Fig. 22.6). This is because most of the inequality is at the alveolar level and thus great variation occurs within individual counting fields. A valuable method of measuring ventilation-perfusion inequality in these instances is by the analysis of expired gas and arterial blood.

We saw in Fig. 22.6 that the arterial oxygen partial pressure is depressed in the presence of ventilation-perfusion ratio inequality because it is loaded with less well oxygenated blood from the well perfused lung base. By contrast, the expired alveolar gas receives a disproportionately high contribution from the apex where the oxygen partial pressure is high. An alveolar-arterial oxygen difference therefore develops, and the magnitude of this difference is a measure of the amount of ventilation-perfusion ratio inequality.

While arterial blood can be collected by puncture, a representative sample of mixed alveolar gas is often impossible to obtain in the diseased lung because of its disturbed pattern of emptying. An alternative is to collect all the expired gas (including the dead space from the bronchi) using a valve-box and a large bag or spirometer and calculate what is called the *ideal alveolar oxygen tension*. This is the value which the alveolar gas would have in the absence of ventilation-perfusion ratio inequality. This calculation is made using the arterial carbon dioxide partial pressure and the alveolar gas equation.

The oxygen partial pressure difference between ideal alveolar gas and arterial blood chiefly reflects those alveoli with an abnormally *low* ventilation-perfusion ratio, that is the alveoli which are underventilated in relation to their blood flow. These alveoli cause the hypoxemia and their presence has the same effect as the admixture of some venous blood with arterial blood. Indeed, it is possible to express their contribution as if a certain proportion of the venous blood bypassed the lung altogether and was then added to the arterial blood. This is called *venous admixture* or wasted blood flow and is calculated from the oxygen partial pressure difference between ideal alveolar gas and arterial blood. Normally, calculated venous admixture is less than 5% of the pulmonary blood flow, but it may rise to 30% or higher in the presence of severe ventilation-perfusion ratio inequality.

The alveoli with an abnormally *high* ventilation-perfusion ratio, that is those which are under perfused in relation to their ventilation, mainly affect carbon dioxide elimination. They behave as if a certain proportion of the inspired gas bypassed the alveoli altogether, that is as if the dead space were increased in size thus resulting in wasted ventilation. Their contribution can be calculated from the carbon dioxide partial pressure of arterial blood and mixed expired gas using the Bohr equation. This gives a value for the *physiologic dead space* which includes not only the volume of the bronchi, but also the so-called alveolar dead space attributable to the over-ventilated alveoli. Normally the physiologic dead space is less than 30% of the tidal volume at rest, but it may rise to 50% or more in the presence of severe disease.

Another technique for measuring ventilation-perfusion inequality is now available. A mixture of six gases having a broad range of solubilities is slowly infused into a peripheral vein and the concentrations of the gases in the arterial blood and expired gas are measured by gas chromatography. From these data it is possible to compute continuous distributions of ventilation-perfusion ratios within the lung.

Normal lungs typically show a narrow distribution with little dispersion of ventilation-perfusion ratios about the normal value of about 1.0 (Fig. 22.7). Older people with apparently normal lungs often show a broadening of the distribution, and different diseases have characteristic distributions of ventilation-perfusion ratios.

An interesting finding with this technique is the impairment of ventilation-perfusion relationships in patients following induction of anesthesia (Duek et al., 1980). Patients with relatively mild chronic obstructive lung disease often develop substantial broadening of their distributions including the development of large amounts of blood flow to lung units

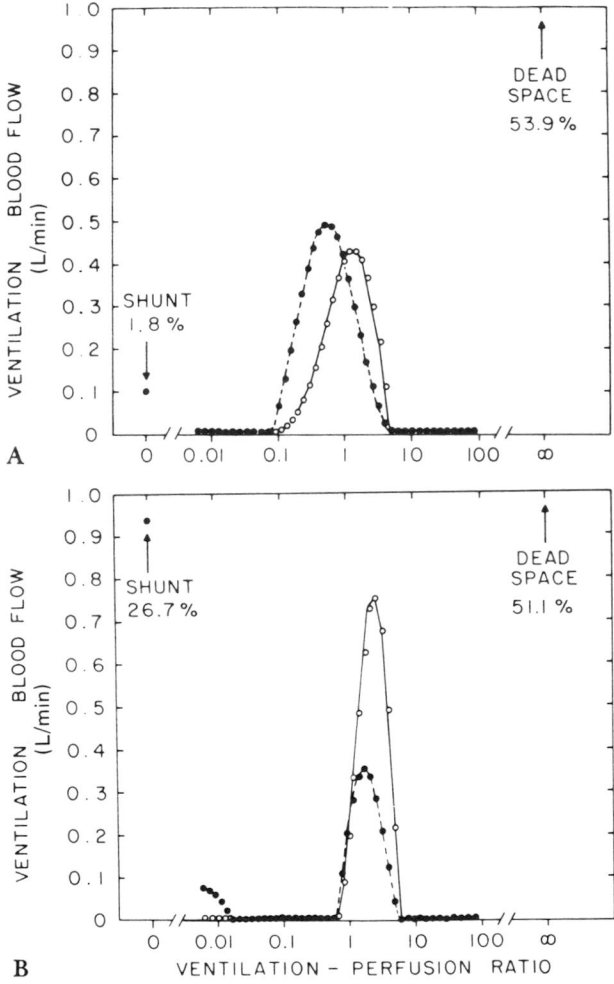

Fig. 22.8 Distribution of ventilation-perfusion ratios in a patient with mild chronic obstructive lung disease before and after induction of anesthesia. Note that prior to induction, the distributions were somewhat broader than that in the normal subject of Fig. 22.7 and there was a small shunt (bloodflow to unventilated lung) of 1.8%. After induction, the shunt increased dramatically to 26.7%. (Reproduced with permission from Duek et al., 1980.)

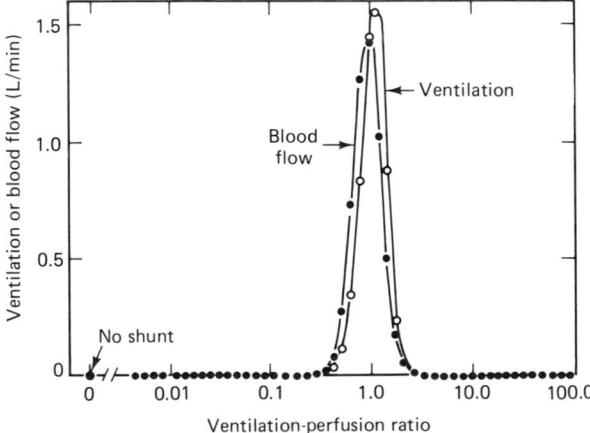

Fig. 22.7 Typical distribution of ventilation-perfusion ratios in a young normal subject. Note that there is little dispersion of ventilation or blood flow around the normal ventilation-perfusion ratio of about 1.0 and that there is no blood flow to unventilated units. (Reproduced with permission from Wagner et al., 1974.)

with low ventilation-perfusion ratios, or unventilated units. Even patients with apparently normal lungs often show an obvious broadening of their distributions of ventilation-perfusion ratios following induction of anesthesia. Figure 22.8 shows a typical example from a patient with mild chronic obstructive lung disease who developed marked worsening of ventilation-perfusion relationships as a result of anesthesia.

REFERENCES

Duek R., Young I., Clausen J., et al. (1980). Altered distribution of pulmonary ventilation and blood flow following induction of inhalational anesthesia. *Anesthesiology*, **52**, 113.

Wagner P.D., Laravuso R.B., Uhl R.R., et al. (1974). Continuous distributions of ventilation-perfusion ratios in normal subjects breathing air and 100% O_2. *J. Clin. Invest.*, **54**, 54.

FURTHER READING

West J.B. (1977). *Regional Differences in the Lung*. New York: Academic Press.

West J.B. (1985). *Ventilation/Blood Flow and Gas Exchange*. 4th edn. Oxford: Blackwell Scientific Publications.

23. Respiratory Function Tests
M. Frye and G. Olsen

Spirometry
    Flow volume loops
Lung volumes
Diffusing capacity
Tests of early airway dysfunction
Interpretation of PFTs
    Preoperative PFTs

Evaluation for the presence of abnormal lung function can assist in the identification of those patients at increased risk of postoperative pulmonary complications. Candidates for preoperative evaluation of pulmonary function include those over the age of 70, patients with known pulmonary disease or history of smoking, dyspnea and cough, obese patients, and patients scheduled for lung resection surgery (Tisi and Gennaro, 1979). Thorough evaluation including history and physical examination, radiologic examination, and laboratory analysis (including arterial blood gas analysis) will usually indicate which patients will require specific pulmonary function tests (PFTs). Many types of PFTs are available. Those most commonly used, and which are most useful, are spirometric tests which measure air flow rates and dynamic lung volumes from maximum inspiration to maximum expiration. Other commonly employed tests will also be described. Although there are no pulmonary function tests which absolutely contraindicate surgery (Gass and Olsen, 1986) their interpretation may identify patients at risk and can aid the anesthestist in preoperative evaluation and subsequent management of the patient.

Pulmonary function testing only identifies physio-logic derangement. These abnormalities are grouped under the terms *obstructive* and *restrictive*. The detection of these physiologic abnormalities as they differ from 'normal' form the basis of pulmonary function test interpretation.

SPIROMETRY

Spirometry is the most frequently performed PFT. It can be virtually diagnostic of some obstructive conditions such as asthma where marked improvement in expiratory flow rate is noted following administration of bronchodilators. Spirometric measurement can be made on instruments as simple as a water-filled, bell-type spirometer with a rotating drum recorder. More complex (and more expensive) electronic flow transducers in which airflow is measured and integrated against time to determine volume are now in vogue. Spirometry with either instrument measures volume per unit time and so determines certain static and dynamic lung volumes as well as air flow rate at various lung volumes. The data are usually presented as volume plotted against time (Fig. 23.1) or as flow

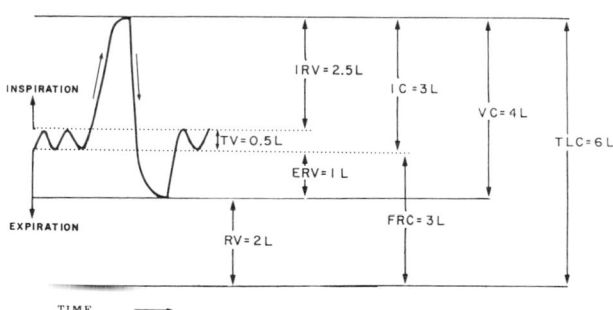

Fig. 23.1 Illustration of the relationship of lung volumes obtained from a spirogram. TV = tidal volume, RV = residual volume, IRV = inspiratory reserve volume, ERV = expiratory reserve volume, IC = inspiratory capacity, FRC = functional residual capacity, VC = vital capacity, TLC = total lung capacity.

against volume (flow-volume loop) discussed later. Spirometry measures lung volumes and flow rates between the position of maximum inspiration termed *total lung capacity* (TLC) to the point of maximum expiration termed *residual volume* (RV). The volume between these extremes is called the *vital capacity* (VC).

Vital capacity is related directly to height and inversely with age. Values are lower in supine than in sitting or standing patients. Values are also lower in processes resulting in ventilatory defects which 'restrict' the lung from reaching normal inspiratory volumes. Conditions occurring commonly in the perioperative period which can do this include pneumonia, atelectasis, muscle weakness, lung resection, poor effort (sedation), pain and ascites. Upper abdominal surgery results in significant short-term decreases in vital capacity probably related to inspiratory diaphragmatic dysfunction (Ford et al., 1983). Vital capacity can also be reduced in obstructive ventilatory defects (eg. emphysema) as well. This results from *encroachment* on the VC by an increased residual volume caused by hyperinflation of the lung (air trapping).

If the patient forcibly exhales his vital capacity as rapidly as possible, the *forced vital capacity* (FVC) is measured. No time limit is applied to this manoeuver, but it should take no more than four seconds (Zamel et al., 1983). Normally, the FVC and VC are equal, but in obstructive ventilatory defects, the FVC may be lower due to air trapping. The rate of air flow during this manoeuver is dependent upon the airway resistance. Airway obstruction is inferred from a reduction of the amount of air that can be expelled during the FVC manoeuver in a set period of time from the onset of the manoeuver, i.e., 0.5, 0.75, 1.0, 2.0 seconds. The set time is designated by subscripts. The most useful is the *forced expiratory volume in one second* (FEV_1) (Fig. 23.2). Normal subjects are able to exhale 85% of

the FVC in one second. This value decreases to 70% with advancing age. FEV_1 is reduced by restrictive ventilatory defects (due to simple reduction in lung volume in general) and obstructive lung diseases such as asthma and emphysema (due to obstruction to expiratory air flow) (Fig. 23.3). To distinguish the two, FEV_1 is compared as a ratio to FVC. In restrictive lung disease, the FEV_1/FVC ratio (expressed as a percentage) is normal since the reduction in FEV_1 is just part of the concentric reduction of all lung volumes. But, in obstructive lung disease, this ratio is severely reduced due to the obstruction to expiratory air flow with a relatively well-maintained VC.

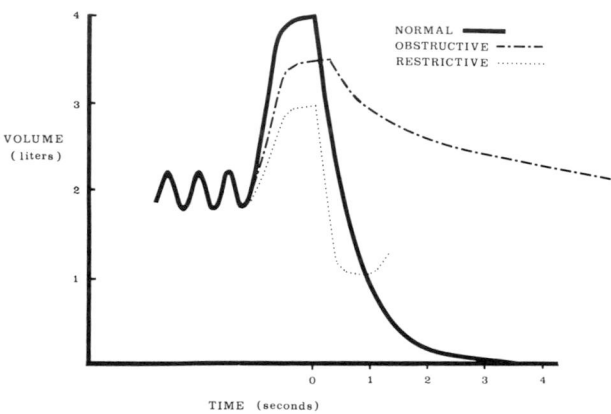

Fig. 23.3 Illustration of the reduction in forced vital capacity and the shapes of the spirogram in restrictive and obstructive ventilatory defects compared to normal (*see* text). Although, the mechanisms are different in obstructive and restrictive disease, the tracings show a reduced FEV_1 in each condition.

The *maximum expiratory flow rate* (MEFR) or peak flow rate (PFR) in liters per minute can be measured from the FVC manoeuver. Peak flow can also be easily measured with a handheld peak flow meter. Values are reduced in obstructive diseases and may rarely be reduced in severe restrictive diseases. Some authors consider this the single best spirometric test because it reflects the ability to produce an adequate cough. Values obtained of less than 200 liters per minute in a surgical candidate suggest an increased risk of postoperative complications (Stein et al., 1962). *Forced expiratory flow rates* (FEF) at specific points in the FVC manoeuver can also be measured and are designated by subscripts. Thus, $FEF_{200-1200}$ is the forced expiratory flow rate between 200 and 1200 ml of expired volume. Similarly, FEF_{25-75} (formerly called the maximal mid-expiratory flow rate or MMFR) is the forced expiratory flow rate in the mid FVC region, i.e. flow from 25–75% of expired volume (*see* Fig. 23.2). Reduction of flow at lower lung volumes (i.e. FEF_{25-75} or FEF_{75-85} is thought by some to represent small airway dysfunction indicative of

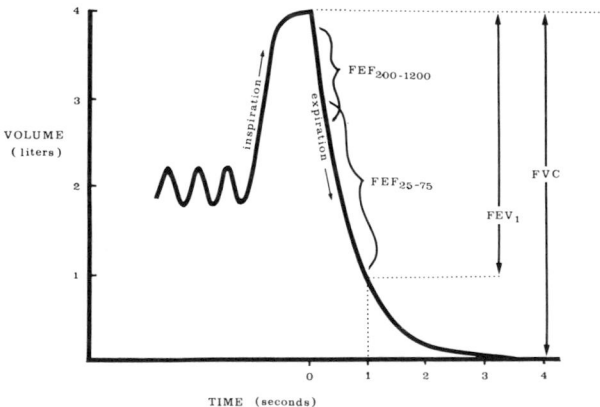

Fig. 23.2 Illustration of a timed spirogram showing the forced vital capacity (FVC) and timed subunits. FEV_1 = forced expiratory volume in one second, FEF_{25-75} = forced expiratory flow between 25% and 75% of the FVC, $FEF_{200-1200}$ = forced expiratory flow between 200–1200 ml of the FVC.

early obstructive airway dysfunction (McFadden et al., 1974). These tests are, however, probably too insensitive and nonspecific and have not fulfilled this role. Since the $FEF_{200-1200}$ is measured at higher lung volumes, the diameter of the airways is greater and, therefore, flow is more influenced by patient effort than by small airway dysfunction.

The maximum volume of air a subject can voluntarily exchange in one minute is the *maximum voluntary ventilation* (MVV), also previously called the maximum breathing capacity (MBC). A normal, healthy, young male has an MVV of about 175 liters per minute. Because high flow rates are involved in the MVV, just as they are in measurement of FEV_1, airway resistance will have a major impact on results. Emphysema patients will have a very low MVV for this reason. In fact, $FEV_1 \times 35$ correlates closely with MVV. Conditions which alter respiratory muscle strength (such as myasthenia gravis and Guillain-Barré syndrome) as well as ailments which limit ribcage movement (like scoliosis and ankylosing spondylitis) will reduce MVV. However, patients with restrictive lung disease can often achieve a normal MVV since they can offset the small breaths they must take due to their stiff thoraces by increasing breathing frequency. The MVV is, unfortunately, very susceptible to reduced effort.

In addition to the MVV, another set of tests reflect respiratory muscle strength. The maximal static inspiratory pressure (PI_{max}) and maximum static expiratory pressure (PE_{max}) are measured against an occluded airway at RV and TLC respectively. These lung volume positions are chosen because they place the respiratory muscles at their most advantageous lengths for each manoeuver. Severe inspiratory muscle weakness is suggested by a PI_{max} of less than -25 cm H_2O (normally near -125 cmH_2O). A severely impaired cough is suggested by a PE_{max} of less than $+40$ cmH_2O (normally $+200$ cmH_2O) (O'Donogue et al., 1976; Latimer et al., 1971).

Flow Volume Loops

Both the inspiratory and expiratory flow-volume relationships can be graphically displayed by what is termed a flow-volume loop (Fig. 23.4). Air flow from TLC is maximal at the beginning of forced exhalation where elastic traction of the alveolar septi on the airway is greatest, expiratory muscle strength is greatest, and airway resistance (R_{aw}) is lowest. Airway resistance increases as forced exhalation proceeds due to the progressive reduction in airway caliber (and elastic retraction) as lung volume falls. R_{aw} is, therefore, greatest at RV. This explains the shape of the flow-volume loop. Flow rate peaks early in expiration and then progressively decreases. At lower lung volumes, where air flow is mostly limited by airway resistance, the flow is said to be *effort independent*. Additional effort, which increases intrapleural pressure, theoretically increases the dynamic compression of the air-

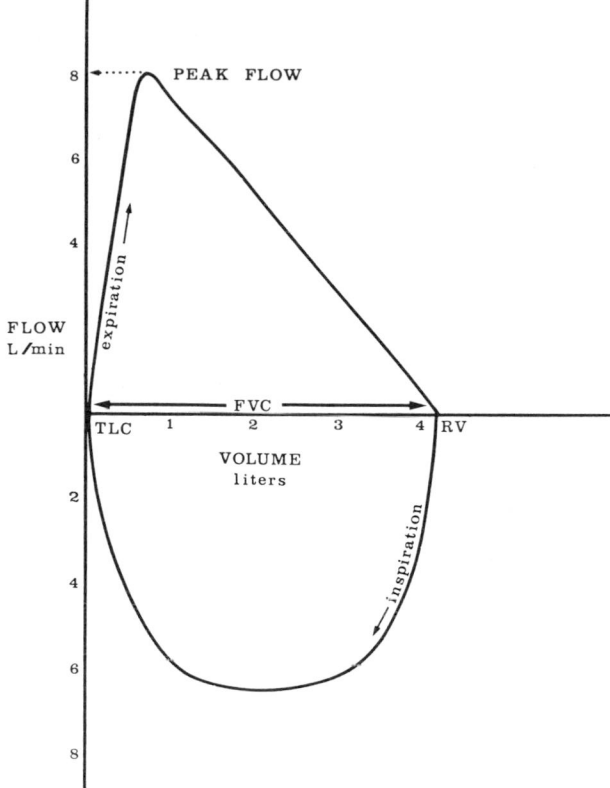

Fig. 23.4 Illustration of a normal flow volume loop. TLC = total lung capacity, RV = residual volume, FVC = forced vital capacity. Measurement of peak expiratory flow is shown.

ways and, therefore, increases airway resistance but fails to increase flow. Thus, the flow-volume loop is very characteristic in emphysema where this phenomenon is accentuated due to the destruction of alveolar walls (Fig. 23.5). The flow-volume loop also has a characteristic shape, in restrictive lung disease, and both intra and extra-thoracic fixed obstructing lesions of the trachea.

LUNG VOLUMES

In addition to the vital capacity which has already been described, several other lung volumes can be measured during spirometry. The *tidal volume* (TV) is the volume of air in a normal quiet breath. The additional maximal volume of air that can be exhaled between the end of tidal expiration to residual volume is the *expiratory reserve volume* (ERV). Likewise, the additional maximal volume of air that can be inhaled from the end of a tidal inspiration is the *inspiratory reserve volume* (IRV). The IRV and TV together make up the *inspiratory capacity* (IC) (*see* Fig. 23.1).

The remaining lung volumes which cannot be obtained from spirometry are measured by a combination of spirometric and inert gas dilution techniques. The *total lung capacity* (TLC) is the total

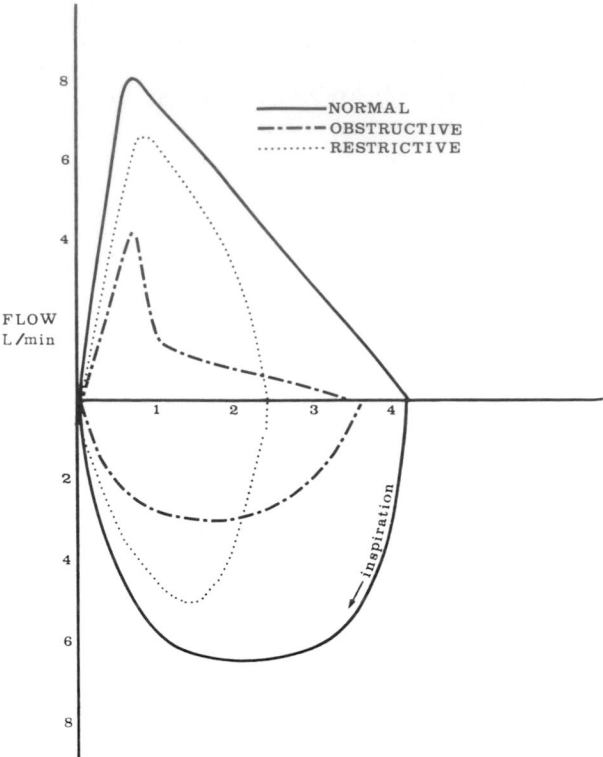

Fig. 23.5 Illustration contrasting a normal flow volume loop to the characteristic flow volume loops of obstructive ventilatory defects and restrictive ventilatory defects. Notice the extremely low flow rates in the obstructive ventilatory pattern.

amount of air in the lungs at maximal inspiration. The volume of air remaining in the lungs after maximal expiration is the *residual volume* (RV). Finally, the volume of air remaining in the lungs at the end of a tidal breath is the *functional residual capacity* (FRC). The FRC represents the *neutral position* between the chest wall, which tends to enlarge, and lung parenchyma which tends to collapse. The FRC is highly reproducible since it is measured at the point at which a subject normally breathes virtually without effort, namely, the end of a tidal breath. The TLC and RV are dependent upon a maximal inspiration or expiration and so are more effort dependent. The measurement of TLC and RV are based on the determination of FRC which is done by either an inert gas dilution technique (Helium dilution or nitrogen washout) or body plethysmography. Once the FRC is known, the TLC and RV are calculated as follows: FRC + IC = TLC and the FRC − ERV = RV. Inspiratory capacity and ERV are determined spirometrically with repeated efforts to ensure maximal values.

In the closed circuit *Helium Dilution Method*, the subject starts at FRC and begins rebreathing from an apparatus containing a known volume and concentration of helium, an inert non-absorbable gas. The exhaled CO_2 is absorbed from the system and oxygen

is added as needed to keep the patient-machine volume constant. After about seven minutes in normal subjects, equilibrium of the helium concentration is reached. The reduction in the concentration of helium from the original concentration is proportional to the volume of air in the lungs at FRC (the starting lung volume) which diluted it. A simple algebraic equation is used to solve for this volume and thus determine the FRC.

$$FRC = \frac{V(He_1 - He_2)}{He_2}$$

In the equation above, V is the volume of the apparatus including the dead-space of the apparatus, He_1 is the initial helium concentration and He_2 is the final helium concentration.

The open circuit *Nitrogen Washout Method* is based on the knowledge that when breathing room air, the concentration of nitrogen in the lungs is 79%. Beginning at FRC, nearly all the nitrogen in the lungs is washed out by having the subject breathe 100% oxygen. All exhaled breaths are collected in a bag, which is then analysed for nitrogen concentration and total volume. The product of nitrogen concentration in the bag (N_2final) and volume of the bag (V_2) will equal the product of FRC (the starting volume) and 79% (the initial concentration of N_2). The volume of FRC is solved in this way.

$$FRC = \frac{V_2 \times N_2 \text{final}}{N_2 \text{initial}}$$

Normally, nitrogen concentration in exhaled breaths at the end of the procedure reaches 2% or less, as measured by a rapid response nitrogen meter. If obstruction is present, the washout may be very slow and may not reach 2% by the end of seven minutes (the usual time for the test). This finding indicates maldistribution of inspired 100% O_2 and non-uniformity of mixing. In disease states where alveolar gas is completely trapped behind occluded airways, the gas dilution techniques will not give an accurate determination of FRC. This inaccuracy can occur in bullous emphysema, asthma, or endobronchial tumours. To determine true total thoracic gas volume (VTG), even in the presence of these diseases, body plethysmography is used.

Body plethysmography is based on Boyle's Law which states that the product of the pressure and volume of a given gas is constant. To perform the test, the subject sits in an airtight chamber, breathing through an airway connected to the outside. The relationship between pressure and volume changes in the chamber is determined by adding a known volume of air into the chamber and noting the increase in pressure. With the subject panting at FRC (a maneuver to keep the larynx widely open), the airway is occluded and pressure at the mouth and inside the box are simultaneously measured. Airway pressure is assumed to be equal to alveolar pressure. The ribcage expands and compresses the air in the chamber and so increases chamber pressure. The change in chamber volume, which is equal to the change in lung volume, is determined by the chamber pressure change. The beginning airway pressure is atmospheric pressure (P_1), and, since the change in lung volume ΔV) and the new airway pressure (P_2) are known, the starting lung volume (FRC) can be calculated. *Airway resistance* (R_{aw}) can also be calculated during the same procedure from changes in air flow and box pressure.

$$V_{TG} = FRC = \frac{P_2 \times (FRC + \Delta V)}{P_1}$$

Elevations of FRC represent hyperinflation which is frequently due to obstructive airway disease but also occurs with advancing age. One disadvantage of a high FRC during anesthesia is that it takes longer to attain the desired alveolar concentration of an inhaled gas due to dilutional factors. Conversely, low FRC invites atelectasis and hypoxemia.

Residual volume, FRC, and TLC are reduced in restrictive lung disease such as interstitial fibrosis and may also be reduced in congestive heart failure and atelectasis. Although RV may be reversibly increased in asthma, it is usually irreversibly increased in emphysema. Elevation of the RV/TLC ratio above the normal value of 20–35% occurs in emphysema at the expense of a reduction in VC. This alone is not diagnostic of emphysema, however, as it is also found in asthma and asymptomatic elderly subjects.

DIFFUSING CAPACITY

Although spirometry and lung volumes provide information concerning the size of the lungs and movement of air, they do not evaluate how well oxygen transfers (diffuses) from alveolar gas to the pulmonary capillary blood. This diffusing capacity depends not only upon the character of the alveolar-capillary membrane (Dm), but also upon the total effective surface area available for gas exchange, the volume of blood in the alveolar capillaries (V_c) the rate of combination of the gas with blood (θ), and cardiac output.

Because diffusing capacity of the lung for oxygen (D_LO_2) is technically difficult to perform, methods using low concentrations of carbon monoxide (CO) are employed. Carbon monoxide diffuses across the alveolar capillary membrane only 0.8 times as rapidly as oxygen, but its hemoglobin affinity is 200 times greater. The uptake of a known amount of carbon monoxide, over a known time period, at a known partial pressure, characterizes the diffusing capacity (D_LCO) in ml/(min·mmHg). The relationship of the factors determining D_LCO are expressed in the equation:

$$\frac{1}{D_LCO} = \frac{1}{D_m} + \frac{1}{\theta V_c}$$

In the *steady state or end-tidal* method, the inspired, expired, and alveolar (end tidal) CO concentrations are measured along with the minute ventilation during quiet steady-state breathing of a CO gas mixture and the D_LCO^{ss} is determined as follows:

$$D_LCO^{ss} =$$

$$\frac{(\text{Insp. \% CO} - \text{Exp. \% CO}) \text{ Minute Ventilation ml/min}}{(\text{End tidal \% CO}) (\text{Baro.Pres.mmHg})}$$

$$= ml/(min \cdot mmHg)$$

The numerator defines the amount of CO taken up in one minute and the denominator defines the CO gradient between alveolus and capillary. End-tidal CO is assumed to be equal to alveolar CO. Because CO has such high affinity for hemoglobin, the capillary/plasma CO partial pressure is virtually zero and so removed from the denominator.

In the *single breath* or *breath holding technique*, D_LCO is determined during a 10 second period of breath-holding at TLC following maximum inspiration (starting from RV) of a known concentration of a CO mixture. Similar values for calculation (inspired volume, inspired and expired CO%) are necessary as with the steady state method. To correct for the inspiratory-expiratory CO difference attributable to dilution from the air already in the patient's lung, a small volume of helium is added to the inspired sample. Since helium is not absorbed, knowing the inspired and expired concentrations of helium allows the determination of that dilution factor and, therefore, the total alveolar volume (V_A) with which the CO is mixed.

$$D_LCO^{SB} = \frac{\text{Insp. Vol} \times \frac{\text{Insp. \% He}}{\text{Exp. \% He}} \times 60}{\text{Baro.Press.(mmHg)} \times \text{time (s)}}$$

$$\times \ln \frac{\text{Insp. CO \%} \Big/ \frac{\text{Insp. \% He}}{\text{Exp. \% He}}}{\text{Exp. CO \%}}$$

The speed of uptake of CO then can be expressed separately and independently of lung volume by dividing the D_LCO by the alveolar volume as determined by the dilution of helium. This value called the K_{CO} or D_L/V_A and represents the diffusing capacity corrected for abnormally low or high lung volumes. The D_L/V_A ratio helps separate a low D_LCO due to actual impaired diffusion of gas from that simply due to reduced alveolar volume. For example, if the remaining lung after pneumonectomy is healthy, the D_L/V_A will be normal, even though D_LCO is reduced proportional to the reduced TLC. Therefore, D_L/V_A represents the functional integrity of the lung volume that is being ventilated.

Conditions resulting in reduced D_LCO and reduced D_L/V_A include emphysema, loss of capillary bed (pulmonary emboli, pulmonary vasculitis) and anemia. An increase in D_LCO accompanies polycythemia and other causes of increase in pulmonary capillary blood volume (left heart failure, exercise, anomalous pulmonary venous return, and left-to-right shunts). Since there is little or no parenchymal destruction in asthma or chronic bronchitis, the D_L/V_A in these conditions is usually normal. In summary, D_LCO is reflective of the lung surface area available for gas exchange, and the D_L/V_A is reflective of the diffusing capacity per liter of ventilated lung volume. Although not routinely used in the preoperative evaluation of pulmonary function, a D_LCO or D_L/V_A of less than 50% of that predicted suggests serious underlying parenchymal dysfunction.

TESTS OF EARLY AIRWAY DYSFUNCTION

Although tests of small airways disease are not as useful in preoperative evaluation of surgical candidates as other pulmonary function tests described, they add to a thorough understanding of lung disease in an earlier stage than usually detected. Measurement of *closing capacity* is such a test. It probably measures the lung volume at which the small (1–5 mm) airways in the dependent portions of the lungs begin to close. To perform the test, pure oxygen is inhaled from RV to TLC. As the breath is slowly exhaled, the concentration of nitrogen at the mouth is measured. The 'first in, last out' phenomenon of air distribution to the apices accounts for the results (Fig. 23.6). Phase I

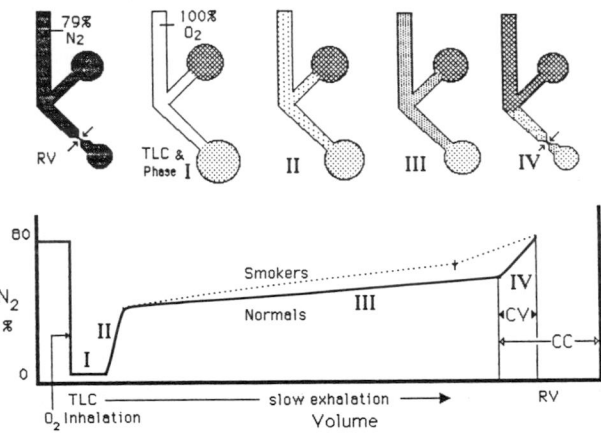

Fig. 23.6 Illustration of the determination of closing volume and closing capacity after inhalation to TLC of 100% O_2. Relative concentrations of N_2 and O_2 in apical and dependent alveoli are depicted during Phase I, II, III, and IV and relate to N_2 concentration in the corresponding phase on the graph (*see* text).

represents pure O_2 exhaled from the dead space of the trachea and airways. In phase II, the alveoli begin to empty. Uniform emptying of alveoli which all contain a mixture of the inhaled O_2 and residual nitrogen left in the alveoli accounts for the gradually rising N_2 concentration of phase III. Because the alveoli at the apices of the lung at RV are larger than those at the bases, the concentration of N_2 in apical alveoli after

the inhalation of pure O_2 to TLC will be higher. When the airways in the dependent areas begin to close, the contribution of N_2 from the apical areas then increases. This is seen as an abrupt rise in nitrogen concentration and indicates the point called the closing capacity (CC). The volume from the CC to RV is the *closing volume*. Increased CC has been noted in smokers and is thought to represent small airways disease. Others feel it represents decreased elastic recoil (Hoeppner et al., 1974), similar to changes accompanying aging; Hoeppner et al., 1974c; Turner et al., 1968). These changes can occur long before reduction in FEV$_1$ and may be a prelude to worsening obstructive lung disease. Whereas the concept of closing volume has merit in explaining atelectasis and hypoxemia at low lung volume, its actual measurement does not appear to be of great value.

The same procedure for measuring the closing capacity can be used in a different way and yield additional information on the presence of small airways dysfunction and maldistribution of ventilation. In the *single breath nitrogen washout*, a line is drawn through phase III. Normally, there is less than 2% increase in N_2 per liter of exhaled volume along this line. Smokers and patients with obstructive airways disease may have a much greater increase in percent N_2 per liter indicating uneven distribution of the inspired oxygen. Buist and Ross, 1973c, (Fig. 23.6). If pure O_2 is inhaled and expiratory N_2 measured in the *multiple breath nitrogen washout* test, an exponential washout curve is normally seen when end tidal N_2 is plotted against cumulative expired volume. Deviation from this normal slope indicates poor ventilation in some areas of the lung.

In larger airways, where resistance to flow is due to convective acceleration and turbulence, flow is dependent upon the density of the gas. Since resistance to flow at 50% VC is mostly due to these larger airways, the maximum flow at 50% of VC ($\dot{V}_{max}50\%$) will increase if a helium-O_2 mixture is breathed. Flow is more laminar in the small airways, and therefore, less density dependent. Due to changes in the small airways in smokers, the effect of small airways resistance will be greater than normal at 50% VC. Therefore, breathing a helium-O_2 mixture will result in a smaller increase in $\dot{V}_{max}50\%$. The lowest lung volume at which breathing a He-O_2 mixture increases flow is called the *volume of isoflow* ($V_{iso}\dot{V}$) and is expressed as a percentage of VC. This volume can be increased in asymptomatic smokers to 25% (normally 10–15%) due to changes in small airways (Dosmann et al., 1975). However, it should be noted that like closing volume, these studies have not proven prognostic of obstructive airways disease.

Alveoli in different areas of lung may empty and fill at different rates due to local differences in compliance and resistance. They are said to have different time constants. Because of this difference, compliance (dynamic) at faster rates of breathing may be reduced. If dynamic compliance during increasing respiratory rates falls to less than 80% of static compliance, it is considered 'frequency dependent'. *Frequency-dependence-of compliance* is thought to be the most specific test of small airways dysfunction.

INTERPRETATION OF PFTs

Interpretation of these multiple tests with their letter abbreviations may strike the uninitiated as an insurmountable task. There are, however, short cuts for deciphering even the most complicated PFT report.

1. Look for the lung volumes (FRC, TLC, RV) first.
   a. If they are above normal ($>120\%$ predicted), consider hyperinflation, possibly secondary to obstructive airways disease.
   b. If they are below normal ($<80\%$ predicted), consider restriction, possibly secondary to lung or chest wall stiffness.
2. Look at spirometry (FVC, FEV_1, FEV_1/FVC, FEF_{25-75}) next.
   a. If the FEV_1, FEV_1/FVC ratio and FEF_{25-75} are reduced, this confirms your suspicion of an obstructive defect.
   b. If the FEV_1, FEV_1/FVC ratio, and FEF_{25-75} are normal, this confirms your suspicion of pure restriction, if lung volume is reduced (1b above).
   c. If hyperinflation is not accompanied by flow rate reduction, or if restriction *is* accompanied by flow rate reductions, consider technical problems or mixed defects.
3. Look last at diffusing capacity D_L/V_A.
   a. If there is hyperinflation and airflow obstruction, a reduced D_L/V_A suggests emphysema, a normal D_L/V_A bronchitis, and an elevated D_L/V_A asthma.
   b. If there is restriction, a reduced D_L/V_A suggests fibrosis/vasculitis, and a normal D_L/V_A suggests a pleural/muscular/chest wall cause of the loss of volume.

Preoperative PFTs

Although some investigators have found certain pulmonary function studies to be more reliable than routine clinical appraisal in predicting postoperative complications. (Stein et al., 1962), the routine use of PFTs in every operative candidate is not indicated. As mentioned in the introduction, history and physical examination will usually identify which patients require PFTs (*see* Table 23.1). Risk of postoperative complications depends not only upon the patient's predisposing medical condition, but also upon the site of surgery. Upper abdominal and lung resectional surgery clearly pose a greater risk than lower abdominal or extra-thoracic surgery (Ford et al., 1983).

The exact risk of postoperative pulmonary complications rises to as high as 100% when FVC is $<70\%$ predicted and FEV_1/FVC ratio is $<65\%$ (Latimer et al., 1971). These complication rates, of course, depend

TABLE 23.1
INDICATIONS FOR PREOPERATIVE PFTS

1. Planned thoracic surgery.
2. Planned abdominal surgery.
3. Morbid obesity.
4. Age >70.
5. Heavy smoking and cough.
6. Known pulmonary disease.

Adapted from Tisi and Gennaro, 1979.

on how 'postoperative complication' is defined. For example, a post-cholecystectomy reduction in lung volume or Pa_{O_2}, which is asymptomatic and does not lengthen hospital stay, could be called a 'finding' rather than a complication. A 'complication', therefore, would indicate a condition which causes symptoms, threatens life, or lengthens hospitalization.

Along with a reduced FVC, a reduction of MVV and FEF_{25-75} to $<50\%$ predicted, suggests a high risk for development of complications (Gracey et al., 1979). The MVV may be predictive, not only because it reflects flow rate and muscle strength, but also reflects intangible characteristics such as stamina and cooperation as well. A peak flow rate of <200 liters per minute is associated with a 66% incidence of postoperative pulmonary complications (Stein et al., 1962). It may be predictive, in part, because it reflects the ability to cough adequately and, therefore, move secretions. Risk is likewise increased if FEV_1 is $<70\%$ predicted. Complication rates can be improved from 60 to 22% if bronchodilators, antibiotics, and chest physiotherapy are instituted preoperatively to patients at increased risk (Gracey et al., 1979; Stein et al., 1970). Patients with carbon dioxide retention (which may not always be suspected clinically) are at markedly increased risk of serious intraoperative and postoperative respiratory difficulties as well (Stein et al., 1962).

Unlike the suggested utility of preoperative PFTs in upper abdominal surgery, their role in open heart surgery is unclear and they may not be predictive of pulmonary complications after cardiovascular surgery (Cain et al., 1979).

There is, however, general agreement that spirometric data can identify patients at high risk of cardiopulmonary complications following lung resection. The routine pulmonary function criteria indicating tolerance of lung resection (up to and including pneumonectomy) include an FEV_1 greater than 2 litres (or greater than 50% of the FVC), an FVC $>50\%$ predicted, MVV $>50\%$ predicted, and RV/TLC ratio $<50\%$ (Olsen et al., 1975). If these criteria are not met, the following *split function* studies are commonly performed before the patient is denied surgery.

Both ventilation, (Kristersson et al., 1972) and perfusion lung radionuclide scans, (Olsen et al., 1974) are predictive of postpneumonectomy pulmonary function. The contribution of each lung can be measured by quantifying the radioactivity from each hemithorax and determining the percentage of the total radioactivity count from each. If pneumonectomy is planned, predicted postoperative FVC and FEV_1 are calculated by multiplying preoperative values by the percentage of total radioactivity emanating from the uninvolved lung. These predicted values correlate well with actual postoperative findings. A predicted postoperative FEV_1 of >0.8 liters is acceptable for surgery (Olsen et al., 1975). Below this level, hypercapnea is more likely and pneumonectomy is not recommended.

A pulmonary vascular resistance above 190 $dyn \cdot s \cdot cm^{-5}$ with exercise may identify increased post thoracotomy operative risk (Fee et al., 1975). In an even more invasive technique, temporary unilateral pulmonary artery occlusion, a balloon-tipped cardiac catheter is used to occlude the pulmonary artery of the lung to be resected (Olsen et al., 1975). High risk and physiologic inoperability are suggested by findings of a Pa_{O_2} <45 mmHg and mean pulmonary artery pressure >35 mmHg on exercise. However, in contrast to findings in these earlier studies, a more recent study suggests that ventilatory insufficiency and pulmonary hypertension do not seem to be the most important physiologic abnormalities uncovered by exercise testing (Olsen et al., 1989). In this study, exercise cardiac index, O_2 delivery and calculated O_2 uptake were the best predictors of intolerance of lung resection. Maximum oxygen uptake on progressive exercise has been suggested as being useful for predicting post thoracotomy risk by other authors as well (Smith et al., 1984). Therefore, surgical intolerance may relate most closely to reduced oxygen transport mechanisms. These studies are not done routinely, however, due to the invasiveness and difficulty of the procedures.

For an overview and more detailed study of pulmonary function testing we suggest several authoritative references (Black and Hyatt, 1969; Comroe et al., 1962; Cotes, 1979; Forster et al., 1986).

REFERENCES

Black L.F., Hyatt R.E. (1969). Maximal respiratory pressures: normal values and relationships to age and sex. *Am. Rev. Respir. Dis.*, **99**, 696.

Buist A.S., Ross B.B. (1973). Quantitative analysis of the alveolar plateau in the diagnosis of early airway obstruction. *Am. Rev. Respir. Dis.*, **108**, 1078.

Cain H.D., Stevens P.M., Adaniya R. (1979). Preoperative pulmonary function and complications after cardiovascular surgery. *Chest*, **76**, 130.

Comroe J.H., Forster R.E., Dubois A.B., et al. (1962). *The Lung*. 2nd edn. Chicago: Year Book Medical Publishers, Inc.

Cotes J.E. (1979). *Lung Function, Assessment and Application in Medicine*. 4th edn. Oxford: Blackwell Scientific Publications.

Dosmann J., Bode F., Urbanetti J., et al. (1975). The use of a helium oxygen mixture during maximum expiratory flow to demonstrate obstruction in small airways in smokers. *J. Clin. Invest.*, **55**, 1090.

Fee J.H., Holmes E.C., Gewirtz H.S., et al. (1975). Role of pulmonary vascular resistance measurements in preoperative evaluation of candidates for pulmonary resection. *J. Thoracic Cardiovasc. Surg.*, **75**, 519.

Ford F.T., Whitelaw W.A., Rosenal T.W., et al. (1983). Diaphragm function after upper abdominal surgery in humans. *Am. Rev. Respir. Dis.*, **127**, 431.

Forster R.E. II, Dubois A.B., Briscoe W.A., et al. (1986). *The Lung, Physiologic Basis of Pulmonary Function Tests*. 3rd edn. Chicago: Year Book Medical Publishers, Inc.

Gass G.D., Olsen G.N. (1986). Preoperative pulmonary function testing to predict postoperative morbidity and mortality. *Chest*, **89**, 127.

Gracey D.R., Divertie M.B., Didier E.P. (1979). Preoperative pulmonary preparation of patients with chronic obstructive disease. *Chest*, **76**, 123.

Hoeppner V.H., Cooper D.M., Zamel N., et al. (1974). Relationship between elastic recoil and closing volume in smokers and non-smokers. *Am. Rev. Respir. Dis.*, **109**, 81.

Kristersson S., Lindell S., Sranberg L. (1972). Prediction of pulmonary function loss due to pneumonectomy using 133-Xe-radiospirometry. *Chest*, **62**, 694.

Latimer R.G., Dickman M., Day W.C., et al. (1971). Ventilatory patterns and pulmonary complications after upper abdominal surgery determined by preoperative and postoperative computerized spirometry and blood gas analysis. *Am. J. Surg.*, **122**, 622.

McFadden E.R., Kiker R., Holmes B., et al. (1974). Small airway disease. An assessment of the tests of peripheral airway function. *Am. J. Med.*, **57**, 171.

O'Donogue W.J., Baker J.P., Bell R.M., et al. (1976). Respiratory failure in neuromuscular disease, management in a respiratory intensive care unit. *JAMA.*, **235**, 733.

Olsen G.N., Block A.J., Swenson E.W., et al. (1975). Pulmonary function evaluation of the lung resection candidate: a prospective study. *Am. Rev. Respir. Dis.*, **111**, 379.

Olsen G.N., Block A.J., Tobias J.A. (1974). Prediction of postpneumonectomy pulmonary function using quantitative macroaggregate lung scanning. *Chest*, **66**, 13.

Olsen G.N., Weiman D.S., Bolton J.W.R., et al. (1989). Submaximal invasive exercise testing and quantitative lung scanning in the evaluation for tolerance of lung resection. *Chest*, **95**, 267.

Smith T.P., Kinasewitz G.T., Tucker W.Y., et al. (1984). Exercise capacity as a predictor of post-thoracotomy morbidity. *Am. Rev. Respir. Dis.*, **129**, 730.

Stein M., Cassara E.L. (1970). Preoperative pulmonary evaluation and therapy for surgery patients. *JAMA*, **211**, 787.

Stein M., Koota G.M., Simon M., et al. (1962). Pulmonary evaluation of surgical patients. *JAMA*, **181**, 765.

Tisi G.M., Gennaro M. (1979). Preoperative evaluation of pulmonary function. *Am. Rev. Respir. Dis.*, **119**, 293.

Turner J.M., Mead J., Wohl M.E. (1968). Elasticity of human lungs in relation to age. *J. Appl. Physiol.*, **25**, 664.

Zamel N., Altose M.D., Speir W.A. (1983). Statement on spirometry (a report on the section on respiratory pathophysiology, ACCP). *Chest*, **83**, 547.

24. Oxygen Therapy
Julian M. Leigh

Oxygen fulfils its metabolic role at the mitochondrial level. The inspired oxygen tension represents the highest values in a descending sequence of oxygen tensions concerned with delivering oxygen to this site (Fig. 24.1).

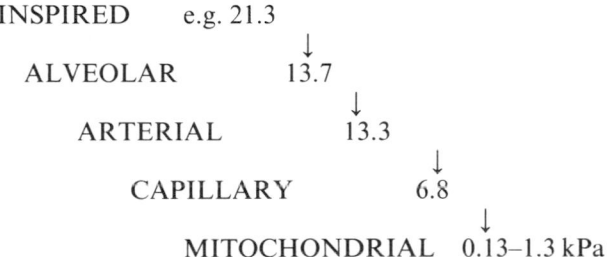

INSPIRED   e.g. 21.3

ALVEOLAR   13.7

ARTERIAL   13.3

CAPILLARY   6.8

MITOCHONDRIAL   0.13–1.3 kPa

Fig. 24.1 The oxygen cascade, with examples of oxygen tension at each stage. Note how small the mitochondrial oxygen tension is.

Various factors operate at each stage in this 'oxygen cascade' to reduce oxygen tension. Should the inspired tension be low or the gradient at any stage be steeper than usual, it may be combated by raising the inspired oxygen tension and thus raising the driving pressure at the beginning of the cascade.

In general, the further down the cascade is the lesion to be treated, then the higher the inspired oxygen tension that is necessary. Campbell (1965) has computed the increases in oxygen content of arterial blood per 1% rise in inspired oxygen concentration, for lesions at different sites (Table 24.1).

The Concept of Tissue Oxygen Availability

It is very useful to consider the total quantity of oxy-

TABLE 24.1
CHANGES IN OXYGEN CONTENT OF ARTERIAL BLOOD FOR
DEFECTS AFFECTING OXYGENATION
(Based on Campbell, 1965)

Lesion	*Changes in O_2 content per 1% rise in inspired oxygen concentration*
Low inspired O_2 concentration	3.0 ml/100 ml
Decreased alveolar ventilation	3.0 ml/100 ml
Venous admixture	0.02 ml/100 ml
Low haemoglobin	0.04 ml/100 ml
CO haemoglobinaemia	0.03 ml/100 ml
Methaemoglobinaemia	0.03 ml/100 ml
Low cardiac output	0.03 ml/100 ml
Poisoning of cell enzymes	0.03 ml/100 ml

gen which is theoretically available to the tissues per minute. This concept was first developed by Richards (1943) and further elaborated by Freeman and Nunn (1963). It is simply the product of arterial oxygen content and cardiac output per minute ($\dot{Q}$):

Available O_2/min =
$$(\text{Hb content} + \text{plasma content}) \times \dot{Q}$$

This expression may be fully formulated as:

Available O_2/min =

$$\left(\frac{1.39 \times \text{Hb} \times Sa_{O_2}}{100} + 0.0225 \times Pa_{O_2} \right) \times \frac{\dot{Q}\,\text{ml}}{100}$$

where,

1.39 = oxygen capacity of haemoglobin in ml/g calculated for a molecular weight of haemoglobin of 64 458.

Hb = measured haemoglobin content in g/100 ml of whole blood.

Sa_{O_2} = percentage oxygen saturation of the haemoglobin in arterial blood.

0.0225 = ml of oxygen dissolved in the plasma of 100 ml of whole blood/kPa applied oxygen tension.

Pa_{O_2} = measured arterial oxygen tension in kPa.

Consideration of some real values helps to highlight the usefulness of this concept, e.g.

Available O_2/min

$$= \left(\frac{1.39 \times 14.5 \times 97.5}{100} + 0.0225 \times 13.3 \right) \times \frac{5000}{100}$$

$$= (19.7 + 0.3) \times 50$$

$$= 985 + 15$$

$$= 1000 \text{ ml/min}$$

Notice how small the plasma contribution is relative to that from haemoglobin, due to the properties of the haemoglobin dissociation curve.

Suppose the patient under consideration has an

oxygen consumption of 250 ml/min. Then his 'coefficient of utilization' of oxygen will be.

$$\frac{250}{1000} \text{ or } 25\%$$

Now, suppose we choose some values of haemoglobin and cardiac output which are lower, but by no means unreasonable, and at the same time permit the arterial oxygen tension to fall to 8 kPa (60 mmHg) (91% saturation); then,

Available O_2/min

$$= \left(\frac{1.39 \times 10 \times 91}{100} + 0.0225 \times 8\right) \times \frac{3000}{100}$$
$$= (12.65 + 0.18) \times 30$$
$$= 379.5 + 5.4$$
$$= 385 \text{ ml/min}$$

If we still assume an oxygen consumption of 250 ml/min then the 'coefficient of utilization' of oxygen has become

$$\frac{250}{385} \text{ or } 65\%$$

If is now obvious that the safety margins are considerably reduced. A further loss of haemoglobin, fall in cardiac output or increase in oxygen consumption, e.g., due to shivering, would place this patient in jeopardy. Such a state of affairs is not uncommon in the early postoperative phase.

Furthermore, where there is a high coefficient of utilization of oxygen, more tissues will be relatively hypoxic necessitating anaerobic glycolysis and thus producing metabolic acidosis. The latter will move the oxyhaemoglobin dissociation curve to the right, i.e., a higher oxygen tension will then be required to produce the same percentage oxygen saturation of haemoglobin. Also, acidosis has a deleterious effect on cardiac contractility and thus on cardiac output. Acidosis therefore has an extremely adverse effect on oxygen availability and may constitute part of a vicious spiral with fatal consequences, if untreated.

A full appreciation of the concepts embodied in the oxygen availability expression and in the 'coefficient of utilization' of oxygen is an invaluable aid to patient management. The relevant points may be summarized:

Factors Reducing Oxygen Availability

1. Low arterial oxygen content

   low Sa_{O_2} $\begin{cases} \text{low} Pa_{O_2} \\ \text{acidosis} \end{cases}$

   low haemoglobin $\begin{cases} \text{anaemia} \\ \text{CO Hb} \\ \text{Met Hb} \end{cases}$

2. Low cardiac output

Factors Increasing Oxygen Requirement
(raising the coefficient of utilization)

1. Shivering
2. Oxygen cost of increased ventilatory effort or tachycardia
3. Pyrexia

Measures to Increase Oxygen Availability

1. Raise arterial oxygen tension
2. Raise haemoglobin content
3. Alleviate acidosis
4. Increase cardiac output

Measures to Reduce Oxygen Requirements

1. Paralysis and IPPV
2. Digitalization
3. Prevention of hyperthermia
4. In extreme circumstances induction of hypothermia, e.g., at 30°C oxygen requirement is 40% of normal

Shifts of the Oxygen Dissociation Curve

Shifts of the oxyhaemoglobin dissociation curve make no difference to *oxygen loading*, provided that the arterial point is on the flat-top segment. Once the arterial point is on the steep segment then oxygen loading is adversely affected by a right shift, as already indicated. Conversely, since oxygen unloading always tends to be on the steep segment, a right shift favours oxygen delivery to the tissues as the haemoglobin is capable of unloading more oxygen at a given P_{O_2}. The position of the steep segment thus reflects the affinity of oxygen for haemoglobin.

It has become fashionable to describe the position of the dissociation curve in terms of a single coordinate, *viz.*, the tension at which 50% saturation of the haemoglobin occurs—the P_{50}—which has a normal value of 3.5 kPa. Thus an increase in P_{50} indicates a low affinity of haemoglobin for oxygen.

Factors which Increase P_{50}

1. An increase in [H^+],
2. An increase in the intracellular organic phosphate ester 2,3-diphosphoglycerate (DPG) which is generated by the anaerobic glycolytic pathway. DPG binds to haemoglobin and reduces its affinity for oxygen. The level of DPG is increased by a fall in intracellular pH and increasing levels of reduced haemoglobin. Thus, increasing oxygen extraction from the erythrocyte favours the production of DPG, and further enhances oxygen release.

All the factors which are concerned in tissue oxygen supply are summarized diagrammatically in Fig. 24.2.

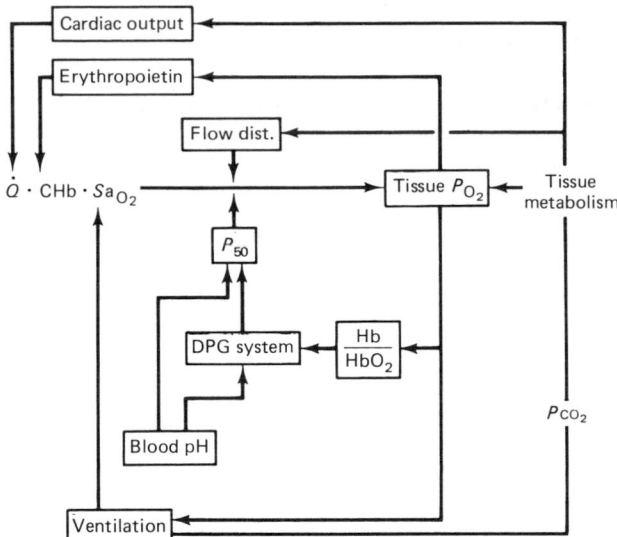

Fig. 24.2 Factors concerned in tissue oxygen supply. Modified from Finch and Lenfant (1972).

ALTERNATIVE OXYGEN TRANSPORT MEDIA

Because of the relatively short shelf life of blood, its antigenicity, the formation of micro-aggregates and the possibility of the transmission of disease, oxygen transporting blood substitutes are of current interest (Faithfull, 1987). Purified crystalline haemoglobin and perfluorochemicals (PFC's) have been investigated.

Crystalline Haemoglobin

Purified crystalline haemoglobin has a shelf life of two years, is not antigenic, and requires no cross-matching. Because it is separated from DPG it has a higher affinity for oxygen with a P_{50} of 14 mmHg (1.9 kPa). Additionally it has a half-life of only four hours being cleared by glomerular filtration. If the haemoglobin is combined by pyridoxalation the P_{50} becomes normal and, if it is also polymerized with glutaraldehyde, the half-life can be prolonged to 25 hours with a P_{50} of 19–22 mmHg (2.5–2.9 kPa) without altering oncotic pressure. Alternatively, pyridoxalated haemoglobin has been encapsulated in liposomes giving a half-life of six hours with a normal P_{50}. These compounds are cleared by tissue binding and reticulo-endothelial uptake. Further developments, however, await clarification of the significance firstly of this endothelial uptake, and secondly, the effect of pure haemoglobin in impairing granulocyte chemotaxis and phagocytosis.

Perfluorochemicals (PFC's)

PFC's are immiscible and are therefore used as emulsions. The pure product can dissolve up to 40 vols. of

O_2%. Commercial products contain 20% PFCs, the rest of the formulation including emulsifiers, heta-starch, electrolytes and glucose. The PFC is supplied frozen and is reconstituted with the other ingredients prior to use.

The PFCs also have a high uptake by the reticulo-endothelial system which may have significance in reducing the ability of this system to deal with infection. PFCs have a higher affinity for oxygen than plasma: O_2 content of 100 ml PFC = 5.5 ml at 550 mmHg (73 kPa). However oxygen transport will depend on the 'fluorocrit'. In practice the dilution in the blood stream means that the patient is 'fluoro-carbonanaemic' and oxygen transport can only be enhanced by very high arterial oxygen tensions. PFC products thus need to be improved.

Micro-circulatory support by PFCs

As blood viscosity varies with shear rate, it is markedly increased under the low flow conditions existing in the micro-circulation in shock states. The viscosity of PFC emulsions is almost independent of shear rate, and so an increased tissue blood flow should be obtained for the same blood pressure. It has been calculated that normal, whole body oxygen flux can be maintained after replacement of 30% of blood volume with commercially available PFC solution. It may be that small particles of PFCs can penetrate deep into hypoxic tissues by-passing sludged cells resulting in re-oxygenation and a renewal of the flexibility of red cell envelopes. PFC may also have useful anti-inflammatory effects by their action on neutrophils and they might promote, for example, increased myocardial salvage and protection against reperfusion syndrome. Protection may also be enhanced in cerebral ischaemia, either local or global. By the same token they may also be useful for acute sickle cell crisis, peripheral vascular disease and intestinal ischaemia. PFCs are also *radio-opaque*, and therefore the oxygenated product may be available in radiology, for example in coronary angiography, and during coronary angioplasty. Additionally, reticuloendothelial uptake facilitates experimental imaging of hepatic and splenic structures.

In conclusion it would appear that modified crystalline haemoglobin will probably be more useful for oxygen transport, whereas PFCs are more likely to be useful for micro-circulatory support.

OXYGEN THERAPY

The object of oxygen therapy is to raise tissue oxygen tension. The only route is the arterial blood. Except for patients on cardio-pulmonary bypass or extracorporeal membrane oxygenator the only access to the arterial blood is via the alveolar-capillary membrane and thence via the inspired gas mixture. Adequate alveolar ventilation is therefore a necessary prerequisite.

A rise in inspired oxygen tension may be achieved either,

1. by raising inspired oxygen concenration (F_{IO_2}),
2. by raising the total atmospheric pressure and thus secondarily affecting P_{IO_2}, or
3. both the above.

Oxygen Therapy at Ambient Pressure is achieved by the application of suitable apparatus to the patient and this chapter deals with the resultant effects on the gas phase. It is not intended to review the history, indications or physiological effects of oxygen therapy. For the historical aspects, the reader is referred to Barach (1962) and Leigh (1974); for the rationale of oxygen therapy to Flenley (1967, 1978) and Campbell and Minty (1978); and for a review of concepts in oxygen transport to Finch and Lenfant (1972).

Basic Requirements

The basic requirements for oxygen therapy equipment were stated by Barach and Eckman (1941) as:

1. Control over oxygen percentage of the inspired gas
2. Prevention of excessive accumulation of carbon dioxide
3. Elimination of resistance to breathing
4. Efficiency and economy in the use of oxygen
5. Adaptability of the apparatus for helium and oxygen therapy, to which one might add, adaptability for administration of gases or vapours for analgesia.

Many devices in current use were not in fact designed to meet these requirements. However, awareness of the performance characteristics of the various devices enables more appropriate selection in a given clinical situation.

With devices which operate on the air admixture principle, the inspired oxygen concentration achieved by a particular oxygen flow may be affected by a variety of factors which differ from patient to patient resulting in *between patient* variation of inspired oxygen concentrations. While the likely range of oxygen concentrations to be expected for a given oxygen flow may be stated by the manufacturer or obtained from the literature, the gas phase performance of such a device in a particular patient under specific clinical conditions cannot necessarily be predicted. Furthermore, since the flow and time characteristics of ventilation are not necessarily constant in a specific patient, there is *within patient* variation of inspired oxygen concentration on a breath to breath basis.

User Demands

The minimum 'user demands' asked of any oxygen therapy system must be: *what is the inspired oxygen concentration?* and *what is the inspired carbon dioxide concentration?* The latter is influenced by that part of the previous expirate which is reinhaled, i.e., the functional apparatus dead space.

These primary considerations are influenced by both patient and device factors. The important patient factors are the inspiratory flow rate and the duration of the expiratory pause. The device factors are physical volume, oxygen flow rate and vent resistance where appropriate.

Ventilatory Flow

An appreciation of the flow pattern of spontaneous ventilation is important when considering the interaction of these various factors. Figure 24.3 shows the

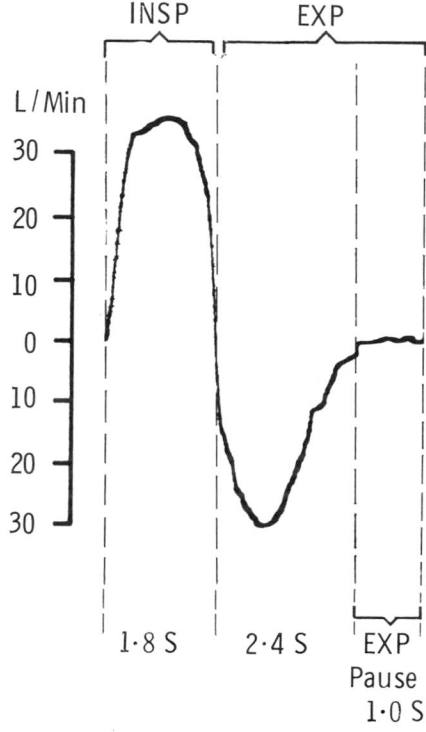

Fig. 24.3 One respiratory cycle from the pneumotachograph of a resting healthy male subject.

flow pattern obtained with a pneumotachograph, of one respiratory cycle of a resting healthy subject. Inspiratory flow is sinusoidal. Expiratory flow reaches a peak in a similar time but then decreases more slowly. There are three time intervals during each cycle, *viz.*, inspiratory time, expiratory time and expiratory pause time. The latter is characterized by 'no flow'. Figure 24.4a is from the same tracing. This may be contrasted with Fig. 24.4b which is from the same subject following exertion. Note the increase in peak inspiratory flow rate and the reduction in inspiratory and expiratory time, with the virtual absence of an

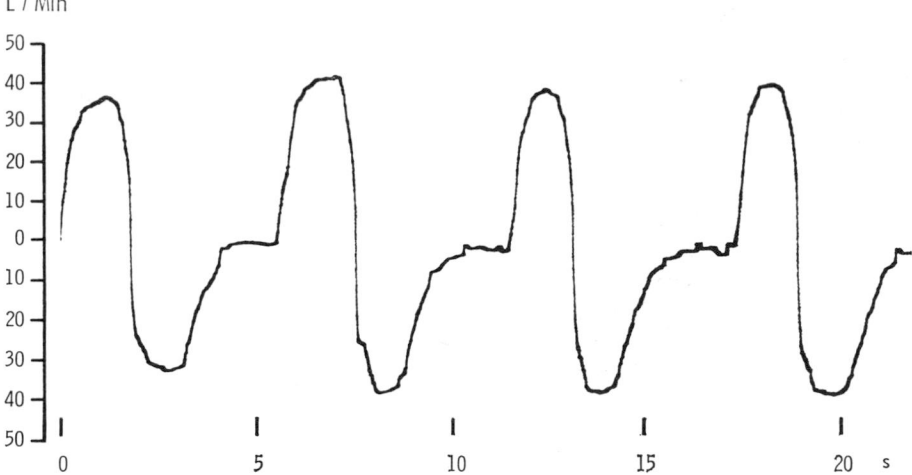

Fig. 24.4a Pneumotachograph of a resting healthy subject.

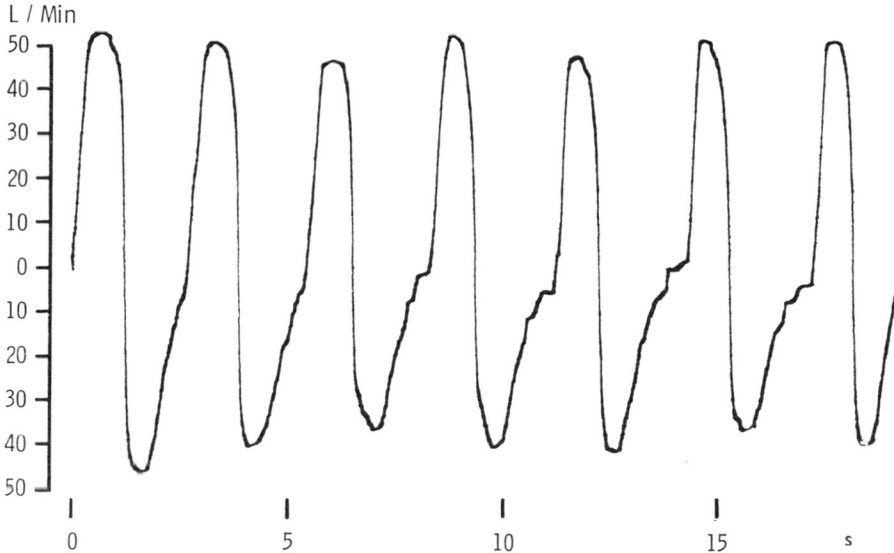

Fig. 24.4b Pneumotachograph of the same subject in a 'breathless' state. Note the increase in peak inspiratory flow rate and the decrease in the time intervals.

expiratory pause. The significance of these changes will be apparent as the discussion progresses.

Methods of Oxygen Therapy

On the basis of an evaluation using the applied theory of the O_2/CO_2 diagram, Leigh (1970) subdivided the methods of oxygen therapy into *fixed performance* and *variable performance* systems. The former will give a controlled oxygen concentration independent of patient factors. The latter constitute air-oxygen admixture systems in which oxygen is supplied at a rate much less than inspiratory flow rate; performance is thus dependent upon their interrelationship with the patient.

Not all the patient and device factors, indicated above, are operative in all the systems which are available for oxygen therapy. It is first necessary to classify fully the mode of operation of the various systems and then consider the role of the operative factors in each case. The classification is based on the technique of expired gas analysis outlined above and is given together with examples of devices in current use in British practice.

Sub-Classification of Devices

Fixed performance systems: independent of patient factors

1. *High Flow*—Ventimasks and other venturi operated devices
2. *Low Flow*—Anaesthetic circuits

Variable performance systems: patient dependent

1. *No capacity system:* inspired oxygen subject to between patient variation: oxygen catheters or nasal cannulae at *low* oxygen flows.
2. *Capacity system:* inspired oxygen subject to both between and within patient variation.
   (a) *Small capacity system:*
      - For O_2 only—catheters or cannulae at higher O_2 flows.
      - For both O_2 and CO_2 (i.e. with rebreathing)—M.C., Harris and Edinburgh masks.
   (b) *Large capacity system:*
      For both O_2 and CO_2 (i.e. with rebreathing)—Pneumask Polymask, Oxyaire, BLB and Portogen.
      Oxygen tent and incubator.

Fixed Performance Systems

The fixed performance devices, when used in the proper manner, supply the predetermined oxygen concentration irrespective of the characteristics of the patient's ventilation.

As inspiratory flow is sinusoidal in character, a fixed concentration system must be capable of delivering the chosen mixture at a rate equal to or greater than peak inspiratory flow rate. When breathing from an anaesthetic circuit this criterion is satisfied since any flow can be met by collapse of the reservoir bag during inspiration. If there were no reservoir bag in a circuit, the fresh gas inflow would have to be greater than or equal to inspiratory flow at all times in order to ensure fixed performance. This state of affairs is precisely that which occurs with the Ventimasks. With anaesthetic circuits, volume demands by the patient are met by collection of gas in the reservoir bag during expiration. Any desired mixture can be given by this technique, but anaesthetic circuits are impractical for clinical oxygen therapy in conscious patients.

Although the high flow system is much less economical, it has distinct advantages, *viz.*, rebreathing is minimized and so is the need for a tight fit to the face.

The high flow system with a variable venturi can be used to provide any required mixture without rebreathing.

Ventimasks have been investigated by Bethune and Collis (1967a) and when oxygen is given at the proper flowrate, functional apparatus dead space is eliminated. Anaesthetic circuits have only been mentioned for completeness since it is with them that anaesthetists habitually give oxygen mixtures. Their functional dead space characteristics are, however, more complex.

Other oxygen therapy devices operating on the venturi principle are available and their performance has been reviewed by Cox and Gillbe (1982). In principle these devices have a smaller mask shell than the Ventimask and are subject to a fall in inspired oxygen if the patient has a high peak flow. Under such circum-

stances this defect can be remedied simply by increasing the oxygen supply to the venturi which increases the total mixture flow to the patient. As the entrainment ratio remains the same, constant performance is assured.

Variable Performance Systems

These may give 21–100% oxygen depending upon the interrelationship of oxygen flow, device factors and patient factors.

No Capacity System. With nasal or transtracheal nasopharyngeal delivery at low oxygen flows, there is not sufficient storage of oxygen in the airway during the expiratory pause significantly to affect the next inspiration. Enrichment is then a pure function of inspiratory flow rate and oxygen flow rate.

In an air-oxygen mixture the total quantity of oxygen present is the sum of:

$$\text{Vol } O_2 \text{ from air} + \text{Vol } O_2 \text{ added}$$

and the concentration of oxygen (F_{IO_2}) in the mixture is given by the ratio of that volume to the total volume:

$$\frac{\text{Vol } O_2 \text{ from air} + \text{Vol } O_2 \text{ added}}{\text{Vol air} + \text{Vol } O_2}$$

therefore

$$F_{IO_2} = \frac{(\text{Vol air} \times 0.2093) + (\text{Vol } O_2 \times 1.0)}{\text{Vol air} + \text{Vol } O_2} \quad \text{(i)}$$

where 0.2093 and 1.0 are the fractional concentrations of oxygen in air and pure oxygen, respectively.

During inspiration tidal volume is acquired as the integral of flow and time. As inspiratory flow is sinusoidal in character (Fig. 24.5) the relation between volume and flow rate is stated by:

$$\text{Vol} = \frac{2Pt}{\pi}$$

where P is peak flow and t is time; or in words—the

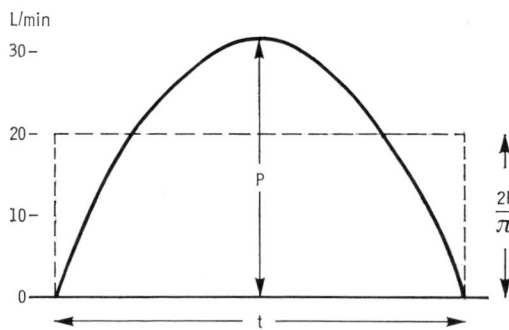

Fig. 24.5 Inspiratory flow wave-form. The area of the rectangle bounded by the broken line is the same as that of the sinusoid and is equal to the inspired volume.

area of the sinusoid is equal to the area of the rectangle of peak flow rate times $2/\pi$ and with the same time base.

In a system where enrichment only occurs during inspiration F_{IO_2} will be given by:

$$\frac{\text{Flow of O}_2 \text{ from air} + \text{flow of O}_2 \text{ added}}{\text{total flow}}$$

By substitution this expression becomes:

$$F_{IO_2} = \frac{\left(\dfrac{2P}{\pi} - O_2 \text{ flow}\right) \times 0.2093 + O_2 \text{ flow}}{\dfrac{2P}{\pi}}$$

Which simplifies to:

$$F_{IO_2} = 0.02093 + 1.242 \left(\frac{O_2 \text{ flow}}{P}\right) \quad \text{(ii)}$$

i.e., oxygen concentration is dependent upon peak flow and added oxygen flow and is independent of the duration of inspiration.

As we are considering a system in which the oxygen flow is small compared to P the breath to breath difference in f_{IO_2} is not marked. A given subject in a steady state therefore receives a reasonably constant F_{IO_2}, given by equation (ii). However, since average peak inspiratory flow rates vary from patient to patient, depending upon physical build and state of the airways, etc., between patient variation in F_{IO_2} occurs.

Since there is no imposed apparatus dead space, rebreathing of carbon dioxide does not occur. In fact the patient's physiological dead space is reduced at all flows (Bethune and Collis, 1967b).

The *oxygen capacity system* is an entirely functional description of nasal and nasopharyngeal delivery at higher oxygen flows. At these flows significant storage of oxygen in the airway occurs during the expiratory pause. However, since the expiratory pause is variable in length a variable volume of oxygen accumulates. Furthermore, as oxygen flow rate increases relative to peak inspiratory flow rate, breath to breath variation in peak flow rate has a more significant effect upon the inspired oxygen concentration. Thus, within patient variation is added to between patient variation. However, the effects of within patient variation are not as marked with these devices as with the large capacity devices.

The flow at which a no capacity system becomes an oxygen capacity system will of course vary from patient to patient but is of the order of 2–3 L/min.

Small Capacity System for Oxygen and Carbon Dioxide

Here apparatus dead space is added in the form of a mask shell. This allows for rebreathing of carbon dioxide and oxygen. While some economy of expired oxygen is achieved some of the fresh oxygen flow is lost through the vent. These masks thus do not provide a quantitative improvement in performance over the previous devices, which deliver oxygen directly into the airway. However, at high flows, they are much more comfortable.

During inspiration, the mask (the volume of which is small relative to tidal volume) empties first *in series* with inspired air so that higher oxygen concentrations are inhaled at the beginning of each inspiration. Figure 24.6 clearly shows this effect. The performance

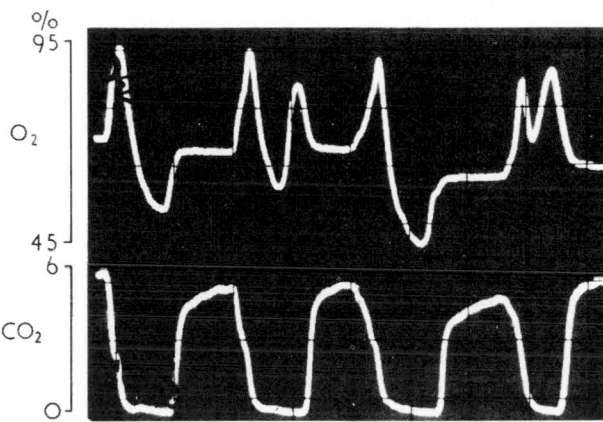

Fig. 24.6 Tidal O_2 and CO_2 measured at the lips with rapid response gas analysers during breathing with an MC mask at 10 L/min. There are four inspirations with four fairly typical CO_2 wave forms, but note that each of the O_2 wave forms rises at the beginning of inspiration towards 100% but falls *within the same inspiration* towards 21% as the inspired flow rate exceeds that of the oxygen inflow. The peak swings *during inspiration* vary from 45–95% and the five end-tidal plateaux show a variation in oxygen concentration of 10% (10 kPa approx.).

of these masks is subject to between patient variation at low flows and both between and within patient variation at high flows in a similar manner to the oxygen capacity system, (*see* Fig. 24.7).

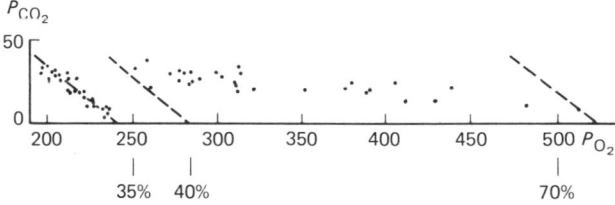

Fig. 24.7 Comparison between fixed performance and variable performance systems. The O_2/CO_2 diagram shows the analysis of separate samples of expiratory gas during the evaluation in five subjects (range of heights 159–196 cm; range of weights 58.5–87.5 kg) of a 35% Ventimask—left hand side—and an MC mask at 5 L/min. The possible scatter of inspired concentrations with the latter device is indicated by the broken 'R' lines and ranges from 40–73%.

Rebreathing and Apparatus Dead Space

Functional apparatus dead space is not the same as the physical volume of the apparatus, being equal to that part of the previous expirate which is re-inhaled. Its value depends upon similar factors to the inspired oxygen concentration and is therefore subject to a similar kind of variation.

It is very important to realize that patients may respond to imposed apparatus dead space by increasing their alveolar ventilation and thus overcoming its effect; or conversely, its imposition may be akin to increasing asphyxia in patients with incipient or actual respiratory failure.

There is, as yet, no accurate quantitative method for measuring tidal volume when wearing an oxygen therapy device, nor is it possible to collect mixed expired gas. Thus functional dead space cannot be measured clinically.

During clinical oxygen therapy, the only reliable estimate of rebreathing would be the continuous presence of carbon dioxide during the end-inspiratory phase of a continuous carbon dioxide trace (e.g., obtained by infrared analysis). A rise in end-tidal or arterial carbon dioxide tension might also occur if there were insufficient compensation by an increase in alveolar ventilation. However, these could also be the result of respiratory depression from some other cause.

This important aspect of oxygen therapy has been well covered by Cotes (1956), Kory et al. (1962), and Bethune and Collis (1967a, b). In particular, the latter authors, using either a model patient-device system or a subject trained to breathe at a constant tidal volume, have elegantly demonstrated the dead space characteristics of the devices under such idealized circumstances.

The following points are of importance and functional dead space or rebreathing will be increased when:

1. Physical volume of the device is large
2. Flow of oxygen delivered is low
3. Expiratory pause is short
4. Inspiratory resistance of the vent is high (the mask is a good fit).

The vent resistance is a function, not only of the cross sectional area of the vent which is placed in the mask deliberately by the designer but also, of that leak area which is added by a poor fit to the face. This latter may be a potent cause of variation in performance.

Large Capacity System

These devices are characterized by the presence of a rebreathing bag (or reservoir bag in the case of the Portogen mask). The Pneumask and Polymask are simply rebreathing bags, while the remainder consist of mask shell plus bag. The Portogen mask has a one-way valve between bag and mask. All these devices have a large volume which empties *in parallel* with inspired air. Inspired oxygen has three sources, *viz.* Fresh oxygen flow which continues throughout the ventilatory cycle; expired gas trapped in the dead space; and air coming through the total vent.

Since expired tidal volume is not constant, the quality of the expirate, i.e., the reciprocally related quantities of carbon dioxide and oxygen, may vary from breath to breath.

The concentrations in the bag just before expiration thus depend upon the quality of the previous expirate, expiratory pause time and the loss of fresh oxygen flow from leaks. The ratio of gas volume taken from the bag to air volume taken through the total vent depends upon the relative flow resistances. The latter will vary with the distending pressure in the bag throughout inspiration. Since the times, volumes, flows and resistances vary, the performance of the devices in this group is exceedingly variable from breath to breath, even in the steady state. It follows that the larger the capacity of the system, the greater is the effect produced by within patient variation of inspired oxygen values.

With the large capacity system it is not too difficult to predict that the shorter the expiratory pause time and the larger the expiratory flow, the less oxygen the patient will get and the more carbon dioxide. In other words, the more the patient requires oxygen therapy, the less well the device will perform at a given oxygen flowrate. 'Breathless' patients should therefore have a high oxygen flowrate. However, a patient with respiratory depression would not be at such a disadvantage with this system.

Oxygen Tent and Incubator

The *oxygen tent* is a large capacity system in which the patient is enclosed. The build-up of oxygen concentration within a tent is an exponential function. However, since both the tent capacity and the leakage are relatively large, the exponential has a long time constant. Only the most elaborately constructed oxygen tents are capable of achieving oxygen concentrations of 50%. This has its advantage, of course, in that carbon dioxide build up is equally limited.

Access to the patient is restricted, so that patient care and oxygen therapy may conflict since the oxygen concentration falls rapidly to ambient on opening the tent. The risk of fire is greatest with this method.

The oxygen tent should be reserved for children who will not tolerate an oxygen mask or catheter. For infants, an *incubator* not only constitutes the only possible method of continuous oxygen therapy but provides a controlled environment in respect of humidity and temperature. Oxygen and carbon dioxide build up is dependent upon the same factors as in the oxygen tent.

In neonatal resuscitation oxygen can only be given by mask or endotracheal tube. Oxygen by intragastric tube may dangerously raise intragastric pressure and only that which leaks back up the oesophagus can contribute to raising the inspired oxygen concentration. Oxygen by glass funnel is ineffective.

Tables 24.2–4 summarize the characteristics of the variable performance systems.

TABLE 24.2

NO CAPACITY SYSTEM

F_{IO_2} subject to between patient variation.
Dead space of patient diminished.

		F_{IO_2}
Peak insp. flow	+	↓
	−	↑
Oxygen flow	+	↑
	−	↓

TABLE 24.3

OXYGEN CAPACITY SYSTEM

F_{IO_2} subject to both between and within patient variation.
Dead space of patient further diminished.

		F_{IO_2}
Peak insp. flow	+	↓
	−	↑
Oxygen flow	+	↑
	−	↓
Expiration pause time	+	↑
	−	↓

TABLE 24.4

CAPACITY SYSTEMS WITH REBREATHING

F_{IO_2} subject to both between and within patient variation.

		F_{IO_2}	F_{IO_2}
Physical volume	+	↑	↑
	−	↓	↓
Oxygen flow	+	↑	↓
	−	↓	↑
Vent resistance	+	↑	↑
	−	↓	↓
Exp. pause time	+	↑	↓
	−	↓	↑
Insp. flowrate	+	↓	↑
	−	↑	↓

Hyperbaric Oxygenation. The quantity of oxygen dissolved in the plasma of whole blood is 0.3 ml/dl per 13.3 kPa (100 mmHg). At pressures of 2.4–3.0 ATA the dissolved oxygen content can amount to about 5.5 ml/dl and in theory the oxygen consumption of the body (5 ml/dl) can be met by the plasma alone.

Hyperbaric oxygen may be given to the patient by giving him 100% oxygen to breathe while inside a pressurized room or by placing him in a small 'tank' pressurized with 100% oxygen. Hyperoxia lowers cardiac output and causes vasoconstriction. The latter can be overcome by vasodilator therapy. The penetration of oxygen into ischaemic tissues is not as great as was originally hoped. However, some arrhythmias occurring after coronary thrombosis may respond to hyperbaric oxygen and there are advocates for the use of hyperbaric oxygen treatment after trauma (Loder 1979). Its uses in medicine have also included treatment of anaerobic infections, carbon monoxide poisoning or sulph- and methaemoglobinaemia, regional ischaemia from primary vascular causes, and of course it is important in the management of decompression sickness.

Central nervous system toxicity of oxygen, in the form of epileptiform fits (Paul Bert effect) is markedly increased at 3 ATA and fits can occur within 2–30 minutes in non-anaesthetized patients. Hyperbaric oxygen therapy is thus usually given to conscious patients at 2–2.5 ATA for treatments of one/two hours interspersed with rest periods. The high pressure conditions introduce the risk of decompression sickness in its various forms not only to patients but also to any personnel who may accompany them within the hyperbaric rooms.

Alternative Sources of Oxygen: Oxygen Concentrators
(Howell, 1985; Easy et al., 1988).

It has always been wasteful that expensively produced medical quality oxygen, which has been extracted from air, is remixed with air for oxygen therapy. It is much cheaper to use an oxygen concentrator to produce oxygen enriched (nitrogen reduced) air. These machines were originally developed for domiciliary oxygen therapy. Air is pumped alternately through two molecular sieve beds containing aluminium silicate crystals. While one is being used to produce oxygen enriched air the other is purged of its nitrogen content (pressure swing absorption). At low flow rates as high as 95% oxygen can be produced for domiciliary use.

In hospitals the use of such a source of O_2 avoids denitrogenation of the lungs as 100% oxygen is rarely if ever mandatory in clinical practice. To cope with swings in demand several concentrators are mounted in parallel.

CONCLUSIONS

Consideration of the factors influencing oxygen availability and oxygen requirements enables a rational approach to oxygen therapy to be adopted.

While it may be argued that what matters to the patient is his resultant arterial oxygen tension, the clinical value of this measurement is severely limited unless it is considered in relation to inspired or ideal alveolar oxygen tension. Since the ideal alveolar oxygen tension depends on inspired oxygen tension and cannot be derived without it, accurate knowledge of and control over inspired oxygen tension should be a fundamental prerequisite of oxygen therapy.

The Ventimasks provide a constant controlled inspired oxygen tension between 24 and 60% without imposing functional apparatus dead space. One can have very little idea of the precise performance of any other device, particularly as capacity and oxygen flows increase. This is particularly important since the risks of possible toxic effects incurred by the over-administration of oxygen may be just as important as not giving enough.

Hyperbaric oxygen therapy is neither widely applied nor firmly established in medicine.

REFERENCES

Barach A.L., Eckman M. (1941). A physiologically controlled oxygen mask apparatus. *Anesthesiology*, **2**, 421.

Barach A.L. (1962). Symposium—inhalational therapy. Historical background. *Anesthesiology*, **23**, 407.

Bethune D.W., Collis J.M. (1967a). The evaluation of oxygen masks. A mechanical method. *Anaesthesia*, **22**, 43.

Bethune D.W., Collis J.M. (1967b). The evaluation of oxygen therapy equipment. Experimental study of various devices on the human subject. *Thorax*, **22**, 221.

Campbell E.J.M. (1965). Methods of oxygen administration in respiratory failure. *Ann. N.Y. Acad. Sci.*, **121**, 861.

Campbell E.J.M., Minty K.B. (1976). Controlled oxygen therapy at 60% concentration—why and how. *Lancet.*, **1**, 1199.

Cotes, J.E. (1956). Reassessment of value of oxygen masks that permit rebreathing. *Brit. Med. J.*, **1**, 269.

Cox D., Gillbe C. (1982). Fixed performance oxygen masks. Hypoxic hazard of low-capacity designs. *Anaesthesia*, **36**, 958.

Easy W.R., Douglas G.A., Merrifield A.J. (1988) A combined oxygen concentrator and compressed air unit. Assessment of a prototype and discussion of its potential applications. *Anaesthesia*, **43**, 37.

Faithfull S. (1987). Oxygen-transporting blood substitutes. *Hospimedica.*, **5**, 45.

Finch C.A., Lenfant C. (1972). Oxygen transport in man. *New Engl. J. Med.*, **286**, 407.

Flenley D.C. (1967). The rationale of oxygen therapy. *Lancet*, **1**, 270.

Flenley D.C. (1978). Clinical hypoxia: causes, consequences, and correction. *Lancet*, **1**, 542.

Freeman, J., Nunn, J.F. (1963). Ventilation-perfuson relationships after haemorrhage. *Clin. Sci.*, **24**, 135.

Howell R.S.C. (1985). Oxygen concentrators. *Brit. J. Hosp. Med.*, **31**, 221.

Kory R.C., Bergmann J.C., Sweet R.D., et al. (1962). Comparative evaluation of oxygen therapy techniques. *J. Am. Med. Assoc.*, **179**, 767.

Leigh J.M. (1970). Variation in performance of oxygen therapy devices *Anaesthesia*, **25**, 210.

Leigh, J.M. (1974). Ideas and anomalies in the evolution of modern oxygen therapy. *Anaesthesia*, **29**, 335.

Loder R.E. (1979). Hyperbaric oxygen therapy in acute trauma. *Ann. Roy. Coll. Surg. Engl.*, **61**, 472.

Richards D.W. (1943–44). The circulation in traumatic shock in man. *Harvey Lect.*, **Series 39**, 217.

25. Physiology of Mechanical Ventilation

H. B. Fairley

A wide variety of techniques have been devised for the maintenance of ventilation in the absence of satisfactory spontaneous breathing. Each has the common objective of producing an intermittent increase in pressure difference across the lungs and airway and, consequently, the first section of this chapter will consider aspects of the mechanics of breathing relative to artificial ventilation.

As a corollary to the mechanics of artificial ventilation, there are changes in the hemodynamics of venous return, or cardiac output and of the pulmonary circulation and its distribution, as well as changes in the distribution of inspired air to the various regions of the lung. Thus, the next two sections will consider the effects of mechanical ventilation on hemodynamics and on ventilation/perfusion relationships.

Finally, special mention will be made of the physiology of mechanical ventilation of patients with respiratory failure due to pulmonary disease.

MECHANICS OF ARTIFICIAL VENTILATION

During normal spontaneous breathing, the work of the respiratory muscles generates a pressure difference, between the pleural 'space' and the upper airway, sufficient to overcome the elastic recoil of the lungs, the resistance of the airways to airflow and the frictional resistance between each tissue component of the lung. In addition work is expended in overcoming elastic and frictional factors in the chest wall. (Rehder and Marsh, 1986).

End-Expiratory Lung Volume (FRC)

Ventilatory failure is commonly associated with a decrease in FRC. This may be due to abnormalities within the lung itself, such as atelectasis, a consolidative process or contusion, or to an abnormality of chest wall posture due, for example, to muscle paralysis. In either case, lung and lung-thorax compliance are decreased and recruitment of alveoli which are underventilated or non-ventilated is an important management objective.

Diaphragm Excursions

In the supine position, the abdominal contents are hydrostatically equivalent to a container of water (Fig. 25.1). The hydrostatic pressure of the abdominal

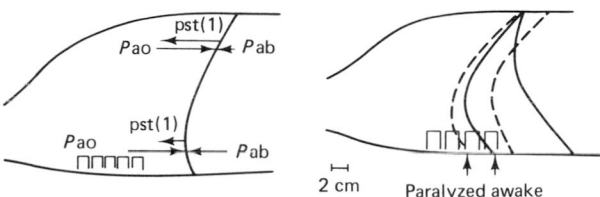

Fig. 25.1 (Left) Pressure differences across diaphragm during positive pressure ventilation. *P*st (1) = *P*ao − *P*ab. *P*ao = airway pressure. *P*st (1) = elastic recoil of lung. (Right) excursions of diaphragm during spontaneous (awake) and passive ventilation. Reproduced with permission from Froese and Bryan (1974).

contents on the diaphragm is therefore greatest posteriorly, and, until recently, it had been believed that the resulting end-expiratory antero-posterior differences in diaphragm muscle stretch were responsible for the greater excursions in the posterior diaphragm during spontaneous respiration. This has now been challenged by demonstration that, in prone subjects, the greater diaphragm motion is still in the dorsal non-dependant area. An inherent difference in regional diaphragm properties is postulated (Krayer et al., 1989).

In contrast during anesthesia and in the paralyzed patient, the shape of the chest wall changes, due to inactivity of the intercostal muscles. The side-to-side diameter of the thorax increases and the antero-posterior diameter decreases. During passive ventilation in the supine position, there is a more even (and therefore abnormal) distribution of diaphragm movement. In the prone position the distribution of ventilation is unchanged from the conscious spontaneous respiration status, with the greater excursions in the dorsal region.

Pulmonary Resistance

The contribution of pulmonary resistance to the actual pressure differences required during IPP ventilation, can only be considered in terms of specific flowrates and lung volumes, since the relationship between pressure and flow is non-linear and the cross-sectional area of the airways is lung volume dependent. Thus, this aspect of the mechanics of IPP ventilation is very much a function of the ventilatory pattern.

A pressure-cycled ventilator, set at rapid flowrates, may cycle early in inspiration since the peak pressure will be related to flowrate and airflow resistance. The delivered volume will increase only when inspiratory flow is reduced to the point where peak pressure is determined primarily by elastic recoil.

HEMODYNAMIC EFFECTS OF IPP

An important mechanical distinction between IPP ventilation and spontaneous breathing is that, although the pressure difference produced during inspiration is positive at the upper airway relative to the pleural cavity in both instances, this is effected by increasing the upper airway pressure first during IPP, and by lowering the pleural pressure first during spontaneous breathing. Thus, regardless of whether greater pressure differentials are necessary during IPP, *mean intrathoracic pressure* will be higher than during spontaneous breathing.

In patients with normal lungs, the increased mean intrathoracic pressure of passive ventilation creates a decrease in right and left ventricular filling. The magnitude of the effect of this on cardiac output depends upon blood volume and the integrity of the sympathetic nervous system control of the peripheral vasculature, particularly the capacitance vessels. The sequence of events is as follows. As airway pressure increases, a proportion of this pressure increase is transmitted to the pleural cavity and, therefore, to the heart and great vessels. If sufficient pressure is applied, pulmonary vascular resistance increases.

On the right side of the circulation, pleural and right atrial pressures increase but their difference (i.e. right ventricular filling pressure) decreases (Cournand et al., 1948). This is counteracted by a decrease in venous compliance, i.e. a homeostatic attempt to maintain a normal distribution between central and peripheral blood volume. It is clear therefore that as mean intrathoracic pressure increases, the consequences in terms of cardiac output will be greatest in the presence of hypovolemia or sympathetic blockade by disease, drugs, or regional anesthesia.

On the left side of the systemic circulation, filling pressure is similarly impaired. Also, the transmural pressure difference between the intra and the extra thoracic aorta causes a decrease in afterload. It follows that, in hyperdynamic states, when heart failure occurs, positive pressure ventilation may be expected to be beneficial. The mechanism by which left ventricular output is reduced by increased intrathoracic pressure is not clear. Decreased preload is certainly one mechanism but it is uncertain whether contractility is also affected (Prewitt et al., 1979;

Haynes et al., 1980; Robotham et al., 1980). Prostaglandins may act as negative inotropic mediators (Dunham et al., 1981).

The effects of lung inflation on the pulmonary vasculature are complex. At abnormally low lung volumes, pulmonary vascular resistance (PVR) is increased. As the lung is inflated, collapsed vessels open and alveolar capillaries are recruited. PVR then decreases. At abnormally high inflation volumes alveolar capillaries are compressed and PVR increases (Roos et al., 1961; Fishman, 1985).

EFFECTS ON VENTILATION/PERFUSION AND PULMONARY GAS EXCHANGE

Currently available data suggest that ventilation/perfusion ratio (V/Q) is abnormally distributed during IPP ventilation. In normal lungs, in the supine position, ventilation is more evenly distributed antero-posteriorly than with spontaneous respiration. The distribution of pulmonary blood flow may be relatively unaltered. Thus, there is a trend towards an increase in both high V/Q (anterior) and very low V/Q (posterior) zones. Reported values for *physiological deadspace* during passive ventilation are frequently similar to awake controls. However, when the decrease in anatomical deadspace due to endotracheal intubation is considered, it is clear that there is a parallel increase in alveolar deadspace (Cooper, 1967). V_D/V_T is constant over a wide range of tidal volumes (Hedley-Whyte et al., 1966; Cooper, 1967). The predictable *changes in pulmonary oxygen exchange* are more complex (Fairley, 1979). In considering the various interrelated factors, the simplest perspective is to *consider the influence of the pattern of ventilation on lung volume*. Underventilation at low tidal volumes results in a progressive decrease in lung compliance and in FRC (Mead and Collier, 1959; Tokics et al., 1987) and an increase in alveolar-arterial oxygen tension difference ($P(A–a)_{O_2}$) (Bendixen et al., 1963). These changes are prevented by large tidal volume ventilation at normocarbia (Fairley, 1966) or by PEEP. The benefit of large tidal volumes is greatest when end-inspiratory lung volume (FRC + tidal volume) exceeds *closing capacity* (Weenig et al., 1974), and these large tidal volumes are therefore important when FRC is decreased below closing capacity. The net effect of these adjustments in tidal volume on shunt-like effect also depends on *inspired oxygen concentration* ($F_{I_{O_2}}$) and on changes in *distribution of pulmonary blood flow*.

At high levels of $F_{I_{O_2}}$, the shunt-like effect of low V/Q regions is minimized (West and Wagner, 1977). Therefore, any favourable readjustment of V/Q distribution by a change to large tidal volume ventilation will be difficult to detect by $P(A–a)_{O_2}$ or Q_S/Q_T (shunt fraction) measurements. As intra-alveolar pressure is increased in ventilated alveoli there may be a parallel increase in regional pulmonary vascular resistance (PVR). Non-ventilated but perfused regions will not be affected in this way and pulmonary blood flow may be redistributed through these unventilated areas (Kanarek and Shannon, 1975; Benumof et al., 1979). The net effect of any given ventilation manoeuvre on $P(A-a)_{O_2}$ therefore also depends on the magnitude of this effect.

Other factors in the interaction between mechanical ventilation and Pa_{O_2} are *hypoxic pulmonary vasoconstriction* and *cardiac output*. Vessels perfusing underventilated alveoli are normally vasoconstricted and thereby minimize the oxygen exchange defect which would otherwise occur. This homeostatic mechanism is opposed by increases in Pa_{O_2}, increased vascular intraluminal pressures (Suter et al., 1975a; Benumof and Wahrenbrock, 1975) and by various pulmonary vasodilator drugs, including many anesthetic agents (Mathers et al., 1977).

In a variety of pulmonary disease states, Q_S/Q_T has been shown to vary directly with cardiac output, probably by a vascular recruitment and decruitment mechanism. This beneficial effect of a decrease in cardiac output on Q_S/Q_T, and therefore on Pa_{O_2}, is opposed by the relationship between mixed venous oxygen content and cardiac output. A decrease in cardiac output causes a decrease in mixed venous oxygen content. At constant Q_S/Q_T this would result in a decrease in Pa_{O_2}. However, *in vivo*, Q_S/Q_T decreases and the net effect on Pa_{O_2} is not predictable.

Inspiratory Waveform

Contemporary practice emphasizes only the importance of features which maintain lung volume, i.e. expiratory transpulmonary pressure, and the interaction between these features and hemodynamics. Many claims have been made in favour of one inspiratory waveform when compared to another and the subject has been reviewed by Baker et al., (1977a, b). There is no evidence that the magnitude of differences observed between inspiratory patterns is clinically important (Fuleihan et al., 1976).

PHYSIOLOGY OF PASSIVE VENTILATION IN PATIENTS WITH PULMONARY DISEASE

Acute Pulmonary Failure in Patients with Previously Normal Lungs

At end-expiration, regional lung volume is determined by the interaction of transpulmonary pressure and regional compliance. In diseased regions, surfactant is frequently decreased and elastic recoil increased. Regional FRC is low and alveoli become unstable. Atelectasis occurs at transpulmonary pressures which would maintain normal alveoli open. Under such circumstances, large tidal volumes may not be sufficient to minimize $P(A-a)_{O_2}$ and a sustained increase in transpulmonary pressure, throughout the respiratory cycle, is frequently necessary. This *positive end-expiratory pressure* (PEEP) causes an increase in FRC

and in lung-thorax compliance, suggesting a recruitment of atelectatic and/or abnormally low volume alveoli. There is usually a parallel increase in Pa_{O_2} (Falke et al., 1972). The time course of this increase in FRC is considerably greater than the length of one inspiration (Fig. 25.2) and one would therefore not

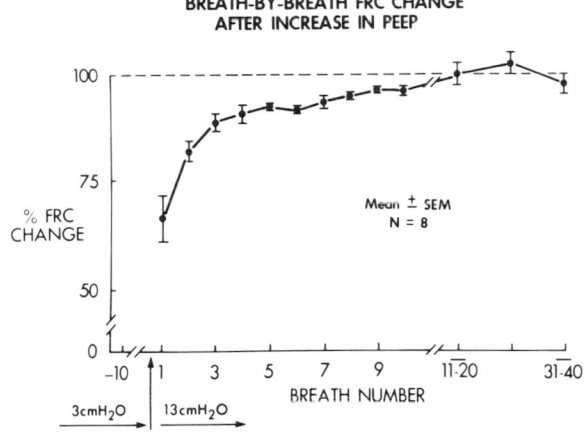

Fig. 25.2 Breath-by-breath increase in FRC following a step increase in end-expiratory pressure of 10 cmH₂O, in thirteen patients with acute pulmonary failure. 66% of the gain in lung volume occurred immediately and 90% was completed in between three and four breaths (16 seconds). After Katz (1981).

expect the transpulmonary pressures created at the peaks of intermittent positive pressure tidal volumes to be fully effective in recruiting this abnormal atelectatic lung (Fig. 25.3).

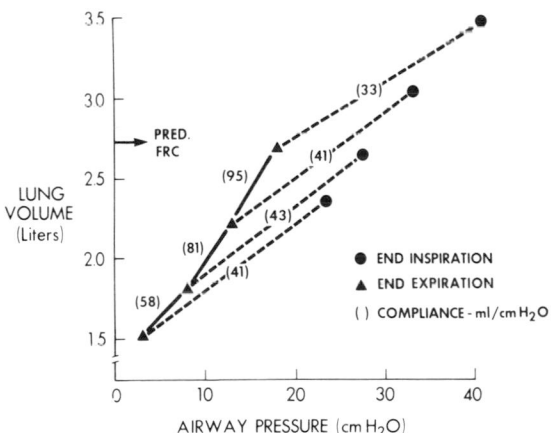

Fig. 25.3 Two point compliance data derived from tidal volumes initiated from FRCs obtained by applying end-expiratory pressure of 3, 8, 15 and 18 cmH₂O, in patients with acute pulmonary failure. The lung volume gained by applying a constant end-expiratory pressure greatly exceeds that gained by comparable pressures during a (transient) tidal volume. The improvement in arterial oxygenation following institution of PEEP correlates with this volume difference. Reproduced with permission from Katz et al. (1981).

Figure 25.4 shows the distensibility of two different types of adult lung-thoraces. In one, in which the lungs were relatively normal, overdistension (as indicated by whole lung-thorax compliance) occurred at a volume increase of 3 litres. In the other, the patient had the adult respiratory distress syndrome (ARDS)

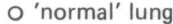

o 'normal' lung
• acute pulmonary parenchymal disease

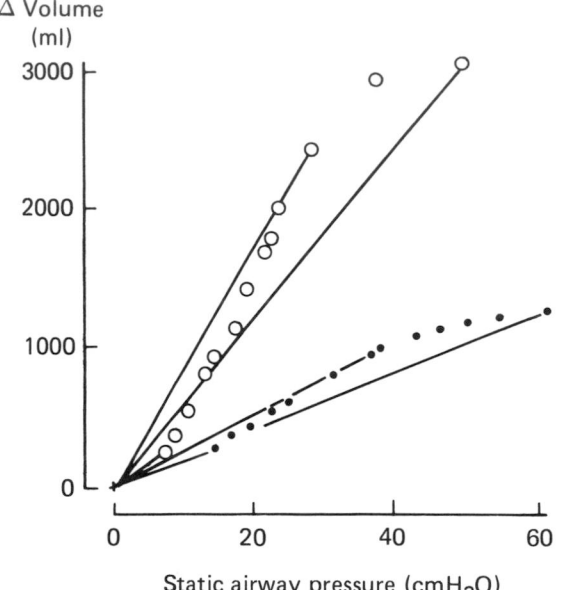

Fig. 25.4 Static pressure-volume points of respiratory system in two patients with respiratory failure. One had neurogenic ventilatory failure without clinical or radiologic signs of pulmonary parenchymal disease (open circles), and the other patient had severe bilateral parenchymal disease (solid circles). Slopes of lines connecting end-expiratory (plus sign) and static end-inspiratory points (open and closed circles) represent C_{Tstat} of total respiratory system, which varies with tidal volume. Reproduced with permission from Suter et al. (1978), *Chest*, **73**, 158.

and comparable overdistension occurred with an added volume of 1 litre or less. Presumably, the two patients' lungs differed both in their compliances and in their initial volumes (FRC). Similarly, one might postulate that, in one, the decrease in FRC resulted from 'collapse' of recruitable air spaces. In the other, a more consolidative process, offering less potential for recruitment, was involved. It can also be seen that a compliance value derived from two points (end-inspiration and end-expiration) can vary for the same lung according to the end-expiratory pressure and tidal volumes selected. This fact can be used clinically to determine the *optimum combination of* PEEP *and tidal volume*, in terms of lung and lung-thorax distensibility (Fig. 25.5).

The effect of PEEP *on cardiac output*, and therefore

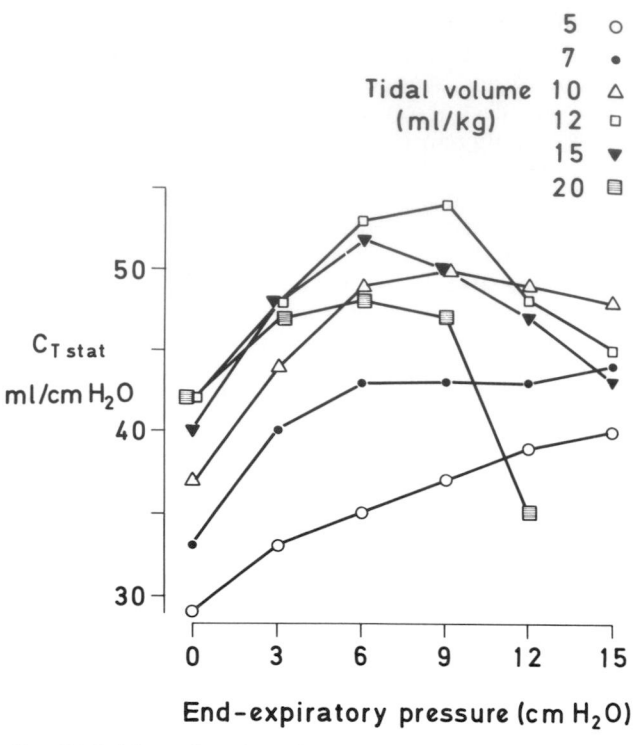

Fig. 25.5 Mean data for 12 patients with acute pulmonary failure. C_{Tstat} is a 'static' lung-thorax compliance obtained by using the airway pressure at the end of a 1.2 second period of zero flow at end-inspiration. Contrast the lowest tidal volume (with apparent continuing recruitment of alveoli at 15 cmH$_2$O PEEP) and the highest tidal volume, with probable overdistension beyond 9 cmH$_2$O PEEP. Reproduced with permission from Suter et al. (1978).

oxygen transport, varies with the zero PEEP (ZEEP) lung volume (Suter et al., 1975b) i.e. the lower the FRC at ZEEP, the greater the level of PEEP at which oxygen transport decreases. This is presumably because low volume lung has a low compliance and transmits a smaller proportion of the airway pressure to the intrapleural space than more normal lungs.

In many cases, oxygen transport is optimal at that point of lung distension at which compliance is greatest (Fig. 25.6). However, as indicated above, the cardiac output effect is dependent on blood volume (Qvist et al., 1975) and other factors. If greater levels of PEEP are necessary to maintain adequate oxygen exchange, 'excessive' lung distension must be permitted and blood volume may have to be increased to offset cardiac output effects.

In patients with very severe ARDS, the pulmonary vascular bed is sufficiently diminished to result in pulmonary hypertension and, ultimately, right ventricular distension. This effect is then exaggerated as airway pressure and, therefore, PVR are increased. With an intact pericardium, this right ventricular enlargement may result in a shift of the interventricular septum to the left, compromising the left ventricu-

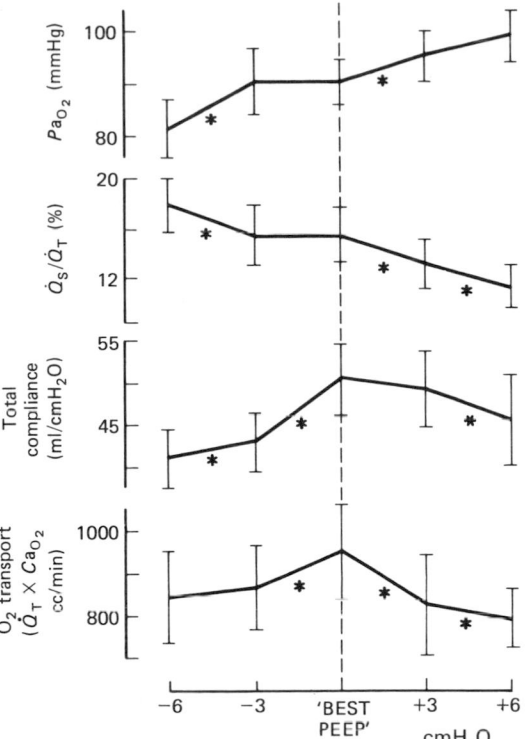

Fig. 25.6 Data from 15 patients (m ± SE) being ventilated for acute pulmonary failure. 'Best PEEP' was empirically chosen as that end-expiratory pressure (for each patient) beyond which oxygen transport decreased. Asterisks represent P < 0.05 between neighbouring values. Reproduced with permission from Suter et al. (1975b).

lar filling (Laver et al., 1979), and therefore decreasing stroke volume.

Intermittent Mandatory Ventilation (IMV)
(Kirby, 1980; Weisman et al., 1983).

This technique of mechanical assistance recognizes a distinction which can be made in most patients, at some part or all of their respiratory failure course. The need for maintenance of lung volume, for correction of a defect in oxygen exchange, does not necessarily co-exist with a defect in the patient's ability to move an adequate minute volume, for pH homeostasis. It is argued that one effect of maintaining optimum lung distension may be to improve compliance, thereby facilitating spontaneous ventilation. Consequently, spontaneous breathing circuits which permit the maintenance of a positive airway pressure have been devised. Using appropriate one-way valving, a volume constant mechanical ventilator is connected in parallel with such a circuit, and the frequency of this ventilator is adjusted to deliver only sufficient (mandatory) breaths to maintain a normal arterial pH. This IMV frequency may vary from zero to a level at which no spontaneous ventilation is inter-

posed, according to the patient's ability to perform adequate ventilatory work. Mean intrathoracic pressure and cardiac output vary directly with the IMV rate.

During spontaneous ventilation, positive pressure may be applied only during expiration (*expiratory positive airway pressure* EPAP or throughout the respiratory cycle (*continuous positive airway pressure* CPAP (Fig. 25.7).

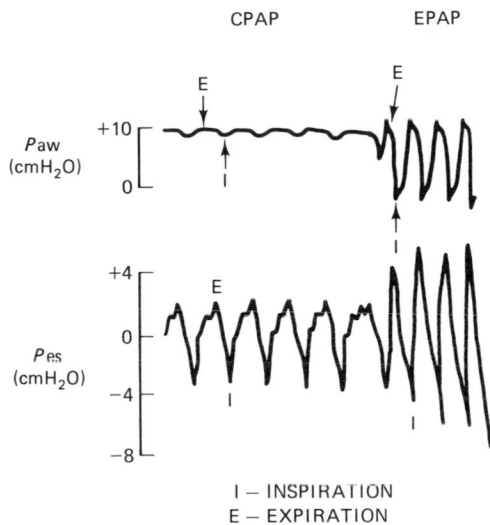

I – INSPIRATION
E – EXPIRATION

Fig. 25.7 Airway (P_{aw}) and esophageal (P_{es}) pressures during spontaneous breathing with continuous positive airway pressure (CPAP) and end-expiratory positive airway pressure (EPAP). Transpulmonary pressure = $P_{aw} - P_{es}$. Note difference in end-expiratory transpulmonary pressure i.e. determinant of FRC. Reproduced with permission from Schlobohm et al. (1981).

CPAP is more comfortable for many patients. Although EPAP results in greater transpulmonary pressure excursions, end-expiratory 'squeezing' occurs. Thus, at comparable end-expiratory pressures, CPAP results in a larger FRC and a smaller $P(A-a)_{O_2}$ than those produced by EPAP (Schlobohm et al., 1981).

Pressure support ventilation is a term for a ventilation mode which functions similarly to manually assisted ventilation. When the machine is triggered by a spontaneous breath, a flow of gas is generated until a preset (pressure support) level of airway pressure is reached. The details vary from one manufacturer to another but, in general, the mode differs from patient-triggered ventilation by maintaining spontaneous respiration while minimizing its work of breathing.

High frequency ventilation (Froese et al., 1987) involves lung ventilation at rapid frequency, usually with tidal volumes less than the anatomical deadspace. In addition to bulk convection of gases, gas exchange also occurs due to inter-regional pendeluft due to time constant inequalities, cardiogenic mixing, molecular diffusion and probably other factors. The two systems which have been used most frequently are high frequency jet ventilation (HFJV) and high frequency oscillation (HFO). The former depends on a venturi principle in an open airway, and the latter on the rapid oscillation of a closed system. Some authors also include conventional mechanical ventilation at low tidal volumes under the HFV heading. At present, the place of HFV in clinical practice is not clear, although a marginal improvement in cardiac output has been demonstrated experimentally, in comparison with conventional ventilation. In patients with a disrupted airway (large broncho-pleural fistula, transected trachea or bronchus) HFJV may be the only method of securing effective gas exchange.

Chronic Obstructive Pulmonary Disease

The overriding problem in ventilating lungs with chronic obstructive pulmonary disease is that produced by the widely differing regional ventilation time constants. The magnitude of the resulting maldistribution of ventilation can be decreased by using as slow an inspiratory flowrate as possible. Expiration is impaired by a combination of defective elastic recoil and airway closure at abnormally large lung volumes. If expiratory time is decreased, air trapping becomes more probable and increased hyperinflation may result in a decrease in cardiac output. Airway closure may be lessened by low-level PEEP. However, PEEP is poorly tolerated (in terms of cardiac output) in this group of patients.

REFERENCES

Baker A.B., Babington P.C.B., Collis J.E., et al. (1977a). Effects of varying respiratory flow waveform and time in intermitent positive pressure ventilation I: Introduction and methods. *Brit. J. Anaesth.*, **49**, 1207.

Baker A.B., Colliss J.E., Cowie R.W. (1977b). Effects of varying respiratory flow waveform and time in intermittent positive pressure ventilation II: Various physiological variables. *Brit. J. Anaesth.*, **49**, 1221.

Bendixen H.H., Hedley-Whyte J., Laver M.B. (1963). Impaired oxygenation in surgical patients during general anesthesia with controlled ventilation. *New Eng. J. Med.*, **269**, 991.

Benumof J.L., Wahrenbrock E.A. (1975). Blunted hypoxic pulmonary vasoconstriction by increased lung vascular pressures. *J. Appl. Physiol.*, **38**, 846.

Benumof J.L., Rogers S.N., Moyce P.R., et al. (1979). Hypoxic vasoconstriction and regional and whole lung PEEP in the dog. *Anesthesiology*, **51**, 503.

Cooper E.A. (1967). Physiological dead space in passive ventilation. *Anesthesiology*, **22**, 90 and 199.

Cournand A., Motley H.L., Werko L., et al. (1948). Physiological studies of the effect of intermittent positive pressure breathing on cardiac output in man. *Am. J. Physiol.*, **152**, 162.

Dunham B.M., Grindlinger G.A., Utsunomiya T., et al. (1981). Role of prostaglandins in positive end-expiratory pressure-induced negative inotropism. *Am. J. Physiol.*, **241**, H783.

Fairley H.B. (1966). The oxygen tightrope. *Can. Anaesth. Soc. J.*, **13**, 98.

Fairley H.B. (1979). The changing arterial oxygen tension-disease or physician? *Anesthesiology*, **51**, 492.

Falke K.J., Pontoppidan H., Kumar A., et al. (1972). Ventilation with end-expiratory pressure in acute lung disease. *J. Clin. Invest.*, **51**, 2315.

Fishman A.P. (1985). Pulmonary circulation. In *Handbook of Physiology*, section 3, vol. I. *Circulation and Non-Respiratory Functions*. Maryland: Bethesda, *Am. Physiol. Soc.*

Froese A.B., Bryan A.C. (1974). Effects of anesthesia and paralysis on diaphragmatic mechanics in man. *Anesthesiology*, **41**, 242.

Froese A.B., Bryan A.C. (1987). High frequency ventilation. *Am. Rev. Respir. Dis.*, **135**, 1363.

Fuleihan S.F., Wilson R.S., Pontoppidan H. (1976). Effect of mechanical ventilation and end-inspiratory pause on blood gas exchange. *Anesth. Analg.*, **55**, 122.

Haynes J.B., Carson S.D., Whitney W.P., et al. (1980). Positive end-expiratory shifts left ventricular diastolic pressure-area curves. *J. Appl. Physiol.*, **48**, 670.

Hedley-Whyte J., Pontoppidan H., Morris M.J. (1966). The response of patients with respiratory failure and cardiopulmonary disease to different levels of constant volume ventilation. *J. Clin. Invest.*, **45**, 1543.

Kanarek D.J., Shannon D.C. (1975). Adverse effect of positive end-expiratory pressure on pulmonary perfusion and arterial oxygenation. *Am. Rev. Res. Dis.*, **112**, 457.

Katz J.A., Ozanne G.M., Zinn S.E., et al. (1981). Time course and mechanisms of lung volume increase with PEEP in acute pulmonary failure. *Anesthesiology*, **54**, 9.

Kirby R.R. (ed.) (1980). Intermittent mandatory ventilation. *Int. Anes. Clinics.*, **18**, May.

Krayer S., Rehder K., Vetterman J., et al. (1989). Position and motion of the human diaphragm during anaesthesia-paralysis. *Anesthesiology*, **70**, 891.

Laver M.B., Strauss W., Pohost G.M. (1979). Right and left ventricular geometry: adjustments during acute respiratory failure. *Crit. Care Med.*, **7**, 509.

Mathers J.M., Benumof J.L., Wahrenbrock E.A. (1977). General anesthetics and regional hypoxic pulmonary vasoconstriction. *Anesthesiology*, **46**, 111.

Mead J., Collier C. (1959). Relation of volume history of lungs to respiratory mechanics in anesthetized dogs. *J. Appl. Physiol.*, **14**, 669.

Prewitt R.M., Sutherland J.B., Dean G.W., et al. (1979). The effect of positive end-expiratory pressure on left ventricular systolic and diastolic volume-pressure characteristics. *Am. Rev. Res. Dis.*, **119**, 161.

Qvist J., Pontoppidan H., Wilson R.S., et al. (1975). Hemodynamic responses to mechanical ventilation with PEEP: the effect of hypervolemia. *Anesthesiology*, **42**, 45.

Rehder K., Marsh H.M. (1986). Respiratory mechanics during anesthesia and mechanical ventilation. In *Handbook of Physiology*, section 3, vol. III. *Mechanics of Breathing*. Maryland: Bethesda. *Am. Physiol. Soc.*

Robotham J.L., Lixfield W., Holland L., et al. (1980). The effects of positive end-expiratory pressure on right and left ventricular performance. *Am. Rev. Res. Dis.*, **121**, 677.

Roos A., Thomas L.J. Jr., Nagel E.L., et al. (1961). Pulmonary vascular resistance as determined by lung inflation and vascular pressures. *J. Appl. Physiol.*, **16**, 77.

Schlobohm R.M., Falltrick R.T., Quan S.F., et al. (1981). Lung volumes, mechanics, and oxygenation during spontaneous positive pressure ventilation. The advantages of CPAP over EPAP. *Anesthesiology*, **55**, 416.

Suter P.M., Fairley H.B., Schlobohm R.M. (1975a). Shunt, lung volume and perfusion during short periods of ventilation with oxygen. *Anesthesiology*, **43**, 617; **45**, 262.

Suter P.M., Fairley H.B., Isenberg M.D. (1975b). Optimum end-expiratory pressure in patients with acute pulmonary failure. *New Engl. J. Med.*, **292**, 284.

Suter P.M., Fairley H.B., Isenberg M.D. (1978). Effect of tidal volume and positive end-expiratory pressure on compliance during mechanical ventilation. *Chest*, **73**, 158.

Tokics L., Hedenstierna G., Strandberg A., et al. (1987). Lung collapse and gas exchange during general anesthesia: effects of spontaneous breathing, muscle paralysis, and positive end-expiratory pressure. *Anesthesiology*, **66**, 157.

Weenig C.S. et al. (1974). Relationship of preoperative closing volume to functional residual capacity and alveolar-arterial oxygen difference during anesthesia and controlled ventilation. *Anesthesiology*, **41**, 3.

Weisman I.M., Rinaldo J.E., Rogers R.M., et al. (1983). Intermittent mandatory ventilation. *Am. Rev. Respir. Dis.*, **127**, 641.

West J.B., Wagner P.D. (1977). Pulmonary gas exchange. In *Bioengineering Aspects of the Lung*. (West J.B. ed.). New York: Dekker.

C. NEUROENDOCRINE SYSTEMS

26. Membrane Physiology
Joan J. Kendig

The structure of cell membranes
  Phospholipid bilayers
  Membrane proteins important in nerve
    function
  Lipid–protein interactions
Events in nerve cell membranes
  Active ion transport
  Electrically gated ion-selective channel state
    transitions
  Transmitter release
  Chemically gated channel state transitions
Summary

This chapter and the following one provide an overview of membrane physiology and the substrates of excitable cell function, with special relation to the anesthetic effects of anesthetic agents. Emphasis is therefore placed on nerve and muscle membrane proteins, their relationship to membrane lipids, and their functional conformation changes which can be correlated with electrical signs of activity.

THE STRUCTURE OF CELL MEMBRANES

Phospholipid Bilayers

The outer membrane of a nerve or muscle cell is less than 6 nm thick, yet most of the important events in excitable cell function occur on or through it. A cell can exist separate from its surrounding environment because of the properties of the amphiphilic molecules which constitute the bulk of the membrane. Hydrophilic portions of such molecules contact the aqueous external milieu and cytoplasm; hydrophobic portions align with each other to form the interior of the membrane. The most common of these molecules are the phospholipids (Fig. 26.1) which align themselves to form a phospholipid bilayer: a sandwich of opposing layers of phospholipids with their polar head groups toward the aqueous interface and their hydrophobic fatty acyl chains meeting in the center. Figure 26.1 represents the concept of the phospholipid bilayer as the structural matrix in which functional proteins are embedded (Singer and Nicholson, 1972).

The structure of a typical phospholipid is also shown in Fig. 26.1. The cell membranes of animal cells are made up of a variety of phospholipids, which differ in the structure and charge of their head groups and the length and conformation of the fatty acyl chains which make up their 'tails.' The charged phospholipid head group enables the outer surface of the bilayer to maintain contact with the aqueous external environment and the aqueous cytoplasm of the cell. The hydrocarbon tails of the fatty acyl chains form an oily interior of the cell membrane, rendering it impermeable to water, ions, and water-soluble biological molecules. The liquid-like interior of the bilayer is in constant motion. Each phospholipid molecule rotates rapidly about its long axis and diffuses laterally in the plane of the bilayer by a process of exchanging position with neighboring phospholipids. The two fatty acyl chains of each phospholipid constantly flex, wag, and rotate to such an extent that the central region of the bilayer has some of the characteristics of a liquid solvent, a property which has considerable importance in anesthetic theory. From the surface to the interior there is a flexibility gradient along the fatty acyl chains; they are most rigid near the polar head groups and most rapidly and randomly moving near the center of the bilayers. There is little coupling between the asymmetric inner and outer halves of the bilayer, which differ in composition; the two halves

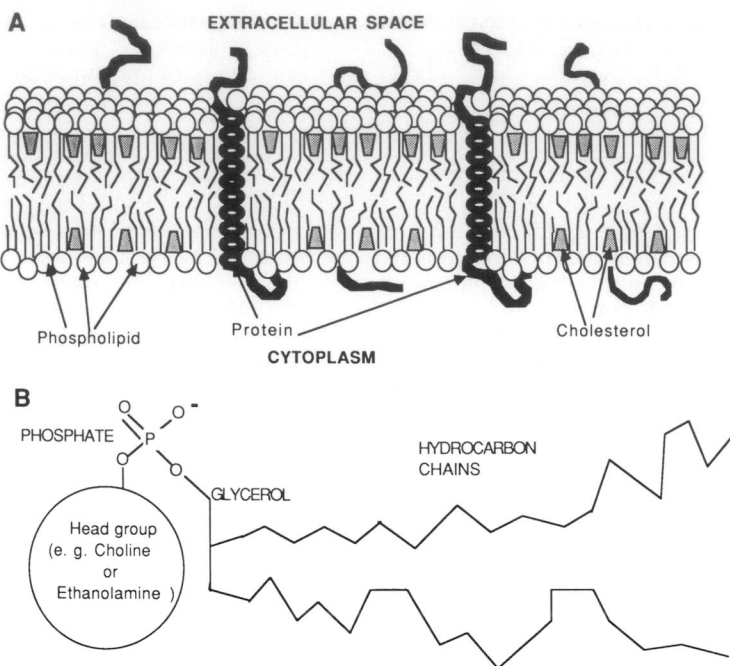

Fig. 26.1 The phospholipid bilayer as the structural matrix of the cell membrane. (A), Phospholipids orient themselves in a double layer to form the bilayer, with polar head groups, represented by circles, facing outward to the aqueous environment of the extracellular space on one side and the cytoplasm on the other. The hydrophobic hydrocarbon chains appose each other, creating an oily liquid-like region in the interior of the membrane. Cholesterol, abundant in natural membranes, confers more rigidity than a pure phospholipid bilayer. Embedded in the membrane are proteins; those shown are intrinsic to the membrane, traversing it completely. Like many intrinsic proteins such as those which form channels for ions, these are shown as having a helical structure in the part which traverses the hydrophobic interior. (B), The detailed structure of a phospholipid. Head groups vary in structure and charge distribution. Some proteins require negatively charged phospholipids, such as phosphatidylserine, for normal function. The phosphate and glycerol links are constant features. Hydrocarbon chains forming the hydrophobic tails of the phospholipid vary in length and saturation; chains with double bonds form kinks which pack less well in a bilayer, resulting in a less ordered, more fluid structure than fully saturated chains.

are held together because they are in their lowest free energy state when water is prevented from contacting the fatty acid chains.

In animal cells, an additional important component of the bilayer is cholesterol (Fig. 26.1). This rigid molecule, abundant in natural membranes, also is an amphiphile with an hydrophilic end exposed to the aqueous layer and an hydrophobic structure embedded in the hydrophobic part of the membrane. It confers additional rigidity on the bilayer, increasing the packing among the outer portions of the phospholipid and rendering this portion of the membrane less fluid and even less permeable than a pure phospholipid bilayer would be (Bretscher, 1985).

The phospholipid bilayer provides physical separation and electrical insulation between the cytoplasm and the aqueous region external to the cell. Proteins with functions restricted to either the interior or exterior compartments of the cell may be bound and organized into multi-subunit complexes on the bilayer surfaces. These proteins are called extrinsic membrane proteins. Intrinsic membrane proteins, on the other hand, are hydrophobic enough to be dissolved within the bilayer or to traverse it with one end in the cytoplasm and the other in the extracellular fluid (*see* Fig. 26.1). Such proteins are capable of acting as transporters for ions and other substances to which the lipid layer is impermeable. In as much as ion concentration gradients and ionic transmembrane currents are important in excitable cell function, these proteins are possible targets for anesthetic actions.

The extent of the 'fluidity' of the membrane phospholipid bilayer is much discussed in anesthetic theory. Early analysis of the actions of anesthetics used bulk hydrophobic solvents such as olive oil or, more recently, octanol as models. These are isotropic fluids, homogeneous in all directions. However, the phospholipids of the membrane bilayer exist in a more ordered anisotropic state. Recent measurement techniques permit a more rigorous analysis of fluidity as it relates to this two-dimensional ordered structure (Stubbs and Smith, 1984). Fluidity, which has been postulated to influence protein function, refers to the physical state of the fatty acyl chains of the bilayer. An increase in fluidity is defined as a decrease in the order parameter (Melchior, 1986) of the bilayer. In pure phospholipid bilayers, fluidity is determined by the unsaturation and length of the chain. Chains with at least one double bond are on average more mobile than fully saturated chains, since the kink caused by the double bond prevents ordered packing between adjacent molecules.

The properties of the lipid bilayer in actual cells complicate any analysis derived from either bulk solvents or homogeneous model bilayers. Besides the asymmetry of the membrane, its heterogeneous content of many different phospholipids, and the high cholesterol content described above, there are additional complications of heterogeneity within the membrane. These include the possible coexistence of areas in a relatively rigid gel phase with the liquid crystal more fluid phase, possible domains of lipids with different properties in the same phase, and the restrictive effects of membrane proteins on nearby lipids.

The existence of lateral phase separations is a property of some phospholipid bilayers that may be important in the regulation and control of the function of intrinsic membrane proteins. Lateral phase separations occur when gel-phase and fluid-phase phospholipids coexist in a membrane. In the fluid-phase, the fatty acid chains are very fluid, there is little cooperative attraction between the fatty acid chains, and the membrane surface area per phospholipid is large (≈ 0.7 nm^2) (Shimshick and McConnell, 1973); in the gel-phase, the fatty acid chains are very ordered, highly cooperative, and the membrane surface area per phospholipid is small (≈ 0.5 nm^2). Phase separations have been considered to facilitate protein function, although the evidence that they exist in mammalian membranes at normal temperature is debatable (Stubbs et al., 1984). The existence of segregated lipid domains in the same liquid crystal phase within the bilayer has been a subject of much debate. There is tentative evidence that in natural membranes they in fact may exist (Melchior, 1986), but the extent to which they do and their importance in providing specific areas whose properties are important to the function of membrane proteins is not proven. More important and more widely recognized is evidence that proteins impose additional heterogeneity of structure on phospholipid bilayers. Transmembrane proteins slow the motion of lipids in contact with them

(Deuticke and Haest, 1987). The uneven shapes of the hydrophobic portions of membrane-intercalated proteins preferentially interact with particular lipid species, creating their own micro-environments of lipids. The charge distribution of the hydrophilic portions of both extrinsic and transmembrane proteins may impose additional requirements for phospholipids with a particular head group, for instance, one with a net negative charge.

Considering the heterogeneity of the membrane and the probable existence of lipid micro-environments within it, measurements of average or bulk membrane fluidity are of questionable relevance in the living animal membrane. In defined experimental membranes, however, lipid properties have been clearly shown to be vital to protein function as outlined below.

Membrane Proteins Important in Nerve Function

In recent years, there has been important progress made in the biochemical characterization of proteins important in excitable cell function. This new information is as yet incompletely correlated with evidence based on electrical signs of protein function to provide an integrated understanding of how these proteins act to regulate cellular activity. Nevertheless, it is now possible to provide solid evidence of the shape and atomic structure of some important membrane proteins to replace the conceptual cartoons derived from functional studies.

The internal ionic composition of all cells is regulated by two types of proteins: those which directly or indirectly use energy to transport ions from one side of a membrane to the other against a concentration gradient, and those which provide a channel which allows a particular ion species to diffuse passively across the impermeable bilayer in the same direction as the concentration gradient. This section will provide examples of each. The regulation of each type of protein is a subject particularly important in anesthesiology. The activity of active ion transport systems is primarily dependent on concentrations of a particular ion species at one or the other membrane surface; Na-K-dependent ATPase and Ca-dependent ATPase are named because of this property. Passive ion-selective channels are regulated in a variety of ways: by changes in transmembrane voltage gradients, by direct action of neurochemicals called transmitters, by ion concentrations at one or the other side of the channel, and by transmitter-activated metabolic cascades. Voltage regulation of sodium channels, direct transmitter activation of the acetycholine receptor channel and β-adrenergic stimulation of adenylate cyclase are presented as examples.

1. **Proteins Involved in Energy-requiring Active Ion Transport: Na-K ATPase.** Sodium-potassium-dependent ATPase is the most familiar of the active ion transport systems, whose activity is primarily re-

sponsible for establishing the inequality in distribution of sodium and potassium between the inside and the outside of the cell. It has been successfully purified as a single protein and placed into artificial bilayers of known constitution. This process, known as reconstitution, is an important technique in analysis of protein function. In the bilayer, which spontaneously forms sealed vesicles, the reconstituted Na-K ATPase hydrolyzes ATP and transports sodium and potassium across the membrane in opposite directions, confirming that this enzyme is the 'sodium pump'. The structure of the pump and its insertion into the membrane is shown in Fig. 26.2. Like a number of functional membrane proteins, it exists as an oligomer with several subunits, all of which traverse the membrane (Stahl and Harris, 1986). Functionally, it possesses binding sites on the external surface for cardiac glycosides, which inhibit pump activity, and on the internal surface for ATP. Although much of the work on the structure of this transmembrane protein is derived from non-neural tissue, it is believed to be fundamentally similar in all cell types, with some differences probable in cardiac glycoside binding sites and in ion affinities. The way the enzyme acts to transport sodium and potassium is also shown in Fig. 26.2. Three sodium ions are extruded from the cell and two potassium ions admitted for every molecule of ATP

hydrolyzed. The ions pass through a channel formed either within or between the subunits. The protein functions as a transporter by undergoing structural changes in response to ion-binding and to phosphorylation; a tentative schema for the enzyme states is shown in Fig. 26.2.

2. **Ion-selective Pores: Na and Ca Channels as Models.** The concept of a channel-forming protein consisting of several subunits, which can exist in a number of different conformations corresponding to different functional states, is generalizable to some passive ion-selective channels. One of the best studied of these is the sodium channel which is responsible for the action potential of peripheral nerves and the fast upstroke of the action potential in heart. Also, for this channel, a great deal of progress has been made in purification and reconstitution into lipid bilayers (Catterall et al., 1986). The biochemical analysis has proceeded far enough to make a structural diagram possible (Fig. 26.3). The components of the multi-subunit protein essential for ion passage and for binding of specific neurotoxins such as tetrodotoxin (TTX) have been identified. The sodium channel also must exist in several conformation states, most of which are 'closed' and do not permit sodium to pass. The prime determinant of the most important transition, from a

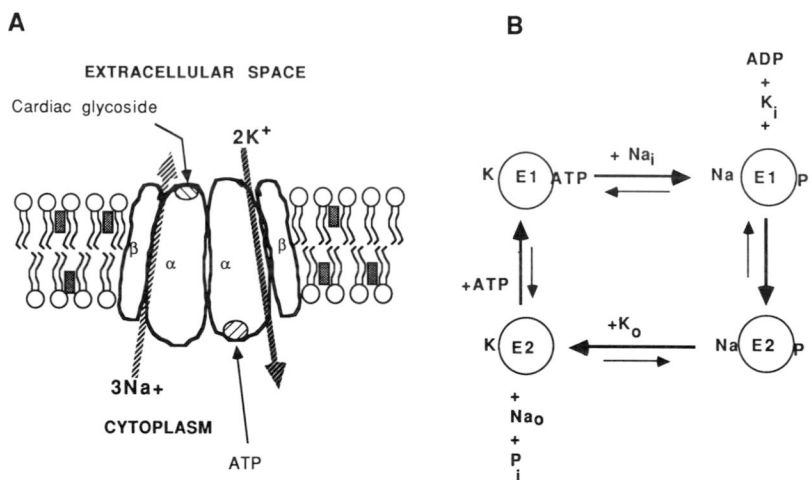

Fig. 26.2 Structure (A) and presumed conformation states (B) of an active ion transport protein, the sodium pump identified with Na^+-K^+-dependent ATPase. This integral membrane protein consists of four subunits, all of which traverse the membrane. Energy from the hydrolysis of ATP, which binds to a site on the inner side of the protein, is used to move Na from the inside to the outside of the cell and K in the opposite direction, with a stoichiometry of 3:2. The ion passage is either between the subunits or within them. On the external side of the protein is a binding site for the cardiac glycoside inhibitors. On the right is a diagram of the conformation changes the enzyme undergoes during transport activity. In response to intracellular Na accumulation, the pump binds intracellular Na, hydrolyzes ATP, and releases K at the cytoplasmic side. The phosphorylated enzyme undergoes a conformation change, E1 to E2, binds extracellular K and releases Na at the extracellular side, together with inorganic phosphate. KE2 bonds ATP and reverts to the E1 conformation to begin the cycle again.

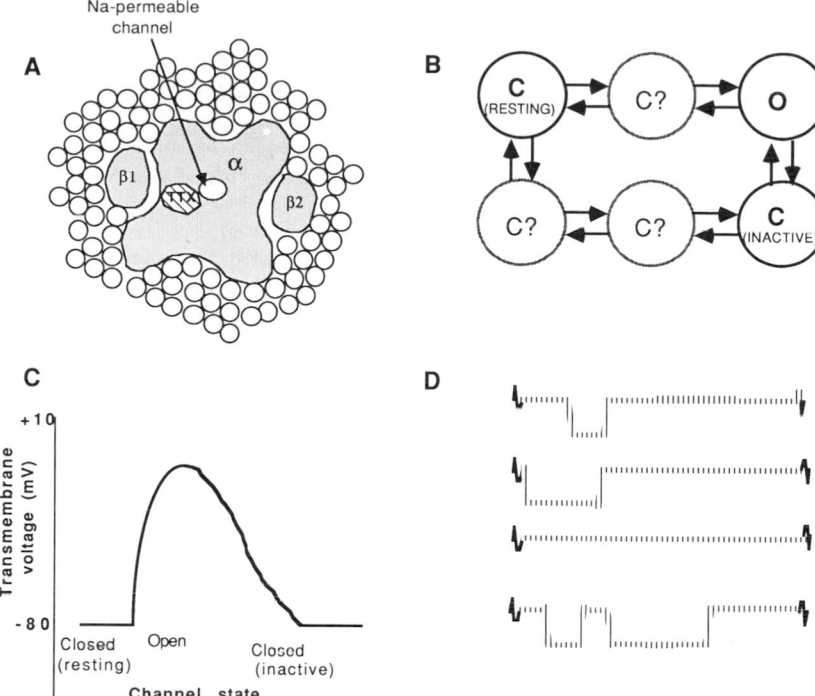

Fig. 26.3 Structure and activity of an important voltage-regulated transmembrane ion channel, the sodium channel responsible for nerve action potentials. (A), view of the channel looking down on the membrane. In the center of the α subunit is the aqueous channel through which sodium ions can cross the membrane. Near it is a binding site for the specific channel blocking agent tetrodotoxin (TTX). The function of the two β subunits is uncertain. (B), channel conformation states. In the closed resting state the channel can respond to a drop in membrane potential by moving (through an unknown number of other closed states) to the open state which permits ion passage. If the membrane remains depolarized the channel moves to a closed inactive state which cannot respond to depolarization by opening. On restoration of the transmembrane potential the channel reverts through an unknown number of closed states to the closed resting state. (C), transmembrane voltage changes and underlying sodium channel state changes during an action potential. (D), activity of a single sodium channel in response to depolarization. Downward deflections are channel openings, baseline is a closed channel. In response to depolarization, this channel opens to a single conducting state; there are no partially conducting channels. This sort of single channel analysis reveals the probability of opening in response to a stimulus and the length of time an average channel stays open, both of which contribute to the properties of the action potential.

closed to an open state permeable to sodium ions, is transmembrane voltage. A drop in voltage gradient causes a measureable movement of charge through the membrane, which must correspond either to a movement of charged particle or to a rearrangement of charge on the protein. Although there is speculation about the identity of this gating charge movement (Salkoff et al., 1987), it is not yet firmly associated with a particular part of the biochemically characterized sodium channel. Likewise, the different conformation states through which the sodium channel must pass are known chiefly from their voltage and time dependence as determined by electrical signs, and have not yet been tied to biochemical evidence of structural changes (Salkoff et al., 1987). Figure 26.3

shows the putative conformational state changes as these have been derived from functional studies, and also the electrical evidence as single channels move from closed to open states.

The calcium channel is also a voltage-gated protein, now known to exist as a variety of subtypes in both brain and in heart, where it is primarily responsible for the plateau phase of the action potential. Eventually it too will be reconstituted and analysed. Much of the progress in sodium channel analysis was made possible by specific toxins such as TTX which bind tightly to sites on the channel, and whose coupling made it possible to retain identification of structurally conserved channel components through destructive purification attempts. The relatively recent discovery of calcium channel blocking agents and activators is providing the same assistance to analysis of this channel (Glossmann et al., 1985).

3. Nicotinic Acetylcholine Receptor Channel (nAChR).

More is known about this transmitter-gated ion channel than about any other neurohumural receptor. It is the postjunctional nicotinic receptor for acetylcholine and for muscle relaxants at the vertebrate neuromuscular junction, coupled to a selective ion-permeable channel. Purification and reconstitution studies, and also techniques derived from molecular genetics have permitted a closer approximation of structure and function than is the case for the sodium channel (Numa, 1986). The nicotinic ACh receptor channel is a pentameric structure composed of five subunits, all of which are intrinsic membrane-spanning proteins (Fig. 26.4). Two, the α subunits, are duplicates; the others are highly homologous. The twin binding sites for acetylcholine and its agonists and antagonists are on the α subunits. It is possible that all five unite to form the channel, which is activated by binding of ACh to the two receptors. The portions of the subunits which traverse the membrane are

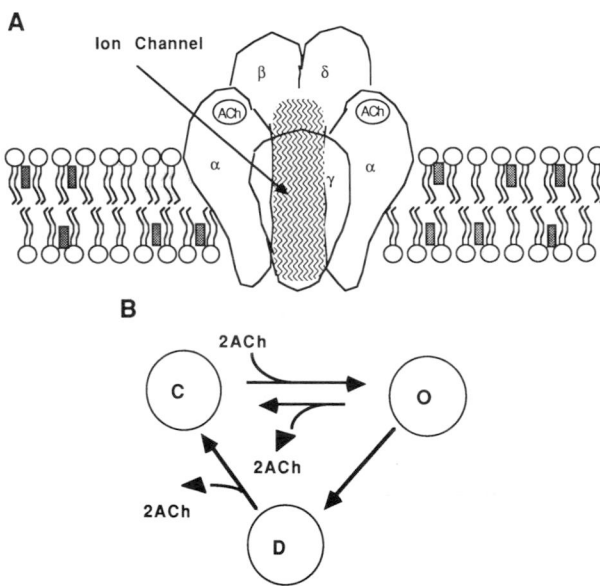

Fig. 26.4 Structure and conformation states of the most-studied transmitter regulated ion channel, the nicotinic acetylcholine receptor (nAChR). (A), the channel is made up of five subunits, all of which traverse the membrane. The paired acetylcholine receptor sites (ACh) are on the homologous α subunits; the ion-permeable channel is at the core of the complex, formed between the subunits. (B), simplified diagram of nAChR state changes during activity. The closed resting channel (C) binds two acetylcholine molecules and opens to allow ion passage (O). Normally ACh is rapidly released and hydrolyzed, and the channel reverts to the resting state. In the continued presence of agonist, however, the channel enters a closed desensitized state (D) with high affinity for ACh.

α-helices, with hydrophobic amino acid residues opposed to the membrane lipid interior (Changeux and Revah, 1987). The details of the portions of the molecule which form the passage for ions are not yet clear; however, to allow ions to pass these parts of the ACh receptor, the channel must maintain an environment with some of the properties of an aqueous solvent.

4. Channels Regulated by Neurohormonally Modulated Intracellular Messengers.

The conformation states of some ion-selective channels are modulated by intracellular concentrations of a variety of neurohormonally regulated 'messengers.' The proteins involved in this complex regulation include transmembrane receptors for transmitter and hormonal ligands, coupled to membrane-bound catalysts identified as GTP-binding proteins. Products of the reactions, including, for instance, cyclic AMP-dependent protein kinase, in turn modify some ion-selective channels by changing their phosphorylation state or by other reactions with the channel. Such a cascade of regulation is shown in Fig. 26.5. Analysis of the transmembrane receptor component of these systems has proceeded furthest with the β-adrenergic receptor coupled to adenylate cyclase shown in Fig. 26.5 (Lefkowitz et al., 1985; Lefkowitz and Caron, 1986); this mode of regulation is shared by other receptors, including adrenergic and muscarinic cholinergic receptors (Hall, 1987; Venter et al., 1986).

Lipid-protein Interactions

Membrane-bound proteins such as the ion transporters require association with lipids in order to function at all, probably because associated phospholipids are required for the protein to assume an active conformation. In attempts to reconstitute purified proteins into defined membranes, it has been found that functional reconstitution often requires a specific membrane composition. For instance, ACh receptor affinity for ligands is influenced relatively little by the surrounding membrane but its ability to function as an ion transporter depends on the presence of considerable cholesterol and is better with phosphatidylethanolamine than with other phospholipids (Fong et al., 1986). Particular proteins may preferentially associate with particular phospholipids within a heterogeneous membrane. In some cases it can be shown that the protein-lipid interaction is very specific, and that the lipid functions as a cofactor in enzyme activity. A more loose association also occurs, in which the protein interacts with a boundary layer of lipids immediately around it, whose maximum number is related to the perimeter area of the protein (Fong et al., 1986). In both cases the ability of the protein to undergo its full range of functional conformation changes depends not only on lipid fluidity but also probably on specific properties of the associated lipids such as charge on the head groups, length of the fatty

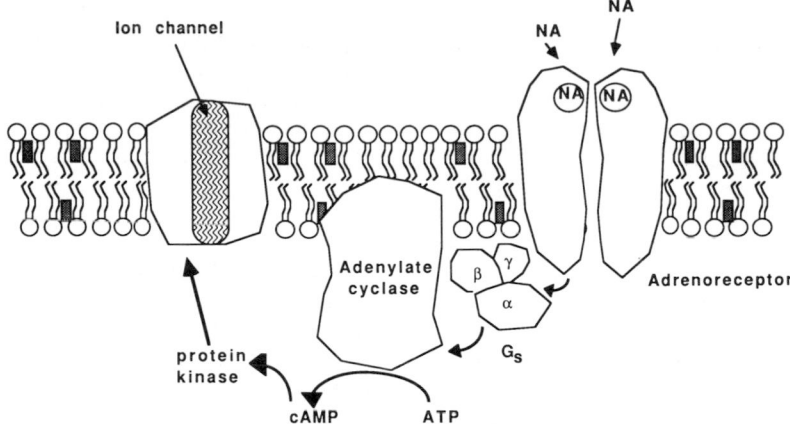

Fig. 26.5 Schema for transmitter receptors indirectly coupled to ion channels through GTP-binding proteins (G proteins). Both α and β catecholamine receptors and the muscarinic acetylcholine receptor are of this type; these receptors display considerable regions of homology among themselves. The β-adrenergic receptor coupled through adenylate cyclase is the most studied of this class, and is shown here. The receptor, which traverses the membrane, is a dimer with a noradrenaline binding site (NA) on each unit. Transmitter binding causes the receptor to activate a stimulatory GTP-binding protein, G_s, which consists of three subunits. G_s activates adenylate cyclase, which converts ATP to cyclic AMP, in turn activating a cyclic AMP-dependent protein kinase, which changes the conformation state of an ion channel. This sequence of events is usually associated with slow modulatory changes in nerve and muscle excitability; potassium-selective channels are the best known channels regulated in this way. There are inhibitory as well as excitatory G proteins, and in some pathways the G-protein subunits act directly on ion channels rather than through cyclic AMP. Other cellular processes are also subject to transmitter-mediated regulation of this type.

acyl chains, and the resulting thickness of the membrane in apposition to the membrane-intercalated portion of the protein. The properties of either the specifically associated or annular boundary lipids are modified in complex ways by the protein; a protein-lipid domain is created with properties different from those of the bulk lipid (Abney and Owicki, 1985). The original fluid-mosaic model of the membrane envisioned proteins floating with relative freedom and mobility within the bilayer, randomly interacting with lipids (Singer et al., 1972). An additional complication is introduced by the demonstration of protein-rich areas of membrane. Proteins are anchored in specific membrane areas by the cytoskeleton and possibly also by intrinsic tendencies to aggregate, creating protein-rich domains which, with their associated lipids, effectively form a phase separation from protein-poor regions.

In many treatments of anesthetic theory, attempts have been made to correlate changes in membrane protein function with changes in lipid fluidity, either continuous increases in motion in the liquid crystalline state or the discontinuous transition from crystalline gel to liquid crystalline state. Discontinuities in the temperature-dependence of protein function, such

as mark a gel-to-liquid phase transition, have often, and sometimes indiscriminately, been taken as evidence of the dependence of protein function on lipid environment. The correlation, however, is reasonable and tempting. In pure lipid systems, activity of membrane Na-K ATPase exhibits definite breaks in its temperature dependence, which can be correlated with the lipid phase transition temperature (Abney et al., 1985) (Fig. 26.6).

In natural membranes, however, the relationship is more complex. In order to investigate the relationship between protein activity and membrane lipid composition, experimental attempts have been made to alter the lipid composition of natural membranes either by attempting to incorporate lipids directly into the cell membranes in culture or by dietary manipulation in the intact animal (Deuticke et al., 1987). Both types of experiments alter bulk lipid composition. Experiments in tissue culture, however, must be analysed cautiously because of artifacts due to the procedure. Dietary modification is successful in changing the lipid composition even of mammalian cells; however, bulk lipid fluidity is less affected, because of compensatory mechanisms which secondarily alter the composition to maintain a given fluidity. Na-K ATPase

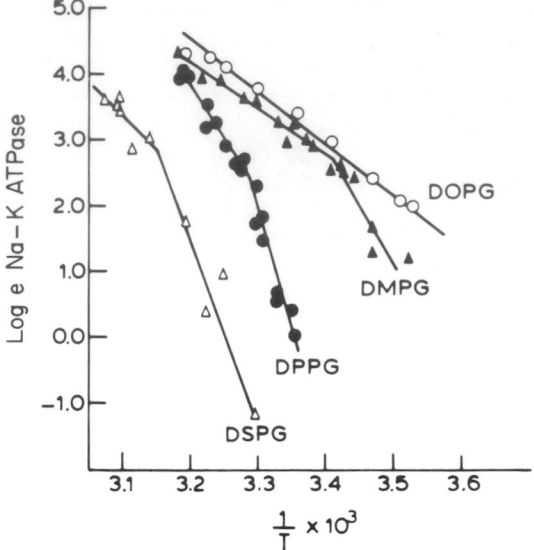

Fig. 26.6 Experimental evidence of the sort used to support the dependence of membrane protein function on properties of the surrounding lipid. Arrhenius plots of rabbit kidney Na-K ATPase activity in four different pure phosphatidylglycerol systems. Temperature dependence of enzyme activity is modified by the lipid surround, and break points in the plot are correlated with the respective lipid phase transition temperatures. DOPG has no transition in this temperature range, and no break was observed in the enzyme activity plot. (Reproduced with permission from Abney and Owicki, 1985; and from Kimelberg and Papabadjopoulox, *J. Biol. Chemistry*, 1974, **249**, 1071).

activity in preparations derived from animals with dietarily modified membranes is altered, but this may be a secondary response to other changes in the cell (Schachter, 1985). In addition to fluidity, specific phospholipid structure is an important prerequisite for protein function. In some enzyme systems, however, lipid requirements appear to be less rigorous than in others, and different lipid properties are important. For instance, charge is important for some Na-K ATPase (Esmann et al., 1985), acyl chain length but not fluidity *per se* for Ca-ATPase (East et al., 1984), fluidity for receptor-stimulated adenylate cyclase (Houslay and Gordon, 1983), and membrane cholesterol content for the nicotinic acetylcholine receptor (Levitzki, 1985).

EVENTS IN NERVE CELL MEMBRANES

The above outline has delineated the basic structure of cell membranes, the structures of some proteins important in excitable cell function, and possible interactions between the lipid bilayer and intrinsic membrane proteins. This section will outline the way membrane proteins make possible the electrical and neurosecretory activity of excitable cells.

Active Ion Transport

The basic condition for excitable cell function is the regulation of intracellular ion content. This is particularly important for three specific ions: sodium, potassium and calcium. The activity of Na-K ATPase, shown in Fig. 26.2, reduces the intracellular content of Na and increases the intracellular concentration of K ion relative to the extracellular fluid. If the membrane were impermeable to both ions, or equally permeable to both, the electrical result would be nil. However, at rest the membrane is more permeable to potassium than to sodium; potassium freely diffuses outward across the membrane in response to its concentration gradient, whereas sodium cannot diffuse inward. The result is an excess of positive charge on the extracellular side of the membrane, rendering the cytoplasmic side negative to the extracellular side by an amount which ranges between 50 and 100 mV, depending on the cell.

The relationship between transmembrane potential and ion permeability is formulated by the well known Nernst equation, given here in a simplified form:

$$V_m = \frac{RT}{F} \ln \frac{P_K[K^+]_o + P_{Na}[Na^+]_o}{P_K[K^+]_i + P_{Na}[Na^+]_i}$$

where V_m is the transmembrane voltage, P_K and P_{Na} are the permeabilities of the two ions, and the bracketed figures are the concentrations of each at the outer (o) and inner (i) surface of the axon membrane.

Ca-dependent ATPase performs a similar function for the calcium ion, extruding it from the cell by transporting it outward across the cell membrane or sequestering the ion in intracellular membrane-bound vesicles, thus reducing normal cytoplasmic calcium concentration to very low levels. Regulation of intracellular Ca is of supreme importance to cell functions; the activity of many proteins is regulated by small transient increases in this ion, which acts as a messenger to trigger cellular responses.

Electrically Gated Ion-selective Channel State Transitions

The best characterized of the voltage sensitive proteins is the sodium channel whose structure is shown in Fig. 26.3. Even before much progress had been made in its molecular characterization, studies on its ion selectivity and the kinetics of both gating charge and ion movement had permitted conclusions to be drawn about its properties and conformation changes.

The sodium channel is responsible for the current which underlies the impulses (action potentials) conducted along peripheral nerves and the axons of central neurons. Figure 26.3 diagrams the relationship between ion channel function and the action potential. As the channels open in response to membrane depolarization, an inward current carried by sodium ions flows and the resulting change in transmembrane potential is reflected by the rising phase of the action potential. Channel inactivation begins to shut off sodium permeability, however, even before the peak of the action potential occurs. The falling phase of the action potential in vertebrate peripheral nerves (Fig. 26.3) is due to the process of inactivation, with a time course slower than that of channel activation.

Repolarization during the falling phase of the action potential in some cells is hastened by the contribution of a second voltage-sensitive ion channel, the potassium channel. In an often-studied axon model, the squid giant axon, the potassium channel contributes much more to membrane repolarization than is the case in vertebrate myelinated fibers (Ritchie, 1979). This channel also responds to depolarization by opening, but with a much slower time course than that displayed by the sodium channel. The resulting increase in permeability is accompanied by an outward current carried by potassium ions. The potassium channel does not normally inactivate; instead, it is closed by the repolarization of the membrane.

The duration and shape of the action potential is due to the balance at each point between the sodium and potassium permeabilities as determined by the overlapping time courses of the conformation changes undergone by the two types of channels.

Transmitter Release

With the exception of electrical connections whose overall importance in central nervous system function has yet to be defined, nerve cells communicate with each other through release of neurohormones (neurotransmitters) at specialized regions of cellular contact (synapses). The process of transmitter release is shown in Fig. 26.7. Nerve terminal depolarization by activity in the presynaptic neuron is followed by an increase in intracellular calcium concentration, as calcium enters through voltage-activated Ca channels. The increased intracellular calcium acts as a catalyst for the process of transmitter release. Transmitter-containing vesicles fuse with the terminal membrane and release their contents into the intercellular cleft, across which the transmitter molecules diffuse to binding sites on receptors in the membrane of the postsynaptic cell.

Chemically Gated Channel State Transitions

1. Fast Excitatory: ACh and Amino Acids. The types of channel changes which may be involved in fast synaptic transmission are shown in Fig. 26.5. This figure illustrates the best understood example of fast transmission, namely that mediated by acetylcholine acting on the nicotinic acetylcholine receptor. This type of receptor-channel complex is found at the neuromuscular junction and in sympathetic ganglia. The permeability increase to both sodium and potassium produces an inward current and a depolarization

of the postsynaptic membrane, which in muscle is sufficient to trigger an action potential in adjacent electrically excitable membrane. The relationship between channel state and postsynaptic electrical response is shown in Figs. 26.4 and 26.7. The opening, triggered by the binding of transmitter to receptor, produces a rapid increase in membrane permeability. Following dissociation of the transmitter from the receptor-channel complex, the channels revert to the closed state. Rapid destruction of the transmitter by acetylcholinesterase present in the synaptic cleft normally removes the transmitter, so that the channels tend to remain closed until a fresh burst of transmitter arrives after release from the presynaptic terminal. There is a third, inactive or desensitized state of the acetylcholine receptor-channel complex which is achieved when acetylcholine or a cholinomimetic agent remains in the synaptic cleft in high concentrations, e.g. in the presence of a cholinesterase inhibitor or with prolonged application of depolarizing neuromuscular blocking agents. The desensitized channel-receptor complex does not open in response to the arrival of a fresh burst of transmitter.

Similar depolarizing ion permeability increases occur in response to the transmitter glutamate, found in the mammalian central nervous system and at some invertebrate neuromuscular junctions. As yet there is not enough evidence about these receptor-channel complexes to compare them in detail to the more familiar acetylcholine-sensitive channel. However, like other channels, they exist as a variety of subtypes, characterized by sensitivity to particular agonists such as NMDA (N-methyl-D-asparate) and kainic acid.

2. The Inhibitory Chloride Channel. A second prominent type of transmitter-sensitive ion channel plays a role in inhibiting, rather than exciting, the postsynaptic nerve cell. The transmitter is γ-aminobutyric acid (GABA), and the open channel is permeable to chloride. The steps in transmitter-receptor coupling and in channel opening are presumed to be similar to those described above for the acetylcholine channel. The response to channel opening is sometimes a membrane hyperpolarization, but a change in membrane potential is not essential to the inhibitory effect of chloride conductance increase. Chloride is normally distributed passively across the cell membrane with a concentration gradient close to electrochemical equilibrium at the resting potential. The effect of a permeability increase to this ion, therefore, is to tend to hold the membrane potential near the resting potential, and thus to prevent the depolarization produced at nearby excitatory synapses. The decrease in membrane resistance when the chloride channels open 'short-circuits' the membrane and reduces the potential change produced by excitatory input.

This rather well-studied channel has received considerable attention in anesthesia-related pharmacology. In addition to the GABA binding site, there is a

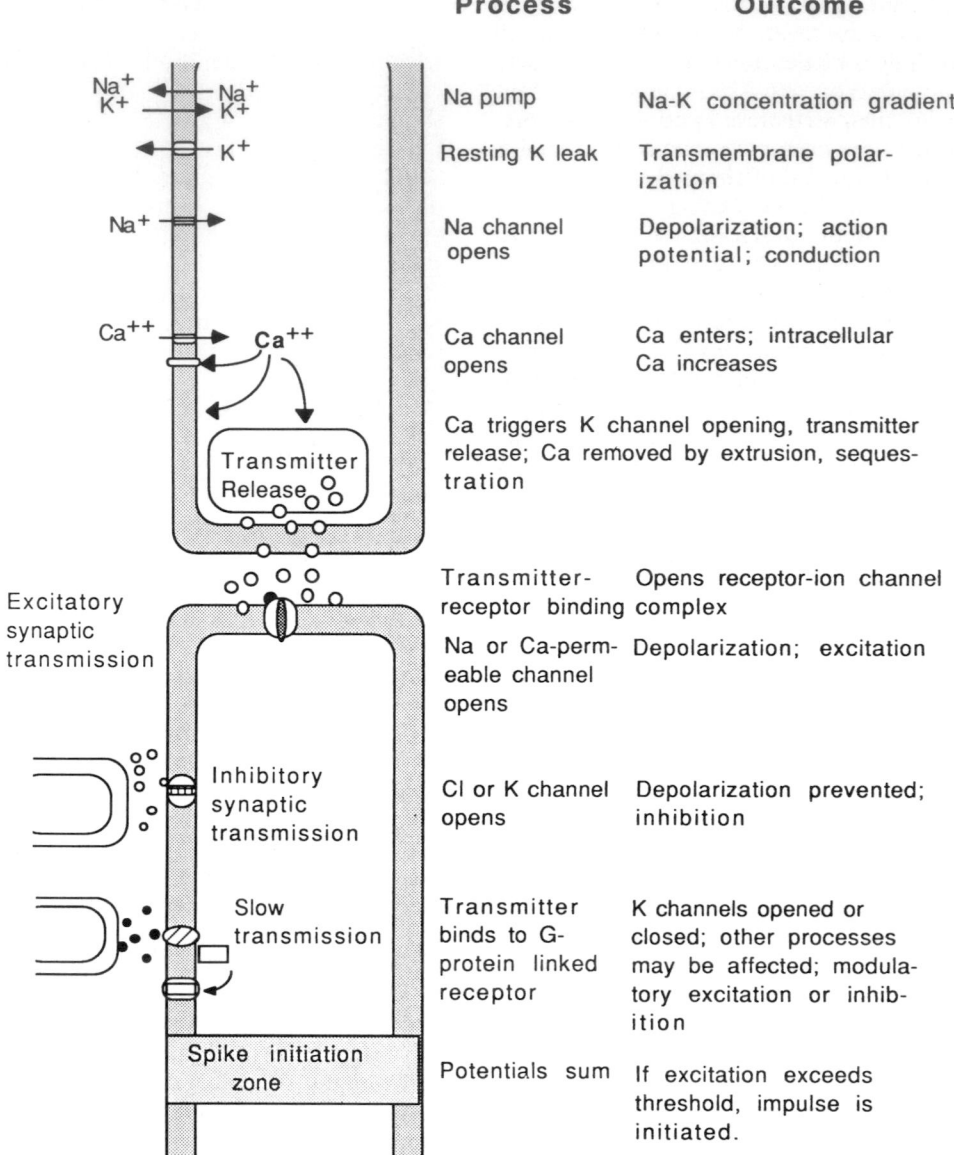

Process	Outcome
Na pump	Na-K concentration gradient
Resting K leak	Transmembrane polarization
Na channel opens	Depolarization; action potential; conduction
Ca channel opens	Ca enters; intracellular Ca increases
	Ca triggers K channel opening, transmitter release; Ca removed by extrusion, sequestration
Transmitter-receptor binding	Opens receptor-ion channel complex
Na or Ca-permeable channel opens	Depolarization; excitation
Cl or K channel opens	Depolarization prevented; inhibition
Transmitter binds to G-protein linked receptor	K channels opened or closed; other processes may be affected; modulatory excitation or inhibition
Potentials sum	If excitation exceeds threshold, impulse is initiated.

Fig. 26.7 Summary of membrane proteins and processes important in nerve and muscle cell excitability. On the left are shown in diagrammatic form two excitable cells at the region of a synapse, the upper presynaptic and the lower postsynaptic. Excitatory synaptic transmission is shown at this synapse, and inhibitory and slow modulatory transmission at two additional synapses. The channel or cellular process is labeled in the center column, and its effect on cellular function on the right.

related binding site on the channel for benzodiazepines. Barbiturates may also bind to this channel and either mimic the transmitter or alter its binding in order to prolong inhibition. The GABA channel is characterized by sensitivity to the convulsant blocking agents picrotoxin and bicuculline. In the central nervous system there is a non-bicuculline sensitive GABA channel, with a receptor site for baclofen, which may operate through the same regulatory mechanism described for catecholamine receptors

below (Andrade et al., 1986). The baclofen channel is now called the GABA-B channel, and the more familiar bicuculline-sensitive channel the GABA-A. The GABA receptor can apparently be coupled to ion-selective channels other than the chloride channel (Alger and Nicoll, 1982).

3. **Catecholamine and Muscarinic Receptors, the Metabolic Cascade, and their Associated Ion Channels.** There has been an explosive growth in the under-

standing of a quite different class of transmitter-regulated changes in excitable cells which are of great importance to the practice of anesthesia, particularly because of their roles in autonomic regulation. These are the processes regulated by adrenergic receptors, separable by their sensitivities to particular agonists into a variety of subtypes, and by the muscarinic cholinergic receptor. All these receptors are intrinsic membrane proteins with considerable homologies to each other, in spite of their distinct pharmacologic differences at the ligand binding site and their often opposite actions on effectors (Hall, 1987; Venter et al., 1986). The adrenergic receptors are probably arranged as dimers in the membrane. Unlike the nicotinic acetylcholine receptor and the GABA receptor, they are not coupled directly to an ion-selective channel. Rather, they form the first link in a chain of reactions such as that shown in Fig. 26.5. The receptors activate excitatory or inhibitory GTP binding proteins, which in turn may regulate ion channels directly or indirectly through adenylate cyclase and cyclic nucleotides or through other cytoplasmic messengers. Commonly the end-stage ion channel known to be subject to modulation by these transmitters is a potassium-selective channel whose tendency to exist in the open state may be either increased or decreased as the ultimate effect of the transmitter (Dunlap et al., 1987). The indirectness of the coupling between the receptor and the ion channel, with the requirement in some cases for build-up of a particular chemical species in the cell, makes the resulting changes in the cell tend to be of a slow, sustained modulatory nature rather than the fast large transients characteristic of the more directly coupled channels. The pharmacologic specificity of the receptor and the different effectors to which it may be linked account for the bewildering variety of effects which characterize autonomic regulation in different tissues.

4. Varieties of Voltage and Ligand-gated Potassium Channels.

The sodium channel of peripheral nerve, the calcium channel, the GABA-linked chloride channel, and the nicotinic acetylcholine receptor channel have all been known for some time. Although subtypes of each have been discovered, in most cases the differences are subtle. In the case of potassium channels, however, it is clear that there are many different types even within the same cell, which are characterized by their marked differences in regulation by transmembrane voltage and time, transmitter, intracellular calcium, or a combination of modes of regulation. The varieties of potassium channels play a role in regulating automaticity in heart, and patterns of discharge in brain. Although potassium channels have been isolated, progress in determining their structures has been slow compared to some other ion channels. Nevertheless, they are of great importance in regulating excitable cell activity, and have been suggested to be important in anesthesia as outlined in the next chapter.

SUMMARY

The growth in knowledge of the molecular biology of excitable cell function has been amazingly fast in the last few years. Not only have many transport proteins been characterized physiologically and their roles in excitation defined, but their structures and their relationship to membrane lipids have been described in considerable detail as well. The next chapter presents considerations of how anesthetic agents may interact with these membrane proteins and their lipid matrix.

Acknowledgements

Preparation of this chapter was supported by NIH grant NS13108 to JJK. The author is indebted to Dr James R. Trudell of the Stanford Department of Anesthesia for a critical reading of the manuscript.

REFERENCES

Abney J.R., Owicki J.C. (1985). Theories of protein-lipid and protein-protein interactions in membranes. In *Progress in Protein-Lipid Interactions*, pp. 1–60. (Watts A., DePont J.J.H.H.M. eds.) Amsterdam: Elsevier.

Alger B.E., Nicoll R.A. (1982). Pharmacological evidence for two kinds of GABA receptor on rat hippocampal pyramidal cells studied *in vitro*. *J. Physiol.*, **328**, 125.

Andrade R., Malenka R.C., Nicoll R.A. (1986). A G protein couples serotonin and GABA$_B$ receptors to the same channels in hippocampus. *Science*, **234**, 1261.

Bretscher M.S. (1985). The molecules of the cell membrane. *Sci. Am.*, **253**, 100.

Catterall W.A., Schmidt J.W., Messner D.J., et al., (1986). Structure and biosynthesis of neuronal sodium channels. *Ann. N. Y. Acad. Sci.*, **479**, 186.

Changeux J.-P., Revah F. (1987). The acetylcholine receptor molecule: allosteric sites and the ion channel. *Trends Neurosci.*, **10**, 245.

Deuticke B., Haest C.W.M. (1987). Lipid modulation of transport proteins in vertebrate cell membranes. *Ann. Rev. Physiol.*, **49**, 221.

Dunlap K., Holz G.G., Rane S.G. (1987). G proteins as regulators of ion channel function. *Trends Neurosci.*, **10**, 241.

East J.M., Jones O.T., Simmonds A.C., et al. (1984). Membrane fluidity is not an important physiological regulator of the (Ca^{2+}-Mg^{2+})-dependent ATPase of sarcoplasmic reticulum. *J. Biol. Chem.*, **259**, 8070.

Esmann M., Watts A., Marsh D. (1985). Spin-label studies of lipid-protein interactions in (Na$^+$,K$^+$)-ATPase membranes from rectal glands of *Squalus acanthias*. *Biochemistry*, **24**, 1386.

Fong T.M., McNamee M.G. (1986). Correlation between acetylcholine receptor function and structural properties of membranes. *Biochemistry*, **25**, 830.

Glossmann H., Ferry D.R., Goll A., et al. (1985). Molecular approach to the calcium channel. In *Advances in Myocardiology*, Vol. 5, pp. 41–76. (Harris P., Poole-Wilson P.A. eds.) New York: Plenum.

Hall Z.W. (1987). Three of a kind: the β-adrenergic receptor, the muscarinic acetylcholine receptor, and rhodopsin. *Trends Neurosci.*, **10**, 99.

Houslay M.D., Gordon L.M. (1983). The activity of adenylate cyclase is regulated by the nature of its lipid environment. *Curr. Top. Membrane Trans.*, **18**, 179.

Lefkowitz R.J., Caron M.G. (1986). Regulation of adrenergic receptor function by phosphorylation. *Curr. Top. Cell Regul.*, **28**, 209.

Lefkowitz R.J., Cerione R.A., Codina J., et al. (1985). Reconstitution of the beta-adrenergic receptor. *J. Membrane Biol.*, **87**, 1.

Levitzki A. (1985). Reconstitution of membrane receptor systems. *Biochimica Biophysica Acta*, **822**, 127.

Melchior D.L. (1986). Lipid domains in fluid membranes: a quick-freeze differential scanning calorimetry study. *Science*, **234**, 1577.

Numa S. (1986). Molecular basis for the function of ionic channels. *Biochem. Soc. Symp.*, **52**, 119.

Ritchie J.M. (1979). A pharmacological approach to the study of sodium channels in myelinated axons. *Ann. Rev. Neurosci.*, **2**, 341.

Salkoff L., Butler A., Wei A., et al. (1987). Genomic organization and deduced amino acid sequence of a putative sodium channel gene in *Drosophila. Science*, **237**, 744.

Schachter D. (1985). Lipid dynamics and lipid-protein interactions in intestinal plasma membranes. In *Progress in Protein-Lipid Interactions*, pp. 231–258. Watts A., DePont J.J.H.H.M. eds. Amsterdam: Elsevier.

Shimshick E.J., McConnell H.M. (1973). Lateral phase separation in phospholipid membranes. *Biochemistry*, **12**, 2351.

Singer S.J., Nicolson G.L. (1972). The fluid mosaic model of the structure of cell membranes. *Science*, **175**, 720.

Stahl W.L., Harris W.E. (1986) Na$^+$,K$^+$-ATPase: structure, function, and interactions with drugs. *Adv. Neurol.*, **44**, 681.

Stubbs C.D., Smith A.D. (1984). The modification of mammalian membrane polyunsaturated fatty acid composition in relation to membrane fluidity and function. *Biochimica Biophysica Acta*, **779**, 89.

Venter J.C., Kerlavage A.R., Fraser C.M. (1986). Alpha and beta adrenergic and muscarinic cholinergic receptor structure. *Biochem. Soc. Symp.*, **52**, 1.

27. Theory of Anesthesia

Joan J. Kendig and J. R. Trudell

Historically, the approaches to a comprehensive theory of anesthesia have evolved from two very different directions. On the one hand, clinicians have probed the observable states of narcosis in man and neurophysiologists have directed their observations to single neurons. On the other hand, biochemists have studied the effects of anesthetics in model systems including olive oil, phospholipid bilayers, single proteins and erythrocyte membranes. The clinician and neurophysiologist can observe many physiological effects of the anesthetic but are only beginning to describe them on a molecular level. The biochemist, in turn, describes the way in which an anesthetic molecule affects the properties of molecules in model membrane systems, but is yet unable to establish the necessary correspondence between these systems and the central nervous system. Theories of anesthesia, using evidence derived from these different sources, have developed into two opposing hypotheses. One is that anesthesia is a unitary phenomenon, fundamentally identical for all agents. The other is that anesthesia is a multi-site phenomenon based on a number of different effects which are to a certain extent agent-specific. These two hypotheses, with their corollaries, are presented in Table 27.1. The logical consequences of each have driven both research and debate in anesthesia since the beginning.

Unlike the pharmacology of other drug classes, structure-activity relationships have little to contribute to anesthetic theory as yet, although they are of undoubted importance (Halsey, 1984). A survey of compounds which produce anesthesia includes large molecules like the steroids, smaller volatile agents such as chloroform, and chemically inert monoatomic agents like xenon. Barbiturates, opiates and the newer intravenous agents present additional divergence in structure. The diversity of structures among anesthetic agents initially suggests that there must be many different ways of producing anesthesia. The varying amounts of narcosis, analgesia, excitation, depression, and convulsive activity characteristic of individual compounds within each class of anesthetics implies an extraordinary sensitivity and complexity in the response of the organism to these drugs.

Despite the structural diversity, there is an excellent correlation between anesthetic potency and ability to dissolve in a hydrophobic solvent (Fig. 27.1). This correlation, first reported by Meyer (1899) and by

TABLE 27.1.
UNITARY AND MULTISITE THEORIES OF ANESTHESIA

	Unitary	*Multisite*
Hypothesis	All anesthetics, both inhalation and intravenous, act in fundamentally the same way	Anesthesia is due to a combination of actions, which may be agent–specific
Corollary	Every anesthetic action relevant to anesthesia must satisfy the Meyer-Overton correlation	Differences between agents of similar hydrophobicity may be relevant to anesthesia
Agent–specific effects	Side effects unrelated to anesthesia	May be part of anesthesia
Pressure reversal	Interpretation as global opposing actions of anesthetics and pressure	Differences between pressure-response curves for different agents interpreted to mean multiple sites
Sources of evidence	Intact animals, model lipid and protein systems	Discrete cellular processes, model systems examined in fine detail

Overton (1901), has been taken to support the hypothesis that there is a single hydrophobic site at which all agents act. In general, studies on model systems, whether lipid or protein, still speak to a unitary hypothesis. Early neurophysiologic studies, based on a limited understanding of the complexity of neuronal processes, also suggested a limited number of target sites for anesthetic action. They thus supported the concept of a single cellular site at which all anesthetics act to produce anesthesia. Studies in neurophysiology of anesthetics, however, now must deal with the greatly increased complexity known to regulate central neuronal activity. A given end point such as decrease in the level of impulse activity can be brought about by changes in more than one of these processes. Anesthetics act on many cellular processes. From the standpoint of cellular neurophysiology, the elegantly simple unitary hypotheses of anesthetic action are presently being forced to give way to multi-site hypotheses, and further to the notion that anesthesia is a somewhat different phenomenon for agents of different structures.

MOLECULAR BASIS OF ANESTHESIA IN MODEL SYSTEMS

Undoubtedly, a discussion of model systems must begin with the pioneering work of Meyer (1899) and Overton (1901). These investigators made the observation that the potency of anesthetics correlated remarkably well with their water to olive oil partition coefficients. Thus, olive oil became the first model for the central nervous system. This correlation, established nine decades ago, is still the best available (Fig. 27.1). Besides the volatile agents, the correlation encompasses substances such as xenon, nitrogen, nitrous oxide and fluorosulphur compounds. Other workers have suggested improvements to this early model system. Ferguson (1939) improved the potency-oil solubility correlation by suggesting that the thermodynamic activity of an anesthetic in a hydrocarbon phase should be substituted for its concentra-

tion. Mullins (1971) proposed that the most important property of an inhalation anesthetic was not its dipole moment, its ability to create or destroy hydrogen bonds, or its stereochemistry, but rather that it was simply the element of volume that the anesthetic occupied in the hydrocarbon phase. Miller et al. (1971) used thermodynamic principles to calculate that the solubility parameter (σ) of the region in which anesthetics act is 9 ± 1; this is close to that of a hydrocarbon phase (benzene = 9.2). Katz and Simon (1977) have characterized additional parameters of the supposed anesthetic site. The usefulness of these thermodynamic approaches is lessened by the implicit assumption that the site of anesthesia is homogeneous enough to be characterized by unique parameters.

There is every reason to believe that the functional site or sites occupied by anesthetics is hydrophobic. The realization of the structural importance of the lipid bilayer focussed early attention on membrane phospholipids as a possible site of anesthesia. The dependence of various proteins on characteristics of their lipid surround is reviewed in the preceding chapter. If anesthetics, in fact, significantly alter lipid properties, then protein properties such as lipid binding and ability to change conformation may be altered as well. Nerve functional proteins may be thought of as operating in a milieu of optimum polarity and viscosity. Any alteration in these characteristics of the proteins' environment due to the presence of drugs, the application of pressure, or change in temperature would alter neuronal membrane protein function, and thus the activity pattern characteristic of a given excitable cell. However, there is considerable argument about whether anesthetics affect membrane lipids sufficiently to account for anesthesia. Measurements of anesthetic effects have focussed on a variety of physical measures of lipid order and disorder. There is no doubt that anesthetics can enter the lipid bilayer, and that their effects in pure phospholipid bilayers are to increase fluidity, acting much like an increase in temperature (Trudell et al., 1973a) (Fig. 27.2). However, there is little agreement on the magnitude of the physical effect of the presence of the anesthetic. Some

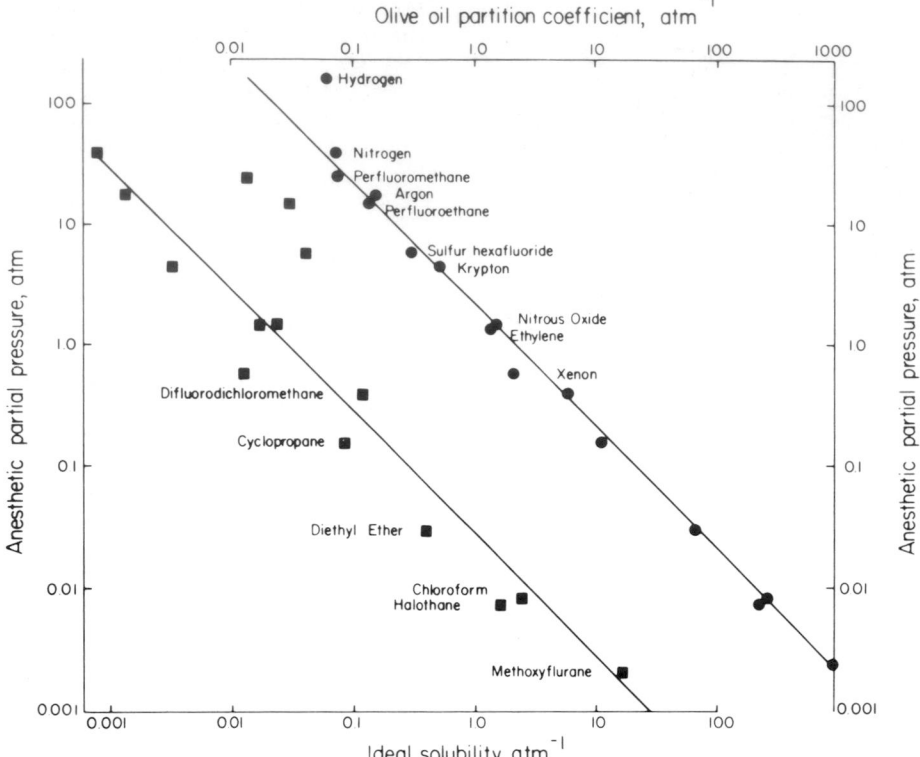

Fig. 27.1 Relationship between anesthetic potency and physical properties of anesthetic agents. Above right: anesthetic partial pressure in atmospheres shows an excellent correlation with solubility in a hydrophobic substance such as olive oil. Below left: anesthetic partial pressure also correlates well with ideal solubility (reciprocal of the vapor pressure). The olive oil correlation was first demonstrated by Meyer (1899) and by Overton (1901), who used it to suggest that the site of anesthetic action was a cellular fatty substance; the modification using ideal solubility was proposed by Ferguson. (Reproduced with permission from Miller, 1985).

studies report it as small or nonexistent at clinical concentrations, equivalent at most to a very small increase in temperature (Franks and Lieb, 1986a); others suggest a more sizeable effect (Trudell et al., 1973a). If lipids exist in different phases in mammals, anesthetic effect may be magnified by a decrease in phase transition temperature such that certain lipids move from the tightly packed gel state to the much looser liquid crystal phase. Anesthetic-induced shifts in phase transition temperature can be demonstrated in defined lipid systems (Trudell, 1977) (Fig. 27.2).

The evidence for the role of lipids in anesthetic effects consists of two types of correlated changes. In the presence of anesthetics, there are parallel changes in lipid fluidity and enzyme activity (Houslay and Gordon, 1983). Also, in many systems anesthetics induce shifts in the break points of Arrhenius plots of activity versus temperature. Since such break points are characteristic of phase transitions, a shift is often taken as evidence that the anesthetic effect is due to a shift in the phase transition temperature of the lipid (Houslay et al., 1983). Such evidence has supported the contention that anesthetics may alter protein func-

tion by acting on lipid surrounds (Fig. 27.3). In addition to these correlations which support a lipid site of action, counter arguments are made to claims that the anesthetic effect on lipids is too small. One argument is that although the structural effect is small, the resulting functional effect may be large (Miller, 1985); the second argument is that anesthetic effects are specific to particular membrane lipids, in particular those closely associated with proteins, and therefore may not be fully expressed in measurements of overall membrane fluidity.

In support of these possibilities, Miller and Pang (1976) showed that lipid composition (the relative proportion of cholesterol, phosphatidylcholine and phosphatidic acid) modulates the ability of an anesthetic to fluidize membranes. Pang et al. (1979) showed that the coupling between increases in permeability and pertubation of membrane structure is strong, the functional changes being an order of magnitude larger than the structural changes. These increases in membrane fluidity take place at clinical anesthetic concentrations which are compatible with those predicted by Meyer and Overton, i.e. 30–

Normal

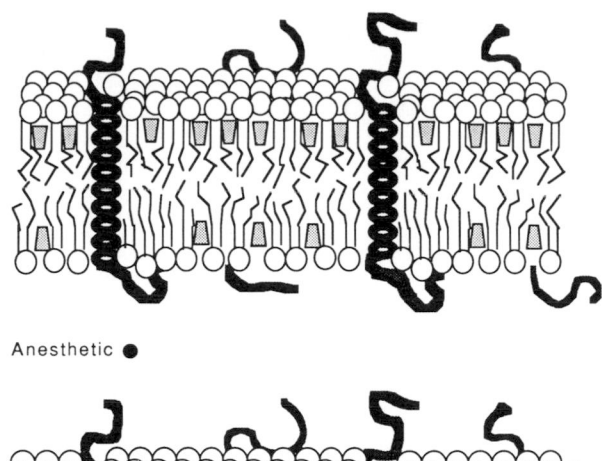

Anesthetic ●

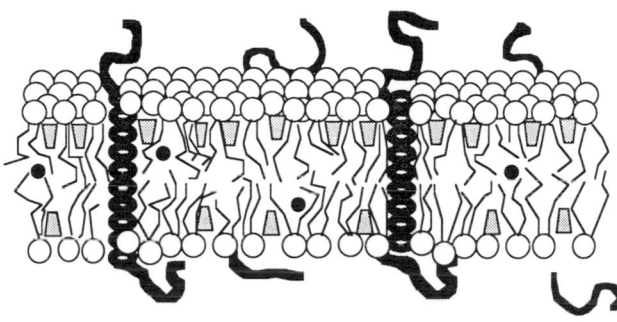

Fig. 27.2 Anesthetic effects on fluidity in the lipid bilayer. Above, the normal relatively ordered bilayer with embedded proteins (for legend *see* Fig. 26.1 of the preceding chapter). Below, anesthetic molecules dissolve in the hydrophobic interior of the bilayer and increase the rate and range of motion of the phospholipids. The result is a less ordered, more fluid bilayer in the liquid crystalline state and a decrease in the temperature at which a given phospholipid moves from the gel phase to the liquid crystal phase. Such effects can easily be demonstrated in model bilayers; whether lipid effects can disturb the function of membrane proteins sufficiently to account for anesthesia is a matter of debate.

60 mmol/L of lipid. The preceding chapter presented the evidence that membranes are in fact heterogeneous with respect to lipid composition, particularly in respect to the lipid surround of proteins. Thus it is possible that important lipid effects are restricted to these domains, and are lost in measurements of bulk fluidity.

Although most studies attempting to implicate lipids in the modulation of protein function have focussed on fluidity, current research on lipid-protein interactions suggests that other properties are also important (*see* preceding chapter). It has been proposed that the effects of apolar anesthetic molecules on the sodium channel can be accounted for by an increase in membrane thickness, whereas polar anesthetics such as alcohols, which might tend to locate near the more polar head group of the bilayer, exert an effect on membrane surface potential (Elliott and Haydon, 1986; Haydon et al., 1986b). Differential ordering and disordering effects of structurally dissimilar agents

have also been reported, dependent on bilayer composition (Miller, 1985). Even structurally similar, anesthetically equipotent isomers exert differential effects on defined lipid bilayers (O'Leary et al., 1986). Thus, although solution in a membrane lipid initially was conceived as a unitary anesthetic hypothesis, exposition of detailed locus and molecule-specific actions within the membrane lipid begins to resemble multi-site theories (Table 27.1).

The alternative possibility to lipid theories is that anesthetics act directly on proteins. The extreme range of molecules that produce anesthesia, from xenon to steroids, would seem to make a protein binding site an unlikely primary site of anesthetic action. Many researchers have proposed that anesthetics directly affect protein function without mediation of the lipid phase (Richards et al., 1978; Richter et al., 1977). Binding of even inert agents to a specific site on a protein was initially demonstrated by Featherstone and Muehlbacher (1963), who demonstrated that xenon links to myoglobin. Until recently, however, there had been no correlation between such binding and functional effects of anesthetics on a protein, distinguishable from possible non-specific effects on associated lipid. This requirement has now been met for the protein luciferase, which in lipid-free preparations is inhibited by anesthetics through site-specific binding (Franks and Lieb, 1986a, b). The ability of anesthetic agents to inhibit luciferase activity correlates well with both lipid solubility and anesthetic potency, showing that the Meyer-Overton correlation also fits a protein site of anesthetic action (Fig. 27.4). The characteristics of anesthetic inhibition support the contention that anesthetics compete with the substrate luciferin by binding to an amphiphilic pocket in the protein. The stoichiometry suggests that two small molecules such as halothane can occupy the site, whereas one larger one, of similar dimensions to luciferin, is sufficient.

The demonstration of size requirement for binding to a specific site on the protein also accounts for another observation important in anesthetic theory. Within a series of hydrocarbons such as alcohols, anesthetic potency increases with chain length and lipid solubility. However, above a given chain length of about 12 carbon atoms, anesthetic potency abruptly decreases. This cut off phenomenon, which can be demonstrated for luciferase inhibition, is logically related to size limitations of the binding site (Franks et al., 1986a). On the other hand, the cut off can also be explained by theories based on solubility in lipid bilayers: above a given chain length, either the anesthetic molecule does not enter the membrane because it cannot fit, or limited aqueous solubility prevents sufficient anesthetic from partitioning into the membrane within the time limits of the experiment (Miller, 1985).

The demonstration of specific anesthetic binding to a site on luciferase, of course, does not show that anesthetics bind to the membrane proteins which underlie nerve function. Direct site-specific actions on

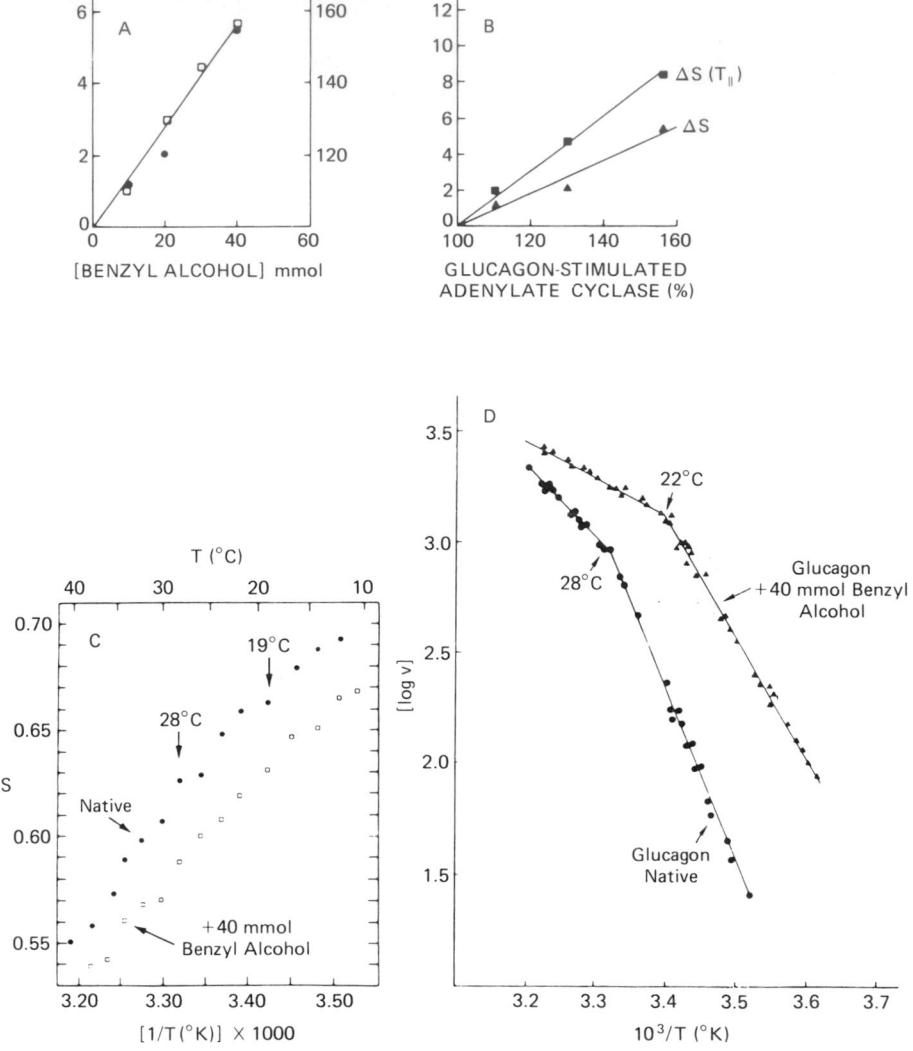

Fig. 27.3 Evidence that a model lipophilic anesthetic molecule, benzyl alcohol, influences protein function through an action on membrane lipids. A. Increasing concentrations of benzyl alcohol increase the activity of glucagon-stimulated adenylate cyclase. B. The increase in adenylate cyclase activity (horizontal axis) is paralleled by an increase in lipid fluidity in the bilayer as measured by decreases in the order parameter (vertical axis). C. Benzyl alcohol shifts the onset of a lipid phase transition temperature downward from 28–22°C. D. The shift in lipid phase transition temperature corresponds to a shift in the break point of the Arrhenius plot of adenylate cyclase activity. (Adapted with permission from Houslay and Gordon, 1980).

a protein important in nerve cell function (the GABA receptor) have been demonstrated for the barbiturates, but it is not clear whether all anesthetics can exert such effects or whether even for barbiturates they are associated with anesthesia (Olsen et al., 1986).

Currently there is no consensus implicating a single region or molecule as the unitary site of action of all anesthetics. Evidence such as the Meyer-Overton correlation, the cut-off phenomenon, and even the

demonstration of saturable volatile anesthetic binding in brain (Evers et al., 1987), is insufficient to discriminate between lipid and protein sites, much less implicate specific lipids or proteins.

BASIS OF ANESTHESIA IN NERVE CELLS

Whether the primary site of anesthetic action be lipid or protein, there is no doubt that the proximal cause of anesthesia must be the modification of the normal

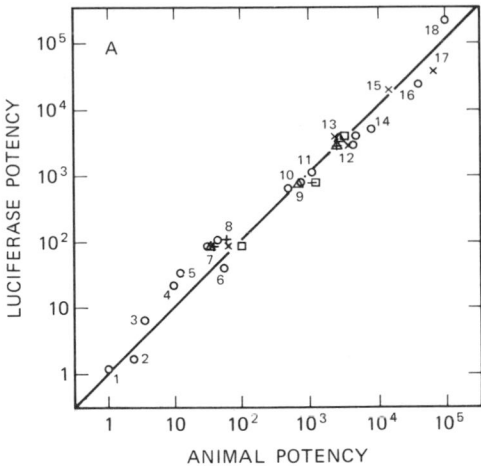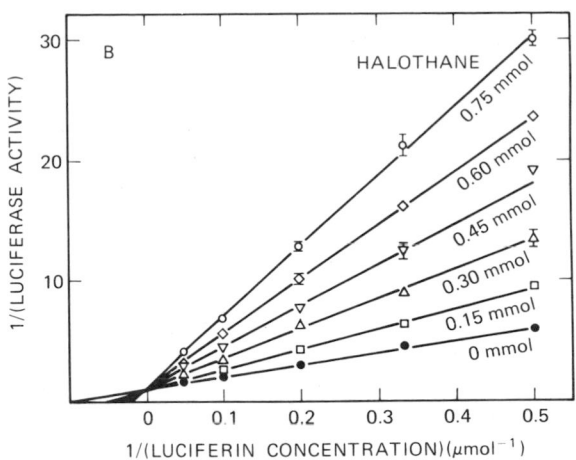

Fig. 27.4 The correlation between lipid solubility and anesthetic potency does not rule out a protein site of action for anesthetics. A. In a lipid-free preparation of the enzyme luciferase, anesthetic potency (horizontal axis) correlates well with ability to inhibit luciferase activity (vertical axis). B. Halothane inhibits luciferase by competing with the substrate luciferin. Inhibition of luciferase (vertical axis) increases as luciferin concentration decreases (horizontal axis). The evidence supports the hypothesis that halothane occupies a specific hydrophobic pocket in the protein. (Adapted with permission from Franks and Lieb, 1984).

activity of some set of functional proteins in excitable cells. A major question then becomes; which functions? Much effort has been expended to identify 'the' site of anesthetic action, a search initially grounded on the assumption that all anesthetics act by exerting their effects on one particular process. Although unitary concepts of anesthetic action are esthetically more pleasing than the alternative of multiple sites, accumulating evidence has begun to support the latter notion. The search for a single site has shown that anesthetics disturb many distinct processes in excitable cells, and the number grows commensurate with new knowledge of the complexity of ion channels and transport systems which regulate the activity of central neurons. The outline of membrane functional proteins presented in the preceding chapter is the presently known set of target sites at which anesthetics may act. The rest of this chapter presents evidence concerning anesthetic action at each: active ion transport systems, voltage-regulated ion channels, excitatory and inhibitory fast transmitter-activated ion channels, and slow metabolically modulated ion channels. Knowledge of these systems themselves is still rapidly expanding, and thus, understanding of anesthetic actions or even a list of anesthetic actions must presently be considered tentative and incomplete.

Resting Potential

1. Active Ion Transport: Na-K-dependent ATPase. The control of resting potential by ion imbalance is outlined in the previous chapter. The active transport system responsible, the sodium pump, regulates resting potential in all cells by this means. In some cells, in addition, the pump contributes directly to resting potential in an electrogenic fashion. Interference with active sodium transport has little immediate effect in large cells in which the electrogenic component of sodium transport is small or negligible, for example the squid giant axon on which much modern experimental neurophysiology is based. In small cells or cells in which the pump is electrogenic, however, reduction in pump activity will lead to a prompt decrease in the electrical potential difference across the cell membrane, or depolarization. Anesthetics have indeed been shown to block active sodium transport (Andersen and Shim, 1971; Helmer et al., 1981; Schwartz, 1968). However, the expected resulting depolarization is not observed in many nerve cells. In central neurons, the effect of anesthetics on transmembrane potential in the resting cell is either inconsistent or there is a net increase, or hyperpolarization (Carlen et al., 1982, 1985; Nicoll and Madison, 1982). Inhibition of sodium transport, therefore, is either of small importance or its effects on resting potential are overshadowed by other anesthetic effects.

2. Active Ion Transport: Ca^{2+} Regulatory Mechanisms. Intracellular calcium concentration is regulated by a variety of buffering mechanisms, including direct active extrusion, sequestration into endoplasmic reticulum, and ion exchange with sodium. Although there is little direct evidence of anesthetic interaction with each of these systems, anesthetics do increase intracellular calcium, possibly by inhibiting sequestration (Vassort et al., 1986). If this is a universal effect on nerve cells, it is one of tremendous importance in light of the role of calcium as a modulator or second messenger in a variety of neuronal processes. One such, a calcium-dependent potassium channel, has received some attention as a possible site of anesthetic action as described below.

3. Ion-selective Channels Operating Near the Resting Potential.

The initial basis of modern electrophysiology was established by the demonstration that nerve and muscle cells are selectively permeable to potassium ions at rest. The resulting conductivity establishes the resting potential in cells such as the squid axon, and any manipulation which alters resting potassium permeability will change resting transmembrane voltage. Early studies made no attempt to separate the resting potassium-permeable channel from the potassium channel activated by depolarization; in fact, there was an assumption of identity. More recently, studies with agents which selectively block voltage-dependent potassium channels have shown no effect on resting conductance, suggesting that the two are at least pharmacologically separable with respect to binding sites for these agents (Chang, 1986). Experiments with anesthetic agents also suggest that the resting and the voltage-dependent potassium channels are distinct; in squid axon, general anesthetics have little effect on resting membrane potential (Armstrong and Binstock, 1964), but do block the voltage dependent potassium channel (Haydon and Urban, 1986a).

Squid axon historically was a fortunate experimental preparation in its simplicity, but ultimately a misleading model neuron, in that both resting and action potentials are made up of a relatively restricted set of ion conductanes compared to most neurons. In central neurons in vertebrates, a vast complexity of ion-selective channels contributes to cellular activity. Among these are calcium-regulated potassium channels, which open in response to increases in intracellular calcium. It has been suggested that a common action of anesthetics is to increase permeability through these channels, leading to a hyperpolarization at rest (Carlen et al., 1985). The evidence that many anesthetics do hyperpolarize some populations of central neurons is suggestive, as is the evidence cited above that anesthetics may increase intracellular calcium concentrations (Vassort et al., 1986), which would tend to activate the channels. The resulting increase in resting potassium conductance would tend to act like inhibition, making it more difficult to excite the cells. However, the consistency of this anesthetic effect, and its possible role in anesthesia, is not yet proven.

Voltage and Transmitter-activated Ion Channels

1. Anesthetic Effects on Channel State Transitions.

For both the sodium channel and the nicotinic acetylcholine receptor (nAChR), there is some evidence, albeit not conclusive, that general anesthetics may act by increasing the rate of transition to a closed state, rather than by the intuitively more obvious mechanism of blocking the passage of ions through the channel. For the sodium channel, this is reflected by an increase in the proportion of channels in the unavailable inactive state (Kendig et al., 1979; Elliott et al., 1986; Haydon et al., 1986b), and an accompanying immobilization of gating charge movement (Fernandez et al., 1982) and increase in rate of decay of sodium currents (Bean et al., 1981). For the acetylcholine channel, the evidence is less clear, and not sufficient to distinguish between a kinetic and a channel-blocking mechanism (Gage et al., 1986). However, as with the sodium channel, anesthetics appear to favor

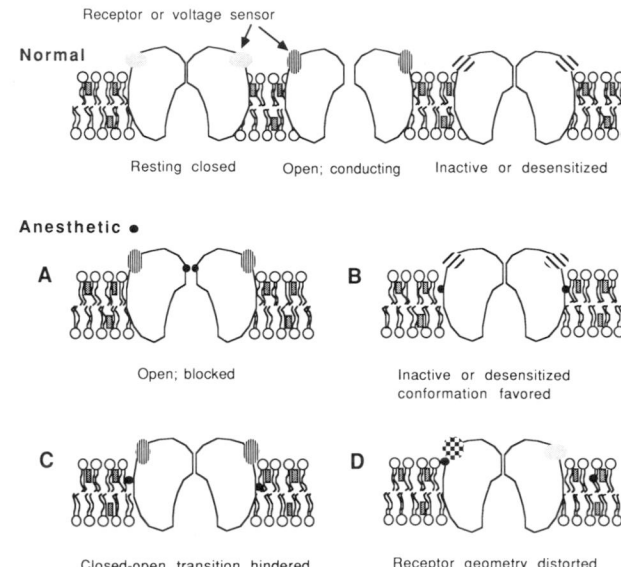

Fig. 27.5 Alternative models for anesthetic inhibition of ion channel function. Top line: in the normal membrane an ion selective channel responds to its trigger (voltage change or transmitter binding) by opening to permit the passage of ions. If the trigger persists, the channel enters an inactive or desensitized closed state. Bottom four modules: in the presence of an anesthetic, channel function is distorted. There are several ways in which this might happen. A. The trigger may operate and the channel open normally, but the anesthetic prevents ion passage by blocking the channel. B. The presence of the anesthetic may favor the transition to or hinder the recovery from a closed state resembling the normal inactive or desensitized state (kinetic mechanism). So far there is insufficient evidence to assign anesthetic effects clearly to block versus kinetic mechanisms of channel inhibition. C. The channel may be triggered normally but the presence of the anesthetic may prevent the conformation change associated with opening. There is no direct evidence for this mechanism, but it is an appealing possible explanation of how anesthetic actions on lipids might interfere with channel function. D. The anesthetic may alter transmitter-receptor binding by occupying the receptor site itself, by allosterically altering the receptor geometry so that binding is altered, or, by a mechanism similar to B, by favoring a channel conformation with an abnormal receptor affinity.

an inactive state of the nAChR channel, increasing the proportion of channels in the high-affinity desensitized state (Firestone et al., 1986). In addition to blocking the channel or favoring a non-conducting conformation state, anesthetics may block transmitter-activated channels by blocking transmitter binding at the receptor site. Alternative models of ion channel block are shown in Fig. 27.5.

2. **Specific Membrane Regions Implicated in Anesthesia.** A schematic of the variety of cellular membrane sites, and the possible actions of anesthetics on them, is presented in Fig. 27.6. Although the sodium current responsible for the upstroke of the action potential in impulse-conducting membrane can be blocked by

anesthetic agents, in the cells in which it can be measured directly the required concentrations for a measurable effect are high. Thus, although it is possible that small-diameter central neurons may be subject to anesthetic effects on this channel, considerations of sensitivity argue against this mechanism playing a significant role in anesthesia. An early study showed that fast excitatory synapses are more sensitive than axons to anesthetic block (Larrabee and Posternak, 1952), and this relative sensitivity has since been documented in comparisons between direct and synaptically evoked responses in brain (Richards et al., 1975). Studies on currents in the postjunctional membrane containing the nAChR receptor suggest that this membrane shares the sensitivity of synaptic

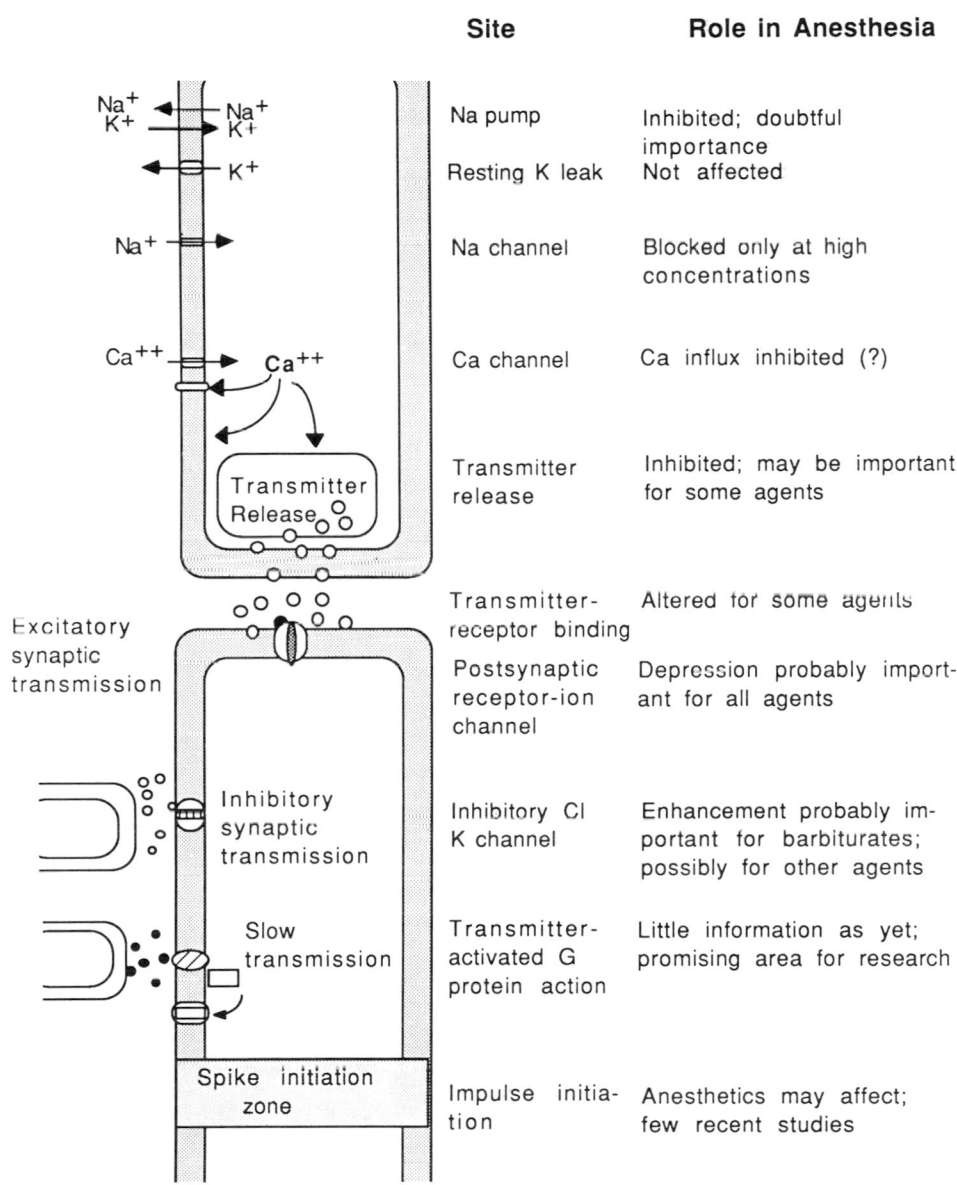

Fig. 27.6 Target sites of anesthetic action in excitable cells, and their possible importance in anesthesia.

transmission as a whole to general anesthetic agents (Gage et al., 1986; Gage and Hamill, 1981). Depression of the postsynaptic response to excitatory transmitter has received much attention as the most accepted of the possible single sites of anesthetic action. Although evidence against single-site theories is increasing, on the grounds of sensitivity depression of postsynaptic transmitter response must presently be considered a probable contributor to anesthesia.

Variably Contributing Additional Mechanisms

1. Potentiation or Mimicry of Inhibition. The evidence that general anesthetics may act somewhat like inhibition by increasing resting conductance in central neurons is presented above. The evidence is also strong that barbiturates, at least, bind to a specific site on the GABA-activated chloride channel and potentiate synaptic inhibition by this means (Barker, 1975; Dunwiddie et al., 1986). Inasmuch as many central neurons are subjected to a powerful tonic inhibitory input, the result of this barbiturate effect is to further limit excitation (Fig. 27.6). The role of this process in anesthesia is uncertain; there has been considerable debate concerning whether enhancement of inhibition is more characteristic of anticonvulsant than of anesthetic barbiturates, or vice versa (MacDonald and Barker, 1978). It is also uncertain whether other general anesthetics share in this property to the same extent as barbiturates, in the absence of a similar well-defined binding site on the channel. There is, however, increasing evidence that they may (Gage and Robertson, 1985).

2. Block of Transmitter Release. Focus on the postsynaptic membrane has diminished the attention paid to the less easily measurable process of transmitter release. Careful studies have shown that general anesthetics depress transmitter release (Matthews and Quilliam, 1964; Weakly, 1969) (Fig. 27.6); however, the role that this mechanism plays in anesthesia is uncertain. It may be that its importance is one of the factors that varies among agents. In mammalian brain, although sensitivity of the entire process of synaptic transmission is apparently universal for all anesthetics, sensitivity to direct application of excitatory transmitter varies (Richards, 1983). The conclusion drawn from these studies is that, at least for some types of agents, depression of transmitter release may play an important part in overall depression of synaptic transmission (Fig. 27.6).

3. Agent-Specific Effects. Various anesthetics produce a variety of different EEG patterns, particularly with respect to seizure-like activity. These can be reproduced in studies on isolated tissue such as hippocampal slice (MacIver and Roth, 1987b), indicating that seizure-inducing agents such as enflurane are exerting different effects from agents such as methoxyflurane. Barbiturate actions on isolated tissue are also

agent-specific (MacIver and Roth, 1987a). There are two ways to consider the importance of such differences among agents. One point of view is that they are side effects unrelated to anesthesia, a point of view consistent with unitary hypotheses of anesthesia (see Table 27.1). The other is that they are inseparable components of the anesthetic action of each agent; anesthesia is thus seen as a constellation of effects, the composition of which differs among agents. This concept corresponds to a multi-site hypothesis of anesthesia (see Table 27.1). A common anesthetic response such as depression of postsynaptic excitation could be brought about by different combinations of actions as shown in Fig. 27.6. The evidence is perhaps strongest that barbiturates may differ from other anesthetics with respect to enhancement of inhibition, and that halothane may differ from other volatile agents in the size of the component due to depression of transmitter release.

Evidence from Pressure Reversal of Anesthesia

The phenomenon of pressure reversal of anesthesia, characterized by a marked increase in anesthetic requirements at hyperbaric pressures tens of atmospheres above normal, has been extensively used as a tool to probe the mechanism of anesthesia. The assumptions underlying its use for this purpose are that all agents act at the same site, which is characterized by specific measures of anesthetic solubility and compressibility, and that in fact pressure actually directly antagonizes the anesthetic effect on this site (see Table 27.1). The universality of pressure reversal for all agents lent support to these assumptions. More recently, however, some studies have shown that the curves relating pressure to anesthetic requirement differ among agents, evidence which has been used to support a multi-site hypothesis of anesthetic action (Halsey et al., 1978; Wardley-Smith and Halsey, 1985) (see Table 27.1). The search for the site of anesthetic-pressure antagonism has revealed a number of anesthetic-pressure interactions on nerve and other cells (Kendig, 1980; Kendig and Grossman, 1986), some indeed antagonistic but others additive, and none as yet is an adequate explanation for pressure reversal of anesthesia at the cellular level. In defined lipid bilayers of various composition, pressure does antagonize the effects of anesthetics on several measures of lipid order (Trudell, 1977; Trudell et al., 1973b; Trudell et al., 1974; Galla and Trudell, 1980). The argument about the relevance of lipid disorder to anesthesia is given above; pressure could also conceivably antagonize anesthetic effects mediated through binding of the anesthetic to a protein.

ANESTHESIA IN THE BRAIN

Sensitive Sites

In similar fashion to the search for a membrane 'site'

of anesthesia, there have been many tests of candidates for the area in the central nervous system whose activity is preferentially altered to bring about anesthesia. Candidates range from cerebral cortex and related hippocampal cortex (Hosick et al., 1971) to various subcortical arousal areas associated with the maintenance of sleep and wakefulness (Darbinjan et al., 1971), and even the spinal cord as it relates to the profound analgesia associated with some anesthetics at subanesthetic concentrations (Kitahata, 1975). The usual dichotomy is the possibility of direct cortical actions of anesthetics, versus some subcortical site such as the reticular formation or the locus coeruleus where anesthetics act to effectively 'deafferent' the cortex and thus indirectly reduce the level of cortical activity. At present, it is not possible to decide between these possibilities. It is possible that anesthetic actions at several levels may contribute to anesthesia; a decrease in cortical sensitivity may occur together with a decrease in input.

Specific Neurotransmitters in Anesthesia

Of agents which produce anesthesia, or at least lessen anesthetic requirement, there is no doubt that opiates act by binding to specific receptors at defined regions in the central nervous system. In the case of opiates, however, the exogenous pharmacology was known long before structurally similar peptides were identified as endogenous neurotransmitters. Other transmitters were first recognized as such, and their roles in modulating anesthesia are only now beginning to be explored.

The evidence that barbiturates and perhaps other anesthetics act in part by enhancing or mimicking the effects of the inhibitory neurotransmitter GABA is presented above. To complete the reasoning that GABA-mimetic effects contribute to anesthesia, it needs to be shown that specific GABA agonists can act as anesthetics. This, in fact, has been demonstrated. Both muscimol and THIP, two GABA-agonists, can induce loss of righting reflex and produce a state resembling anesthesia (Cheng and Brunner, 1985). Imperfect as such evidence is, it is consistent with the possibility that enhancement of GABA inhibition may in fact contribute to anesthesia.

The second neurotransmitter system which has been associated with anesthesia is that activated by α_2 adrenergic agonists. These have been known for some time as sedatives and antihypertensives. One, clonidine, was shown to prolong barbiturate sleep time in a fashion antagonized by a specific antagonist (Mason and Angel, 1983). Clonidine also lowers volatile anesthetic requirement, and its use for this purpose has been reported in clinical studies (Ghignone et al., 1987; Flacke et al., 1987). Thus activation of some α_2 receptor pathway may also contribute to anesthesia, although clonidine by itself is not capable of producing anesthesia. The site where clonidine acts has not

been identified with certainty, although some studies implicate the locus coeruleus. It also remains to be seen whether anesthetics act to mimic or enhance α_2 agonist effects on neural tissue, as is the case for GABA.

SUMMARY

Currently, understanding anesthetic action in terms of events at the cellular and molecular level is in a state of transition. Earlier elegant unitary hypotheses have given way to some extent to evidence that even within the lipid bilayer effects on lipid properties are agent-specific and multiple. There is increasing evidence at the cellular level that there are detailed anesthetic interactions with a variety of distinct processes important in neuronal function, and that these also are not completely congruent among agents of different types. The ultimate effect, however, a shift in the level of cortical activity, may be uniform, although brought about by slightly different means for each agent.

REFERENCES

Andersen N.B., Shim C.Y. (1971). Sodium transport and anesthetic requirements in the toad. *Anesthesiology*, **34**, 338.

Armstrong C.M., Binstock L. (1964). The effects of several alcohols on the squid giant axon. *J. Gen. Physiol.*, **48**, 265.

Barker J.L. (1975). CNS depressants: effects on postsynaptic pharmacology. *Brain Res.*, **92**, 35.

Bean B.P., Shrager P., Goldstein D.A. (1981). Modification of sodium and potassium channel gating kinetics by ether and halothane. *J. Gen. Physiol.*, **77**, 233.

Carlen P.L., Gurevich N., Durand D. (1982). Ethanol in low doses augments calcium-mediated mechanisms measured intracellularly in hippocampal neurons. *Science*, **215**, 306.

Carlen P.L., Gurevich N., Davies M.F., et al., (1985). Enhanced neuronal K+ conductance: a possible common mechanism for sedative-hypnotic drug action. *Can. J. Physiol. Pharmacol.*, **63**, 831.

Chang D.C. (1986). Is the K permeability of the resting membrane controlled by the excitable K channel? *Biophys. J.*, **50**, 1095.

Cheng S-C., Brunner E.A. (1985). Inducing anesthesia with a GABA analog, THIP. *Anesthesiology*, **63**, 147.

Darbinjan T.M., Golovchinsky V.B., Plehotkina S.I. (1971). The effects of anesthetics on reticular activity. *Anesthesiology*, **34**, 219.

Dipple I., Houslay M.D. (1978). The activity of glucagon stimulated adenylate cyclase from rat liver plasma membrane is modulated by the fluidity of its lipid environment. *Biochem. J.*, **174**, 179.

Dunwiddie T.V., Worth T.S., Olsen R.W. (1986). Facilitation of recurrent inhibition in rat hippocampus by barbiturate and related nonbarbiturate depressant drugs. *J. Pharmacol. Exper. Ther.*, **238**, 564.

Elliott J.R., Haydon D.A. (1986). Mapping of general anaesthetic target sites. *Nature*, **319**, 77.

Evers A.S., Berkowitz B.A., d'Avignon D.A. (1987). Correlation between the anaesthetic effect of halothane and saturable binding in brain. *Nature*, **328**, 157.

Featherstone R.M., Muehlbacher C.A. (1963). The current

role of inert gases in the search for anesthesia mechanisms. *Pharmacol. Rev.*, **15**, 97.

Ferguson J. (1939). The use of chemical potentials as indices of toxicity. *Proc. R. Soc. London. Series B: Biol. Sci.*, **127**, 387.

Fernandez J.M., Bezanilla F., Taylor R.E. (1982). Effect of chloroform on charge movement in the nerve membrane. *Nature*, **297**, 150.

Firestone L.L., Sauter J.F., Braswell L.M., et al., (1986). Actions of general anesthetic on acetylcholine receptor-rich membranes from *Torpedo Californica*. *Anesthesiology*, **64**, 694.

Flacke J.W., Bloor B.C., Flacke W.E., et al. (1987). Reduced narcotic requirement by clonidine with improved hemodynamic and adrenergic stability in patients undergoing coronary bypass surgery. *Anesthesiology*, **67**, 11.

Franks N.P., Lieb N.R. (1984)., **310**, 599.

Franks N.P., Lieb W.R. (1986a). The pharmacology of simple molecules. *Arch. Toxicol.*, Suppl. **9**, 27.

Franks N.P., Lieb W.R. (1986b). Do direct protein/anesthetic interactions underlie the mechanism of general anesthesia? In *Molecular and Cellular Mechanisms of Anesthetics*, pp. 319–329. (Roth S.H., Miller K.W., eds.) New York: Plenum.

Gage P.W., Hamill O.P. (1981). Effects of anesthetics on ion channels in synapses. In *International Review of Physiology*, *Vol. 25*, pp. 1–45. (Porter R. ed.) Baltimore: University Park Press.

Gage P.W., McKinnon D., Robertson B. (1986). The influence of anaesthetics on postsynaptic ion channels. In *Molecular and Cellular Mechanisms of Anesthetics*, 139–153. (Roth S.H., Miller K.W. eds.) New York: Plenum.

Gage P.W., Robertson B. (1985). Prolongation of inhibitory postsynaptic currents by pentobarbitone, halothane and ketamine in CA1 pyramidal cells in rat hippocampus. *Br. J. Pharmacol.*, **85**, 675.

Galla H.J, Trudell J.R. (1980). Asymmetric antagonistic effects of an inhalation anesthetic and high pressure on the phase transition temperature of dipalmitoyl phosphatidic acid bilayers. *Biochim. Biophys. Acta*, **599**, 336.

Ghignone M., Calvillo O., Quintin L. (1987). Anesthesia and hypertension: the effect of clonidine on perioperative hemodynamics and isoflurane requirements. *Anesthesiology*, **67**, 3.

Gordon L.M., Sauerhaber R.D., Isgate J.A., et al. (1980). The increase in bilayer fluidity of rat liver plasma membranes achieved by the local anaesthetic benzyl alcohol affects the activity of intrinsic enzymes (1980). *J. Biol. Chem.*, **255**, 4519.

Halsey M.J. (1984). A reassessment of the molecular structure-functional relationships of the inhaled general anaesthetics. *Br. J. Anaesth.*, **56**, 9S.

Halsey M.J., Wardley-Smith B., Green C.J. (1978). The pressure reversal of general anaesthesia—a multi-site expansion hypothesis. *Br. J. Anaesth.*, **50**, 1091.

Haydon D.A., Urban B.W. (1986a). The actions of some general anaesthetics on the potassium current of the squid giant axon. *J. Physiol.*, **373**, 311.

Haydon D.A., Elliott J.R., Hendry B.M., et al. (1986b). The action of nonionic anesthetic substances on voltage-gated ion conductances in squid giant axons. In *Molecular and Cellular Mechanisms of Anesthetics*, pp. 267–277. (Roth S.H., Miller K.W. eds.) New York: Plenum.

Helmer P., Rusy B., Bittar E. (1981). Sensitivity to halothane of the sodium efflux in single barnacle muscle fibers. *J. Pharmacol. Exper. Ther.*, **217**, 248.

Hosick E.C., Clark D.L., Adam N., et al. (1971). Neurophysiological effects of different anesthetics in conscious man. *J. Appl. Physiol.*, **31**, 892.

Houslay M.D., Gordon L.M. (1983). The activity of adenylate cyclase is regulated by the nature of its lipid environment. *Curr. Top. Membrane Trans.*, **18**, 179.

Katz Y., Simon S.A. (1977). Physical parameters of the anesthetic site. *Biochim. Biophys. Acta*, **471**, 1.

Kendig J.J. (1980). Anesthetics and pressure in nerve cells. In *Molecular Mechanisms of Anesthesia*, pp. 59–68. (Fink B.R. ed.) New York: Raven Press.

Kendig J.J., Courtney K.R., Cohen E.N. (1979). Anesthetics: molecular correlates of voltage- and frequency-dependent sodium channel block in nerve. *J. Pharmacol. Exper. Ther.*, **210**, 446.

Kendig J.J., Grossman Y. (1986). Homogeneous and branching axons: Differing responses to anesthetics and pressure. In *Molecular and Cellular Mechanisms of Anesthetics*, pp. 333–353. (Roth S.H., Miller K.W. eds.) New York: Plenum Press.

Kitahata L.M. (1975). Modes and sites of analgesic action of anesthetics on the spinal cord. *Int. Anesthesiol. Clinics*, **13**, 149.

Larrabee M.G., Posternak J.M. (1952). Selective action of anaesthetics on synapses and axons in mammalian sympathetic ganglia. *J. Neurophysiol.*, **15**, 91.

MacDonald R.L., Barker J.L. (1978). Different actions of anticonvulsant and anesthetic barbiturates revealed by use of cultured mammalian neurons. *Science*, **200**, 775.

MacIver M.B., Roth S.H. (1987a). Barbiturate effects on hippocampal excitatory synaptic responses are selective and pathway specific. *Can. J. Physiol. Pharmacol.*, **65**, 385.

MacIver M.B., Roth S.H. (1987b). Enflurane-induced burst firing of hippocampal CA 1 neurons. *Br. J. Anaesth.*, **59**, 369.

Mason S.T., Angel A. (1983). Anaesthesia: the role of adrenergic mechanisms. *Eur. J. Pharmacol.*, **91**, 29.

Matthews E.K., Quilliam J.P. (1964). Effects of central depressant drugs upon acetylcholine release. *Br. J. Pharmacol.*, **22**, 415.

Meyer H.H. (1899). Zur theorie der alkoholnarkose. I. Mit welch Eigenshaft der Anasthetika bedingt ihre narkotische Wirkung? *Archiv. für Experimentelle Pathologia Pharmakologie*, **42**, 109.

Millar K.W. (1981). In *Burger's Medicinal Chemistry*, 4 edn., P. 623. John Wiley and Sons.

Miller K.W. (1985). The nature of the site of general anesthesia. *Int. Rev. Neurobiol.*, **27**, 1.

Miller K.W., Pang K.Y. (1976). General anesthetics can selectively perturb lipid bilayer membranes. *Nature*, **263**, 253.

Miller K.W., Paton W.D.M., Smith E.B., et al. (1971). Physico-chemical approaches to the mode of action of general anesthetics. *Anesthesiology*, **36**, 339.

Mullins L.J. (1971). Anesthetics. In *Handbook of Neurochemistry*, Vol. VI, pp. 395–421. (Lajtha A. ed.) New York: Plenum.

Nicoll R.A., Madison D.V. (1982). General anesthetics hyperpolarize neurons in the vertebrate central nervous system. *Science*, **217**, 1055.

O'Leary T.J., Ross P.D., Levin I.W. (1986). Effects of anesthetic tetradecenols on phosphatidylcholine phase transitions. *Biophys. J.*, **50**, 1053.

Olsen R.W., Fischer J.B., Dunwiddie T.V. (1986). Barbiturate enhancement of gama-aminobutyric acid receptor binding and function as a mechanism of anesthesia. In *Molecular and Cellular Mechanisms of Anesthetics*, pp. 165–177. (Roth S.H., Miller K.W. eds.) New York: Plenum.

Overton E. (1901). *Studien uber die Narkose Zugleich ein Beitrag zur Allgemeinen Pharmacologie*. pp. 1053–1059. Jena: G. Fischer.

Pang K.Y., Chang T.L., Miller K.W. (1979). On the coupling between anesthetic-induced membrane fluidization and cation permeability in lipid vesicles. *Mol. Pharmacol.*, **15**, 729.

Richards C.D. (1983). Actions of general anaesthetics on synaptic transmission in the CNS. *Br. J. Anaesth.*, **55**, 201.

Richards C.D., Martin K., Gregory S., et al. (1978). Degenerate perturbations of protein structure as the mechanism of anesthetic action. *Nature*, **276**, 775.

Richards C.D., Russell W.J., Smaje J.C. (1975). The action of ether and methoxyflurane on synaptic transmission in isolated preparation of the mammalian cortex. *J. Physiol.*, **248**, 121.

Richter J., Landau E.M., Cohen S. (1977). The action of volatile anesthetics and convulsants on synaptic transmission: a unified concept. *Mol. Pharmacol.*, **13**, 548.

Schwartz E.A. (1968). Effect of diethylether on sodium efflux from squid axons. *Curr. Mod. Biol.*, **2**, 1.

Trudell J.R. (1977). A unitary theory of anesthesia based on lateral phase separations in nerve membranes. *Anesthesiology*, **46**, 5.

Trudell J.R., Hubbell W.L., Cohen E.N. (1973a). The effect of two inhalation anesthetics on the order of spin-labeled phospholipid vesicles. *Biochim. Biophys. Acta*, **291**, 321.

Trudell J.R., Hubbell W.L., Cohen E.N. (1973b). Pressure reversal of anesthetic-induced disorder in spin-labeled phospholipid vesicles. *Biochim. Biophys. Acta*, **291**, 328.

Trudell J.R., Payan D.G., Chin J.H., et al. (1974). Pressure induced elevation of phase transition temperature in dipalmitoyl-phosphatidylcholine vesicles: An electron spin resonance measurement of the enthalpy of phase transition. *Biochim. Biophys. Acta*, **373**, 151.

Vassort G., Whittembury J., Mullins L.J. (1986). Increases in internal Ca^{2+} and decreases in internal $H+$ are induced by general anesthetics in squid axons. *Biophys. J.*, **50**, 11.

Wardley-Smith B., Halsey M.J. (1985). Mixtures of inhalation and I.V. anaesthetics at high pressure: a test of the multi-site hypothesis of general anaesthesia. *Br. J. Anaesth.*, **57**, 1248.

Weakly J.N. (1969). Effect of barbiturates on 'quantal' synaptic transmission in spinal motoneurones. *J. Physiol.*, **204**, 63.

28. Physiology of the Electro-encephalogram
W. Hoffman and B. Grundy

The purpose of this chapter is to define the electrophysiological mechanisms by which the electroencephalogram (EEG) is generated and to delineate how the EEG may be interpreted clinically to evaluate cerebral pathophysiology and the effects of anesthetics. The relationship of the EEG to neuronal and brain electrical activity will also be established. This will aid the clinician in using the EEG to obtain a better understanding of patient status.

ELECTROPHYSIOLOGY OF THE NEURON

The mechanisms by which neurons produce electrical activity in the brain depend primarily on the ability to maintain ionic gradients across the nerve cell membrane. The membrane, which is approximately 80–100 angströms thick, consists of a bimolecular layer of lipids (Fig. 28.1). The polar component of each lipid chain faces the interior of the cell or the extracellular space. Protein layers are present on both the inside and the outside of the cell membrane, oriented in close proximity to the polar regions of the lipid layer. The physico-chemical nature of the neuronal cell membrane gives the membrane high capacitance; this enables the membrane to maintain an electrochemical gradient, which allows nerve cell activity (Robertson, 1962). Movement of ions across the cell membrane occurs through negatively or positively charged aqueous channels, which allow selective permeability to ionic constituents (Fig. 28.2). Recent evidence sug-

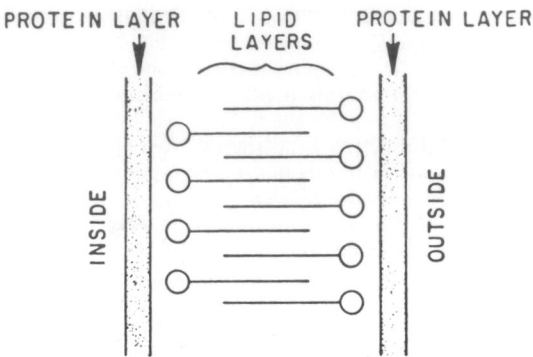

Fig. 28.1 Molecular characteristics of the neuronal cell membrane. The bimolecular layer of lipids has polar components facing the inside and outside of the cell which are closely associated with the protein layers. The lipid characteristics of the membrane produce a barrier to ion movement and provide high capacitance. Reproduced with permission from C. Eyzaguirre, S.J. Fidone (1975).

gests that ion channels are composed of proteins arranged as bundles of α helices that span the membrane and have specific peptide sequences characterizing selective channels and receptors (Lear et al., 1988).

Electrochemical Gradients

The neuron produces an electrical gradient across the cell membrane by maintaining an intracellular ionic

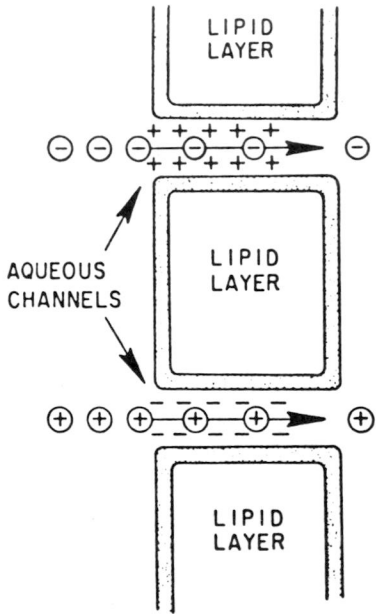

Fig. 28.2 A view of the cell membrane showing aqueous channels which allow selective conductance of positive and negative ions. These channels can be opened and closed by biochemical processes that alter the gating potential at each pore. Reproduced with permission from C. Eyzaguirre, S.J. Fidone (1975).

composition that is markedly different from that in the extracellular space. The intracellular concentration of sodium (Na^+) (Fig. 28.3) is maintained at a low level, with respect to the extracellular space, by a sodium ion pump that uses metabolic energy to extrude Na^+ from the cell as fast as it leaks in. Potassium (K^+) is maintained at a higher intracellular than extracellular concentration by an active energy-requiring process called the *potassium ion pump*. Chloride (Cl^-) is distributed passively across the cell according to its electrochemical gradient and it is generally not necessary to postulate the presence of a chloride ion pump. Proteins provide a net negative charge within the intracellular space.

Although the nerve cell maintains an electrochemical gradient across the cell membrane by active (ionic pump) and passive (ion-selective aqueous channels) processes, the number of positively and negatively charged ions on each side of the membrane is equal (Davson, 1970). This principle of electrical neutrality is upheld in spite of the fact that the neuron maintains a negative potential of 70–90 mV inside the cell with respect to the extracellular space. This occurs because the resting potential of the nerve cell is a membrane phenomenon produced by the movement of a negligibly small number of ions compared with the intracellular and extracellular concentrations. The movement of ions such K^+ and Cl^- produces a separation of charge across the cell membrane and a resting membrane potential. While the sodium pump is primarily responsible for the electrochemical gradient from the inside to the outside of the cell, the higher conductance and movement of K^+ and Cl^- across the cell membrane provide the electrical charge for the resting membrane potential (Eyzaguirre and Fidone, 1975). The ratio of the intracellular to extracellular ionic concentrations may be used to calculate an equilibrium potential. This is the membrane potential at which K^+, or Cl^- will have no tendency to move either into or out of the cell. These equilibrium potentials may be calculated under normal physiologic conditions and at body temperature (38°C) using the Nernst equation:

$$\text{EMF (millivolts)} = -61 \log_{10} \frac{\text{concentration inside}}{\text{concentration outside}}$$

For a membrane permeable only to potassium:

$$
\begin{aligned}
E_{K^+} &= -61 \log_{10} [K_i]/[K_0] \\
&= -61 \log_{10} [140\,\text{mEq/L}]/[4\,\text{mEq/L}] \\
&= -94\,\text{mV}
\end{aligned}
$$

For a membrane permeable only to sodium:

$$
\begin{aligned}
E_{Na^+} &= -61 \log_{10} [Na_i]/Na_0] \\
&= -61 \log_{10} [14\,\text{mEq/L}]/142\,\text{mEq/L}] \\
&= +61\,\text{mV}
\end{aligned}
$$

Each of these ions contributes to the resting membrane potential according to its equilibrium potential and its permeability across the cell membrane. The

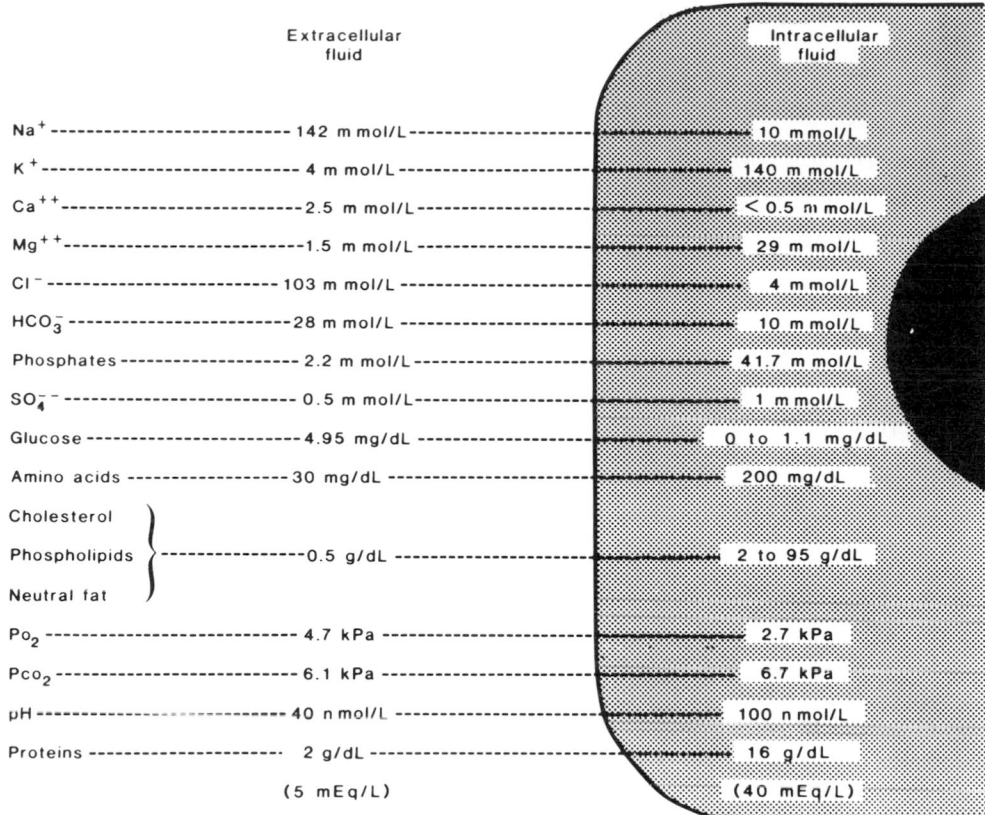

Fig. 28.3 Chemical constitutents inside and outside the cell membrane. Ionic components contribute to the electrical gradient. The neurone actively maintains potassium (K^+) inside the cell and sodium (Na^+) outside the cell. Chloride (Cl^-) is passively distributed according to the electrochemical gradient produced by proteins inside the cell and the distribution of positive charge across the cell membrane. Reproduced with permission from A.C. Guyton (1986).

membrane potential can then be calculated using the Goldman equation. For two positive ions, K^+ and Na^+, and one negative ion, $Cl^- = -61$

$$E = -61 \log_{10} \frac{P_K[K_i] + P_{Na} + [Na_i] + P_{Cl}[Cl_0]}{P_K[K_0] + P_{Na}[Na_0] + P_{Cl}[Cl_i]}$$

where P represents the permeability of each respective ion. Potassium contributes primarily to the resting membrane potential because Cl^- concentration differences passively follow the membrane potential and because the conductance of Na^+ across the membrane is very low.

Depolarization

Depolarization or hyperpolarization may occur across the neuronal membrane when the conductances of Na^+ and K^+ are altered. This may occur as a local membrane effect, such as that produced by neurotransmitters (Katz, 1961). The change in potential decays as it moves across the cell, away from the point of depolarization. Neuronal membrane depolarization may also accur when a theshold membrane

potential is reached (Fig. 28.4) and an increase in membrane Na^+ conductance produces an action potential. Subsequently, K^+ conductance increases and repolarization is seen. An action potential can be propagated throughout the cell and axonal membrane without a decay in the potential due to the active changes in Na^+ and K^+ conductance.

ELECTROPHYSIOLOGY OF THE ELECTROENCEPHALOGRAM

Several potential electrical sources of cortical EEG have been identified. Neuronal depolarization in subcortical regions does not contribute significantly to surface EEG because of their distance from scalp electrodes. This is due to the electrical nature of brain tissue, which restricts volume conduction of current and produces a rapid reduction of voltage as a function of distance (Cooper et al., 1965). It is also unlikely that action potentials of cortical neurons have more than a minimal effect on EEG because the time scale of their occurrence is much shorter than that of EEG waves. Furthermore, anesthetic techniques that

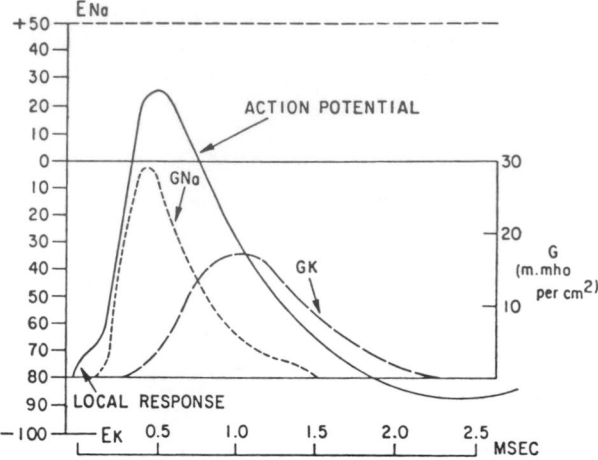

Fig. 28.4 Action potential, as recorded from inside the neurone, which shows simultaneous membrane conductance (G) changes. Initial local response on the cell membrane, as produced by neurotransmitters, with increases in sodium conductance (GNa), in movement of the ions into the cell and in the cell membrane potential. Later, inactivation of sodium conductance, combined with an increase in potassium conductance (GK) and movement to the outside, returns the membrane potential to normal levels. Reproduced with permission from C. Eyzaguirre, S.J. Fidone (1975).

suppress cortical neuronal action potentials do not abolish EEG (Li and Jasper, 1953). A more likely source of EEG recorded from the scalp is the slower depolarization and hyperpolarization that occur along the dendritic tree and neuronal cell body, which are graded summations of multiple excitatory and inhibitory postsynaptic potentials. Calvet et al. (1964), identified three levels within the cortical layers of the cat that generate cortical potentials. The first is at a superficial level, which derives primarily from dendritic sources and leads to surface negativity. Second source, which is deeper in the cortical layers, arises from dendritic and soma components and produces surface positivity. A third, more generalized cortical component also derives from soma and dendritic structures and produces slow wave potentials that are negative at the cortical surface.

Source and Spread of EEG Potentials

Pyramid cells are a major source of EEG potentials. Ball et al., (1977), found, by recording cortical EEG with both depth and surface electrodes, that current dipoles could be demonstrated with depth electrodes, whereas recordings from surface electrodes 2 mm apart were very similar and showed no phase reversal (Fig. 28.5). As a depth electrode was advanced from

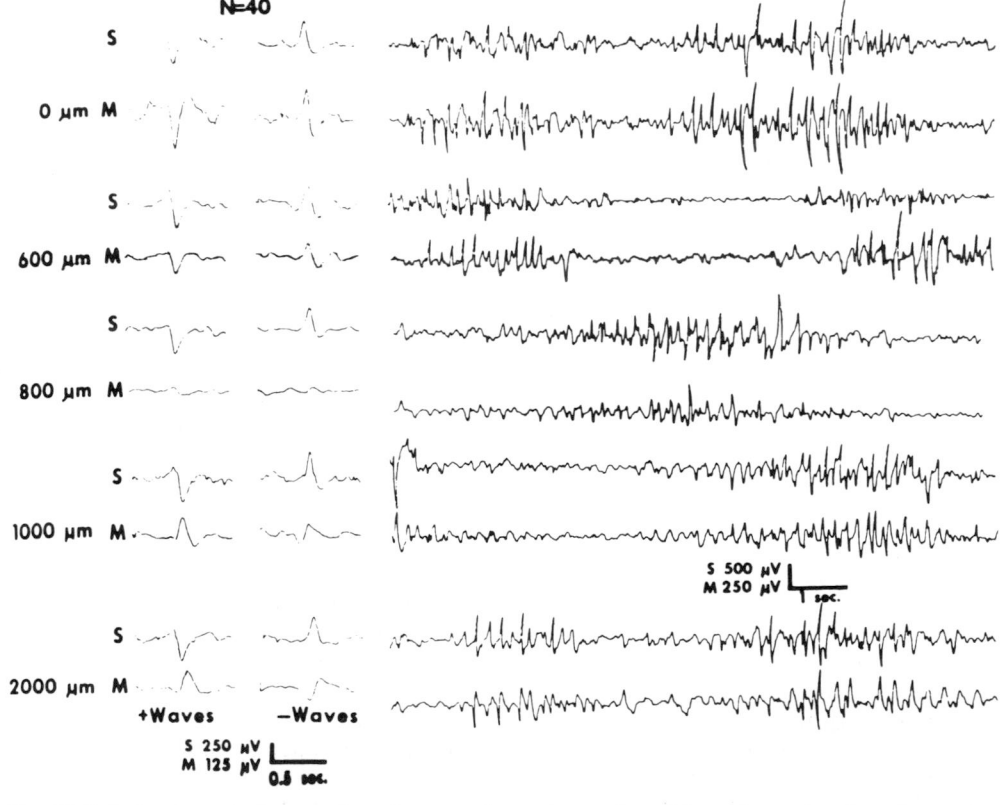

Fig. 28.5 Left, averaged recording from surface electrodes (S) and depth microelectrodes (M) obtained from cortical spindle activity (right). The isopotential point of 800 μm and a phase reversal at greater depths indicate that cortical pyramidal neurones provide the primary current flow for cortical surface electrical activity. Reproduced with permission from G.J. Ball, P. Gloor, C.J. Thompson (1977).

the cortical surface toward the depth of the brain, an isopotential point was located at a depth of about 800 μm. Upon still deeper insertion of the microelectrode, a phase reversal was observed. The orientation of the current dipoles detected with depth electrodes, perpendicular to the cortical surface, produces much smaller field potentials between electrodes placed on the surface of the brain. The pyramidal cells in the granular layer of the cortex, with their long dendritic trees oriented perpendicularly to the cortical surface, are the only neurons that could account for this pattern of recordings.

Because volume conduction of current and the spread of potentials is limited through brain tissue, cortical potential changes can be localized to within 1–2 mm when brain tissue electrodes are used. In contrast, the skull and scalp allow the passive spread of current from neuronal electrical activity. Scalp electrodes measure the sum of potential changes from brain tissue within 2–2.5 cm of the electrode (DeLucchi et al., 1962). For this reason, localized depolarization involving small segments of cortical tissue may be lost in scalp recordings due to general activity of surrounding tissue. However, if cortical activity is synchronous over several square centimeters of tissue, this is well transmitted to scalp electrodes.

As indicated above, it is likely that excitatory and inhibitory postsynaptic potentials involving the pyramidal soma and dendritic tree are primarily responsible for EEG wave potentials (Creutzfeldt et al., 1966). The question then arises as to whether this coherent postsynaptic activation arises from subcortical pacemakers or from intracortical associations. Attempts to isolate the cortex surgically by brain-slicing techniques suggest that the cortex can generate spontaneous activity, which includes spindles (Andersen and Andersson 1968). Other studies have shown, however, that abolition of spontaneous cortical neuronal activity by means of anesthesia does not abolish slow wave activity of the cortex (Li et al., 1953), but that removal of subcortical thalamic regions does not abolish spontaneous EEG (Kristiansen and Courtois, 1949). These results suggest that subcortical mechanisms are the primary pacemakers of EEG activity. The work of Morison and Dempscy (1942), indicates that sensory input produces a primary cortical response, which is mediated by specific thalamic nuclei. The primary response is followed by a generalized cortical activation, mediated by nonspecific thalmic nuclei. Continuous stimulation of nonspecific thalamic nuclei produces progressive cortical activation by recruiting effects. The waxing and waning of spontaneous EEG is probably mediated by alternating excitatory and inhibitory input from subcortical regions. It has been suggested that distributor cells located within nonspecific thalamic nuclei mediate cortical activity by alternating excitation and inhibition of specific thalamic nuclei that connect directly to cortical regions (Andersen and Sears, 1964). Brain transection studies have shown that the reticular formation is of primary importance in maintaining the desynchronized, irregular EEG seen in the awake state (Bremer, 1935). This activation is produced by general sensory input and is mediated by connections to nonspecific thalamic nuclei.

Electrode Placement

In order to evaluate field potential changes on the scalp, it is necessary to relate electrode positions to anatomic structures of the brain. The arrangement of EEG electrodes on the scalp is called a montage. In bipolar scalp recordings, electrical differences are measured between two electrodes, both of which are likely to detect EEG potentials. Bipolar electrode arrangements are usually oriented anterior to posterior or transversely with respect to the surface of the brain and may be referred to as parasagittal or coronal bipolar electrode chains. Potential differences between these electrodes represent an algebraic sum of the electrical activity seen at each electrode, and much of the EEG signal may be lost if both electrodes simultaneously record the same activity. Phase reversal of an EEG signal between channels in a bipolar electrode chain localizes that signal to the area of the common electrode.

Another method of electrode placement is to use a common reference point, such as one ear or linked ears, against which the EEG signal from other active electrodes may be referred. This allows the relative evaluation of potential changes at each active electrode with respect to a common reference point. The common reference is usually placed in close proximity to the head to minimize direct current shifts, but at a point at which EEG activity is minimal. The common reference allows the simultaneous evaluation of relative potentials at each of several active electrodes. It also allows the rejection of spurious electrical activity that may occur at both electrodes, but which has no relation to EEG activity. It is possible, however, that both common and active electrodes see similar potential changes related to EEG, or that a signal may be seen at the common reference, which bears no relation to the EEG signal at the active site. In these cases that actual EEG signal can be distorted.

Another method of electrode derivation is the average reference. In this case, the active scalp electrodes are connected through equal resistance to provide an average reference. The EEG signal from each active electrode is than related to a floating average of activity derived from all active electrodes. The Hjorth source derivation is similar to this, except that the active signal from each electrode is not included in the average reference calculation but is compared with an average source of surrounding electrodes. This provides a less active reference electrode and allows local potential changes or cortical generators to be more easily evaluated (Cooper et al., 1980).

In each type of recording, a standard placement of electrodes is desirable. For this purpose, the International 10–20 System (Jasper, 1958) allows for precise placement of electrodes and comprehensive coverage of the cortical surface. This system of electrode placement uses bony landmarks of the head to generate a series of lines, based on measurements of the distance from nasion to inion and from one preauricular point to the other, as well as a measurement of head circumference. Electrodes are placed where lines intersect at intervals of 10% or 20% of line length (Fig. 28.6). Electrodes placed at these points allow signal localization and comparisons of EEG recordings among patients.

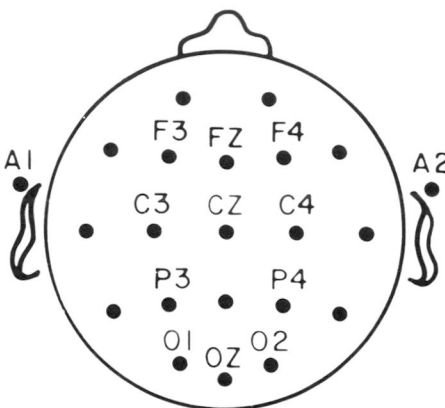

Fig. 28.6 Schematic diagram showing the 10–20 International system for electroencephalographic (EEG) electrode placement. A typical montage of electrodes uses a distribution of these reference points on the scalp to localize the EEG signal according to cortical regions. Note that odd numbers are on the left, even number on the right, 'Z' in the midline. Reproduced with permission from B.L. Grundy (1983).

Obtaining a Clear Signal

In order to obtain accurate, reliable recording of EEG in the clinical setting, it is necessary to isolate and amplify brain electrical activity but to exclude inappropriate noise interference. Noise from biological sources as well as motion artifact and electrical and other sources of interference should be eliminated or minimized at the source to the greatest extent possible. Electrodes must be well secured, and electrode impedances must be low and balanced. Physiological EEG is most apparent over a frequency range of 1–50 Hz, and filters are used to help exclude activity outside this frequency range. Electroencephalographic activity can be separated into four frequency components: delta (δ) (0–< 4 Hz), theta (θ) (4–< 8 Hz), alpha (α) (8–< 13 Hz) and beta (β) (13–50 Hz). Each of these components may have physiological significance.

These *frequency bands* are somewhat arbitrary and do not always correspond exactly to the *physiologic rhythms* nominally in these frequency ranges. For

example, α rhythm is characteristic of the alert waking state in the adult with eyes closed. It is most prominent occipitally and is attenuated by eye opening or startling. A rhythm showing these characteristics but with a frequency of 7–7.5 Hz is known as a 'slow α variant' rather than θ rhythm. Theta rhythm is seen in children and young adults, particularly with hyperventilation. Delta rhythm is typical of metabolic encephalopathy or normal slow wave sleep. Beta activity is seen during mental performance of mathematical calculations or in the alert state with eyes open. Frontal β rhythms are typical in patients chronically treated with barbiturates or benzodiazepines and may persist as long as two weeks after these drugs are withdrawn.

There is no substitute for the experienced encephalographer in interpreting EEG, but several methods of signal analysis show promise in facilitating systematic interpretation, quantitation, and statistical analysis of EEG. Most popular of these is power spectral analysis. Analogue EEG is collected, filtered to exclude activity outside the frequency range of interest, and digitally sampled at a rate greater than twice the highest frequency of the filtered analog signal. This is called the Nyquist frequency. For example, if it is desired to analyse EEG over a frequency range of 1–50 Hz, the Nyquist frequency for digital sampling would be greater than 100 Hz. Inadequate sampling rates for analog-to-digital conversion may distort the signal by making harmonics of higher frequencies appear to be frequencies in the range of interest. A timed epoch of digitized EEG, usually 2–4 seconds, can be analysed by using a Fourier analysis to provide a graph of power of the signal as a function of the frequency components. (Power is approximately equivalent to the square of the amplitude). These techniques are of value because they provide a display of EEG that is reproducible, relatively free of interpreter variability, and much more compact than the standard paper record. Some data, such as spike activity, is lost in this processing, and much artifact may be included.

MAGNETOENCEPHALOGRAPHY

Among new recording techniques that analyse the source of neuronal electrical currents, the magnetoencephalogram (MEG) is the most promising. Synchronized electrical currents generated by cortical neurons produce magnetic fields, which can be measured outside the skull (Weinberg et al., 1986). Neuromagnetic fields detected by the MEG are not attenuated or distorted by the resistive barrier of the skull and scalp, as is EEG; therefore, neuronal current sources in the three-dimensional space occupied by the brain can be accurately localized and mapped (Cohen, 1972). While the EEG and MEG measure different aspects of currents (Cuffin and Cohen, 1979), theoretically, the two types of measurements may be related. When activity during consciousness and sleep was measured simultaneously by MEG and EEG, both showed the same peak frequency for α rhythms, particularly at 10 Hz (Hughes et al., 1976). The correlation between MEG and EEG in awake α patterns does not occur in sleep patterns. Sleep spindles are poorly presented by MEG and the most common MEG rhythm observed during sleep is θ (4–5 Hz).

It is apparent that EEG and MEG present different data when similarly prepared and correlated. Some of the present problems associated with MEG include difficulty in interpreting secondary current sources and nonstationary current fields, and difficulty with the three-dimensional modality of magnetic fields within the brain (Nunez, 1986). If these problems are overcome, MEG has the potential for enabling a holistic analysis of current sources and waves within the brain.

CLINICAL EVALUATION WITH EEG

In the normal awake adult, the dominant EEG frequency is α in 75–90% of the cases. A β rhythm may occur 7% of the time and an irregular or θ frequency 5–7% of the time. A normal amplitude of 10–50 μV is present in each of these frequencies approximately 80% of the time, with high or low-amplitude variants occurring at other times. With aging (greater than 65 years), α activity generally slows and the incidence of a slow variant of α (7–8 Hz) increases. Beta activity increases with aging, as does the incidence of irregular slowing of EEG frequency and focal abnormalities. Focal δ and θ waves in geriatric patients may suggest an impairment of local cerebral perfusion and metabolism, even when clinical signs of impairment are not present (Fig. 28.7).

Epilepsy

Epilepsy may be defined as hyperactive or hypersynchronous neuronal discharges within the brain. The overactive state of neuronal function is thought to arise from an imbalance of the normal excitatory mechanisms that relay information from lower centers to the cortex, and which produce arousal, and inhibitory mechanisms that provide feedback inhibition and allow focusing of cortical function on specific sensory input. Feedback inhibitory interneurons have been identified in the brain, which utilize gamma-amino butyric acid (GABA) as a neurotransmitter (Fonnum and Storm-Mathisen, 1969; Kiloh et al., 1981). Benzodiazepine receptors interact with the GABA receptor to increase chloride conductance and decrease neuronal excitability. Both GABA and benzodiazepine receptors have been identified in cortical and subcortical tissue and have been proposed to be primarily involved in controlling neuronal excitability in the onset of epilepsy (Penfield and Jasper, 1947).

Clinically, epilepsy may be characterized as being either cortical or subcortical in origin. Subcortical epilepsy reportedly originates from cortical-activating mechanisms located in the reticular formation and intralaminar nuclei of the thalamus (Gastaut and Fischer-Williams, 1957). This concept is supported by experiments showing that electrical or chemical stimulation of these areas produces epileptic-like cortical activity (Jasper and Droogleever-Fortuyn, 1947). Grand mal epilepsy is one type of subcortical epilepsy (Fig. 28.8). The EEG preceding a grand mal seizure shows low-voltage, fast β activity. This is followed by high-voltage spikes of 8–12 Hz that coincide with the tonic phase of the seizure, and which quickly decay into short rows of spike activity, separated by slow

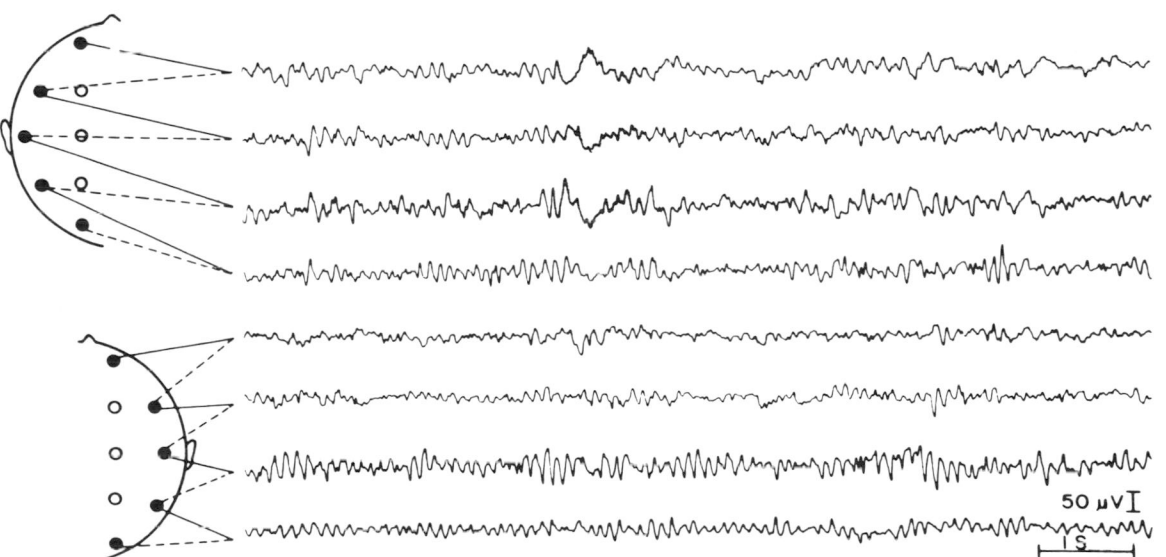

Fig. 28.7 Electroencephalographic record showing abnormal, sporadic, left temporal slow waves observed in a 61-year-old subject with no clinical manifestations of the condition. Reproduced with permission from R. Spehlmann (1981).

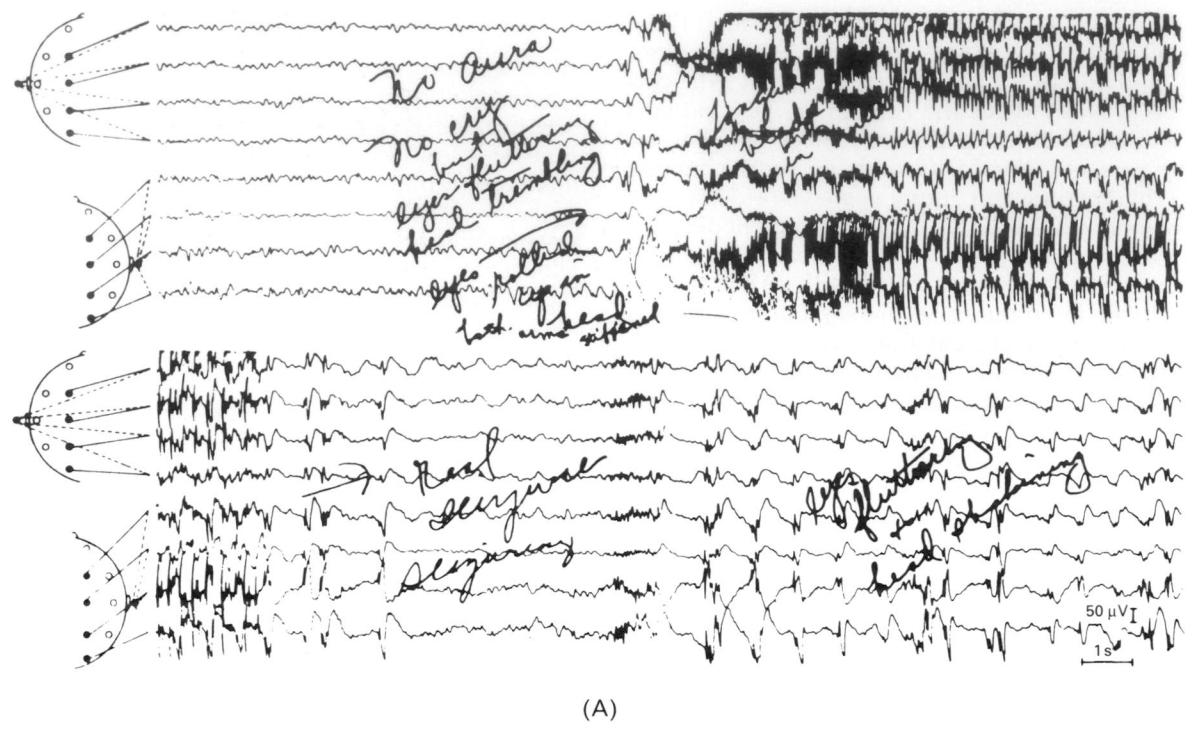

(A)

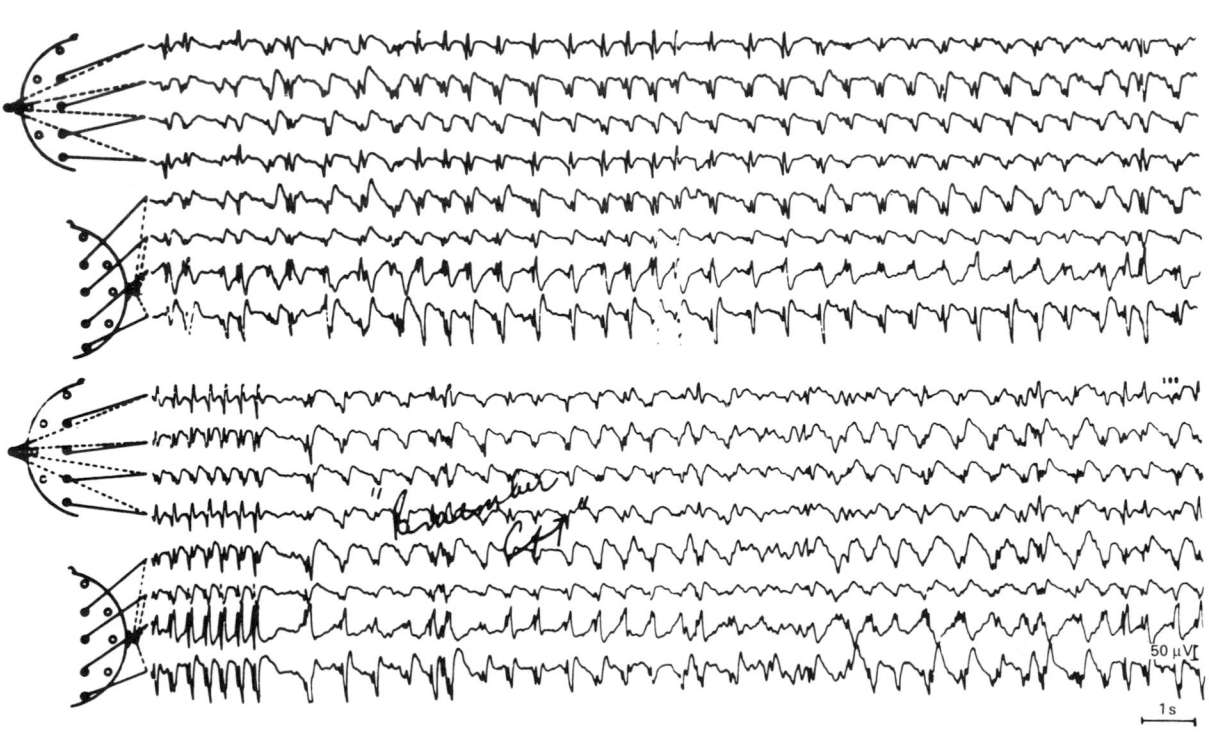

(B)

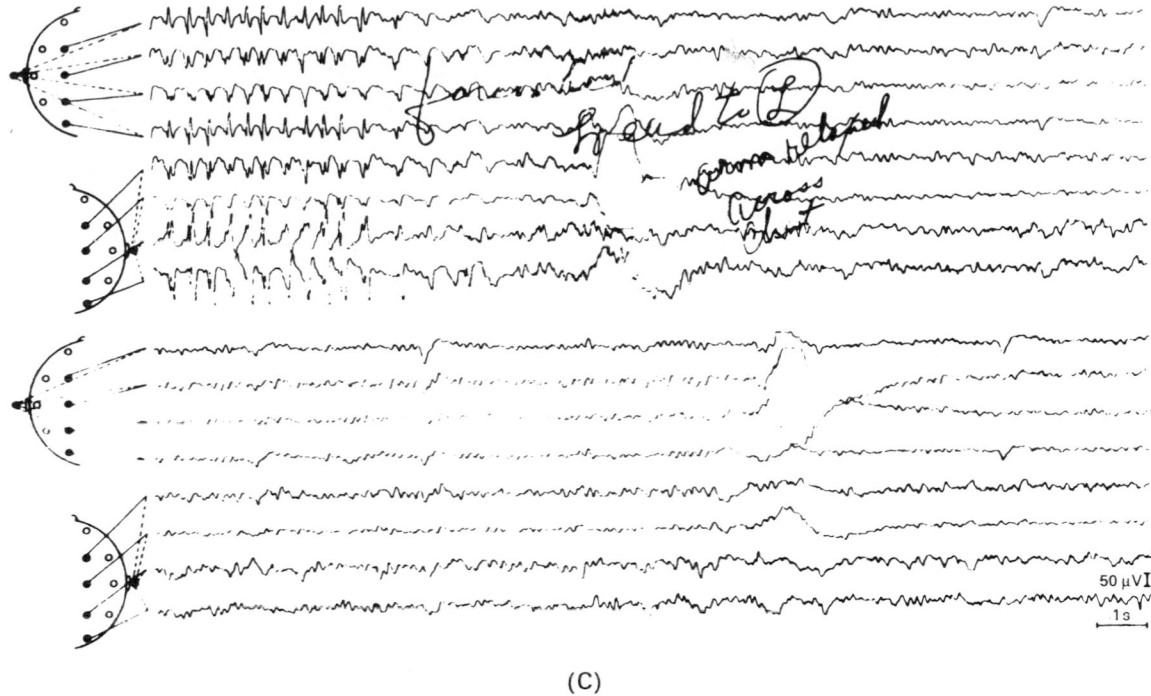

(C)

Fig. 28.8 (A), Generalized tonic-clonic seizure in an 18-year-old girl with a life-long history of major and minor generalized seizures. *Top*: Pattern of slight drowsiness, suddenly interrupted by intermittent spikes and movement artifacts at the onset of a rhythm of generalized repetitive spikes of increasing amplitude and decreasing frequency, which lasts about 10 seconds. Technician's comments read: 'No aura, no cry, but eyes fluttering, head trembling, eyes rolled up in head, both arms stiffened. Tongue blade in mouth'. This represents the tonic phase of the tonic-clonic seizure. *Bottom*: Spikes begin to be interrupted by slow waves. This signals the beginning of the clonic phase, which starts with rhythmical high-amplitude polyspike-and-wave and spike-and-wave complexes at about 1 Hz. Technician's notes read: 'Real seizure, seizuring. Eyes fluttering + head shaking'. (B), Continuation of the generalized seizure shown in Fig. 28.8A. High amplitude spike-and-wave discharges continue during clonic phase. Top part is continuous with the bottom part of Fig. 28.8A. Technician's note reads: 'Remember Cat', indicating that the technician was testing the patient's ability to remember a test word; the patient later did not recall anything. (C), End of the generalized seizure. Top part is continuous with bottom part of Fig. 28.8B. The end of the high-amplitude generalized bisynchronous spike-and-wave complexes represents the end of the clonic phase of the seizure. This is followed by slow waves, movement artifacts, and gradual return of normal background activity. Technician's notes read: 'Head to left, arms relaxed across chest'. This was a mild generalized seizure. More violent seizures are usually followed by postictal depression of amplitude and longer lasting slow waves of lower frequency. Violent seizures can usually not be recorded completely because the recording electrodes become dislodged. Reproduced with permission from R. Spehlmann (1981).

1.5–3 Hz waves that coincide with the clonic phase of grand mal seizures. Finally, the EEG becomes quiescent with slow δ activity, while the patient becomes flaccid. This slow activity corresponds to clinical postictal depression and may persist for several hours.

Petit mal seizures are also subcortical in origin. They are seen in children, rather than in adults, and may be precipitated by hyperventilation or by hypoglycemia. The EEG pattern seen with petit mal consists of bilateral and generalized spike and wave activity, which occurs at a rate of 3–4 per second (Fig. 28.9). Most attacks of petit mal are accompanied by slight myoclonic twitchings that are often restricted to the eyelids. Myoclonic epileptic attacks, also sub-

cortical, are accompanied by myoclonic jerkings that are bilateral and symmetrical (Janeway et al., 1967). The EEG pattern during these attacks resembles the spike and wave pattern of petit mal, but the spikes are usually multiple rather than single. Myoclonic attacks occur frequently in cases of subcortical epilepsy and have been regarded as smaller episodes of grand mal (Gastaut et al., 1957).

Localized or focal EEG seizure patterns are most likely to be of cortical origin (Symonds, 1959). A variety of pathological processes can lead to hypersensitivity of cortical foci, which probably involves chronic dendritic depolarization of pyramid neurons (Ward, 1961). Seizure activity within these cortical

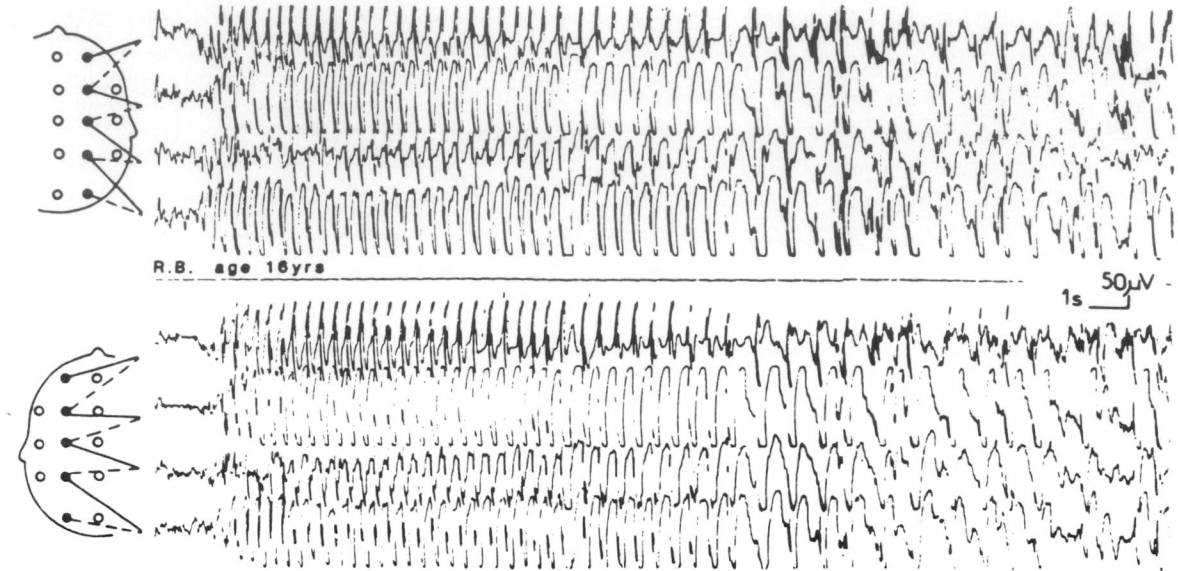

Fig. 28.9 High-amplitude 3–4 sec, generalized, seizure activity in a 16-year-old patient. Reproduced with permission from H. Gastaut, B.G. Zifkin, E. Mariana et al. (1986).

foci may then spread both locally and to other associated cortical regions by means of recruitment (Fig. 28.10) (Ralston, 1958). The interictal discharges of epileptogenic foci are accompanied by strong inhibitory patterns in surrounding cortical tissue. With the onset of seizure activity, the EEG pattern shows a transition from sporadic interseizure activity to rhythmical spikes or sharp waves, usually at a rate of 10–12 Hz. As the attack develops clinically, this rate may decrease to as low as 2 Hz. In psychomotor epilepsy,

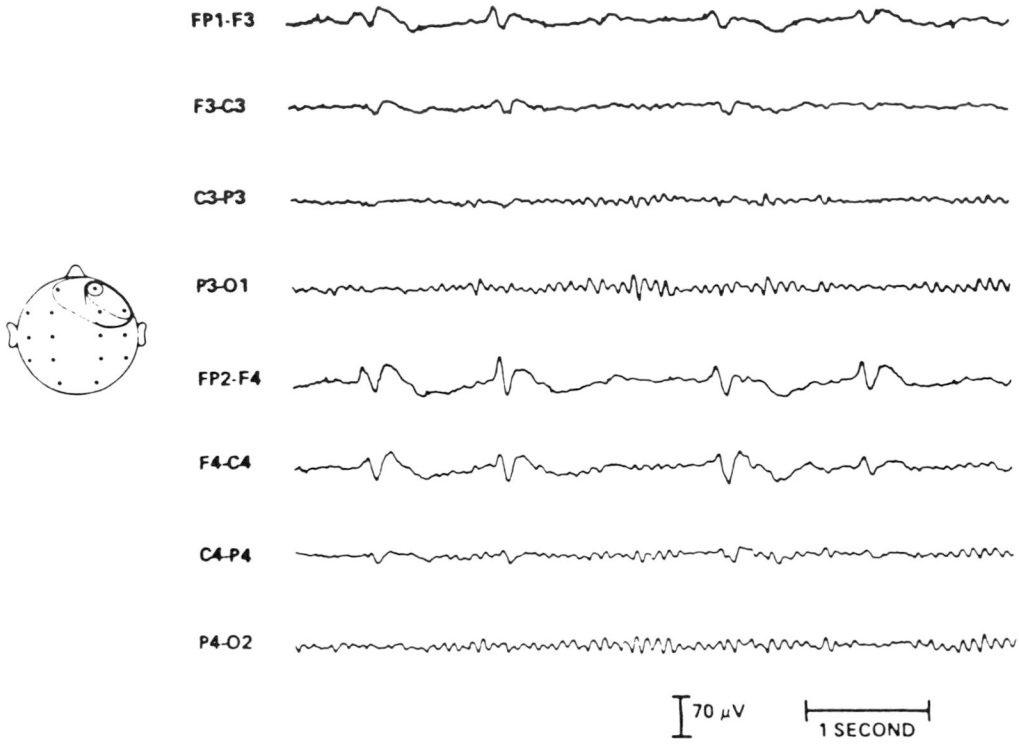

Fig. 28.10 Spike and wave activity indicating focal seizure pattern in the right frontal cortex with spread of this activity to left and posterior regions. Reproduced with permission from E. Wyllie, H. Luders, H.H. Morris et al. (1986).

the epileptic focus is most often located in the temporal lobe. Often the seizure activity spreads bilaterally to mirror foci in the opposite cortex by means of commissural connections. Additional bilateral recruitment of epileptic activity may also accur by association with subcortical generators, which makes the diagnosis of primary focal epilepsy more difficult (Ralston, 1958).

Tumors

Tumor tissue in the brain is not active in generating electrophysiological signals. EEG abnormalities that occur as a result of a tumor are produced primarily because of the space-occupying effect of the tumor and the possible compromise of blood flow to surrounding tissue. Early reports describe EEG slowing with cerebral tumors (Walter, 1936). The distribution of this slowing within the montage of EEG electrodes may provide information on the site of the tumor (Fig. 28.11). Slow activity that is bilaterally symmetrical, synchronous, and rhythmic is quite often associated with infratentorial tumors, due to the displacement and distortion of subcortical centrencephalic structures (Bagchi et al., 1961). Intracranial pressure is often increased with these tumors, due to obstruction of cerebrospinal fluid flow, but this is not likely to be the source of EEG abnormalities. Supratentorial tumors involving subcortical structures may produce widespread EEG abnormalities due to the distortion of centrencephalic structures. This distortion may be unilateral or bilateral and depends on the location of the tumor. Cortical tumors may produce focal δ activity or spikes as a result of direct pressure, induction of edema, or vascular insufficiency in local neurons. Delta activity may be due to a lack of input from subcortical sites (Elul, 1972). This activity may

be continuous or episodic and quite often occurs somewhat lateral and anterior to the site of the tumor (Arfel and Fischgold, 1961). Cerebral abscesses and chronic subdural hematomas often produce similar slowing of EEG due to their space-occupying effects. Similarly, EEG amplitude is usually depressed with a subdural hematoma, due to the compression of cortical neurones and to the increased distance between the cortex and the scalp electrodes.

Cerebral Trauma

Acute head injury may be associated with both short and long-term changes in EEG, which depend on the severity of the injury and which provide a prognosis for eventual recovery. Experimentally, head injury produces an immediate reduction in EEG amplitude (Williams and Denny-Brown, 1941). This is followed by a generalized slowing of EEG to δ activity. The rapidity of recovery of the EEG from this state depends on the severity of the head injury and correlates roughly with the clinical evaluation. In mild head injury in humans, there is a generalized slowing of EEG to θ or δ activity, which usually resolves to a normal EEG pattern within 10 minutes (Ulett, 1955). In severe head injury, the extent and persistence of EEG attenuation depends on the degree of injury; marked attenuation is associated with coma and, most often, with eventual death. EEG amplitude attenuation usually changes to a slowing of activity within 1–2 days. The extent of this slowing depends on the degree of head injury and the prognosis for the patient is poor if the dominant EEG activity is 4 Hz or lower (Dawson et al., 1951). From this state the EEG eventually returns to a normal pattern if the patient recovers, which may require several days to several months. Quite often, localized head injury may also

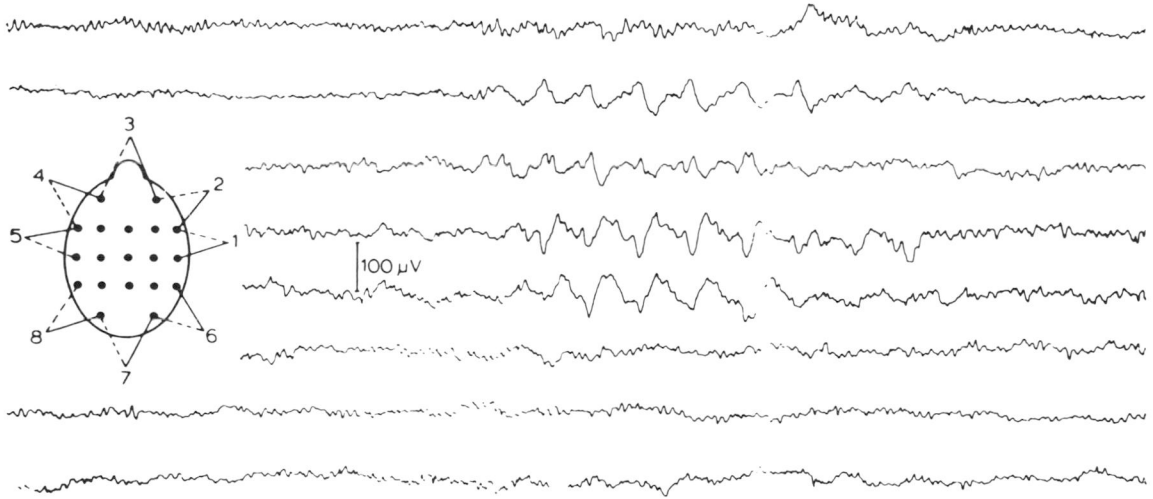

Fig. 28.11 Glioblastoma, left frontal region. Man aged 24 years with headaches for 3 months. EEG: bilateral rhythmical delta discharge in frontal regions, more evident on left side. More 10Hz rhythm in right temporal region than in left. Reproduced with permission from L.G. Kiloh, A.J. McComas, J.W. Osselton et al. (1981).

be associated with focal EEG attenuation and slowing with post-traumatic epilepsy (Kaufman and Walker, 1949). Epilepsy may be prefaced by high-amplitude spiking activity and may occur several days to several weeks after the injury.

Cerebrovascular Disease

Cerebrovascular disease may produce ischemia and neuronal damage by infarction or by brain hemorrhage. The extent and degree of the ischemia and associated brain edema may produce widespread or localized changes in EEG, which depend on the neuronal mechanisms that are affected. Infarction of the brainstem may produce no observable changes in EEG unless portions of the mesencephalic tegmentum and the reticular activating system are damaged (Titeca, 1965). In these cases, normal EEG is replaced by bilaterally synchronous slow wave activity. Pontine infarction can produce 'alpha coma', with widespread symmetrical α activity not reactive to eye opening—a pattern essentially similar to the EEG seen in the normal adult during halothane anesthesia (Fig. 28.12). Cerebrovascular insufficiency involving the vertebrobasilar and posterior cerebral arterial branches may also produce a decrease in EEG amplitude and a slowing of activity, particularly in regions of the temporal and occipital cortex.

Unilateral occlusion of the internal carotid artery may produce little change in EEG if clinical signs of cerebral ischemia are not apparent. This is due to the ability of the contralateral arterial system to produce adequate blood flow and oxygenation to the affected cortex through the circle of Willis. When carotid occlusion is accompanied by cerebral arterial disease, a diffuse slowing to θ or δ EEG and a decrease in amplitude may be observed throughout the ipsilateral cortex (Roger et al., 1961). Focal slowing and decreases in amplitude are usually most apparent in the temporal or frontotemporal regions (Fig. 28.13) (Solomon, 1966) or in parieto-occipital areas—the watershed areas of the anterior and middle cerebral arteries. When cerebrovascular accidents affect specific areas of the cortex, the slowing and diminution of EEG may be more focal. Focal δ activity may be apparent within a few hours of the infarction. Surrounding cortical tissue may also show slowing to θ activity, which may be associated with perifocal edema (Lavy et al., 1964). In some cases in which the lesion affects thalamic regions, the slowing of EEG and the decrease in amplitude may be apparent over the entire cortex with little localization. This depression in EEG activity correlates with a decrease in cortical metabolic activity and can be considered a selective, remote cortical effect due to thalamic injury, which is called diaschisis (Feeney and Baron, 1986). The extent to which EEG is affected throughout the cortex correlates with the state of consciousness. If EEG changes are unilateral and particularly focal in nature, consciousness is often preserved. Resolution of EEG abnormalities usually occurs over a period of several weeks, particularly if the abnormalities are focal in nature. Long-term, there is a good correlation between the persistence of EEG slowing and decreased regional cerebral blood flow (Ingvar, 1967). Clinically, the correlation between recovery of function and resolution of EEG abnormalities is not precise. EEG may recover over a period of time with little

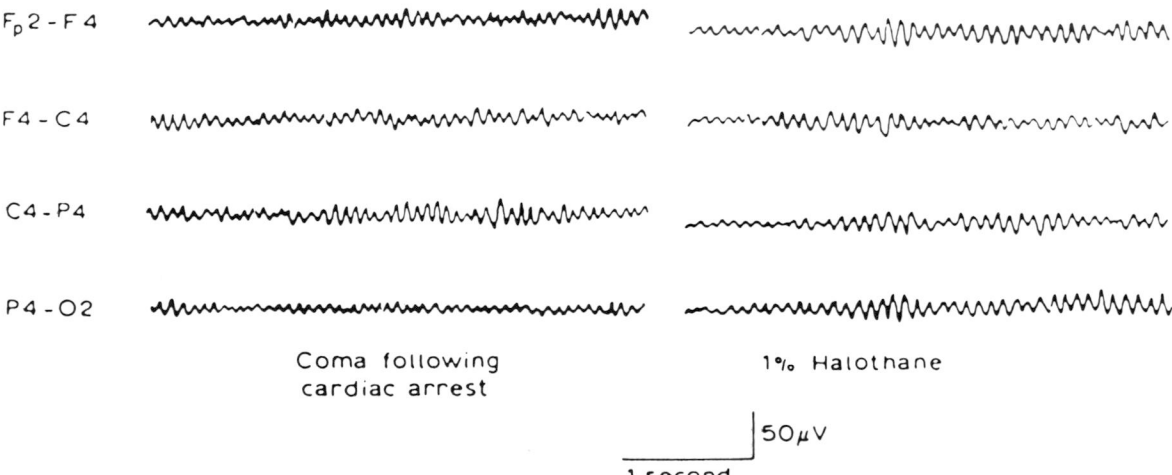

Fig. 28.12 Irreversible and reversible 'alpha coma' produced by cardiac arrest and halothane, respectively. This sort of sustained rhythmic sinusoidal activity secondary to ischemic damage is maximal 2–4 days after the cardiopulmonary arrest and can also be in the θ and β range. Depending on its concentration, halothane can also produce EEG patterns identical to those seen in 'theta coma' and 'beta coma.' The alveolar concentration of halothane producing the alpha-like rhythm above is about 1%. Bipolar EEG derivations where F_P2 is right frontal pole, F4 right frontal, C4 right central, P4 right parietal, and O2 right occipital electrode placement. Reproduced with permission from J.J. Stockard, R.G. Bickford (1981).

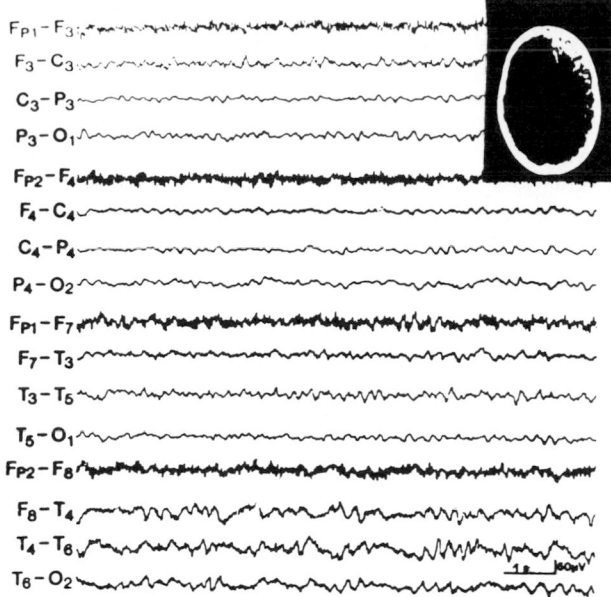

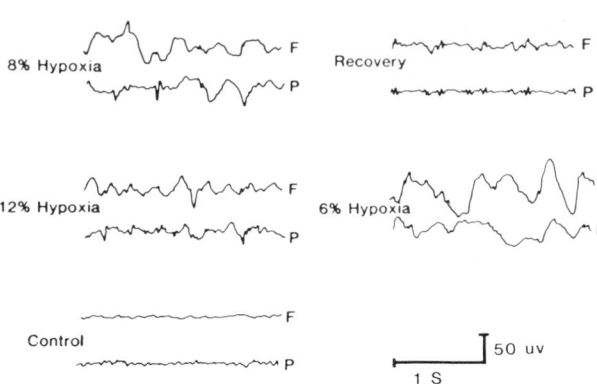

Fig. 28.14 Experimental record from a cat showing bipolar frontal (F) and parietal (P) electroencephalographic (EEG) changes with progressive hypoxia. EEG changed from low-amplitude fast activity during control to high-amplitude δ activity during hypoxia, with some recovery toward normal values when the animal was reoxygenated.

Fig. 28.13 Electroencephalogram showing continuous high-amplitude slow wave (θ–δ) activity in the right hemisphere produced by cerebrovascular insufficiency. Computed tomograph showed a large stroke-related lesion, which involved the right hemisphere. Reproduced with permission from N. Schaul, L. Green, R. Peyster et al. (1986).

improvement in clinical symptoms. On the other hand, as with head injury, the state of consciousness and clinical symptoms may improve rapidly following a cerebrovascular accident while EEG slowing continues over a much longer period.

Acute cerebral ischemia, as during carotid endarterectomy, does not change the EEG until regional flow falls to about 20 ml/(100 g · min), approximately 40% of normal. Although the EEG may be flat at less than about 18 ml/(100 g · min), neurons are viable (but quiescent) until flow is further compromised to 10 ml/(100 g · min), when potassium begins to leak out of the cells. Thus, the EEG alone cannot distinguish between levels of ischemia that endanger neurons and lesser levels of ischemia where nerve cells are quiet but viable. Since viability cannot be determined, ischemia must be corrected as rapidly as possible (Grundy and Heros, 1986).

Hypoxia

The electroencephalogram rapidly reflects altered cerebral function during hypoxia (Fig. 28.14). Lack of oxygen initially produces frontal α rhythms. Delta waves appear as consciousness is lost. The EEG changes of hypoxia are more pronounced in younger subjects, but all subjects show clinical and EEG changes when arterial oxygen saturation falls below 65% (Planques et al., 1965). With increasing hypoxia the EEG frequency slows progressively (Brazier,

1948), but the sequence is not recorded at all electrodes on the scalp. There is a correlation between cerebral venous oxygen tension and EEG activity during hypoxia (Schaertlin, 1961), but this does not persist in the post-hypoxic phase. High-energy phosphates in the brain are rapidly depleted during acute hypoxia, and the EEG reflects these changes. The EEG ceases when cortical creatinphosphate is 1–1.5 μmol/L that is 70–80% μmol/L below normal (Schmahl et al., 1966). Using microfluorometric techniques to continuously record local levels of pyridine nucleotides, Chance and Schoener (1962) and Chance and Pring (1968) found EEG silence when pyridine nucleotides fell 80% (70% with gradual onset of hypoxia). At an inspired oxygen concentration of 6%, EEG bursts and short silent periods appear but cortical creatinphosphate is still nearly normal. Though the energy potential of the brain may be normal and electrical activity may still be absent, as in severe hypercarbia, the electroencephalogram cannot be maintained when creatinphosphate is very low.

Changes in the energy state of the brain have been correlated with electrophysiologic activity of the brain and changes in membrane function. EEG suppression occurs before adenosine triphosphate (ATP) changes, and sodium pump failure is seen after ATP depletion in both ischemia (Naritomi et al., 1988; Crockard et al., 1987) and hypoxia (Milito et al., 1988). Fluorometric measurement of changes in cytosolic free calcium in hypoxia showed that cytosolic calcium increased 20 seconds before EEG silence and decreased 7 seconds before restoration of EEG with reoxygenation (Uematsu et al., 1988). This suggests that the change in electrical activity may be related to the rise in cytosolic calcium. Calcium antagonists may have cerebral protective effects (Hossmann et al., 1983; Forsman et al., 1986; Abe et al., 1988), and some of these agents have been shown to accelerate the post-ischemia restoration of high-energy phosphates in cerebral cortex (Bielenberg et al., 1987).

Hypocarbia

Hyperventilation slows EEG frequencies and increase EEG amplitudes (Gibbs, 1940), effects being more pronounced in the young. The fundamental α rhythm is not reduced, but lower frequency components are increased (Morrice, 1956). Davis and Wallace (1942) found that 3 minutes of hyperventilation slowed the EEG to a dominant frequency of 4–6 Hz and that 100% oxygen lessened the slowing. Hyperventilation and hypocarbia decrease cerebral blood flow, but after the cerebral venous P_{O_2} becomes less than 19 torr, no further decrease in cerebral blood flow occurs with progressive hypocarbia (Noell and Schneider, 1944). Forced hyperventilation cannot decrease cerebral blood flow by more than 40% (Kety and Schmidt, 1948), this limit presumably imposed by cerebral vasodilatation in response to pH changes produced by ischemia and subsequent hypoxia. Total cerebral oxygen consumption does not change during hyperventilation sufficient to produce a 30% drop in cerebral blood flow, so that the EEG and neurologic changes seen with hyperventilation do not seem to be due to cerebral hypoxia. Yet local changes in cerebral blood flow with localized hypoxia may occur with overbreathing, and cortical tissue lactate does increase by as much as five times (Weidner, 1969) while high-energy phosphates are little affected. Though there is no clear correlation between EEG frequency spectrum and cerebral flow, there is a parallel change between EEG and cortical lactate.

Hypercarbia

Moderate hypercarbia produces an arousal pattern in the EEG (Gerard et al., 1936) that is more pronounced in the young (Rossen et al., 1963). Concentrations of carbon dioxide above 25% cause a decrease, then disappearance of rapid EEG activity (Wyke, 1957), and high-voltage, 3-Hz activity is increasingly dominant at carbon dioxide concentrations above 30%. After 2–5 minutes at 80% carbon dioxide, the EEG is silent, though high-energy phosphates are essentially stable. Hypercarbia produces changes in the EEG tracing seen during anesthesia. It can suppress seizure activity seen with halogenated ethers (Stockard et al., 1973).

Hypotension

With sudden, complete cessation of blood flow, the EEG becomes flat and cortical creatinphosphate becomes less than 1% of control in less than 2 minutes (Doring and Gerlach, 1957). In healthy persons, autoregulatory mechanisms maintain cerebral blood flow near normal when perfusion pressure drops as low as 60–70 torr (Lassen, 1959). Clinical symptoms and EEG changes appear when cerebral blood flow falls to 50% of normal (Finerty et al., 1954). Patients with impaired autoregulatory mechanisms suffer significant decreases in cerebral blood flow and associated EEG changes at higher pressures (Kety et al., 1950). Changes produced by cerebral ischemia are less homogeneous than those produced by arterial hypoxia, and lesions cluster in arterial boundary zones (Levy et al., 1975). That portion of the cortex supplied by the middle cerebral artery seems especially vulnerable. Hypercarbia may exacerbate this problem (Eklof et al., 1973); unperfused and well-perfused areas of cortex may coexist.

Hypotension may alter EEG patterns seen during general anesthesia. Beecher et al. (1938) saw EEG signs of deepening anesthesia when cats receiving diethyl ether were subjected to hypotension. But Bellville and Artusio (1956) saw no EEG change when trimethaphan was used to produce systolic blood pressure of 60–80 torr during cyclopropane anesthesia. On-line EEG monitoring can be used to identify periods of neuronal compromise during hypotension. This would seem especially valuable in those patients with compromised autoregulation of cerebral blood flow.

Hypoglycemia

Insulin-induced hypoglycemia produces concurrent loss of consciousness and loss of EEG α rhythm (Himwich et al., 1939). EEG slowing leading to δ activity is seen with progressive cerebral depression from lack of glucose (Aizawa, 1957). This EEG slowing is accompanied by fluxes of sodium into the brain and potassium out of the brain as active transport mechanisms fail (Meyer et al., 1962). Homeostasis and EEG activity are re-established with glucose administration, but if the hypoglycemia is prolonged, severe permanent brain damage may result. Neuronal damage is more likely to occur if hypoxia and hypoglycemia coexist than in the presence of either insult alone.

ANESTHESIA AND THE ELECTROENCEPHALOGRAM

The purpose of anesthesia is to produce analgesia and to depress the brain so that sensations of pain and awareness of surgical procedures are suppressed. Anesthetics designed for this purpose produce a change in EEG that may be related to the level of anesthesia. Increasing doses of most anesthetics produce progressive stages of anesthesia (Guedel, 1920): euphoria, agitation or excitation, deeper stages of sleep, and finally, a stage of anesthesia that is deep enough to enable painless surgery. Induction of anesthesia coincides with a decrease in α and an increase in β activity, which corresponds to the clinical stage of activation. This may be related to generalized cortical activation due to loss of normal inhibition. As the depth of anesthesia increases, EEG frequency decreases until a slow-wave pattern in the δ or θ range occurs. If anesthetic depth is further increased at this stage, a very deep level of surgical sleep is produced, which coincides with a pattern of burst suppression on the EEG and with near-maximal depression of cerebral metabolic activity. A further increase in anesthesia will produce complete cortical electrical silence and a flat EEG.

To some extent, stages of anesthesia with several different agents produce similar general patterns of EEG change. For this reason, the pattern of EEG changes with anesthesia can, in some settings, be considered an indication of anesthetic depth. However, not all anesthetics produce the same maximal state of cerebral depression. For example, high doses of some anesthetics, such as barbiturates and isoflurane, can produce complete electrical silence at the cortex, while others, such as halothane or narcotics, only substantially slow the EEG. Furthermore, anesthetics can produce excitatory changes as well as inhibitory changes in EEG activity, and, at least in epileptic patients, one part of the brain may be depressed by anesthesia at the same moment that another region is excited (Fig. 28.15).

Inhalation Anesthetics

Earlier reviews of the effects of anesthetics on the electrical activity of the brain were comprehensive when written and are still valuable (Clark and Rosner, 1973; Rosner and Clark, 1973; Stockard and Bickford, 1981). Halothane is one of the commonly used inhaled anesthetics. EEG changes coincide with the metabolic, depressant effects of halothane in the cerebrum. If anesthetic levels of halothane are inspired, initially there is a shift from dominant, unanesthetized α activity to rapid β activity. As anesthesia deepens, the frequency slows until, at deep surgical anesthesia, high-amplitude δ and θ activity predominate (Oshima et al., 1981). Reports suggest that deep halothane anesthesia may further suppress EEG to burst suppression or to quiescence (Gain and Paletz, 1957), but this may be more a function of the toxic action of halothane at these levels, rather than a strictly anesthetic effect (Bassell et al., 1982).

Enflurane is an inhaled agent with anesthetic actions similar to halothane, although it is absorbed more rapidly. During anesthetic induction, the dominant frequency is lost and β activity increases; surgical anesthesia is marked by high-voltage δ and θ activity, as with halothane (Bassell et al., 1982; Levy,

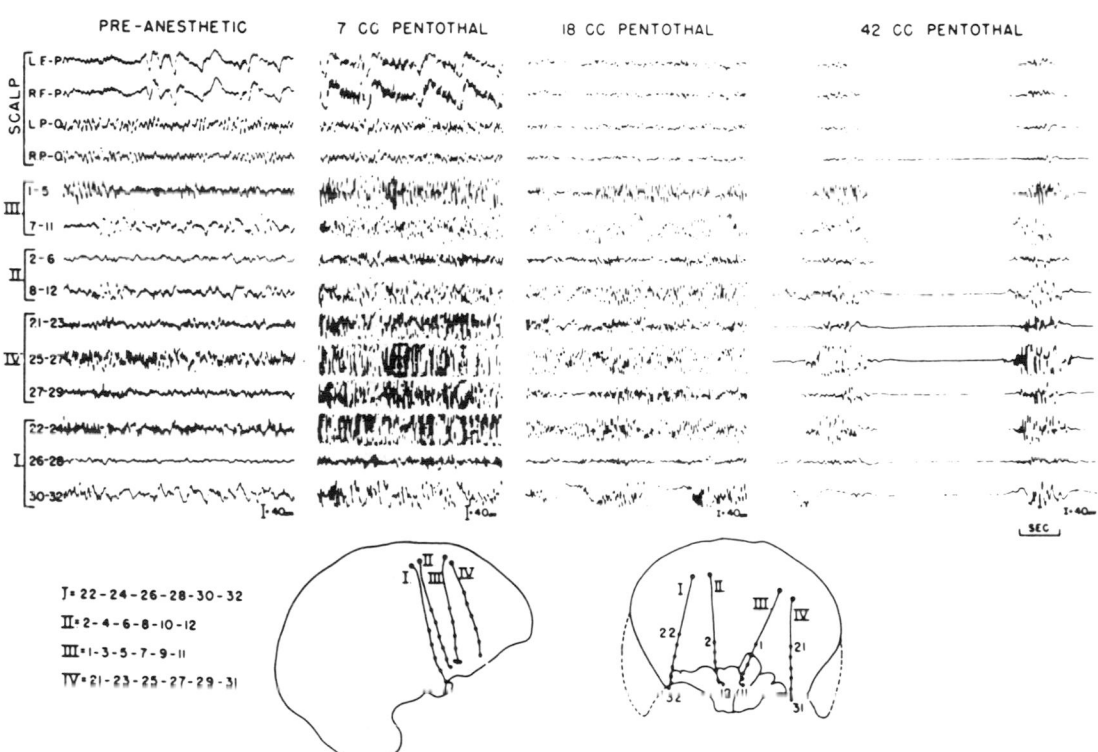

EFFECT OF PENTOTHAL ON SCALP AND DEPTH ELECTROGRAMS

Fig. 28.15 Depth recording in an epileptic patient receiving thiopental intravenously in a concentration of 25 mg/ml. The location of the depth electrodes is shown in A–P (anterior/posterior) and lateral X-ray views. Note the overall similarity in pattern but the individual channel differences, particularly in the depth. Reproduced with permission from J.J. Stockard, R.G. Bickford (1981).

1986). With higher concentrations of enflurane, spiking activity may occur (Moorthy et al., 1980). This may be followed by a generalized seizure pattern, with occasional tonic-clonic muscle activity, which is typical of grand mal seizure (Stockard et al., 1973). Seizures with enflurane are most likely when it is the sole anesthetic in a patient who is hyperventilated at deep levels of anesthesia (Fig. 28.16).

Isoflurane is an inhaled anesthetic that provides more effective cerebral metabolic depression, less cerebrovasodilatation, and less increase in intracranial pressure than halothane provides. These characteristics have made it popular for neurosurgical anesthe-

sia. The effect of isoflurane on the EEG during anesthetic induction is similar to that of halothane. The primary difference between the cerebral effects of the two agents lies in the more complete cerebral metabolic depression with isoflurane at deep anesthetic levels and the associated burst suppression of EEG during surgical anesthesia, with complete supression of electrical activity at high, nontoxic concentrations (Fig. 28.17) (Newberg et al., 1983).

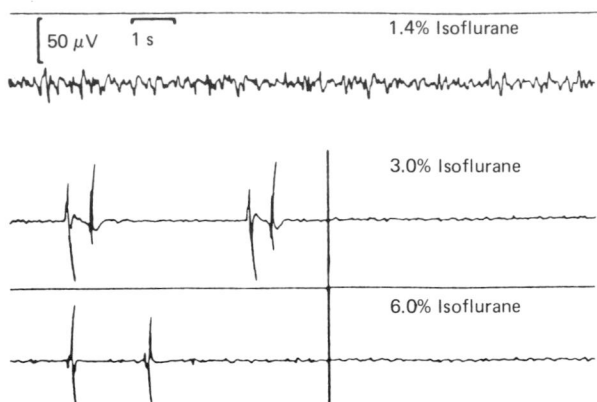

Fig. 28.17 Electroencephalogram of a dog given isoflurane at increasing concentrations. An anesthetic pattern is seen at 1.4% isoflurane, which changes to rhythmic spikes separated by isoelectric silence at 3% and 6%. Reproduced with permission from L.A. Newberg, J.H. Milde, J.D. Michenfelder (1983).

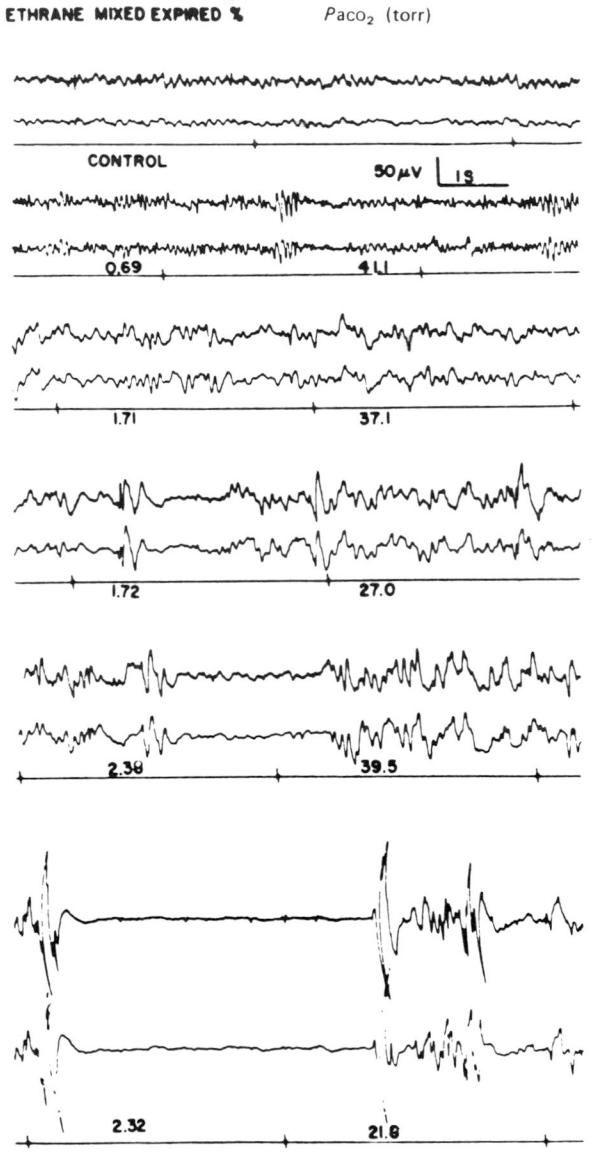

Fig. 28.16 Effect of increasing depth of enflurane concentration and changes in Pa_{CO_2} in humans. Note spiking activity at high enflurane concentration and low Pa_{CO_2}. Reproduced with permission from D.L. Clarke, E.C. Hosick, B.S. Rosner (1971).

Intravenous Anesthetics

Barbiturates given for rapid intravenous induction of anesthesia, such as thiopental, produce a level of anesthesia that generally depresses brain activity. After intravenous injection, thiopental quickly passes across the blood-brain barrier and rapidly equilibrates in brain tissue. The anesthetic effect of short-acting barbiturates, such as thiopental, is usually brief (7–8 minutes) because of redistribution of the drug to less well-perfused tissues, such as muscle and fat. Other barbiturates may have longer anesthetic action due to differences in lipid solubility, dissociation, and plasma protein binding.

With slow intravenous injections of barbiturate, EEG changes are similar to those with other anesthetics (Pichlmayr et al., 1984). An initial phase of EEG activation is seen, with an increase in amplitude in all frequency ranges. This changes to a dominant rhythmic, high-amplitude δ and θ activity as the depth of anesthesia increases. The EEG pattern may progress to burst suppression or to quiescence with additional drug (Quasha et al., 1981; Todd et al., 1984) (Fig. 28.18). EEG changes are closely linked to the cerebral metabolic depressant effects of barbiturates (Kassel et al., 1980). As the depth of anesthesia decreases, the EEG slowly recovers α and β activity,

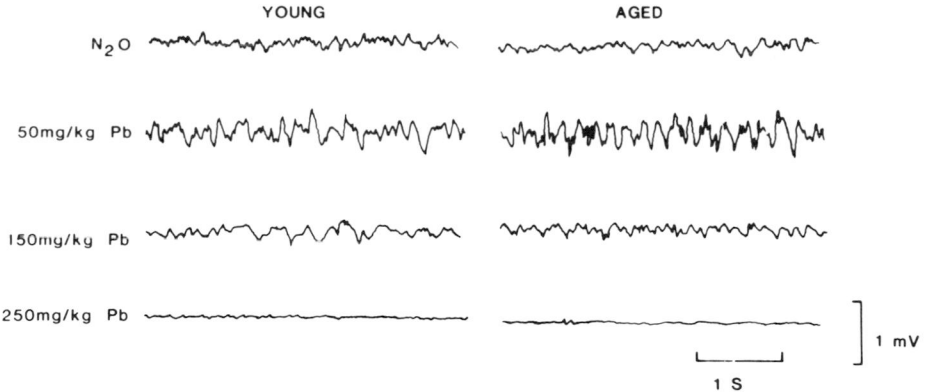

Fig. 28.18 Electroencephalographic (EEG) records in young and aged rats showing effects of increasing phenobarbital anesthesia. Activity changes from low-amplitude fast activity with nitrous oxide ventilation to high-amplitude slow waves and is depressed to isoelectric EEG at the highest dose. Reproduced with permission from V.L. Baughman, W.E. Hoffman, D.J. Miletich et al. (1986).

while slow-wave activity decreases. With fast, intravenous injections of thiopental for induction, the initial stages of EEG pass quickly, and synchronous high-amplitude δ and θ activity commonly coincides with anesthesia within 1–2 min. The EEG slowly returns to a nonsynchronous pattern, with α and β activity occurring over 7–8 min as anesthesia lightens. The effect of barbiturates on EEG over time depends on the method of drug administration, lipid solubility, dissociation, and plasma protein binding of the particular barbiturate compound, as well as on tissue perfusion and metabolism in the patient.

In contrast to barbiturates, ketamine is a dissociative anesthetic that stimulates cerebral metabolism. Following intravenous or intramuscular injection, ketamine disrupts the normal EEG pattern and high-amplitude θ activity (4–7 Hz) coincides with anesthesia. Secondary patterns of β activity may also be observed periodically that coincide with θ activity. This pattern slowly returns to normal over 20–40 min as the patient recovers. As with barbiturates, EEG effects depend on the dose and method of anesthetic administration. The θ EEG rhythm and cerebral metabolic activation seen with ketamine are thought to be due to suppression of normal cortical inhibition and to secondary activation of subcortical rhinencephalic structures.

Narcotics are important in anesthesia. They can be used to supplement the effects of other anesthetic agents by providing analgesia and deeper anesthesia with minimal concomitant cardiovascular depression. More recently, narcotics have been used as a primary anesthetic agent for major surgical procedures (Sebel et al., 1981). Synthetic opioids such as fentanyl, sufentanil, and alfentanil have a rapid onset and a relatively brief duration of action, qualities that facilitate control of anesthetic depth. (Some anesthetists, however, doubt that narcotics alone can be relied upon for complete anesthesia in all patients.)

During induction with anesthetic doses of narcotics, α activity slows and β activity ceases in the EEG within 1–2 min (Scott et al., 1985). Diffuse θ and some δ activity follow rapidly. Within 5 min of induction, high-amplitude δ activity is dominant and is synchronized in a high percentage of patients (Fig. 28.19).

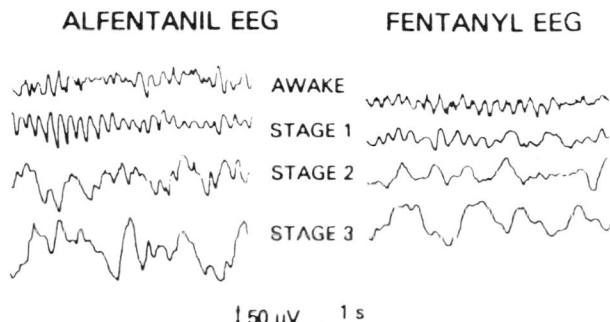

Fig. 28.19 Electroencephalographic (EEG) stages for alfentanyl and fentanyl. Activity changes from mixed α and β activity during awake state to high-amplitude δ activity at stage 3 with both anesthetics. Reproduced with permission from J.C. Scott, K.V. Ponganis, D.R. Stanski (1985).

These changes slowly reverse 15–20 min after induction; δ activity becomes lower in amplitude and irregular, while θ activity increases. If additional doses of narcotics are not given, α and β activity slowly return. Sharp-wave and spiking EEG have been observed with sufentanil and fentanyl (Bovill et al., 1982) and supraclinical doses of these drugs produce seizure-like activity in animals (Fig. 28.20) (Keykhah et al., 1985). Measurements of brain metabolism during anesthesia with fentanyl or sufentanil show that these narcotics depress metabolic activity, but not

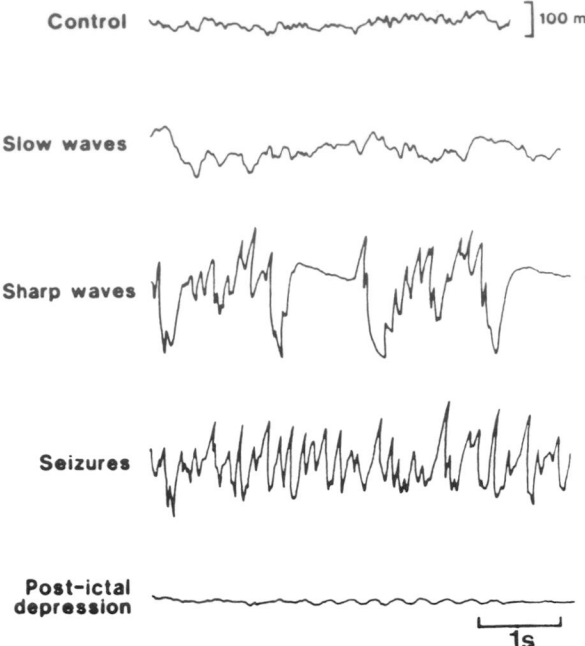

Fig. 28.20 Representative records of electroencephalographic (EEG) changes in rats with increasing sufentanil doses. Anesthetic EEG pattern changes to sharp waves and seizure activity with elevated doses of sufentanil. Reproduced with permission from M.M. Keykhah, D.S. Smith, C. Carlsson et al. (1985).

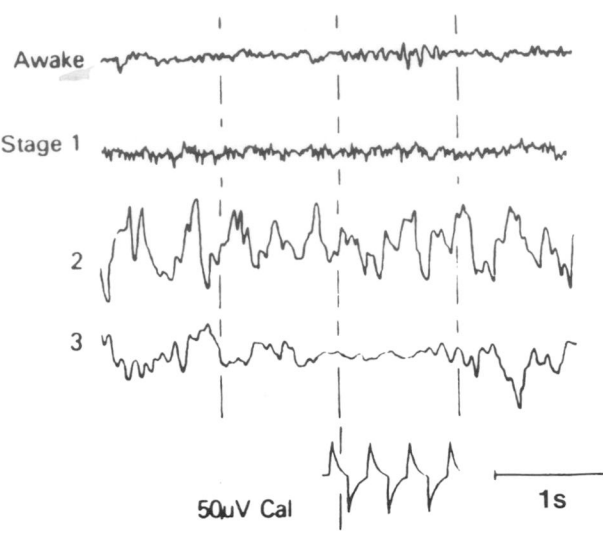

Fig. 28.21 Electroencephalographic progression with increasing etomidate dose. Activation of β activity is seen in stage 1, which reverts to high-amplitude, low-frequency waves and periods of quiescence at stage 3. Reproduced with permission from J.R. Arden, F.O. Holley, D.R. Stanski (1986).

to the same extent as barbiturates or potent inhalational anesthetics (Bovill et al., 1982). The absence of maximal brain metabolic or EEG suppression with high doses of narcotics indicates that the mechanism of anesthesia is different from that with other anesthetic drugs. It is likely that these agents, like ketamine, do not depress neuronal activity in general but act more specifically at limbic and other subcortical sites to dissociate afferent sensory activity from conscious cortical function.

Etomidate is a relatively new anesthetic agent that produces anesthesia by depressing neuronal metabolic function but provides little analgesia (Doenicke et al., 1982). This drug is unusual in that it suppresses brain metabolism and EEG substantially but has little effect on cardiovascular function. This is probably because the primary site of action of etomidate is at neuronal GABA receptor sites, which modulate brain metabolic electrical function. Following anesthetic induction with etomidate, electrical activity of all frequencies initially increases with transient neuronal excitation (Pichlmayr et al., 1984). This pattern quickly reverts to high-amplitude, slow-wave activity with loss of α and β waves. As anesthesia deepens, synchronous δ activity becomes dominant (Fig. 28.21) (Doenicke et al., 1982; Arden et al., 1986). An overdose of etomidate manifests as further depression of EEG to burst suppression or quiescence (Milde et al., 1985). Reversal of anesthesia occurs quickly with eto-

midate; the phases of anesthesia are passed through in reverse order and dominant α activity returns in 8–10 min.

In summary, we have shown how neuronal and brain electrical activity produce EEG signals, how these signals are collected, and what changes occur in normal, pathophysiological, and anesthetic states. The availability of computerized techniques of digital EEG evaluation, such as spectral analysis, allows quantification with less variability due to interpretation. However, an experienced encephalographer should always be present during EEG recording in order to confirm the validity of the signal and to detect abnormal EEG, such as μ waves, which signal analysis may not detect. New, sophisticated methods, such as the magnetoencephalogram, have the potential to specifically localize brain magnetoelectrical signals throughout the brain without the limitations of surface scalp recording.

REFERENCES

Abe I., Kogure K., Watanabe T. (1988). Prevention of ischemic and postischemic brain edema by a novel calcium antagonist (PN200-110). *J. Cerebr. Blood Flow Metab.*, **8**, 436.

Aizawa T. (1957). Cerebral circulation and metabolism in coma. *Psychiat. Neurol. Jap.*, **59**, 943.

Andersen P., Andersson S.A. (1968). *The Physiological Basis of the Alpha Rhythm*. New York: Appleton-Century-Crofts.

Andersen P., Sears T.A. (1964). The role of inhibition in the phasing of spontaneous thalamocortical discharge. *J. Physiol.*, **173**,, 459.

Arden J.R., Holley F.O., Stanski D.R. (1986). Increased sensitivity to etomidate in the elderly: initial distribution versus altered brain response. *Anesthesiology*, **65**, 19.

Arfel G., Fischgold F. (1961). EEG signs in tumours of the brain. In *Electroencephalography and Cerebral Tumours*. *Electroencephalogr. Clin. Neurophysiol.*, Suppl. **19**, 36.

Bagchi B.K., Kooi K.A., Selving B.T., et al. (1961). Subtentorial tumours and other lesions: an electroencephalographic study of 121 cases. *Electroencephalogr. Clin. Neurophysiol.*, **13**, 180.

Ball G.J., Gloor P., Thompson C.J. (1977). Computed unit-EEG correlations and laminar profiles of spindle waves in the electroencephalogram of cats. *Electroencephalogr. Clin. Neurophysiol.*, **43**, 330.

Bassel G.M., Cullen B.F., Fairchild M.D., et al. (1982). Electroencephalographic and behavioural effects of enflurane and halothane anaesthesia in the cat. *Br. J. Anaesth.*, **54**, 659.

Baughman V.L., Hoffman W.E., Miletich D.J., et al. (1986). Effects of phenobarbital on cerebral blood flow and metabolism in young and aged rats. *Anesthesiology*, **65**, 500.

Beecher H.K., McDonough F.K., Forbes H. (1938). Effects of blood pressure changes on cortical potentials during anesthesia. *J. Neurophysiol.*, **1**, 324.

Bellville J.W., Artusio J.F. Jr. (1956). Effect of Arfonad on anesthetic requirements during cyclopropane anesthesia. *Anesthesiology*, **17**, 347.

Bielenberg G.W., Beck T., Sauer D., et al. (1987). Effects of cerebroprotective agents on cerebral blood flow and on postischemia energy metabolism in the rat brain. *J. Cerebr. Blood Flow Metab.*, **7**, 480.

Bovill J.G., Sebel P.S., Wauquier A., et al. (1982). Electroencephalographic effects of sufentanil anaesthesia in man. *Br. J. Anaesth.*, **54**, 45.

Brazier M.A.B. (1948). Physiological mechanisms underlying the electrical activity of the brain. *J. Neurol.*, **11**, 118.

Bremer F. (1935). Cerveau isole et physiologie du sommeil. *Seanc. Soc. Biol.*, **118**, 1235.

Calvet J., Calvet M.C., Scherrer J. (1964). Etude stratigraphique corticale de l'activite EEG spontanee. *Electroencephalogr. Clin. Neurophysiol.*, **17**, 109.

Chance B., Pring M. (1968). Logic in the design of the respiratory chain. In *Biochemie des Sauerstoffs*. (Hess B., Staudinger H. eds.) Berlin: Springer.

Chance B., Schoener B. (1962). Correlation of oxidation-reduction changes of intracellular reduced pyridine nucleotide and changes in the electroencephalogram of the rat in anoxia. *Nature*, **195**, 956.

Clark D.L., Hosick E.C., Rosner B.S. (1971). Neurophysiological effects of different anesthetics in unconscious man. *J. Appl. Physiol.*, **31**, 884.

Clark D.L., Rosner B.S. (1973). Neurophysiologic effects of general anesthetics: I: electroencephalogram and sensory evoked responses in man. *Anesthesiology*, **38**, 564.

Cohen D. (1972). Magnetoencephalography: detection of the brain's electrical activity with a super conductive magnetometer. *Science*, **199**, 81.

Cooper R., Osselton J.W., Shaw J.C. (1980). *EEG Technology*, 3rd edn. Boston: Butterworths.

Cooper R., Winter A.L., Crow H.J., et al., (1965). Comparison of subcortical, cortical and scalp activity using chronically indwelling electrodes in man. *Electroencephalogr. Clin. Neurophysiol.*, **18**, 217.

Creutzfeldt O.D., Watanabe S., Lux H.D. (1966). Relations between EEG phenomenon and potentials of single cortical cells. *Electroencephalogr. Clin. Neurophysiol.*, **20**, 19.

Crockard H.A., Gadian G.D., Frackowiak R.S.J., et al. (1987). Acute cerebral ischaemia: concurrent changes in cerebral blood flow, energy metabolites, pH, and lactate measured with hydrogen clearance and ^{31}P and ^{1}H nuclear magnetic resonance spectroscopy. II. changes during ischaemia. *J. Cerebr. Blood Flow Metab.*, **7**, 394.

Cuffin B.N., Cohen D. (1979). Comparison of the magneto-encephalogram and electroencephalogram. *Electroencephalogr. Clin. Neurophysiol.*, **47**, 132.

Davis H., Wallace W.M.L. (1942). Factors affecting changes produced in the electroencephalogram by standardized hyperventilation. *Arch. Neurol. Psychiatr.*, **47**, 606.

Davson H. (1970). *A Textbook of General Physiology*, 4th edn Boston: Little, Brown.

Dawson R.E. Webster J.E., Gurdjiian E.S. (1951). Serial electroencephalography in acute head injuries. *J. Neurosurg.*, **8**, 613.

DeLucchi M.R., Garoutte B., Aird R.B. (1962). The Scalp as an Electroenceophalogram. *Electroencephalogr. Clin. Neurophysiol.*, **14**, 191.

Doenicke A., Loffler B., Kugler J., et al. (1982). Plasma concentration and E.E.G. after various regimens of etomidate. *Br. J. Anaesth.*, **54**, 393.

Doring H.J., Gerlach E. (1957). Saureloscliche Phosphor-verbindungen des Gehirns unter dem Einfluss von Anoxie, Ischaemic und Narkotischen Stoffen. *Naunyn-Schmiedeberg's Aach. Exp. Path. Pharmak.*, **232**, 271.

Drift J.H.A. Van der (1961). Ischemic cerebral lesions. *Angiology*, **12**, 401.

Eklof B., MacMillan V., Siesjo B.K. (1973). The effect of hypercapnic acidosis upon the energy metabolism of the brain in arterial hypotension caused by bleeding. *Acta Physiol. Scand.*, **87**, 1.

Elul R. (1972). The genesis of the EEG. *Int. Rev. Neurobiol.*, **15**, 227.

Eyzaguirre C., Fidone S.F. (1975). The bases of excitation. In *Physiology of the Nervous System*, 2nd edn , pp. 7–19, Chicago: Year Book Medical.

Feeney D.M., Baron J.C. (1986). Diaschisis. *Stroke*. **17**, 817.

Finnerty F.A., Witkin L., Fazekas J.F. (1954). Cerebral haemodynamic during cerebral ischaemia induced by auto hypotension. *J. Clin. Invest.*, **33**, 1227.

Fonnum J., Storm-Mathisen J. (1969). GABA synthesis in the rat hippocampus correlated to the distribution on inhibitory neurons. *Acta Physiol. Scand.*, **76**, 35A.

Forsman M., Fleischer J.E., Milde J.H., et al. (1986). The effects of nimodipine on cerebral blood flow and metabolism. *J. Cerebr. Blood Flow Metab.*, **6**, 763.

Gain E.A., Paletz S.G. (1957). An attempt to correlate the clinical signs of fluothane anesthesia with the electroencephalographic levels. *Can. Anaesth. Soc. J.*, **4**, 289.

Gastaut H., Fischer-Williams M. (1957). Etude Electro-encephalographic study of syncope, its differentiation from epilepsy. *Lancet*, **2**, 1018.

Gastaut H., Fischer-Williams M. (1959). The physiopathology of epileptic seizures. In *Handbook of Physiology*, pp. 329–346. (Field J., Magoun H.W., Hall V.E. eds.) Washington: American Physiological Society.

Gastaut H., Zifkin B.G., Mariana E., et al. (1986). The long-term course of primary generalized epilepsy with persisting absences. *Neurol.*, **36**, 1021.

Gerard R.W., Marshall W.H., Saul L.J. (1936). Electrical

activity of the cat's brain. *Arch. Neurol. Psychiatr.*, **36**, 675.

Gibbs F.A., Williams D., Gibbs E.L. (1940). Modification of the cortical frequency spectrum by changes in CO_2, blood sugar and O_2. *J. Neurophysiol.*, **3**, 49.

Grundy B.L. (1983). Intraoperative monitoring of sensory-evoked potentials. *Anesthesiology*, **58**, 72.

Grundy B.L., Heros R. (1986). Ischemic cerebrovascular disease. In *Controversies in Neuroanesthesia and Neurosurgery*, pp. 1–76. (Matjasko J., Katz J. eds.) Orlando: Grune and Stratton.

Guedel A.E. (1920). Signs of inhalation anesthesia. A fundamental guide. In *Inhalation Anesthesia*, pp. 10–52. (Guedel A.E. ed.) New York: Macmillan.

Guyton A.C. (1986). *Textbook of Medical Physiology*, 7th edn, p. 7 Philadelphia: W.B. Saunders, Co.

Himwich H.E., Frostig J.P., Fazekas J.F., et al. (1939). The mechanism of the symptoms of insulin hypoglycemia. *Am. J. Psychiatr.*, **96**, 371.

Hossmann K.A., Paschen W., Cuba L. (1983). Relationship between calcium accumulation and recovery of cat brain after prolonged cerebral ischemia. *J. Cerebr. Blood Flow Metab.*, **3**, 246.

Hughes J.R., Hendrix D.E., Cohen J., et al. (1976). Relationship of the magnetoencephalogram to the electroencephalogram. Normal wake and sleep activity. *Electroencephalogr. Clin. Neurophysiol.*, **40**, 261.

Ingvar D.H. (1967). The pathophysiology of occlusive cerebrovascular disorders. *Acta Neurol. Scand.*, **43**, Suppl. 31, 93.

Janeway R., Ravens R.J., Pearce L.A., et al. (1967). Progressive myoclonus epilepsy with lafora inclusion bodies. *Arch. Neurol.*, **16**, 565.

Jasper H.H. (1958). The ten twenty electrode system of the international federation. *Electroencephalogr. Clin. Neurophysiol.*, **10**, 371.

Jasper H., Droogleever-Fortuyn J. (1947). Experimental studies on the functional anatomy of petit mal epilepsy. *Res. Publ. Ass. Nerv. Ment. Dis.*, **26**, 272.

Kassel N.F., Hitchon P.W., Gerk M.K., et al. (1980). Alterations in cerebral blood flow, oxygen metabolism, and electrical activity produced by high dose sodium thiopental. *Neurosurgery*, **7**, 598.

Katz B. (1961). How cells communicate. *Sci. Am.*, **205**, 209.

Kaufman I.C., Walker A.E. (1949). The electroencephalogram after head injury. *J. Nerv. Ment. Dis.*, **109**, 383.

Kety S.S., King B.D., Horvath S.M., et al. (1950). The effects of an acute reduction in blood pressure by means of differential spinal sympathetic block on the cerebral circulation of hypotensive patients. *J. Clin. Invest.*, **29**, 402.

Kety S.S., Schmidt C.F. (1948). The effects of altered arterial tensions of carbon dioxide and oxygen on cerebral blood flow and cerebral oxygen consumption of normal young men. *J. Clin. Invest.*, **27**, 484.

Keykhah M.M., Smith D.S., Carlsson C., et al. (1985). Influence of sufentanil on cerebral metabolism and circulation in the rat. *Anesthesiology*, **63**, 274.

Kiloh L.G., McComas A.J., Osselton J.W., et al. (1981). *Clinical Electroencephalography*, 4th edn. London: Butterworths.

Kristiansen K., Courtois G. (1949). Rhythmic electrical activity from isolated cerebral cortex. *Electroencephalogr. Clin. Neurophysiol.*, **9**, 265.

Lassen N.A. (1959). Cerebral blood flow and oxygen consumption in man. *Physiol. Rev.*, **39**, 183.

Lavy S., Carmon A., Schwartz A. (1964). Depression of electrical cortical activity in acute cerebrovascular acidents. *Confinia Neurol.*, **24**, 349.

Lear J.D., Wasserman Z.R., DeGrado W.F. (1988). Synthetic amphiphilic peptide models for protein ion channels. *Science*, **240**, 1177.

Levy W.J. (1986). Power spectrum correlates of changes in consciousness during anesthetic induction with enflurane. *Anesthesiology*, **64**, 688.

Levy D.E., Brierly J.B., Silverman D.G., et al. (1975). Brain hypoxia initially damages cerebral neurons. *Arch. Neurol.*, **32**, 450.

Li C.L., Jasper H.H. (1953). Microelectrode studies of the electrical activity of the cerebral cortex in the cat. *J. Physiol.*, **121**, 117.

Meyer J.S., Gotoh F., Tazaki Y., et al. (1962). Regional cerebral blood flow and metabolism *in vivo*. Effects of anoxia, hypoglycemia, ischemia, acidosis, alkalosis and alterations of blood P_{CO_2}. *Arch. Neurol.*, **7**, 560.

Milde L.N., Milde J.H., Michenfelder J.D. (1985). Cerebral functional, metabolic, and hemodynamic effects of etomidate in dogs. *Anesthesiology*, **63**, 371.

Milito S.H., Raffin C.N., Rosenthal M., et al. (1988). Potassium ion homeostasis and mitochondrial redox activity in brain: relative changes as indicators of hypoxia. *J. Cerebr. Blood Flow Metab.*, **8**, 155.

Moorthy S.S., Reedy R.V., Paradise R.R., et al. (1980). Reduction of enflurane-induced spike activity by scopolamine. *Anesth. Analg.*, **59**, 417.

Morrice J.K.W. (1956). Slow wave production in the EEG with reference to hyperpnoea, carbon dioxide and autonomic balance. *Electroencephalogr. Clin. Neurophysiol.*, **8**, 49.

Morison R.S., Dempsey E.W. (1942). A study of thalamo-cortical relations. *Am. J. Physiol.*, **135**, 281.

Naritomi H., Sasaki M., Kanashiro M., et al. (1988). Flow thresholds for cerebral energy disturbance and Na^+ pump failure as studied by *in vivo* ^{31}P and ^{23}Na nuclear magnetic resonance spectroscopy. *J. Cerebr. Blood Flow Metab.*, **8**, 16.

Newberg L.A., Milde J.H., Michenfelder J.D. (1983). The cerebral metabolic effects of isoflurane at and above concentrations that suppress cortical electrical activity. *Anesthesiology*, **59**, 23.

Noell W., Schneider M. (1944). Uber die Durchblutung und die Sauerstoffversorgung des Gehrins. IV, Mitteilung. Die Rolleder Kohlensaure. *Pflugers Arch. Ges Physiol.*, **247**, 514.

Nunez P.L. (1986). The brain's magnetic field: some effects of multiple sources on localization methods. *Electroencephalogr. Clin. Neurophysiol.*, **63**, 75.

Oshima E., Shingu K., Mori K. (1981). E.E.G. activity during halothane anaesthesia in man. *Br. J. Anaesth.*, **53**, 65.

Penfield W., Jasper H. (1947). Highest level seizures. *Res. Pubs. Assoc. Nerv. Ment. Dis.*, **26**, 252.

Pichlmayr I., Lips U., Kunkel H. (1984). *The Electroencephalogram in Anesthesia. Fundamentals, Practical Applications, Examples.* New York: Springer-Verlag.

Planques J., Grezes-Rueff C., Bolinelli R., et al. (1965). Cerebral tolerance of chronic anoxia. *Electroencephalogr. Clin. Neurophysiol.*, **19**, 608.

Quasha A.L., Tinker J.H., Sharbrough F.W. (1981). Hypothermia plus thiopental: prolonged electroencephalographic suppression. *Anesthesiology*, **55**, 636.

Ralston B.L. (1958). Mechanisms of transition of interictal

spiking foci into ictal seizure discharges. *Electroencephalogr. Clin. Neurophysiol.*, **10**, 217.

Robertson J.D. (1962). The membrane of the living cell. *Sci. Am.*, **206**, 64.

Roger J., Naquet R., Gastaut H., et al. (1961). Electroencephalographic and electrocardiographic manifestations provoked by carotid compression in cerebral circulatory insufficiencies. In *Cerebral Anoxia and the Electroencephalogram*, (Gastaut H., Meyer J.S. ed.) Springfield: Thomas.

Rosner B.S., Clark D.L. (1973). Neurophysiologic effects of general anesthetics: II: sequential regional actions in the brain. *Anesthesiology*, **39**, 59.

Rossen R., Simonson E., Baker J. (1963). Electroencephalogram during hypercapnia. *Arch. Neurol.*, **8**, 373.

Schaertlin C.E. (1961). Polargraphische messung der sauerstoffspannung im hirnblut bei hypoxie. *Helv. Physiol. Pharmacol. Acta*, **19**, 255.

Schmahl F.W., Betz E., Dettinger E., et al. (1966). Energiestoffwechsel der Gross Hirnrinde und Electroencephalogram bei Sauerstoffmangel. *Pflugers Arch. Ges. Physiol.*, **292**, 46.

Schaul N., Green L., Peyster R., et al. (1986). Structural determinants of electroencephalographic findings in acute hemispheric lesions. *Ann. Neurol.*, **20**, 703.

Scott J.C., Ponganis K.V., Stanski D.R. (1985). EEG quantitation of narcotic effect: the comparative pharmacodynamics of fentanyl and alfentanil. *Anesthesiology*, **62**, 234.

Sebel P.S., Bovill J.G., Wauquier A., et al. (1981). Effects of high-dose fentanyl anesthesia on the electroencephalogram. *Anesthesiology*, **55**, 203.

Solomon S. (1966). Evaluation of carotid artery compression in cerebrovascular disease: an electroencephalographic clinical correlation. *Arch. Neuro.*, **14**, 165–70.

Spehlmann R. (1981). *EEG Primer.* New York: Elsevier/North Holland Biomedical Press.

Stockard J.J., Bickford R.G. (1981). The neurophysiology of unaesthesia. In *A Basis and Practice of Neuroanaesthesia.* pp. 3–49. (Gordon E. ed.) New York: Elsevier/North-Holland.

Stockard J.J., Bickford R.G., Smith N.T., et al. (1973). Structure-activity relationships of ether, fluroxene, isoflurane and enflurane. *Electroencephalogr. Clin. Neurophysiol.*, **34**, 713.

Symonds C. (1959). Excitation and inhibition in epilepsy. *Brain*, **82**, 133.

Titeca J. (1965). Contribution of EEG to the study of hemiplegias of vascular origin. *J. Belg. Med. Phsy. Rhum.*, **11**, 89.

Todd M.M., Drummond J.C., Sang H. (1984). The hemodynamic consequences of high-dose methohexital anesthesia in humans. *Anesthesiology*, **61**, 495.

Uematsu D., Greenberg J.H., Reivich M., et al. (1988). *In vivo* fluorometric measurement of changes in cytosolic free calcium from the cat cortex during anoxia. *J. Cerebr. Blood Flow Metab.*, **8**, 367.

Ulett G.A. (1955). Clinical and experimental studies of mild head injuries. *Electroencephalogr. Clin. Neurophysiol.*, **7**, 496.

Ward A.A. (1961). The epileptic neurone. *Epilepsia*, **2**, 70.

Walter W.G. (1936). The location of cerebral tumours by electroencephalography. *Lancet*, **2**, 305.

Weidner A. (1969). Energiestatus der Grosshirnrinde der Katze Wahrend Passiver Hyperventialtion. Inaugural Dissertation, Marburg.

Weinberg H., Brickett P., Coolsma F., et al. (1986). Magnetic localisation of intracranial dipoles: simulation with a physical model. *Electroencephalogr. Clin. neurophysiol.*, **64**, 159.

Williams D., Denny-Brown D. (1941). Cerebral electrical changes in experimental concussion. *Brain*, **64**, 223.

Wyke B.D. (1957). Electrographic monitoring of anaesthesia. I. neuropharmacological aspects. *Anaesthesia*, **12**, 157.

Wyke B.D. (1957). Electrographic monitoring of anaesthesia. II. clinical and experimental studies of cerebral function during barbiturate narcosis. *Anaesthesia*, **12**, 259.

Wyllie E., Luders H., Morris H.H., et al. (1986). Ipsilateral forced head and eye turning at the end of the generalized tonic-clonic phase of versive seizures. *Neurology*, **36**, 1212.

29. Pain: Theory and Management
K. Budd

Pain is an unpleasant sensory and emotional experience associated with actual or potential tissue damage, or described in terms of such damage. All pain perception depends upon the transmission of impulses through pathways within the nervous system from the site of the stimulus to the higher centres of the brain where they may impinge upon our consciousness and be interpreted. The principal parts of the nervous system involved in this process are:

- Receptors in the skin and other organs
- Peripheral nerves
- Neuronal aggregates in the spinal cord and associated fibre tracts
- The brainstem and thalamus
- The limbic system
- The cerebral cortex
- Other parts of the brain indirectly involved.

THEORIES OF PAIN
(Perl, 1980)

Intensive theory. This theory denies the existence of specialization in receptors and central neurons. The theory suggests that sense organs and their central connections are normally excited by non-noxious stimulation and participate in sensations other than pain, however, when overstimulated they yield an unusually strong response which is interpreted by the higher centres as pain.

Pattern concept. This is a derivative of the Intensive Theory and suggests that pain results not from activating specialized sense organs but from a particular combination of responses originating in individual, unspecialized sensory receptors or else from the composite activity reaching the central nervous system from a particular region. The 'Gate Control Theory' is a variation of the pattern concept.

Specificity theory. This postulates that some sense organs are specifically adapted (specialized) to detect and signal the advent of noxious stimulation. Consequently, activity in this system leads to the appreciation of the sensation of pain, whereas activity generated by those sense organs involved with non-noxious stimulation plays little or no role in the primary production of the painful sensation.

PAIN RECEPTORS AND PERIPHERAL CONDUCTION

The skin and subcutaneous tissues contain a variety of receptors of a varying degree of complexity. Pain perception is almost certainly mediated by the simple, free nerve endings. These are the terminations of the unmyelinated and finely myelinated afferent nerves having their cell bodies in the posterior (dorsal) root ganglia of the spinal cord. These nerve endings are present in the dermis and many of them penetrate into the epidermis. The concentration of nerve endings varies from one region of the skin to another and in certain parts of the body they are present in thousands per square centimetre.

In addition to pain, these nerve endings will subserve other sensory modalities and will exhibit marked differences in specificity of response. The thermoreceptors, responding only to heating or cooling, will, for example, differ among themselves in their patterns of response within relatively narrow ranges of temperature.

The nerve endings which respond to painful stimulation are known as nociceptors. (Fig. 29.1). Some

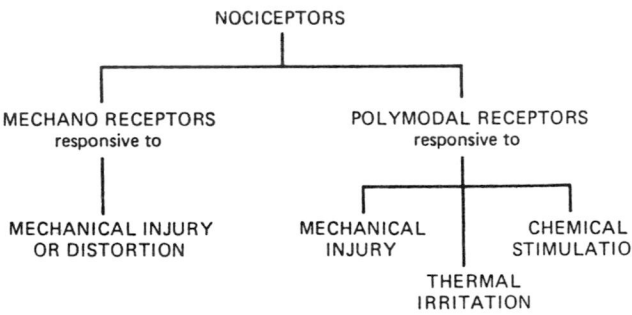

Fig. 29.1 Receptors.

nociceptors respond mainly to mechanical (e.g. crush) injury whereas others, polymodal nociceptors, are responsive to noxious heat and chemical irritation as well as mechanical injury. The chemical stimulation may be exogenous (e.g. acid burn) or from endogenous agents such as histamine, kinins and 5–hydroxytryptamine (serotonin) released into the tissue during processes such as inflammation, infection or following trauma. Prostaglandins, notably PGE_2, released or synthesized in response to this process will intensify the pain by sensitizing the tissues to the endogenous chemicals and may also stimulate nociceptors directly.

Receptors similar to those innervating the skin are found in muscle and the viscera. Their response differs however, and they will produce pain of a dull, vague nature following distension, stretch or traction and will not respond to burning, crush or incision. Central representation of somatic and visceral nociception may be different thus accounting for some of the paradoxical differences between these two types of pain.

It is important to realize that whilst most pain is generated by the stimulation of the nociceptors, so-called nocigenic pain, there are alternative modes of pain production. It may occur due to damage to a peripheral nerve or central nerve pathway—neurogenic pain, or by the conversion of a psychological or psychopathological experience into a physical symptom—somatization—engendering psychogenic pain. Damage to or changes within the sympathetic nervous system may also cause pain—sympathetically mediated or maintained pain.

Afferent Conduction

The nerve fibres of which the nociceptors are the terminal portion are relatively small in cross section and comprise finely myelinated Aδ fibres, 1–4 µm in diameter conducting at 5–45 m/s and the unmyelinated C fibres, diameter 0.25–1.5 µm conducting at 0.5–2.0 m/s. Other modalities of sensation are transmitted in the rapid, myelinated Aβ fibres of 5–15 µm diameter at 30–100 m/s.

Any noxious stimulus may produce multiple firings not only in the nociceptive fibres but also in others which are specific for other modalities of sensation. When a painful stimulus such as a pin prick, is applied to the skin, firing commences in both Aδ and C fibres in addition to the larger fibres transmitting non-painful modalities of sensation. The relatively rapid transmission within the Aδ fibres generates the characteristic sharp, immediate pain to be followed by the duller and more prolonged pain due to the slower transmission of impulses in the polymodal C fibres; hence the description of fast and slow pain.

Aδ generated pain is well localized whereas C fibre pain is poorly localized and the persistence of the latter fibres firing after the stimulus has been removed may be due, at least in part, to the release of histamine, kinins, prostaglandins and other biologically active substances and their presence in the tissues following injury.

The threshold for pain perception in man is relatively constant (approx. 44–45°C applied to the skin), contrary to popular belief, and is physiologically mediated whereas pain tolerance or response is very variable, psychologically mediated and affected and changed by many factors, e.g. age, personality, etc.

PATHWAYS IN THE SPINAL CORD

Virtually all the sensory input from the body or vis-cera enters the spinal cord through its dorsal roots although some 30% of the ventral root fibres are unmyelinated C nociceptive afferents having their cell bodies in the dorsal root ganglia (Fig. 29.2).

The cells of the dorsal horn are arranged in six laminae stratified in a dorsal-ventral direction, running the entire length of the cord (Figs. 29.2 and 29.3). This cytoarchitecture was first described by Rexed in 1952 who also delineated four other laminae in the intermediate and ventral horn parts of the cord.

Lamina I corresponds to the marginal zone and laminae II and III to the substantia gelatinosa and these receive the majority of the Aδ and C nociceptive fibre input.

Large Aβ low-threshold mechanoreceptor primary afferents enter in the medial portion of the dorsal root, medial to the dorsal horn and pass without synapse up the dorsal columns (Fig. 29.2). Aβ fibres from skin give off collaterals which enter the dorsal horn from the medial side and ramify in several laminae. The C fibres enter via both dorsal and ventral roots to ramify mainly in the substantia gelatinosa. Aδ nociceptor axons also enter through the lateral portion of the dorsal root and ramify in laminae I, II and V.

Each lamina may receive not only its own direct input but also that from neighbouring laminae. If the activity of these latter is high an additive process will develop influencing contiguous laminae or transmitting directly to adjacent cord levels or higher centres. Consequently, a lamina which receives a direct peripheral input is dominated by that input but is also influenced or modulated by the converging information coming from more dorsally or even ventrally placed laminae. Thus, lamina V receives small Aδ fibres activated by pinprick and hot and cold receptors, whilst the large cells of the marginal zone (Lamina I) receive only noxiously generated activity. The information from these two zones of spinal grey is transmitted through spinothalamic fibres to the same thalamic nucleus (ventroposterior) which receives dorsal column impulses relayed through the medial lemniscus. If, however, the periphery is stimulated more intensely activating both Aδ and C fibres, the neurones of lamina V will receive convergent excitation from the substantia gelatinosa in addition to direct excitation from Aδ peripheral afferents. This will bring about a degree of excitation sufficient to activate neurons in the deeper laminae VII and VIII resulting in cephalad transmission of information through spinoreticular axons which form the majority of fibres ascending in the anterolateral quadrant of the spinal cord (Bowsher, 1957).

GATE CONTROL THEORY

The term 'Gate Control' is now applied to the rapidly acting mechanisms which accept and control the passage of impulses from the afferent fibre input to cells which may then trigger the various effector systems

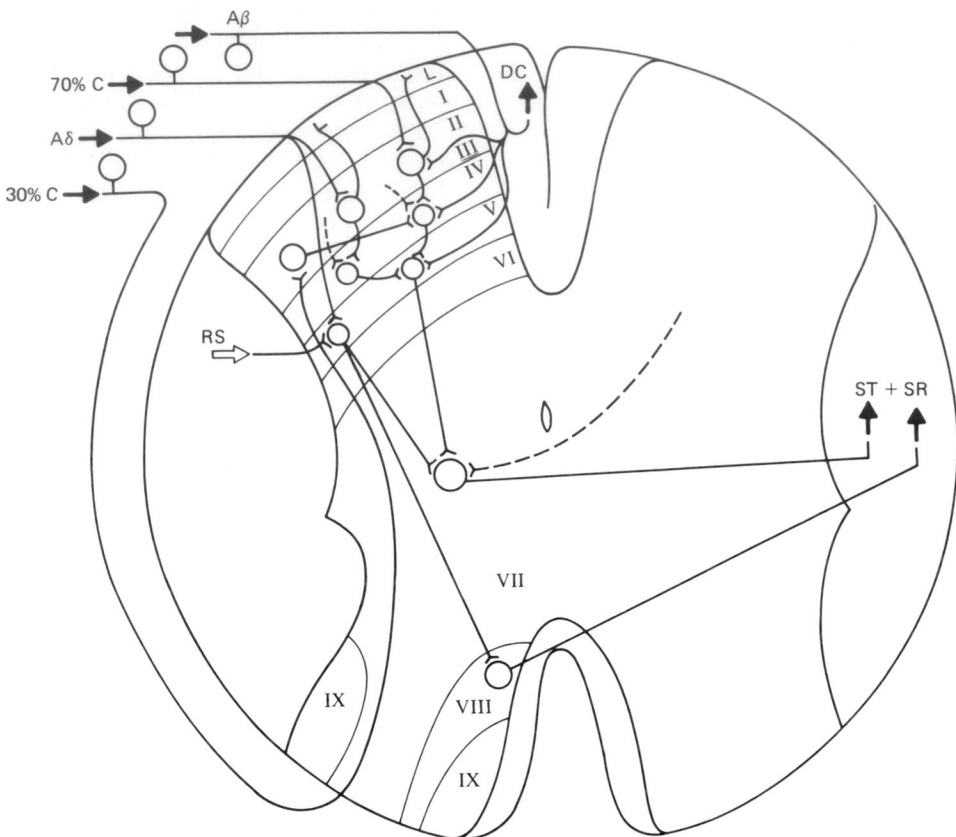

Fig. 29.2 Aβ, Aδ, and C fibre input to cord. Spinothalamic (ST), Spinoreticular (SR) and Dorsal Column (DC) output. Rexed laminae indicated by Roman numerals. Note: 30% afferent C fibres enter by ventral horn. Descending inhibitory reticulo-spinal connection (RS) to lamina V.

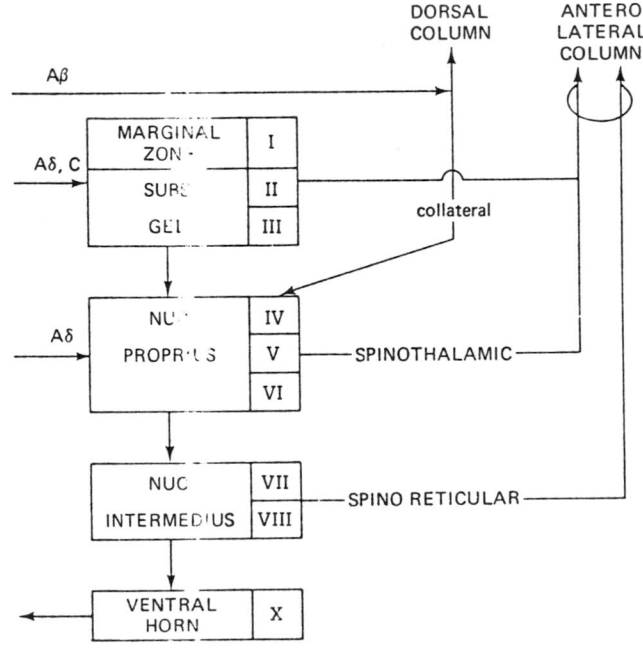

Fig. 29.3

and evoke sensation (Melzack and Wall, 1965; Wall, 1978).

It is possible that the distribution of afferent impulses in the spectrum of the peripheral nerve is monitored by the cells of the substantia gelatinosa which act like a gate. They determine whether or not sufficient activity is forwarded to fire the secondary neurones (Transmission or 'T' cells) in the pain pathway deeper in the dorsal horn (Wall, 1979).

Aβ fibres (Fig. 29.4) are activated by light touch, scratch, vibration and rubbing and have a lower threshold than do the Aδ and C fibres. Even allowing for this low threshold, they have a tendency to adapt to their environment and become dormant unless continuously stimulated. If this activity is maintained, the cells of the substantia gelatinosa will be positively stimulated which will, in turn, lead to inhibition of the effector or 'T' cells, thus blocking the onward progression of noxious impulses entering in the Aδ and C fibres.

If, however, an increase of peripheral stimulation by heavier pressure, pinprick, temperature above the painful threshold (45°C) and noxious stimuli occurs, activity will be increased in the Aδ and C fibres such

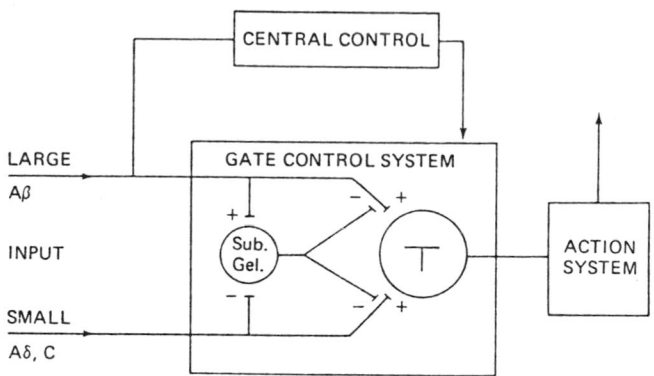

Fig. 29.4 Gate control theory—diagrammatic representation.

that their effect upon the substantia gelatinosa cells may be sufficient to overcome the inhibitory effects of the Aβ input and 'open the gate' allowing the level of activity in the 'T' cells to rise above their firing threshold and thus the noxious stimulus to be passed into the central nervous system, possibly to be appreciated as pain.

Consequently, there is continual interaction between these two afferent systems, facilitatory and inhibitory, and the onward progression of the noxious stimulus depends on which system predominates at any time. The gate control is, however, dominated by descending influences from the brain, collectively known as 'central control' which can override the delicate regulating mechanisms at spinal cord level. Melzack (1973) believes a central biasing mechanism exists in the brainstem reticular formation which exerts a tonic inhibitory influence on all levels of the somatic projection system.

The central control appears to have the facility to alter the setting of the 'gate' in the substantia gelatinosa and this would explain why voluntary or emotional behaviour can augment or supress pain. It must be emphasized, however, that cellular function in the cord is not rigid and unchanging; there is a marked degree of plasticity of function, especially under pathological conditions.

Following tissue or nerve damage, foreign substances, e.g. kinins, peptides, are absorbed by the unmyelinated C fibres which transport them centrally to the cord where they induce physiological changes in cellular circuitry to unmask normally ineffective synapses thereby altering the receptive areas controlled by the A fibres. Both pre and post-synaptic inhibitions decline in association with the receptive field changes (Woolf and Wall, 1982) Cells in laminae I and II show contrasting responses in that some will fire for a prolonged period after only a brief peripheral stimulus whilst others will habituate, slow repeated stimuli producing an initial response that rapidly fades with each repetition. This habituation is spatially specific in that if one part of the receptive field habituates, a movement of the stimulus to a new

place in the receptive field will immediately produce a response. The receptive fields also show amoeboid properties, moving to accommodate stimuli outside the normal territory. Also stimulation via the dorsolateral funiculus will cause the receptive field to expand. (Dubisson et al., 1979). Finally, if an area of the body is deprived of its nerve supply thus functionally deafferenting cells in the dorsal horn which previously responded to stimulation of this area, after a short period these cells begin to respond to stimuli applied to other areas with intact nerve supply. Some change has occurred by which non-innervated cells have expanded their receptive fields to incorporate innervated peripheral structures. (Devor and Wall, 1981).

Whilst the gate control theory does not provide a total explanation, it forms a basis for much theoretical and practical investigation. It makes allowance for the high degree of specialization of receptor fibre units, explains the interaction of two main afferent fibre systems and emphasizes the importance of central screening, selection of patterned information and descending control.

It has pointed the way for treatment of some forms of pain by methods which stimulate the large myelinated fibres, e.g. transcutaneous electrical neural stimulation (TENS), segmental acupuncture, and can offer an explanation for the hyperalgesia and lancinating pains of post herpetic neuralgia, thought to be due to a disproportionately large destruction by the virus of the Aβ fibres allowing Aδ and C fibres greater access to central pathways. Hence, minimal stimulation of the affected areas will give rise to intense pain of both Aδ (sharp) and C (dull) varieties.

Nevertheless, there are important reservations about the theory including the lack of conclusive evidence of patterned feedback in the dorsal horn, or of the precise identity of the 'T' cells. The theory does not account for an apparent discrepancy between the intensity and duration of stimulus and the sensation of pain evoked by it. This is particularly noticeable in some of the neuralgias where severe pain may follow a trivial stimulus in spite of there being no significant sensory modality deficit and an intact large fibre state. It is possible that this phenomenon is due to a mass synchronous discharge in the motor systems of the spinal cord spilling into sensory areas (Crue, 1975), or repetitive epileptiform activity by sensory neurones on the afferent side. This latter is underlined by the clinical benefit of treating neuralgias with anticonvulsant drugs.

SPINAL ASCENDING PATHWAYS

The spinal ascending pathways may be conveniently divided into two; oligosynaptic (few synapses) and multisynaptic.

Oligosynaptic System

This comprises two principal pathways in relation to

pain; the lateral spinothalamic tract and the extero-ceptive (as opposed to proprioceptive) fibres of the dorsal columns. Both are rapidly conducting and the dorsal column fibres in particular, because of their organized mapping, carry precise information about the localization of the painful stimulus. The classical spinothalamic tract is now known to be a composite tract comprising spinotectal, spinoreticular, spino-rubral and spinovestibular pathways. Consequently, few fibres in this tract reach the thalamus directly (Fig. 29.5).

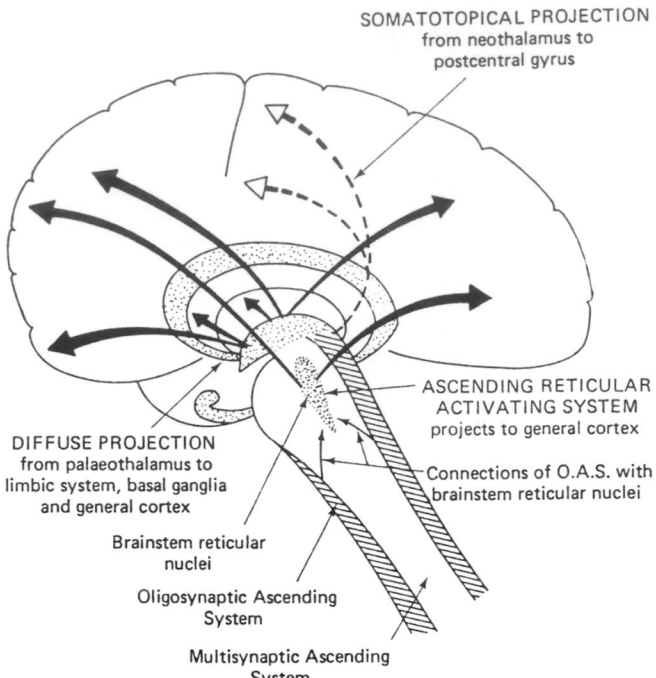

Fig. 29.6 The higher projections of the oligosynaptic and multisynaptic ascending systems.

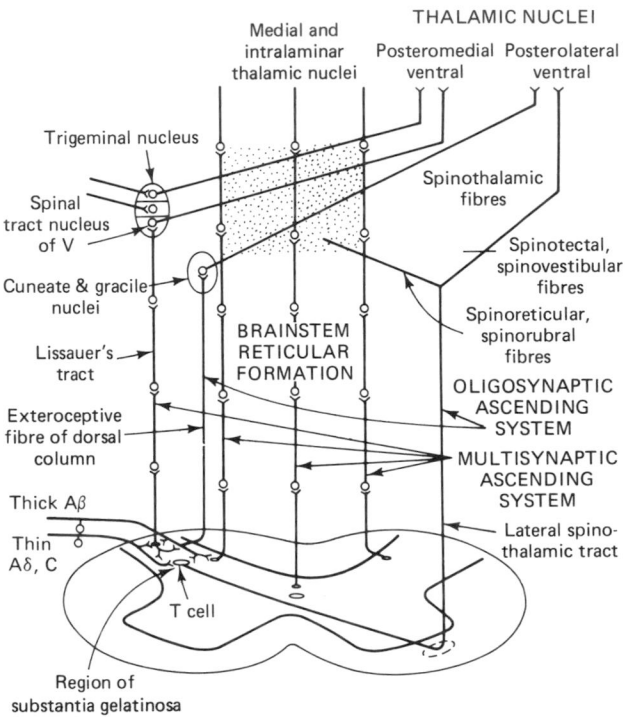

Fig. 29.5 Ascending pathways associated with the transmission of stimuli appreciated as pain.

Degeneration studies show that fibres in this tract end for the most part, in the recticular formation of the brainstem. Lesser numbers terminate in the corpora quadrigemina and periaqueductal grey matter of the midbrain and in two distinct thalamic cell groups, the ventrobasal complex and the intralaminar nuclei. Although the spinothalamic and spinoreticular are separate and independent systems they intermingle in the spinal cord. The former, after relay in the ventrobasal thalamus, is projected somatotopically to the first and second somatosensory areas in the postcentral gyrus and parietal operculum respectively (Figs. 29.6 and 29.7). Fibres of the spinoreticular tract, after relay in the reticular formation, are projected to the intralaminar thalamus, the hypothalamus and limbic system. The intralaminar thalamus projects diffusely to the whole non-primary cortex as well as to the corpus striatum in a point to point

fashion. Functionally, the spinothalamic tract carries a number of discriminative somatic sensations including pinprick but excluding true pain, whereas the spinoreticular is responsible for a spectrum of protopathic sensations ranging from itch to agony (Bowsher, 1979).

Multisynaptic System

This system consists of a spinal reticular core, known as the fasciculi proprii, together with Lissauer's tracts. The spinal reticular core is composed of long chains of neurones which extend upwards to the brain-stem reticular formation. The cell bodies and synapses in this chain lie within the boundaries of the grey matter and the axons span a number of segments in either direction. The origin of the neurons in the fasciculi proprii is from the margin of the whole central grey matter.

Lissauer's tracts carry the axons of the substantia gelatinosa cells on each side of the cord. These will travel to three segments in either direction before reentering their zone of origin to synapse with other nerve cells. In the medulla the substantia becomes continuous with the nucleus of the spinal tract of the trigeminal nerve which subserves pain arising in the face.

The fibres of the spinal reticular core reach the medial and intralaminar thalamic nuclei after relays in the brainstem reticular formation, whilst Lissauer's tract fibres eventually reach the posteromedial ventral nucleus of the thalamus. Both of these components of

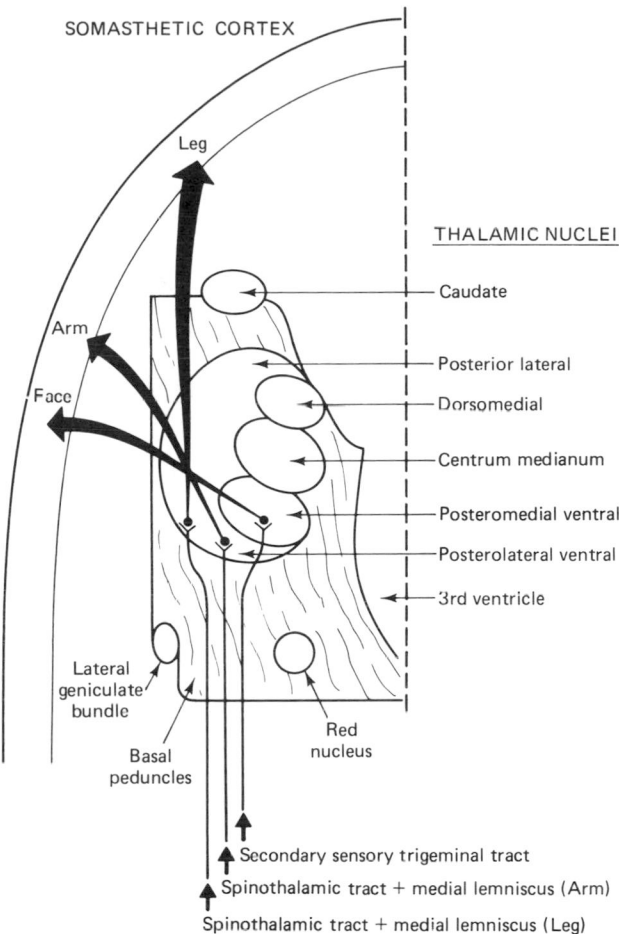

SOMASTHETIC CORTEX

THALAMIC NUCLEI

Caudate

Posterior lateral

Dorsomedial

Centrum medianum

Posteromedial ventral

Posterolateral ventral

3rd ventricle

Lateral geniculate bundle

Basal peduncles

Red nucleus

Leg

Arm

Face

Secondary sensory trigeminal tract

Spinothalamic tract + medial lemniscus (Arm)

Spinothalamic tract + medial lemniscus (Leg)

Fig. 29.7 Afferent pathways through the thalamus—coronal section.

DESCENDING CONTROL

It is now well established that ascending information in all sensory systems is modulated by centrifugal influences from the brain. In the somatosensory system, such downstream control is exerted via pathways descending in the white matter of the cord. Such descending controls originate in the cortex, diencephalon and brainstem, the last having great importance in the context of pain.

Inhibition of nociceptive messages in dorsal horn neurons has been reported to originate in the mesencephalic periaqueductal grey matter, in some of the raphe nuclei which contain serotonergic descending neurons, in the locus coeruleus (noradrenergic

neurons) and in part of the reticular formation (Fig. 29.8).

Both endogenous and exogenous opioids have been suggested to (1) activate the descending serotonergic inhibitory pathway via the same neuronal opioid receptors, possibly located in the periaqueductal grey and (2) directly inhibit spinal transmission by binding

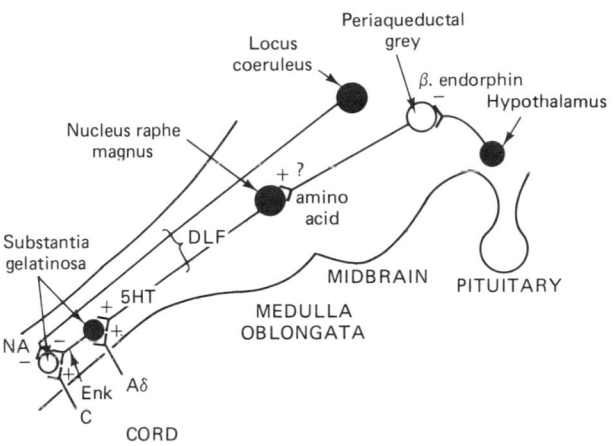

Periaqueductal grey

Locus coeruleus

β. endorphin

Hypothalamus

Nucleus raphe magnus

amino acid

Substantia gelatinosa

DLF

5HT

MIDBRAIN

MEDULLA OBLONGATA

PITUITARY

NA

Enk

Aδ

C

CORD

Fig. 29.8 Descending inhibitory pathways.
NA = noradrenaline; ENK = enkephalin
5HT = 5-hydroxytryptamine
DLF = dorsolateral funiculus
C = endorphin.

the multisynaptic system lack somatotopic organization and the passage of information to supraspinal levels is relatively slow. Whereas the oligosynaptic system is thought to localize the site of pain and warn of its presence, the multisynaptic system is thought to underline the diffuse persistent quality of the fully appreciated pain (Hannington-Kiff, 1974).

to opioid receptors in the dorsal horn (Zimmerman, 1979). In this latter situation, nociceptive information is transmitted by the primary afferent neuron to the first synapse and the information is conveyed to the next cell by the release of a neurotransmitter into the synapse. Occupation of the presynaptic opioid receptors with enkephalin released from the interneurone or by systemically administered opioid drugs will inhibit the release of the primary nociceptive transmitter (neurokinin A, neuropeptide K) (Fleetwood-Walker et al., 1988) and hence block the onward passage of the noxious signal (Fig. 29.9). The central action of opioids in the periaqueductal grey triggers descending mechanisms which result in the inhibition of neurotransmission in the dorsal horn in a similar manner.

In a parallel biochemical mode, certain secondary analgesic drugs, e.g. antidepressants, tranquillizers, anticonvulsants, are thought to exert their inherent analgesic effect by reducing the rate of presynaptic reuptake of neurotransmitter substances within the brain (Budd, 1978). The analgesic effects of brain stem electrical stimulation and the microinjection of opioids in this area have been said to be due to descending inhibition in the spinal cord being generated by these manoeuvres and also to inhibitory influences upon certain systems in the brainstem, e.g. the gigantocellular reticular formation, the forebrain and the limbic structures.

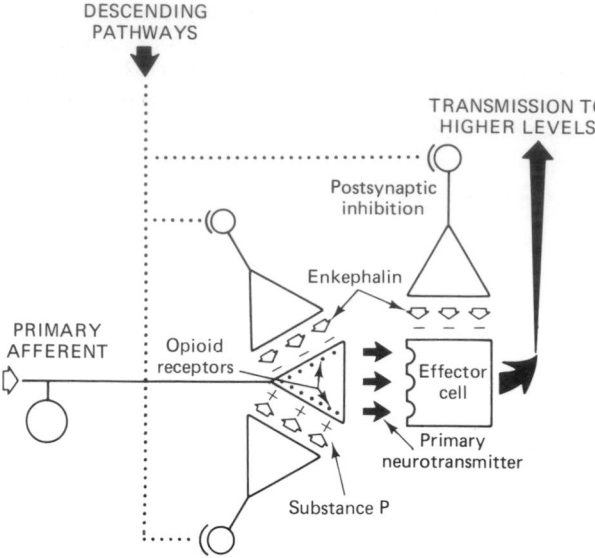

Fig. 29.9 Schematic representation of the first sensory synapse. Sites of modification of the afferent nociceptive impulse.

DESCENDING PATHWAYS

In the brain stem there exists a neural system which when activated results in the production of analgesia. The central component of this system is situated in the periaqueductal and periventricular structures of the brainstem, a fact which has been shown by the effectiveness of electrical stimulation and microinjections of morphine in producing profound analgesia. The periaqueductal grey receives an inhibitory β-endorphinergic projection from the cells in the infundibular region of the hypothalamus, which by inhibiting the inhibitory neurons within the periaqueductal grey activate other similarly placed neurons which project to the nucleus raphe magnus in the midline of the medullary reticular formation. The neurons in this nucleus are serotonergic and their axons descend in the dorsolateral funiculus of the cord to end in synaptic contact with enkephalinergic interneurons on the border between lamina I and the substantia gelatinosa in the spinal grey matter (*see* Fig. 29.8).

Other inhibitory noradrenergic neurons in the midbrain (locus coeruleus) and medulla project to the cord and directly inhibit nociceptive transmission neurones in the pain pathway. The evidence for a dopaminergic involvement in the descending systems is less well documented. Dopamine depletion or blockade of receptors, even in the case of analgesia produced by central electrical stimulation, results in only partial blockade of the analgesic effect indicating that a dopaminergic pathway is not the exclusive route descending to the cord.

Interactions with other monoaminergic transmitters must take place for complete depletion of these agents with drugs such as tetrabenazine or reserpine, results in an almost total blockade of the anal-gesia produced by morphine or central electrical stimulation. The output of the descending control system is further confused as the periaqueductal region receives diverse inputs from numerous brain areas and is involved in various emotional, motivational and sensory systems. Little is known of the specific organization of these external inputs and their ultimate effect upon descending influences.

THE TREATMENT OF PAIN

Pain is classically divided into two categories, acute pain and chronic pain.

Acute pain—acts as a warning to the organism that its integrity is threatened and avoiding action should be taken. It is relatively short lived and is frequently self-limiting or can be dealt with or treated by conventional methods. Examples are postoperative pain, renal and biliary colic, dental abscess, bony fractures, etc.

Chronic pain—has gone beyond the stage of being valuable to the organism and detracts from the quality of life to a greater or lesser extent. It may produce psychological changes in the sufferer, accentuate existing psychopathology and, in the case of chronic pain due to malignant disease, cause a foreshortening of life. In contrast to acute pain, chronic pain rarely limits its own duration, may be difficult to treat because of the multifactorial aetiology and therapy may encompass a large number of modalities both conventional and unconventional. Examples are trigeminal neuralgia, post herpetic neuralgia, back pain, the pain from malignant disease.

In the treatment of acute pain, analgesic drugs are most commonly used. In the majority of cases, agents of low analgesic efficacy given once or twice by mouth will be sufficient to control the pain. e.g. paracetamol, aspirin, codeine. For more severe or prolonged discomfort, regular doses of orally administered analgesics can be graded and titrated according to the patients response. In situations where pain is severe, high efficacy analgesics of the opioid variety may need to be administered by mouth or by alternative routes. These include intravenous injection, which has the advantage of rapid onset and the facility for accurate titration of dose to response, intramuscular injection, sublingual, epidural and intrathecal injection, and the use of infusions or intermittent administration by pump intravenously or by catheter placed in the epidural or intrathecal space. Commonly used analgesics include morphine, diacetylmorphine (heroin), papaveretum, pethidine, buprenorphine and phenazocine.

In the immediate postoperative period and during parturition, the use of inhalational analgesics may be of value. Nitrous oxide in a 50% mixture with oxygen (Entonox) may be administered intermittently for specific pain producing manoeuvres e.g. physiotherapy, dressings, removal of stitches, or at the beginning of each labour pain. Other inhalational agents have been used such as trichlorethylene and methoxyflurane but because of their smell and other side effects have fallen out of favour.

The use of regional local anaesthetic techniques is well described to prevent noxious impulses reaching the spinal cord. These may be single injections or continuous infusions and more recently opioid analgesics have been used epidurally or intrathecally for post-operative pain relief. Noninvasive techniques such as transcutaneous electrical neural stimulation (TENS) have a place in postoperative and labour pain control. By means of low frequency pulses of electricity the large nerve fibres can be stimulated to increase their input into the dorsal horn and there, theoretically at least, 'close the gate.' By even less well understood modes of action, analgesia can be achieved in numerous situations by such diverse techniques as acupuncture, hypnosis, biofeedback, massage, manipulation, heat and cold.

The treatment of chronic pain is a much more difficult problem not only because of the often multifactorial aetiology of the condition, the variation of the presenting symptom complex sometimes hourly, the degrees of psychological involvement but also because of the personal variation in response to therapy of whatever kind, and the possibility of a hidden secondary gain influencing the outcome in either the short or long-term. In general, the treatment of chronic pain can be divided into three main categories:

1. Drug therapy
2. Physical therapy—destructive or stimulatory
3. Miscellaneous.

Drug Therapy

Primary analgesics
  Opioids
    e.g. morphine, diamorphine, phenazocine, buprenorphine, levorphanol, codeine.
  Non-steroidal anti-inflammatory agents
    e.g. aspirin, naproxen, piroxicam, ibuprofen, paracetamol.
  Others
    e.g. nefopam, benzydamine, nitrous oxide.
Secondary analgesics
  Psychoactive drugs
    e.g. Antidepressants
          Anxiolytics
          Anticonvulsants
          Steroids
          Muscle relaxants
          Some cytotoxic agents
          Catecholamine blocking agents
          Metabolic blockers
          Calcium antagonists
          Opioid antagonists.
Drugs given over variable periods of time are usually prescribed to be administered by mouth (orally, sub-lingually, buccally). They may also be used rectally, transcutaneously, by the use of depot preparations or intravenously, epidurally or intrathecally via an external or internalized pump.

Physical Therapy

Destructive methods
  Nerve cutting by surgery,
  Radio frequency lesion,
  Neurolytic chemicals
    e.g. phenol, alcohol,
  Tractotomy, thalamotomy, rhizotomy, cordotomy by surgery, or laser
  Radiotherapy
  Cryolesions
  Thermal lesions of ganglia, tracts, thalamus

Stimulatory methods
  Heat, cold, massage, manipulation
  Transcutaneous electrical neural stimulation
  Percussion, vibration
  Dorsal column electrical stimulation
  Deep brain electrical stimulation
  Acupuncture, acupressure.

Miscellaneous

  Psychotherapy
  Biofeedback
  Operant conditioning
  Hypnosis
  Group behavioural therapy
  Occupational therapy.

All of the above methods may be used alone or in combination. For a more detailed and complete description, the relevant textbooks should be consulted.

FUTURE DEVELOPMENTS

The future of the therapy of pain presents an interesting challenge. There will be the refining of techniques in current use and certain developments of these but the major advances are most likely to come in the area of therapeutics and the application of drugs.
The main avenues of change will be:

1. The modulation of activity of the endogenous opioid agents and their systems.
2. Pharmacological modification of transmission of impulses within the central nervous system by affecting the secretion, reuptake and metabolism of neurotransmitter substances or the mimicking of their actions with synthetic agents.
3. Development of opioid agents acting at all the opioid receptors with the teasing out of the molecular configuration which after binding with the appropriate receptor produces analgesia alone with no other effects.

REFERENCES

Bowsher D. (1957). Termination of the central pathway in man: the conscious appreciation of pain. *Brain*, **80**, 606.

Bowsher D. (1976). Role of the reticular formation in response to noxious stimulation. *Pain*, **2**, 361.

Bowsher D. (1979). *What has the Spinothalamic Tract to do with Pain?* Paper read to the Intractable Pain Society of Great Britain and Ireland.

Budd K. (1978). Psychtropic drugs in the treatment of chronic pain. *Anaesthesia*, **33**, 531.

Crue B.J. (1975). *Pain Research and Treatment.* p. 62, New York: Academic Press.

Devor M., Wall P.D. (1981). Plasticity in the spinal cord sensory map following peripheral nerve injury in rats. *Brain Res.*, **1**, 679.

Dubisson D., Fitzgerald M., Wall P.D. (1979). Ameboid receptive fields of cells in laminae 1, 2 and 3. *Brain Res.*, **177**, 376.

Fleetwood-Walker G.M., Hope P.J., Mitchell R., et al. (1988). Effects of agonists selective for NK-1, NK-2 and NK-3 receptors on somatosensory transmission in superficial dorsal horn. *Regul. Peptides*, **22**, 67.

Hannington-Kiff J.G. (1974). *Pain relief.* p. 10. Oxford: Heinemann Medical Books.

Melzack R. (1973). *The Puzzle of Pain.* p. 166. London: Penguin Books Ltd.

Melzack R., Wall P.D. (1965). Pain mechanisms: a new theory. *Science*, **150**, 971.

Perl E.R. (1980). Afferent basis of nociception and pain. p. 19. In *Pain* (ed. Bonica J.J.) New York: Raven Press.

Wall P.D. (1978). The gate control theory of pain mechanism. A re-examination and restatement. *Brain*, **101**, 1.

Wall P.D. (1979). The role of the substantia gelatinosa as a gate control. In *Pain.* (ed. Bonica J.J.) New York: Raven Press.

Woolf C.J., Wall P.D. (1982). Chronic peripheral nerve section diminishes the primary afferent A-fibre mediated inhibition of rat dorsal horn neurones. *Brain Res.*, **242**, 77.

Zimmerman M. (1979). Peripheral and central nervous mechanisms of nociception, pain and pain therapy. In *Advances in Pain Researches and Therapy.* (ed. Bonica J.J.) New York: Raven Press.

30. The Endocrine and Metabolic Responses to the Stresses of Anesthesia and Surgery

B. Chernow and T. Higgins

Causes of perioperative stress
    The stress response—endocrine and
        metabolic manifestations
Stress responses to anesthesia
    Responses to specific anesthetic agents
    Responses to regional anesthesia
Future horizons

Hormones mediate much of the body's homeostatic response to stress. The circulating concentrations of the so-called 'fight or flight' hormones norepinephrine (noradrenaline), epinephrine (adrenaline), cortisol and growth hormone increase in response to most acute stresses. The plasma levels and activities of these and other hormones and minerals vary following different stressful situations. Although the stressors have existed for centuries, the availability of sensitive and specific hormonal assays are relatively new (within the last three decades). For this reason, the endogenous 'stress responses' continue to be defined. Newer anes-thetic-analgesic approaches have permitted a reduction in the perioperative stress experienced by patients.

Evidence is accumulating (Anand et al., 1987; Yeager et al., 1987) to support the concept that modulation of the stress response may improve outcome from surgery. In this chapter, the term 'stress response' is used to mean all stress-induced changes in circulating hormone and mineral concentrations during the perioperative period. This chapter details the causes of perioperative stress, the stress-induced hormonal and metabolic changes and methods used to reduce the stress response. Emphasis is placed upon the effects of anesthetics and analgesics on these responses.

CAUSES OF PERIOPERATIVE STRESS

Perioperative anxiety, induction of anesthesia, endotracheal intubation, vascular cannulation, surgically-induced tissue trauma, visceral pain, and the process of recovery from surgery are each stressful and contribute to the responses discussed below. In addition to these expected perioperative events, unwanted complications (such as sepsis, hemorrhage, hypothermia, pneumonia, pneumothorax, etc.) may also alter the measurable stress responses.

The level or degree of each stressful component is probably central to the amount of observed hormonal or metabolic change. Higher grades of surgical stress are reflected perioperatively by increased circulating concentrations of stress hormones (Chernow et al., 1987a). Patients undergoing 'minor' surgery (such as inguinal hernia repair or laparoscopy) have no measurable perioperative increases in plasma norepinephrine, epinephrine, cortisol, thromboxane, serum thyroxine, tri-iodothyroxine or angiotensin converting enzyme values in comparison with perioperative concentrations (Chernow et al., 1987a). On the other hand, moderate surgical stress (e.g. cholecystectomy) causes transient (observed at 1 hour but not 24 hours postoperative) surgery-related increases in plasma cortisol, epinephrine and norepinephrine values, compared to preoperative values. Major surgical stress (for example, colectomy) causes higher and more prolonged increases in these variables (Chernow et al., 1987a).

With the use of preoperative sedation (diazepam), general anesthesia (sodium pentothal, isoflurane, nitrous oxide, oxygen) and neuromuscular blockade (pancuronium bromide), patients undergoing neck explorations (for thyroid or parathyroid disorders) have no intraoperative increases (compared to preoperative) in plasma cortisol, adrenocorticotrophin (ACTH) or epinephrine concentrations (Udelsman et al., 1987). However, intermittent increases in plasma norepinephrine concentrations as well as consistent increases in plasma renin activity are seen (Udelsman et al., 1987). These patients show large increases in cortisol, ACTH and epinephrine during and following reversal of neuromuscular blockade and during extubation. Thus, the period of recovery from surgical stress may be as important as, if not more important than, the time of surgery itself.

The provision of local anesthesia, with or without epinephrine, provokes a minimal stress response. In a double-blind, randomized trial in humans, local dental anesthesia (inferior alveolar nerve block using lidocaine) with or without epinephrine caused no clinically important increases in heart rate, blood pressure or plasma norepinephrine concentrations (Chernow et al., 1983). In that study, the effect of anesthesia *per se* was investigated without the confounding variable of surgery. Although epinephrine-containing local anesthetics do raise plasma epinephrine concentrations (Chernow et al., 1983; Barber et al., 1985; Cioffi et al., 1985), the plasma epinephrine threshold beyond which hemodynamic actions are manifest, is not achieved. Local anesthesia prior to minor surgery (Cioffi et al., 1985) and the addition of preoperative sedation (Goldstein et al., 1982), limit the stress response to such procedures.

In addition to the stresses listed above, many medications, including anesthetics (*see below*), alter the stress response. Obviously, surgical trauma to endocrine organs directly affects endocrine function (Maruyama et al., 1987). It is impossible to list all of the potential stressors which trigger the perioperative stress response; however, those described here seem to be the predominant offenders.

The Stress Response—Endocrine and Metabolic Manifestations

The circulating concentrations of the 'traditional'

stress hormones (norepinephrine, epinephrine, cortisol, growth hormones and glucagon) increase after moderate and major surgery (Chernow et al., 1987a; Hakanson et al., 1984; Chernow et al., 1985), but not after minor surgery (Chernow et al., 1987a). As a consequence of these surgery-induced hormonal changes, hyperglycemia, postoperative increases in free fatty acids and variations in plasma insulin values are commonly observed after moderate and major surgery. Antidiuretic hormone, ACTH, cortisol, renin and angiotensin concentrations increase in the circulation following major surgical procedures such as open-heart surgery (El-Etr et al., 1981). Serum prolactin concentrations increase, while progesterone levels decrease in women following surgical stress (Soules et al., 1980). In men, serum testosterone levels decrease, while luteinizing hormone (LH) concentrations increase after surgery (Aono et al., 1976).

Whether stress-induced changes are appropriate, pathologic, or adaptive is unclear. For example, the illness-induced alterations in thyroid function may be adaptive (the likely answer) or perhaps they reflect a type of tissue hypothyroidism (Smallridge et al., 1985). Other changes, such as hemorrhagic-induced, and positive-end-expiratory pressure (PEEP) induced increases in plasma catecholamine concentrations (Chernow et al., 1984, 1986) are adaptive and occur in order to compensate for reductions in cardiac output due to hemorrhage and PEEP, respectively.

Stress-induced metabolic alterations are as common as hormonal changes. Energy expenditure and the metabolic cost of breathing may be markedly altered in postoperative patients (Savino et al., 1985). Illness-induced increases in free fatty acids contribute to the ionized hypocalcemia (Zaloga et al., 1987) that is seen in many critically ill postoperative patients. This part of the stress response is detrimental since physiologic response to endogenous vasoactive substances and exogenous medications are commonly Ca-dependent in their action. Expected responses will be blunted in the setting of hypocalcemia (Chernow et al., 1987b).

The degree of the endocrine and metabolic stress responses and the physiologic manifestations of these responses may be age-dependent. For example, Bullington et al. (1987) showed that although the elderly have a more marked plasma catecholamine response to endotracheal intubation, they have less of an intubation-related increase in heart rate than younger persons. Arnetz (1985) found an inverse relationship between age and surgery-induced increases in serum prolactin levels. The stress responses are clearly evident in the very young (Anand et al., 1987; Chernow et al., 1982b; Rehulka and Kraus, 1986) and probably decrease with age (Bullington et al., 1987; Arnetz, 1985).

STRESS RESPONSES TO ANESTHESIA

The metabolic and hormonal responses to surgery are

minimized when afferent neuronal transmission is blocked with extradural anesthesia (Engquist et al., 1977) or splanchnic nerve blockage (Shirasaka et al., 1986). Opiate anesthesia also reduces the stress response when opiates are administered in dosages high enough to provide central inhibition of hormonal secretion (George et al., 1974). All other anesthetic techniques have the potential to modify the stress response to trauma; however, some anesthetics may provoke hormonal secretion even in the absence of surgical stimulation.

The intravenous and inhaled anesthetics have a relatively minor influence on stress-hormone secretion compared to the effect of surgery itself (Oyama, 1980; Tarhan et el., 1971). Perhaps more important than the anesthetic agents administered is the mode of ventilation, since continuous positive pressure ventilation (CPPV) results in an increased antidiuretic hormone (ADH) response and a decrease in free-water clearance compared to intermittent positive pressure ventilation, or spontaneous ventilation with or without continuous positive airway pressure (Hemmer et al., 1980). Positive-end-expiratory pressure (PEEP) increases plasma renin, aldosterone and antidiuretic hormone (Annat et al., 1983). In experimental animals, graded levels of PEEP result in progressive increases in plasma norepinephrine levels, which correlate inversely with changes in cardiac output, and are rapidly reversible (Chernow et al., 1986). These PEEP-induced increases in sympathetic activity may have additional end-organ effects; however, more study is needed in this area.

Responses to Specific Anesthetic Agents

Sodium thiopentone (Pentothal) and methohexitone (Brevital) are ultra-short acting barbiturates used as anesthetic induction agents. Barbiturates nonspecifically depress the central nervous, cardiovascular, respiratory and renal systems. In subanesthetic doses, these drugs may actually cause an increased sensitivity to somatic pain. It is presumed that such a paradoxical response would be accompanied by an increase in circulating stress hormone concentrations.

Benzodiazepines, particularly midazolam, diazepam and lorazepam, are useful premedicants and induction agents, and appear to decrease the stress response in man (Goldstein et al., 1982).

Etomidate, an intravenous non-narcotic anesthetic, has caused concern amid reports of increased mortality in intensive care patients receiving this agent (Ledingham and Watt, 1983). Experimental data suggest etomidate inhibits cortisol secretion in response to stress via inhibition of 11 B-hydroxylase and cholesterol cleavage enzymes (Prezioai, 1983). In healthy human females, the use of etomidate results in the inhibition of cortisol secretion for 24 h without altering the blood glucose, lactate or plasma free fatty acid concentrations (Lacoumenta et al., 1986b). Propofol,

a newer intravenous anesthetic, does not prevent adrenocortical secretions of cortisol and aldosterone in response to surgical stress or ACTH stimulation at a single dose of 2.5 mg/kg (Fragen et al., 1988). Information is not yet available on endocrine responses to continuous propofol infusion.

Ketamine is a dissociative anesthetic frequently employed in pediatric anesthesia, and in patients in shock presenting for emergency surgery. In contrast to the other intravenous anesthetic agents, it causes increases in cerebral blood flow and oxygen consumption, cardiovascular stimulation via the central sympathetic nervous system, and increases in plasma epinephrine and, to a lesser degree, norepinephrine levels (Zsigmond and Domino, 1980; Chernow et al., 1982a).

Nitrous oxide produces sympathetic stimulation, increased plasma catecholamine and corticosteroid levels when given alone, or in combination with other inhaled agents (Winter et al., 1972; Smith et al., 1970).

Inhalational anesthetics, such as halothane, enflurane and isoflurane, tend to blunt the surgically-induced increases in plasma norepinephrine (Roizen and Horrigan, 1979b). Changes in blood glucose and lactate, and plasma cortisol, insulin and catecholamine levels are similar when halothane is used at either 1.2 or 2.1 MAC (Lacoumenta et al., 1986a). Halothane anesthesia during seven hours without surgery does not affect the plasma cortisol concentration or urinary catecholamine excretion (Von Werder et al., 1970). Halothane anesthesia alone induces marked prolactin release, with only minor further elevation seen with the onset of surgery (Malatinsky et al., 1986). Ether and cyclopropane, which are seldom used in the United States, both exert a stimulatory effect on the sympathetic nervous system and on the adrenal cortex (Kehlet, 1982).

Succinylcholine is a depolarizing muscle relaxant commonly administered prior to endotracheal intubation. It is hydrolyzed by the liver and by plasma pseudocholinesterase, and subsequently is metabolized to succinic acid and choline. Its duration of action may be prolonged in the presence of insufficient or atypical pseudocholinesterase. Lower pseudocholinesterase activity has been described with liver disease, pregnancy and drug therapy. Succinylcholine causes the release of potassium from skeletal muscle, and in certain conditions (burns, trauma, prolonged immobilization, peripheral paralysis, long-standing intra-abdominal infection) the rise may be sufficient to cause hyperkalemic cardiac arrest. This metabolic side effect is, therefore, a drug-induced problem and is *not* a consequence of the stress response.

The non-depolarizing neuromuscular blocking agents (d-tubocurarine, pancuronium, metocurine, gallamine, vecuronium and atracurium) are thought to combine with the acetylcholine receptor without activation. The pharmacokinetics and pharmacodynamics of these agents differ, particularly with regard to the mode of elimination and duration of action. These characteristics are well-reviewed elsewhere (Miller and Savarese, 1986). Pancuronium and gallamine both cause tachycardia, which has been attributed to a vagolytic effect, but may in fact be a sympathomimetic effect (Domenech, 1976). Plasma norepinephrine levels decrease following pancuronium administration (Roizen et al., 1979a). Enhanced neuromuscular blockade occurs with magnesium sulfate therapy, an effect that is only partly antagonized by calcium (Ghoneium and Long, 1970).

The administration of high dose narcotics has been studied extensively as to its efficacy in providing 'stress-free' anesthesia for open-heart surgery. In contrast to potent inhalational or balanced nitrous oxide-narcotic-relaxant anesthesia, intravenously administered morphine (2–4 mg/kg) or fentanyl (50–200 µg/kg) blunt or eliminate the initial endocrine-metabolic responses to open-heart surgery, as evidenced by urinary catecholamines (Stanley et al., 1975), plasma glucocorticoids, antidiuretic hormone (Lacoumenta et al., 1986a), aldosterone, renin, glucose and lactate levels (Kehlet, 1982). High-dose narcotic anesthesia for abdominal surgery has similar initial effects (Haxholdt et al., 1981). However, the inhibitory effect of high-dose narcotics on the stress response appears to be transient and effective only while high concentrations are maintained in the blood and tissues (Dubois et al., 1982), and this inhibition does not carry over into the postoperative period (Brandt et al., 1978; Walsh et al., 1981).

Responses to Regional Anesthesia

Regional anesthesia is most practical for patients undergoing lower abdominal, pelvic and lower extremity operations, and the studies of this technique pertain primarily to operative procedures in these sites. Spinal or epidural anesthesia alone produces minor and inconsistent changes in plasma cortisol, free fatty acids, glucose, lactate, prolactin, growth hormone, FSH and LH levels (Kehlet, 1982). Low spinal anesthesia has no effect on plasma norepinephrine, epinephrine, or mean arterial pressure, while thoracic dermatome spinal anesthesia (high enough to cause a fall in mean arterial pressure) causes suppression of arterial plasma norepinephrine and epinephrine levels (Pflug and Halter, 1981).

When looking at the hormonal responses to surgical stress, either low or high spinal anesthesia effectively blocks the surgery-induced increases in plasma norepinephrine, epinephrine, growth hormone and cortisol concentrations observed under conventional inhalational anesthesia (Pflug et al., 1981). Epidural anesthesia (to T4–T6 dermatome) combined with general anesthesia abolishes the rise in plasma cyclic AMP and reduces the stress-induced increases in plasma glucose and cortisol levels compared to general anesthesia alone (Madsen et al., 1977). Regional anesthesia blocks the surgically-induced in-

creases in plasma prolactin, ACTH, glucose and growth hormone and further decreases the minor diminution in FSH and LH seen in female patients (Kehlet, 1982). If blood pressure changes do not occur, regional anesthesia also blocks the operative-associated changes in aldosterone and renin (Kehlet, 1982). These studies support the intuitive logic that preventing transmission of afferent nerve impulses from the surgical site to the central nervous system is a more efficient method of blocking the stress response than central obtundation by conventional general anesthesia.

Data obtained from the administration of epidural opioids supports the concept that it is sympathetic blockade, rather than simply pain relief, that mitigates the stress response to the surgical procedure. While epidural administration of either bupivacaine or morphine produces pain relief and blunting of the cortisol response, plasma epinephrine and norepinephrine concentrations are unchanged after the local anesthetic. The administration of epidural opioids, however, blunts the rise in plasma norepinephrine compared to a control group. While epidural opioids are less effective than epidural local anesthetics in blunting the immediate stress response to surgery, it has been concluded that postoperative pain is an important factor in the hormonal response to surgery since extradural opioids have been found to suppress the endocrine response in the late postoperative period. (Rutberg et al., 1984). In contrast, others have concluded that the relief of pain *per se* does not have a major influence on the catabolic response to abdominal surgery as determined by urinary excretion of cortisol, catecholamines and nitrogen (Hjortso et al., 1985). Intravenous bupivacaine, in concentrations comparable to those observed during regional anesthesia, has a positive chronotropic and arterial vasoconstrictive effect, with only quantitatively minor changes observed in plasma epinephrine levels, and little effect on norepinephrine levels, blood glucose, plasma cortisol, or free fatty acids (Hasselstrom et al., 1984).

FUTURE HORIZONS

The most important concerns of investigators in this area are threefold: first, to extend our knowledge about what variables are altered in the stress response to surgery; second, to learn how best to modulate these responses; and third, to define the value or harm resulting from modulation of the stress response. It remains unclear which hormone best defines the stress response, serves as a predictor of clinically important and—organ responses such as wound healing, infection, immunology and cellular function (Tonnesen et al., 1984; Hole and Unsgaard, 1983). Preliminary studies support the concept that reduction in stress as marked by urinary cortisol excretion, is associated with improved outcome in high risk patients (Yeager et al., 1987). Efforts should continue to link outcome with modification of the stress response.

REFERENCES

Anand K.J.S., Sippell W.G., Aynsley-Green A. (1987). Randomized trial of fentanyl anesthesia in preterm babies undergoing surgery: effects on the stress response. *Lancet*, 1, 243.

Annat G., Viale J.P., Bui Xuan B., et al. (1983). Effect of PEEP ventilation on renal function, plasma renin, aldosterone, neurophysins and urinary ADH, and prostaglandins. *Anesthesiology*, 58, 136.

Aono T., Kurachi K., Miyata M., et al. (1976). Influence of surgical stress under general anesthesia on serum gonadotropin levels in male and female patients. *J. Clin. Endocrinol. Metab.*, 42, 144.

Arnetz B.B. (1985). Endocrine reactions during standardized surgical stress—the effects of age and methods of anesthesia. *Age and Ageing*, 14, 96.

Barber W.B., Smith L.E., Zaloga G.P., et al. (1985). Hemodynamic and plasma catecholamine responses to epinephrine-containing perianal lidocaine anesthesia. *Anesth. Analg.*, 64, 924.

Brandt M.R., Korshin J., Prange Hansen A., et al. (1978). Influence of morphine anesthesia on the endocrine-metabolic response to open heart surgery. *Acta Anaesthesiol. Scand.*, 22, 400.

Bullington J., Rigby J., Pinkerton M., et al. (1987). The effects of age on the adrenergic response to endotracheal intubation. *Anesth. Analg.*, 66, S23.

Chernow B., Lake C.R., Coyle J., et al. (1982a). The effect of ketamine on catecholamine levels in plasma, urine and CSF. *Crit. Care Med.*, 10, 600.

Chernow B., Rainey T.G., Heller R., et al. (1982b). Marked stress hyperglycemia in a child. *Crit. Care. Med.*, 10, 696.

Chernow B., Balestrieri F., Ferguson C.D., et al. (1983). Local dental anesthesia with epinephrine—minimal effects on the sympathetic nervous system or on hemodynamic variables. *Arch. Intern. Med.*, 143, 2141.

Chernow B., Lake C.R., Barton M., et al. (1984). Sympathetic nervous system sensitivity to hemorrhagic hypotension in the subhuman primate. *J. Trauma*, 24, 229.

Chernow B., Anderson D.M. (1985). Endocrine responses to critical illness. *Semin. Resp. Med.*, 71, 1.

Chernow B., Soldano S., Cook D., et al. (1986). Positive end-expiratory pressure increases plasma catecholamine levels in non-volume loaded dogs. *Anaesth. Intens. Care*, 14, 421.

Chernow B., Alexander H.R., Smallridge R.C., et al. (1987a). Hormonal responses to graded surgical stress. *Arch. Intern. Med.*, 147, 1273.

Chernow B., Zaloga G.P., Malcolm D., et al. (1987b). Glucagon's chronotropic action is calcium dependent. *J. Pharmacol. Exper. Ther.*, 241, 833.

Cioffi G.A., Chernow B., Glahn R.P., et al. (1985). The hemodynamic and plasma catecholamine responses to routine restorative dental care. *JAMA*, 111, 67.

Domenech J.S., Garcia R.C., Sasiain J.M.R., et al. (1976). Pancuronium bromide: an indirect sympathomimetic agent. *Br. J. Anaesth.*, 48, 1143.

Dubois M., Pickar D., Cohen M.,et al. (1982). Effects of fentanyl on the response of plasma beta-endorphin immunoreactivity to surgery. *Anesthesiology*, 57, 468.

El-Etr A.A., Glisson S.N., Balasarawathi K. (1981). Endocrine changes during anesthesia and cardiopulmonary bypass. *Cleve. Clin. Quarter.*, 48, 132.

Engquist A., Brandt M.R., Fernandes A., et al. (1977). The blocking effect of epidural anesthesia on the adrenocortical and hyperglycaemic response to surgery. *Acta Anaesthesiol. Scand.*, 21, 330.

Fragen R. J., Weiss H.W., Molteni A. (1988). Adrenocortical effects of Diprivan (Propofol), Etomidate and Pentothal. *Seminars in Anesthesia*, 7, 1085.

George J.M., Reier C.E., Lanese R.R., et al. (1974). Morphine anesthesia blocks the cortisol and growth hormone response to surgical stress in humans. *J. Clin. Endo. Metab.*, 38, 736.

Ghoneim M.M., Long J.P. (1970). The interaction between magnesium and other neuromuscular blocking agents. *Anesthesiology*, 32, 23.

Goldstein D.S. (1982). Circulatory plasma catecholamine, cortisol, lipid and psychological responses to a real-life stress (third molar extractions): effect of diazepam sedation and inclusion of epinephrine with the local anesthetic. *Psychosom. Med.*, 44, 259.

Hakanson E., Rutberg H., Jorfeldt L., et al. (1984). Endocrine and metabolic responses after standardized moderate surgical trauma: influence of age and sex. *Clin. Physiology*, 4, 461.

Hasselstrom L.J., Morgensen T., Kehlet H., et al. (1984). Effects of intravenous bupivacaine on cardiovascular function and plasma catecholamine levels in humans. *Anesth. Analg.*, 63, 1053.

Haxholdt O.S., Kehlet H., Dryberg V. (1981). Effect of fentanyl on the cortisol and hyperglycemic response to abdominal surgery. *Acta Anaesthesiol. Scand.*, 25, 434.

Hemmer M., Viquerat C.E., Suter P.M., et al. (1980). Urinary antidiuretic hormone excretion during mechanical ventilation and weaning in man. *Anesthesiology.*, 52, 395.

Hjortso N.C., Christensen N.J., Anderson T., et al. (1985). Effects of the extradural administration of local anaesthetic agents and morphine on the urinary excretion of cortisol, catecholamines and nitrogen following abdominal surgery. *Br. J. Anaesth.*, 57, 400.

Hole A., Unsgaard G. (1983). The effect of epidural and general anesthesia on lymphocyte functions during and after major surgery. *Acta Anaesthesiol. Scand.*, 27, 135.

Kehlet H. (1982). The modifying effect of general and regional anesthesia on the endocrine–metabolic response to surgery. *Reg. Anesth.*, 7:S38.

Lacoumenta S., Paterson J.L., Burrin J., et al. (1986a). Effects of two differing halothane concentrations on the metabolic and endocrine responses to surgery. *Br. J. Anaesth.*, 58, 844.

Lacoumenta S., Paterson J.L., Myers M.A., et al. (1986b). Effects of cortisol suppression by etomidate on changes in circulating metabolites associated with pelvic surgery. *Acta Anaesthesiol. Scand.*, 30, 101.

Ledingham I., Watt I. (1983). Influence of sedation on mortality in critically ill multiple trauma patients. *Lancet*, 1, 1270.

Madsen S.N., Brandt M.R., Engquist A., et al. (1977). Inhibition of plasma cyclic AMP, glucose and cortisol response to surgery and epidural analgesia. *Br. J. Surg.*, 64, 669.

Malatinksy J., Vigas M., Jurcovicova J., et al. (1986). The patterns of endocrine response to surgical stress during different types of anesthesia and surgery in man. *Acta Anesth. Belg.*, 37, 23.

Maruyama K., Muneyuki M., Kojima T., et al. (1987). Changes in serum glucose and serum growth hormone levels during pituitary surgery. *Anesth. Analg.*, 66, 746.

Miller R.D., Savarese J.J. (1986). Pharmacology of muscle relaxants and their antagonists. In *Anesthesia*, 2nd edn.

New York: Churchill Livingstone. Chapter 27, pp. 889–944.

Oyama T. (1980). The influence of general anesthesia and surgical stress on endocrine function. *Contemp. Anesth. Pract.*, **3**, 173.

Pflug A.E., Halter J.B. (1981). Effect of spinal anesthesia on adrenergic tone and the neuroendocrine responses to surgical stress in humans. *Anesthesiology*, **55**, 120.

Prezioai P. (1983) Etomidate, sedatives, and neuroendocrine changes. *Lancet*, **1**, 276.

Rehulka J., Kraus M. (1986). Regulation of liver corticoid metabolism during early postnatal life—effects of surgical stress. *Physiologia Bohemoslovaca*, **35**, 211.

Roizen M.F., Forbes A.R., Miller R.D., et al. (1979a). Similarity between effects of pancuronium and atropine on plasma norepinephrine levels in man. *J. Pharmacol. Exp. Ther.*, **211**, 419.

Roizen M.F., Horrigan R.W. (1979b). Anesthetic dose that blocks adrenergic response to incision. *Anesthesiology*, **51**, S141.

Rutberg H., Hakanson E., Anderberg B., et al. (1984). Effects of the extradural administration of morphine, or bupivacaine, on the endocrine response to upper abdominal surgery. *Br. J. Anaesth.*, **56**, 223.

Savino J.A., Dawson J.A., Agarwal N., et al. (1985). The metabolic cost of breathing in critical surgical patients. *J. Trauma*, **25**, 1126.

Shirasaka C., Tsuji H., Asoh T., et al. (1986). Role of the splanchnic nerves in endocrine and metabolic response to abdominal surgery. *Br. J. Surg.*, **73**, 142.

Smallridge R.C., Chernow B., Snyder R., et al. (1985). Angiotensin-converting enzyme activity—a potential marker of tissue hypothyroidism in critical illness. *Arch. Intern. Med.*, **145**, 1829.

Smith N.T., Eger E.I., Stoelting R.K., et al. (1970). The cardiovascular and sympathomimetic responses to the addition of nitrous oxide to halothane in man. *Anesthesiology*, **32**, 410.

Soules M.R., Sutton G.P., Hammond C.B., et al. (1980). Endocrine changes at operations under general anesthesia: reproductive hormone fluctuations in young women. *Fertility and Sterility*, **33**, 364.

Stanley T.H., Philbin D.M., Coggins C.H. (1969). Fentanyl-oxygen anesthesia for coronary artery surgery: cardio-vascular and antidiuretic hormone responses. *Can. Anaesth. Soc. J.*, **26**, 168.

Stanley T.H., Isern-Amaral J., Lathrop G.D. (1975). Urine norepinephrine excretion in patients undergoing mitral or aortic valve replacement with morphine anesthesia. *Anesth. Analg.*, **54**, 509.

Tarhan S., Fulton R.E., Moffitt E.A. (1971). Body metabolism during general anesthesia without superimposed surgical stress. *Anesth. Analg.*, **50**, 915.

Tonnesen E., Huttel M.S., Christensen N.J., et al. (1984). Natural killer cell activity in patients undergoing upper abdominal surgery: relationship to the endocrine stress response. *Acta Anaesth. Scand.*, **28**, 654.

Udelsman R., Norton J.A., Jelenich S.E., et al. (1987). Responses of the hypothalamic-pituitary-adrenal and renin-angiotensin axes and the sympathetic system during controlled surgical and anesthetic stress. *J. Clin. Endocrinol. Metab.*, **64**, 986.

VonWerder K., Stevens W.C., Cromwell T.H., et al. (1970). Adrenal function during long-term anesthesia in man. *Proc. Soc. Exp. Bio. Med.*, **135**, 854.

Walsh E.S., Paterson J.L., O'Riordan J.B.A., et al. (1981). Effect of high-dose fentanyl anaesthesia on the metabolic and endocrine response to cardiac surgery. *Br. J. Anaesth.*, **53**, 1155.

Walsh J., Puig M.M., Loritz M.A., et al. (1987). Premedication abolishes the increase in plasma beta-endorphin observed in the immediate postoperative period. *Anesthesiology*, **66**, 402.

Winter P.M., Hornbein T.F., Smith G. (1972). Hyperbaric nitrous oxide anesthesia in man: determination of anesthetic potency and cardiorespiratory effects. Abstracts of Scientific Papers. p. 103. ASA meeting.

Yeager M.P., Glass D.D., Neff R.K., et al. (1987). Epidural anesthesia and analgesia in high risk surgical patients. *Anesthesiology*, **66**, 729.

Zaloga G.P., Willey S., Tomasic P., et al. (1987). Free fatty acids alter calcium binding: a cause for misinterpretation of serum calcium values and hypocalcemia in critical illness. *J. Clin. Endocrinol. Metab.*, **64**, 1010.

Zsigmond E.K., Domino E.F. (1980). Clinical pharmacology and current uses of ketamine. In *Trends in Intravenous Anesthesia*, pp. 283–328. (Aldrete J.A., Stanley T.H., eds.) Chicago: Year Book Medical Publishers.

D. METABOLIC PROCESSES

31. Nutrition and Metabolism

V. Marks and C. M. Williams

All vital processes require energy which is obtained from the chemical reactions performed by living cells. In the animal kingdom, the principal mechanism for the liberation of energy is the gradual oxidation of metabolic substrates. In some tissues, such as striated muscle, energy requirements may be met anaerobically by glycolysis—but only for short periods.

Ingested food is the fundamental source of all energy for vital processes. When food is consumed in excess of energy requirements, the surplus may be incorporated into the fabric of the body. When food intake is insufficient to meet energy requirements, the deficit is made good by utilizing pre-existing metabolic stores, e.g. glycogen and triglycerides, or in extremes tissue protein.

Metabolic processes resulting in the breakdown of tissue are referred to as *catabolic*; those concerned either with construction or deposition of these metabolic stores are termed *anabolic*. In the healthy adult subject of constant weight, anabolism and catabolism proceed simultaneously at approximately equal rates, so that there is neither a net gain nor a net loss in body tissues which are, nevertheless, maintained in a state of constant flux.

After ingestion, food is digested to a form in which it can be absorbed and transported to the cells of the body. Through an intricate series of biochemical reactions, it can be utilized by the cells for energy requiring processes such as the synthesis of proteins and other structural elements, muscular contraction, nervous conduction, transport of substances across membranes and glandular secretion. The ability to 'capture' energy and divert it into physiologically 'useful' pathways is a function of intracellular transfer mechanisms. These occur in conjunction with respiratory enzyme systems in the mitochondria of the cells. The most important transfer systems are the NAD-NADH and NADP-NADPH nucleotides; the cytochromes and the flavoproteins.

Even under 'ideal' conditions only a small and variable proportion of the energy liberated by oxidative processes can be utilized by the cell for maintaining vital processes. Excess energy is lost as heat. It has been calculated that the overall loss accounts for up to 75% of the energy released from ingested foodstuffs; only 25% being available for use in functional systems. Ultimately, all of the energy produced in the body—with the exception of the relatively small amount utilized as mechanical work—will be dissipated as heat so that the measurement of heat production can be used to provide an estimate of energy expenditure.

METABOLISM

Metabolic Rate

The term metabolism, in its broadest sense, includes all the chemical reactions involved in growth, development and maintenance of both the physiological and nutritive state of an individual. Basal metabolism or basal metabolic rate (BMR), is used to describe the minimal amount of heat produced by a fasting person, physically and mentally at rest in a room at 20°C. It represents the energy required to maintain essential body function and includes the energy required for maintenance of chemical and electrical gradients, and for the transport of essential molecules against concentration gradients. It provides for the maintenance of cardiac contraction, skeletal muscle tone and the continuation of reabsorption and secretory processes of the kidney. Basal metabolic rate may be measured by direct calorimetry in which the heat produced by an individual in a closed container (calorimeter) is measured by the rise in temperature of water circulating on the exterior of the chamber. A more convenient measure of basal metabolic rate is provided by the technique of indirect calorimetry using the Benedict-Roth Spirometer. Assuming a *respiratory quotient* (RQ), or *respiratory exchange ratio* (RER) of 0.82, oxygen consumption is measured and energy expenditure calculated from a knowledge of the proportions of carbohydrate and fat contributing to the metabolic processes (an RQ of 0.82 indicates 60% of energy provision from carbohydrate and 40% from fat). For a very accurate determination of metabolic rate, it is necessary to measure urea excretion as well, since proteins, in contrast to carbohydrates and fat are incompletely oxidized. From this value, the amount of oxygen consumed and carbon-dioxide produced as a result of amino-acid oxidation may be calculated. When this is subtracted from total O_2 consumed and

CO_2 produced, an accurate figure for RQ can be derived from which energy expenditure can be calculated. Formerly, measurement of basal metabolic rate by indirect calorimetry and its expression as a percentage of the mean for healthy individuals of similar age and size (expressed in terms of surface area), was widely used as a test of thyroid and other endocrine gland function. This method has now been superseded by more precise measures of circulating thyroid hormone levels, together with measurements of the regulatory hormones TRH and TSH.

The ready availability of stable isotopes of oxygen (^{18}O) and hydrogen (^2H) in recent years and improvements in techniques for their analysis, has allowed the development of the doubly labelled water method for measuring energy expenditure. A loading dose of water labelled with the stable isotopes, deuterium and ^{18}O is given. Deuterium is eliminated from the body as water alone; ^{18}O, however, is eliminated both as water and carbon dioxide. The difference between elimination rates of the two isotopes provides a measure of carbon dioxide production. If the respiratory quotient is known, oxygen consumption and therefore energy expenditure can be measured. The technique is noninvasive and because it does not require the continuous measurement of gaseous exchange, can be used to assess energy expenditure over long periods of time and under a variety of conditions.

Resting Metabolic Expenditure

A less precise but more practical measure of energy expenditure frequently used in clinical settings is that of *resting metabolic expenditure* (RME) or *resting energy expenditure* (REE). This is a measure of energy expenditure in individuals in a resting condition, in a post-absorptive state under conditions of thermoneutrality. RME is estimated to be approximately 10% higher than BMR and includes the thermic affect of food, (specific dynamic action).

RME can be calculated using the Harris-Benedict equations, as follows:

For men:

RME (kcal/day) =
$$66.4730 + 13.7516(W) + 5.0033(H) - 6.7550(A)$$

For women:

RME (kcal/day) =
$$65.5095 + 9.563(W) + 1.8496(H) - 4.6756(A)$$

Where W = present weight in kg, H = height in cm; A = age in years.

It is of particular value in calculating average energy requirements of individuals receiving specialized nutritional support in the form of enteral and parenteral feeding. The individual figure for RME is used plus additional correction factors which allow for degree of activity and the catabolic state of the patient (Table 31.1).

TABLE 31.1
CORRECTION FACTORS FOR PREDICTING ENERGY
REQUIREMENTS IN HOSPITAL PATIENTS*

Clinical condition	Correction factor
Fever	$1.0 + 0.13$ per °C
Elective surgery	1.0–1.2
Peritonitis	1.2–1.5
Soft tissue trauma	1.14–1.37
Multiple fractures	1.2–1.35
Major sepsis	1.4–1.8
Thermal injury	
0–20% +	1.0–1.5
20–40%	1.5–1.85
40–100%	1.85–2.05

* Total energy requirement is predicted by product of correction factors × RME.
+ Percent body surface area burned.
After Silberman and Eisenberg, 1982.

METABOLIC SUBSTRATES

The main constituents of diet that provide energy are fats, carbohydrates and to a lesser extent, proteins. After complete oxidation these yield 38.9, 17.2 and 17.2 kJ (9.3, 4.1 and 4.1 kcal) per gram respectively.

The composition of diets varies enormously according to political, cultural and individual preferences. Consequently, the contribution to the total metabolic energy pool made by each type of nutrient cannot be stated except in the most general terms. It has been suggested that in Western society, where three meals a day constitute the dietary norm, carboyhdrates contribute about 45%, fats 42% and protein about 13% to the total energy pool.

In some individuals, alcohol is an important additional source of energy; each gram (1.25 ml) of pure alcohol providing 7 kilocalories after complete oxidation to carbon dioxide and water. In Britain roughly 6% of total energy intake is derived from alcohol, but in some individuals it may provide as much as 50% of their daily energy intake.

The regulatory mechanisms of fat, carbohydrate and protein metabolism are closely interrelated both inside and outside the cell. It is nevertheless convenient to consider each of these dietary constituents independently though it must be stressed that this approach has been adopted so as to facilitate description.

Carbohydrates

The polysaccharides (starch and dextrins) and the disaccharides, sucrose and lactose, comprise the main digestible carbohydrates of the diet. The polysaccharides consist of polymers of the simple sugar glucose and contribute approximately 50% of the total carbohydrate intake. Approximately 25% is contributed by sucrose, a disaccharide comprised of glucose and fructose, and 10% by lactose, which consists of equal proportions of glucose and galactose.

Before they can be absorbed in the gut, polysaccharides and disaccharides must be converted to their constituent sugars, glucose, galactose and fructose. The starches are digested in the duodenal lumen to liberate glucose and maltose. Maltose, sucrose and lactose are then cleaved to their respective monosaccharide constituents by the action of specific membrane-bound disaccharidases at the mucosal surface. The hydrolyzed sugars are transported across the mucosal membrane by carrier-mediated mechanisms. Glucose and galactose share a common carrier system which has been shown to be energy and sodium dependent and which transports the sugars against a concentration gradient. Fructose is not actively transported and enters the mucosal cell by a process termed facilitated diffusion. It is now recognized that the process of digestion and absorption of carbohydrates is not completely efficient and a proportion of starch and certain sugars (e.g. fructose, sorbitol, raffinose) escape digestion and absorption. In the colon, these carbohydrates are fermented by colonic bacteria to the short-chain fatty acids (SCFA) which, following absorption, may contribute to whole body energy provision.

From the above discussion it can be appreciated that the major carbohydrate entering the portal system following digestion is the simple sugar, glucose. Glucose is the most important carbohydrate of the body and is a major source of energy for all cells and tissues. Except under extraordinary circumstances, e.g. prolonged fasting, glucose is the sole metabolic fuel for cells of the central and peripheral nervous systems. For this, and other reasons, the maintenance of a constant blood glucose concentration is a vital homeostatic function. Apart from certain pathological conditions, the circulating blood glucose concentration is maintained within narrow limits (3–10 mmol/L) and the whole body glucose pool rarely fluctuates outside the limits of 5–20 g of glucose. These limits are maintained despite enormous fluctuations in the supply and demand for glucose and are achieved by a number of homeostatic mechanisms, the most important of which are autoregulatory and are either neurally or hormonally mediated.

The liver plays a central role in the regulation of glucose homeostasis and following a carbohydrate meal much of the glucose entering from the portal circulation is converted to glycogen, the form in which glucose is stored in the liver. Glucose is also converted to triglycerides (fat) in the liver and these are transported to adipose tissue where they are stored. The first step in the metabolic transformation of glucose is conversion to glucose-6-phosphate by the enzyme hexokinase, this reaction takes place immediately upon entry of glucose into the cell, so that effectively no free glucose is found in the intracellular compartment. Dietary galactose must also be converted to glucose-6-phosphate before it can take part in intracellular processes. Fructose must be metabolized to either dihydroxyacetone-phosphate and glyceraldehyde-3-phosphate, or to fructose-6-phosphate before it can enter the glycolytic pathway. Because of the high activity of the enzymes which carry out these transformations neither fructose nor galactose is normally demonstrably present in peripheral blood, even after a large meal.

Complex carbohydrates of foods which escape digestion and absorption are termed dietary fibre. The major unavailable carbohydrates include cellulose, hemicellulose, lignin, pentosans, gums and pectins. Although gums and pectins are not strictly fibrous in nature, they exert similar effects to the fibrous, insoluble plant cell wall components and are therefore included in the term dietary fibre. Until recently these components of the diet were regarded as unavailable sources of energy, which if eaten in sufficient quantities, could exert a laxative effect. It is now clear that these dietary constituents produce alterations in gastrointestinal function through effects on gastric emptying, intestinal mobility and absorption of the products of digestion; such actions have profound effects on the rate of disposition of digested nutrients.

Feeding studies have shown that certain types of fibre reduce the rise of blood glucose and insulin concentrations following a carbohydrate meal and lower serum lipid concentrations in individuals with hyperlipidaemia. The mechanism of these effects is not yet clearly understood and the different types of dietary fibre differ considerably in their ability to ameliorate the rise in glucose and insulin concentrations following a carbohydrate load. Certain types of fibre, most notably the gums, have been shown to induce metabolic changes by binding to and inhibiting the absorption of substances from the gut e.g. bile acids and certain lipid components of the diet. The observed effects of dietary fibre on gastrointestinal transit time and carbohydrate and lipid metabolism suggested that their increased consumption may be of benefit in the treatment of patients with diabetes and hyperlipidaemias. A number of studies of diabetic and hyperlipidaemic subjects have supported this observation, but large amounts of the gum must be fed in order to achieve beneficial effects.

Epidemiological observations have led to the hypothesis, which is unproven, that many diseases of modern civilization including coronary heart disease, diverticular disease and cancer of the large bowel, can be attributed to the fibre-depleted diets consumed in Western society. Nevertheless, these observations provide the basis for recommendations made in several recent reports on diet and health for increased consumption of dietary fibre by the population as a whole.

Fats and Fatty Acids

Dietary fats consist of triglycerides, cholesterol and phospholipid of which triglycerides comprise by far the greatest component. Triglycerides consist of three long-chain fatty acids esterified with glycerol. In the duodenal lumen triglycerides are hydrolyzed by the action of pancreatic lipase to form mono and diglycerides as well as constituent fatty acids and glycerol. By the action of bile salts these form micellar structures which are absorbed across the mucosal membrane by passive diffusion. Within the mucosal cell, these breakdown products of triglyceride hydrolysis are re-esterified to form triglyceride. Reformed triglycerides combine with the carrier protein β lipoprotein polypeptide (or apoprotein) and small amounts of cholesterol and phospholipid to form chylomicrons. These pass from the serosal surface of the mucosal cell into the lymphatic system and enter the general circulation via the thoracic duct. Chylomicrons may be taken up and used directly by peripheral tissues; this uptake is dependent upon the action of the enzyme lipoprotein lipase, present on the capillary walls of blood vessels supplying peripheral tissues e.g. skeletal muscle, heart and adipose tissue. Lipoprotein lipase hydrolyzes chylomicron triglycerides to form fatty acids and glycerol and its activity is enhanced by insulin and the intestinal hormone GIP (gastric inhibitory polypeptide). The fatty acids liberated by lipoprotein lipase are rapidly taken up and used as important sources of energy by most cells of the body. In adipose tissue they are esterified with glycerol phosphate (formed from glucose) and deposited as triglyceride within the adipocyte. Successive removal of triglyceride from the chylomicron particle results in a triglyceride-poor lipoprotein referred to as a chylomicron 'remnant'.

Chylomicrons are also rapidly removed by the liver where they are reconstituted to form lipoprotein structures containing varying proportions of protein, triglycerides, cholesterol and phospholipid. Table 31.2

TABLE 31.2
AVERAGE LIPID AND PROTEIN COMPOSITION OF PLASMA
LIPOPROTEINS

Component	Average composition %			
	Chylomicrons	VLDL	LDL	HDL
Protein	2	9	21	50
Triglycerides	84	54	11	4
Cholesterol	2	7	8	2
Cholesterol esters	5	12	37	20
Phospholipids	7	18	22	24

shows the different types of lipoproteins found in the plasma and their approximate compositions, and compares them with chylomicrons.

VLDL is the major lipoprotein synthesized in the liver. It is released into the circulation where it acts as a circulating store of fatty-acids. Uptake and utilization of fatty acids released from VLDL is dependent upon the action of lipoprotein lipase, in a similar manner to that of the chylomicrons. Cleavage and removal of triglyceride fatty acids from VLDL results in the formation of a VLDL 'remnant' which may be removed by the liver. If the VLDL 'remnant' remains in the circulation, further hydrolysis and removal of triglyceride leads to the formation of the LDL particle. The HDL fraction is synthesized in and secreted by, the liver, and is largely concerned with the regulation of reverse cholesterol transport i.e. the removal of excess cholesterol from peripheral tissues and transport to the liver.

In recent years interest has centred around the measurement of circulating concentrations of various lipoprotein fractions; high concentrations of the LDL fraction have been linked with an increased propensity to atherosclerosis and coronary heart disease whilst levels of the HDL fraction have been demonstrated to be inversely related to risk of this disease. Recent evidence has implicated chylomicron and VLDL 'remnants' in the pathogenesis of atherosclerosis. Abnormalities in the lipid composition of chylomicron and VLDL remnants have been observed in subjects with diabetes mellitus, and may explain the greater propensity to atherosclerosis which is evident in this disease.

The relationship between amounts and types of dietary fat, atherosclerosis and coronary heart disease, has also received much attention in recent years. Much of this interest stems from animal and human studies which have shown that feeding diets rich in saturated fatty acids increases circulating cholesterol concentrations whilst increased consumption of poly- and mono unsaturated fatty acids has the reverse effect.

An association between dietary fat and the aetiology of coronary heart disease is based largely on comparisons of international figures for fat consumption in different countries and the incidence of coronary heart disease in these countries; such comparisions provide some support for an involvement of dietary components, particularly dietary fat, in the aetiology of this disease. These studies, and others which have investigated the relationship between various dietary constituents and the incidence of degenerative diseases, have led to suggestions that the increased incidence of diseases such as diabetes mellitus, obesity, diverticular disease and coronary heart disease, are due to alterations in diet which have occurred in Western populations in the past century. This has led to recommendations for population reductions in the consumption of certain dietary constituents, e.g. fat, and increased consumption of others, e.g. dietary fibre. Whether such recommendations are more appropriately directed at individuals at increased risk of these diseases remains a controversial issue.

Appreciation of the role of dietary fatty acids in physiological and biochemical processes remains incomplete. It has long been known that two 18 carbon fatty acids, i.e. linoleic and linolenic acid, are essential to man. Enzymes necessary for the insertion of a double bond between the methyl end of the fatty acid and carbon number nine, are absent in animals but present in plant systems. Consumption of plant products provide the only source of these essential fatty acids. Estimates of requirements vary but recommended figures for the intake of these fatty acids lie between 2 and 10 g per day. Although animals are unable to synthesize linoleic and linolenic fatty acids, they can readily transform these products into 20 and 22 carbon fatty acids with 3, 4 and 5 double bonds.

Transformation of linoleic acid results in the production of two important 20 carbon fatty acids dihomo-γ-linolenic and arachidonic acids. Linolenic acid may undergo chain elongation and desaturation to a series of fatty acid products, the most important of which is eicosapentanoic acid. This latter pathway is particularly active in marine animals so that fish provide a rich source of eicosapentanoic acid. Interest in these three fatty acids—arachidonic, dihomo-δ-linolenic and eicosapentanoic, lies in the fact that they have been shown to act as precursors for the synthesis of prostaglandins (eicosanoids), (Fig. 31.1). Prostaglandins appear to be involved in inflammation and in cardiovascular, renal and gastrointestinal physiology. Disturbances in their rates of production in certain tissues have been implicated in a number of pathological conditions including rheumatoid arthritis, breast cancer and thrombosis. Arachidonic acid is the precursor of the most active members of this family of compounds. Interest has centred around thromboxane (TXA_2) and prostacyclin (PGI_2) which have been shown to possess potent pro (TXA_2) and anti (PGI_2) platelet aggregatory properties. Disturbances in their relative rates of production by platelets (TXA_2) and endothelial cells (PGI_2) is thought to play a part in thrombus formation. Complex interrelationships exist between the metabolism of the 20 carbon

atom precursors of the prostaglandins, and dietary fatty acid modification has been shown to cause alteration in membrane phospholipid fatty acid composition, prostaglandin synthesis and cell function. The most notable example of this is the increased blood clotting time which is observed on feeding large amounts of fish oils (EPA) to human subjects. The precise mechanism of this effect and other consequences of dietary fatty acid manipulation remain to be elucidated.

Proteins

Proteins are an essential dietary constituent for man; essentially arising as a result of an inability to synthesize certain amino acids which form constituent parts of structural and functional proteins of the body. Before they can be absorbed, proteins undergo digestion in the duodenum and jejunum by the action of proteases, secreted by the pancreas, and also by membrane bound tri and dipeptidases. By the actions of these enzymes all dietary proteins are broken down to single amino acids, and dipeptides and tripeptides, prior to absorption. Transport across the luminal membrane is dependent upon a number of stereospecific carrier systems, shared by a number of different amino acids. Depending on the particular amino acid, transport may be active, occurring against a concentration gradient and dependent upon the presence of sodium (e.g., tryptophan), or passive, with no uptake against a concentration gradient (e.g., glycine). Amino acids are transported from the mucosal cell via the portal circulation, whence they are conveyed to the tissues of the body. Free amino acids are converted into tissue proteins; amino acids present in excess of requirements for growth and tissue repair are rapidly metabolized by intricate metabolic steps involving transamination and deamination, to provide energy yielding substrates. The release of amines and synthesis of urea in the liver is a consequence of

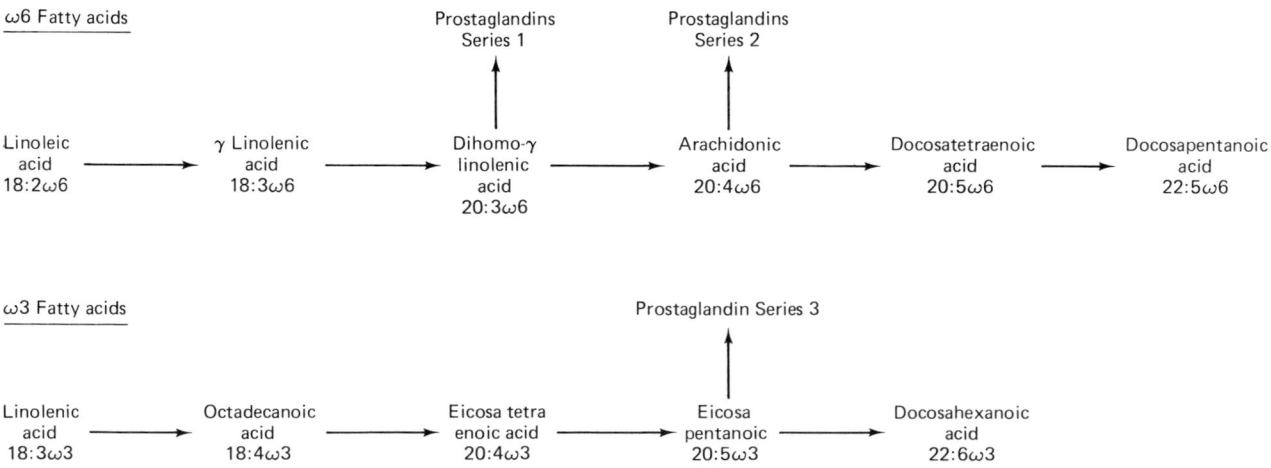

Fig. 31.1 Pathway of linoleic and linolenic acid metabolism; relationship to prostaglandin production.

the metabolism of amino acids to energy yielding substrates. Rates of urea excretion are usually fairly stable; significant increases only occur when a very high protein diet is fed (when protein intake greatly exceeds requirements for protein synthesis) or when there is marked breakdown of tissue protein, for energy provision and gluconeogenesis, or in response to injury.

The major purpose of dietary protein is to provide essential amino acids for growth and tissue repair. In the adult, eight amino acids are required as essential components of the diet, these are isoleucine, leucine, lysine, methionine, phenylalanine, threonine, tryptophan and valine. In infants and young children there is an additional requirement for arginine and histidine. Protein requirements are clearly greatest for the rapidly growing child and in the pregnant or lactating woman. In the adult, dietary protein is necessary to maintain optimal rates of synthesis of rapid turnover proteins, e.g., transport proteins, hormones and enzymes and to maintain the structural integrity of rapidly dividing cells (e.g., mucosal cells, skin and the RBC). Even in apparently inert tissues, e.g., muscle, constituent proteins are constantly undergoing synthesis, breakdown and re-synthesis. Although the rate of protein turnover is less rapid than in the visceral protein compartment, the relatively greater mass of muscle means that a considerable proportion of dietary amino acids are used to maintain optimal rates of protein turnover in this tissue. It is calculated that muscle contributes approximately 80% to whole body protein turnover and that a significant proportion of basal energy requirements are directed towards the maintenance of muscle protein turnover.

During periods of food deprivation or starvation, amino acids are released from muscle protein to provide substrates for hepatic gluconeogenesis and to provide for the internal energy requirements of muscle cells themselves. It would appear that the net release of amino acids which occurs in fasting, is due to a reduction in the rate of muscle protein synthesis, rather than an increase in the rate of protein breakdown in this tissue. In some states of trauma, and particularly when there is an associated sepsis, release of amino acids from muscle, and muscle mass depletion, is particularly marked. This exaggerated catabolism of muscle protein appears to be due to an active breakdown of muscle protein; in certain states whole body protein synthesis may also be increased, but because breakdown exceeds synthesis, net loss of muscle protein mass occurs. The increased losses of amino acids which are observed during fasting and trauma are reflected in increased excretion of urinary nitrogen (mostly urea). Negative nitrogen balance is therefore the net consequence of excessive protein catabolism over anabolism and reflects a loss of lean tissue from the body. During starvation a series of complex endocrinological and metabolic adaptations occur which serve to minimize these losses. The major component of this adaptive response is an increased capacity to synthesize and utilize ketone bodies which are products of hepatic fatty acid oxidation. The most notable adaptation occurs in the brain, which normally has an obligate requirement for glucose, since nerve cells are unable to utilize fatty acids. Within a few days of fasting the increased capacity of the brain to utilize ketones reduces the requirement for glucose (synthesized via gluconeogenesis from amino acids). This reduced demand for glucose reduces the influx of substrate amino acids from muscle with a consequent reduction in the degree of muscle protein catabolism and negative nitrogen balance. In the average normal adult this adaptive mechanism reduces the loss of nitrogen in the urine from 12 g/d on the first day of starvation to less than 5 g/d after five to six days. These adaptive mechanisms do not appear to operate in critically ill patients and lean tissue losses are more exaggerated and sustained than in the fasted state. The reasons for this and possible methods for encouraging adaptation are the subject of intensive research.

OTHER NUTRIENTS

Carbohydrates, fats and proteins make up the bulk of the diet but small amounts of other essential nutrients must also be provided to ensure optimal nutritional health. These include the vitamins, minerals and trace elements which perform a multitude of essential functions within the body. Failure to provide these micronutrients in adequate amounts results in the manifestation of specific, well defined deficiency syndromes. Lack of sufficient thiamine, for example, leads to disturbances in carbohydrate metabolism which results in impaired energy provision in the nervous system and can cause marked neurological disturbances and even permanent damage.

Vitamins

A number of vitamins have been recognized to be essential in man. These include the fat soluble vitamins A, D, E and K and the water soluble vitamins C and those of the B group, including riboflavin, thiamine, B_6, nicotinic acid, folic acid, B_{12}, biotin and pantothenic acid. The precise biochemical and physiological functions of all these vitamins have not yet been elucidated though quite a lot is known about some of them. Some, for example, thiamine, nicotinic acid and riboflavin, act as essential cofactors for enzymes concerned with energy transformations within the cell. Others, such as folic acid and vitamin B_{12} (hydroxycobalamin), are involved in the synthesis of nucleic acids. Vitamin A (retinol) is involved in normal vision as it forms a component part of the visual pigment rhodopsin. This vitamin also plays an important role in the normal differentiation of epithelial cells. Skin and mucosal manifestations of vitamin A deficiency are thought to be a consequence of disturbances in normal epithelial cell formation.

Functions of other vitamins including vitamin C and vitamin E are less well established. In the case of the latter, vitamin deficiency syndromes are virtually unknown in man probably because of the wide distribution of vitamin E in normal foods.

The likelihood of vitamin deficiencies arising within a population are dependent upon the distribution of vitamins in commonly eaten foods, methods of food processing, cooking and storage and the presence of individuals with a higher than normal requirement for the vitamin. The elderly represent a vulnerable group with respect to vitamin C intake, since fresh foods containing this vitamin may not be regularly consumed by elderly individuals who may also have a higher requirement for vitamin C. Vitamin D deficiency is not uncommon in individuals of Asian origin living in the UK. The reason for this greater susceptibility may be due to genetic, cultural and dietary factors. The Asian diet, particularly that of the weaning child, is relatively poor in vitamin D and calcium, and rickets has been observed in children of Asian families living in Britain where exposure to sunlight is limited. There is some dispute as to the true essentiality of vitamin D in man. Cholecalciferol, the precursor for the synthesis of vitamin D within the human body, can be formed by the action of ultraviolet light upon the skin; the cholecalciferol so formed then undergoes transformation to the biologically active metabolite of vitamin D (1, 25 dihydroxycholecalciferol) by successive hydroxylations in the liver and the kidney. Some forms of hepatic and renal disease are associated with a defect in this transformation; children with chronic renal disease being maintained by haemo or peritoneal dialysis, for example, may require dietary supplements of vitamin D to prevent the development of rickets.

Minerals and Trace Elements

Minerals required in amounts exceeding 200 mg/d include sodium, potassium, phosphorus, calcium, magnesium and smaller amounts of the trace elements are required ranging from recommended intakes of 15 mg/d for iron to 3 mg/d for copper. Trace elements proven to be essential nutrients in man and whose lack in the diet has been shown to be associated with specific deficiency syndromes include iron and zinc although proven deficiencies of the latter are extremely rare.

Other minerals which have been shown to be necessary in animals and are known to be involved in metabolic processes or form structural components of body tissues include iodine, cobalt, selenium, manganese, molybdenum, silicon and vanadium.

The minerals and trace elements support a wide range of functions in man. Sodium and potassium maintain excitability of nerve and muscle cells and are important determinants of osmolality and fluid balance. Calcium is a major component of bone and also determines muscle excitability and the release of hormones from secretory cells. Iron is a major component of the respiratory and muscle pigments, haemoglobin and myoglobin, and of the cytochrome proteins which regulate electron flow in the respiratory chain. Zinc is a cofactor for a large number of metabolic enzymes and is involved in protein synthesis. Deficiency of iron is one of the commonest of all nutritional deficiency syndromes and although inadequacies in zinc intake are said to be not uncommon in the UK, convincing evidence is still lacking. A number of studies have shown that zinc supplementation improves the healing of leg ulcers and surgical wounds, but only if a low serum zinc concentration is present. Serum zinc is however known to be an unreliable index to total body zinc status.

This example serves to illustrate an important nutritional principle in relation to supplementation with micronutrients. Improvements in general health and alleviation of specific defects in response to supplementation can only be achieved if inadequate nutrient status is present. Assessment of vitamin, mineral and trace element status should therefore be carried out prior to supplementation. This is however extremely difficult if not impossible to do at the present time, except in the most general terms or when gross deficiencies are present. Because of the interactions between different trace elements, e.g., iron, zinc and copper, care should be taken to ensure that balanced doses of appropriate supplements are provided. Mega dose supplementation with vitamins and minerals has no place in the treatment of diseases whose aetiology is not associated with inadequate intake of, or increased requirements for, that particular nutrient except in specific illnesses where a pharmacologic effect is sought.

TOTAL PARENTERAL NUTRITION

The past few years have seen major advances in the formulation of artificial feeding regimes which have occurred along with improvements in techniques for their administration. These changes, together with a better understanding of the metabolic consequences of severe illness, have greatly improved nutritional support of those patients who are unwilling to eat, or are unable to eat, digest and absorb, sufficient normal foods to meet their nutritional requirements. Patients in whom the gastrointestinal tract is functional, but in whom anorexia or swallowing difficulties preclude normal feeding, may be provided with a liquid enteral diet administered by means of a nasogastric tube. Those in whom the gastrointestinal tract is non-functional or for whom nutritional requirements cannot be met by tube feeding, may require the provision of nutrients via the intravenous route (parenteral nutrition).

Parenteral feeding regimes provide carbohydrate (normally glucose), fat (triglycerides) and protein (as individual amino acids) along with necessary vitamins and minerals. Because of the hypertonic nature of most intravenous feeds they must be administered via a central venous catheter so that they can be rapidly diluted by the high rate of blood flow in the vein. The large diameter of the vessel used (usually the superior vena cava) reduces the tendency to thrombosis formation which tends to occur when the highly irritating feeding solutions are infused into smaller veins. Most centres now administer all components of the feed together; these are mixed under sterile conditions and delivered at a continuous rate from a single three-litre bag under gravity or by infusion using a constant infusion pump.

The aim of parenteral nutrition is to meet the energy and protein requirements of the individual such that lean tissue losses are minimized. Vitamin and mineral provision is also important since depletion of tissue reserves of these essential nutrients may be accelerated under the catabolic conditions of serious illness. Energy and protein requirements should be calculated on an individual basis with reference to estimates of energy expenditure and measurements of urinary nitrogen losses. Vitamin and mineral requirements may be provided in the form of standard solutions of constant composition. Recent recommendations have been made for vitamin and trace element provision during intravenous feeding: these are mostly higher than the figures recommended for healthy individuals and are designed to meet heightened tissue requirements and prevent whole body depletion. Electrolytes: i.e. Na^+, K^+ and Cl^-, may be provided in a standard form along with the dextrose and amino acid solution but many patients require modification to these amounts, depending upon endocrinological factors and renal function, and losses occurring via the gastrointestinal tract (GIT), and from burns and wounds.

Amino acids are provided in the form of a mixture of essential and non-essential amino acids. Although various modifications in the amino acid profiles for parenteral nutrition have been suggested, there is no good evidence that any of these have significant advantages in terms of improvements in nitrogen balance. At the present time most commercially available amino acid mixtures correspond to those amino-acids found in egg protein. This protein consists of 51% essential amino acids, is of high biological value and is used as a reference protein against which the biological value of other dietary proteins is assessed.

Energy is provided in the form of both carbohydrate and fat; the aim should be to meet the individuals energy requirement in the form of these two nutrients alone. This is referred to as the non-protein energy component of the feed. At one time it was considered inadvisable to administer fats intravenously to traumatized patients, particularly those with sepsis, since it was thought to lead to deposition of fats in the liver and the formation of fatty thromboembolism. This is now thought not to be the case, indeed, excessive provision of glucose is thought to be responsible for the development of some of these side-effects. Provision of energy as fat has other advantages in that its high energy density means that a greater amount of energy can be provided in a relatively small volume. This can offer considerable advantages to patients in whom fluid restriction is advantageous. Fat suspensions, unlike glucose solutions, are isotonic and can be administered via a peripheral line if necessary. The provision of energy as fat may also offer certain metabolic advantages. Increased rates of fat oxidation enhance the hepatic synthesis of 'ketone bodies'. As already mentioned, increased ketone body production may be metabolically advantageous by reducing the rate of amino acid based gluconeogenesis in the liver. Ketone bodies have also been suggested to directly suppress protein breakdown in skeletal muscle.

Various means of manipulating these metabolic processes are being investigated in the parenteral feeding of critically ill patients.

Medium chain fatty acids (MCT) are known to be more readily oxidized and converted to ketones than long chain fatty acids found in most intravenous feeds. Carnitine, a co-factor in fatty acid metabolism, may also accelerate the rate at which fatty acids are converted to ketone bodies and an increased loss of carnitine is reported to occur in traumatized subjects. The potential value of both MCT and carnitine in intravenous feeding needs further investigation.

In practice, most feeding regimes are formulated such that an equal proportion of energy is derived from carbohydrate and fat sources. A minimum amount of carbohydrate (100–150 g) must be provided to ensure sufficiency of glucose for metabolism by cells of the brain and the erythron, with an obligatory requirement for glucose. It is also required to maintain optimal rates of fatty acid utilization.

HORMONAL AND NEURAL CONTROL OF ENERGY METABOLISM

The hormonal and neural control of energy metabolism is complex. It involves a large number of hormones of which insulin, glucagon, growth hormone, ACTH, cortisol, TSH, thyroxine, adrenaline and various intestinal factors, such as GIP (glucose dependent insulinotropic peptides), are amongst the most important. Contrary to former belief, the endocrine system does not function independently, but is closely integrated with, and partly controlled by, the autonomic nervous system.

Insulin

Insulin is the most important single hormone controlling metabolic processes. It not only regulates glucose metabolism but also controls the metabolism of both lipids and amino acids. The most impressive action of insulin concerns its ability to lower the blood glucose concentration. It does this by a dual mechanism—on the one hand by increasing glucose uptake in the peripheral tissues, particularly by striated muscle and adipose tissue, and on the other by decreasing hepatic glucose output.

It has been shown that most mammalian cells do not permit free entry of glucose in an indiscriminate manner. Instead, there is an active transcellular transport mechanism which only acts on sugars of a particular chemical structure. This is now known to be the case with the insulin-secreting β-cells of the pancreatic islets. However, the cells of the liver remain unique among mammalian cells in that they appear not to have a stereospecific transport system. The most highly differentiated cells of the body, namely the neurons and the most lowly, namely the erythrocytes, share the distinction of having a specific sugar transport mechanism which is independent of insulin. Most other cells including those of muscle, connective and adipose tissue exhibit an extremely low rate of transcellular glucose transport in the absence of insulin; in effect they are insulin-dependent. Thus, when insulin is present, glucose enters the cell readily from the ECF and becomes available for intracellular metabolism.

There is evidence that insulin has an action upon the metabolism of glucose by the brain. Recent studies have also raised the possibility that a neural mechanism originating from a hypothalamic insulin-sensitive receptor is involved in the regulation of hepatic glucose production. However, insulin itself appears to be relatively unimportant for normal brain function. The disastrous effects of insulin overdosage are for example not due to insulin *per se* but to hypoglycaemia as the brain, unlike most other tissues of the body, has an almost absolute requirement for glucose for the provision of energy. Nervous tissue cannot utilize free fatty acids for this purpose although it has been shown that during prolonged starvation adaptation does occur so that ketones may be utilized as well as, or instead of, glucose.

The biological half-life of insulin in the blood is very short; in the region of 2–5 minutes but its biological actions may persist for longer. This explains the reactive hypoglycaemia that occasionally develops when glucose infusions are terminated abruptly. Under these conditions, insulin released during the phase of hyperglycaemia continues to exert its effect even after the stimulus for further insulin secretion has ceased. Fortunately hypoglycaemia produced in this way is rarely sufficiently severe to cause symptoms as it would otherwise seriously limit the clinical usefulness of intravenous glucose infusions. A similar situation sometimes occurs spontaneously in mild diabetics, who, 3–5 h after eating a meal, may experience slight to moderate symptoms of spontaneous hypoglycaemia.

In the liver, insulin decreases gluconeogenesis and glycogenolysis and encourages glycogen synthesis. In the absence of insulin, gluconeogenesis and glycogenolysis increase and glucose pours out of the liver into the ECF. Since the glucose so liberated is also inhibited from entering the peripheral tissues it can go nowhere except to increase the concentration in the glucose pool. This causes a rise in the blood glucose concentration and eventually leads to spillage in the urine. In itself this is not unduly harmful in the short term although it is extremely wasteful of protein which has to be broken down to provide the glucose precursors used by the liver for gluconeogenesis. What is far more harmful, is the steep rise in plasma ketones which causes the profound acid-base disturbance so characteristic of diabetic ketoacidosis. Prolonged hyperglycaemia does result in certain complications of poorly controlled diabetes mellitus notably retinopathy and possibly nephropathy.

The synthesis of fats and their release from adipose tissue is under hormonal control. Insulin promotes triglyceride synthesis not only by stimulating fatty acid synthesis but also by increasing the availability of glycerolphosphate. For thermodynamic reasons glycerol liberated by lipolysis cannot be utilized within adipose tissue cells for resynthesizing triglyceride. Instead 'energy rich' glycerolphosphate formed during the metabolic conversion of glucose must be used. Because glucose cannot enter the adipose tissue cell except in the presence of insulin, one consequence of insulin deficiency is that lipolysis is unopposed by re-esterification. As a result, there is a large net increase in fatty acid release from the adipose tissue cells. The liberation of free fatty acids from adipose tissue is hastened by any mechanism that increases intracellular lipolysis by activating the hormone-dependent lipase present in the adipose tissue cells. Enzyme dependent lipase activity is decreased by insulin and by prostaglandins but increased by most other hormones. It is still unknown which of these are important physiologically, but current evidence suggests that glucagon, adrenaline and noradrenaline, released locally from sympathetic nerve terminals, are probably the most important.

The main determinant of insulin secretion is the concentration of glucose in the blood perfusing the pancreatic islets; a high concentration of glucose in the blood stimulating insulin secretion; a low concentration inhibiting it. However, in addition to the direct action of glucose, subtle interactions between the β-cells and the secretory products of the adjacent glucagon and somatostatin containing cells also modify the pattern of insulin secretion. Furthermore, many other factors such as ketone bodies, amino acids, gut hormones and the autonomic nervous system affect insulin secretion. Sympathomimetic drugs, for example, adrenaline and noradrenaline, and sympathetic nervous activity, which predominantly activate α-adrenergic receptors, inhibit insulin secretion whilst those that mainly influence β-adrenergic receptors and stimulate adenylate cyclase potentiate insulin release. Consequently, any stress, whether physical or mental, that non-specifically activates the sympathetic nervous system leads to the inhibition of insulin secretion unless α-adrenergic blockade is imposed artificially. Excessive sympathetic nervous activity is in fact one of the factors responsible for 'stress-induced' diabetes.

Glucagon

If insulin is the main anabolic hormone of the body then glucagon secreted from the adjacent α cells of the pancreatic islets can paradoxically lay claim to being one of the main catabolic hormones, at least under stressful conditions since it is also one of the main stimulators and regulators in insulin secretion.

The best known effect of glucagon is the rapid stimulation of hepatic glycogenolysis and glucose release from the liver. Since glucagon does not directly increase peripheral glucose uptake this action leads to a rise in blood glucose concentration. Advantage is taken of this fact therapeutically in the use of glucagon for raising the blood glucose concentration of patients with hypoglycaemia due to overtreatment with insulin or sulphonylureas, and in whom, for some reason, glucose itself cannot be given by mouth. Glucagon has no immediate hyperglycaemic action when the liver glycogen reserves are low as in the patient with alcohol induced hypoglycaemia, hepatocellular necrosis or acute starvation.

Glucagon stimulates insulin secretion by a direct action on the β-cells of the pancreatic islets and promotes lipolysis in adipose tissue. These actions are probably as important physiologically, as implied above, as its better known hyperglycaemia properties. Glucagon also promotes gluconeogenesis and accelerates amino acid metabolism by the liver. One consequence of this is that urea production is increased. Indirectly therefore, glucagon increases protein breakdown in the body and increases nitrogen waste. These actions of glucagon have led some authors to conclude that hyperglucagonaemia may contribute to the metabolic abnormalities of diabetes mellitus but the evidence is inconclusive.

When administered parenterally to the non-stressed, non-fasting individual, the lipolytic effect of glucagon is masked by its marked insulinotropic action. In other words, glucagon is so potent a stimulus to insulin secretion that under the conditions of pharmacological experimentation its ability to mobilize fatty acids from adipose tissue by increasing intracellular lipolysis is more than overcome by the increase in insulin secretion. If stimulation of insulin secretion is blocked by sympathetic nervous activity, however, glucagon can increase lipolysis and produce a rise in plasma free fatty acids, even in normal individuals.

Glucagon secretion is inhibited by high concentrations of free fatty acids in the blood, by hyperglycaemia and, above all, by hyperinsulinaemia. Indeed, insulin seems to be essential for glucose to exert its inhibitory effect on glucagon secretion. In the absence of insulin, as in the insulinoprivic diabetic, glucose does not suppress glucagon secretion even at very high concentrations and plasma glucagon levels are elevated. Somatostatin is another important inhibitor of glucagon secretion and has been extensively used in pharmacological experiments to try and assess the role of glucagon in the manifestation of hyperglycaemia. The relevance of these experiments to physiological and pathological conditions is, however, dubious and highly speculative.

Effects of Other Hormones on Energy Metabolism

Although many other hormones, apart from insulin and glucagon, are involved in the control of energy metabolism, in very few of them is the association as direct or as active as with the pancreatic hormones. The gut hormones, of which more than 20 different types are now recognized, play a vital role in controlling digestion and absorption of nutrients. Glucose-dependent insulinotropic peptide (GIP), is the dominant hormone among this group and appears to be the major insulinotropic hormone responsible for the greater stimulation of insulin secretion observed with oral than intravenous glucose administration. Carbohydrates and fats are both potent stimulators of GIP secretion. Hypersecretion of GIP in response to excessive nutrient intake, has been suggested as a primary step in the aetiology of obesity, with hyperinsulinaemia and subsequent development of insulin-resistant diabetes, as a long-term consequence of this defect. GIP also appears to have direct metabolic effects on peripheral tissues, most notably adipose tissue where it activates lipoprotein lipase; but further investigation of these actions are required before the overall significance of this hormone in determining the rate and extent of nutrient disposition can be fully appreciated.

Thyroid hormones play an important role in setting the general level of metabolic activity; a notable feature of these hormones is their potentiating effect on the action of the catecholamines. Although the molecular basis of this action is not clearly understood, recent evidence suggest that thyroid hormones may act to enhance the rate of interaction of catecholamine receptors with adenylate cyclase by actions on the guanine-nucleotide binding protein which couple the receptor-enzyme unit.

The role of cortisol and growth hormone in determining metabolic events is also poorly understood. Both these hormones act in a 'permissive' capacity, enhancing the catabolic actions of hormones such as glucagon and catecholamines, however the effects of growth hormone may not be direct since its major action appears to be mediated by the insulin like growth factors (somatomedins), a group of small molecular weight substances which are produced in the liver and other tissues and are concerned with regulation of cellular growth.

In the past, much importance was attached to the metabolic effects of adrenaline; comparatively less attention was given to those of noradrenaline, the neurohormone released at sympathetic nerve terminals. Noradrenaline is a potent stimulator of lipolysis in adipose tissue and causes marked elevation of free fatty acid concentrations. It has been implicated not only in the regulation of substrate availability during stress and starvation, but also in the control of body temperature via influences on brown adipose tissue (BAT) thermogenesis. Noradrenergic stimulation of brown adipose tissue in experimental animals leads to hypertrophy and a decrease in the degree of uncoupling of mitochondria. Noradrenergic stimulation of brown adipose tissue (BAT) during cold exposure is thought to be an important determinant of temperature regulation in hibernating animals and in new-born infants. A similar mechanism has been suggested to play a part in the homeostatic response to overfeeding and the maintenance of a constant body weight in humans, although evidence for this remains speculative. A possible role of BAT in the development of malignant hyperthermia has also been suggested but has been little studied to date.

FURTHER READING

Bloom S.R., Polak J.M. (eds.). (1981). *Gut Hormones*. London: Churchill Livingstone.

Dickerson J.W.T., Lee H.A. (1988). *Nutrition in the Clinical Management of Disease*. London: Edward Arnold.

Karran S.J., Alberti K.G.M.M. (eds.). (1980). *Practical Nutritional Support*. London: Pitman Medical.

Woolfson A.M.J. (ed.). (1987). *Biochemistry of Hospital Nutrition*. London: Churchill Livingstone.

Richards J.R., Kinney J.M. (eds.). (1977). *Nutritional Aspects of Care in the Critically Ill*. London: Churchill Livingstone.

Foa P.P., Bagaj J.S., Foa N.L. (eds.). (1977). *Glucagon: Its role in Physiology and Clinical Medicine*. New York: Springer-Verlag.

Newsholme E.A., Start C. (1973). *Regulation in Metabolism*. London: Wiley.

Bondy P.K., Rosenburg L.E. (eds.). (1980). *Metabolic Control and Disease*. Philadelphia: Saunders.

Marks V., Rose F.C. (2nd edn.). (1981). *Hypoglycaemia*. Oxford: Blackwell.

Ellenberg M., Rifkin H. (3rd edn.). (1983). *Diabetes Mellitus Theory and Practice*. New York: Medical Examination Publishing Co.

Lands W.E.M. (ed.). (1985). *Biochemistry of Arachidonic Acid Metabolites*. Boston, Dordrecht, Lancaster: Martinus Nijhoff.

Silberman H., Eisenberg D. (eds.). (1982). *Parenteral and Enteral Nutrition for the Hospitalized Patient*. Norwalk, Connecticut: Appleton-Century-Crofts.

Fischer J.E. (1983). *Surgical Nutrition*. Boston: Little, Brown and Co.

Coward W.A., Prentice A.M., Murgatroyd P.R., et al. (1984). *Measurement of CO_2 Production and Water Production Rates in Man using ^2H, ^{18}O-Calorimeter and Isotope Values*. Workshop on Human Energy Metabolism, Wageningen.

32. Parenteral Nutrition
H. Lee

It is clear that nutritional support for many critically ill patients is sadly neglected. In the current era of high technology with ever improved ventilator care, better monitoring techniques, the use of continuous arteriovenous haemofiltration, plasmaphoresis, it is surprising how often the patient wastes away behind the very improved techniques to keep him alive. It is still true today, as it was twenty years ago, that starvation does occur in the midst of plenty, often in the mistaken belief that nutritional support of patients is of secondary importance or, if acknowledged that it is required, it is too difficult to administer.

One of the most gratifying advances over the last ten years has been the resolution of many of the features of the metabolic response to trauma and infection and the ability to treat these problems. Whereas a decade ago there was a tendency to overtreat with parenteral nutrition, it is now recognized that many patients can do remarkably well by nasogastric (or naso-enteric) feeding through fine bore tubes with comprehensively prepared and economically viable commercial feeds and the only absolute contra-indication to enteral nutrition is, in fact, total gastrointestinal failure.

Nutritional support implies recognition of the need that it is comprehensive and meets all nutritional/metabolic requirements of a patient, i.e., nitrogen, energy, water, electrolytes, vitamins and essential biological elements whilst, at the same time, taking careful note of whatever end-organ failure the patient may be suffering from. To delay nutritional support in those patients requiring it is inevitably going to lead to more morbidity and mortality and the arguments hitherto used that, say, parenteral nutrition is expensive, do not stand scrutiny when the costs of looking after, in a hospital bed, patients with increased morbidity or even mortality are considered. Many studies have comprehensively shown that nutritional support enhances wound healing, enables the patient to better combat infection, reduces the length of hospital stay and is cost effective.

THE METABOLIC RESPONSE TO INJURY

It is not the purpose of this chapter to describe in great detail the metabolic response to injury, trauma or infection, but rather to highlight the main features upon which the basis of nutritional support can be rationalized. Ever since Cuthbertson's work in the 1930s which showed an increased nitrogen output as a result of fractured femurs, a vast amount of work has been undertaken to identify various responses in the scenario of altered metabolism following trauma. Although traditionally divided into an ebb phase, followed by a flow phase, there is some suggestion that there is a very early flow phase lasting but a few hours (Frayn, 1987) followed by the ebb phase (semidormant metabolic phase) for 12–14 h, followed then by the true catabolic phase i.e., flow phase, which may last for weeks or months depending upon other intercurrent problems afflicting the patient, e.g., repeated anaesthetics, repeated infections, wound dehiscence or prolonged pain. Basically, during the ebb phase, body temperature and oxygen consumption are relatively decreased, there is an out-pouring of circulating catecholamines with relative suppression of insulin secretion. In the flow phase, there are a number of inter-related reactions which, depending on their relative preponderance, bring about a near equilibrium (homeostatic) situation. The initial reaction is associated with salt and water retention (the effects of antidiuretic hormone and aldosterone). There is then an increase in oxygen consumption, an increased resting metabolic expenditure, increased gluconeogenesis and usually increased lipolyis. The latter usually occurs in some 80% of patients—i.e., early (within 24 h) keto-adaptation. This causes increasing levels of circulating glucagon, cortisol and growth hormone with relatively decreased circulating catecholamines, usually raised serum insulin concentrations, although with relative target organ resistance, i.e., stress diabetes, all culminating, unless treated, in negative nitrogen balance.

The individual's fuel reserves are limited, thus the glycogen stored in the liver and muscle is rapidly utilized within 12–18 h, energy is then derived from ketone (acetoacetate and β-hydroxybutyric acid) body formation as a result of lipolysis (the better the keto adaptation the less severe the degree of negative nitrogen balance), and then there is a rapid dissolution of muscle mass resulting in breakdown of amino acids, the amino moieties being transferred to the liver by the alanine shuttle and the nitrogen segments degraded to urea and the carbon fractions converted to glucose (gluconeogenesis).

In careful turnover studies, it has been shown that in some patients there is truly an increased catabolic rate, whilst in others, there is a diminished synthetic rate. Such research studies are not easily brought to the bedside, but this should not inhibit the clinician from determining what is happening to his patient. What is certain is that if a catabolic patient is not given exogenous nutrient substrates, then he must necessarily undergo a process of self-cannibalism leading to well known negative nitrogen balance.

Negative Nitrogen Balance

Unfortunately, when conducting ward rounds and assessing patient needs, rarely is any attempt made to determine whether a patient is in negative nitrogen balance or not. Even the word 'starvation' seems demeaning and is rarely used for fear of later repercussions. How strange, therefore, that infection is readily recognized by a rise in temperature, the patient sweating and may be feeling and looking hot, an increased white cell count, but clinicians often seem unable to recognize malnutrition in the midst of plenty or may be simply avoiding the subject of nutritional support altogether.

Negative nitrogen balance has many features

TABLE 32.1

Catabolic Status	
Moderate catabolism	10–14 g nitrogen/d i.e. urea appearance rate (UER) of 294–420 mmol/d† (based on 24 h urine urea measurement)*
Moderately severe catabolism	14–24 g nitrogen/d (UER of 420–756 mmol/d)
Hypercatabolic	> 24 g nitrogen/d (UER > 756 mmol/d)

Notes
† Based on 70 kg body weight.
* Maybe considerably elevated by gastrointestinal haemorrhage, absorpotion of haematomata or from necrotic tissue. In these situations expect urea: creatinine ratio divergence.

(McEntee et al., 1986; Lee, 1988b), the most commonly recognized of which are loss of weight (although rapid weight changes always reflect alterations in fluid balance), increased susceptibility to infection because of impaired immunocompetence, poor wound healing with an increased rate of wound dehiscence, e.g., anastomosis after gastrointestinal surgery or superficial wounds, hypoalbuminaemia with consequent peripheral oedema and poor capillary circulation (this impairs wound healing and may lead to skin necrosis and bed sores), noticeable mental apathy and globally increased morbidity and mortality. All these aspects of negative nitrogen balance in the non-nutritionally supported patient are exacerbated by intercurrent infection, by pain from injuries and by further surgical intervention (the 'nil by mouth' phenomenon). Further, for each degree centigrade increase in temperature there is a 12% increase in basal metabolic rate.

Although much work has been done at the bedside with respect to calorimetry and measuring oxygen consumption and carbon dioxide production, this is not readily available in all district hospitals. Therefore, some handle should be sought by which to assess negative nitrogen balance. One can either take the simplistic approach (McEntee et al., 1986) and say that all patients will require 0.2 g of nitrogen/kg body weight and 30–35 kcal/kg of body weight per day and not bother to measure or, alternatively, to use the 24 hour urine urea excretion rate as a marker. In this way, patients can be divided into groups of catabolism (*see* Table 32.1) on the basis of using the urea excretion rate formula (Table 32.2).

There is absolute agreement that in the immediate post trauma or surgical situation every effort must be made to restore blood gas equilibrium, the peripheral circulation, fluid (blood and plasma) and electrolyte requirements (Lee, 1988a). If after 3 days a patient is not able to take oral nutrition voluntarily or by nasogastric tube then not to give total parenteral nutrition (TPN) is tantamount to poor medical practice. It can be readily appreciated from Table 32.2 that it is not unusual for patients to be breaking down 15–20 g of nitrogen/d. However, two important points must be remembered. The total urea excretion rate can be markedly increased as a result of protein released from (a) areas of necrotic tissue (b) from absorption of large haematomata (c) absorption of blood following gastrointestinal haemorrhage. Secondly, there is absolutely no point in pursuing urea nitrogen excretion rates above 24 g/d for to infuse greater amounts than about 22–24 g of nitrogen per day is to exceed the metabolic capacity of the liver to usefully anabolize such amino acids, hence deamination rates will increase and simply add to an already high urea excretion rate. Thus, in such patients one can only reduce the degree of nitrogen balance negativity, not obviate it, and it would be metabolic folly to attempt to do so.

Starvation

Many of the early studies on the value of parenteral nutrition lacked credibility because there was a failure to differentiate between carefully adapted starvation where an individual may lose up to 60% of his initial body weight over weeks or months before finally succumbing, and the rapid flow phase following acute injury where if an individual loses more than 30% of his initial body weight then survival is remote. This is a long standing observation which many clinicians still fail to grasp. Sheer clinical acumen clearly reveals the rate at which some patients literally waste away over a short period of 2–3 weeks. Such wasting is often compounded, not only by inanition and failure to provide substrates but also by the use of drugs, e.g., steroids which can increase the albumen catabolic rate

TABLE 32.2
ASSESSMENT OF DAILY NITROGEN LOSSES AND REQUIREMENTS

Observation Urine urea nitrogen = 80% of total urine nitrogen across a wide range of urea excretion.

1 g urea (16.6 mmol urea) = 28/60 g nitrogen (mol.wt urea = 60)
Total body water (unisex figure) = 60% body wt in kg
Urea is equally distributed through body water.
Thus (a) 24 h urine urea in g $\times$ 28/60 $\times$ 6/5* = X $\times$ 0.56 = (A)g
    (b) measure proteinuria if any = Y $\times$ 4/25† = (B)g
    (c) Correction for any rise in blood urea (B.U.) assuming no change in body weight in kg
    Rise in B.U. over 24 h = Zg
Zg $\times$ 60% body wt. $\times$ 28/60 = Z $\times$ body wt. $\times$ 0.28 = (C)g
(A) + (B) + (C) = nitrogen loss

* Correct for untreated patients and those receiving synthetic crystalline amino acids as nitrogen source.
† 1 g nitrogen = 6.25 g protein.
Note: This formula takes no account of extrarenal losses e.g. enterocutaneous fistula losses, excessive vomiting, skin exfoliation.
1 litre of fistula fluid may contain up to 2–4 g nitrogen/day.

by 15%, or other drugs which actually interfere with amino acid metabolism, e.g., tetracycline, oxytetracycline, which interfere with incorporation of amino acids into nucleic acid synthesis and other drugs that may cause hepatic insufficiency e.g., rifampicin, erythomycin. Furthermore, inherent liver damage related to initial trauma and/or hypoxaemia can severely compromise the liver's ability to synthesize protein.

Sepsis

In the past decade a considerable amount of excellent research work has shown that comprehensive TPN in severely infected patients is very valuable. There has been a school of thought that suggested that less nitrogen should be given and more energy provided, the latter only as carbohydrate. Numerous studies now show the validity of supplying both carbohydrate and fat on an equienergetic basis to such patients and that they can tolerate up to 20 g of nitrogen/d (Roulet et al., 1983; Dahn et al., 1984; Nanni et al., 1984). Clearly, all clinicians recognize that in the critically ill patients with multiple end organ failure in whom normal substrate metabolism is lost, no matter what TPN/enteral nutrition (EN) support is given, survival is not likely to be guaranteed.

ASSESSMENT OF NUTRITIONAL STATUS
(Burgert and Anderson, 1979; Neale and Elia, 1986; Goodinson and Dickerson, 1988)

This has to be done just as diligently as seeking the source of infection and treating with appropriate antibiotics and ensuring then that the antibiotics are effective. In the accompanying Table 32.3 are a list of the most commonly used parameters to make an assessment of a patient's nutritional profile. Not all these measurements can be used in every clinical situation and, furthermore, no one single test itself indicates malnutrition. However, hopefully, if TPN is started soon enough in patients likely to require nutritional support, then the initial measurements may not show any evidence of malnutrition and subsequent evaluation would simply confirm that sufficient TPN/EN had been given to the individual.

The most useful measurements are weight (in kilograms), skinfold thickness, midarm muscle circumference, serum albumin and visual appraisal of the patient. None of these parameters are difficult to undertake, or require elaborate equipment; moreover they are readily reproducible by interested members of the attendant team. Once such baselines have been obtained then it is customary to weigh the patient daily, measure the skinfold thickness and midarm muscle circumference once weekly and, at least twice

TABLE 32.3
SUGGESTED MEASUREMENTS FOR ASSESSING NUTRITIONAL STATUS

Tests for malnutrition	Equipment required	Result in malnutrition
1. *Body weight in kg and recent loss	Various scales	> 10%
2. *Triceps skin fold thickness (TST) Fat energy reserves	Holtain skin fold calipers	< 10 mm in males < 13 mm in females
3. *Mid-arm muscle circumference (MAMC) Muscle protein reserves (MAMC = arm circumf. − π(TST))	Tape measure in cm	< 23 cm in males < 22 cm in females
4. *Serum albumin (visceral protein)	Routine lab. test	< 35 g/litre
5. Serum transferrin ⎱ short half-life Complement C₃ ⎰ proteins	Routine lab. test	< 2 g/litre (not reliable)
6. *Retinol binding protein Thyroxine binding pre-albumin	Special tests	
7. Urinary hydroxyproline	Special test	†Collagen turnover
8. Lymphopaenia	Routine lab. test	< 1.2 × 10⁹/litre
9. Plasma amino acid profile	Specialized tests	Changing valine/glycine ratio
10. Urine 3 methylhistidine	Specialized tests	Increased muscle breakdown
11. Hair root morphology	Tweezers and microscopy	More telogens and dysplastic hairs
12. Finger dynamometry	Dynamometer and interested clinician	Diminished power
13. Skin responses to intradermal injections of antigenic material	e.g. DNCB, candida	Skin anergy (time consuming and little value)
14. *Visual assessment of patient	Eyes! and clinical acumen	

* The most useful tests. Do nos. 1 and 14 daily; nos. 2, 3, 4 and 6 twice weekly (e.g. Mon. and Thurs, as a routine).
(From Lee, 1988b.)

weekly, assess serum albumin. In some centres, routine measurements of 3-methylhistidine are available—this metabolite is non-recyclicable and is derived from muscle breakdown (8.2 µmol/L = 1 g nitrogen breakdown).

Most hospitals in the UK now have District Nutritional Support Teams which are multidisciplinary comprising surgeons, physicians, pharmacists, nutritionists and nurses. Any clinician who is in doubt about what is required can call upon their services without relinquishing his control over a patient's overall management. Having decided, therefore, that a patient requires nutritional support, it has to be decided whether or not the gastrointestinal tract is functional, and that it can be approached by a nasogastric fine bore tube, naso-enteric or even fine bore jejunostomy tube, bearing in mind that some patients may have quite prolonged gastric atony although the small bowel is functional. The absolute indication for parenteral nutrition is gastrointestinal failure and here it is mandatory that appropriate angio access is obtained for prolonged feeding in such patients.

A central venous catheter is required for TPN. It is important to stress, however, that such insertions should only be undertaken with those who have experience with these techniques, not only in terms of inserting the central catheter but in fashioning a subcutaneous tunnel. Although hitherto it has been customary to state that the central venous feeding line should be used only for TPN, with the advent of triple lumen central catheters, it is now possible to give other agents to patients, e.g., antibiotics and cytotoxic agents through the same central venous access point.

There are two alternative approaches. One is by inserting an Abbott flexible drum catheter peripherally so that its tip ends centrally thereby allowing normal TPN regimens. The author has previously reported on such catheters being left *in situ* for 2 or 3 weeks at a time without any untoward side effects. Alternatively, there are now available comprehensive peripherally administered nutrient solutions whereby fat, carbohydrate and amino acids can be delivered through distal access sites. These solutions have a low osmolality, thereby substantially reducing the incidence of aseptic thrombophlebitis. There is absolutely no place, however, for giving peripheral isotonic amino acids alone in such patients. This latter practice is, in fact, no more than giving expensive sterile water.

THERAPEUTIC MODIFICATION TO METABOLIC RESPONSE TO TRAUMA

Over the years the search has continued in vain to seek therapeutic agents that might modify the metabolic response to trauma. Beta blockers have been used without success and likewise various muscle relaxants. More recently, an approach with naftidofuryl (Praxilene) was conducted on a large number of patients (Jackson et al., 1984) and, again, no metabolic benefits found.

The only successful approach to modification of the response has been by elevating the environmental temperature which has been particularly valuable with burns patients. It has been convincingly shown that nursing patients naked in a raised environmental temperature reduces the metabolic rate and the latent heat for evaporation of water from skin (environmental temperature should be 30–32°C). Hormone therapy with insulin and growth hormone have only met with very limited and non-confirmed metabolic improvement in such patients.

Nutritional Support

Over the past 20 years there have been many swings of the pendulum concerning the ideal energy substrate. In the 1960's the debate was whether glucose was superior to fructose, whether sorbitol, xylitol, ethanol or any of these in combination had anything to offer over the ideal physiological substrate glucose. Then there was a vogue for giving vast amounts of glucose intravenously and covering this with equally high doses of insulin which really only had the effect of maintaining normoglycaemia but little other evidence of improved anabolic effect. In the 1970's the arguments then were whether it was physiological or even prudent to give a fat emulsion intravenously and particularly in those patients with sepsis. There were also divergent opinions about the total amount of energy that should be given and it was quite common to give 3000–3500 kcal daily. The excellent work of Hill and his associates (MacFie et al., 1981) finally put to rest any opinion other than that the ideal amount of energy recommended was 30–35 kcal/kg of body weight per day for most patients. There is rarely a need, therefore, to exceed 2200 kcal/d. The only rare exception to this is in patients with severe widespread burns. As mentioned above, there is absolutely no doubt that the equienergetic provision of energy from carbohydrate and fat is the ideal in septic patients who can utilize such energy preferentially as opposed to being given glucose only. Further, there had been a tendency to give far too much nitrogen to patients but the rule is now that there is very rarely a need to exceed 22–24 g nitrogen daily.

Debates have occurred as to whether specialized amino acid solutions are required for patients with, say, severe muscle trauma, those with liver disease, or those with renal disease. Since branched chain amino acids are preferentially metabolized in muscle, there was a theory to suggest that amino acid solutions with an increased proportion of branched chain amino acids, e.g., leucine, isoleucine and valine would produce better nitrogen balance results than the basic profile amino acids. However, this has not been borne out in practice. As for acute renal failure, such patients can now be dialysed frequently or, even better, receive continuous arteriovenous haemofiltration (CAVH) whereby they too can benefit from standard amino acid preparations. There is absolutely no evidence whatsoever to suggest that giving these patients essential amino acid solutions only has any advantageous effects over full profile preparations.

With liver failure patients it has been suggested, particularly following the uncontrolled work of Fischer and colleagues (Freund and Fischer, 1981), that solutions high in branched chain amino acid solutions (the old F080 formulation) would not only result in more rapid resolution of coma but also improve their metabolic status. However, controlled studies (Rossi-Fanelli et al., 1982) have not borne this out. It is reasonable to suggest that decompensated cirrhotic patients who are already hypoproteinaemic may benefit from a solution with slightly higher concentrations of branched chain amino acids but for patients with fulminant hepatitis this has little value (Crossley and Williams, 1986).

There has been considerable discussion as to whether patients with acute pancreatitis can or should receive normal profile TPN formulations. Here the worry has been that intravenous infusions of fat emulsions might stimulate pancreatic lipase enzyme release or maybe amino acids stimulate proteolytic enzymes. There is no evidence to support this view and, indeed, recent studies have shown TPN treated pancreatitis patients faired better than those not so treated (Tandon, 1986).

Many clinicians have been concerned that TPN regimens containing a fat emulsion may lead to an increased incidence of pulmonary insufficiency. The evidence for this is very poor indeed. Before jumping to the conclusion that a so-called 'white lung' is due to the infusion of lipid, it is important to exclude such problems as pulmonary oedema, intercurrent chest infections and/or disseminated intravascular coagulation. It is our firm policy to infuse energy from glucose and fat sources on an equienergetic basis for any patient who may be on a ventilator.

There are many advantages to be obtained by giving equienergetic ratios of fat and carbohydrate (Table 32.4). It is no longer acceptable practice to give glucose only regimens covered with equally high amounts of soluble insulin.

With respect to amino acid solutions these should be full profile amino acids with all eight essential amino acids, the two semi-essentials, histidine and cystine and also a balanced profile of non-essential amino acids. There are many such amino acid solutions available commercially with very little to choose between them either in terms of efficacy in acquiring positive nitrogen balance or in the absence of side-effects. They vary little in their electrolyte content and any extra electrolytes can usually be added to a standard 3 L bag TPN regimen. It is the author's view that each District General Hospital should have a limited number of TPN regimens available in its pharmacy, these to be clearly described on the nutritional support prescription chart so that clinicians get to know best how to handle a few limited formulations. There can be little justification for having a vast array of

TABLE 32.4

SUGGESTED ENERGY REGIMEN FOR A 70 kg MAN SUPPLYING 8.4 MJ (2000 kcal) WHO RARELY NEEDS MORE PER DAY, DERIVED ON 50% BASIS EACH FROM GLUCOSE AND FAT

Glucose	50% solution + potassium (usually 60 mmol/L) ± soluble insulin
	500 ml (28 ml/h as continuous infusion via central catheter)
	250 g glucose 4.2 MJ (1000 kcal) per 24 h
	3.57 g/kg body weight per day
	0.15 g/(kg · h) (well within tolerance limits)
Fat	20% soya bean oil emulsion (Intralipid)
	500 ml (allow 6–8 hours fat-free infusion period before morning blood sample)
	100 g fat-triglyceride 4.2 MJ (1000 kcal) per 24 hours (note extra kcal from glycerol)
	1.43 g/kg body weight per day
	0.06 g/(kg · h)

Advantages over glucose-only regimen

Small energy volume	1000 ml
Low energy osmolar load	86 mosm/h^{-1}
Energy loss (per urine) per day	Less than 5%

- Need to add soluble insulin rare
- Metabolically remain within individual energy substrate tolerance limits
- Improved protein weight gain as opposed to water and fat gain
- Less risk of hypercarbia and respiratory compromise
- Diminished oxygen required
- Overall less respiratory effort and risk of myocardial 'strain'
- Less chance of inducing fatty liver
- Essential in septic patient
- Monitoring made easier

amino acid solutions in the pharmacy which cannot be cost effective nor improve clinical education in this area. As indicated above, TPN implies comprehensive nutritional support and the guidelines for this are shown in Table 32.5.

TABLE 32.5

Guidelines for comprehensive parenteral nutrition

1. Scrupulous, aseptic technique for insertion and after-care of catheter (central or peripheral).
2. Immediate chest X-ray to check catheter correctly located.
3. Correct patient assessment using anthropometric, biochemical and physiological measurements.
4. Nitrogen (full profile amino acid solution) 0.2–0.25 g/kg body weight.
5. Energy 30–35 kcal/kg body weight.
6. Energy (kcal):nitrogen (g) ratio 140:1 (catabolic patients); up to 180:1 less catabolic.
7. Derive energy equally from glucose and fat. Do not exceed 700 g glucose per day.
8. Give energy and nitrogen simultaneously—gives best anabolic effect.
9. Nitrogen (g):potassium (mmol); magnesium (mmol), phosphorus (mmol) ratios of 1:5–7; 1:1; 1:0.5.
10. Water-soluble vitamins from onset (protect from light); after 2 weeks fat soluble vitamins.
11. Essential biological elements zinc, copper, selenium, chromium, ? manganese, molybdenum, essential fatty acids.
12. HPPF, plasma or blood for immediate restoration of serum oncotic pressure or haemoglobin concentration.
13. Folinic acid 5 mg daily.
14. Use IV feeding line for nutritional purposes only whenever possible.
15. Mobilize patient as soon as possible—promotes anabolism.
16. Reassess and recalculate requirements (do *not* speculate).
17. Monitor constantly and appropriately.

PRACTICAL CONSIDERATIONS
(Lee, 1986; Hopkinson and Davis, 1987)

The whole delivery of TPN has been much simplified with the advent of 3 L bags, most of which have an average volume of 3.5 L. Most district pharmacies will justifiably demand, that the days prescription for a 3 L bag regimen is received by 10 a.m. and they also be informed that adequate angio access is already *in situ* (there should also be a rule that if a new angio access site has just been placed, then radiological proof of its correct positioning should be available). TPN regimens for hospital patients should be infused over a 24 h period and this will usually require the assistance of constant volumetric infusion pumps. If TPN is required, then it is worth giving it accurately over timed intervals and the use of pumps is recommended.

Although 1 L bottles of amino acids, carbohydrate and fats are available, and can readily be used, the 3 L bag has much to recommend it. In specialized areas such as liver failure, renal failure, severe trauma, the clinician should not feel reticent about approaching his local Nutritional Support Team for advice.

Although the argument is often put forward that 3 litre volumes cannot be tolerated by many patients, in practice this is rarely the case. However, with high carbohydrate concentration solutions and also amino acid solutions, up to 24 g/L, the volume of the infusion can be reduced to as little as 2 to 2.5 L. In conclusion, therefore, glucose and a fat emulsion (in the UK soya bean emulsion) are the only two energy substrates to be considered and then there is a choice from a number of full profile crystalline L amino acid preparations. Trace element solutions are now available, which include selenium and chromium and are commercially prepared. There are also comprehensive vitamin preparations.

Monitoring

Once TPN has been started then it is mandatory that its effectiveness is monitored (Lee, 1988b). The degree of monitoring and the frequency will depend upon the underlying condition of the patient being treated. Nevertheless, there are basic daily requirements. These include careful weighing, comprehensive fluid balance charts, blood urea and electrolytes, including glucose, simple blood gas measurements and alternate day full blood count. If the patient has hepatic insufficiency then alternate day or twice weekly prothrombin ratio should be measured. If hyponatraemia is discovered, then the possibility of drugs causing antidiuretic hormone (ADH) release or ADH hypersecretion as a result of cardiothoracic or cerebral complications should be sought and with hypernatraemia the question of sodium overloading with certain antibiotics considered (Lee, 1988a).

Hyperkalaemia is a rare occurrence unless potassium conserving diuretics are being given to a patient with moderate renal insufficiency. However, hypokalaemia is not infrequent, as often there is a tendency to underestimate potassium requirements. If the serum potassium is below 3 mmol/L, then a rule of thumb observation is that there is a 10% deficiency in total body potassium and this deficit can be corrected by working on a unisex replacement figure of 42 mmol/kg of body weight. Such repletion should be attempted over a 24–36 h period usually with ECG monitoring.

Once TPN has been started weekly anthropometric measurements of skinfold thickness and midarm muscle circumference are required and certainly once or twice weekly measurements of serum albumin. Again, twice a week measurement of 24 h urine urea excretion rate is sensible to make sure that the initial assessments are keeping in line with requirements, whilst, simultaneously, ensuring that the factors that may artifically augment the urea appearance rate have not significantly changed. Weekly liver function tests should be undertaken and likewise measurements of serum zinc, copper and magnesium. Assuming that selenium supplements are made *ab initio* at 400 nmol/d then there is no need for this special measurement. As mentioned earlier, with initial careful assessment of the patient, and using a limited number of modern nutrient substrates, then the number of metabolic complications following TPN have been dramatically reduced (Table 32.6).

Most of the metabolic complications now seen with TPN are not directly related to the TPN regimen itself. They either relate to underlying alteration in hepatic function and/or renal function and may be associated with respiratory tract infections. This does not imply that TPN regimens cause an alteration in end-organ function, but rather the underlying disease maybe associated with sepsis which has altered the metabolic handling of safe solutions.

Simple fluid overload can rarely be attributed to TPN itself. Likewise, hyper and hyponatraemia are usually due to other extraneous causes. As for hypokalaemia, this may well be the result of inadequate provision of potassium with a TPN regimen or excessive losses associated with nasogastric aspiration or profuse diarrhoea. Unless zinc, copper and selenium supplements are given early in TPN regimens then it is possible that deficiencies may occur (Shenkin, 1986; 1987). As for vitamins, it is a simple basic rule to say

TABLE 32.6
POSSIBLE COMPLICATIONS OF TPN

Problem	Possible cause
Metabolic	
Metabolic acidosis; lactic acidosis	Fructose*, sorbitol*, ethanol*, carbohydrate combinations; infection; liver or renal insufficiency
Metabolic alkalosis	Gastric aspiration; inadequate potassium supplements
Hyperosmolar dehydration syndrome	Hypertonic glucose; sorbitol
Hyperuricaemia	Fructose, sorbitol, xylitol*
Oxalaemia and oxaluria	? Xylitol
Hypertriglyceridaemia	Excess glucose; sorbitol; fat emulsion
Hyperlipidaemia	Excess fat emulsion; bacterial infection or toxaemia
Hypophosphataemia	Phosphorus free glucose regimens
Essential fatty acid deficiency	Fat free regimen
Hyperammonaemia	Protein hydrolysate solution
Folate metabolism disturbance	Ethanol, methionine
Hypercarbia	Excess glucose provision
Fatty liver	Excess glucose provision
Eczematous rash (acrodermatitis enteropathica)	Zn deficiency
Bone marrow hypoactivity (red and white cell series)	Cu deficiency
Altered cerebration	Poorly designed amino acid solutions, hypophosphalaemia; hypokalaemia
Hyponatraemia	Water overload, rarely inadequate sodium provision
Hypercalcaemia	Amino acid solution ? mechanism
Bleeding diathesis	Vitamin K deficiency
Vascular access	
Thrombosis	Hypertonic solution via short peripheral catheter
Infection, septicaemia, endocarditis	Poor technique
Catheter embolus	Avoid catheters with sharp needle casings
Damage to structures during central venous catheterization (e.g. nerve injury, haematoma haemorrhage, pneumothorax)	Poor technique; inexperience

* It is strongly recommended that glucose and a fat emulsion (Intralipid) are the ONLY energy sources ever used.
(From Lee 1988b).

that all fat and water soluble vitamins should be added from the beginning to any TPN regimen since their individual measurements are difficult to undertake and few District General Hospitals have such facilities.

In the past, there have been many lists of complications concerning angio access techniques but again, it is my view these are minimal provided expert insertion of these catheters is insisted upon.

PARENTERAL NUTRITION FOR SPECIFIC END-ORGAN FAILURE
(Lee, 1986c)

Clearly, there are specialized requirements in paediatric i.v. nutrition which is beyond the scope of this chapter. However, for adult TPN, it is my view that the currently available energy and nitrogen substrates for TPN are suitable for almost all adult conditions requiring TPN (McEntee et al., 1986). Patients with acute renal failure can be fed intravenously using normal solutions provided they are regularly dialysed or they can have CAVH which maintains the milieu interieur near normal and therefore permits almost normal metabolic utilization of substrates (Lee and Talbot, 1989). As for liver failure patients, this question is not yet resolved though it does appear that for the decompensated cirrhotic patient amino acid solutions augmented with branched chain amino acids may be preferable though in fulminant hepatitis there is no such need. For patients with gastrointestinal or pulmonary failure standard solutions are suitable. Although in the past, specialized solutions have been recommended for patients in cardiac failure, this is no longer necessary, though care must be taken to avoid fluid overload.

There will be diabetics who appear in the Intensive Care Unit requiring TPN and for them a standard regimen will be required though this may need additionally appropriate continuous infusions of insulin according to blood (not urinary) sugar measurements. Although formerly it was considered inappropriate to use soya bean oil emulsions (Intralipid) in the treatment of diabetics hyperlipidaemia, this is no longer the case. Much of the hypertriglyceridaemia previously reported in such patients was not due to infusion of fat emulsion but rather to excessive glucose infusion with inadequate insulin dosage and thus conversion of glucose to triglycerides.

There are now a number of patients who, having been started on TPN, then graduate to long-term home TPN management. According to the current UK HTPN Registry about 1–2 patients per million population will require this treatment per year. In approximately 50% of these, such treatment will be unnecessary by the end of one year because normal bowel function will have been restored (Yule, 1981; Lee, 1987).

For these patients, once it has been realized they have been on continuous TPN for, say 6–8 weeks and are not making further progress with respect to gastrointestinal tract function, then attempts should be made to get them on to HTPN. This is not a difficult task, bearing in mind that many patients with chronic renal failure go home on regular haemodialysis treatment or chronic ambulatory peritoneal dialysis (CAPD). It is the author's particular approach with such patients that they are taught to mix their own solutions in a 3 litre bag at home after an initial training period in hospital usually lasting between 2 and 3 weeks. Thus far, in 17 patients treated this way over the past 10 years, none have had any sepsis problems related to home prepared TPN bags, there has been no inappropriate self administration of drugs or loss of angio access sites due to poor technique. If home TPN patients are managed by commercial enterprise, this may cost up to £30 000 per year, though many clinicians can get the treatment cost down to the region of £18 000–20 000 per year by the do-it-yourself method. Indeed, one General Practitioner has claimed to get the cost down to between £15 000–18 000 per year. Nevertheless, the point about home TPN is that provided a certain number of patients can be afforded total bowel rest, yet maintained nutritionally replete, then the underlying condition may well resolve so that home treatment may later stop. This is totally different from, say, chronic renal failure where patients are maintained by home HD or CAPD and the only way forward is by renal transplantation.

As far as protein sparing peripheral intravenous isotonic amino acid therapy is concerned this is now 'a dead duck'. However, peripheral i.v. nutrition may be given with full comprehensive TPN regimens comprising amino acids, fat and carbohydrate with preparations having an osmolar load not exceeding 600 mosmol/L.

With respect to cancer patients, here again, a word of caution is required. Though it has been shown in a number of studies that cancer patients skin allergy can be reversed by appropriate TPN, nevertheless one must be cautious as to whether TPN for such patients actually prolongs worthwhile life. In the US there has been a particular proliferation of home TPN arrangements for cancer patients (Daly and Dudrick, 1981; Copeland et al., 1983; Lee, 1986b). In the UK a more considered approach has been adopted, because there is insufficient evidence to show that TPN *per se* is the panacea for these patients. On the other hand, if malnutrition appears to be an obstacle to giving specific cytotoxic and/or radiotherapy treatment to such patients then, of course, TPN should be given and malnutrition and/or anorexia should not be made an excuse for not providing what otherwise may be successful specific treatment. Nevertheless, in the UK at the time of writing cancer patients receiving TPN remain a small proportion of the total, whereas in the US home TPN accounts for some 80% of the total. The UK HTPN Registry adopt an entirely different attitude.

ENTERAL NUTRITION

The only absolute indication for TPN is gastro-intestinal failure. However, where the gut is functional, and by that is meant the small intestine, then a number of approaches are possible. These include sip feeding, fine bore nasogastric feeding, fine bore naso-enteric feeding or fine bore jejunostomy feeding. The wherewithal to deliver enteral feeding has improved dramatically in the past 10 years (Lee, 1988d; Russell 1986; Tandon, 1986). There are now comprehensive lists of preparations available (ACBS approved) and all of these can be administered by a fine bore tube. Most District General Hospitals have a specialist nurse who can insert fine bore tubes, although this should be well within the remit of junior medical hospital staff. The container for delivery of comprehensive nutrition may be 1 litre or 1.5 litre size plastic triangular receptacle, bottle or simple cannister. The fine bore tubes may be left *in situ* for up to 1 month. These are well tolerated by patients and, what is more, allows them to return home earlier than hitherto. The amount of monitoring with enteral nutrition is much less than with parenteral nutrition and, of course, the complications with respect to the 'access site' are naturally far less. Nevertheless, the indications for enteral nutrition are no less serious than those for parenteral nutrition. The same initial assessments are required and, to a more or less degree, the same monitoring. Overall, metabolic complications are infrequent with enteral nutrition and there are very few access site complications.

CONCLUSION

There can no be longer be any justification for a patient in hospital to experience 'starvation in the midst of plenty'. The methods for TPN and EN have now been dramatically rationalized, are safe and capable of easy monitoring. It is no longer tenable for any clinician to say he could not feed his patient because (a) the wherewithal was not available (b) the technique is too complicated or (c) the complication rate not merited. It is my unreserved view that all patients requiring nutritional support in hospital, provided they are recognized early, can be maintained by some method of nutritional delivery programme.

REFERENCES

Burgert S.L., Anderson C.F. (1979). An evaluation of upper arm measurements used in nutritional assessment. *Am. J. Clin. Nutr.*, **32**, 2136.

Copeland E.M., Dudrick S.J., Daly J.M., et al. (1983). Nutritional changes in neoplasia. In *Surgical Nutrition*, Chap. 15, pp. 515–534. (Fischer J.M. ed.). Boston, Toronto: Little, Brown & Company.

Crossley L.R., Williams R. (1986). Nutrition in liver failure. In *Proceedings of the XIII International Congress of Nutrition, pp. 663–665*. (Taylor T.G., Jenkins N.K. eds.) London: John Libbey.

Dahn M.S., Kirkpatrick J.R., Blasier R. (1984). Alterations in the metabolism of exogenous lipid associated with sepsis. *J. Parent. Ent. Nutr.*, **8**, 169.

Daly J.M., Dudrick S.J. (1981). Results of intravenous nutrition in cancer patients. In *Clinical Surgery International 2. Nutrition and the Surgical Patient*. Chap. 12, pp. 191–196. (Hill G.L. ed.). Edinburgh: Churchill Livingstone.

Frayn K.N. (1987). Fuel metabolism during sepsis and injury. *Intensive Ther. Clin. Monitor.* **8**, 174.

Freund H.R., Fischer J.E. (1981). Hepatic failure. In *Clinical Surgery International 2. Nutrition of the Surgical Patient*. Chap. 13, pp. 201–218. (Hill G.L. ed.). Edinburgh: Churchill Livingstone.

Goodinson S.M., Dickerson J.W.T. (1988). Assessment of nutritional status. In *Nutrition in the Clinical Management of Disease*. 2nd edn. (Dickerson J.W.T., Lee H.A. eds.). Chap. 21, pp 456–485. London: Edward Arnold.

Hopkinson R., Davis A. (1987). A guide to parenteral feeding. *Care Crit. Ill.*, **3**, 64.

Jackson J.M., Khawaja H.T., Weaver P.C., et al. (1984). Naftidrofuryl and the nitrogen, carbohydrate and lipid responses to moderate surgery. *Br. Med. J.*, **289**, 581.

Lee H.A. (1986a). Practical aspects of intravenous feeding. In *Clinical Nutrition in Gastroenterology*. Chap. 6, pp. 85–96. (Heatley R.V., Losowsky M.S., Kelleher J. eds.). Edinburgh: Churchill Livingstone.

Lee H.A. (1986b). Problems of nutrition in cancer patients. In *Head and Neck Oncology*, pp. 279–284. (Bloom H.J.G., Hanham I.W.F. eds.). Raven Press.

Lee H.A. (1986c). An overall view of nutrition in organ failure. In *Proceedings of the XIII International Congress of Nutrition*, pp. 674–677. (Taylor T.G., Jenkins N.K. eds.). London: John Libbey.

Lee H.A. (1987). Paediatric HTPN—a facility in need of rationalization. *Intensive Ther. Clin. Monitor.*, **8**, 194.

Lee H.A. (1988a). Fluid balance and parenteral feeding. In *General Anaesthesia*. 5th edn. Chap. 101, pp. 89–110. (Nunn J.F., Utting J.E., Brown B.R. eds.). London: Butterworth Scientific.

Lee H.A. (1988b). Parenteral Nutrition. In *Nutrition in the Clinical Management of Disease*. 2nd edn. Chap. 23, pp. 496–511. (Dickerson J.W.T., Lee H.A. eds.). London: Edward Arnold.

Lee H.A. (1988c). The nutritional management of renal disease. In *Nutrition in the Clinical Management of Disease*, 2nd edn. Chap. 12, pp. 262–279. (Dickerson J.W.T., Lee H.A. eds.). London: Edward Arnold.

Lee H.A. (1988d). Enteral feeds. In *Nutrition in the Clinical Management of Disease*, 2nd edn. Chap. 22, pp. 486–495. (Dickerson J.W.T., Lee H.A. eds.). London: Edward Arnold.

Lee H.A., Talbot S.T. (in press). Nutrition in renal failure. *Nutr. Res: Rev.*

Macfie J., Smith R.C., Hill G.L. (1981). Glucose or fat as a non-protein energy source? A controlled clinical trial. *Gastroenterology*, **80**, 103.

McEntee G.P., Moran K., Duignan J.P., et al. (1986). Monitoring nitrogen losses in parenteral nutrition. *Parenteral Ther.*, **7**, 124.

Nanni G., Siegel J.H., Coleman B., et al. (1984). Increased lipid fuel dependence in the critically ill septic patient. *J. Trauma.*, **24**, 14.

Neale G., Elia M. (1986). Nutritional assessment. In *Clinical Nutrition in Gastroenterology*. Chap. 4, pp. 48–71. (Heatley R.V., Losowsky M.S., Kelleher eds.). Edinburgh: Churchill Livingstone.

Rossi-Fanelli R., Riggio O., Cengiano C., et al. (1982). Branched amino acids *vs* lactulose in the treatment of hepatic coma. A controlled study. *Dig. Dis. Sci.*, **27**, 929.

Roulet M., Detsky A.S., Marliss E.B., et al. (1983). A controlled trial of the effect of parenteral nutritional support on patients with respiratory failure and sepsis. *Clin. Nutr.*, **2**, 97.

Russell R.I. (1986). Enteral feeding. In *Clinical Nutrition in Gastroenterology*. Chap 7, pp. 97–114. (Heatley R.V., Losowsky M.S., Kelleher J. eds.). Edinburgh: Churchill Livingstone.

Shenkin A. (1986) A comparison of the enteral and parenteral provision of micronutrients. In *Proceedings of the XIII International Congress of Nutrition*, pp. 677–680. (Taylor T.G., Jenkins N.K.). London: John Libbey.

Shenkin A. (1987). Essential trace elements during intravenous nutrition. *Intensive Ther. Clin. Monitor.*, **8**, 38.

Tandon R.K. (1986). Nutritional support in pancreatic failure. In *Proceedings of the XIII International Congress of Nutrition*. pp. 669–671. (Taylor T.G., Jenkins N.K. eds.). London: John Libbey.

Yule A.G. (1981). Results of intravenous nutrition in gastroenterological patients. In *Clinical Surgery International 2. Nutrition and the Surgical Patient*. Chap. 12, pp. 196–201. (Hill G.L. ed.). Edinburgh: Churchill Livingstone.

FURTHER READING

Grant A., Todd E. eds. (1982). *Enteral and Patenteral Nutrition: A Clinical Handbook*. Oxford: Blackwell Scientific Publications.

Howard A., McLean Baird I. eds. (1983). *Advances in Clinical Nutrition*. London: John Libbey.

Johnston I.D.A. ed. (1983). *Advances in Clinical Nutrition*. Lancaster: M.T.P. Press Ltd.

Sherwood Jones E. ed. (1982). *Intensive Care*. Lancaster: M.T.P. Press Ltd.

Weinsier R.L., Butterworth C.E. (1981). *Handbook of Clinical Nutrition*. London: C.V. Mosby Company.

33. Cellular Metabolism
N. Soni

Energetics
ATP
   Mechanisms of ATP production
The mitochondrion
Pathways
   Catabolism
   Carbohydrates
   Oxidation of fat
   Amino acids
   Tricarboxylic cycle
   Lactic acidosis; lactic accumulation,
     anaerobic respiration and acidosis
   Respiratory quotient
Regulation of metabolism
   Calcium/calmodulin messenger system
   Cyclic AMP system
   Protein kinase C
Energy and exercise
   Anaerobic threshold
Ischaemia and cell death
   The role of calcium
   Oxygen free radical formation
   Excitotoxic damage
   Reperfusion injury
   Conclusion

While a certain knowledge of the metabolic pathways has been a requisite part of anaesthetic training, recent developments in the understanding of the pathophysiology of conditions such as ischaemia or septic shock, have given these pathways a more immediate clinical relevance.

The term 'cellular metabolism' refers to the wide range of enzymatic reactions occurring within a cell. These reactions are not isolated events, but are part of an integrated, purposeful mechanism that results in the cell being a functional unit. Each such metabolic unit has three main categories of activity. The first is the breakdown of various substrates to provide a convenient energy source. The second is the production of building materials from substrate sources either by breaking them down or by converting them into suitable forms. The third activity is the integration of the substrates and building materials into both small and large molecules required both for cellular function and for growth of the cell and of the organism-biosynthesis. This somewhat simplistic overview encompasses all the catabolic, anabolic and conversion functions of 'metabolism'. This chapter will concentrate on the production of usable energy within the cell. This is achieved by the formation of high energy phosphate bonds. The feedback mechanisms which regulate the production of these high energy bonds and the pathways through which they are produced are considered as part of a homeostatic mechanism to sustain adequate energy levels in the cell (Fig. 33.1).

ENERGETICS

In discussing the activities involved in cellular metabolism, it is important to be aware of the basic concepts of bio-energetics. During cell metabolism, energy production and utilization is a dynamic process. The first law of thermodynamics states that energy is neither created nor destroyed so during a

EXOGENOUS SUBSTRATES / DIET

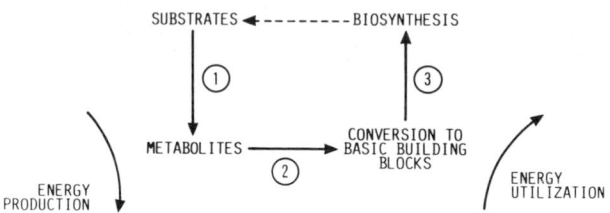

Fig. 33.1 Cellular metabolism. 1 = substrates used to produce energy. 2 = metabolites converted to usable building blocks. 3 = building blocks used to synthesize larger molecules (biosynthesis). These complex molecules can, if necessary be used to produce energy.

chemical reaction the total energy at the end of the reaction must be the same as at the beginning. Looking at this in simple terms, it can be seen that the sum of the energy contents of the products and the energy released in other forms should be equal to that of the reactants. The difference between energy of the reactants and the products is termed the free energy change of the reaction— ΔG.

ΔG = free energy of products − free energy of
reactants.

In the context of cellular metabolism, this free energy can then be used to perform work or can be released in the form of heat. For example, the chemical reactions in the oxidation of glucose result in an energy difference of 680 kcal/mol between the reactants and the products. This is the free energy change, ΔG and, if collected, this energy can be used for energy-requiring cell functions. Catabolism, or the breakdown of substrates, results in the production of a large amount of free energy. A series of enzymatic reactions are used as a means of harnessing and temporarily storing this free energy by producing high energy phosphate bonds. The term, high energy bond, refers to the free energy held in the reactant which is released or made available when for example ATP becomes ADP during a reaction.

ADENOSINE TRIPHOSPHATE (ATP)

ATP is found throughout the animal and plant kingdom. Plants use light as the source of free energy which can be harnessed to produce ATP, while in the animal kingdom it is the free energy produced by the breakdown of substrates that is incorporated for ATP production. ATP is a nucleotide that consists of molecules of adenine, ribose and three phosphate groups. To form ATP from ADP requires the attachment of the third phosphate and this requires an energy input of 15 kcal/mol for the reaction to proceed. Conversely, when ATP becomes ADP there is a significant release of free energy (approx. 12 kcal/mol). It is this free energy which is utilized in order that other reac-

tions in the cell can proceed. In the cell, ATP and ADP exist in equilibrium, dependent on the rate of production and utilization of ATP.

Actual production of ATP occurs in several sites and by several different mechanisms. ATP is formed from glycolysis, from oxidative phosphorylation, from creatine phosphate utilization and myokinase activity. Glycolysis, creatine phosphate hydrolysis and myokinase all occur in the cytoplasm and produce ATP. Oxidative phosphorylation and, to some extent, creatine phosphate hydrolysis occur in the mitochondria. These are the main sites for ATP production, and in aerobic cells approximately 90% of all ATP production occurs in the mitochondria. Erythrocytes are an exception, as there are no mitochondria, and all energy production takes place in the cytoplasm.

Mechanisms of ATP Production

The first two mechanisms to consider are glycolysis and oxidative phosphorylation. Glucose is converted to pyruvate with limited ATP production (2 ATP). The pyruvate can then enter the tricarboxylic cycle or be converted to lactate. Under anaerobic conditions, ATP is produced by the breakdown of glucose through to lactate but, in the presence of oxygen, the pyruvate and lactate can enter the tricarboxylic acid cycle and utilize oxidative phosphorylation with a much higher yield of ATP (38 ATP/glucose). This is also the common end-pathway for other substrates, such as fats and amino acids. The mechanism by which oxidative phosphorylation can produce molecules of ATP will be considered in more detail below, but the result is to produce a significantly larger yield of ATP than can be produced under anaerobic conditions.

At least two further mechanisms should also be considered. The first is in muscle, which may require large quantities of energy rapidly. There is a mechanism within the cytoplasm for the rapid production of ATP. This is the so-called creatine/creatine phosphate energy shuttle. This mechanism which occurs in muscle, heart and brain cells uses a high energy phosphate bond formed in creatine phosphate which can be 'stored' in the cytoplasm. Under situations where the ADP concentration rises, a reaction can occur where a phosphate bond is donated to the ADP from the creatine phosphate resulting in the formation of new ATP. This is not a new source of ATP, but merely a storage mechanism; this will be discussed below. The other mechanism of note is the ability of ATP to be produced from ADP in the presence of myokinase. This involves the reaction of two molecules of ADP to produce one molecule of ATP and one molecule of AMP. This reaction results in the formation of one molecule with a higher energy bond and one with a lower energy bond. (Hochachka, 1985). Two of these mechanisms will be discussed in more detail.

Creatine/Creatine Phosphate Shuttle

The amount of ATP in a cell at any particular time is not enough to act as a significant energy store and may be rapidly depleted if the demand is too large, as may occur in muscle cells during exercise. Creatine phosphate is a means by which high energy bonds are stored in the cytoplasm and can be used to produce ATP rapidly. Creatine phosphate is formed in the mitochondrion and then moved to the cytoplasm.

The association of creatine phosphokinase with the enzyme ATPase allows the rapid production of ATP at the site of its utilization. This is achieved by the ADP present reacting with the creatine phosphate to produce ATP and creatine. The reaction is mediated by cytosolic creatine kinase. The main substrate is ADP, which increases rapidly as ATP is utilized and the rising concentration of ADP encourages further formation of ATP. Creatine phosphokinase isoenzymes are found in the cytosol of muscle, heart and brain. The isoenzymes are also found in the mitochondria where their function is the manufacture of creatine phosphate using ATP and creatine. A feedback mechanism operates whereby the rate of formation of creatine phosphate increases as free creatine increases. The resultant creatine phosphate can move easily by shuttle to its site of utilization. The shuttle serves as a store, a messenger system and a transport mechanism for intracellular energy (Bessman and Carpenter, 1985).

Oxidative Phosphorylation and the Respiratory Chain

This is the intramitochondrial mechanism by which the majority of ATP is produced under aerobic conditions. It is the common endpoint for most metabolic pathways.

As substrates are metabolized through the various pathways redox reactions occur. In these reactions, the electrons are transferred from the electron donor (reducing agents) to an electron acceptor (oxidizing agents). Generally, this is done by the transfer of hydrogen, usually in a dehydrogenase reaction. This occurs at a number of sites in the pathway. At each of these sites, there are one of four groups of electron carriers which can bind the free hydrogen atoms. These are the pyridine linked dehydrogenases (NAD and NADP co-enzymes), flavin linked dehydrogenases (FAD and FMN), iron/sulphur proteins and cytochromes. This type of reaction can be demonstrated by NAD^+.

If NAD^+ binds with one hydrogen molecule then as one of the electrons neutralizes the charge on NAD^+, the proton and the other electron bind to the molecule to produce NADH, which is uncharged leaving one proton H^+. This molecule, NADH, is acting as an electron carrier.

$$NAD^+ + H_2 \rightarrow NADH + H^+$$

(2 electrons in the NADH)

The purpose of the carrier molecule is to transport these electrons/protons to the respiratory chain. The respiratory chain consists of an arrangement of molecules within the inner mitochondrial membrane along which the electrons pass (Fig. 33.2).

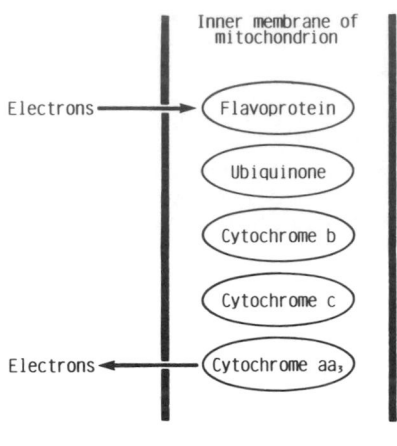

RESPIRATORY CHAIN:

Fig. 33.2 The respiratory chain. Electrons pass along a series of carrier molecules producing a 'current'.

The overall reaction which occurs along the chain is the reduction of oxygen to water. This liberates a large quantity of free energy. The series of reactions occurring in the chain serve to harness the release of energy at each step in the chain, so that ATP can be produced.

The mechanism by which this is believed to occur is termed the chemiosmotic theory of respiration. In the respiratory chain there is a series of carefully arranged molecules which have the ability to accept and transfer electrons. The electrons appear to have a cyclical pathway in the chain passing outwards across the inner membrane and then back to the inner surface again. The flux of electrons through the respiratory chain produces an electric current, or energy, which is then used to allow hydrogen ions to move across the membrane (translocate) via specific carrier molecules in the chain. This facilitates the movement of hydrogen ions from inside the matrix of the mitochondria across the inner membrane, and produces an electrochemical gradient, associated with a decreasing pH on one side of the membrane and an increasing pH on the other. The electron transfer can be seen as a form of 'pump' across the membrane creating a gradient. The electrochemical gradient created allows the movement of hydrogen back down this gradient and this ion transfer releases energy which is then linked by a molecule called F_1-F_0 ATPase complex to the production of ATP. Therefore, the number of ATP molecules produced is dependent on the number of protons translocated. It should be emphasized that the specific mechanisms involved in these reactions are complex and still require further elucidation (Mitchell, 1974; Hatefi, 1985) (Fig. 33.3).

There are several different types of electron carrier which are found at the various sites in the metabolic pathways. These carriers, which collect the protons and electrons being produced, have different values when they are presented to the respiratory chain. NADH is able to produce three molecules of ATP as its electrons pass through the chain, but $FADH_2$, which is a similar molecule, results in the production of only two molecules of ATP. This is in part because it enters the respiratory chain at a different point from NADH. The third carrier molecule is NADPH. It consists of an NADH and an additional phosphate bond so that the actual value of NADPH, in terms of molecules of ATP which can be produced, is four. Structurally, there is little difference from NADH but, in fact, while NADH is largely concerned in the pathways associated with degradative metabolism, NADPH is predominantly found in those pathways which link metabolic degradation to biosynthetic systems.

In this section, we have seen how the respiratory chain can be used to generate an electrochemical gradient by the movement of protons from inside the mitochondrion outwards across the inner membrane. This outward movement of protons or proton trans-

location is an energy-yielding reaction in that potential energy is held by the gradient. As the protons flow down the gradient back into the inner mitochondrion this energy is coupled to the production of ATP by the F_1-F_0 ATPase complex.

This occurs in the mitochondrion and is isolated from the cytoplasm. The structure and function of the mitochondrion should be considered in more detail.

THE MITOCHONDRION

Mitrochondria are the power houses of the cell. It is here that oxidative phosphorylation, which is the most efficient form of energy production available within the cell, takes place. As the centres which produce ATP, the mitochondria are often to be found located close to the sites which use ATP most frequently. However, they may also be found closely associated with sites at which substrates are stored. They essentially consist of two membranes, the inner one being convoluted with a large number of folds called cristae. The inner membrane is the site of the respiratory chain and is intimately involved with oxidative phosphorylation. The outer membrane, in contact with the cytoplasm, contains a number of enzymes some of which are involved with producing the substrates for use in the metabolic pathways

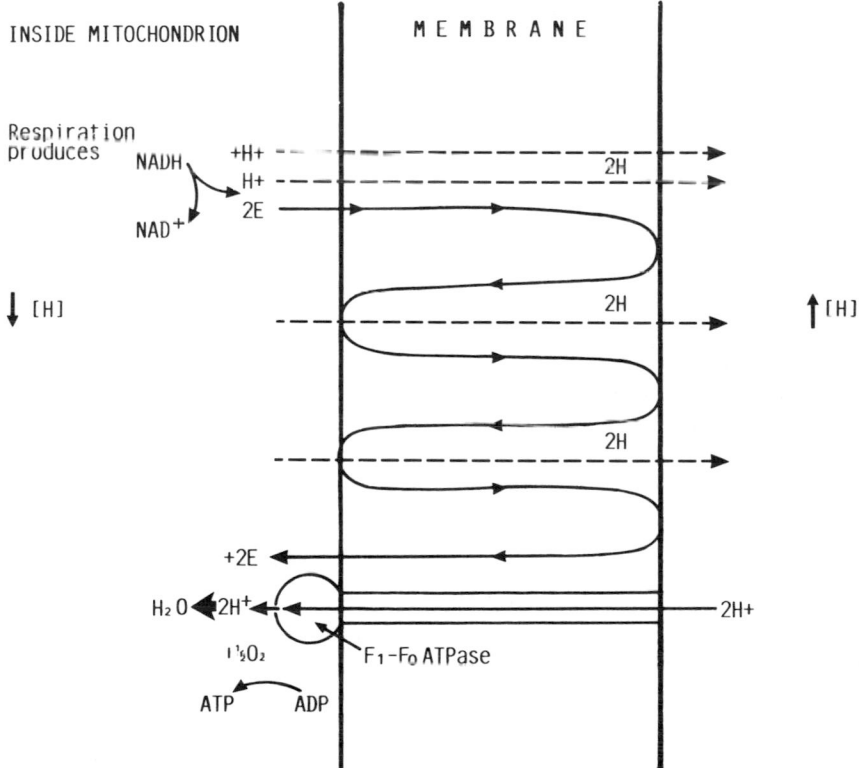

Fig. 33.3 The respiratory chain functionally uses the current to extrude protons and thereby generate a gradient across the membrane. Each pair of protons then pass back down the gradient via F_1–F_0 ATPase to produce ATP.

within the mitochondria. These pathways themselves are often situated in the matrix within the mitochondria. For the mitochondria to function under normal conditions, with the membranes separating the inner contents from the cytoplasm, there obviously have to be mechanisms by which various substrates can pass across the membranes into the matrix. These have been termed translocation systems. For ATP to be formed, it is essential that phosphate can pass into the mitochondria. This translocation is effected by the use of the energy from the proton gradient which occurs in the mitochondria. The phosphate carrier system is also linked to systems which allow other molecules to exchange across the membrane. Examples of this would be the exchange of dicarboxylates (malate, fumarate) or the exchange of isocitrate and citrate.

While the substrates obviously need a system by which they can be transported into the mitochondrion, it is also important to consider that the reducing equivalents formed inside the mitochondrion may also be required for metabolic functions outside. There are appropriate mechanisms by which NADH, for example, can be transported across the mitochondrial membrane. Similarly, excess reducing equivalents produced in the cytosol can be moved into the mitochondrion by carriers in specific shuttle systems.

PATHWAYS

In the preceding sections, the concept of energetics, the way in which ATP is used as an energy unit and the mechanism by which it is produced have been discussed. In the following section, the actual pathways through which substrates are metabolized are described. It is essential to try to view each individual pathway as part of an integrated system, the purpose of which is the formation of usable energy.

Catabolism

In general terms, catabolism can be considered as a break-down of dietary components to very specific substrates which can be used in the cellular pathways to produce energy. The three main types of substrate are proteins, polysaccharides and lipids. These are broken down in the gastrointestinal tract or elsewhere into amino acids, hexoses and pentoses, fatty acids and glycerols. The polysaccharides proceed via glycolysis to pyruvate and then either enter the tricarboxylic cycle (TCA) or are metabolized to lactate. Lactate can enter the TCA cycle easily. Fatty acids are metabolized to acetyl CoA and thence to the TCA cycle. Amino acids feed into the TCA cycle at various sites. Consequently there is, in effect, an end common pathway in the presence of oxygen (Fig. 33.4).

Carbohydrates

Glucose can be utilized readily by cells. There are two pathways, glycolysis and the hexose monophosphate

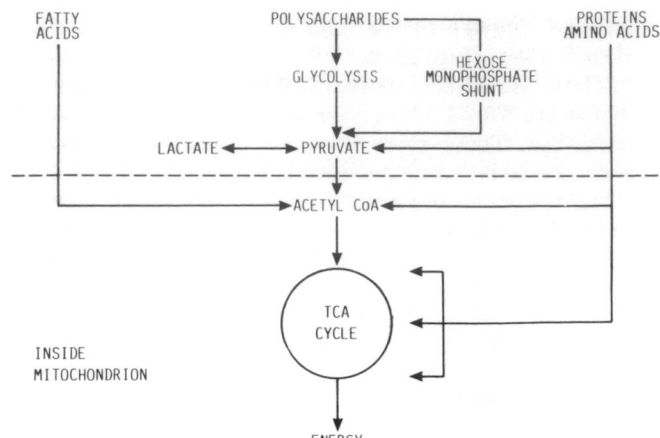

Fig. 33.4 The metabolic pathways. A common pathway inside the mitochondria.

shunt. Glycolysis describes the pathway from glucose to pyruvate/lactate although, for completeness, the production of glucose from glycogen is included. Three regulatory enzymes are mentioned: *Hexokinase* primes glycolysis which is inhibited by glucose-6-phosphate; *Phosphofructokinase* is stimulated by ADP, AMP and inhibited by ATP; *Pyruvate kinase* which is inhibited by other substrates like fatty acids. These three regulate the activity of the glycolysis pathway (Fig. 33.5).

$$\text{Glucose} \dashrightarrow \rightarrow \relbar\joinrel\relbar \text{pyruvate} + 2\,\text{ATP}\,(+2\,\text{NADH})$$
$$\text{Pyruvate} \dashrightarrow \rightarrow \relbar\joinrel\relbar \text{lactate} \qquad (-2\,\text{NADH})$$

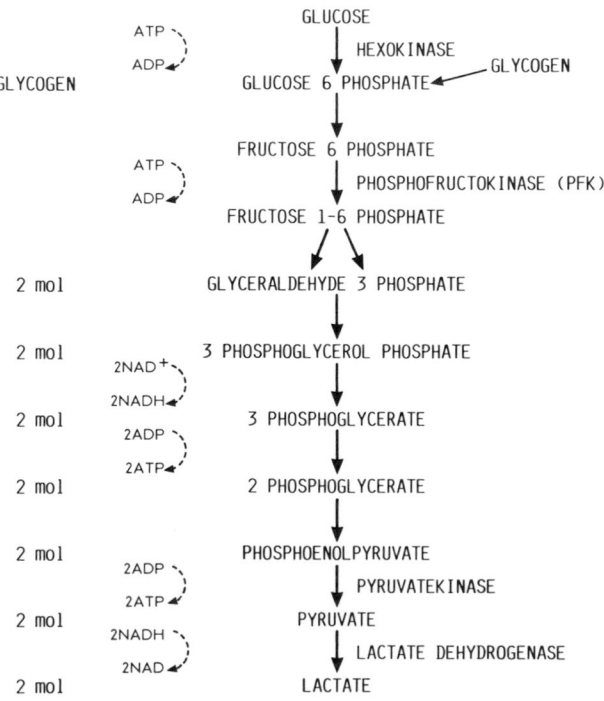

Fig. 33.5 Glycolysis. Note 1 molecule of glucose forms 2 molecules of glyceraldehyde-3-phosphate and hence 2 molecules of lactate.

Hexose Monophosphate Shunt

The hexose monophosphate shunt is the alternative extramitochondrial oxidative pathway. This pathway is found where the cell is involved in synthesizing activities, specifically fat and steroid synthesis, and is used to generate NADPH in the cytoplasm. It can also be used to convert pentoses to hexoses for glycolysis or vice versa for the production of nucleic acids. The production of cytoplasmic NADPH is of particular significance in erythrocytes. NADPH acts as a reducing agent to maintain glutathione in a reduced state. This is important in minimizing the oxidation of haemoglobin to methaemoglobin by oxidizing agents such as hydrogen peroxide which may be formed during oxygen transport.

Oxidation of Fat

There are large fat stores in the body. Fatty acids from these stores are transported attached to albumin and are absorbed into the cell. In the cytoplasm the fatty acid is esterified with CoA to produce fatty acyl CoA (a reaction which requires ATP). Fatty acyl CoA then binds to carnitine, a carrier molecule in the mitochondrial membrane, which transports the acyl group across the membrane. Once in the mitochondrion, the carnitine is displaced by intramitochondrial CoA producing acyl CoA which can then be oxidized, (acyl is RC=0).

Free Fatty Acid (FFA) + CoA + ATP →
$\qquad$ → acyl CoA + ADP $\qquad$ (cytoplasm)
Acyl CoA + carnitine → acyl carnitine
$\qquad$ (mitochondrial membrane)
Acyl carnitine + CoA → acyl CoA + carnitine
$\qquad$ (intramitochondrial)

The acyl CoA is then oxidized. Each reaction results in the splitting off of two carbon atoms as acetyl CoA and the production of one $FADH_2$ (2 ATP) and one NADH (3 ATP). The acetyl CoA enters the citric acid cycle while the residual acyl CoA recycles through the reaction (Fig. 33.6).

The remaining acyl CoA can recycle through the same pathway producing one acetyl CoA molecule for each cycle, which can then pass through the tricarboxylic cycle. Each cycle also produces one $FADH_2$ and one NADH which can be used to produce ATP ($FADH_2$ → 2 ATP, ADH → 3 ATP)

For example:
a 16 carbon fatty acid being oxidized will produce 8 acetyl CoA and 7 $FADH_2$ and 7 NADH.

The 8 acetyl CoA produce 96 ATP via the TCA cycle.

Total energy production in the mitochondrion is 131 ATP but 2 ATP are required in the cytoplasm to activate the fatty acid so net production is 129 ATP.

In this oxidation a total of 23 molecules of O_2 are used and produce 16 molecules of CO_2. This gives a respiratory quotient of about 0.7.

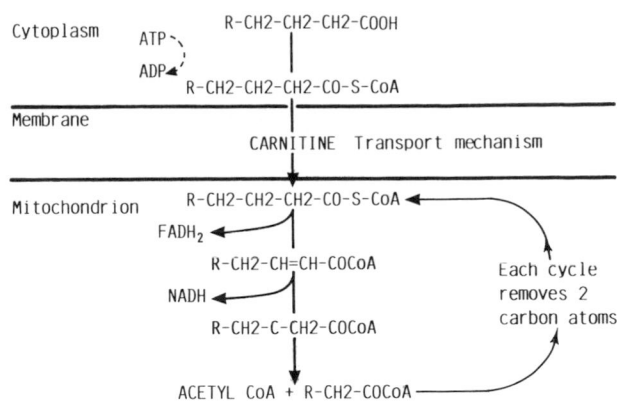

Fig. 33.6 Fat metabolism. Each cycle removes two carbon atoms. R value falls by 2 carbons.

Ketone Bodies

If large amounts of fat are oxidized the rate of production of acetyl CoA will increase. The TCA cycle utilizes acetyl CoA in combination with oxaloacetic acid. If there is a shortage of glucose, and therefore a relative deficiency of oxaloacetic acid, a relative excess of acetyl CoA will arise. The excess acetyl CoA is then diverted to form ketone bodies in the liver mitochondria.

Acetyl CoA + acetyl CoA + H_2O → acetoacetate
Acetoacetate + NADH + H → B-hydroxybutyrate

The ketone bodies can diffuse out of the mitochondria and into the bloodstream. In the peripheral tissues and more especially the brain, these can be converted to acetyl CoA and be utilized in the TCA cycle. This is of use in some situations where the supply of intracellular glucose may be limited. These include starvation and carbohydrate free diets and, in these circumstances, energy production can be maintained using the ketones. In diabetes there is a lack of intracellular glucose and excessive production of ketone bodies occurs.

It is important to remember that carbohydrate can be converted to fat, but fat cannot form glucose.

Amino Acids

Protein absorbed by the body can be used in a variety of ways. It can be broken down to amino acids to be reassimilated as protein, used as a nitrogen source for a wide range of molecules, e.g. nucleic acids, cytochromes or haem, or can be metabolized through the tricarboxylic cycle. The amino acids can enter the cycle at several sites, (Fig. 33.7). This occurs when normal glucose stores are depleted. There is always a requirement for glucose and as fats cannot be converted to glucose, the only source available is from the amino acid pool. The amino acids are metabolized in a variety of ways. Some, such as aspartic acid or glutamic acid, are 'glucogenic' as glucose can be pro-

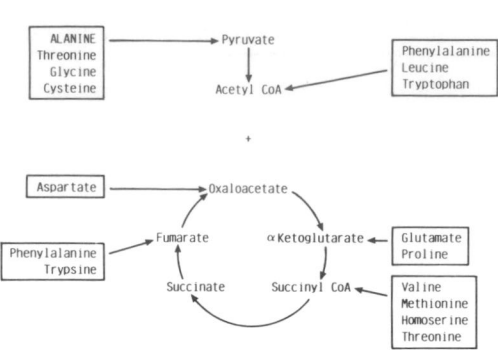

Fig. 33.7 Amino acid metabolism.

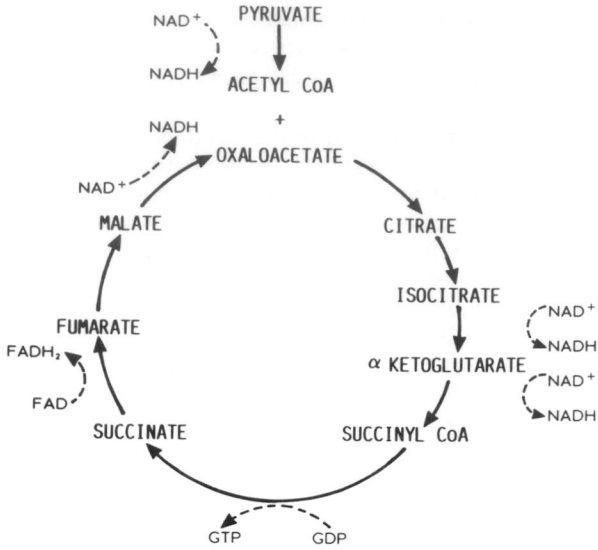

Fig. 33.8 The tricarboxylic acid cycle.

duced. This is because their metabolic pathway ends at pyruvate which can be used as a glucose substrate while others, like leucine, yield only acetyl CoA which can be used to produce ketones but not glucose, and are 'ketogenic', i.e. Pathways to pyruvate are glucogenic; pathways to acetyl CoA are ketogenic.

Tricarboxylic Cycle (TCA)

As can be seen from the pathways described, there is a final common pathway for glucose, fats and amino acids. Glycolysis can only liberate a small part of the available energy in glucose during metabolism to lactate. Total conversion to CO_2 and H_2O through the TCA cycle results in a far greater yield, provided there is adequate oxygen. This cycle occurs in the inner compartment of the mitochondrion.

The TCA cycle and ATP production by the respiratory chain are both oxygen dependent. During one cycle 3 NADH, 1 $FADH_2$ and 1 GTP are formed. The NADH and $FADH_2$ are coupled to ATP production through the respiratory chain (Fig. 33.8).

The overall reaction is:

$$Pyruvate + O_2 \rightarrow CO_2 + H_2O + 4\,NADH + FADH_2 + GTP$$

The value of the reaction in terms of ATP equivalents formed:

4 NADH is equivalent to 12 ATP;
1 $FADH_2$ is equivalent to 2 ATP
GTP is an ATP equivalent.
A total of 15 ATP equivalents.

Lactic Acidosis; Lactate Accumulation; Anaerobic Respiration and Acidosis

Lactic acidosis is often thought to be a consequence of anaerobic respiration and it may well be indirectly; but it is worth considering how the acidosis develops.

In aerobic respiration there is a net utilization of H^+ ions, as glucose is used to produce ATP.

$$Glucose + [38\,MgADP] + [38\,Pi] + 6O_2 + 30.4H^+ \rightarrow [38\,MgATP] + 6CO_2 + 44H_2O$$

i.e. hydrogen ions are, in fact, used at a rate of approximately 0.8 H^+ per ATP produced, and as ATP is hydrolyzed hydrogen ions are produced at a rate of 0.8 H^+ per ATP. Therefore, if respiration matches the hydrolysis of ATP, there is no net increase in hydrogen ions (Busa and Nuccitelli, 1984).

Anaerobic respiration does not produce hydrogen ions in the production, through metabolism, of lactate, nor is there utilization of hydrogen ions.

$$glucose + 2\,ADP + 2\,Pi \rightarrow 2\,ATP + 2\,lactate + 2\,H_2O$$

However, when ATP is hydrolyzed to ADP the result is the production of H^+:

$$ATP + H_2O \rightarrow ADP + Pi + H^+$$
(One hydrogen/ATP hydrolyzed)

In anaerobic respiration the net result of coupled respiration and ATP hydrolysis is:

$$glucose \rightarrow 2\,lactate + 2\,ATP \rightarrow 2\,ADP + 2H^+ + 2\,Pi + 2\,lactate$$

i.e. the production of hydrogen ions.

This is not lactic acid, but the production of lactate, a versatile substrate; and hydrogen ions. These may well associate to produce lactic acid, but it is conceptually different from lactic acid production. In the presence of oxygen, the lactate can be rapidly utilized in the TCA cycle and the hydrogen ions assimilated in the production of ATP (Mizock, 1987).

In a variety of aerobic circumstances the coupling of respiration and ATP hydrolysis may not be 1:1. If ATP is being rapidly utilized there may be a rapid accumulation of hydrogen ions. Therefore, even with aerobic respiration, an acidosis could develop if ATP hydrolysis is occurring faster than ATP production (Busa and Nuccitelli, 1984).

'Lactic acidosis' is often monitored in clinical practice. Several biochemical parameters can be measured. These include the serum lactate and also the lactate/pyruvate (L/P) ratio. This may be misleading, as the presence of lactate does not necessarily indicate an acidosis. The serum lactate is an end point measurement of lactate metabolism and is the balance of production, both normal and abnormal, and utilization. Similarly, the L/P ratio is an indicator of the amount of anaerobic metabolism occurring, but again as multiple variants affect both lactate and pyruvate concentration, the value derived needs careful interpretation.

Respiratory Quotient

This is the ratio of CO_2 produced to oxygen consumed per unit time. The different substrates each have different RQs. If the oxygen uptake can be accurately measured and also CO_2 production, then an estimate of which substrate is being used can be made. Difficulties arise for several reasons. It is difficult to accurately measure gas utilization or production in the clinical setting, although this can now be achieved. A steady state is needed as a period of increased CO_2 production, acidosis or alkalosis can all alter the value. The most important consideration is that it is an end point determination dependent on several sources. While catabolism of fat, sugar and amino acid are all represented, so are fat synthesis and other anabolic processes. Interpretation of the final RQ must be made very cautiously. (Normal values; glucose 1.0, fat 0.7, amino acid 0.8.)

REGULATION OF METABOLISM

Cellular metabolism is controlled at many levels, but three specific areas can be considered. Substrates and metabolites within the cell, regulatory enzymes in the metabolic pathways and exogenous influences, such as hormones, acting on the cell surface—all interact to regulate cell function.

Substrate availability, pH, ATP/ADP ratio and the presence of oxygen all influence metabolism. In various circumstances the type of substrate available to the cell may alter and this may then result in an activation of a pathway. An example of this occurs in spermatozoa, where, in some species, the addition of lactate or pyruvate to the environment results in increased respiration in the cells (Halangk et al., 1985). Similarly, the oxidation of lactate may be inhibited in the presence of fatty acids and, in this situation, gluconeogenesis is enhanced (Mandel, 1985).

pH appears to have marked importance, and small changes in pH can affect the cell in a number of ways. These include interaction with calcium binding to calmodulin, which results in modification of this second messenger system. The function of cyclic AMP may be affected as there is also a local influence on enzyme activity within the metabolic pathway. As the intracellular pH is not constant and reflects the balance between hydrogen ion utilization and production, which is dependent on the metabolic state of the cell, a role for pH in regulation of metabolism would be expected (Busa et al., 1984).

ADP is a 'metabolite' which, as its concentration rises, reflects increased utilization of ATP. This rise is usually accompanied by a fall in ATP concentration and, therefore, the ratio of ADP/ATP indicates the energy status of the cell. This ratio influences several of the pathways. An increase in ADP stimulates ATP production by both glycolysis (phosphofructokinase activity) and oxidative phosphorylation while, if there is excess ATP, then the rate limiting enzymes in the glycolytic pathway are inhibited. This helps to maintain a steady state of ATP availability and is a 'feedback system'.

The availability of oxygen also influences the production of energy, but has little effect on ATP utilization. Oxidative phosphorylation decreases at low oxygen tension and this is probably due to the sensitivity of cytochrome c oxidase, within the respiratory chain, to hypoxia. As oxygen tension falls and cytochrome c becomes reduced and non-functional, the production of ATP by oxidative phosphorylation decreases and the ADP/ATP ratio increases. This stimulates ATP production, but by other pathways (Wilson and Erecinska, 1986).

The role of the regulatory enzymes within the pathways must be considered. This includes the rise of ADP activating both phosphofructokinase and pyruvate kinase which stimulates glycolysis. Similarly, ADP activates isofructokinase in the TCA cycle increasing the rate at which oxidative phosphorylation progresses under aerobic conditions.

Metabolism is also affected by exogenous influences, such as hormones. These usually act via second messengers. Three intracellular mechanisms are of particular importance. Cyclic AMP and calcium/calmodulin are both mechanisms by which hormones exert short-acting effects in the cell, while calcium activated protein kinase probably has a similar mechanism of action, but produces protracted effects. These processes will be discussed in more detail below.

It is important to realize that all these mechanisms interact. For example, a change in pH influences free cytosolic calcium and subsequent binding to calmodulin. It may also influence the cyclic AMP system as well as affecting various enzyme activities, thereby modulating intracellular metabolism. While each 'feedback' system may be relatively simple, their dynamic interaction is complex.

Calcium-Calmodulin Messenger System

Extrinsic control of the cell is mediated by hormones which act on surface receptors and trigger a secondary messenger system in the cell. Among other functions, the calcium messenger is intimately involved in the control of glycogenolysis. A hormone, e.g. adrenaline, acts on the surface of the cell and the membrane generates inositol 1, 4, 5, triphosphate via phospholipase C. This induces the release of Ca^{2+} from the endoplasmic reticulum. The rise in Ca^{2+} concentration causes increased calcium binding to the protein, calmodulin, which is a subunit, in this instance, of phosphorylase b kinase. The phosphorylase kinase increases its activity catalyzing the conversion of phosphorylase b to a, thereby increasing the rate of glycogenolysis.

As a result, a small rise in cytosolic free calcium has far reaching consequences. However, the intracellular calcium concentration is kept remarkably constant by several mechanisms. The intracellular calcium concentration is low compared with the external concentration, so that there is a tendency for calcium to move down a concentration gradient into the cell. However, there is control of calcium movement across the plasma membrane as well as a method by which the mitochondria act as a temporary buffer or sump for cytosolic calcium. The plasma membrane has both a calcium pump and a sodium/calcium pump by which calcium is extruded. The mitochondrion has a calcium pump which drives calcium into the mitochondrion where is it stored as a calcium phosphate complex. All of these pumps are ATP dependent and consume energy (Fig. 33.9).

Cyclic AMP System

The other main system uses cyclic AMP as a secondary messenger. A hormone, e.g. glucagon, interacts with a surface receptor and activates adenyl cyclase. This results in an increase of cyclic AMP and this, in turn, increases the activity of cyclic AMP dependent protein kinase. Phosphorylase kinase is activated and converts phosphorylase b to a. Glycogen breakdown increases. This result is similar to the calcium system described above and the two mechanisms are complementary (Fig. 33.10).

Protein Kinase C

A third system is a calcium activated protein kinase, protein kinase C, which is dependent on phospholipid 'association' in order to function. When in contact with the phospholipid, the enzyme becomes sensitive to the presence of calcium. The role of this system has yet to be determined, but it would appear that it is associated with cell responses that are then sustained,

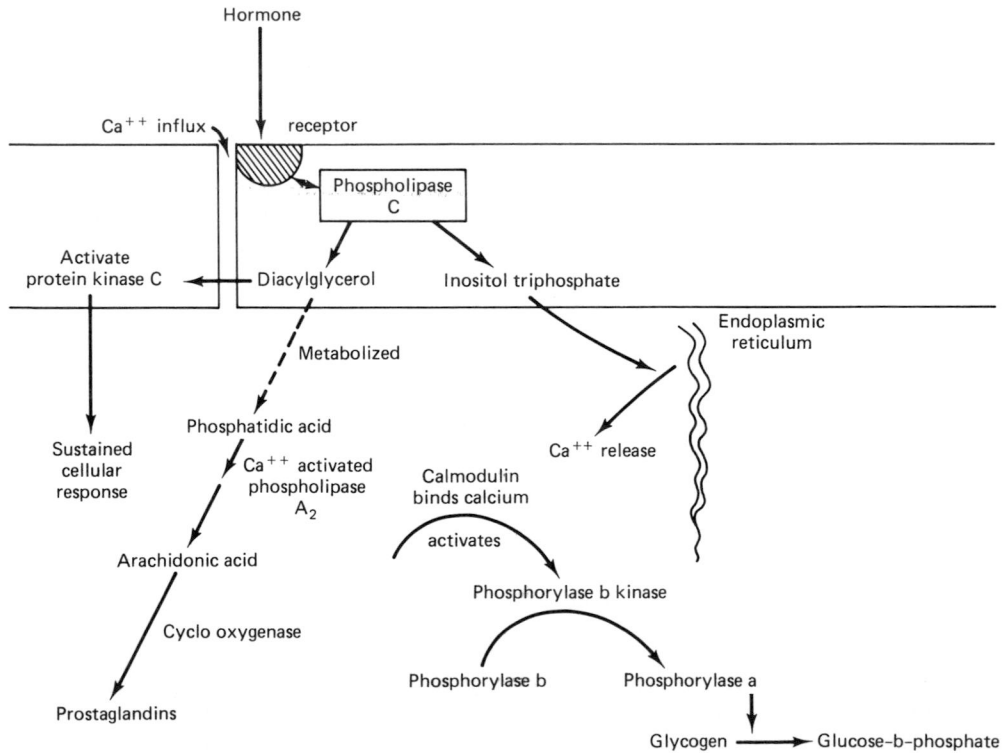

Fig. 33.9 Calcium messenger system. Calcium release from the endoplasmic reticulum and flux into the cell result in increased free cytosolic calcium. This binds to calmodulin and activates protein kinase. Calcium is also involved in prostaglandin synthesis.

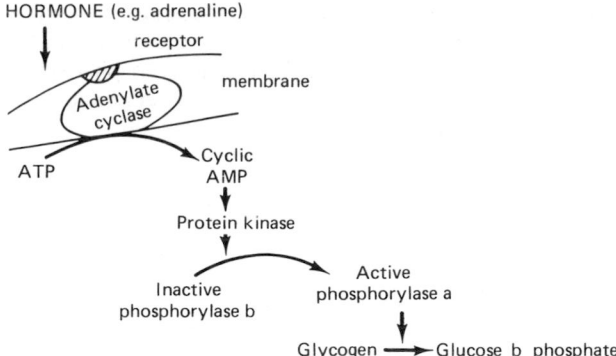

Fig. 33.10 Cyclic AMP messenger system. Mediated by protein kinases.

in contrast to the rapid reversibility of the calmodulin system. It is integrated with both the cyclic AMP and calmodulin systems (Rasmussen, 1986).

ENERGY AND EXERCISE

The changes in energy production and utilization occurring during exercise can be used to illustrate the dynamic integration of these metabolic pathways and their controls.

In the resting state there is adequate ATP, a stable ADP/ATP ratio and a low concentration of ADP. This sustains the glycolytic pathway and oxidative phosphorylation at a low level of activity which is adequate for basal ATP turnover. Contrary to the traditional view, there is good evidence to suggest that even at rest, under aerobic conditions, there is active continuous lactate production (Mazzeo et al., 1986). This lactate is either oxidized or used for glucose or glycogen manufacture. The low serum lactate under normal circumstances represents the balance between production and clearance.

As exercise commences ATP is hydrolyzed producing energy, ADP and inorganic phosphate (Pi). As a result, the concentration of ATP is reduced and ADP increased and consequently the ADP/ATP ratio changes. This not only increases the rate of oxidative phosphorylation, but also the activity of phosphofructokinase (PFK) and creatine phosphokinase (CPK) stimulating glycolysis and creatine phosphate mobilization respectively. All three mechanisms increase ATP production. In the cytoplasm CPK and pyruvate kinase (PK) compete for ADP, but CPK has the higher affinity for ADP. Therefore a small rise in the concentration of ADP preferentially activates CPK and creatine phosphate is utilized. If ADP concentration rises further, due to increasing ATP utilization, then PK is activated and glycolysis is fully mobilized. In this way the enzyme affinities act to integrate ATP production by the two different mechanisms.

A number of fuels are used by the cell. These include endogenous stores of high energy bonds such as creatine phosphate, as well as endogenous substrates such as glycogen and amino acids. Exogenous substrates such as glucose, glycogen, fatty acids and amino acids, can be used. Substrate uptake into the cell may be enhanced under some circumstances, as occurs with exercise (Haworth and Berkoff, 1986). However, a very important endogenous and exogenous fuel for oxidative metabolism is lactate. Large quantities of lactate are formed in some muscle cells especially those involved in rapid response, e.g. fast twitch cells, which can then be utilized as an oxidative substrate in other muscle cells. Therefore, in this circumstance, the value of glycolysis is the rapid supply of an oxidative substrate, lactate, which can be used by other cells, as well as the ATP production from the process.

As exercise continues, the requirement for ATP may exceed production from both creatine phosphate stores and oxidative phosphorylation or, alternatively, these pathways may be rate-limited by oxygen availability. Under these circumstances, anaerobic production of ATP becomes an important back-up system. The production of lactate by glycolysis will increase still further and will outstrip its oxidative utilization, resulting in the accumulation of lactate both in the cell and in the bloodstream.

Following exercise, there is what has been termed an 'oxygen debt' but this is a misleading expression. In effect, the cell will be in a depleted energy state. The ADP concentration will be high and ATP low. This is corrected by ATP production via oxidative phosphorylation. Similarly, creatine phosphate levels need to be replenished. The primary substrate is lactate which is oxidized, accounting for a large proportion of the lactate utilization post exercise. Lactate carbon atoms can also be traced into glycogen and amino acids so that there are several other potential pathways for the lactate (Brooks and Gaesser, 1980). During this time the oxygen requirement is high but this continues long after the lactate has been utilized, and probably constitutes ongoing oxidative metabolism to replenish stores. It is also used for the synthesis of glycogen and probably some amino acids to replenish those used as substrate during exercise.

As can be seen from this discussion, the interpretation of serum lactate levels requires caution as it reflects an endpoint of an equilibrium between production and utilization (Mazzeo et al., 1986; Hochachka, 1985).

Anaerobic Threshold

The anaerobic threshold is defined as the level of work or O_2 consumption just below that at which metabolic acidosis and the associated changes in gas exchange occur. Essentially, as the ATP requirement exceeds that which can be supplied by oxidative metabolism, there is an increase in the utilization of the anaerobic pathways. This may be due to increased ATP use or to inadequate oxygen supply.

As the proportion of ATP produced by glycolysis increases and ATP hydrolysis continues, there is an accumulation of hydrogen ions (an acidosis) which is buffered by the bicarbonate system leading to the production and excretion of CO_2. There is a rapid increase in the ratio of CO_2 production to O_2 consumption (RQ). Under normal circumstances the RQ is about 0.8, but at the anaerobic threshold it can increase to well over 1.0. Other measurements which correlate with the anaerobic threshold and can be used clinically are the end tidal CO_2, which remains constant at the point at which end tidal O_2 rises, and the rise in minute ventilation which occurs simultaneously. This point correlates with biochemical values such as blood lactate or pyruvate/lactate ratio and therefore can be used as an investigative tool clinically (Wasserman et al., 1973). Reliable measurement of expired gas concentration requires sophisticated equipment which has only recently become available, so the actual clinical value of the anaerobic threshold has yet to be established.

ISCHAEMIA AND CELL DEATH

The loss of the blood supply to the tissue results in the cell being deprived of oxygen and metabolic substrates, and also the accumulation of toxic metabolites which under normal circumstances are removed by the bloodstream. The consequences can be described as a number of interrelated chains of events which culminate in cell death. While energy depletion has a central role, the death of a cell is a result of multisystem failure and there is no single mechanism or event which can be identified as the specific point beyond which the changes are irreversible.

Initially, the supply of both oxygen and other substrates fail. The fall in oxygen tension in the cell produces many effects. One specific result is the reduction of cytochromes c, a, a_3 (*see* respiratory chain Fig. 33.2 p. 382). Reduced a_3 inhibits the respiratory chain and this uncouples oxidative phosphorylation, and reduces ATP production. In some creatures, such as turtles, this cytochrome can be reoxidized even after protracted hypoxia, while in mammals it becomes irreversible within minutes, (Lutz et al., 1984). Enzymes associated with the cytochromes, e.g. cytochrome c oxidase, are also inhibited by falling cellular oxygen tension as well as a multitude of other enzymes, especially oxidases. The net result is a reduction in ATP production, relative to utilization, and a consequent rise in ADP concentration. With inhibition of the tricarboxylic cycle, fatty acid oxidation also ceases and fatty acids and acyl CoA accumulate. If the ischaemia is not total and some oxygen is available or, alternatively, reperfusion occurs, these substrates can be diverted along other pathways which may still be functional. These include the cyclooxygenase or lipoxygenase pathways which produce prostaglandins and leukotrienes. The potentially detrimental consequences of this 'aberrant' mechanism have yet to be fully evaluated (Meyer et al., 1987). Ongoing energy requirements are met by local supplies of ATP or from stored sources such as creatine phosphate. Glycolysis is initially enhanced and so glucose utilization increases. The lack of supply of substrate to the cell limits the ability of this pathway to sustain ATP levels. In the heart, hypoxia and substrate starvation appears more detrimental than hypoxia alone, implying that the ability to produce some energy is important (Isselhard et al., 1980). In other tissue, such as the brain, this is not necessarily the case. It has been suggested that the association of hyperglycaemia, indicating adequate substrate, with incomplete ischaemia results in worsened damage. This is possibly because the increased acidosis from sustained anaerobic metabolism may be more damaging than energy depletion. In this situation, substrate starvation might be beneficial (Kraig et al., 1985) (Siesjo, 1988).

As a consequence of these events, the cell becomes critically depleted of ATP and ATP-dependent mechanisms start to fail. The sodium/potassium and calcium ion pumps in the cell membrane become less efficient affecting membrane permeability. There is a net influx of sodium and efflux of potassium. Calcium also moves down its concentration gradient into the cell with implications to be discussed below. Enzyme systems including those involved in glycolysis will fail. The hydrogen ions produced by ongoing ATP hydrolysis, anaerobic metabolism and accumulating fatty acids all contribute to a rapidly deteriorating intracellular acidosis. As the pH falls, intracellular enzyme systems fail and, at values around 6.5, glycolysis is inhibited and, at 6.0 ceases completely (Rotin et al., 1986). The ADP and AMP may in these circumstances either pass out of the cell through the leaky membrane or be broken down to hypoxanthine. In the severely hypoxic cells in which most of the adenine nucleotides are broken down, they can no longer regenerate ATP even if oxygen became available. In the less damaged cells, hypoxanthine will accumulate in the cytosol. The implications of hypoxanthine production will be discussed below.

These various events are part of the biochemical changes in the ischaemic cell. It is a picture of a multitude of energy dependent processes failing because of total energy depletion.

From a clinical viewpoint, there is considerable interest in potentially reversible pathophysiological mechanisms involved in ischaemic damage. Three specific mechanisms are discussed. The first is calcium mediated cell damage; the second is the role of oxygen free radicals, and the third excitatory receptors (Siesjo, 1988; Krause, 1988).

The Role of Calcium

Under normal circumstances, the calcium concentration in the cytosol is much less than outside the cell and is finely controlled. Calcium can be taken up by both the mitochondria and the endoplasmic reticulum or be extruded from the cell by an ATP dependent Na-Ca antiport system. By these means the cytosol concentration is kept at its normal level. Influx of calcium through calcium channels or release from the endoplasmic reticulum results in changes in the cytosolic concentration, and this has a messenger function affecting intracellular enzymes.

In postmortem cell studies high concentrations of calcium can be found intracellularly, especially in the mitochondria. The phenomenon known as the 'calcium paradox' may demonstrate a deleterious effect of intracellular calcium flux. This occurs when isolated heart tissue is incubated in a calcium free medium and then, at a later stage, calcium is added. There is a massive influx of calcium into the cells and the cells subsequently die. Calcium appears to be implicated in the cell death. It is also known that an increase in cytosolic free calcium can alter the activity of calmodulin modulated enzymes, activate phospholipase A and C (which can damage membrane phospholipid), affect Na–K ATPase, and hence ATP production and, as the mitochondrial calcium increases, uncouple oxidative phosphorylation. In contractile cells an influx of calcium may trigger contraction and increase ATP utilization see Table 33.1. Considering all these potential consequences, it is reasonable to assume that uncontrolled calcium influx may be detrimental and this would appear to complement the circumstantial evidence mentioned above.

TABLE 33.1
EFFECTS OF INCREASING INTRACELLULAR CALCIUM

1. Activation of phospholipase A_2
2. Activation of nucleases
3. Conversion of xanthine dehydrogenase to xanthine oxidase
4. Release of excitatory neurotransmitters.

However, establishing the role of these calcium mediated events in ischaemia has been difficult. Abnormal mitochondrial respiration with normal intracellular calcium, and normal respiration despite increasing calcium, have both been demonstrated (Wilson et al., 1983). Furthermore, absence of extracellular calcium increases susceptibility to anoxia. Also calcium blockade has been shown to be protective against ischaemia in contractile tissue, but is less convincing in non-contractile tissue. This implies that the calcium blockade, by decreasing the activation of myofibrils, reduces contractile energy requirement, thus conserving ATP rather than preventing damaging calcium influx. Measured changes in cytosolic free calcium do not correlate with ischaemic damage and large changes associated with physiological events such as cell fertilization do not result in cell damage (Cheung et al., 1986). Therefore, the direct evidence

identifying calcium as the damaging agent in ischaemia has not yet been found.

In conclusion, the role of calcium in ischaemic injury has yet to be clearly defined, although it almost certainly contributes to some of the damaging mechanisms.

Oxygen Free Radical Formation

Oxygen free radical formation is the other mechanism implicated in ischaemic damage. Under normal circumstances, ATP and its derivatives are either broken down to adenine nucleotides or degraded initially to hypoxanthine and then to uric acid. This is achieved using the enzyme xanthine oxidase (xanthine acceptor oxidoreductase) (Charlat et al., 1987; Kaminski et al., 1986). This enzyme exists in at least two forms. At normal oxygen tension almost all of it is in a dehydrogenase form with a reaction:

$$\text{hypoxanthine} + H_2O + NAD^+ \rightarrow$$
$$\text{uric acid} + NADH + H^+$$

At low oxygen tension, it is rapidly changed by a calcium mediated reaction into xanthine oxidase. This enzyme uses molecular oxygen as a substrate even at low oxygen tension.

$$\text{Hypoxanthine} + H_2O + 2\,O_2 \rightarrow$$
$$\text{uric acid} + 2\,O_2^- + 2H^+$$

The oxygen free radical formed is highly reactive and potentially destructive. In the normal cell there are always a small number of free radicals produced, but they are easily dealt with by cell enzymes, superoxide dismutase and catalase. If large quantities are produced, the cell defences are overwhelmed and damage ensues. The superoxide attacks the phospholipid membrane, degrades collagen and may disrupt lysosomes causing extensive intracellular damage. The mitochondrial membrane is also vulnerable to free radicals (Parks et al., 1983; Bulkley, 1983).

During an ischaemic episode, depletion of cell energy reserves results in the failure of membrane pumps and while potassium moves out of the cell, sodium and calcium move in. Hypoxanthine accumulates as a consequence of the degradation of adenine nucleotides. A low oxygen tension and the calcium influx enhance xanthine oxidase activity. If oxygen is available, superoxide is formed and damage results. If there is true anoxia, oxygen radicals will not form, but the stage is set for reperfusion injury if an oxygen supply is regained (Lehninger, 1980), (Fig. 33.11).

Excitotoxic Damage

A third mechanism has been postulated. Recently three new receptors for excitatory amino acids have been identified. These are the kainate (K), quisqualate (Q) and N methyl D aspartate (NMDA) receptors which are found throughout the central nervous

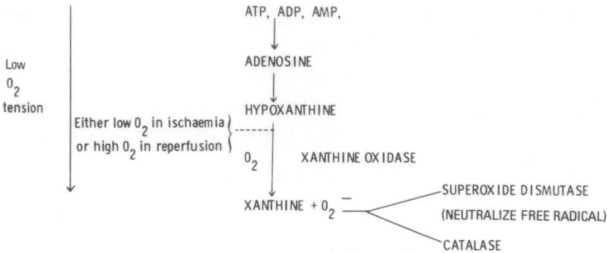

Fig. 33.11 Oxygen free radical formation. At low oxygen tension xanthine oxidase is formed. This catalyzes the breakdown of hypoxanthine (purine metabolite) to xanthine with the formation of oxygen free radical formation. If the oxygen supply returns to normal, reperfusion, then increased free radical production may occur.

system. There is evidence to suggest that in ischaemia extracellular aspartate and glutamate increase. These activate K and Q receptors which mediate sodium channels so that there is sodium influx. The NMDA receptors which gate ion channels are also activated and permits calcium influx. The influx of calcium may mediate further intracellular calcium movements and be associated with effects such as disaggregation of microtubules, proteolysis and protein phosphorylation all of which lead to membrane dysfunction and ultimately cell death. The role of these receptors requires further evaluation (Siejso, 1988).

Reperfusion Injury

Cell survival depends on reperfusion and restoration of substrate supply. Paradoxically, the increased availability of oxygen, which is fundamental to cell survival, may result in the activation of potentially damaging mechanisms. This is an area of considerable interest in relation to cardioplegia, organ transplantation and organ salvage following ischaemic or hypoxic insults. In each situation cellular damage may be accentuated during the reperfusion phase. Some of the potential problems which result when the oxygen supply is restored almost certainly relate to oxygen free radical formation.

Hypoxanthine accumulation and xanthine oxidase activation, which occur with hypoxia, facilitate the creation of free radicals, which can then injure the cellular structures. The main effect is to cause lipid peroxidation, mediated by a perferryl radical, which results in membrane damage. This oxygen radical formation is accelerated by the increased availability of oxygen associated with reperfusion. Other oxidases, cyclooxygenase and lipoxygenase, can also produce free radicals or, alternatively, can metabolize available free fatty acids to produce prostaglandins and leukotrienes. These may have multiple effects including alteration of the microcirculation affecting blood and substrate supply and changes in membrane integrity which may allow rapid calcium influx. This calcium influx may be detrimental in terms of uncon-trolled enzyme activation or, alternatively, stimulation of myofibril contraction which utilizes ATP. There are, of course, a number of other major factors, including acid base balance, substrate supply and the availability of adenine nucleotides in the cell which may influence cell or organ viability (Ernster, 1988).

The main thrust of research in this area appears to be towards methods of maintaining intracellular energy reserves, blocking calcium influx to avert potential calcium mediated problems and either preventing the formation of oxygen free radicals or minimizing their detrimental effects.

CONCLUSION

In this chapter the mechanisms of energy production and utilization have been summarized. As the understanding of basic cell function increases, the potential diagnostic and therapeutic interventions acting at cellular level will also increase. This is already seen in the use of calcium antagonists and xanthine oxidase inhibitors as well as in modifications of the approach to areas such as parenteral nutrition. These are exciting developments in the management of a variety of pathophysiological states and it is inevitable that cellular energetics will have an increasing importance in clinical practice.

REFERENCES

Bessman S.P., Carpenter C.L. (1985). The creatine-creatine phosphate energy shuttle. *Ann. Rev. Biochem.*, **54**, 831.

Brooks G.A., Gaesser G.A. (1980). End points of lactate and glucose metabolism after exhausting exercise. *J. Appl. Physiol.*, **49**, 1057.

Bulkley G.B. (1983). The role of oxygen free radicals in human disease processes. *Surgery*. **94**, 408.

Busa W.B., Nuccitelli R. (1984). Metabolic regulation via intracellular pH. *Am. J. Physiol.*, **246**, R409.

Charlat M.L., O'Neill P.G., Egan J. M., et al. (1987). Evidence for a pathogenic role of xanthine oxidase in the stunned myocardium. *Am. J. Physiol.*, **252**, H566.

Cheung J.Y., Bonventre J.V., Malis C.D., et al. (1986). Calcium and ischaemic injury. *New Engl. J. Med.*, **314**, 1670.

Ernster L. (1988). Biochemistry of reoxygenation injury. *Crit. Care Med.*, **16**, 947.

Halangk W., Bohnesack R., Frank K., et al. (1985). Effect of various substrates on mitochondrial and cellular energy state of intact spermatazoa. *Biomed. Biochem. Acta*, **44**, 411.

Hatefi Y. (1985). The mitochondrial electron transport and oxidative phosphorylation system. *Ann. Rev. Biochem.*, **54**, 1015.

Haworth R.A., Berkoff H.A. (1986). The control of sugar uptake by metabolic demand in isolated adult rat heart cells. *Circ. Res.*, **58**, 157.

Hochachka P.W. (1985). Fuels and pathways as designed systems for support of muscle work. *J. Exp. Biol.*, **115**, 149.

Isselhard W., Schorn B., Hugel W., et al. (1980). Experimental aspects of myocardial protection during cardiac arrest. Cardioplegia symposium: St. Thomas Hospital/ The Royal Society.

Kaminski Z.W., Pohorecki R., Ballast C.L., et al. (1986). Three forms of xanthine; acceptor oxidoreductase in rat heart. *Circ. Res.*, **59**, 628.

Kraig R.P., Pulsinelli W.A., Plum F. (1985). Heterogenous distribution of hydrogen and bicarbonate during complete brain ischaemia. *Prog. Brain Res.*, **63**, 155.

Kravse G.S., White B.C., Aust S.D. et al., (1988). Brain cell death following ischaemia and reperfusion: a proposed biochemical sequence. *Crit. Care Med.*, **16**, 714.

Lehninger A.L. (1980). *Biochemistry*, 2nd edn. Cardioplegia Proceedings of the Royal Society, London. London: Worth.

Lutz P.L., McMahon P., Rosenthal M., et al. (1984). Relationships between aerobic and anaerobic energy production in turtle brain in situ. *Am. J. Physiol.*, **247**, R740.

Mandel L.J. (1985). Metabolic substrates cellular energy production and the regulation of proximal tubular transport. *Ann. Rev. Physiol.*, **47**, 85.

Mazzeo R.S., Brooks G.A., Scoeller D.A., et al. (1986). Disposal of blood lactate in humans during rest and exercise. *J. Appl. Physiol.*, **60**, 232.

Meyer F.B., Sundt T.M., Yanagihara T., et al. (1987). Focal cerebral ischaemia *Mayo Clin. Proc.*, **62**, 35.

Mitchell P. (1974). Vectorial chemistry and the molecular mechanics of chemiosmotic coupling; power transmission by proticity. *Biochem. Soc.* Transact; 9th Ciba Medal Lecture, **4**, 398.

Mizock B.A. (1987). Controversies in lactic acidosis. *JAMA*, **258**, 497.

Parks D.A., Bulkley G.B., Granger D.N. (1983). Role of oxygen free radicals in shock, ischaemia and organ preservation. *Surgery*, **94**, 431.

Rasmussen H. (1986). The calcium messenger system. *New Engl. J. Med.*, **314**, 1094.

Rotin D., Robinson B., Tannock I.F. (1986). Influence of hypoxia and an acid environment on the metabolism and viability of culture cells; potential implications for cell death in tumours. *Cancer. Res.*, **46**, 2821.

Siesjo B.K. (1988). Mechanisms of ischaemic brain damage. *Crit. Care Med.*, **16**, 954.

Wasserman K., Whipp B.J., Koyl S.N., et al. (1973). Anaerobic threshold and respiratory gas exchange during exercise. *J. Appl. Physiol.*, **35**, 236.

Wilson D.R., Arnold P., Burke T., et al. (1983). Sequential changes in mitochondrial function in ischaemic acute renal failure in the rat. *Kidney Int.*, **23**, 209.

Wilson D., Erecinska M. (1986). The oxygen dependence of cellular energy metabolism. *Adv. Med. Biol.*, **194**, 229.

34. Acid-base Balance
J. Norman

Terminology and fundamentals
  The role of water
  Sampling of body fluids
Regulation of the blood acid-base state
  Defence against changes in P_{CO_2}
Assessment of acid-base disorders
  Indices available
  Acid-base charts
Significance of changes in pH

Acid-base balance is concerned with hydrogen ions, with their concentration and regulation and with the effects of changes in their concentration. One of the characteristic features of living bodies is their capacity to cope with large amounts of hydrogen ions in any day. Thus, an adult human may excrete some 15 000 mmol of carbonic acid a day and with its associated hydrogen ions and some 50–150 mmol of phosphoric and sulphuric acids each day in the urine. In addition there may well be internal transfers of 1000 mmol of lactic acid from muscle to the liver and kidneys. Finally, of course, oxidative phosphorylation in generating ATP depends on the ability of mitochondria to pump hydrogen ions across membranes.

Given these vast movements, it is perhaps not surprising that the body has developed mechanisms which keep the internal environment reasonably con-stant in terms of the intensity of the acidity of the fluids. Claude Bernard recognized this need for homeostasis over one hundred years ago. This chapter is designed to review the fundamental concepts of acid-base balance, the controlling mechanisms, the assessment of disorders and the implications of changes in acid-base state.

TERMINOLOGY AND FUNDAMENTALS

Whilst acids and bases can be defined in a number of ways, the Brönsted definitions suffice for clinical purposes. An *acid* is a substance which tends to loose an hydrogen ion and a *base* a substance which tends to gain an hydrogen ion. The stronger the losing or gaining tendency, the stronger is the acid or base. Acids and bases usually exist in pairs with the base accepting the hydrogen ion from the acid. Depending on the relevant conditions such chemical reactions are reversible and proceed both ways.

$$Acid \rightleftharpoons H^+ + Base$$
$$HCl \rightarrow H^+ + Cl^-$$
$$H_2CO_3 \rightleftharpoons H^+ + HCO_3^-$$
$$H_2O \rightleftharpoons H^+ + OH^-$$

Some substances can act as bases in some circumstances and acids in others. Thus, bicarbonate is the conjugate base for carbonic acid but is the conjugate acid for carbonate ions:

$$HCO_3^- \rightleftharpoons H^+ + CO_3^{2-}$$

Proteins and amino acids often have both acidic and

basic side groups and the overall 'acid' character will depend on the prevailing conditions.

The strength of an acid or base solution is measured using a scale of pure numbers—the pH scale. Small numbers indicate strongly acid conditions and large ones basic conditions. Theoretically the pH scale is related to what the chemists call the *activity* of the hydrogen ions present:

$$pH = -\lg a \, H^+$$

where 'a' refers to the activity. In turn the activity is related to the concentration of the hydrogen ions as expressed on a molar scale. In dilute solutions the relationship is on a one-to-one basis but in concentrated solutions this is not so. But in practice this fine distinction can be ignored and we assume:

$$pH = -\lg [H^+]$$

or the equivalent

$$pH = 1/[H^+]$$
$$pH = \lg (1/[H^+])$$

To calculate hydrogen ion concentration from pH the equation is altered to:

$$[H^+] = 10^{-pH}$$

The range of hydrogen ion concentrations found in the body is large: this was one of the reasons why Sorensen introduced the pH notation. In extracellular fluid and blood the concentration is low and is expressed in nanomoles/litre. Table 34.1 gives some pH values and the equivalent concentrations.

TABLE 34.1

pH units	Hydrogen ion concentration nmol L^{-1}
3	1 000 000
6	1000
7	100
7.1	80
7.4	40
7.7	20
8	10
9	1

There are occasional academic discussions as to whether we should use pH or hydrogen ion concentration. Note that whilst pH can be defined in terms of hydrogen activity, in practice it is measured by reference to solutions whose pH values are defined but whose hydrogen ion concentration or activity is not. Thus one can take one's choice. It is perhaps also worth noting that the effects of changes in acidity are more directly related to the logarithmic scale than to the direct scale.

The Role of Water

Water is an acid dissociating to a small extent into hydrogen and hydroxyl ions:

$$H_2O \rightleftharpoons H^+ + OH^-$$

The extent of the dissociation is small. At room temperature some 55.6 moles of water (1 litre) give 100 nmol each of hydrogen and hydroxyl ions. At body temperature the dissociation is a little larger—some 158 nmol of each ion are produced. Thus at room temperature the pH will be 7.0 units and at 37°C 6.8 units. Neutrality (where the concentrations of hydrogen and hydroxyl ions are equal) exists at these pH values.

Sampling of Body Fluids

It is possible to measure the acid-base state of almost any body fluid. In clinical practice it is usual to attempt to obtain a representative sample of extracellular fluid. Whilst mixed venous blood does provide such a sample, because we are often also interested in the state of oxygenation, it is customary to obtain an arterial blood sample. In handling such samples it is important to avoid any mixing with air, to use only heparin in a low concentration (not more than 1000 i.u./ml) and to analyse the sample as soon as possible. If any delay in analysis is expected the sample should be kept cool in a mixture of ice and water. Conventional venous blood samples, often taken when a tourniquet is used, are not helpful and should only be used to give crude indices of the metabolic state of the patient.

Other body fluids such as cerebrospinal fluid, urine and gastric juice may also be studied to determine acidity. The principles of measurement of pH are dealt with elsewhere in this volume.

REGULATION OF THE BLOOD ACID-BASE STATE

In normal health the arterial blood pH is maintained within a narrow range of between 7.36 and 7.44 ($[H^+]$ between 44 and 36 nmol/L). There are four mechanisms which contribute to this stability.

Buffer Systems. A buffer system is a mixture of either a weak acid and its conjugate base or of a weak base and its conjugate acid. In blood the important buffers are the bicarbonate/carbonic acid system, the dihydrogen phosphate/monohydrogen phosphate system and the proteins both in plasma and in the red cells. Of these, the bicarbonate/carbonic acid system is the most important. The main effect of any buffer pair is to minimize the change in pH seen when strong bases or acids are added that would occur in their absence. How does this occur?

Imagine a closed flask contains 1 litre of pure water. At room temperature the pH will be 7.0 ($[H^+]$

100 nmol/L). If we add 10 mmol of a strong acid (e.g. HCl) to this litre the acid dissociates completely to give a hydrogen ion concentration of 10 mmol/L and the pH becomes 2.0. The acidity has increased 100 000-*fold*. Alternatively adding 10 mmol of a strong base (e.g. NaOH) would reduce the hydrogen ion concentration to 1 picomol/L and the pH would be 12.

What happens if we have a buffer pair present? Imagine the flask starts with a bicarbonate concentration of 24 mmol/L and a carbonic acid concentration of 1.2 mmol/L. In this flask (now at 37°C) the following reactions can occur:

$$H_2CO_3 \rightleftharpoons H^+ + HCO_3^-$$

An equilibrium is reached and by applying the Law of Mass Action we arrive at the Henderson equation:

$$[H^+] = K_D \frac{[H_2CO_3]}{[HCO_3^-]}$$

K_D is the dissociation constant and has a value of 800 nmol/L.

Hasselbach in 1916 used the pH notation to derive the Henderson-Hasselbach equation:

$$pH = pK + lg\,[HCO_3^-]/[H_2CO_3]$$

For carbonic acid the pK is 6.10 units. For our flask with the bicarbonate at 24 mmol/L and the carbonic acid at 1.2 mmol/L the hydrogen ion concentration comes out at 40 nmol/L and the pH at 7.4. The importance of these calculations lies in remembering that the acidity is determined by the balance between the two elements of the buffer pair. To change the acidity, one or both concentrations must change or, more accurately, the ratio must change.

We can now see what happens when we add the 10 mmol of either strong acid or strong base. With the 10 mmol of hydrochloric acid the following occurs:

$$HCl + HCO_3^- \rightarrow Cl^- + H_2CO_3$$

The 10 mmol of acid react with 10 of the 24 mmol of bicarbonate reducing that concentration to 14 mmol/L and increasing the carbonic acid concentration to 11.2 mmol/L. The hydrogen ion concentration is given by the new balance and is 640 nmol/L and the pH 6.20. Thus with the buffer the change in acidity is markedly reduced—from a 100 000-*fold* change to a 16-*fold* one.

Adding the base gives the following reaction:

$$NaOH + H_2CO_3 \rightarrow NaHCO_3 + H_2O$$

But there are only 1.2 mmol of carbonic acid present and only 1.2 mmol of the base will be neutralized. Thus the final concentration of hydroxyl ions will be 8·8 mmol/L and the pOH (corresponding to the pH) will be 2.06. The pH is then given by:

$$pH = 13.6 - pOH$$

and comes out at 11.54. Thus the bicarbonate/carbonic acid system is not very effective in buffering a

large amount of strong base—in the circumstance of this flask. Other buffer systems behave similarly.

Carbon Dioxide. In addition to the large amount of water present in the body, there is, in life, an almost inexhaustible supply of carbon dioxide. The resting production is some 200 ml/min which is approximately 9 mmol/min. Thus we have the capacity to keep a reasonably constant pressure of carbon dioxide in the blood and hence a constant carbonic acid concentration:

$$CO_2 + H_2O \rightleftharpoons H_2CO_3$$

Let us examine what happens if in our model we change it to keep the carbonic acid concentration constant as 1.2 mmol/L. Adding the 10 mmol of hydrochloric acid will still reduce the bicarbonate concentration to 14 mmol/L but the excess carbonic acid will be eliminated and the concentration remain at 1.2 mmol/L. The new hydrogen ion concentration becomes 68 nmol/L and the pH 7.17. We have gained an extra unit in keeping the pH constant. If we add the 10 mmol of sodium hydroxide, we now have much better buffering for although the bicarbonate concentration will increase to 34 mmol/L, the carbonic acid concentration remains at 1.2 mmol/L. The new hydrogen ion concentration becomes 28 nmol/L and the pH 7.55. Thus, in life, the presence of a large production of carbon dioxide and the ability of the lungs to remove it and keep the carbonic acid concentration relatively constant improved the ability to maintain a constant pH. Figure 34.1 illustrates the effectiveness of the bicarbonate/carbonic acid system in defending the body against the changes produced by strong acids or bases.

Physiological Control. The body adds further refinements to control pH even more accurately. The carbon dioxide tension in arterial blood, and hence the carbonic acid concentration can be modified. Chemoreceptors in the carotid and aortic bodies are sensitive to changes in pH as well as to changes in P_{CO_2} and P_{O_2}. An acid pH will stimulate the receptors to produce an increase in alveolar ventilation and hence a reduction in P_{CO_2}; an alkaline pH has the opposite effect. The reflex occurs quickly.

Elimination Mechanisms. These three mechanisms are the first line of defence against changes in pH. The kidney also acts to control pH, usually by eliminating and excreting any offending strong acid or base. The time course is somewhat longer but, together with the liver's capacity to metabolize many organic acids to carbon dioxide, acts to eliminate the problems.

Defence Against Changes in P_{CO_2}

The preceding discussion has illustrated the vital role of carbon dioxide and bicarbonate in defending the acid-base state of the body. But carbonic acid is itself

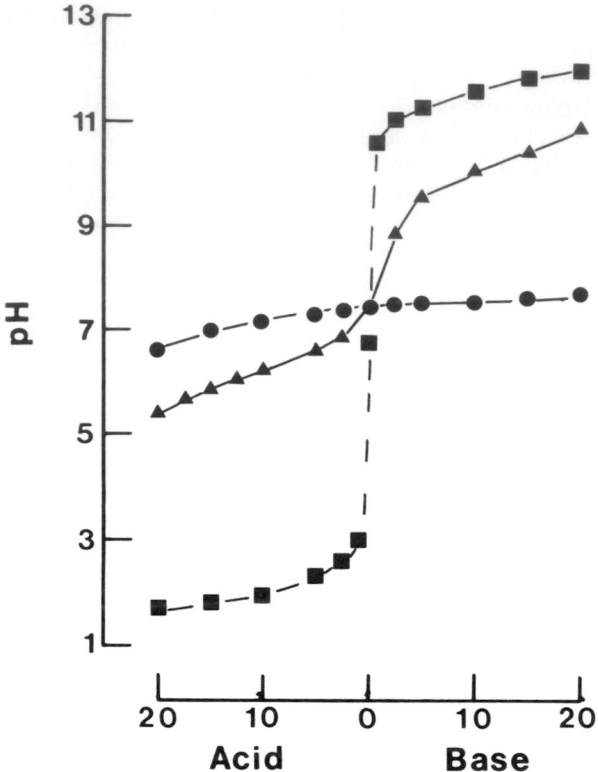

Fig. 34.1 Titration curves showing the effects of adding concentrations (mmol/L) of strong acid or base on the pH of (a) water (■), (b) a closed mixture of sodium bicarbonate (24 mmol/L) and carbonic acid (1.2 mmol/L) (▲) and (c) an open mixture containing sodium bicarbonate (24 mmol/L) and a fixed concentration of carbonic acid (1.2 mmol/L) (●). The bicarbonate carbonic acid system acts as a buffer; physiological control of the carbonic acid concentration improves its efficiency.

an acid. How does the body react if there are changes in carbonic acid levels due perhaps to respiratory failure or to overventilation? Firstly, it must be remembered that a buffer system cannot act as a buffer for one of its constituents. Thus for the carbonic acid/bicarbonate pair a ten-*fold* change in P_{CO_2} will produce a ten-*fold* change in hydrogen ion concentration and a one unit change in pH. This is, of course, the basis on which the Severinghaus P_{CO_2} electrode works in measuring P_{CO_2}. The defence in the body is the presence of other buffer pairs whose dissociation constants are less than those of the carbonic acid/bicarbonate pair (i.e. their pK values are higher). The phosphates and in particular the proteins form such buffers. Their action diminishes the changes seen when P_{CO_2} changes.

Haemoglobin is especially important in having a role here. It transports oxygen, carbon dioxide and defends against the acid forming properties of carbon dioxide. Oxyhaemoglobin is a stronger acid than reduced haemoglobin. Thus in the tissues when oxygen is unloaded, the weaker acid, reduced haemo-

globin, can pick up some of the hydrogen ions formed when carbon dioxide reacts with water. This is the Christiansen, Douglas and Haldane effect.

ASSESSMENT OF ACID-BASE DISORDERS

The assessment of acid-base disorders has probably caused more confusion than anything else in this branch of clinical chemistry. Some of the difficulties have arisen because the measurements necessary are not always easy. In earlier days it was easier to measure the bicarbonate (or carbon dioxide concentration) in serum; later it became possible to estimate P_{CO_2} fairly easily. The pioneering work of Astrup and Siggaard-Andersen some thirty years ago led to systems which give measurements of the pH and P_{CO_2} of blood, using small samples and virtually at the bedside. The recent developments in microprocessors allow these measurements to be processed to give a bewildering array of indices which should but may not reduce the confusion otherwise likely.

A second source of confusion arose because some indices were developed as a result of changes induced in blood outside the body i.e. *in vitro*. Sadly what happens to blood when its P_{CO_2} is changed *in vitro* does not necessarily happen when the changes occur *in vivo*. A chemical diagnosis was easy, a pathophysiological one much less so. Further treatment based on the chemical diagnosis may well be inappropriate. However, what is not well established are the likely changes seen in life with the common disorders. How one looks at them, depends on one's point of view. This review will present some of the alternatives.

One final word of caution is needed. The measuring systems are very good, provided they are properly maintained and their performances checked regularly. Most provide primary measurements of pH, P_{CO_2}, P_{O_2} and haemoglobin concentrations. The other indices coming out of the microprocessors use these measurements. It must be remembered that any errors in the primary measurements or in the algorithms will accumulate. Even the simple use of the Henderson-Hasselbach equation to calculate one prime factor from measurements of the other two can produce gross errors. In practice pK is not necessarily constant!

Indices Available

pH measurements are made routinely and can be converted to hydrogen ion concentrations. If the pH is less than 7.35 ([H^+] concentration > 45 nmol/L) an *acidaemia* is present. If the pH is greater than 7.44 ([H^+] < 35 nmol/L) then an *alkalaemia is present*.

There are two main routes which produce changes. Either respiratory factors alter leading to changes in P_{CO_2} and carbonic acid levels or other stronger acids and bases are present. The first set of changes are termed *respiratory* and the second *metabolic*. Metabolic is perhaps an unfortunate term because the main product of metabolism is carbon dioxide. However it has been in use for many years and it does act to lump together all the other causes. Purists may prefer the term *non-respiratory*.

Respiratory Indices

The only one used is the P_{CO_2}. Increases above 6 kPa (45 mmHg) are associated with a *respiratory acidosis* and decreases below 4.7 kPa (35 mmHg) a *respiratory alkalosis*. Note the use of the words acidosis and alkalosis—they differ from acidaemia and alkalaemia and indicate a change that is normally, but not always, expected to produce the associated change in acidity. Remember that P_{CO_2} may change as part of the compensatory change for the addition of a strong acid or base.

Metabolic Indices

There are far too many of these but the following list gives some that may help. Ideally if there is an excess of lactic acid in the blood then we should measure that directly. This is not necessarily easy and alternatives can be used.

The Anion Gap. In serum the sodium concentration is of the order 140 mmol/L, the potassium 4.0 mmol/L, the chloride some 110 mmol/L and the bicarbonate some 24 mmol/L. The difference between the sum of the two cations and the two anions is some 10 mmol/L and is called the anion gap. It is due to the presence of other anions (notably proteins). If the gap is increased then some other anion is present which will almost certainly be an acid. The anion gap is a useful screen to detect such a presence and can be assessed using routine blood chemistry.

Plasma Bicarbonate Ion Concentration. The normal value is 24 mmol/L and can be calculated from the pH and P_{CO_2}. In metabolic acidosis the value falls and it rises in metabolic alkalosis. Unfortunately, respiratory disorders also change it—it will rise with renal compensation in respiratory acidosis and fall with a respiratory alkalosis.

Alkali Reserve and Carbon Dioxide Combining Power. These are two interesting indices which were the first proposed to standardize for the respiratory state of the patient. In both the serum was equilibrated with a P_{CO_2} of 5.3 kPa. In the first the plasma bicarbonate concentration was measured and in the second the total carbon dioxide in serum determined. The normal values would be 24 and 25.2 mmol/L respectively. By controlling the P_{CO_2} any changes would be likely to be due to a metabolic cause.

Standard Bicarbonate was introduced as an alternative. Here whole blood was equilibrated with a normal P_{CO_2} and the plasma bicarbonate concentration de-

rived. The limitation is that it uses an *in vitro* technique and is not completely isolated from respiratory changes. The reason is that whole blood has a high concentration of haemoglobin which makes it a more powerful buffer than most tissue fluids. Hence blood *in vivo* behaves as a weaker buffer than *in vitro* and the pH changes and bicarbonate ion changes are greater *in vivo*.

Buffer Base was introduced to sum up the concentrations of all the buffering anions present in blood. Changes in P_{CO_2} would alter the distribution but not the total concentration of buffers present.

Base Excess was introduced as a further refinement of buffer base to measure the difference between the actual buffer base value and that expected for the haemoglobin concentration. Anaemia affects buffer base values. Base excess is normally between -2 and $+2$ mmol/L.

Non-Respiratory pH was introduced to deal with the problem of the difference between *in vivo* and *in vitro* behaviour. It is based on experiments establishing what changes will occur if P_{CO_2} is altered acutely in man. From a chart of such changes (Fig. 34.2) it is

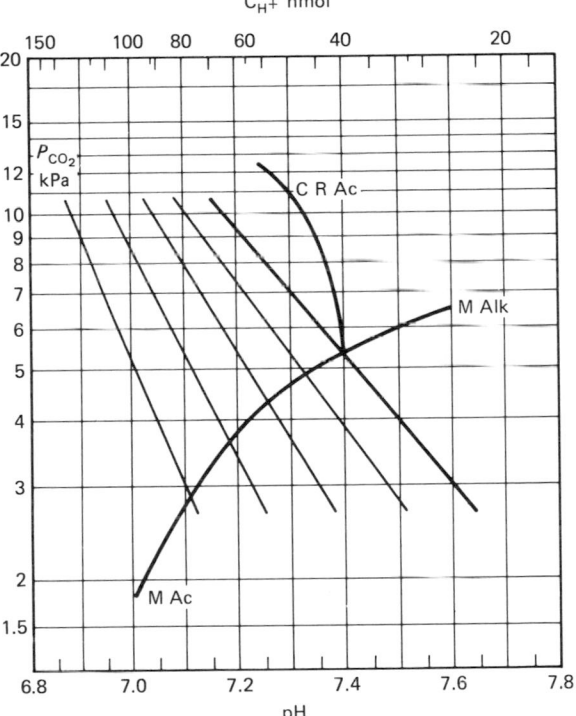

Fig. 34.2 pH P_{CO_2} diagram showing the common patterns of acid-base disorder. The diagonals show the changes in pH expected with acute changes in P_{CO_2} for varying degrees of metabolic acidosis (Stoker et al., 1972). The line labelled CRAc shows the average of changes seen with chronic respiratory failure. MAc and MAlk show the types of changes to be expected in patients with metabolic acidosis and alkalosis.

TABLE 34.2

INDICES OF ACID-BASE BALANCE

Index	Normal	Respiratory		Metabolic	
		Acidosis	Alkalosis	Acidosis	Alkalosis
ph	7.37–7.43	↓	↑	↓	↑
P_{CO_2} (kPa)	4.9–5.9	↑	↓	↓	↑
Plasma bicarbonate (mmol/L)	22–28	↑	↓	↓	↑
Standard bicarbonate (mmol/L)	22–28	—*	—*	↓	↑
Buffer base (mmol/L)	46–52	—*	—*	↓	↑
Base excess (mmol/L)	−2–+2	—*	—*	↓	↑
Non-respiratory pH	7.37–7.43	—	—	↓	↑

* No changes seen in *in vitro* experiments. *In vivo*, changes may occur.

possible to back project to see what pH would be found were the P_{CO_2} to be normalized *in vivo*. The normal value is 7.4 and a metabolic acidosis would be associated with low pH values, an alkalosis with high values. Table 34.2 summarizes the indices available together with their normal ranges and the changes likely in acid-base disorders.

Acid-base Charts

Much of the difficulty in interpreting acid-base results disappears if one of the various charts relating two of the three main variables are used. The value of the charts lies in showing the interrelationships between the variables, e.g. how much change in pH will follow a change in P_{CO_2}. The second value lies in following trends with serial blood samples. Restoration towards normality is satisfying whilst departures from predicted paths should arouse suspicions that other factors need consideration. Figures 34.3 and 34.4 show two such charts on which are superimposed the common pathways associated with respiratory and metabolic disorders.

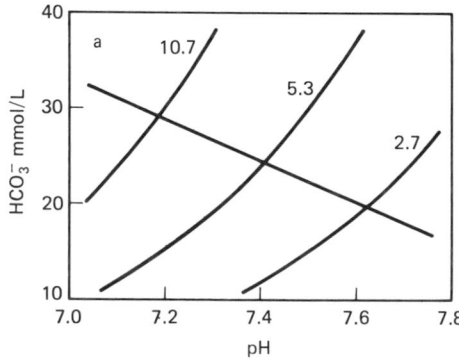

Fig. 34.4 The Davenport acid-base diagram has pH values on the abscissa; values to the left of 7.4 indicate an acidaemia, the right an alkalaemia. The diagonal shows the changes to be seen in normal blood when the P_{CO_2} is altered. These are the normal buffer lines. Values of pH and plasma bicarbonate or pH and P_{CO_2} to the left of and below these lines indicate a metabolic acidosis; to the right and above, a metabolic alkalosis.

SIGNIFICANCE OF CHANGES IN pH

Patients whose pH values lie well outside the normal range are likely to be ill and are at risk of dying. Nevertheless, it is important to remember that an acidosis or an alkalosis is not necessarily dangerous but rather that the underlying cause may be. Patients do survive having pH values as low as 6.8 and as high as 7.8. Exercising athletes may lower their pH to values of 7.0. The causative oxygen debt and lactic acidosis resolve following the end of the exercise. A patient in cardiac failure from a myocardial infarct may also have a lactic acidosis and a similarly low pH. His prognosis is, of course, much worse. Thus acid-

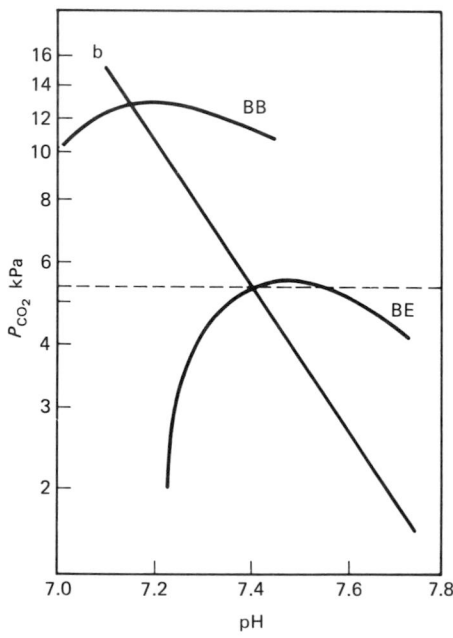

Fig. 34.3 This is the Siggaard-Anderson acid-base diagram. The Siggaard-Anderson chart has the lines for base excess (BE) and buffer base (BB) marked.

base disturbances in blood should be looked at first as indicators that suggest there may be underlying problems. Treatment should be directed at these problems first. It is rare for agents such as sodium bicarbonate or an acid to be needed as the initial therapy for a metabolic problem. An exception could be that artificial ventilation may be the treatment for an acute respiratory acidosis in a patient following anaesthesia and surgery.

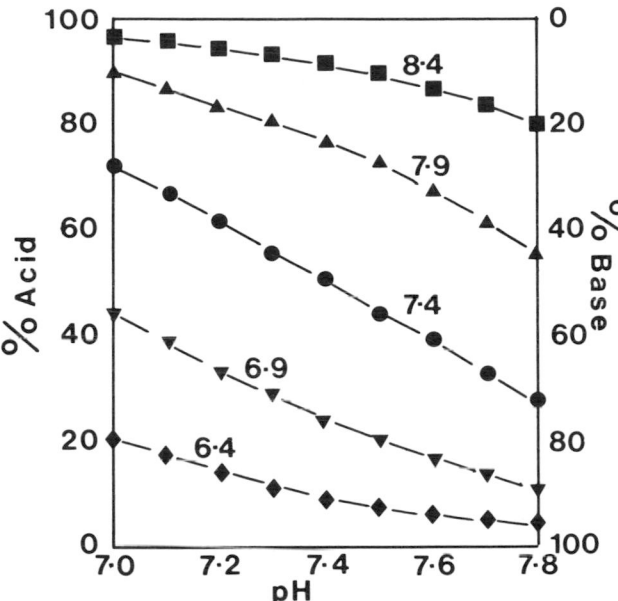

Fig. 34.5 Effect of changing pH and pK on the proportion of a buffer pair, protein or drug to be found in the acid or base form. pK values are shown above each line. In the pH range encountered in anaesthesia if a drug has a pK of 7.4 changing pH from 7.1 to 7.7 reduces the proportion in the acid form from 67% to 33%. For a drug with a pK of 6.4 the corresponding change is from 16% to 5%.

Changes in pH can have some important effects on enzyme activity and on the distribution of proteins and drugs. Most enzyme activity will be at an optimum at some specific pH and marked changes will alter the effects of the enzymes. Changes in pH act as controllers for some enzyme acivity.

The distribution of drugs in the body may also be affected by changes in pH. Many drugs are either weak acids or bases and the relative fractions in each form will depend on the pH and the pK of the drug concerned. Figure 34.5 illustrates this and shows that marked changes can be seen when the pH is close to the pK value. Transfer of drug is usually in the non-ionized form and when there are marked differences in pH across a boundary there can be marked differences in the concentrations of active drug in two compartments.

Other effects of changes in pH include changes on the interactions of haemoglobin with oxygen by changing the P_{50}. An acidosis can help delivery of oxygen to the tissues and an alkalosis hinder it. Additional specific effects are deal with elsewhere in this book.

FURTHER READING

There are several excellent monographs on acid-base balance. The following list contains some which may be regarded almost as historical but nevertheless contain much that is sound.

Davenport H.W. (1958). *The ABC of Acid-Base Chemistry*. Chicago: University Press.
Filley G.F. (1971). *Acid-Base and Blood-Gas Regulation*. Philadelphia: Lea and Febiger.
Gardener M.L. (1978). *Medical Acid-Base Balance: The Basic Principles*. London: Balliere Tindall.
Hainsworth R. (ed.). (1986). *Acid-Base Balance*. Manchester: Manchester University Press.
Peters J.P., Van Slyke D.D. (1932). Clinical Chemistry. Baltimore: Williams and Wilkins.

35. The Liver and Anesthesia
L. Strunin

Liver blood flow
  Measurement of hepatic blood flow
  Anesthetic factors influencing blood flow
Drug metabolism
  Non-depolarizing neuromuscular blocking
    agents
  Opioids
  Intravenous induction agents
  Volatile anesthetic agents
*Anesthesia in the patient with liver
    dysfunction*
  Jaundice as the presenting symptom
  Disorders of blood coagulation
  Renal failure after operation
  Chronic liver disease
  Anesthetic considerations
  Viral hepatitis
Acute liver failure
  Investigation and management of the
    multisystem disorders

The liver in a normal man weighs some 1500 g and is perfused at a rate of 1 ml/g of liver tissue/min, representing some 25% of the cardiac output. The liver has a vital role in metabolism and in the control of carbohydrate, protein and fat which are essential to most body processes. In the event of liver cell failure there may be gross disturbance of blood glucose and lactate concentrations, an inability to synthesize proteins concerned with blood clotting and a low serum albumin concentration. As well as prolonged metabolism of drugs, energy substrates may be unavailable and there may be secondary effects on other organs of the body such as the kidney and brain.

In addition to normal metabolism and the biotransformation of many exogenously administered drugs the liver also has a major excretory role in the production of bile. A further aspect of bile secretion is the production of bile salts which are essential for the absorption of fat and fat soluble vitamins, in particular vitamins A and K from the gut. Disorders of bilirubin metabolism lead to the retention of bilirubin in the serum and the clinical appearance of jaundice, in addition there may be a deficiency in the absorption of vitamin K resulting in reduced prothrombin production.

Anesthesia and anesthetic agents may interfere with many aspects of liver function. In addition, preexisting disease may be influenced detrimentally by the combination of surgery and anesthesia. Of particular importance are changes in liver blood flow, drug metabolism and the potentially toxic effects of anesthetic agents on the liver cell. Before embarking on anesthesia in patients with liver disease a full hepatic assessment should be made. This includes a careful history, with specific questions concerning drug and alcohol intake and exposure to the risk of viral infections, clinical examination of the patient as well as a review of liver function tests. Such tests, unfortunately, are somewhat crude and inexact, and only begin to show changes when there is considerable deterioration of liver function. Clinical examination of the patient may be proportionately of more importance than the results of any one 'specific' liver function test.

Asymptomatic changes in liver function tests are not uncommon (Hulcrantz et al., 1986). A common finding with many of these patients is that they are obese, or have increased alcohol consumption or diabetes mellitus. Liver biopsy (the best method of determining a diagnosis) reveals a significant number with either chronic active hepatitis or cirrhosis. In these patients, the most likely outcome following anesthesia and surgery is that there will be no major detrimental changes in hepatic function except those related to the extent of the operation and other factors, e.g. blood transfusion (Strunin and Davies, 1983).

LIVER BLOOD FLOW

The splanchnic blood flow (SBF) perfuses the gastrointestinal tract, spleen, pancreas, gall bladder, omentum and liver. With the exception of the liver, all the splanchnic organs initially receive an arterial blood supply and then their venous drainage passes to the liver via the portal vein. The liver's blood supply is in two parts, 70% from the portal vein and the remaining 30% from the hepatic artery. In practice the SBF may be accounted for by the flow of blood in the portal vein and hepatic artery. Measurement of hepatic blood flow (HBF) is more usual than measurement of SBF and the two terms are usually considered as interchangeable (Cooperman, 1972); liver blood flow (LBF) may be used as an alternative to HBF.

Grayson and Mendel (1965) described the splanchnic blood supply in terms of two low pressure and one high pressure zones supplying three main parallel resistances. In normal health the portal vein is responsible for the majority of the blood flow to the liver, but the hepatic artery supplies some 50% of the hepatic oxygen requirement. However where there is portal hypertension and obstruction to portal vein blood flow the hepatic artery blood flow is increased. In addition, portasystemic shunts open, e.g. around the esophagus as varices. The increased hepatic arterial blood flow was the rationale for portacaval anastomosis, without necessarily decreasing total liver blood flow to an unacceptable low level. However, it should be noted that the results of surgically induced portasystemic shunts are poor and many centers have moved to injection sclerotherapy for the management of esophageal varices (Westaby et al., 1982).

Measurement of Hepatic Blood Flow

The original method of estimating hepatic blood flow (EHBF) used the Fick principle and employed bromsulphthalein (BSP) as the indicator. BSP is not ideal as some of it undergoes enterohepatic circulation and in patients with a raised serum bilirubin there may be inadequate extraction of BSP from the circulation. As an alternative indicator indocyanine green (ICG) is more suitable as it is cleared from the plasma almost exclusively by the liver and enterohepatic circulation is negligible. However both BSP and ICG rely on good hepatocyte function for their uptake from the plasma. In the presence of liver disease, where there is reduction in biliary flow or biliary obstruction or severe hepatocellular disease the clearance of both BSP and ICG may be markedly impaired, yet liver blood flow may be relatively normal. In these circumstances the Kupffer cells may still be active, and since these cells are part of the reticuloendothelial system, they will readily take up colloidal particles. Hepatic blood flow can be estimated using the following formula:

$$EHBF = K \times BV$$

where BV is blood volume and K (the peripheral disappearance rate constant) = 0.693 divided by $T_{1/2}$—the time required for the indicator concentration to fall to half the initial value. Various colloidal particles have been used such as radioactive colloidal gold, denatured albumin labelled with ^{131}I and colloidal particles of chromic phosphate labelled with ^{32}P. Blood sampling or an external gamma counter placed over the liver are used to detect the indicator. Other methods of estimating hepatic blood flow include the clearance of ^{85}Kr or ^{133}Xe using an external gamma counter over the liver and in the experimental animal electromagnetic flowmeters around the portal vein and hepatic artery. Electromagnetic flowmeters have also been used in man at the time of a laparotomy. Despite the various indicators available for measurement of HBF in man, most studies have been done in animal models or human volunteers, either conscious or under general anesthesia; very little data is available on changes in liver blood flow during anesthesia and surgery, particularly in patients with liver disease.

Anesthetic Factors Influencing Liver Blood Flow

Blood flow in the splanchnic bed and to the liver is related directly to perfusion pressure and inversely to vascular resistance. A reduction in systemic arterial pressure to the order of 80 mmHg will not result in any significant change in hepatic blood flow. Below this value, however, autoregulation fails and in addition to a reduction in hepatic arterial blood flow, portal venous and therefore total hepatic blood flow will all decrease as the systemic arterial pressure decreases. In can be seen therefore that a reduction in liver blood flow could be due to a decrease either in the portal vein or hepatic artery perfusion pressure. These in turn could be due to reduced systemic arterial or increased hepatic venous pressure.

The splanchnic vascular bed and the hepatic artery are richly innervated by the sympathetic nervous system and contain both α and β adrenergic receptors. Therefore any factor which increases sympathetic nervous activity will affect splanchnic vascular resistance and liver blood flow (Table 35.1). In general terms all

TABLE 35.1
FACTORS AFFECTING LIVER BLOOD FLOW

	Splanchnic vascular resistance	*LBF*
Hypoxia	Increased	Reduced
Hypercarbia (a)	Increased	Reduced
α stimulation	Increased	Reduced
β blockade	Increased	Reduced
Ganglion blockade	No change	Reduced
β stimulation	Reduced	Increased
N$_2$O, suxamethonium and hypercarbia	Increased	Reduced
Halothane and hypercarbia	Reduced	Increased
Methoxyflurane and halothane (b)	—	Reduced (? direct effect on hepatic artery)

(a) Not all authors agree on hypercarbia reducing LBF (*see* Hughes et al., 1979).
(b) The alleged direct effect of these agents on the hepatic artery has been observed during coeliac angiography (Alfery and Benumof, 1981); it is not clear whether catheter spasm, the radio-opaque dye or the agents themselves are responsible.

anesthetic techniques, including spinal and extradural blockade, reduce liver blood flow either as a result of decreased perfusion pressure or splanchnic vasoconstriction. However, a study of hepatic blood flow, measured by a colloidal gold technique, showed that the main determinant of the extent of the alteration in splanchnic blood flow during anesthesia and surgery was surgical trauma (Gelman, 1976). In patients undergoing herniorrhaphy or excision of a breast tumour EHBF decreased to 82% and 76% respectively, while in patients undergoing partial gastrectomy or cholecystectomy, EHBF decreased to 48% and 42% respectively of its initial value. Anesthesia, in these cases was with either diethyl ether or halothane, and these led to a decrease in EHBF 88% and 84% of the initial values.

The decrease in liver blood flow seen with all anesthetic techniques is also accompanied by decreased oxygen uptake by the splanchnic organs. Comparisons of the ratios between these two variables show that changes in arterial carbon dioxide tension are very relevant (Table 35.2). The fact that all ratios are less than unity suggest the possibility of hypoxic conditions occurring within the liver during anesthesia.

TABLE 35.2
SPLANCHNIC CIRCULATION DURING ANESTHESIA

Anesthetic	R	Type of ventilation
Halothane	0.85	Spontaneous
Halothane	0.82	Controlled
N$_2$O-curare	0.82	Controlled
Cyclopropane	0.79	Controlled
N$_2$O-curare	0.59	Hyperventilation
Methoxyflurane	0.55	Controlled

Ratio (R) of change in blood flow during anesthesia to change in oxygen consumption. (R = 1: equal reduction of both SBF and splanchnic oxygen consumption; R <: residual oxygen consumption in excess of remaining perfusion.)

In patients with normal liver function it is unlikely that the reduction in liver blood flow associated with any anesthetic technique or surgical procedure will have detrimental effects. However, in the patient with pre-existing liver disease any decrease in liver blood flow may be detrimental. It therefore seems sensible that in such patients the anesthetic technique used should be the one that has the least effect on the splanchnic circulation and liver blood flow. From the available information it would seem that a spinal or extradural anesthetic will reduce blood flow in proportion to the decrease in mean arterial pressure produced. For general anesthesia, an oxygen-nitrous oxide, relaxant, opioid sequence with IPPV to normocapnia would seem to have the least effect on splanchnic vascular resistance and liver blood flow.

Of the currently used volatile anesthetic agents halothane has been most studied (see Table 35.1). Both hypo and hyper-ventilation seem undesirable. Hypoxia and hypotension, by causing sympathetic stimulation, will increase splanchnic vascular resistance and thereby reduce liver blood flow. Enflurane and isoflurane appear to be similar in their effects to halothane (Gelman, 1986). However, their influence on hepatic artery blood flow (HABF) appears to be less; although this latter data is derived from animal models (Hughes et al. 1980; Gelman, 1986) and may not be applicable in humans. In theory, enflurane and isoflurane may preserve oxygen supply to the liver better than halothane. This assumes that in a given circumstance HABF is capable of increasing. Even so, the extent of pre-existing disease and the surgical procedure are probably much more relevant in determining any detrimental outcome as far as postoperative liver problems are concerned than the anesthetic technique used.

DRUG METABOLISM

The liver is the major organ of drug metabolism and is capable of dealing with a wide variety of drugs using a limited number of relatively simple processes. Phase I reactions act on the lipid soluble drug and by either oxidation, reduction or hydrolysis may convert the drug in question directly to a water soluble metabolite which can then be excreted in either the urine or bile. Phase II reactions concern conjugation and act either on the drug itself or after a phase I reaction and again produce a water soluble metabolite which may be excreted. Most anesthetic drugs are metabolized by oxidation but recently attention has focused on the reductive pathway, particularly for volatile anesthetic agents. Factors which may affect metabolism of drugs include, inherited abnormalities of drug metabolizing enzymes, age, sex, liver blood flow, volume of distribution, pre-existing liver disease and interactions between drugs.

The capacity of the liver to metabolize drugs may be increased. This occurs because the drug metabolizing enzyme complexes may be induced by a wide variety of substances including barbiturates and in particular phenobarbital. Under these circumstances there is an increase in the amount of microsomal enzymes and cytochromes involved in drug metabolism in the smooth part of the endoplasmic reticulum of the hepatocytes. Enzymatically induced animal models in combination with hypoxia have been used for the study of the metabolism of volatile anesthetic agents, in particular with reference to potential hepatotoxicity (Stock and Strunin, 1985).

Non-depolarizing Neuromuscular Blocking Drugs

It is well recognized the patients with liver damage may require increased doses of non-depolarizing neuromuscular blocking drugs and exhibit apparent resistance. This was first described for curare and more recently for pancuronium. The explanation of the resistance is not entirely clear and does not seem to be related to the low pseudocholinesterase concentration sometimes found in liver disease, or to alteration in protein binding. In patients with cirrhosis the probable explanation is the increase in the distribution volume of pancuronium as a result of the liver disease (Duvaldestin et al., 1985). However in patients with total biliary obstruction, where liver cell function may be relatively normal a prolonged effect of steroid muscle relaxants may occur. This may reflect the lack of the biliary route of excretion in these patients (Somogyi et al., 1977). However, Westra et al. (1981) have demonstrated that steroidal muscle relaxants are less readily taken up by the liver cells in the presence of infused taurocholate and chenodeoxycholate. This effect is not seen with the non-steroidal based neuromuscular blocking agents.

Vecuronium has a high biliary clearance (Bencini et al., 1986) in contrast to other non-depolarizing neuromuscular blocking drugs. In the presence of cholestasis (biliary obstruction) there is a prolonged elimination phase, but as hepatic uptake is rapid and this probably accounts for the normal short action of vecuronium (Lebrault et al., 1986). Surgical manipulation of the liver and biliary tract may affect the clearance of vecuronium and possibly prolong its action (Bencini et al., 1986). In patients with cholestasis, cirrhosis or hepatic failure the muscle relaxant of choice is probably atracurium. It is independent of hepatic metabolism, as it undergoes non-enzymatic breakdown in plasma and is excreted in the urine (Miller, 1986).

Since hepatic disease may be accompanied by renal dysfunction, any neuromuscular blocking drug may have an increase in its elimination time. Monitoring of neuromuscular activity, avoidance of incremental doses and facilities for postoperative ventilation are essential for the management of patients with liver disease given neuromuscular blocking drugs.

Opioids

In cirrhotic patients morphine elimination time is increased due to a decrease in hepatic extraction ratio or heptatic blood flow; renal impairment may be an additional factor but cholestasis does not interfere with morphine pharmacokinetics (McQuay and Moore, 1984; Shelly et al., 1986; Mazoit et al., 1987). Most hepatology texts indicate that morphine is unsuitable for cirrhotic patients, claiming profound and prolonged effects of conventional doses. Although some of this is explicable by altered pharmacokinetics, the presence of 'coma factors' due to hepatic dysfunction may compound the normal action of morphine or other opioids (Corall and Williams, 1986).

Intravenous Induction Agents

Of the currently available intravenous induction agents none are dependant on biliary excretion for their elimination. However, the elimination phase is prolonged if liver blood flow is reduced in cirrhotic patients (Van Been et al., 1983) although increased doses may be required for such patients due to increased volume of distribution there may be a prolonged recovery, particularly if infusion techniques are used (Thompson et al., 1986; Grounds et al., 1987). Thiopentone illustrates all these difficulties; etomidate has no advantages (Van Been et al., 1983); propofol has yet to be assessed (Grounds et al., 1987); benzodiazepines may have extremely prolonged action, and only small doses should be administered. Oxazepam and lorazepam are to be preferred (Corall et al., 1986).

Volatile Anesthetic Agents

All volatile anesthetics undergo biotransformation primarlly to non-volatile substances by oxidative metabolism. These are then excreted in the bile and urine and may be present in small amounts for several weeks after anesthesia. Of the currently used ethane vapours, 20%, 3% and less than 0.5% of halothane, enflurane and isoflurane are metabolized respectively. In addition, reductive metabolism of halothane may occur giving rise to both volatile and non-volatile metabolites.

The reductive metabolic pathway has been extensively investigated as a possible mechanism for unexplained hepatitis following halothane (UHFH) exposure. Animal models using enzyme induction and hypoxia do demonstrate hepatic damage after single exposure to halothane; damage also occurs with other agents including thiopentone and fentanyl and may reflect the effects of hypoxia, compounded by the drugs, rather than a direct action of the drug itself. Therefore the relevance of these studies to the human experience is unclear (Stock et al., 1985). In particular, UHFH is usually associated with multiple exposures to halothane, often at short intervals, and factors such as hypoxia, hypotension, enzyme induction, viral infection and blood transfusion have to be ruled out. A genetic predisposition to UHFH has been proposed and a guinea pig model developed (Lind et al., 1987). An immune response to the metabolites of halothane has been proposed to explain the development of UHFH (Stock et al., 1985).

Although there appears to be no contraindication to the use of halothane in patients with liver disease, where the cause is known and does not relate to a previous halothane anesthetic, the medicolegal climate in many parts of the world is such that halothane is no longer used for such patients. Liver damage has been reported following the use of both enflurane and isoflurane (Eger et al., 1986; Brown and Gandolfi, 1987; Carrigan and Straughen, 1987; Stoelting, 1987; Stoelting et al., 1987). At present, it is believed that these cases represent drug association only and it has yet to be proven that the drugs caused the liver damage directly or as a result of some other interaction (Eger et al., 1986; Stoelting, 1987). Since isoflurane has been least associated with liver dysfunction it is currently the volatile agent of choice in patients with hepatic dysfunction.

ANESTHESIA IN THE PATIENT WITH LIVER DYSFUNCTION

Patients may present for anesthesia and surgery with many forms of liver disease and the exact diagnosis may not be clear. The degree of liver dysfunction, the presence or absence of jaundice and the presence of viral infection must be assessed and the clinical examination of the patient is also relevant (Strunin, 1978).

Jaundice as the Presenting Symptom

Jaundice is a clinical observation and occurs when serum bilirubin exceeds 20 μmol/L. Such an increase may be associated with disorders of bilirubin metabolism or may be evidence of cellular liver disease. Many causes of jaundice are not amenable to surgical treatment and unnecessary diagnostic laparotomies may be avoided by careful questioning of the patient concerning drug history, alcohol intake, or evidence of chronic liver disease or viral infection. The major deciding factors for surgery in jaundiced patients are shown in Table 35.3. In particular, ultrasound (Table 35.4) should be used as the determining pathway for further diagnostic tests or therapeutic manoeuvers such as: endoscopic retrograde cholangiopancreatography and papillotomy (ERCP), percutaneous transhepatic cholangiography (PTC) and magnetic resonance imaging MRI.

TABLE 35.3
DECIDING FACTORS FOR SURGERY IN JAUNDICED PATIENTS

Symptom or sign	Likely diagnosis
Abdominal pain	Gallstones
Fever, rigors	Cholangitis, hepatic abscess
Enlarged gallbladder	Intrahepatic, neoplastic obstruction
Aids to Diagnosis	*Inference of Results*
Leucocytosis	Cholangitis, gallstones
Increased transaminases normal alkaline phosphatase	Hepatocellular damage
Increased alkaline phosphatase normal transaminases	Biliary obstruction
Abdominal radiograph	Gallstones, gas in biliary tree indicating a fistula
Oral, I.V. or percutaneous cholangiogram or ultrasound scan	Indication of site of biliary obstruction
Liver biopsy	Differentiation of intra- and extra-hepatic cholestasis
Liver scintiscan	Liver tumor

TABLE 35.4
USE OF ULTRASOUND TO DETERMINE DIAGNOSTIC TESTS

Diagnostic test

1. Ultrasound indicates space occupying lesions, consider abscess, cyst, tumour, proceed to liver biopsy.
2. Ultrasound shows nondilated ducts, proceed to liver biopsy and/or ERCP.
3. Ultrasound shows dilated ducts, proceed to PTC or ERCP.
4. Ultrasound shows portal/hepatic vein obstruction, proceed to arteriography/phlebography.
5. Ultrasound accompanied by CAT scanning and MRI.

Disorders of Blood Coagulation

A prolonged prothrombin time may occur in the jaundiced patient and results from the lack of absorption of vitamin K from the gut due to the absence of bile salts. Other clotting factors also require the presence

of vitamin K and therefore complex blood coagulation problems may occur. Furthermore, if there is concomitant hepatocellular disease, defective synthesis may also lead to a lack of clotting factors. Such defective synthesis is associated with a low serum albumin concentration in patients with liver disease.

All jaundiced patients should receive a course of parenteral vitamin K therapy before anesthesia and surgery. If prothrombin activity does not return to normal, it is indicative of hepatocellular damage and fresh frozen plasma infusion may be helpful in reducing the risk of severe hemorrhage during surgery or diagnostic procedures.

Renal Failure after Operation

Postoperative renal failure is a well recognized complication of obstructive jaundice. The probable cause is excess circulating endotoxin produced from the patients own bowel flora, caused by the reduction in bile salts resulting from the biliary obstruction. During anesthesia and surgery there is a reduction in renal vascular perfusion and the stage is set for acute renal failure (Bailey, 1976). This complication is potentially avoidable by taking the following steps. Patients should be adequately rehydrated prior to surgery, consideration should be given to biliary drainage percutaneously preoperatively, antibiotic therapy should be instituted, and finally adequate urine output should be maintained before, during and after the operation by fluid infusion and, if necessary, by administration of mannitol (Table 35.5).

TABLE 35.5
PREVENTION OF POSTOPERATIVE RENAL FAILURE IN THE PATIENT WITH BILIARY OBSTRUCTION

Serum bilirubin (μmol/L)	Management
Over 20	Urinary catheter: monitor urine output 1. If urine volume greater than 50 ml/h, no action 2. If urine output less than 50 ml/h, fluid loading and mannitol 5 or 10% until adequate diuresis
Over 140	Preoperative: fluid loading, antibiotics and urinary catheter Fluid loading plus mannitol 5–10% to maintain urine volume above 50 ml/h. Continue regime pre and postoperatively up to 36 h

Chronic Liver Disease

Chronic liver disease, hepatocellular disease or cirrhosis are often used to describe the same thing. Cirrhosis is a pathological term and describes the changes which occur in the liver, produced by a number of etiological factors

Compensated chronic liver disease is compatible with a complete feeling of wellbeing, and when symptoms do occur they are usually vague. One of the most useful signs of cirrhosis is the presence of spider naevi on the skin of the face, arms and upper torso. A constant feature of the condition is increased resistance to flow of blood in the portal venous system, resulting in portal hypertension and the development of collateral venous channels. These latter are most commonly found around the umbilicus, at the lower end of the esophagus (esophageal varices) and in the rectum. In the later stages of chronic liver disease there may be progressive signs of impending renal failure. Other observations which suggest that chronic liver disease has become decompensated include jaundice, edema, ascites, a flapping tremor of the hands and changes in the patient's neurological state progressing to coma. A change in size or shape of the liver may indicate that a hepatoma has developed. The three major complications which may occur in the cirrhotic patient are encephalopathy, ascites and gastrointestinal hemorrhage. Other problems include infection, jaundice and vitamin deficiency.

Patients with chronic liver disease may present for anesthesia and surgery either for procedures unrelated to their liver dysfunction or as a result of complications such as gastrointestinal bleeding. A grading system should be used (Table 35.6) to assess liver

TABLE 35.6
GRADING OF SEVERITY OF LIVER DISEASE
(Pugh et al., 1973)

Clinical and biochemical measurement	Points scored for increasing abnormalities		
	1	2	3
Encephalopathy (grade)	None	1 & 2	3 & 4
Bilirubin (µmol/L)	< 25	24–40	> 40
Albumin (g/L)	35	28–35	< 28
Prothrombin time (sec prolonged)	1–4	4–6	> 6

Using this system patients who score 5–6 points are considered good operative risks (Grade A); 7, 8 or 9 moderate (Grade B); and patients with 10–15 poor operative risks (Grade C).

function in such patients with a view to determining their 'fitness for anesthesia'. In general, only patients in Grade A should be considered as suitable. It may be possible to improve the liver function of patients with chronic liver disease where some acute episode, such as gastrointestinal hemorrhage, has produced a deterioration. In these circumstances, protein restriction may restore the patient's liver function to its previous state and subsequently reduce the risk of problems during anesthesia and surgery. Similarly,

administration of vitamin K may improve prothrombin activity.

Anesthetic Considerations

The neurological response of the patient to analgesic or sedative drugs used for premedication may be a useful guide as to what will happen in the postoperative period. Hydrocortisone hemisuccinate should be given by intramuscular injection if the patient is on steroid therapy. Fluid balance should be assessed particularly in the severely jaundiced patient.

All anesthetic techniques, both regional and general will decrease liver blood flow. In the patient whose liver function is already compromised further damage may occur regardless of anesthetic choice. As already indicated above, halothane is not contraindicated, but the dose should be adjusted in accordance with the patient's cardiovascular system. Suitable anesthetic techniques for major surgery in patients with chronic liver disease and the treatment of bleeding esophageal varices have been described (Ward et al., 1975; Ward et al., 1976). Most often, fentanyl is the opioid of choice along with isoflurane if a volatile supplement is needed, atracurium is preferred for muscle relaxation.

Viral Hepatitis

Viral hepatitis may be associated with liver dysfunction ranging from a mild disturbance, with or without jaundice, to acute liver failure. Recovery may be complete with immunity to further infection, or the patient may be left a symptomless carrier of the virus or with chronic liver disease. A number of different viruses can cause hepatitis, for example, cytomegalovirus or the Epstein-Barr virus of glandular fever, but most cases are related to either hepatitis A (HAV), hepatitis B (HBV) or non-A non-B virus (NANB) infection. With the exception of NANB serological screening can determine infection with hepatitic viruses and identify carriers. In view of the association between HBV, NANB and HIV (human immunodeficiency virus the causative agent of acquired immune deficiency syndrome-AIDS) infection, patients should be considered as potentially infectious to others for all viruses until proven otherwise. Indeed, many infection control systems are based on the premise that all body fluids and secretions are potentially infectious and sensible precautions should be taken with all patients, since carriers cannot always be identified.

HBV is of concern since infection with this virus may be followed by a carrier state, chronic liver disease, and the development of hepatoma (primary carcinoma of the liver). NANB has also been shown to be associated with the development of a carrier state and chronic liver disease. In countries with blood bank screening programmes NANB is now the commonest cause of post-transfusion hepatitis (PTH).

During anesthesia and surgery, the major anxiety with regard to HBV and NANB is the risk of spread of the infection to theater personnel. The viruses are transmitted primarily parenterally. The infectivity of patients for HBV may be assessed by measuring the surface antigen (HBsAg) associated with HBV infection. A further antigen, the 'e' antigen, which is derived from the core of the hepatitis B virus, may also be present and indicates a high degree of infectivity. As indicated above any patient may be infected, but a number of high risk groups have been identified (Strunin, 1986). Since these patients may present at any time for anesthesia and surgery it is suggested that a routine be followed so as to avoid any contamination.

The number of personnel in the operating theater should be kept to a minimum and disposable caps, masks, gowns, gloves and overshoes worn as appropriate. For the anesthetist the wearing of gloves may make the placement of intravenous needles more difficult. Unnecessary injections and blood sampling should be avoided. Clearly marked bags should be available so that every disposable item that comes into contact with the patient may be incinerated. Nondisposable anesthetic items may be sterilized where appropriate by heating, ethylene oxide or the use of proprietary bleach solutions.

In the event of inadvertent contamination with infected material, the person at risk should be tested for HBsAg and antibody (anti-HBs), if the latter test is available and the results obtainable within a few hours. As soon as it is established that infected material was involved the recipient, unless previously vaccinated or unless shown to have anti-HBs, should receive a dose of specific hyperimmune anti-HBs serum. Ideally this should be done within 48 hours of exposure; and this should be followed by a second dose one month later. Physicians most commonly aquire HBV in the course of their professional activities as a result of needle sticks. Therefore, it is unlikely that gloves, gowns or other protective devices that can be pierced by a needle will be protective. All anesthetists should consider vaccination as the only rational protection against HBV. The vaccines available, either human or recombinant DNA derived are both safe and effective. Nevertheless, since HBV vaccination does not protect against NANB precautions should still be taken with body fluids from patients. The risk of acquiring HIV infection during anesthetic practice seems extremely low, and will be further reduced by the care taken in avoiding HBV and NANB.

Patients with compensated liver disease who have chronic HBV or NANB infection are unlikely to suffer further deterioration of their liver function other than that attributable to the extent of their pre-existing liver dysfunction and subsequent surgery. However, if the patient is in the incubation period of acute viral hepatitis or has active disease, anesthesia and surgery may be extremely hazardous and should be postponed if possible (Powell-Jackson et al., 1982; Aranha and Greenlee, 1986).

ACUTE LIVER FAILURE

Patients with chronic liver disease often develop hepatic failure in the terminal phase of their illness. The prognosis here is poor because of the underlying irreversible liver damage and the single most common cause in the United Kingdom is alcohol abuse.

Acute liver failure, sometimes called fulminant hepatic failure (FHF) occurs in a small group of patients and by definition is a clinical syndrome that occurs as a result of massive necrosis of liver cells in a patient who has had no previous evidence of liver disease. It is characterized by the onset of a severe progressive encephalopathy and a mortality rate as high as 80–90% in those patients who develop signs of grade four coma (the patient is unrousable and may or may not respond to noxious stimuli). However patients with FHF who recover do so completely and are unlikely to develop chronic liver disease.

The common causes of FHF are, paracetamol overdose, viral hepatitis, and UHFH (Corall et al., 1986). In most patients the diagnosis of acute liver failure is not difficult; the patient is deeply jaundiced, comatose and has other clinical signs related to acid-base, cardiac, renal, metabolic and hematological disturbances. The liver is small and the peripheral stigmas of underlying chronic liver disease are absent. The transaminases are markedly raised and often greater than 2000 i.u./L. Alkaline phosphatase concentration and albumin levels may be relatively normal. The most striking feature is a markedly prolonged prothrombin time.

Management of FHF requires close cooperation between many departments and ideally patients should be admitted to a specialized unit (Ward et al., 1977; Corall et al., 1986). Since viral hepatitis is a common cause of the condition all patients should be screened for the presence of hepatitis B surface antigen.

Investigation and Management of the Multisystem Disorders

Acid-base disturbances are common and hyperventilation is a constant feature during the early stages of coma. Hypoxia is a frequent finding and results from decreased respiration due to depression of the respiratory center as the condition progresses, pulmonary edema, infection or intrapulmonary shunting occurs. Oxygen therapy and IPPV with positive end expiratory pressure may be necessary.

Renal disturbances including hyponatremia and hypokalemia are seen in about 50% of patients at some time in their illness. In addition about half of the patients with FHF develop renal failure.

Hypoglycemia can develop rapidly in acute liver failure and lead to irreversible brain damage. Blood glucose levels should be monitored frequently and complication may be avoided by infusion of 10% dextrose intravenously.

As liver function deteriorates synthesis of clotting factors declines. This is manifested as a prolonged prothrombin time and depressed circulating levels of fibrinogen and other clotting factors. Daily infusions of fresh frozen plasma are indicated, although these only partially correct clotting defects and bleeding may occur from esophageal varices. If the gastric pH can be maintained above 5.0 by prophylactic ranitidine therapy, hemorrhage from the upper gastrointestinal tract may be prevented.

The common modes of death in patients with FHF are encephalopathy, cerebral edema and infection. Use of conventional supportive therapy does improve the overall mortality in FHF but it is unlikely that any such maneuvers have any real effect on either encephalopathy or cerebral edema. At present the cause of encephalopathy of FHF remains speculative. However, it is probably due wholly or partly to an accumulation of compounds that arise because of a failure of the liver to detoxify its normal metabolic products particularly those resulting from protein catabolism.

The survival of patients with FHF may be improved by management in a center designed for treatment of such patients (Corall et al., 1986). Effective antidote treatment of paracetamol poisoning in the first 14 hours will prevent FHF. Charcoal hemoperfusion, aggressive treatment of cerebral edema including intracranial pressure monitoring are proven methods of reducing mortality in acute liver failure.

REFERENCES

Alfery D.D., Benumof J.L. (1981). Hepatic blood flow alterations during anesthesia and surgery. In *Anesthesia and the Patient with Liver Disease* (Burnell Brown Jr. F.A. ed.), Philadelphia: Davis Company.

Aranha G.V., Greenlee H.B. (1986). Intraabdominal surgery in patients with advanced cirrhosis. *Arch. Surg.*, **121**, 774.

Bailey M.E. (1976). Endotoxin, bile salts and renal function in obstructive jaundice. *Br. J. Surg.*, **63**, 774.

Bencini A.F., Scaf A.H.J., Sohn Y.J., et al. (1986). Hepatobiliary disposition of vecuronium bromide in man. *Br. J. Anaesth.*, **58**, 988.

Brown B.R. Jr., Gandolfi A.J. (1987). Adverse effects of volatile anaesthetics. *Br. J. Anaesth.*, **59**, 14.

Carrigan T.W., Straughen W.J. (1987). A report of hepatic necrosis and death following isoflurane anesthesia. *Anesthesiology*, **67**, 581.

Cooperman L.H. (1972). Effects of anesthetic on the splanchnic circulation. *Br. J. Anaesth.*, **44**, 967.

Corall I., Williams R. (1986). Management of liver failure. *Br. J. Anaesth.*, **58**, 234.

Duvaldestin P., Lebrault C., Cahuvin M. (1985). Pharmacokinetics of muscle relaxants in patients with liver disease. *Clin. Anesth.*, **3**, 293.

Eger EI. II., Smuckler E.A., Ferrel L.D., et al. (1986). Is enflurane hepatotoxic? *Anesth. Analg.*, **65**, 21.

Ferrier C., Marty J., Bouffard J., et al. (1985). Alfentanil pharmacokinetics in patients with cirrhosis. *Anesthesiology*, **62**, 480.

Gelman S. (1976). Disturbances in hepatic blood flow during anesthesia. *Arch. Surg.*, **111**, 881.

Gelman S. (1986). Effects of anesthetics on splanchnic circulation. In *Cardiovascular Actions of Anesthetics*, pp. 126–61. (Altura B.M., Halevy S. eds.). Basel: Karger.

Grayson J., Mendel D. (1965). *Physiology of the Splanchnic Circulation* Baltimore: Williams and Wilkins.

Grounds R.M., Lalor J.M., Lumley J., et al. (1987). Propofol infusion for sedation in the intensive care unit: preliminary report. *Br. Med. J.*, **294**, 397.

Haberer J.P., Shoeffler E., Couderc E., et al. (1982). Fentanyl pharmacokinetics in anesthetised patients with cirrhosis. *Br. J. Anaesth.*, **54**, 1267.

Hughes R.L., Campbell D., Fitch W. (1980). Effects of enflurane and halothane on liver blood flow and oxygen consumption in the greyhound. *Br. J. Anaesth.*, **52**, 1079.

Hulcrantz R., Glauman H., Lindberg G., et al. (1986). Liver investigation in 149 asymptomatic patients with moderately elevated activities of serum aminotransferases. *Scand. J. Gastroenterol.*, **21**, 109.

Lebrault C., Duvaldestin P., Henzel D., et al. (1986). Pharmacokinetics and pharmacodynamics of vecuronium in patients with cholestasis. *Br. J. Anaesth.*, **58**, 983.

Lind R.C., Gandolfi A.J., Brown B.R., Jr. et al. (1987). Halothane hepatotoxicity in guinea pigs. *Anesth. Analg.*, **66**, 222.

Mazoit J., Sandouk P., Zetlaovi P., et al. (1987). Pharmacokinetics of unchanged morphine in normal and cirrhotic subjects. *Anesth. Analg.*, **66**, 293.

McQuay H., Moore A. (1984). Be aware of renal function when monitoring morphine. *Lancet*, **2**, 284.

Miller R.D. (1986). Pharmacokinetics of atracurium and the nondepolarising neuromuscular blocking agents in normal patients and those with renal or hepatic dysfunction. *Br. J. Anaesth.*, **58**, 22S.

Powell-Jackson P., Greenway B., Williams R. (1982). Adverse effects of exploratory laparotomy in patients with suspected liver disease. *Br. J. Surg.*, **68**, 449.

Pugh R.N.H., Murray-Lyon I.M., Dawson J.L., et al. (1973). Transection of the oesophagus for bleeding oesophageal varices. *Br. J. Surg.*, **60**, 646.

Shelly M.P., Cory E.P., Park G.R. (1986). Pharmacokinetics of morphine in two children before and after liver transplantation. *Br. J. Anaesth.*, **58**, 1218.

Somogyi A.A., Shanks C.A., Triggs E.J. (1977). Clinical pharmacokinetic of pancuronium bromide. *Eur. J. Clin. Pharmacol.*, **10 (s)**, 367.

Stock J.L., Strunin L. (1985). Unexplained hepatitis following halothane. *Anesthesiology*, **63**, 424.

Stoelting R.K. (1987). Isoflurane and postoperative hepatic dysfunction. *Can. J. Anaesth.*, **34**, 223.

Stoelting R.K., Blitt C.D., Cohen P.J., et al. (1987). Hepatic dysfunction after isoflurane anesthesia. *Anesth. Analg.*, **66**, 147.

Strunin L. (1978). Preoperative assessment of the patient with liver dysfunction. *Br. J. Anaesth.*, **50**, 25.

Strunin L. (1986). Viral hepatitis. In *Anesthesiology* pp. 95–101. (Stanley T.H., Petty W.C. eds.). Dordhrecht: Martinus Nijhoff.

Strunin L., Davies J.M. (1983). The liver and anaesthesia. *Can. Anaesth. Soc. J.*, **30**, 208.

Thompson I.A., Fitch W., Hughes R.L., et al. (1986). Effects of certain IV anaesthetics on liver blood flow and hepatic oxygen consumption in the greyhound. *Br. J. Anaesth.*, **58**, 69.

Van Been H., Manger F.W., Van Boxtel C., et al. (1983). Etomidate anaesthesia in patients with cirrhosis of the liver: pharmacokinetic data. *Anaesthesia*, **38**, 61S.

Ward M.E., Adu-Gyamfi Y., Strunin L. (1975). Althesin and pancuronium in chronic liver disease. *Br. J. Anaesth.*, **47**, 1199.

Ward M.E., Davies T.D.W., Strunin L. (1976). Anaesthesia for injection of bleeding oesophageal varices. *Ann. R. Coll. Surg. Engl.*, **58**, 315.

Ward M.E., Trewby P.N., Williams R., et al. (1977). Acute liver failure. *Anaesthesia*, **32**, 228.

Westaby D., Macdougal B.R.D., Williams R. (1982). *Variceal Bleeding*. London: Pitman Books Ltd.

Westra P., Houwertjes M.C., Wesseling H., et al. (1981). Bile salts and neuromuscular blocking agents. *Br. J. Anaesth.*, **53**, 407.

36. Anaesthesia and the Kidney

Michael Cousins and G. Skowronski

Applied anatomy and physiology of the kidney are briefly reviewed. This includes an account of: renal blood flow, glomerular filtration rate, juxtaglomerular apparatus, renal autoregulation and intrarenal blood flow distribution, tubular transport mechanisms, solute handling in proximal tubule, function of Loop of Henle and distal tubule system. This section concludes with a summary of changes in tubule fluid along the length of the nephron.

Acute effects of anaesthesia are reviewed in detail. Indirect effects include those on circulatory and sympathetic nervous systems, autoregulation, endocrine systems such as those involving atrial natriuretic peptide anti-diuretic hormone, adrenaline and noradrenaline, renin, angiotensin and aldosterone. Direct effects of anaesthesia on renal function have now been confirmed both *in vitro* and *in vivo*.

Delayed direct nephrotoxicity of anaesthetics relates predominantly to methoxyflurane (MOF) and its metabolism to inorganic fluoride. Other factors are: MOF dose, genetics, age, enzyme induction, obesity, other nephrotoxic drugs. Clinical implications are presented. Enflurane nephrotoxicity is rare but aetiologic factors are similar to the foregoing. Isoflurane and halothane are not nephrotoxic.

A consideration of the influence of anaesthetic management on the incidence and severity of postoperative acute renal failure, concludes the review.

Introduction

Before considering the effects of anaesthesia on the kidney, it is necessary to review briefly its applied anatomy and physiology (Sullivan and Grantham, 1982; Pitts, 1965; Hawker, 1982; Bastron and Deutsch, 1976).

APPLIED ANATOMY OF THE KIDNEY

Anatomy of the Renal Vasculature

Each main renal artery divides into several interlobar arteries. These divide again to form the arcuate arteries, which run in the boundary between renal cortex and medulla. The arcuate arteries send numerous parallel branches, the interlobular arteries, out towards the renal surface. From the interlobular arteries are derived the glomerular afferent arterioles. The glomerular capillaries coalesce to form glomerular efferent arterioles, which then branch again to form the peritubular capillary network (Fig. 36.1).

This arrangement of two capillary beds in series, separated only by the efferent arterioles is unique to the renal circulation. Blood flowing through the glomerular capillaries has a high hydrostatic pressure, thus favouring filtration. However, in the peritubular capillary network, colloid osmotic pressure is high following filtration of protein-free fluid in the glomeruli, and hydrostatic pressure is low. This favours reabsorption of peritubular interstitial fluid (*vide infra* in Fig. 36.4).

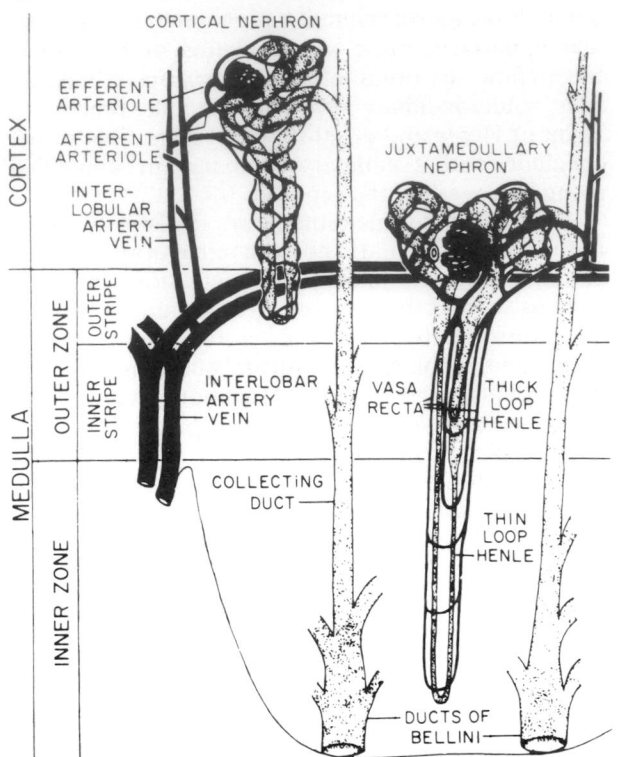

Fig. 36.1 Blood supply of kidney. Note vasa recta looping deep into medulla, beside Loop of Henle of juxtamedullary nephron. Note cortical nephron's blood supply. (Reproduced with permission from R.F. Pitts, 1965. *Physiology of the Kidney and Body Fluids*. Chicago: Year Book Medical).

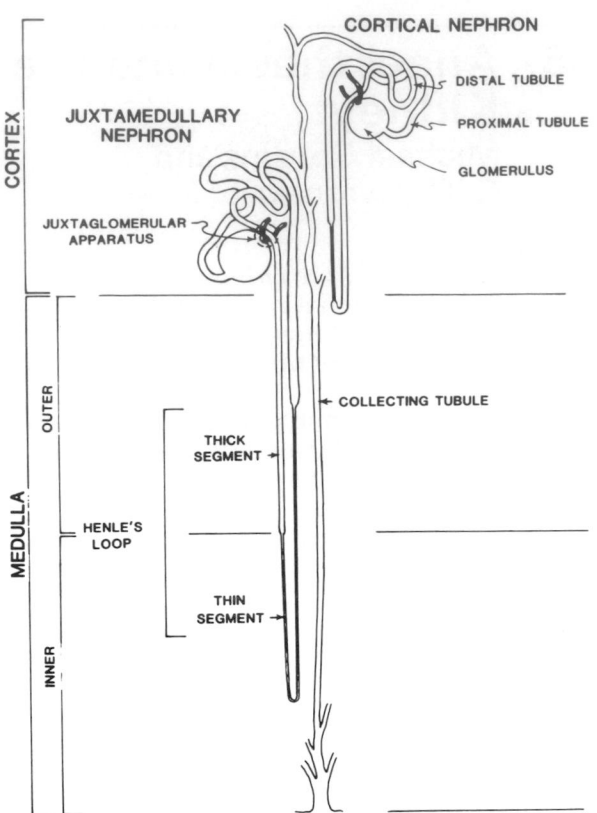

Fig. 36.2 Summary of nephron components. (Reproduced with permission from L.P. Sullivan, J.J. Grantham, 1982. *Physiology of the Kidney*. Philadelphia: Lea & Febiger.)

In the juxtamedullary region, efferent arterioles branch after leaving the glomeruli. Some of these branches contribute to the peritubular capillary networks surrounding Loops of Henle and collecting ducts in the outer medulla; other branches form bundles of vessels, the vasa recta, which make no contact with proximal tubular tissue, as is the case elsewhere in the renal cortex, but penetrate deep into the medulla before further branching.

Renal Tubular Anatomy

The glomerular filtrate flows from the glomerular capsule (Bowman's capsule) into the proximal tubule, which consists of a convoluted (pars convoluta) and a straight segment (pars recta). Detailed examination of proximal tubular cell types actually reveals three segments rather than two: S_1, the proximal portion of the pars convoluta, S_2, the distal pars convoluta and proximal pars recta, and S_3, the distal pars recta.

From the pars recta, tubular fluid enters the Loop of Henle, consisting of an initial thin segment, which conducts urine towards or into the medulla, followed by a thick ascending segment. At the end of this thick ascending portion, the distal tubule begins, and comes into contact with the glomerulus from which it origin-

ated, and with the afferent and efferent arterioles connected to that glomerulus. These three structures at this point form the juxtaglomerular apparatus which is responsible for the regulation of renal blood flow, and is to some extent involved in the control of systemic arterial blood pressure (Fig. 36.2).

The juxtaglomerular apparatus is characterized by a number of specialized cells. The distal tubular epithelium in this region shows large columnar cells, which make up the macula densa. These cells are in intimate contact with granular cells lining the afferent and efferent arterioles, and also with a group of cells known as the lacis or polkissen (polar cushion), which occupy the space between the three structures (Fig. 36.3 and *vide infra* Fig. 36.12). The distal convoluted tubule is functionally and structurally an area of transition between the Loop of Henle and the collecting duct, which runs directly from the cortex through the medulla, opening at a papilla into the renal pelvis.

The juxtamedullary nephrons have a number of special features. These include larger glomeruli, long proximal tubules and long Loops of Henle which extend deep into the renal medulla. The renal medulla therefore consists of the collecting ducts, the long Loops of Henle derived from the juxtamedullary nephrons, and the parallel long vascular Loops of the vasa recta, and these latter two structures produce a

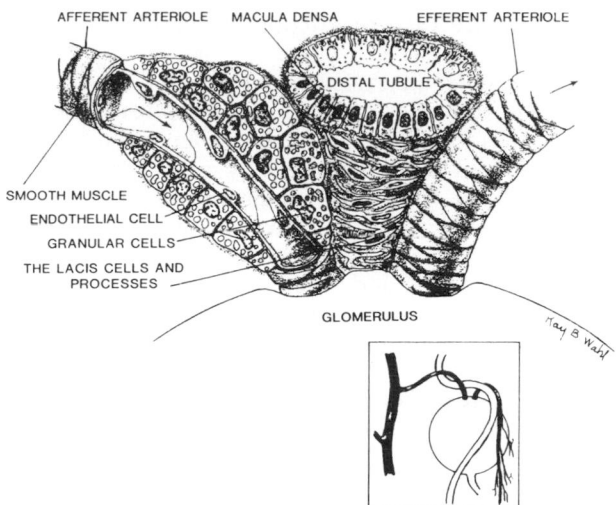

AFFERENT ARTERIOLE   MACULA DENSA   EFFERENT ARTERIOLE

DISTAL TUBULE

SMOOTH MUSCLE
ENDOTHELIAL CELL
GRANULAR CELLS
THE LACIS CELLS AND
PROCESSES

GLOMERULUS

Fig. 36.3 Juxtaglomerular apparatus of inner cortical juxtamedullary nephron. (Reproduced with permission L.P. Sullivan, J.J. Grantham, 1982. *Physiology of the Kidney*. Philadephia: Lea & Febiger.)

uniquely hypertonic extracellular fluid which has a major influence on the composition of urine flowing through the collecting ducts (*see* Fig. 36.2).

APPLIED PHYSIOLOGY OF THE KIDNEY

Introduction

Although the kidneys receive 25% of the cardiac output, they represent only 0.4% of total body mass. Yet they are the prime organs in maintaining the homeostasis of the milieu interieur. In the adult, close to 180 L of glomerular filtrate pass into the proximal nephron each day, equivalent to 60 times the plasma volume. However, glomerular filtration rate (GFR) varies greatly during any 24 h period (range: 10–200, mean 125 ml/min in average sized adults). Over 99% of the glomerular filtrate is reabsorbed together with the other essential substances, either passively or by energy requiring processes. It is not surprising that the kidney has one of the highest oxygen consumptions per gram of tissue of any major body organ (6 ml/(100 g·min)). The reabsorption of sodium accounts for over half of the oxygen consumption. In contrast to other tissues, oxygen consumption varies with blood flow and the arteriovenous oxygen content difference of 1–2 ml/100 ml does not change with alterations in blood flow. Thus, the magnitude of blood flow determines the filtration rate, amount of sodium presented for reabsorption, work to be done and consequent oxygen consumption.

Renal Blood Flow and Glomerular Filtration

The sites of greatest vascular resistance in the renal vascular tree, and therefore the most important con-

trol areas, are the glomerular afferent and efferent arterioles. Under normal circumstances, glomerular blood flow is controlled so that about 20% of the glomerular plasma flow is filtered into the tubules.

The major force favouring filtration in the glomerulus is the capillary hydrostatic pressure (Pgc), which depends on the cardiac output, the systemic arterial blood pressure, and the state of contraction or relaxation of the afferent and efferent arterioles (Fig. 36.4).

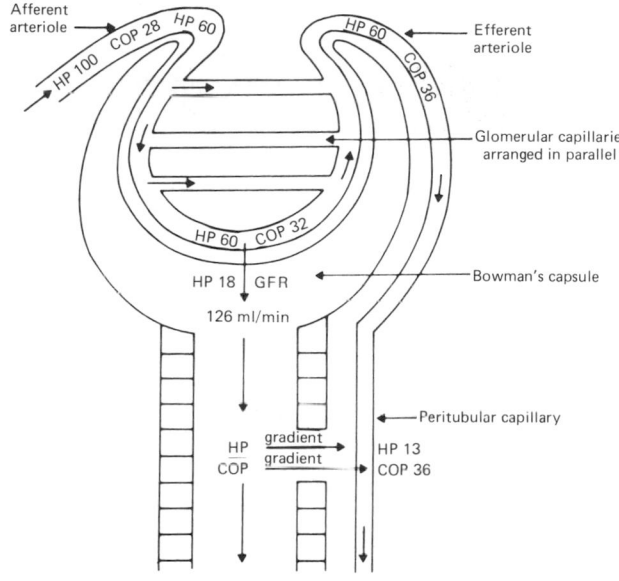

Fig. 36.4 Forces involved in glomerular filtration. HP = hydrostatic pressure in mmHg. COP = colloid osmotic pressure in mmHg. GFR = glomerular filtration rate. Also shown are the forces favouring reabsorption in the proximal convoluted tubule. (Reproduced with permission R.W. Hawker, 1982. *Notebook of Medical Physiology. Renal and Body Fluids*. Edinburgh: Churchill Livingstone.)

This is opposed by the colloid osmotic pressure (πb) of the blood, and the capsular or tubular hydrostatic pressure (Pt). Thus, the net filtration pressure (Pf) can be expressed as:

$$Pf = Pgc\text{-}Pt\text{-}\pi b$$

The filtration pressure falls along the length of the glomerular capillary as the plasma colloid osmotic pressure rises, due to filtration of protein-free fluid from the capillary. This rise in colloid osmotic pressure becomes less as glomerular blood flow increases, and therefore the net filtration pressure increases with increasing renal blood flow. As blood flows through the remainder of the renal vasculature, hydrostatic pressure gradually falls as colloid osmotic pressure rises. This favours reabsorption of fluid into the bloodstream, from the peritubular capillary bed onwards (Fig. 36.5).

The glomerular filtration rate depends not only on

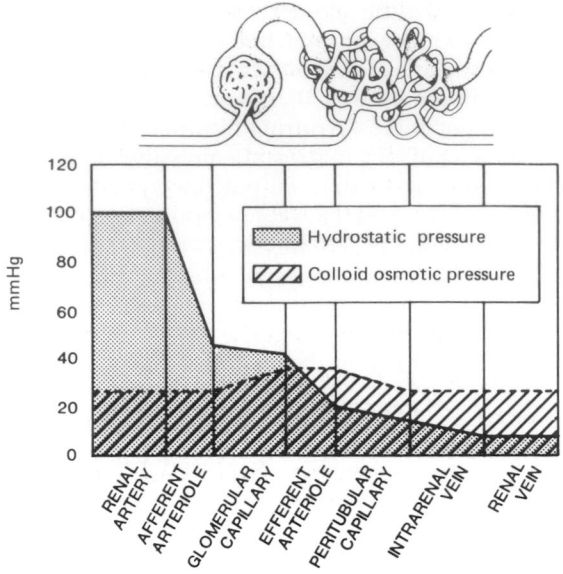

Fig. 36.5 Hydrostatic and colloid osmotic pressures within the renal vasculature. (Reproduced with permission L.P. Sullivan, J.J. Grantham, 1982. *Physiology of the Kidney*. Philadelphia: Lea & Febiger.)

the filtration pressure, but on the glomerular capillary permeability, which is 10–100 times that of capillaries elsewhere, and the total glomerular capillary surface area. Either or both of these may be reduced in disease states. The product of the latter two variables is the filtration coefficient (Kf).

The Juxtaglomerular Apparatus and the Renin/Angiotensin System

The resistance provided by the afferent and efferent arterioles is low compared to that offered by the arterioles of other organs, and as a consequence, in health, there is always some blood flow in all the renal capillaries, rather than the intermittent opening and closing of individual capillaries which occurs elsewhere in the body (vasomotion).

Sympathetic vasoconstrictor fibres arising from T4-L1 spinal segments, passing via the coeliac plexus, innervate both arterioles and the smooth muscle of the initial portions of the vasa recta. Parasympathetic fibres also innervate the arterioles, and probably pass via the renal hilum. Their function is unknown.

Both α and β adrenergic receptors are present in the arterioles, but α receptors greatly outnumber β, and both adrenaline and noradrenaline at all dose levels produce vasoconstriction. The mechanism by which low dose adrenaline increases urine flow and osmolality in septic shock is currently not known.

Dopamine is present in high concentrations in the renal cortex and there appear to be specific receptors for it. Its physiological role is not known, but pharmacologically, small doses of dopamine cause vasodilatation, mediated by specific receptors, while larger doses produce vasoconstriction, mediated by α adrenergic receptors.

The granular juxtaglomerular cells which synthesize, store and release renin, are specialized smooth muscle cells found mainly in the media of the afferent arteriole, and are innervated by renal sympathetic nerve endings. Major stimuli leading to renin release include a fall in renal perfusion pressure, a rise in the sodium concentration of tubular fluid in the region of the macula densa, and stimulation of the renal sympathetic nerves. The receptors which mediate the latter are β-adrenoreceptors, and this explains the inhibitory action of β-blocking drugs upon renin release. A range of other factors and drugs also affect renin release and these include (Stokes, 1983): decreased renal perfusion pressure; increased sodium or chloride concentration in the macula densa; sympathetic stimulation via β adrenoceptors; whole body sodium depletion; hypokalaemia; upright posture; decreased circulating angiotensin II level.

Renin acts within the general circulation as a specific proteolytic enzyme, which cleaves a decapeptide, angiotensin I, from renin substrate, a glycoprotein synthesized in the liver. Angiotensin I has almost no pressor activity, but cleavage of a further two amino acids by angiotensin converting enzyme (ACE), predominantly in the lung, but also in peripheral vascular beds, results in the vasoactive metabolite angiotensin II.

Angiotensin II has a direct vasoconstrictor effect, with some 50 times the potency of noradrenaline, but with a half-life of only 30 s. In the renal circulation it produces falls in blood flow, glomerular filtration rate, and sodium excretion. Angiotensin II also stimulates sodium retention by stimulating aldosterone production in the adrenal medulla, stimulates autonomic ganglia, produces complex effects on autonomic outflow areas in the hindbrain, and stimulates drinking and antidiuretic hormone release.

Renal Autoregulation

In the absence of extrinsic neural and hormonal influences, renal blood flow (RBF) and glomerular filtration rate (GFR) are maintained relatively constant over a range of mean arterial pressure of approximately 80–180 mmHg (Fig. 36.6). It is clear that this effect is mediated by changing arteriolar tone, especially in the afferent arteriole, but the mechanism by which this occurs remains poorly understood. Elegant micropipette techniques suggest that each nephron is somehow able to control the GFR of its own glomerulus, and this is termed 'tubulo-glomerular feedback'. The macula densa is believed to be central to this phenomenon, but neither the signal detected by the macula densa nor the mechanism by which it responds are known.

Several extrarenal factors superimpose major influences upon this autoregulatory mechanism. The central blood volume modulates both RBF and, under physiological circumstances, GFR. In sodium

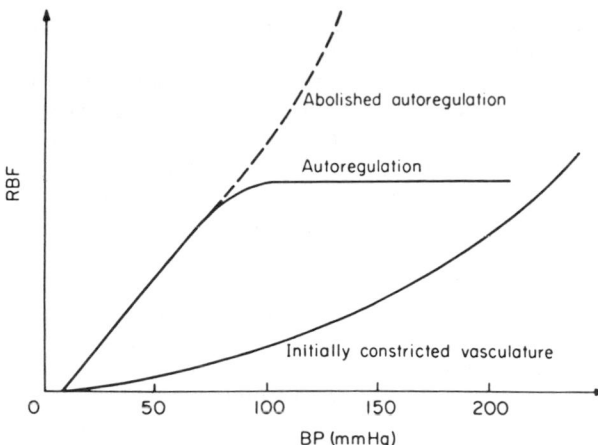

Fig. 36.6 Autoregulation of renal blood flow (RBF). Pressure-flow relationship in renal artery under normal conditions (autoregulation), in the absence of auto-regulation (e.g. 2 MAC halothane), and associated with an initially constricted vasculature (e.g. high dose adrenaline or haemorrhage). Note that at the same arterial blood pressure (BP), RBF is markedly lower with an initially vasoconstricted vasculature. (Reproduced with permission K. Thurau, A. Levin, 1971. The renal circulation, In *The Kidney*, Vol. III, Rouiller C., Muller A.E. eds. New York: Academic Press.)

depletion, hypovolaemia and low cardiac output states, renin release and angiotensin synthesis are stimulated, leading to a reduction in RBF and, to a lesser extent, GFR. However, evidence for a major role of angiotensin in the regulation of RBF and GFR under physiological conditions is not strong.

Atrial natriuretic peptide (atriopeptin, ANP) is a recently identified 28 amino acid peptide which is intimately involved in renal and cardiovascular homeostasis. It produces an increase in glomerular filtration with marked natriuresis and diuresis, and inhibits aldosterone secretion and ADH release. ANP also appears to be a potent directly-acting generalized vasodilator and a selective renal vasodilator; it can suppress elevated renin levels, and may have central effects on the hypothalamus which influence cardiovascular and renal function.

A 126 amino acid prohormone is stored in perinuclear granules within atrial cardiocytes. The primary stimulus for cleavage of the prohormone and release of ANP is atrial stretch, and plasma levels can be increased by volume expansion, some vasoconstrictors, immersion in water, atrial tachycardia, and high salt diets. Thus, ANP appears to be the mediator of an important feedback mechanism in which fluid and electrolyte accumulation leads to increased atrial stretch, ANP secretion, and excretion of the extracellular volume load. Conversely, hypovolaemia would lead to inhibition of ANP secretion (Needleman and Greenwald, 1986).

Increased circulating levels of adrenaline also reduce RBF to a greater degree than GFR. Prosta-glandin E2 production by the kidney is increased under circumstances of renal vasoconstriction, and may modulate the vasoconstrictive effect.

Intrarenal Blood Flow Distribution

Most of the renal blood flow (90%) is received by the highly vascular cortex. The factors which control intrarenal blood flow distribution are not known. However it has been suggested that sustained reduction in renal cortical perfusion, to a level where glomerular filtration ceases, may be a critical factor in the pathogenesis of acute renal failure (ARF).

In some patients with renal failure, Hollenberg et al. (1968) reported that the rapid flow compartment, as determined by a [85]Kr-washout renal arteriography technique, was markedly reduced. This was thought to represent cortical blood flow, and seemed to be markedly reduced or absent in patients with acute renal failure secondary to hypotension or nephrotoxins but was only reduced in proportion to total RBF in patients with chronic renal failure. The results of experimentation in this area remain contradictory, and neither the significance nor mechanism of such changes are understood.

TUBULAR FUNCTION

Broadly there are four major methods by which the tubules handle endogenous and exogenous substances; all are based on the three basic functions of the nephron; filtration, reabsorption and secretion (Fig. 36.7).

Tubular Transport Mechanisms

Passive diffusion is the simplest type of tubular transport. Net movement of solutes occurs in the direction of concentration, osmotic, or electrical gradients, which are created by various transport mechanisms. In the case of weak acids and bases, gradients are established by alterations in tubular pH. As a weak base moves from the slightly alkaline blood to an acid tubular fluid, it tends to become the ionized, lipid-insoluble form, which is relatively non-diffusible, and tends to remain trapped in the urine (diffusion trapping). The non-ionized form therefore tends to continue to move down its concentration gradient from blood to urine. Procaine is an example of a solute whose excretion may be affected in this way. The converse is illustrated by phenobarbitone, a weak acid, largely present in unionized form in blood, whose excretion is slowed by the presence of an acid urine, and favoured by an alkaline urine.

Some solutes pass through membranes more rapidly than could be explained by passive diffusion alone, and in some of these cases it is thought that temporary bonding to a carrier substance in the cell membrane results in facilitated diffusion. Still other

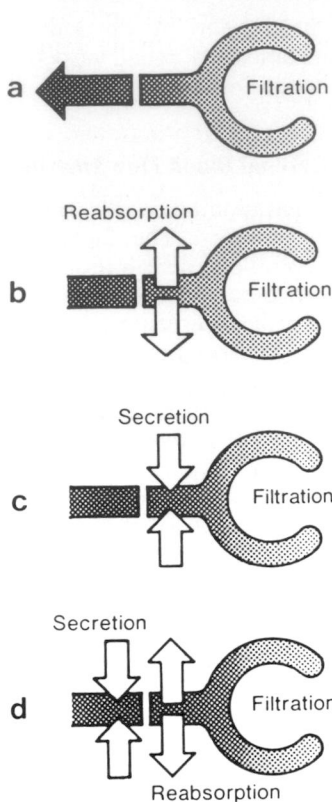

Fig. 36.7 Summary of tubular functions. (a) Filtration only, e.g. inulin, gallamine. (b) Filtration and reabsorption proximally, e.g. sodium, glucose. (c) Filtration and secretion proximally, e.g. para-aminohippuric acid. (d) Filtration, reabsorption proximally, and secretion distally, e.g. potassium ions.

solutes are transported by carriers against electrochemical gradients, by processes requiring energy expenditure, and this is termed 'active transport'. Both these carrier mediated types of transport demonstrate the properties of specificity, competition and saturation.

Some of these mechanisms are capacity-limited, i.e. they have a relatively fixed rate of transport regardless of the concentration gradient (glucose transport is an example). Other mechanisms are *gradient-limited* (e.g. sodium transport in the distal tubule). A transport mechanism tends to be gradient-limited when the tubular epithelium is relatively permeable to that substance, i.e. when there is a strong tendency for back diffusion. In the case of sodium transport, this tendency is limited by passive reabsorption of water accompanying reabsorbed sodium, which keeps tubular and plasma sodium concentrations roughly equal. Gradient-limited mechanisms are also affected by the flow rate of tubular fluid, i.e. their performance is improved when tubular flow is high.

In some cases, an active transport mechanism may drive the movement of a second solute. For instance, in the proximal tubule, active reabsorption of sodium facilitates the reabsorption of glucose. Such mechan-

isms are referred to as 'cotransport' systems. When movement of the second solute occurs in the same direction as the first, this is known as a symport system; when a cotransport system is used to exchange substances across a membrane, as in the case of the Na-K pump, this is referred to as an antiport system.

Solute Handling in the Proximal Tubule

Urea is freely filtered at the glomerulus, but is also passively reabsorbed in the proximal tubule and collecting ducts (Fig. 36.7b). The rate of reabsorption is facilitated when urine flow down the tubule is low, and *vice versa*. This explains the rise of blood urea in oliguric states. Urea may be actively secreted into the urine by the pars recta of the proximal tubule, but the quantitative significance of this is uncertain. There is a high concentration of urea in the medullary interstitium, and this plays an important osmotic role in the concentration of urine by the countercurrent process.

Organic anions, of which para-amino hippurate is the experimental prototype, are extensively but reversibly protein-bound, and therefore poorly filtered at the glomerulus. Free organic anions are actively secreted mainly into the S_2 portion of the proximal tubule, and this promotes further unbinding from protein (Fig. 36.7c). Examples include not only a range of endogenous substances, but many drugs including penicillins, cephalosporins, diuretics, and salicylates. Passive reabsorption of these substances may occur in the distal nephron, when there is an appropriate pH, as discussed above.

The excretion of organic cations is less well understood. Again, some are protein-bound and therefore poorly filtered, but the major transport mechanism appears to be active secretion in the proximal tubules. Substances in this category include catecholamines, atropine, morphine, and cimetidine.

The main system of sodium reabsorption is the Na-K ATPase pump of the proximal tubule (Fig. 36.7b). Sodium is pumped out of the tubule cells into the paracellular spaces and interstitium in exchange for potassium. This pump system, together with the high permeability for sodium of the luminal cell membrane of the proximal tubular cell, favours net reabsorption. Passive osmotic movement of water with sodium serves to offset the tendency toward back-diffusion. In the early part of the proximal tubule, symport mechanisms provide for simultaneous reabsorption of glucose and amino acids with sodium. Most chloride reabsorption is passive in association with the active transport of sodium. It is now recognized that active transport mechanisms also exist for chloride and a Na-Cl symport has been suggested (Herbert et al., 1981).

Bicarbonate is effectively reabsorbed in the proximal tubule by means of the carbonic anhydrase system which secretes hydrogen ions into tubular fluid, with the formation of CO_2 and water from the bicarbonate therein, while new bicarbonate, together with sodium, is secreted into the renal cortical interstitium.

The net result of all the above processes is that 60–70% of the glomerular filtrate is reabsorbed in the proximal tubule, with only minor changes in composition, largely due to concurrent passive reabsorption of water.

Function of the Loop of Henle and Distal Tubule Systems

The Loop of Henle and the vasa recta function under the now well-known countercurrent principle. This process is most efficient in the juxtamedullary nephrons and its function is firstly to reabsorb a further 15–20% of solute and water from the nephron, but much more importantly, to set up a major osmotic gradient in the renal medulla so that further reabsorption of water can take place in the collecting duct. The descending limb of the Loop of Henle possesses no

known active transport mechanisms. However, because there is a gradient in sodium, chloride and urea as the Loop descends further into the medulla, there is progressive flow of water out of the Loop into the surrounding interstitium, and eventually into the vasa recta (Fig. 36.8). Both the ascending segment of the thin limb and the thick segment are responsible for the creation of this medullary osmotic gradient. The nature of the responsible transport mechanism is uncertain. Initially it was believed that an active reabsorption mechanism for sodium was involved. There is some evidence, however, to suggest that active chloride reabsorption also takes place, and recent experimental data strongly supports the existence of an ATPase dependent sodium-chloride symport (Herbert et al., 1981).

A countercurrent mechanism also exists in the renal medulla for urea, resulting in a very high urea concentration in the inner medulla. This urea concentration gradient occurs because water reabsorption takes

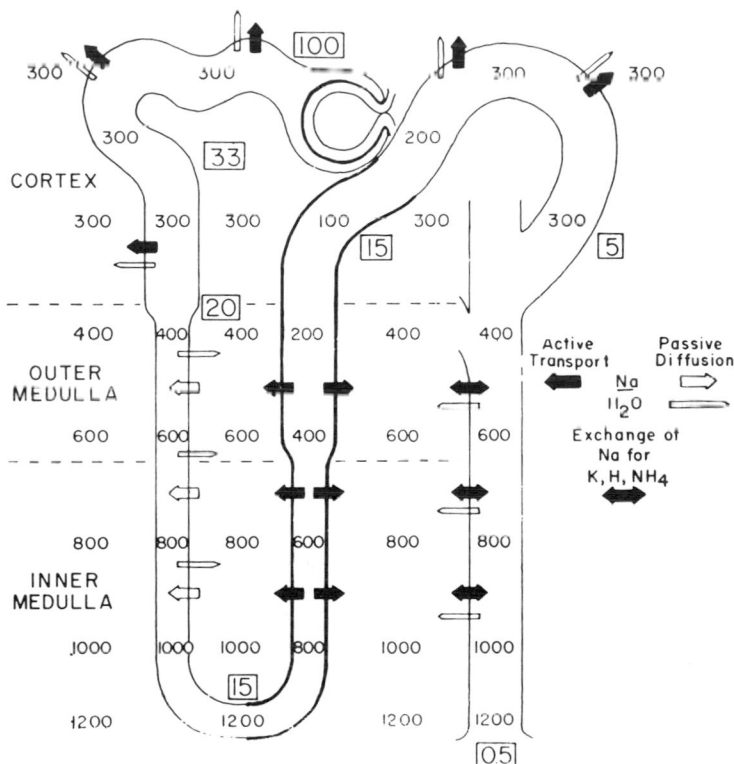

Fig. 36.8 Countercurrent mechanism. Summary of active (solid thick arrows) and passive (open, thick arrows) movement of sodium along the course of the nephron. Movement of water is shown by open, narrow arrows. Note the ascending limb of the Loop of Henle is impermeable to water. Concentrations of tubular fluid and interstitial fluid are given in mosmol/kg; large boxed numerals are estimated percent of glomerular filtrate remaining within the tubule at each level. There is now evidence that chloride may be actively pumped in this region with sodium following passively. (Reproduced with permission R.F. Pitts, 1965 *Physiology of the Kidney and Body Fluids*. Chicago: Year Book Medical Publishers.)

place more rapidly than urea reabsorption in the ascending limb and distal tubule, resulting in progressive concentration of urea in the tubules, and a gradient of urea concentration favouring its reabsorption into the medullary interstitium from the collecting ducts. Medullary interstitial urea thus contributes significantly to the countercurrent mechanism and to the osmotic reabsorption of water in the Loop of Henle and the collecting duct.

The distal tubule functions as an extension of the thick ascending limb. Active salt transport continues with control mediated by aldosterone, and, as permeability to water is low, there is progressive dilution of tubular fluid to 80–100 mosmol/kg. The distal portion of the tubule is sensitive to ADH, which raises its water permeability, resulting in a further 5–8% passive reabsorption of water in this region.

The collecting duct is poorly permeable to electrolytes and water, and further active transport mechanisms exist for the active removal of salts. However, in the presence of ADH, the duct can become freely permeable to water, and thus the composition of the residual 10% (20 L) of the glomerular filtrate can be adjusted to yield urine of volume and composition appropriate to the maintenance of the milieu interieur.

The urine concentrating mechanism thus depends upon active transport mechanisms in the ascending limb of the Loop of Henle, the countercurrent arrangement of tubules and blood vessels and the low inner medullary blood flow (50 ml/(100 g·min)). This permits an increase in osmolality in the medullary interstitium from 300 mosmol kg^{-1} at the corticomedullary junction to 1200 mosmol kg^{-1} at the inner medulla. Equilibration of collecting duct fluid with this high osmolality depends upon the action of ADH (Fig. 36.8).

Summary of Changes in Tubule Fluid Along Length of Nephron

It is helpful to compare the concentrations of various substances in the tubule fluid to those in plasma, along the length of the nephron (Fig. 36.9, *see* also Fig. 36.5). For example fluid in the proximal tubule is iso-osmotic with plasma, becomes hyperosmotic at the medullary tip of the Loop of Henle, is hypo-osmotic as it reaches the distal tubule and then may become hyperosmotic in the collecting duct under the influence of ADH. Another way of viewing these changes is to consider the fraction of the filtered substances remaining in the tubule fluid as it passes down the nephron (Fig. 36.10).

RENAL EFFECTS OF ANAESTHESIA

The observed major effects of anaesthesia and surgery on renal function and body fluid homeostasis have been assumed to be due to indirect circulatory and neuroendocrine responses. However, anaesthetic

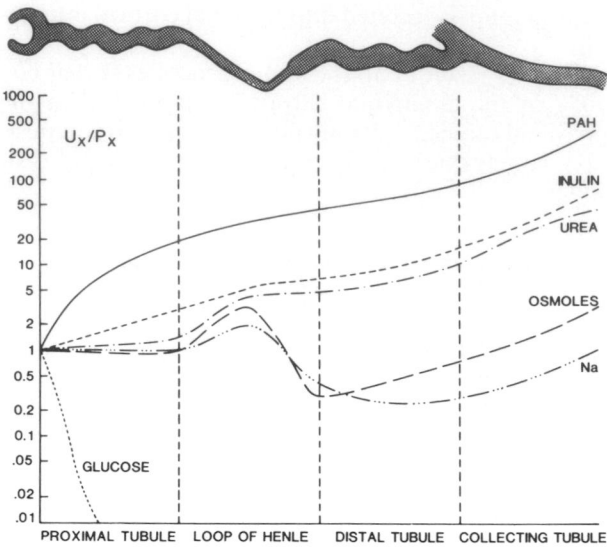

Fig. 36.9 Summary of changes in urine to plasma concentration ratio (Ux/Px) of various substances along the nephron. Note that the ordinate is a Log scale. (Reproduced with permission L.P. Sullivan, J.J. Grantham, 1982. *Physiology of the Kidney*, Philadelphia: Lea & Febiger.)

agents also have direct effects on renal function which may be acute, or delayed, as exemplified by the delayed toxicity which has been reported after methoxyflurane anaesthesia. This section will discuss the combined effects of anaesthesia and surgery upon renal function and fluid-electrolyte homeostasis in

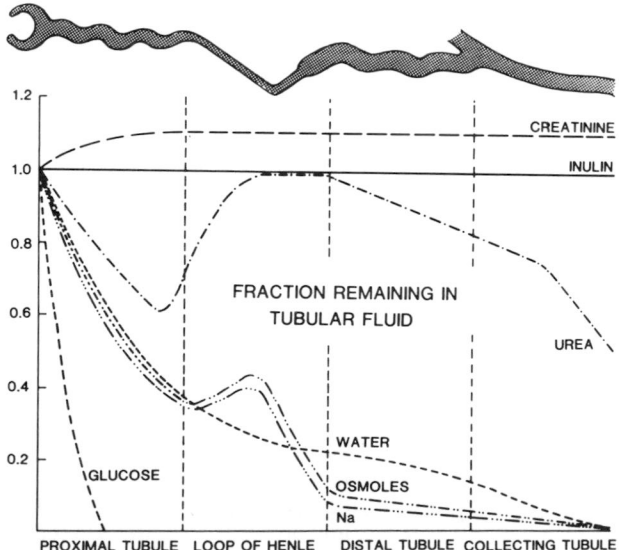

Fig. 36.10 Summary of changes in fractions of substances remaining in tubular fluid along the length of the nephron (Reproduced with permission L.P. Sullivan, J.J. Grantham, 1982. *Physiology of the Kidney*. Philadelphia: Lea & Febiger.)

normal man, anaesthetic problems of patients with renal disease having been described in other reviews (Mazze and Cousins, 1981; Mazze, 1977). Mention will also be made of renal effects of drug interactions which may occur between anaesthetics and therapeutic agents such as antibiotics and enzyme-inducing drugs.

ACUTE EFFECTS OF ANAESTHETICS ON RENAL FUNCTION

The earliest reports of the effects of anaesthesia on renal function were from Pringle and his colleagues in 1905 (Pringle et al., 1905). They reported the effects of ether anaesthesia on water and non-protein nitrogen excretion in eight patients undergoing a variety of minor and major surgical procedures. Urine flow averaged 50 ml/h on the day prior to surgery, fell to 1.2 ml/h during the operation, and returned toward normal postoperatively.

In surgical patients without renal disease, all general anaesthetic agents temporarily depress renal function with urine flow, glomerular filtration rate (GFR), renal blood flow (RBF), and electrolyte excretion being reduced. This consistent and generalized depression of renal function has been attributed to many factors, including the type and duration of surgical procedure, the physical status of the patient, especially that of the cardiovascular and renal systems, preoperative and intraoperative blood volume, fluid and electrolyte balance, the choice of anaesthetic agent and the depth of anaesthesia (Seitzman et al., 1963; Boba and Landmesser, 1965; Mazze and Barry, 1967; Deutsch et al., 1966, 1967, 1968). Changes in renal function following spinal and epidural anaesthesia have been reported to parallel the degree of sympathetic blockade and therefore the amount of hypotension produced (Kennedy et al., 1970; Kennedy, 1969). In most cases the changes in renal function associated with anaesthesia and surgery revert spontaneously. At the termination of short uncomplicated procedures RBF and GFR usually return to normal within a few hours. When surgery is more extensive and anaesthesia prolonged, secondary effects related to the endocrine system may be manifested by impairment of the ability to promptly excrete a waterload or conversely, inability to produce a concentrated urine (Mazze and Cousins, 1973a; Cousins and Mazze, 1973b). The depression in renal function caused by anaesthetic agents may be due to their direct or indirect effects.

Indirect Circulatory Effects

During general anaesthesia RBF may be depressed as a consequence of renal vasoconstriction, systemic hypotension, or both. Drugs causing the greatest increase in catecholamine excretion, such as cyclopropane and diethyl ether, tend to support systemic blood pressure, but in so doing cause a marked increase in renal vascular resistance, decrease in RBF and depression of renal function (Deutsch et al., 1967). This catecholamine effect may be accentuated in the presence of hypovolaemia. Halothane and thiopentone, although not causing a catecholamine response, are associated with a moderate increase in renal vascular resistance (Deutsch et al., 1968), as blood is diverted from the kidney to compensate for hypotension induced by myocardial depression and peripheral vasodilatation. Renal blood flow and GFR fall with these agents, but not as much as with anaesthetic agents that stimulate catecholamine release.

Some evidence suggests that circulating catecholamines may cause a redistribution of renal blood flow with a marked reduction occurring in cortical perfusion (Truniger et al., 1971). Redistribution is prevented by α-adrenergic blockade, but not by denervation of the kidney or by prophylactic administration of mannitol. Thus it is possible that administration of anaesthetic 'supplementary' drugs with α adrenergic block activity, such as droperidol, may result in the smallest changes in renal haemodynamics.

The mean blood pressure at which an injurious reduction of RBF occurs has not been precisely determined in man. Studies in dogs show a reduction in RBF with changes in distribution of cortical blood flow at a mean arterial blood pressure of 70 mmHg (Rosen et al., 1968) during haemorrhagic shock. In this situation of increased sympathetic tone there is systemic vasoconstriction which includes the kidney. This may be associated with very low RBF at blood pressures which would usually be in the autoregulatory range for RBF (*see* Fig. 36.6). Unfortunately, conclusive information is not available concerning renal blood flow and distribution of flow during vasodilatory hypotension in man such as is produced by ganglion blocking and other 'hypotensive' drugs (Westermark, 1969; Moyer and McConn, 1956). (*see* Fig. 36.6).

Indirect Sympathetic Nervous System Effects

As noted above, under a wide variety of normal and abnormal physiologic conditions, RBF is regulated to maintain stability of GFR. With increasing stress, RBF decreases significantly, however, filtration fraction (GFR/RBF) increases, GFR thereby remaining constant, suggesting efferent renal arteriolar constriction. Finally, during severe stress, GFR also decreases. Judged by their depressant effect on RBF and GFR, general anaesthesia, syncope, pain, severe exercise and haemorrhage represent severe stress. It has been assumed that the major renal effects of these diverse stimuli are mediated via sympathetic nervous system stimulation. Some evidence indicates that general anaesthesia may have important direct effects (*see below*).

Evidence for the role of the sympathetic nervous system in the renal effects of anaesthetics was provided by Berne's classic experiments in dogs with one normal and one denervated kidney (Berne, 1952). Prior to induction of pentobarbitone or chloralose anaesthesia, RBF and GFR of the denervated and normally innervated kidneys were the same. However, following induction of anaesthesia, RBF and GFR on the normally innervated side decreased while no changes were seen on the denervated side. Changes in the normally innervated kidney appear to have been due to increased vasoconstrictor tone caused by anaesthesia. This finding is supported by clinical and animal studies which report that spinal or epidural anaesthesia may produce minimal alterations in renal function provided blood pressure is maintained by measures such as infusion of balanced salt solutions (Fig. 36.11, Table 36.1) (Kennedy et al., 1970; Kennedy, 1969; Runciman et al., 1984). Complete deafferentation of the operative site and prevention of the release of catecholamines and other renal vasoconstrictive substances may also be important factors in preventing a deleterious redistribution of cortical blood flow (Truniger et al., 1971).

Autoregulation

In some studies, autoregulation has been reported to be abolished by the inhalation anaesthetics. For example, under halothane anaesthesia, decreases in RBF and GFR of 50% or more occur in patients with stable mean arterial blood pressures above 80 mmHg (Habif et al., 1951). Evidence of maintenance of autoregulation under anaesthesia was obtained in animals anaesthetized with pentobarbitone or chloralose (Ochwadt, 1961). Autoregulation was also studied in the isolated perfused kidney connected to the circulation of a dog anaesthetized with halothane 1 MAC. Over a range of mean perfusion pressures of 75–150 mmHg 1 MAC halothane did not interfere with autoregulation of blood flow (Bastron and Deutsch, 1976; Bastron and Kaloyanides, 1974). In contrast, *in vivo* studies in a sheep model with chronically implanted intravascular catheters have shown marked interference with renal autoregulation under anaesthesia with 2 MAC halothane (Runciman et al., 1984) (*see* Table 36.1).

Indirect Endocrine Effects

Endocrine effects on renal function during anaesthesia are closely tied to the circulatory effects discussed above. Most important in regulating urine volume is anti-diuretic hormone (ADH). Renin, angiotensin, aldosterone, adrenaline, and noradrenaline also play important roles in electrolyte excretion and regulation of renal blood flow.

Abnormalities in ADH Secretion

Although there are some conflicting data (Bachman, 1955), the weight of evidence now indicates that opioid drugs and general anaesthetic agents are re-

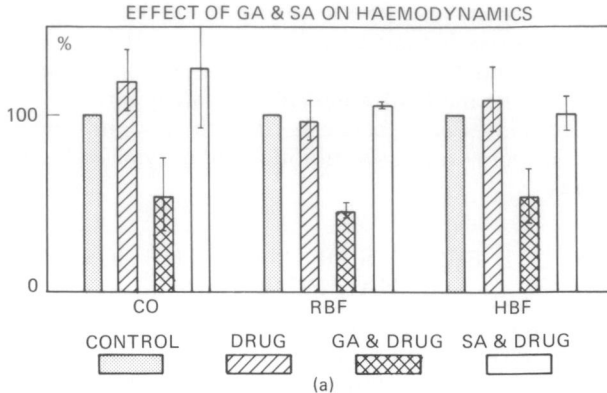

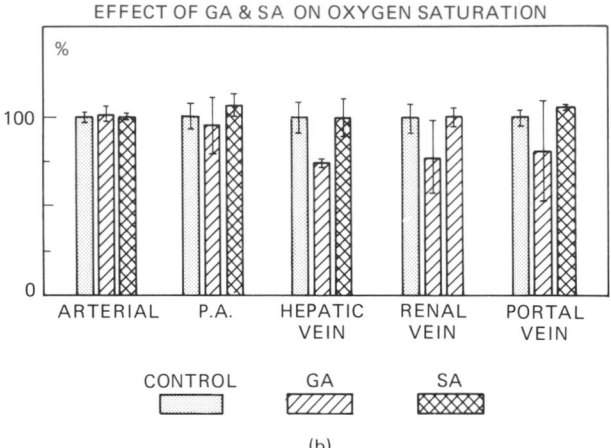

Fig. 36.11 (a) and (b): Effects on kidney of general anaesthesia with halothane compared to spinal anaesthesia. Data were obtained from a sheep preparation with chronic vascular catheters, which permitted direct determination of blood flow through and oxygen and marker drug extraction across, the kidney. General anaesthesia (GA) = halothane 1% at normoxia. Spinal anaesthesia (SA) = T_4 level produced by 0.5% tetracaine. The mean value of each variable during *control* (free standing no drugs), *drug* (marker drug for CO, RBF, HBF), *general anaesthesia*, *spinal anaesthesia* studies has been expressed as a percentage of the mean value of the corresponding variable during the control period on the same day. The mean and S.D. of the percentage are shown. There were significant reductions in renal blood flow and renal vein oxygen tension with GA but not with SA. Drug = control drug study; GA + drug = general anaesthesia study; SA + drug = subarachnoid anaesthesia study; CO = cardiac output; RBF = renal blood flow (sodium ^{125}I-iodohippurate infusion and renal vein, artery sampling); HBF = hepatic blood flow (IOH infusion and hepatic, portal vein sampling). (Reproduced with permission from W.B. Runciman, L.E. Mather, A.H. Ilsley et al., 1984. A sheep preparation for studying interactions between blood flow and drug disposition: III Effect of general and spinal anaesthesia on regional blood flow and oxygen tensions. *Br. J. Anaesth.*, **56**, 1251.)

sponsible for increased release of ADH (Bastron et al., 1976). As discussed above, this results in increased reabsorption of water from the collecting ducts and

TABLE 36.1*
EFFECTS OF GENERAL ANAESTHESIA ON HAEMODYNAMICS, INDICATOR KINETICS AND CEFOXITIN ELIMINATION

	Control-drug study		General anaesthesia (GA)-drug study		
	Control	+ Cefoxitin	Control	+ GA	+ GA + Cefoxitin
Haemodynamics					
Cardiac output (L/min)	4.3 (0.5)*	4.5 (0.3)	5.2 (0.1)	2.3 (0.3)	3.4 (0.1)
Liver blood flow (L/min)	1.7 (0.2)	1.9 (0.3)	1.6 (0.3)	0.78 (0.08)	0.97 (0.20)
Kidney blood flow (L/min)	0.59 (0.04)	0.59 (0.02)	0.50 (0.03)	0.31 (0.07)	0.37 (0.02)
Indicator kinetics					
Extraction ratio of IOH at the kidney	0.62 (0.04)	0.60 (0.01)	0.71 (0.04)	0.54 (0.12)	0.40 (0.03)
Clearance† (ml/min)	364 (11)	355 (9)	361 (13)	161 (5)	146 (5)
Cefoxitin elimination					
Extraction ratio of the kidney		0.58 (0.05)			0.30 (0.05)
Clearance† (ml/min)		344 (29)			110 (27)

*Mean (standard deviation)
†Clearance = extraction ratio × flow

EFFECTS OF SPINAL ANAESTHESIA ON HAEMODYNAMICS, INDICATOR KINETICS AND CEFOXITIN ELIMINATION

	Control-drug study		Spinal anaesthesia (SA)-drug study		
	Control	+ Cefoxitin	Control	+ SA	+ SA + Cefoxitin
Haemodynamics					
Cardiac output (L/min)	4.8 (0.2)**	5.0 (0.5)	4.8 (0.5)	4.4 (0.3)	6.3 (1.0)
Liver blood flow (L/min)	ND†	ND	ND	ND	ND
Kidney blood flow (L/min)	0.69 (0.03)	0.69 (0.06)	0.58 (0.06)	0.69 (0.03)	0.61 (0.08)
Indicator kinetics					
Extraction ratio of IOH at the kidney	0.82 (0.02)	0.76 (0.01)	0.81 (0.05)	0.77 (0.01)	0.75 (0.03)
Clearance (ml/min)	560 (23)	525 (40)	471 (26)	530 (16)	457 (47)
Cefoxitin elimination					
Extraction ratio of the kidney		0.77 (0.02)			0.78 (0.05)
Clearance (ml/min)		528 (42)			478 (74)

*Mean (standard deviation)
†Not determined
**Reproduced from Regional Anaesthesia Suppl 7:523, 1982 with permission of J. B. Lippincott Co.

the elaboration of a concentrated urine. The combination of this effect with the decreased GFR associated with the use of inhalation general anaesthetics is a major potential cause of the concentrated urine and water retention which may follow general anaesthesia (Bastron et al., 1976).

Preoperative depletion of extracellular fluid is a potent stimulus to ADH release and this may be reduced by administration of crystalloid solutions preoperatively (Barry et al., 1964). However, neurogenic stimuli due to anxiety or pain and drug induced stimulation of ADH release are unlikely to be affected. Also, haemodynamic changes resulting from blood loss and intermittent positive pressure ventilation may trigger ADH release via baroreceptors (Fig. 36.12).

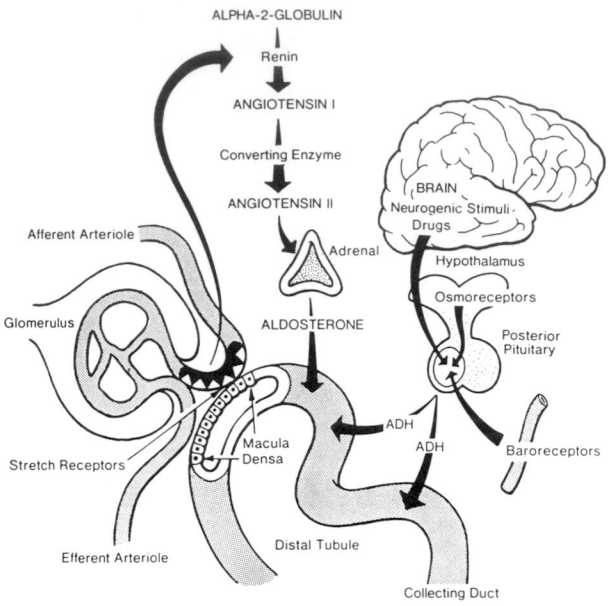

Fig. 36.12 Overview of hormonal control of kidney function.

Syndrome of Inappropriate ADH Secretion (S.I.A.D.H.).

A sustained and inappropriately elevated secretion of ADH may occur following major surgery for malignancies, such as those of lung and brain (Bartter and Schwartz, 1967). This inappropriate secretion of ADH from such tumours results in hyponatraemia and low serum osmolality despite persistent excretion of a hypertonic urine. This is associated with restlessness, disorientation, stupor, or convulsions. Improvement follows restriction of water intake. Similar abnormalities are sometimes attributed to the so called 'sick cell syndrome' in ill elderly patients, however the validity of such a diagnosis is now questioned (Bichet and Schrier, 1982). Persistence of the usual elevation of ADH following anaesthesia in otherwise healthy patients may rarely result in a clinical picture similar to S.I.A.D.H. although usually less severe. This should be regarded as an exaggerated physiological response, however, in very severe cases, death may result. It is not known if any anaesthetic agent poses a significantly greater risk of the occurrence of this condition.

Diabetes Insipidus.

The production of large volumes of urine despite rising serum osmolality sometimes follows neurosurgical procedures, particularly hypophysectomy and posterior fossa operations. Unlike diabetes insipidus of renal origin, diabetes insipidus due to neurogenic causes is responsive to exogenous vasopressin (ADH).

Adrenaline and Noradrenaline

Both adrenaline and noradrenaline produce marked renal vasoconstriction, especially of afferent arterioles, with a decrease in RBF and, to a lesser degree, GFR. Sodium, chloride and potassium excretion are depressed, probably due to the decreased filtered load or to increased reabsorption from the tubules. Antidiuresis may occur following administration of adrenaline and noradrenaline, and Eranko et al. (1953), have suggested that ADH may be responsible. It is difficult to determine how much of the renal effect of anaesthetic agents such as ether and cyclopropane is due to the increase in catecholamines which they provoke and how much to their other systemic effects.

Renin-angiotensin

An additional hormonal pathway capable of affecting renal function is the renin-angiotensin system. Control of renin release is complex and is influenced by several factors which are in turn affected by the administration of anaesthesia. Sodium content of tubular fluid in the macula densa region, catecholamine levels, sympathetic nervous impulses, and intraluminal pressure of afferent arterioles are probably all involved (Bastron et al., 1976; Vander, 1967).

Deutsch et al (1967), have reported increased renin activity in two non-operated subjects anaesthetized with cyclopropane and two with halothane. In contrast, three of four subjects anaesthetized with morphine, thiopentone, nitrous oxide and muscle relaxants showed a decrease in renin activity. The authors suggest that a fall in renin activity might explain the relatively greater reduction in GFR than in RBF observed with this technique in comparison with cyclopropane or halothane. However, the number of patients is too small and the data too fragmentary for firm conclusions to be drawn. In patients undergoing cardiac surgery, under nitrous oxide and high dose morphine anaesthesia, renin levels in peripheral venous blood increase with surgical stimulation but not with drug administration (Bailey et al., 1975). Other events during anaesthesia and surgery may alter renin release and thus it is difficult to attribute altered renin levels to anaesthesia *per se*. Such events include: sodium loading or depletion, altered sympathetic tone and renal perfusion, changes in RBF and distribution of RBF.

Aldosterone

Aldosterone, one of the hormones controlling sodium excretion, is formed in the zona glomerulosa of the adrenal cortex. Its release is primarily dependent upon the juxtaglomerular apparatus (*see* Fig. 36.12), as discussed elsewhere in this review. It has been suggested that anaesthetics alter the response of atrial and other baroreceptors to changing blood pressures (Prys-Roberts, 1980). However detailed studies of the effects of anaesthetics on sodium metabolism are not available.

Despite anaesthesia induced aldosterone release and the sodium retention it produces, it is well known that serum sodium concentration falls following general anaesthesia and surgery. This dilutional hyponatraemia has been ascribed to dominance of ADH effect, liberation of endogenous sodium-free water from oxidation of fat, and over administration of sodium-free fluids. Indeed, the postoperative patient has in the past been thought to be intolerant to sodium administration and the practice of infusing small volumes of sodium-free fluid developed. The recent reversal of this view is discussed below.

Mechanical Ventilation and the Kidney

The effects of respiratory support upon the kidney are difficult to assess because different methods of ventilation, nutritional state, blood gases, acid-base status, temperature and haematocrit all may profoundly affect renal function (Priebe and Hedley-White, 1984). In addition, mechanical support probably produces a number of alterations in renal function as a direct consequence of its effects on the cardiovascular system as a whole. These include increases in renal and hepatic venous pressure, altered atrial filling pressures, falling arterial pressure and cardiac output. Similarly, changes in renal function due to hypoxia and acidosis are probably mediated directly by their effects on the cardiovascular system.

Glomerular and Tubular Function

Mechanical ventilation with PEEP usually results in a fall in glomerular filtration rate, urinary sodium excretion and urine output, while the effect on free water clearance and osmolar clearance are somewhat variable. Mechanical ventilation without the addition of PEEP generally has less effect upon renal function, while the use of spontaneous ventilation with CPAP has variable effects, possibly more dependent on the extent of underlying lung pathology than the use of CPAP, the most significant alterations occurring when the lungs are normal and little change being seen when the lungs are severely diseased.

Renal Blood Flow

Renal blood flow is usually decreased during respiratory support. However, it has been suggested that the fall in urine output and sodium excretion seen clinically are more related to intrarenal blood flow redistribution from the outer to the inner cortex (Hall et al., 1974).

Neuroendocrine Changes

Mechanical ventilation with PEEP always promotes ADH secretion and raised ADH levels (although other mechanisms may also contribute to the production of concentrated urine in this setting). This rise in ADH activity may be related to falling cardiac output or blood pressure or rising intracranial pressure but the precise mechanism is not understood. It cannot be prevented by bilateral cervical vagotomy and carotid sinus denervation in dogs, and pulmonary J-receptors, plasma renin activity, transmural left atrial pressure, serum osmolality and cortical levels all appear not to be involved (Bark et al., 1980).

Mechanical ventilation also causes stimulation of the renin-angiotensin system. Again, the underlying mechanism is unclear. The response still occurs in denervated kidneys, yet can be blocked by β-blocking drugs. Thus, some intrarenal mechanism involving β receptors appears to be involved. (Priebe et al., 1984).

Renal sympathetic stimulation during mechanical ventilation decreases RBF, sodium excretion, GFR and urine output. Because there is no change in filtration fraction, the likely mechanism is afferent arteriolar vasoconstriction.

Direct Effects of Anaesthetics on Renal Function

Direct effects of anaesthetic agents on renal function are obscured by the marked indirect haemodynamic and endocrine effects considered above. In the isolated toad bladder, cyclopropane and nitrous oxide gave rise to dose-dependent stimulation, and halothane to dose-dependent inhibition, of active sodium transport. Ether produced a biphasic response with initial stimulation being followed by inhibition of ion transport (Andersen, 1966). These studies suggest that such effects could occur in the renal tubule.

In an effort to elucidate the mechanism of the above responses, Andersen performed additional experiments in bladders from toads previously treated with reserpine, α or β adrenergic blocking agents and with adrenaline. Cyclopropane was used as the test gas (Andersen, 1967). In untreated bladders, cyclopropane produced a dose-dependent stimulation of sodium transport, while in reserpinized bladders and those treated with α blockers, cyclopropane produced dose-dependent inhibition of sodium transport. β blockers had no effect upon the bladder response to cyclopropane. Andersen suggested that the inhibition of sodium transport by anaesthetic agents may be a direct effect whereas anaesthetic-induced catecholamine release caused a stimulation of sodium transport mediated via α receptors. Confirming his earlier studies, Andersen then showed that methoxyflurane, a non-catecholamine releasing agent, caused dose-related depression of sodium transport in untreated bladders. This effect gradually reversed after discontinuation of the anaesthetic. Studies in goldfish tubules reported depressed organic acid transport with some anaesthetics. In rabbit kidney slices, Bastron et al., 1974), reported dose related depression of PAH accumulation with methoxyflurane, halothane, enflurane, fluroxene and diethyl ether (Bastron et al., 1974, 1976). Other *in vitro* studies showed that PAH uptake in suspensions of proximal tubules was decreased at 1 MAC levels of halothane and methoxyflurane (Bastron et al., 1976).

If indeed anaesthetics alter PAH extraction by the kidney, these results cast considerable doubt on the validity of studies using PAH clearance as a measurement of RBF in the absence of knowledge of renal vein PAH concentration. These concerns are borne out by recent studies where direct measurements of blood flow through, oxygen consumption by, and drug extraction across kidneys were made in a sheep model with chronically implanted vascular catheters (Runciman et al., 1984). Anaesthesia with 2 MAC halothane/40% oxygen/nitrogen balance and normocarbia resulted in decreases in renal blood flow to 50% of awake control values, with significant reductions in renal vein oxygen tensions. Intrinsic renal clearance (clearance corrected for changes in RBF) of a perfusion limited drug cleared by the kidney (cefoxitin) was markedly reduced (*see* Table 36.1). These changes persisted for some hours after anaesthesia. In comparison, spinal anaesthesia caused only very minor changes (*see* Table 36.1). Iodohippurate, handled in a similar manner to PAH by the kidney, showed considerable variation in extraction ratio from day to day, within animals and between animals (Runciman et al., 1984). It now seems clear that PAH extraction cannot be assumed to be constant in 'control' measurements or under anaesthesia. The finding of marked reductions in intrinsic clearance of marker drugs is clear evidence of a direct effect of anaesthetics on tubular function.

Summary of Acute Renal Effects of Anaesthetics

In many of the above studies, it is impossible to dissect out the role of anaesthesia *per se* from other factors such as anxiety, pain, surgical stimulus or blood loss. Thus comparison of the many studies in patients during surgery shows wide variation in reported renal effects (*see* Hawker, 1982). In healthy volunteers pretreated with 4% fructose/water, receiving 1.5% halothane, Deutsch et al. (1966) reported that a 19% reduction in GFR and a 38% reduction in RBF occurred. In patients prior to surgery, Cousins and Mazze reported similar changes in GFR and RBF at 1 MAC halothane, isoflurane and enflurane (Cousins et al., 1976, Mazze et al., 1974a) (Table 36.2). Renal effects of anaesthesia do appear to be dose related and are favourably influenced by adequate repletion of extracellular fluid. Spinal anaesthesia has only minimal effects on RBF, GFR and oxygen consumption and does not influence the intrinsic clearance of marker drugs (*see* Table 36.1). Intravenous induction agents have rarely been studied in a manner that permits clear definition of their effects on the kidney (Priano, 1982), in the absence of other anaesthetics. In humans thiopentone is reported to decrease renal plasma flow in association with an increase in renal vascular resistance. However this is a very old study, using PAH clearance with the potential problems noted above (Habif et al., 1951b). In some centres continuous thiopentone infusion is now used as the sole anaesthetic and in this situation peripheral resistance is increased, however precise measurements of renal function have not been made with different steady state blood concentrations of thiopentone. Diazepam decreases RBF, GRF and urine flowrate, probably in a dose-related manner (Priano, 1982).

TABLE 36.2
EFFECTS OF ANAESTHESIA ON RENAL FUNCTION

Subjects	Fluid status	Anaesthetic	Conc.	RBF	GFR	FF	References
				\multicolumn{3}{c}{% Change}	
Patients during surgery	ECF depleted	Halothane	0.5–1% +	61	48	34	Mazze et al. (1963)
		Halothane	1.2–3% +	69	58	26	
	ECF depleted	Halothane	0.5–1% +	12	8	4	Barry et al. (1964)
		Halothane	1.2–3% +	47	40	10	
Patients prior to surgery	ECF depleted	Halothane	1 MAC + +	—	30	—	Mazze et al. (1974a)
		Enflurane	1 MAC + +	23	20	10	Cousins et al. (1976)
		Isoflurane	1 MAC + +	50	36	4	Mazze et al. (1974a)
Volunteers unoperated	ECF depleted	Halothane	1.5% +	38	19	39	Deutsch et al. (1966)
		N_2O	30% +	36	27	23	Deutsch et al. (1968)
		Narcotic					
		Curare					

+ Inspired Concentrations
+ + End Alveolar Concentrations

Ketamine appears to produce smaller changes in RBF compared to other IV induction agents, particularly in situations of hypovolaemia (Idval et al., 1980; Priano, 1983). The new agent propofol has been studied in a sheep model with chronic vascular catheters, under conditions of continuous infusion. Renal blood flow and GFR were unaltered. Renal extraction of cefoxitin was decreased 33% but recovered within 9 h of anaesthesia; this effect was probably due to a temporary decrease in energy dependent transport of cefoxitin by the kidney. Opioid drugs in 'supplementary doses' during anaesthesia produce small but significant decreases in RBF, GFR and urine flow. These changes appear to be similar with morphine, meperidine and fentanyl (Priano and Vatner, 1981a,b; Hunter et al., 1980; Priano, 1983).

It is not known whether the effects of anaesthesia are greater in diseased kidneys, although from first principles this would seem likely. Current opinion favours reduction of inner cortical blood flow as the initiating factor in acute tubular necrosis; the influence of anaesthetics on these changes is unknown. Finally it is now reported that hypoxia *per se* is capable of reducing renal cortical blood flow. In the surgical patient under anaesthesia complex factors may operate such as combined blood loss and hypoxia. Only direct measurements of GFR, RBF and oxygen consumption by the kidney can resolve these complex issues and point to the optimal management of patients at risk from a renal viewpoint. In the absence of sophisticated measurements, the clinician is well served by the monitoring of hourly urine flow rate and measurement of urine sodium concentration at appropriate intervals.

DELAYED RENAL EFFECTS OF ANAESTHETICS: DIRECT NEPHROTOXICITY

The kidney is particularly susceptible to damage from drugs or toxins because of its rich blood supply and increased concentration of compounds in renal tubular cells during reabsorption or secretion. Because of the countercurrent mechanism, medullary concentration of specific compounds is possible to a degree not found in the interstitial fluids of other tissues of the body. The amount of damage produced by nephrotoxins depends upon many factors such as the duration and intensity of exposure, the degree of toxin binding to plasma protein and tissues other than kidney, the degree and duration of binding to renal tissue, and the rapidity of renal or extrarenal elimination. Toxic damage to the kidney may be either acute or chronic, may predominantly affect glomerular or tubular function, or cause generalized renal damage. Toxicity can be manifested by anuria, oliguria or polyuria. An extensive review of the subject of toxic nephropathy has been written by Schreiner (1972).

ANAESTHETIC METABOLISM AND RENAL TOXICITY

Until the early 1960's, volatile anaesthetics were believed to be inert compounds not metabolized in the mammalian body. In 1964, using isotopically-labelled anaesthetics, it was shown that rats metabolize diethyl ether, chloroform and methoxyflurane to carbon dioxide, and halothane and methoxyflurane to chloride ions (*see* Van Dyke and Ward, 1973).

Interest in the metabolism of volatile anaesthetics was greatly stimulated by the finding that renal dysfunction after methoxyflurane anaesthesia is caused by a metabolite of this agent (Cousins et al., 1974). Simultaneously, a toxic metabolite was implicated in the hepatic necrosis caused by fluroxene and by chloroform in laboratory animals (Cascorbi and Singh-Amaranath, 1973; Brown et al., 1974).

The impact of studies such as these can be seen from the current trend toward the use and development of anaesthetics which undergo minimal metabolism (Cousins et al., 1982). Clinical experience so far supports the enhanced safety of these agents with regard to organ toxicity.

The following brief discussion will be limited to four clinically important volatile anaesthetics—methoxyflurane, enflurane, isoflurane and halothane. Although use of methoxyflurane has diminished in the last decade, it is included here because studies relating its metabolism to nephrotoxicity brought about a change in attitude of anaesthetists towards anaesthetic toxicity (Fig. 36.13). Furthermore, because the nephrotoxic fluoride ion is formed (in lesser amounts) during metabolism of other volatile anaesthetics, the problem of renal toxicity is not exclusive to methoxyflurane. A more detailed review of the renal toxicity of inhalation anaesthetics has been given (Cousins et al., 1973, 1982).

METHOXYFLURANE

Methoxyflurane is now rarely used. However the history of investigation of its renal toxicity now represents the most precisely documented example of anaesthetic toxicity in general and renal toxicity in particular.

In humans, over 50% of net absorbed methoxyflurane is metabolized, mostly with the formation of fluoride, dichloroacetic acid and methoxydifluoroacetic acid. Postoperative urinary oxalate excretion represents only about 7% of absorbed methoxyflurane (Yoshimura et al., 1976). In 1966, sixteen cases of postoperative renal dysfunction, characterized by diuresis and poor response to a vasopressin challenge, were reported in a group of 94 patients who had received methoxyflurane (Crandell et al., 1966). Despite the high incidence of toxic effects observed in this study, defects in its design as well as widespread acceptance of the safety of methoxyflurane left most

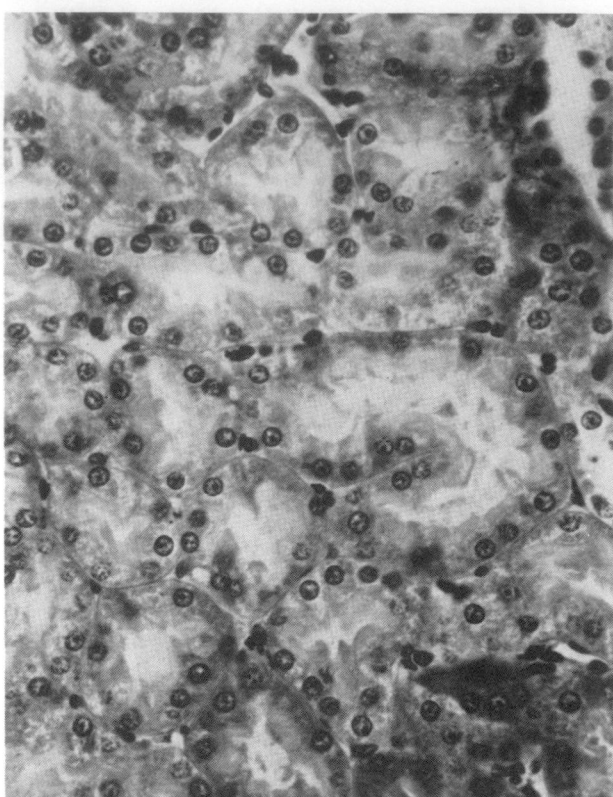 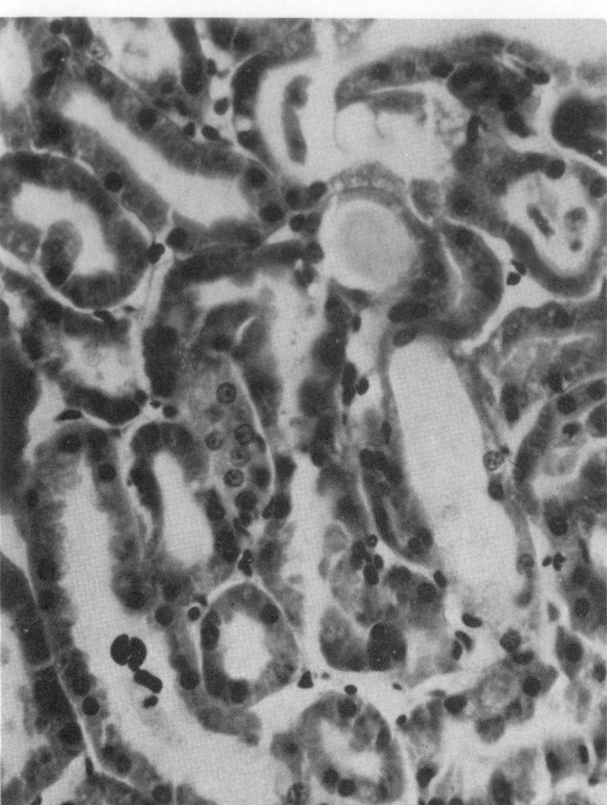

Fig. 36.13 Methoxyflurane (MOF) nephrotoxicity. Light microscopy of proximal convoluted tubules of renal cortex of Fischer 344 rats. Haematoxylin and eosin × 500. *Left*: Normal kidney. Note tall columnar cells of proximal tubules, generous brush borders and small lumina. *Right*: Kidney from rat anaesthetized with 0.75% MOF for 6 h. Acute tubular necrosis is present. Note widespread dilatation of tubules with marked reduction of height of cells and intraluminal slough of necrotic cells. (Reproduced with permission R.I. Mazze, M.J. Cousins, J.C. Kosek, 1972. Dose related methoxyflurane nephrotoxicity in rats. A biochemical and pathologic correlation. *Anaesthesiology*, **36**, 571.)

anaesthetists unconvinced that the results were applicable to the general patient population. Another early report of 20 cases of renal dysfunction in 180 patients given methoxyflurane also made little impression. Over the next five years, a number of reports of renal toxicity associated with methoxyflurane appeared, but it was not until 1971 that Mazze et al. reported the results of a randomized, prospective study which left no doubt as to the nephrotoxicity of this anaesthetic.

A report in 1970 described a case of methoxyflurane nephrotoxicity associated with high levels of fluoride in serum and urine. In 1973, peak serum levels of fluoride and urinary oxalate were found to correlate with renal dysfunction in patients receiving methoxyflurane (Cousins et al., 1973). It was pointed out that the observed symptoms were unlikely to be caused by oxalic acid, but indirect evidence indicated that fluoride could be responsible for the polyuric renal insufficiency. The observation of calcium oxalate deposition in the kidneys of patients suffering renal failure after methoxyflurane anaesthesia suggested the possibility that this was a contributing factor to the renal lesion. Cousins et al., 1974, subsequently reported that fluor-

ide is primarily responsible for methoxyflurane nephrotoxicity in an animal model. In Fischer 344 rats, administration of fluoride, in an amount sufficient to simulate the urinary fluoride excretion following a nephrotoxic dose of methoxyflurane, produced polyuric renal failure and morphological changes similar to those seen after methoxyflurane. On the basis of the same dose of methoxyflurane, injection of a stoichiometric equivalent quantity of oxalic acid produced no abnormalities. Ten times this dose of oxalic acid resulted in anuric renal failure and morphological changes unlike those due to methoxyflurane (Cousins et al., 1974) (Figs. 36.14 and 36.15). Thus, it appears that oxalic acid does not play a major role in the polyuric renal failure caused by methoxyflurane. It is, however, possible that calcium oxalate deposition may contribute to the lesion, especially in the case of the less common post-methoxyflurane chronic renal failure.

Hollenberg et al. (1968) for example, described three cases of irreversible acute oliguric renal failure after methoxyflurane in which oxalate deposition was prominent. A case of generalized oxalosis after meth-

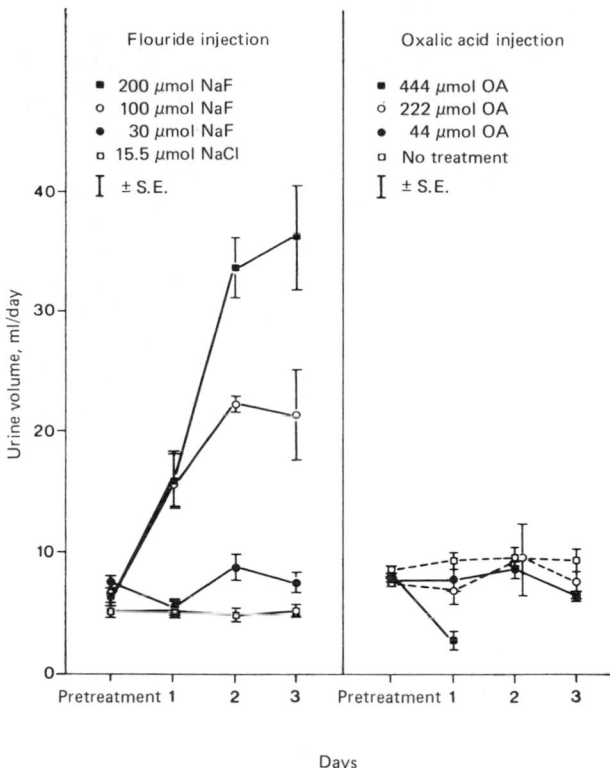

Fig. 36.14 Aetiology of methoxyflurane nephrotoxicity. Comparison of injections of stoichiometrically equivalent doses of sodium fluoride (NaF) or oxalic acid (OA) to simulate the urinary excretion of NaF and OA resulting from low, medium and high doses of MOF. Daily urine volume (mean + SE) before and after treatment. Dose-related polyuria occurred after NaF, and was similar in magnitude to low, medium and high doses of MOF. OA treatment did not cause polyuria. Treatment with 444 µmol (40 mg) of oxalic acid resulted in oliguria. (Reproduced with permission from M.J. Cousins, R.I. Mazzo, J.C. Kosek et al., 1974. The etiology of methoxyflurane nephrotoxicity. *J. Pharmacol. Exp. Ther.*, **190**, 530.)

oxyflurane has also been reported. The patient had pre-existing renal insufficiency, and phenobarbitone had been administered preoperatively. Methoxyflurane—nitrous oxide was administered for about three hours. At autopsy, calcium oxalate crystals were found in the kidney, thyroid, bronchus, heart and retina. Increased metabolism and renal insufficiency may have led to high plasma oxalate levels in this patient (*see* Cousins et al., 1982).

Clinical Features of Methoxyflurane Nephrotoxicity

In a randomized, prospective clinical study, Cousins and Mazze (1973a), reported details of changes in renal function at increasing doses of methoxyflurane (MOF) (Figs. 36.16, 36.17). Subclinical toxicity occurred after 2.5–3 MAC hours of MOF (serum $F^- > 50\,\mu mol/L$). This was manifested by delayed return to maximum preoperative urine osmolality,

unresponsiveness to vasopressin (ADH) administration and elevated serum uric acid concentration. Mild clinical toxicity occurred after 5 MAC hours of MOF (Serum $F^- > 90\,\mu mol/L$). In addition to the abnormalities noted above, there was hypernatremia, serum hyperosmolality, polyuria, and low urine osmolality. The latter two abnormalities were evidence of a water losing nephropathy and this was confirmed by the failure to respond to ADH (*see* Fig. 36.17). Urine osmolality also failed to respond to a water load, confirming the presence of both a diluting and a concentrating defect in renal tubules. This would result in inability to compensate for fluid restriction or a fluid overload. Frank clinical toxicity was present at 7 MAC hours MOF (Serum F^- 80 to $175\,\mu mol/L$). Abnormalities in serum and urine variables were more pronounced than at lower MOF doses and thirst and polyuria added difficulty to postoperative management.

Predisposing Factors in Methoxyflurane Nephrotoxicity

Dose
A dose-response relationship exists for methoxyflurane nephrotoxicity in man (Cousins et al., 1973a), and an animal model (Mazze et al., 1972). Parameters indicative of renal dysfunction correlate with dose of methoxyflurane (MAC-hours). Although nephrotoxicity was observed at peak serum fluoride levels above $50\,\mu mol/L$ it should be borne in mind that this peak level is only an indicator of total kidney exposure (concentration × time) to fluoride. Prolonged exposure of the kidney to concentrations of serum fluoride as low as $25\,\mu mol/L$ may result in nephrotoxicity (Plummer et al., 1985).

Genetic Factors
Although Fig. 36.15 indicates a strong dose-response relationship, considerable individual variation is apparent in both peak serum fluoride concentration after a given dose of methoxyflurane and degree of nephrotoxicity observed at each fluoride level. This indicates individual variation in both extent of methoxyflurane metabolism and renal sensitivity to fluoride, presumably due in part to genetic factors. Animal experiments provide evidence of genetic differences in both metabolism and organ sensitivity. Of six inbred rat strains, only Fischer 344 rats developed renal toxicity after anaesthesia for 3 h with 0.5% methoxyflurane (Mazze et al., 1973c). The susceptibility of this strain was due to both a high rate of methoxyflurane biotransformation and a high renal sensitivity to fluoride.

Age
Peak serum fluoride levels in paediatric patients (mean age 10.2 years) were found to be lower than

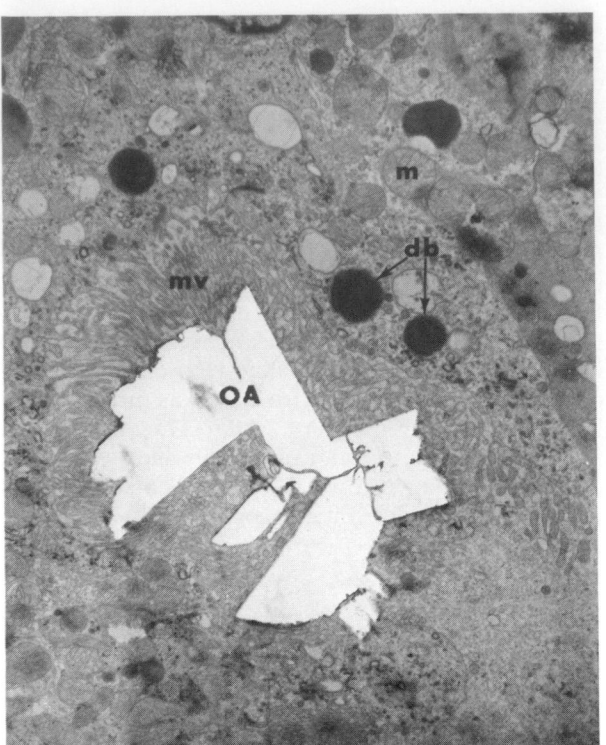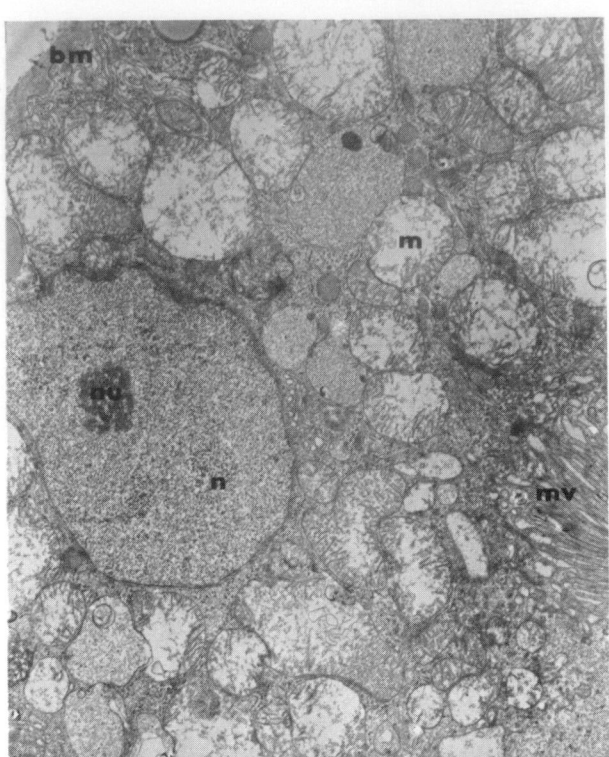

Fig. 36.15 Aetiology of methoxyflurane nephrotoxicity. Proximal convoluted tubule cells from renal cortex of Fischer 344 rats. Electron micrographs × 1347. *Left*: Tubule cells from rat injected with 444 μmol (40 mg) of oxalic acid, 24 h later. Note large oxalate crystals (OA) completely occupying tubule lumen. However, despite this dose, ten times higher than the equivalent OA from high dose MOF, mitochondria (m) are essentially normal. *Right*: Tubule cell from rat anaesthetized with 0.5% MOF for 3 h, 24 h later. Note marked mitochondrial swelling with disruption of the cristae and rupture of mitochondria. db = dense bodies; n, nucleus; nu, nucleolus; mv = microvilli; bm, basement membrane. (Reproduced with permission from M.J. Cousins, R.I. Mazze, J.C. Kosek et al., 1974. The etiology of methoxyflurane nephrotoxicity. *J. Pharmacol. Exp. Ther.*, **190**, 530.)

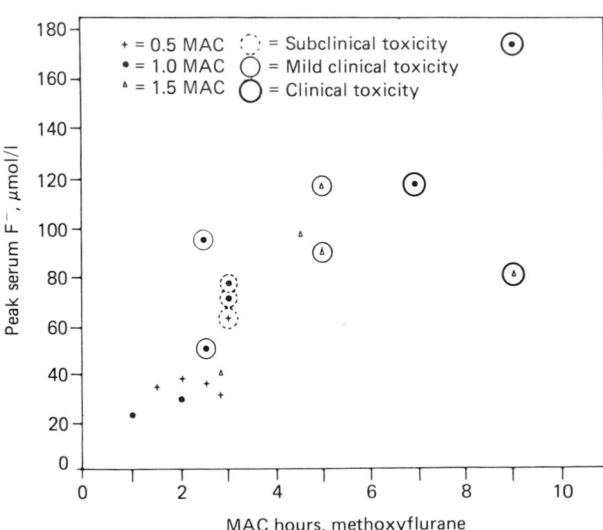

Fig. 36.16 Dose response relationship of methoxyflurane nephrotoxicity in man. (*see* text). (Reproduced with permission from M.J. Cousins, R.I. Mazze, 1973. Methoxyflurane nephrotoxicity. A study of dose response in man. *JAMA*, **225**, 1611.)

those reported in adults after similar exposure to methoxyflurane (Stoelting and Peterson, 1975). This could be due to lower rates of methoxyflurane biotransformation or to altered fluoride pharmacokinetics (e.g. increased deposition in bone). No cases of methoxyflurane nephrotoxicity have been reported in children.

Enzyme Induction

Factors which increase methoxyflurane metabolism increase the risk of nephrotoxicity. Treatment of rats with the mixed-function oxidase inducer phenobarbitone increases methoxyflurane metabolism (Van Dyke and Wood, 1973), and exacerbates nephrotoxicity (Cousins et al., 1974) (Fig. 36.18). Treatment with 3-methylcholanthrene, an inducer of cytochrome P-448, does not result in increased microsomal metabolism of this anaesthetic. Administration of isoniazid, or other compounds containing the hydrazine moiety, to rats results in increased rates of microsomal metabolism of methoxyflurane and other halogenated ether anaesthetics to inorganic fluoride (Rice et al., 1980b;

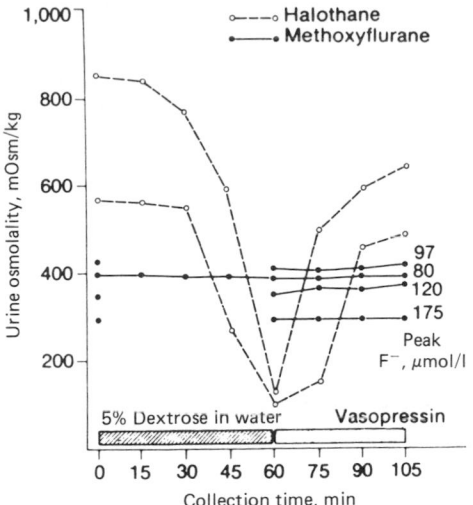

Fig. 36.17 Methoxyflurane nephrotoxicity. Vasopressin infusion tests in four patients with polyuric renal dysfunction following methoxyflurane. Note that these patients do not respond to a water load (diluting defect) or to a vasopressin challenge (concentrating defect). In comparison two patients following halothane showed marked reductions in urine osmolality after a water load and normal increases in urine osmolality with vasopressin. (Reproduced with permission from M.J. Cousins, R.I. Mazze, 1973. Methoxyflurane nephrotoxicity. A study of dose response in man. *JAMA*, **225**, 1611.)

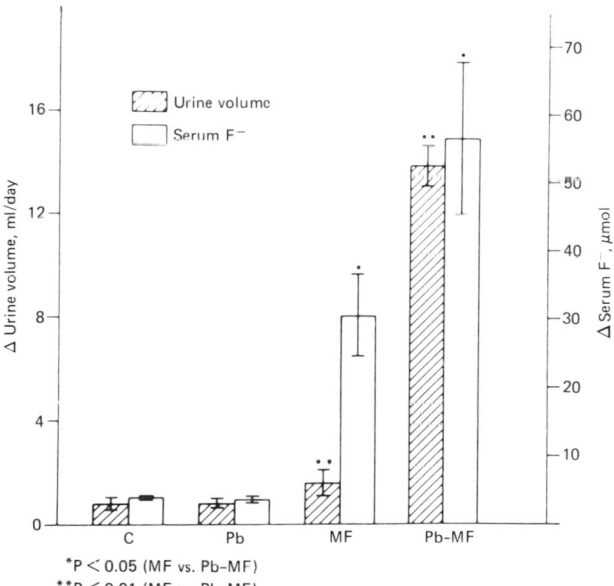

*P < 0.05 (MF vs. Pb-MF)
**P < 0.01 (MF vs. Pb-MF)

Fig. 36.18 Effect of enzyme induction. Changes in serum inorganic fluoride (F⁻) concentrations and urine volume, mean + SE. C = control, no treatment; Pb = phenobarbitone 25 mg/kg twice daily for 4 days; MF = methoxyflurane 0.25% for 1.5 hours; Pb-MF = phenobarbitone preceeding MOF. (Reproduced with permission from M.J. Cousins, R.I. Mazze, J.C. Kosek et al., 1974. The etiology of methoxyflurane nephrotoxicity. *J. Pharmacol. Exp. Ther.*, **190**, 530.)

Fish and Rice, 1979a). Although the hepatic microsomal content of total cytochrome P-450 is not increased, a specific form of the cytochrome may be induced (Rice et al., 1980b).

Presumably, mixed-function oxidase induction with appropriate agents increases methoxyflurane metabolism in man, but only indirect evidence is available to support this hypothesis. In the case of generalized oxalosis after methoxyflurane described by (*see* Cousins et al., 1982), although complicating factors were present, phenobarbitone may have resulted in increased methoxyflurane metabolism. Cases involving other anaesthetics (*see* 'enflurane') suggest that the increased anaesthetic metabolism caused by isoniazid in rats may also occur in man.

Other Nephrotoxic Drugs

Administration of other nephrotoxic drugs increases the likelihood of methoxyflurane nephrotoxicity. Treatment of rats with both gentamicin and methoxyflurane results in greater renal impairment than does treatment with either drug alone (Barr et al., 1973). These two drugs also exert a synergistic effect on the kidney in humans. Severity of methoxyflurane nephrotoxicity was apparently aggravated as a result of commencement of gentamicin therapy in the postoperative period (Mazze and Cousins, 1973b) (Fig. 36.19). Tetracycline, a potentially nephrotoxic drug, has also been implicated as an exacerbating factor in methoxyflurane renal failure (Proctor and Barton, 1971).

Obesity

Young et al. (1975) reported that obese patients developed higher serum fluoride levels during, and 2 h after, methoxyflurane anaesthesia than do non-obese patients. Although it might be postulated that fat may serve as a depot for methoxyflurane, resulting in prolonged metabolism and sustained fluoride levels, in this study obese patients did not have higher serum fluoride levels 1–3 days post-anaesthesia. However, Young et al. compared their data from obese patients with data reported elsewhere for non-obese patients. Caution was recommended in the administration of methoxyflurane to obese patients.

Clinical Implications for use of Methoxyflurane

1. MOF dose of 2–2.5 MAC hours should not be exceeded.
2. To achieve the lowest possible MOF concentration it should not be administered, for surgery, without anaesthetic adjuvants.
3. Blood pressure changes cannot be relied upon to guide anaesthetic depth, because of the marked cardiovascular stability of MOF.
4. Uncalibrated vaporizers should not be used for MOF.

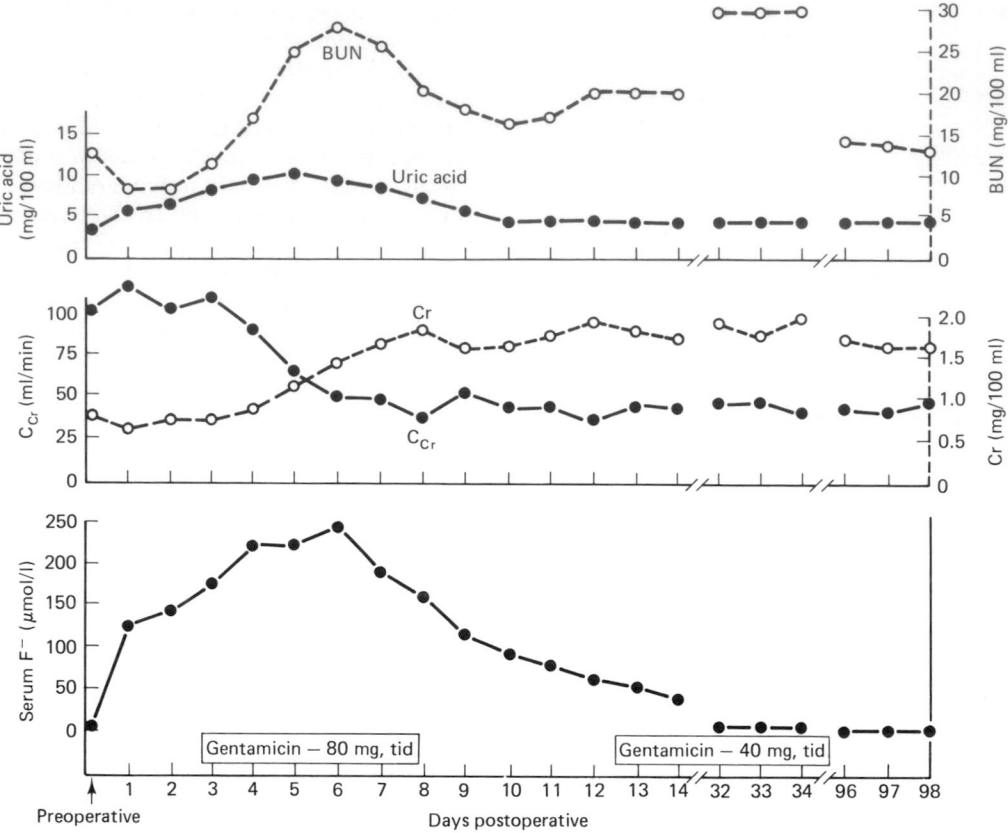

Fig. 36.19 Combined nephrotoxicity of gentamicin and methoxyflurane. Biochemical findings in a patient who developed nephrotoxicity due to the combined effects of methoxyflurane (MOF) and gentamicin. Following MOF mild nephrotoxicity occurred which rapidly increased in severity when gentamicin therapy was commenced. Note that when a second course of gentamicin was required no nephrotoxicity resulted. Preop = preoperative values; BUN = blood urea nitrogen; C_{Cr} = creatinine clearance; F^- = serum inorganic fluoride. (Reproduced with permission from R.I. Mazze, M.J. Cousins, 1973. Combined nephrotoxicity of gentamicin and methoxyflurane anaesthesia in man. *Br. J. Anaesth.*, **45**, 394.)

5. MOF should not be used in the presence of other nephrotoxic drugs, in patients with impaired renal function or in those undergoing surgery with an added risk of renal complications.
6. Today methoxyflurane use is largely restricted to low-doses for analgesia or sometimes for short-term supplementation of a balanced anaesthetic technique. It remains the volatile anaesthetic with greatest analgesic properties.

ENFLURANE

Conclusive proof of methoxyflurane nephrotoxicity in 1974 and emerging evidence of halothane hepatotoxicity has resulted in a sharp increase in the clinical use of enflurane, with a corresponding decrease in halothane use (Cousins et al., 1982). Enflurane is metabolized in man to fluoride ion, difluoromethoxy-difluoroacetic acid and an unidentified acidic metabolite (Cousins et al., 1976; Miller and Gandolfi, 1980a;

Burke et al., 1981). Enflurane metabolism is approximately one twentieth that of methoxyflurane and one tenth that of halothane. In a study in humans, about 83% of administered enflurane was exhaled unchanged and 2.4% recovered as urinary metabolites.

Due to its minimal metabolism and rapid excretion via the lungs, serum fluoride levels after enflurane are lower than those observed after methoxyflurane anaesthesia. After 2.7 MAC hours of enflurane, serum fluoride concentration peaked at 22 μmol/L 4 h post-anaesthesia (Cousins et al., 1976), (Fig. 36.20). However, some individuals may metabolize enflurane much more extensively. In a reported case of post-operative renal failure, serum fluoride concentration was 93.6 μmol/L on the second day after six hours of 1% enflurane (total dose = 3.5 MAC-hours) (Loehning and Mazze, 1974). Increased enflurane metabolism and impaired fluoride excretion may have contributed to this high level. Clearly, where potential exacerbating factors, such as prolonged anaesthesia, administration of other nephrotoxic drugs, enzyme

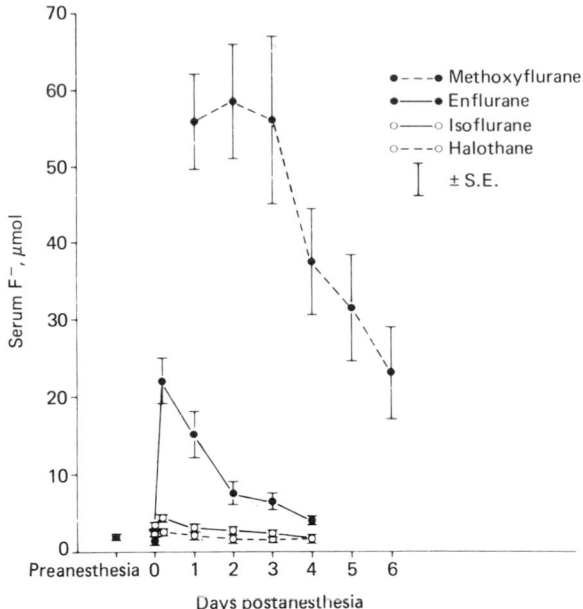

Fig. 36.20 Serum inorganic fluoride (F⁻) concentrations prior to and following anaesthesia with various inhalation anaesthetics. Note the marked and sustained increases in F⁻ following methoxyflurane. After enflurane anaesthesia peak F⁻ occurs earlier and declines much more rapidly. (Reproduced with permission from M.J. Cousins, L.R. Greenstein, B.A. Hitt et al., 1976. Metabolism and renal effects of enflurane in man. *Anesthesiology*, **44**, 44.)

induction or obesity are present, the possibility of fluoride nephrotoxicity must be considered.

Enflurane Dose

The effect of prolonged enflurane anaesthesia on renal function has been studied in rats and man. In Fischer 344 rats, 6–10 h of 2.5% enflurane resulted in renal dysfunction similar to that in another group receiving 1.5 h of 0.25% methoxyflurane (Barr et al., 1974). Peak serum fluoride levels were similar in the two groups.

Renal effects of enflurane in man are dose-dependent. In patients receiving a mean of 2.7 MAC hours of enflurane, renal function was not impaired 24–28 h postoperatively (Cousins et al., 1976). Blood chemistry of volunteers receiving 9.6 MAC hours of enflurane indicated minimal changes in renal function at 24 h and 5 days (Eger et al., 1976). However, in a similar study in which renal function was assessed by maximum urine osmolality in response to vasopressin, impairment was observed 24 h but not 5 days postanaesthesia (Mazze et al., 1977).

Enflurane and Other Nephrotoxic Drugs

As is the case with methoxyflurane, administration of the nephrotoxin gentamicin to rats can exacerbate the renal effects of enflurane. Fischer 344 rats receiving gentamicin, 25 mg/kg twice daily for 9 days, followed by 1 MAC enflurane for 6 h, exhibited more pronounced morphological changes in the kidney and greater urine volumes than did animals receiving either gentamicin or enflurane alone (Cousins et al., 1978). With lower doses of gentamicin (5 mg/(kg·d) for 15 days) and enflurane (2% for 2 h), no synergistic effect was observed in rats with surgical induced renal insufficiency (Fish et al., 1979b). Rats with surgically induced kidney damage, but not receiving gentamicin, developed only mild and reversible changes in renal function after 6 h of 2% enflurane (20 days earlier, these animals had received 2 h of 2% enflurane) (Sievenpiper et al., 1979). These changes were probably not due to fluoride, as animals receiving 1% halothane instead of enflurane reacted in a similar manner.

Evidence relating to a combined effect of enflurane and nephrotoxic drugs in humans is lacking, but this could be due to caution in the use of enflurane in patients thought to be at risk. Enflurane anaesthesia has, however, been associated with renal dysfunction in several patients with pre-existing renal disease (Loehning et al., 1979); Eichhorn et al., 1976).

Enzyme Induction

Treatment of rats with the mixed-function oxidase inducing agent, phenobarbitone, results in the increased metabolism of enflurane by the hepatic microsomal fraction *in vitro* (Greenstein et al., 1975; Hitt et al., 1977; Ivanetich et al., 1979). However, phenobarbitone treatment does not affect enflurane metabolism or nephrotoxicity *in vivo* (Barr et al., 1974). Similarly, in a group of 102 surgical patients classified according to drug history, no differences were found in peak serum fluoride concentration after enflurane between control patients and those taking miscellaneous drugs, ethanol or drugs known to cause enzyme induction (phenobarbitone, phenytoin) (Dooley et al., 1979).

As mentioned earlier, the rate of metabolism of halogenated ether anaesthetics is increased in hepatic microsomes prepared from isoniazid-treated rats (Rice et al., 1980b). This effect is also observed *in vivo*. Isoniazid-treated Fischer 344 rats exposed to 2% enflurane became polyuric and excreted increased fluoride relative to similarly exposed rats not treated with isoniazid (Rice and Mazze, 1980a). Isoniazid has a similar effect in man. Almost half of 20 patients taking isoniazid prior to enflurane anaesthesia had unusually high peak serum fluoride concentrations postanaesthesia (over 100 μmol/L in three patients) (Mazze et al., 1982). It was suggested that susceptibility to this effect of isoniazid may be related to acetylator phenotype. As the hydrazine moiety is responsible for the inducing effect (Fish et al., 1979a), enflurane should be used with caution in patients taking drugs containing this group. Alcohol has also been shown to enhance enflurane metabolism in rats (Van Dyke,

1983), but the clinical significance of this finding has not been investigated.

Obesity

Obesity also contributes to elevated fluoride levels after anaesthesia. Cousins et al. (1976), reported an obese patient who had a peak serum fluoride concentration of 52 µmol/L after 4 MAC hours of enflurane. After similar exposures to enflurane, serum fluoride concentrations were higher in obese than in non-obese patients (28 versus 17 µmol/L (Bentley et al., 1979; Miller et al., 1980b). The rate of increase of serum fluoride levels during and after 2 MAC hours of enflurane in obese patients (5.5 µmol/(L·h)) was twice that in a non-obese group (2.5 µmol/(L·h)). These differences were apparently due to more rapid biotransformation of enflurane in the obese group.

Renal Ischaemia

Using the isolated perfused kidney, Rice et al. (1987) confirmed that, at normal perfusion rates, 50 µmol/L inorganic fluoride was nephrotoxic. In comparison, 30 min of complete 'warm' renal ischaemia, followed by normal perfusion was associated with increased sensitivity to the nephrotoxic effects of inorganic fluoride. In this situation the isolated perfused kidney was sensitive to the nephrotoxic effects of inorganic fluoride at concentrations of 25 µmol/L (Rice et al., 1987). This raises the possibility that patients suffering episodes of renal ischaemia may be susceptible to developing nephrotoxicity following enflurane anaesthesia.

Overall, there appears to be little risk of fluoride nephrotoxicity after moderate doses of enflurane in the absence of risk factors. Reports of enflurane nephrotoxicity are rare, despite the fact that risk factors (obesity, gentamicin therapy, prolonged anaesthesia) are presumably present in a large number of enflurane administrations. Enflurane is excreted more rapidly than methoxyflurane, and this results in fluoride levels peaking earlier and returning to baseline levels more quickly in comparison to methoxyflurane (Cousins et al., 1976; Barr et al., 1974). Thus, for the same peak serum fluoride concentration, exposure of the kidney to fluoride is more prolonged after methoxyflurane than after enflurane (*see* Fig. 36.20).

ISOFLURANE

Although synthesized soon after enflurane, clinical introduction of isoflurane was delayed until 1981. This was partly due to initial difficulty in purifying the drug but also to subsequently disproven studies reporting carcinogenicity. Isoflurane, an isomer of enflurane, is metabolized to inorganic fluoride and trifluoroacetic acid both in rats and man (Cousins et al., 1973c; Hitt et al., 1974; Holaday et al., 1975; Mazze et al., 1974b). As studies with enflurane have shown the difluoro-

methyl group to be metabolically stable, biotransformation of isoflurane is likely to proceed by initial attack at the chlorine-bearing carbon.

Isoflurane is metabolized to a lesser extent than other clinically used volatile anaesthetics. In humans, almost the entire dose is exhaled unchanged, less than 0.2% is excreted as urinary metabolites (Holaday et al., 1975). Fischer 344 rats also metabolized isoflurane minimally, serum fluoride concentration reaching only 6.5 µmol/L after 4 MAC hours and 7.3 µmol/L after 15 MAC hours of isoflurane (Cousins et al., 1973c) (preanaesthetic values are 2–3 µmol/L).

Due to the minimal extent of metabolism of isoflurane, fluoride nephrotoxicity has not been associated with its use in man (Mazze et al., 1974a) or rats (Cousins et al., 1973c). In humans, peak serum fluoride concentrations average 4.4 µmol/L (twice the preanaesthetic value), well below the nephrotoxic threshold, after 1.2–5.3 MAC hours of isoflurane (Mazze et al., 1974a) (*see* Fig. 36.20).

In obese rats with surgically induced chronic renal insufficiency, inorganic fluoride levels were approximately 20 µmol/L (Fish et al., 1987). This is below the nephrotoxic threshold in normal kidneys, however it is close to the nephrotoxic threshold for inorganic fluoride in kidneys exposed to ischaemia (Rice et al., 1987). The clinical significance of these studies in animals remains to be determined.

INFLUENCE OF ANAESTHETIC MANAGEMENT ON THE INCIDENCE AND SEVERITY OF POSTOPERATIVE ACUTE RENAL FAILURE

A number of aetiological factors, acting singly or in combination, must be considered when evaluating a patient who develops postoperative acute renal failure (ARF) (Table 36.3). The factors most commonly encountered are those which act by reduction of RBF to produce renal ischaemia. These are the most amenable to modification by sound anaesthesia practice. The predominantly vascular aetiology of this type of ARF (Oken et al., 1966; Hollenberg et al., 1968) has led to the use of the term 'vasomotor nephropathy'. Reduction of RBF to 50–70% normal results in sustained afferent arteriolar constriction and renal cortical ischaemia. It now seems that decreased glomerular permeability, tubular back leak of filtrate and tubular obstruction are merely secondary phenomena. An important consequence of ischaemia and hypoxia may be swelling of vascular epithelial cells resulting in obstruction of microvasculature. This may prevent re-establishment of blood flow, even if the initial insult is effectively treated—the 'no-reflow phenomenon' (Bastron et al., 1976). It seems likely that the renin-angiotensin system plays a powerful role in the production of renal cortical ischaemia via afferent arteriolar constriction. Improvement in RBF will often result in an increase in urine output, and prevent or ameliorate the development of ARF, but it

TABLE 36.3
AETIOLOGICAL FACTORS IN ACUTE RENAL FAILURE

1. *Vasomotor nephropathy* (*Acute tubular necrosis* {*ATN*}).
   Post ischaemic
     Hypovolaemic shock
     Cardiogenic shock
     Septic shock
     Iatrogenic (e.g. excessive use of diuretics)
   Nephrotoxic
     Haemoglobin pigments (especially myoglobin)
     Uric acid
     Anaesthetics (especially methoxyflurane)
     Antibiotics (e.g. aminoglycosides)
     Radiographic dyes
     Dextran 40

2. *Acute interstitial nephritis*
     Penicillin
     Sulphonamides

3. *Renal vascular injury*
     Malignant hypertension
     Arterial embolism
     Septic embolism (e.g. endocarditis)

4. *Acute on chronic renal failure*

5. *Acute glomerulonephritis*

6. *Renal dysfunction in systemic disease*
     Vasculitides
     Collagen diseases

by no means follows that any intervention which improves urine output will be ultimately beneficial to the oliguric patient. For example, administration of frusemide intravenously might maintain a normal or increased urine output, but hypovolaemia might be exacerbated, leading to a reduction in GFR and RBF.

During ischaemia the enzyme xanthine dehydrogenase is converted to xanthine oxidase (XO) (Pearson et al., 1987) by proteolysis and ATP is metabolized to hypoxanthine (HX). At reperfusion, XO combines with its substrate HX, in the presence of molecular oxygen, to generate superoxide radicals and hydrogen peroxide, which react with cell protein, lipid and DNA to cause cellular and organ injury. Excessive oxygen free radical (superoxide) production during or after renal ischaemia episodes may play a part in the development of postoperative renal failure. This is supported by studies which report that superoxide dismutase, a scavenger of superoxide, and allopurinol, an inhibitor of xanthine oxidase, are protective after renal ischaemia (Hansson et al., 1986). It is interesting to speculate that the renal damage produced by the toxic metabolite inorganic fluoride could have additive effects on cellular constituents to those produced by superoxide radicals and hydrogen peroxide resulting from ischaemia.

There was previously controversy concerning the use of sodium containing fluids in surgical patients (Hayes et al., 1959; Shires et al., 1961; Shires, 1964; Roth et al., 1969; Middleton et al., 1969). Most clinicians now agree that some salt containing solution is beneficial in major surgery, with the amount infused proportional to the degree of surgical trauma (Thompson et al., 1968; Moore and Shires, 1967). However, it is necessary to assess the response to intravenous fluids by measurement of urine volume and content, as well as by non-renal parameters such as left atrial pressure and auscultation of lung bases.

Whenever anaesthesia is proposed in a patient considered to have a high risk of developing postoperative ARF (Dawson, 1965; Barry et al., 1961; Sawyer et al., 1963; Schreiner, 1972; Baxter and Maynard, 1968) (*see* Table 36.4) the following strategies should be considered:

TABLE 36.4
'AT RISK' SITUATIONS FOR THE KIDNEY

1. Cardiopulmonary bypass or surgery of the aorta (Thompson et al., 1968) or renal vessels.
2. Major biliary tree surgery (Dawson, 1965).
3. Procedures in which large volumes of blood may be transfused.
4. Hypovolaemic hypotension (Barry et al., 1961).
5. Lengthy or extensive surgical procedures in older patients. (ARF Mortality <50% at <40 years, >80% above 80 years age).
6. Surgery in patients with pre-existing renal disease (Sawyer et al., 1963).
7. Obstetric complications such as abruptio placentae (Schreiner, 1972).
8. Major trauma (Baxter and Maynard, 1968).
9. Transfusion of mismatched blood (Baxter and Maynard, 1968).
10. Cardiac or hepatic failure (Bastron and Deutsch, 1976).
11. Rhabdomyolysis and Myoglobinuria (Bastron and Deutsch, 1976) (e.g. Prolonged coma, Malignant Hyperthermia).
12. Septicaemia (Bastron and Deutsch, 1976).

1. *Bladder catheterization* and measurement of hourly urine volume and urine sodium concentration are the only practical means of following renal function intraoperatively, and should be regarded as mandatory in any high risk case. Mechanical patency of the urine drainage system should be checked whenever unexpected 'oliguria' occurs. Periodic determination of urine sodium concentration may occasionally be helpful.

2. *Maintenance of an adequate circulating blood volume* and an adequate cardiac output are clearly the most important means available for maintaining RBF and GRF. Continuous arterial and central venous pressure (CVP) monitoring should be considered in high risk patients, and pulmonary artery catheterization is indicated where closer

monitoring of cardiovascular function is required (e.g. cardiac or respiratory failure associated with pre-existing renal disease), or when measurement of CVP is unreliable (e.g. chronic lung disease, cardiac disease). Low atrial blood pressure is a potent stimulus for renal vasoconstriction (Kahl et al., 1974) and renal blood flow may be improved by 50–100% at any given arterial pressure by acute elevation of atrial pressures which are below normal (Kahl et al., 1974; Mason and Ledsom, 1974). Aggressive preoperative volume loading may be beneficial (Bush et al., 1981) and certainly extracellular volume depletion due to preoperative fasting should be prevented by an appropriate regimen of intravenous fluids.

3. *Inotropic drugs.* In those patients with a low cardiac output—despite an adequate intravascular volume, renal function can undoubtedly be improved by catecholamine infusion (Goldberg et al., 1977; Leier et al., 1978). While the specific renal effects of dopamine have been widely publicized, clinical data suggests that the effect of inotropes on the systemic circulation dominate any direct effect on the renal vasculature. Therefore, systemic rather than renal considerations dictate the choice of any particular agent.

At low doses by infusion 1–2 µg/min epinephrine increases cardiac output and reduces systemic vascular resistance, because its action on β receptors dominates over effects on α receptors. As dosage is increased action on α receptors increases and eventually intense vasocontriction results (> 10 µg/min). Dobutamine was designed to overcome the problems of tachycardia with isoprenaline, while retaining positive inotropic effects (Sakamoto and Yamada, 1977; Goldberg et al., 1977). In practice dobutamine in a dose of 5–15 µg/(kg·min) has effects similar to epinephrine given at a rate of 1–3 µg/min in the adult. Dopamine, in doses of 0.5–3 µg/(kg·min) has unique effects on dopaminergic receptors in the renal vasculature, resulting in improved renal perfusion and a diuretic response (Goldberg et al., 1977), some of which may be tubular in origin (Hilberman et al., 1984). At doses of 3–10 µg/(kg·min) β adrenergic stimulation results in increased cardiac output. At doses of 15–20 µg/(kg·min) α adrenergic stimulation occurs, with increased vascular resistance. However responses in individual patients vary, and in practice dopamine infusion rate is carefully adjusted in the range 0.5–15 µg/(kg·min) while monitoring cardiac output and indices of renal function. It should be recognized that evidence is currently lacking that prophylactic use of dopamine alters the course of incipient acute renal failure in humans.

4. *Vasodilators.* Although nitroprusside causes renal vasodilatation in isolated kidneys, its effects in intact animals and man have varied. The factors responsible for this may include low left atrial blood pressure leading to reflex renal vasoconstriction, a decline in renal perfusion pressure beyond the autoregulatory range, and reflex increases in cardiac output in response to vasodilatation. In patients with severe congestive heart failure, vasodilatation with captopril may worsen RBF and renal function. However sometimes a combination of inotropic drugs and vasodilators may improve cardiac function and renal perfusion.

5. *Diuretics.* Clinical studies in the 1960's (Seitzman et al., 1963; Barry et al., 1961; Porter et al., 1967) suggested that large doses of mannitol were effective in preventing renal failure in patients undergoing aortic aneurysm surgery, and cardiac valve replacement. It is possible that the main action of mannitol in these studies was as a volume expander. The current status of diuretics in protection from ARF is similar to that of steroids in shock—there is strong experimental evidence that diuretics significantly protect kidneys when given before an ischaemic insult (Cronin et al., 1978; de Torrente et al., 1978) but both clinical and experimental data relating to diuretics given after oliguria ensues are disappointing. It is often claimed that the administration of high dose diuretics predisposes to the development of non-oliguric ARF which has a better prognosis than the oliguric form. There appear to be few scientific data to either support or contradict this claim.

The administration of diuretics for the prevention of renal failure remains a widespread practice. It is important to remember that unrecognized hypovolaemia may be worsened by large doses of diuretics, and the question of toxicity, particularly ototoxicity and nephrotoxicity of frusemide, should be borne in mind.

6. *Other approaches.* Promising experimental data are available for a number of agents which may have a role in preventing the onset of ARF. These include Adenosine triphosphate (ATP) (Siegel et al., 1980), Magnesium chloride (Siegel et al., 1980), β-blocking drugs (Stowe et al., 1978) and calcium antagonists (Schanne et al., 1979). The role of spinal and epidural blockade in patients 'at risk' needs to be defined, however, favourable effects re-

TABLE 36.5

INVESTIGATIONS WHICH MAY BE HELPFUL IN DISTINGUISHING PRE-RENAL OLIGURIA (PRO) FROM ACUTE RENAL FAILURE (ARF)

	PRO	*ARF*
Urinary sodium concentration (mmol/L)	< 20	> 40
Urinary osmolality (mosmol/kg)	> 550	< 350
Urine/plasma osmolar ratio	$> 2:1$	$< 1.1:1$
Urine/plasma urea ratio	$> 20:1$	$< 10:1$
Urine/plasma creatinine ratio	$> 40:1$	$< 10:1$
Urinary sediment (casts)	Non-cellular	Cellular

ported in normal kidneys (Kennedy et al., 1970; Kennedy, 1969; Runciman et al., 1984) indicate the need for further studies.

7. *Persistent Oliguria*. In those patients in whom oliguria persists it is important to distinguish prerenal oliguria from established ARF. Table 36.5 lists those diagnostic features which are the most helpful in this regard.

REFERENCES

Andersen N.B. (1966). Effect of general anaesthetics on sodium transport in the isolated toad bladder. *Anesthesiology*, **27**, 304.

Andersen N.B. (1967). Synergistic effect of cyclopropane and epinephrine on sodium transport in toad bladder. *Anesthesiology*, **28**, 438.

Bachman L. (1955). The antidiuretic effects of anaesthetic agents. *Anesthesiology*, **16**, 939

Baily D.B., Miller E.D., Kaplan J.A., et al. (1975). The renin–angiotensin–aldosterone system during cardiac surgery with morphine-nitrous oxide anaesthesia. *Anesthesiology*, **42**, 538.

Bark H., Le Roith D., Nyska M., et al. (1980). Elevations in plasma ADH levels during PEEP ventilation in the dog: mechanisms involved. *Am. J. Physiol.*, **239**, 474.

Barr G.A., Mazze R.I., Cousins M.J., et al. (1973). An animal model for combined methoxyflurane and gentamicin nephrotoxicity. *Br. J. Anaesth.*, **45**, 306.

Barr G.A., Cousins M.J., Mazze R.I., et al. (1974). A comparison of the renal effects and metabolism of enflurane and methoxyflurane in Fischer 344 rats. *J. Pharmacol. Exp. Ther.*, **188**, 257.

Barry K.G., Cohen A.C., Knochel J.P., et al. (1961). Mannitol infusion II. The prevention of acute renal failure during resection of an aneurysm of the abdominal aorta. *New Engl. J. Med.*, **264**, 967.

Barry K.G., Mazze, R.I., Schwartz, F.D. (1964). Prevention of surgical oliguria and renal-haemodynamic suppression by sustained hydration. *New Engl. J. Med.*, **270**, 1371.

Bartter F.C., Schwartz E.B. (1967). The syndrome of inappropriate secretion of antidiuretic hormone. *Am. J. Med.*, **42**, 790.

Bastron R.D., Deutsch S. (1976). *Anaesthesia and the kidney*. New York: Grune and Stratton.

Bastron R.D., Kaloyanides G.J. (1974). Effects of methoxyflurane (MOF) on PAH uptake by rabbit kidney tissue slices. *Am. J. Physiol.*, **227**, 460.

Baxter C.R., Maynard D.R. (1968). Prevention and recognition of surgical renal complications. In *Clinical Anaesthesia*, pp. 322–333. Philadelphia: F.A. Davis.

Bentley J.B., Vaughan R.W., Miller, M.S., et al. (1979). Serum inorganic fluoride levels in obese patients during and after enflurane anesthesia. *Anesth. Analg.*, **58**, 409.

Berne R.M. (1952). Haemodynamics and sodium excretion of denervated kidney in anaesthetized and unanaesthetized dog. *Am. J. Physiol.*, **171**, 148.

Bichet D., Schrier R.W. (1982). Evidence against concept of hyponatraemia and 'sick cells'. *Lancet*, **1**, 742.

Boba A., Landmesser C.M. (1965). Renal complications after anaesthesia and operation. *Anesthesiology*, **26**, 240.

Brown B.R., Sipes I.G., Sagalyn A.M. (1974). Mechanisms of acute hepatic toxicity: chloroform, halothane and glutathione. *Anesthesiology*, **41**, 554.

Brown C.B., Ogg C.S., Cameron J.S. (1981). High dose furosemide in acute renal failure: a controlled trial. *Clin. Nephrol.* **15**, 90.

Burke T.R., Branchflower R.V., Lees D.E., et al. (1981). Mechanism of defluorination of enflurane. Identification of an organic metabolite in rat and man. *Drug Metab. Disposit.* **9**, 19.

Bush H.L., Huse J.B., et al. (1981). Prevention of renal insufficiency after abdominal aortic aneurysm resection by optimal volume loading. *Arch. Surg.*, **116**, 1517.

Cascorbi H.F., Singh-Amaranath A.V. (1973). Modification of fluroxene toxicity. *Anesthesiology*, **38**, 454.

Cousins M.J., Greenstein L.R., Hitt B.A., et al. (1976). Metabolism and renal effects of enflurane in man. *Anesthesiology*, **44**, 44.

Cousins M.J., Fulton A., Haynes W.D.G., et al. (1978). Enflurane nephrotoxicity and pre-existing renal dysfunction. *Anaesth. Intens. Care*, **6**, 277.

Cousins M.J., Plummer J., Hall P. de la M. (1982). Volatile anaesthetic metabolism and acute toxicity. In *Reviews on Drug Metabolism and Drug Interactions* (Beckett A.H., Garrod J.W. eds.) London, Freund, **4**: 49.

Cousins M.J., Mazze R.I. (1973a). Methoxyflurane nephrotoxicity. A study of dose response in man. *JAMA*, **225**, 1611.

Cousins M.J., Mazze R.I. (1973b). Anaesthesia, surgery and renal function. Immediate and delayed effects. *Anaesth. Intens. Care*, **1**, 355.

Cousins M.J., Mazze R.I., Barr G.A., et al. (1973c). A comparison of the renal effects of isoflurane and methoxyflurane in Fischer 344 rats. *Anesthesiology*, **38**, 557.

Cousins M.J., Mazze R.I., Kosek J.C., et al. (1974). The etiology of methoxyflurane nephrotoxicity. *J. Pharmacol. Exp. Ther.*, **190**, 530.

Crandell W.B., Pappas S.G., MacDonald A. (1966). Nephrotoxicity associated with methoxyflurane anaesthesia. *Anesthesiology*, **27**, 591.

Cronin R.D., de Torrente A., Miller P.D., et al. (1978). Pathogenic mechanisms of early norepinephrine–induced acute renal failure: Functional and histological correlates of protection. *Kidney Int.*, **14**, 115.

Dawson J.L. (1965). Postoperative renal function in obstructive jaundice: effect of a mannitol diuresis. *Br. Med. J.*, **1**, 82.

de Torrente A., Miller P.D., Cronin R.E., et al. (1978). Effects of furosemide and acetylcholine in norepinephrine–induced acute renal failure. *Am. J. Physiol.*, **235**.

Deutsch S., Goldenberg M., Stephen G.W., et al (1966). Effects of halothane anaesthesia on renal function in normal man. *Anesthesiology*, **27**, 793.

Deutsch S., Hickler R.B., Pierce E.C., et al. (1967). Changes in renin activity of peripheral venous plasma during anaesthesia. *Fed. Proc.*, **26**, 2.

Deutsch S., Pierce E.C., Jr., Vandam L.D. (1967). Cyclopropane effects on renal function in normal man. *Anesthesiology*, **28**, 547.

Deutsch S., Pierce E.C. Jr., Vandam L.D. (1968). Effects of anaesthesia with thiopental, nitrous oxide and neuromuscular blockers on renal function in normal man. *Anesthesiology*, **28**, 184.

Dooley J.R., Mazze R.I., Rice S.A., et al. (1979). Is enflurane defluorination inducible in man? *Anesthesiology*, **50**, 213.

Eger E.I., Calverley R.K., Smith N.T. (1976). Changes in blood chemistries following prolonged enflurane anaesthesia. *Anesth. Analg.*, **55**, 547.

Eichhorn J.H., Hedley–Whyte J., Steinman T.I., et al. (1976). Renal failure following enflurane anesthesia. *Anesthesiology*, **45**, 557.

Eranko O., Karvonen M.J., Laamanen A., et al. (1953). The antidiuretic action of adrenaline and noradrenaline in the water–loaded dog. *Acta Pharmacol. Toxicol.*, **9**, 345.

Fish M.P., Rice S.A. (1979a). Isoniazid metabolites and anesthetic metabolism. *Anesthesiology*, **51**, S256.

Fish K.J., Sievenpiper T.J., Rice S.A., et al. (1979b). Enflurane and gentamicin in chronic renal failure. *Anesthesiology*, **51**, S262.

Fish K.J., Rice S.A., Margary J. (1987). Isoflurane metabolism in obese rats with chronic renal insufficiency. *Anesthesiology*, **67**, A303.

Goldberg L.I., Hsieh Y.Y., Rosnekov L. (1977). Newer catecholamines for treatment of heart failure and shock: an update on dopamine and a first look at dobutamine. *Prog. Cardiovasc. Dis.*, **19**, 327.

Greenstein L.R., Hitt B.A., Mazze R.I. (1975). Metabolism *in vitro* of enflurane, isoflurane and methoxyflurane. *Anesthesiology*, **42**, 420.

Habif D.V., Papper, E.M., Fitzpatrick H.F., et al. (1951). The renal and hepatic blood flow, glomerular rate and urinary output of electrolytes during cyclopropane, ether and thiopental anaesthesia, operation and the immediate postoperative period. *Surgery*, **30**, 241.

Hall S.V., Johnson E.E., Hedley-White J. (1974). Renal hemodynamics and function with continuous positive pressure ventilation in dogs. *Anesthesiology*, **41**, 452.

Hansson R. (1986). Kidney protection by pretreatment with free radical scavengers and allopurinol: renal function at recirculation after warm ischaemia in rabbits. *Clin. Sci.*, **71**, 245.

Hawker R.W. (1982). *Notebook of medical physiology. Renal and body fluids*. Edinburgh: Churchill Livingstone.

Hayes M.A., Byrnes W.P., Goldenberg I.S., et al. (1959). Water and electrolyte exchanges during operation and convalescence. *Surgery*, **46**, 123.

Herbert S.C., Culpepper R.M., Andreoli T.E. (1984). NaCl transport in mouse medullary thick ascending limbs. 1. Functional nephron heterogeneity and ADH–stimulated NaCl co–transport. *Am. J. Physiol.* (Renal Fluid Electrolyte Physiol 10): F412.

Hilbermann M., Maseda J., Stinson E.B., et al. (1984). The diuretic properties of dopamine in patients after open-heart operation. *Anesthesiology*, **61**, 489.

Hitt B.A., Mazze R.I., Beppu W.J., et al. (1977). Enflurane metabolism in rats and man. *J. Pharmacol. Exp. Ther.*, **203**, 193.

Hitt B.A., Mazze R.I., Cousins M.J., et al. (1974). Metabolism of isoflurane in Fischer 344 rats and man. *Anesthesiology*, **40**, 62.

Holaday D.A., Fiserova–Bergerova V., Latto I.P., et al. (1975). Resistance of isoflurane to biotransformation in man. *Anesthesiology*, **43**, 325.

Hollenberg N.K., Epstein M., Rose S.M., et al. (1968). Acute oliguric renal failure in man: evidence for preferential cortical ischemia. *Medicine*, **47**, 455.

Hunter J.M., Jones R.S., Utting J.E. (1980). The effect of anaesthesia with nitrous oxide in oxygen and fentanyl on renal function in the artificially ventilated dog. *Br. J. Anaesth.* **52**, 343.

Idval J., Aronsen F., Stenberg P. (1980). Tissue perfusion and distribution of cardiac output during ketamine anesthesia in normovolemic rats. *Acta Anaesth. Scand.*, **24**, 257.

Ivanetich K.M., Lucas S.A., Marsh J.A. (1979). Enflurane and methoxyflurane. Their interaction with hepatic cytochrome P-450 in vitro. *Biochem. Pharmacol.*, **28**, 785.

Kahl F.R., Flint, J.F., Szidon J.P. (1974). Influence of left atrial distention on renal vasomotor tone. *Am. J. Physiol.*, **226**, 240.

Kennedy W.F. (1969). Effects of spinal and peridural block on renal and hepatic function. In *Regional Anesthesia. Clinical Anesthesia Series*, Vol. 2 (Bonica J.J. (ed.).) Philadelphia: F.A. Davis.

Kennedy W.F., Everett G.D., Cobb L.A., et al. (1970). Simultaneous systemic and hepatic hemodynamic measurements during high spinal anesthesia in normal man. *Anesth. Analg.*, **49**, 1016.

Leier C.V., Heoan P.T., Huss P., et al. (1978). Comparative systemic and regional hemodynamic effects of dopamine and dobutamine in patients with cardiomyopathic heart failure. *Circulation*, **58**, 466.

Loehning R.W., Mazze R.I. (1974). Possible nephrotoxicity from enflurane in a patient with severe renal disease. *Anesthesiology*, **40**, 203.

Mason J.M., Ledsom J.R. (1974). Effects of obstruction of the mitral orifice or distension of the pulmonary vein-atrial junctions on renal and hind-limb vascular resistance in the dog. *Circ. Res.*, **35**, 24.

Mather L.E., Selby D.G., Runciman W. B. (1987). Pharmacology of propofol (Diprivan). *Anaesth. Intens. Care*, **15**, 112.

Mazze R.I. (1977). Critical care of the patient with acute renal failure. *Anesthesiology*, **47**, 138.

Mazze R.I., Barry K.G. (1967). Prevention of functional renal failure during anaesthesia and surgery by sustained hydration and mannitol infusion. *Anesth. Analg.* **46**, 61.

Mazze R.I., Calverley R.K., Smith N.T. (1977). Inorganic fluoride nephrotoxicity: prolonged enflurane and halothane anesthesia in volunteers. *Anesthesiology*, **46**, 265.

Mazze R.I., Cousins M.J. (1973a). Renal toxicity of anaesthetics: With specific reference to nephrotoxicity of methoxyflurane. *Can. Anaesth. Soc. J.*, **20**, 64.

Mazze R.I., Cousins M.J. (1973b). Combined nephrotoxicity of gentamicin and methoxyflurane anaesthesia in man. *Br. J. Anaesth.* **45**, 394.

Mazze R.I., Cousins M.J. (1981). Renal diseases. In *Anesthesiology in Unusual Diseases*. (Katz J., Benumof J., Kadis L.B. (eds).) Philadelphia: W.B. Saunders.

Mazze R.I., Cousins M.J., Barr G.A. (1974a). Renal effects and metabolism of isoflurane in man. *Anesthesiology*, **40**, 536.

Mazze R.I., Cousins M.J., Kosek J.C. (1972). Dose related methoxyflurane nephrotoxicity in rats. A biochemical and pathological correlation. *Anesthesiology*, **36**, 571.

Mazze R.I., Cousins M.J., Kosek J.C. (1973c). Strain differences in metabolism and susceptibility to the nephrotoxic effects of methoxyflurane in rats. *J. Pharmacol. Exp. Ther.*, **184**, 481.

Mazze R.I., Hitt B.A., Cousins M.J. (1974b). Effects of enzyme induction with phenobarbital on the *in vitro* and *in vivo* defluorination of isoflurane and methoxyflurane. *J. Pharmacol. Exp. Ther.*, **190**, 523.

Mazze R.I., Shue G.L., Jackson S.H. (1971). Renal dysfunction associated with methoxyflurane anaesthesia. A randomised prospective clinical evaluation. *JAMA*, **216**, 278.

Mazze R.I., Schwartz F.D., Slocum H.C., et al. (1963). Renal function during anesthesia and surgery. I. The effects of halothane anaesthesia. *Anesthesiology*, **24**, 279.

Mazze R.I., Woodruff R.E., Heerdt M.E. (1982). Isoniazid–

induced enflurane defluorination in humans. *Anesthesiology*, **57**, 5.

Middddleton E.S., Mathews R. Shires T. (1969). Radiosulphate as a measure of the extracellular fluid in acute haemorrhagic shock. *Ann. Surg.*, **170**, 174.

Miller M.S., Gandolfi A.J. (1980a). Enflurane biotransformation in humans. *Life Sci.*, **27**, 1465.

Miller M.S., Gandolfi A.J., Vaughan R.W., et al. (1980b). Disposition of enfluane in obese patients. *J. Pharmacol. Exp. Ther.*, **215**, 292.

Moore F.D., Shires G.T. (1967). Moderation. *Ann. Surg.*, **166**, 300.

Moyer J.H., McConn R. (1956). Renal haemodynamics in hypertensive patients following administration of pendiomide. *Anesthesiology*, **17**, 9.

Needleman P., Greenwald J.E. (1986). Atriopeptin: A cardiac hormone intimately involved in fluid, electrolyte and blood pressure homeostasis. *New Engl. J. Med.*, **314**, 828.

Ochwadt B. (1961). Relation of renal blood supply to diuresis. *Prog. Cardiovasc. Dis.*, **III**, 501.

Oken D.E., Arce M.L., Wilson D.R. (1966). Glycerol–induced haemoglobinuric acute renal failure in the rat. Micropuncture study of the development of oliguria. *J. Clin. Invest.*, **45**, 724.

Pearson J.D., Beckman J.S., Freeman B.A., et al. (1987). Characterization of xanthine dehydrogenase conversion to xanthine oxidase during renal ischemia. *Anesthesiology*, **87**, A305.

Pitts R.F. (1965). *Physiology of the kidney and body fluids.* Chicago: Year Book Medical Publishers.

Plummer J.L., Cousins M.J., Hall P. de la M. (1982). Volatile anaesthetic metabolism and acute toxicity. *Rev. Drug Metab. Drug Interac.*, **12**, 49.

Plummer J.L., Hall P., Jenner M.A., et al. (1985). Hepatic and renal effects of prolonged exposure of rats to 50 ppm methoxyflurane. *Acta Pharmacologica et Toxicologica*, **57**, 176.

Porter G.A., Kloster F.E., Herr R.J., et al. (1969). Renal complications associated with valve replacement surgery. *J. Thorac. Cardiovasc. Surg.*, **53**, 145.

Priano L.L. (1982). Alteration of renal hemodynamics by thiopental, diazepam and ketamine in conscious dogs. *Anesth. Analg.*, **61**, 853.

Priano I.L. (1983). Effect of high dose fentanyl on renal hemodynamics in conscious dogs. *Can. Anaesth. Soc. J.*, **30**, 10.

Priano L.L. (1983). Renal hemodynamic alterations following administration of thiopental, diazepam or ketamine to conscious hypovolemic dogs. *Adv. Shock Res.*, **9**, 173.

Priano L.L., Vatner S.F. (1981a). Morphine effects on cardiac output and regional blood flow distribution in conscious dogs. *Anesthesiology*, **55**, 236.

Priano L.L., Vatner S.F. (1981b). Generalised cardiovascular and regional hemodynamic effects of meperidine in conscious dogs. *Anesth. Analg.* **60**, 649.

Priebe H.J., Hedley-White J. (1984). Respiratory support and renal function. In *The Kidney in Anaesthesia* (Priebe H.J. (ed.)). *Int. Anesth. Clin.*, **22**, 203.

Pringle H., Maunsell R.C.B., Pringle S. (1905). Clinical effects of ether anaesthesia on renal activity. *Br. Med. J.*, **2**, 542.

Proctor E.A., Barton F.L. (1971). Polyuric acute renal failure after methoxyflurane and tetracycline. *Br. Med. J.*, **4**, 661.

Prys–Roberts C. (ed) (1980). *The Circulation in Anaesthesia.* Oxford: Blackwell Scientific Publications.

Rice M.J., Southard J.H., Hjelmhaugh J.A., et al. (1989). The effects of fluoride ion on the ischemic and nonischemic canine kidney. *Anesthesiology*, **67**, A304.

Rice S.A., Mazze R.I. (1980a). Serum and urinary F⁻ levels and renal function following enflurane anesthesia in isoniazid treated rats. *Fed. Proc.*, **39**, 998.

Rice S.A., Sbordone L., Mazze R.I. (1980b). Metabolism by rat hepatic microsomes of fluorinated ether anesthetics following isoniazid administration. *Anesthesiology*, **53**, 489.

Rosen S.E.M., Hollenberg N.K., Dealy J.B., et al. (1968). Measurement of the distribution of blood flow in the human kidney using the intra-arterial injection of ¹³³Xe: relationship to function in the normal and transplant kidney. *Clin. Sci.*, **34**, 287.

Roth E., Lax L., Maloney J.V. Jr. (1969). Ringer's lactate solution and extracellular fluid volume in the surgical patient. A critical analysis. *Ann. Surg.* **169**, 149.

Runciman W.B., Mather L.E., Ilsley A.H., et al. (1984). A sheep preparation for studying interactions between blood flow and drug disposition: III Effects of general and spinal anaesthesia on regional blood flow and oxygen tensions. *Br. J. Anaesth.*, **56**, 1251.

Sakamoto T., Yamada T. (1977). Hemodynamic effects of dobutamine in patients following open heart surgery. *Circulation*, **55**, 525.

Sawyer K.C., Sawyer R.B., Robb W.C. (1963). Postoperative renal failure. *Am. J. Surg.*, **106**, 668.

Schanne F.A.X., Kane A.B., Young E.E., et al. (1979). Calcium dependence of toxic cell death: A final common pathway. *Science*, **206**, 700.

Schreiner G.E. (1972). Toxic nephropathy due to drugs, solvents and metals. In *Drugs Affecting Kidney Function and Metabolism*, pp. 248–280. Sydney: S. Karger.

Seitzman D.M., Mazze R.I., Schwartz F.D., et al. (1963). Mannitol diuresis: A method of renal protection during surgery. *J. Urol.*, **90**, 139.

Shires T. (1964). Shock and metabolism. *Surg. Gynecol. Obstet.*, **124**, 284.

Shires T., Williams J., Brown F. (1961). Acute change in extracellular fluids associated with major surgical procedures. *Ann. Surge.*, **154**, 803.

Siegel N.J., Glazier W., Chaudry I.II., et al. (1980). Enhanced recovery from acute renal failure by the postischemic infusion of adenine nucleotides and magnesium chloride in rats. *Kidney Int.*, **17**, 338.

Sievenpiper T.S., Rice S.A., Mazze R.I. (1979). Renal effects of enflurane anesthesia in Fischer 344 rats with pre-existing renal insufficiency. *J. Pharmacol. Exp. Ther.*, **211**, 36.

Stoelting R.K., Peterson C. (1975). Methoxyflurane anesthesia in pediatric patients: evaluation of anesthetic metabolism and renal function. *Anesthesiology*, **42**, 26.

Stokes G.S. (1983). The renin–angiotensin system—its physiology and role in disease states. *Anaesth. Inten. Care*, **11**, 369.

Stowe N., Emma J., Magnusson M., et al. (1978). Protective effect of propanolol in the treatment of ischemically damaged canine kidneys prior to transplantation. *Surgery*, **84**, 265.

Sullivan L.P., Grantham J.J. (1982). *Physiology of the kidney.* Philadelphia: Lea and Febiger.

Thompson J.E., Vollman R.W., Austin D.J., et al. (1968). Prevention of hypotensive and renal complications of aortic surgery using balanced salt solution—thirteen year experience with 670 cases. *Ann. Surg.*, **167**, 767.

Truniger B., Rosen S.M., Grandchamp A., et al. (1971). Redistribution of renal blood flow in haemorrhagic hypotension: Role of renal nerves and catecholamines. *Europ. J. Clin. Invest.*, **1**, 277.

Vander A.J. (1967). Control of renin release. *Physiol. Rev.* **47**, 359.

Van Dyke R.A. (1983). Enflurane, isoflurane and methoxyflurane metabolism in rat hepatic microsomes from ethanol–treated rats. *Anesthesiology*, **58**, 221.

Van Dyke R.A., Wood C.L. (1973). Metabolism of meth-

oxyflurane: release of inorganic fluoride in human and rat hepatic microsomes. *Anesthesiology*, **39**, 613.

Westermark L. (1969). Haemodynamics during halothane anaesthesia in the cat. *Acta Anaesth. Scand. Suppl.*, **35**.

Yoshimura N., Holaday D.A., Fiserova-Bergerova V. (1976). Metabolism of methoxyflurane in man. *Anesthesiology*, **44**, 372.

Young S.R., Stoelting R.K., Peterson C., et al. (1975). Anesthetic biotransformation and renal function in obese patients during and after methoxyflurane or halothane anesthesia. *Anesthesiology*, **42**, 451.

37. Immunological Aspects of Anaesthetic Practice
B. Walton

Basic immunology
    Non-specific resistance mechanisms
    The complement system
Specific immunity
    Antibody-mediated responses
    Antibodies
    Cell mediated responses
    Theories of specificity
    Co-operation
Transplantation and malignancy
    Autoimmunity
    Hypersensitivity
    In vitro assessment of immune reactions
The effects of anaesthesia and surgery on immune status
    Practical implications of depression of immune status
Adverse reactions to drugs
    Intravenous anaesthetic agents
    Inhalational anaesthetic agents

Anaesthesia and immunology are sciences which overlap in two main areas. Firstly, it is clear that exposure to the 'insult' of anaesthesia and surgery engenders alterations in many facets of immune status—with possible practical implications in relation to the ability to fight infections and malignancy in the postoperative period. Secondly, rare adverse reactions to both intravenous and inhalational anaesthetic agents may sometimes be immunologically mediated.

Discussion of these topics will follow a summary of basic concepts in immunology in health and disease intended for the anaesthetist keen to remind himself of some of the essentials of this complex subject. This brief summary is derived from several excellent stand-

ard texts, and for further reading, Roitt, et al., (1985) for example, is recommended.

BASIC IMMUNOLOGY

The term 'immunity' implies ability to recognize and protect against foreign substances (known as antigens). Molecules capable of eliciting an immune response are usually proteins, although smaller molecules can act as a 'hapten' and achieve antigenic status by combining with a protein. Protection involves a variety of non-specific resistance mechanisms which inter-relate with specific immune responses. Two basic features of immune responses are memory and specificity. Initial exposure to an antigen evokes specific antibody production (primary response), and the antigen is eliminated by contact with these antibodies. The primary response leaves the host prepared for further exposure to the same (or, sometimes, closely related) antigen. Re-exposure results in a more rapid and profound secondary response. Normal immunity also implies an ability to distinguish between endogenous proteins (so-called 'self' and 'non-self'). Failure of this mechanism results in antibodies directed against host tissues—and these auto-antibodies may be responsible for a wide variety of autoimmune diseases. While responses to antigens usually offer protection against the environment, extension of these responses can cause host tissue damage ('allergy' or 'hypersensitivity').

Non-Specific Resistance Mechanisms

The host non-specifically protects against foreign organisms in a variety of ways. For example, the action of ciliated epithelium clears the respiratory tract and many ingested organisms are killed by gastric acid. Acids in sweat and sebaceous secretions are bactericidal, as are lysosymes present both in secretions and in the granules of polymorphonuclear leucocytes and macrophages (phagocytes). Thick mucous secretions on the surface of some cells non-specifically retard the entry of viruses and, once inside cells, viral replication is inhibited by the production of interferon. The efficiency of phagocytes is enhanced by the local inflammatory response to infection or injury. Increased capillary permeability allows phagocytes to congregate and, as a result of the local exudation of properdin and complement, phagocytosis is encouraged.

The Complement System

The complement system consists of at least nine plasma proteins (designated C1–C9). When activated, the system augments and encourages many immune responses. The major biological effects of complement result from the breakdown (or conversion) of component C3, which can be converted (into C3a and C3b) by activation of either of two pathways (Fig. 37.1). The *classical* pathway for complement

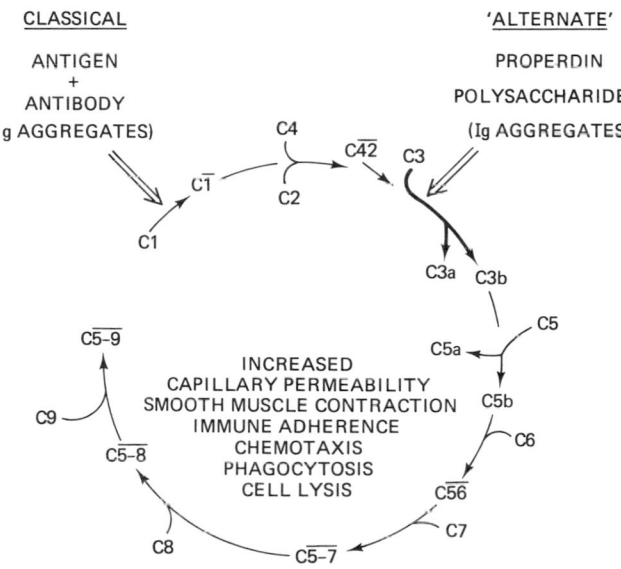

Fig. 37.1 The complement system.

activation usually involves antigen-antibody complexes, although the pathway can be 'triggered' by immunoglobulin aggregates, and components C1, C4 and C2 are involved (and consumed). The conversion of C3 can also be activated via an '*alternate*' or '*properdin*' pathway—independent of components C1, C4 and C2, and *not* requiring antigen-antibody complex formation. Endotoxin, bacterial wall polysaccharides and immunoglobulin aggregates are capable of activating complement via the alternate pathway, as are several drugs. Amplification of C3 conversion via this route results from a positive feedback loop involving the major C3 cleavage product C3b. Following conversion of C3 (by either pathway), an 'attack sequence' results from the sequential involvement of further complement components in an amplifying 'cascade', with the ultimate formation of a complex molecule (C5–9) capable of cell membrane damage.

The rate of complement activation is regulated by several mechanisms. The positive feedback loop already mentioned is balanced by regulation resulting both from the inherent rapid decay of several components and the involvement of inhibitor and inactivator molecules.

The biological results of complement activation include the release of anaphylatoxins (causing vasodilatation and increased capillary permeability), enhancement of immune adherence (important for phagocytosis), the release of histamine and chemotactic factors and cell lysis. Furthermore, the complement system plays a part in the induction of specific immune responses. Although complement augments many host protection mechanisms, activation may result in damage to host tissues. Thus, cell destruction following incompatible blood transfusion, drug induced thrombocytopenia and immune complex diseases all involve complement activation with, in the latter example, the attraction of phagocytes to the site of complex deposition.

Assay of complement component and breakdown product levels in serum has allowed recognition of patterns of pathway activation in various diseases. For example, in systemic lupus erythematosis, classical pathway activation is manifest by low levels of C1, C4 and C2, whereas Gram negative bacteria activate complement via the 'alternate' pathway, leaving classical pathway components intact. Finally, levels of C3 and its products have been monitored in relation to adverse reactions to intravenous agents in an attempt to identify the mechanisms responsible.

SPECIFIC IMMUNITY

The entry of antigen into the body may initiate specific immune responses involving either free (humoral) antibody production or sensitized lymphocytes with antibody-like molecules on their surface. Both these responses relate to populations of small lymphocytes which are necessary for the primary responses to an antigen and carry 'memory'. Small lymphocytes can be separated into two morphologically similar populations, both derived from the same stem cells and designated B and T lymphocytes (Fig. 37.2).

Antibody Mediated Responses

B lymphocytes are so-called because, in the chicken, they are dependent on a rectal lymphoid organ—the Bursa of Fabricius (equivalent to Peyers patches or, possibly, bone marrow in man). They are formed in the haemopoietic organs and, on contact with an antigen, proliferate and become a population of *specific* antibody-secreting plasma cells. Different classes of antibody may be produced, with differing biological activities, all with the same specificity for the antigen concerned.

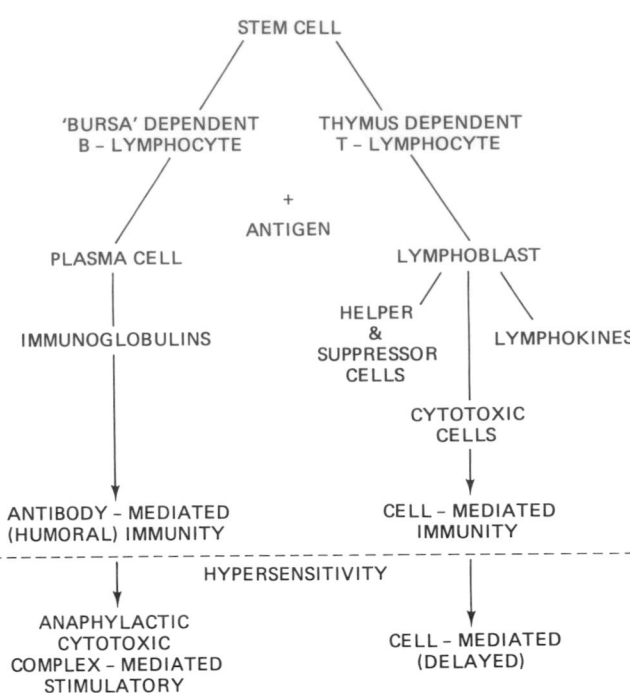

Fig. 37.2 Specific immunity and hypersensitivity.

Antibodies

Antibodies or immunoglobulins are large molecular weight proteins originally defined by electrophoretic mobility as gamma globulins. Each consists of four polypeptide chains, two heavy and two light, held together by disulphide bridges. Each antibody has heavy chains of one to five types—resulting in five different classes of immunoglobulin (IgG, M, A, D and E), and the molecule is shaped somewhat like the letter Y. The 'foot' of the Y is the so-called Fc (fragment crystallizable) portion, which is responsible for various biological activities (such as complement activation). The 'arms' of the Y form the so-called Fab (fragment antigen-binding) portion, and swing apart at their junction (hinge) with the Fc portion to combine with antigen. The classes of immunoglobulin have differing physiological roles. Thus IgG antibodies diffuse into the interstitial fluid, neutralize bacterial toxins and play a major role in humoral defence against invading organisms. They can cross the placenta and offer protection in early life. IgA antibodies are present predominantly in surface secretions and afford initial protection against organisms in the respiratory and gastrointestinal tracts. IgM antibodies are large molecules which remain in the blood. They appear early as part of the primary response to infections, fix complement and are active in agglutination and cytolysis. This class includes anti-A and anti-B, typhoid and WR antibodies. The function of IgD is unclear although they may be lymphocyte receptors. IgE antibodies (homocytotropic or reaginic) are bound to mast cells. On contact with antigen mast cell degranulation occurs, and the resultant release of histamine and other vasoactive amines causes increased capillary permeability and encourages the accumulation of blood-borne defence elements. Their physiological role may involve protection against parasites.

Cell Mediated Responses

Cell mediated immune responses result from activation of T lymphocytes by antigen. T lymphocytes proliferate within and are dependent upon the thymus gland. When activated, these cells do not become antibody secreting plasma cells but transform into active lymphoblasts with several important roles. They may become cytotoxic and attack target cells in, for example, foreign grafts. Groups of activated T lymphocytes (designated 'helper' or 'suppressor' lymphocytes) encourage and regulate B lymphocyte activity, and release a number of active substances (lymphokines) which influence the activity of other cell groups. It is thought that the recognition of an antigen by T lymphocytes is more complex than the mere matching of antigen to portions of antibody molecules on the lymphocyte surface, and may involve appropriate genetic predisposition. Thus, the possession of certain genes of the mixed histocompatibility system may predispose the host to the development of various immunologically mediated diseases.

Theories of Specificity

There have been several theories advanced to explain how lymphocytes can respond appropriately to contact with an enormous variety of antigens. An initial 'instructive' theory suggested that contact with an antigen resulted in the production of antibodies modelled to match the 'template' of the antigen concerned. In other words, antibodies were thought to be produced *non-specifically* but later become specific as a *result* of antigen contact. However, this approach has been discarded in favour of the 'clonal selection' theory. It is now thought that the genetic apparatus carries all information needed to synthesize various antibodies. Lymphocytes are thought able to respond to one particular antigen which matches antibody receptor molecules on the cell surface. Activation of the lymphocyte causes proliferation to form a 'clone' of identical cells, all specifically sensitized to the antigen concerned—with results depending on whether a B or a T lymphocyte was initially involved. It was believed that all necessary information for antibody production was present in the 'germ line' of an animal, and that each lymphocyte merely expressed a tiny part of the information. However, it is now considered more likely that lymphocyte precursors carry a basic immunoglobulin gene which undergoes random mutation during cell differentiation.

Cooperation

Specific immune responses and non-specific resistance

mechanisms are intimately inter-related. Thus the attachment of specific antibody to bacterial cell walls encourages phagocytosis. 'Processing' of antigen by macrophages and subsequent presentation to lymphocytes stimulate more active B and T cell involvement. The activation of complement by antigen-antibody complexes promotes phagocytosis, lysis of bacteria and neutralization of toxins. In addition, phagocytosis of virus particles may be promoted by initial neutralization by serum antibodies. Finally, there is extensive cooperation between the two limbs of specific immunity, particularly in the presence of low antigen concentrations.

TRANSPLANTATION AND MALIGNANCY

Genetically determined foreign substances on the surface of transplanted cells are responsible for immune reactions against them. The most important are antigens of the ABO system and the major histocompatibility (MHS) system. The latter antigens are coded for in the so-called MHS region of the chromosome, with various sub-loci coding for serologically determined (SD, formerly HLA—human leucocyte antigen) and lymphocyte determined (LD, formerly MLC—mixed lymphocyte culture) antigens. It is thought that SD and LD antigens stimulate B and T lymphocytes respectively, with graft rejection involving both humoral and cell mediated reactions.

Tumours also exhibit transplantation antigens, the host responses to which are known as immunosurveillance. It is thought that a cell responsible for a tumour may be a mutant possessing at least one 'foreign' antigen. Recognition of this antigen by a T lymphocyte results in proliferation to form a 'clone' of sensitized lymphocytes which attack the tumour cells. If a tumour develops in man, the implication is that the tumour has, in some way, escaped from immunosurveillance. Some tumours may be more antigenic than others, resistance to host defence mechanisms may result from incomplete eradication of the tumour in the first instance, or the rate of growth of the tumour may be sufficient to overwhelm host defences. In addition, several factors may decrease the ability of the host to mount an adequate defence against tumour antigens. Thus there may be genetic variability in host response, immunosuppressive drugs may have been given (for example, following transplantation) and, in many patients with malignant disease, non-specific depression of both 'limbs' of specific immunity may be seen. Although defence against tumour cells is mainly the prerogative of T lymphocytes, other cells may be 'triggered' by tumour surface antigens (in the presence of antibodies and complement) to become killer cells and take part in cytotoxic attack.

Natural killer (NK) cells are a subpopulation of lymphocytes (distinct from B lymphocytes, T lymphocytes or macrophages) which are capable of attacking tumour cells, virus infected cells, or even some normal target cells. This activity does not require the previous processing of a specific antigen and is controlled by suppressor monocytes and enhanced by interferon. NK cells play an important part in the elimination of blood-borne tumour cells and low NK activity is associated with an increased incidence of metastases.

Autoimmunity

The term autoimmunity implies that immune responses are directed against the host's own tissues as a result of failure to differentiate between 'self' and 'non-self'. It was originally thought that any lymphocytes capable of responding to endogenous antigens were eliminated and that autoimmunity developed only as a result of a 'forbidden clone' of lymphocytes arising by somatic mutation. However, it now seems more likely that such lymphocyte activity against 'self' antigens is suppressed by various control mechanisms (for example, suppressor T lymphocytes) and that autoimmune disease results from failure of these controls. A local inflammatory response, amplified by humoral factors such as complement (activated by antigen-antibody complexes), causes cells to congregate at the site of antibody deposition, and tissue damage results. Phagocytosis proceeds and the release of lysozymes causes tissue digestion. The importance played by inflammation in autoimmune disease is underlined by the efficacy of steroid therapy in many cases.

Autoantibody production is seen most commonly in genetically predisposed individuals; it may be initiated by infection or tissue damage, and a wide spectrum of autoimmune diseases may result. Organ specific diseases may be associated with circulating antibodies directed only against the organ concerned. An example is Hashimoto's thyroiditis, a disease with strong familial links, in which anti-thyroid antibodies are found. Myasthenia gravis is thought to be caused by an antibody directed against acetycholine receptors on the post-synaptic membrane. On the other hand, some organ specific autoimmune diseases are associated with a variety of non-specific autoantibodies as, for example, primary biliary cirrhosis, in which antimitochondrial antibodies are found. Finally, there are the non-organ-specific diseases such as systemic lupus erythematosus, in which a variety of non-specific autoantibodies are seen and tissue damage is widespread.

Hypersensitivity

Hypersensitivity or allergy may be considered extensions of either B or T lymphocyte activity resulting in host tissue damage. Humoral (antibody-mediated) hypersensitivity reactions fall into three main categories: Type I (anaphylaxis), Type II (cytotoxicity), and Type III (complex mediated).

Type I hypersensitivity (anaphylaxis) results from the degranulation of mast cells and the release of mediators including histamine and serotonin. The clinical syndrome reflects widespread smooth muscle contraction and increased capillary permeability. Immunoglobulins, usually of the IgE class (reagins) attach to the surface of mast cells and, on contact with antigen, cause degranulation. The term 'atopy' describes localized Type I reactions to extrinsic antigens (allergens) such as pollen or house dust mite. The syndromes asthma and hay fever result from contact between allergens and IgE bound to cells in the bronchial or nasal muscosae. IgE mediated histamine release does not usually involve complement, although complement may occasionally be involved in histamine release due to reaginic antibodies of the IgG class.

Type II (cytotoxic) reactions occur when circulating antibodies contact cell-surface antigens. Encouraged by complement activation, phagocytosis and cell lysis proceed. Examples include transfusion reactions, in which isohaemagglutinins (usually IgM) are directed against red cell surface antigens, and cytotoxicity against transplants caused by antibodies directed against cell surface antigens.

Type III (complex-mediated) reactions result from the deposition of antigen-antibody complexes, with local inflammation, histamine release, increased capillary permeability and tissue damage. Complement activation causes cell lysis, and platelet aggregation results in vasoactive amine release. Other enzyme systems, including the coagulation and fibrinolytic systems are activated, as are kinins (vasoactive peptides chemotactic for polymorphonuclear leucocytes). The formation of microthrombi leads to local ischaemia. If the antibodies are present in excess, the complexes tend to be confined to the site of antigen entry—for example, actinomycosis. Alternatively, widespread syndromes, such as serum sickness, result from the generalized deposition of complexes seen in cases of antigen excess.

Another minor category of antibody-mediated hypersensitivity is also recognized—Type V (stimulatory) reactions occur when an antibody stimulates a cell rather than destroying it. An example is long acting thyroid stimulator (LATS), an autoantibody which stimulates thyroid cell surface receptors that usually respond to thyroid stimulating hormone (TSH), and produces thyrotoxicosis.

Extension of T lymphocyte responses may result in Type IV (cell mediated) hypersensitivity. Examples include cell mediated reactions to infections (caseation in tuberculosis and granulomatous skin lesions in leprosy) and dermatitis related to chemicals, metals and antibiotic ointments. Activated T lymphocytes release a number of lymphokines, including migration inhibition, monocyte chemotactic and skin reactive factors, which encourage the accumulation of phagocytes, and increase the intensity of local inflammation and tissue damage.

In Vitro Assessment of Immune Reactions

A brief summary of some commonly used *in vitro* methods for assessing immune reactions is included here. For more detail, readers are referred to standard texts on this subject (for example, Gell and Coombes, 1975). Antigen-antibody reactions can be identified by various precipitation techniques in agar gel and by combining antibody with radiolabelled antigen. Both direct and indirect immunoflourescence allows antibodies to be visualized microscopically—techniques commonly used to detect autoantibodies. The complement fixation test detects either antigen or antibody if the other is known. If complement is fixed during an antigen-antibody reaction, none remains to cause lysis of indicator red blood cells by antibody. Two commonly used *in vitro* tests for cell mediated immune reactions are lymphocyte transformation (LTT) and leucocyte (or macrophage) migration inhibition (MIT) tests. Both depend on *in vitro* recognition of antigens by sensitized lymphocytes. In the LTT, the lymphocytes transform into blasts and the transformation is monitored microscopically by the uptake of tritiated thymidine into the transforming cells. In the MIT, the release of lymphokines by the sensitized lymphocytes on contact with antigen inhibits the migration of either normal leucocytes or guinea pig macrophages from the open end of a capillary tube. The areas of migration are mapped by planimetry, and comparisons of migration areas in the presence or absence of putative antigen provides evidence for cell mediated reactions. The LTT can also be performed with the non-specific mitogen phytohaemagglutinin (PHA—a bean extract). Variations of lymphocyte response to standard doses of PHA are used to monitor changes in lymphocyte reactivity in the perioperative period, following drug administration.

THE EFFECTS OF ANAESTHESIA AND SURGERY ON IMMUNE STATUS

Early workers noticed that leucocytosis was commonly seen following exposure to surgery under diethyl ether anaesthesia, and the anaesthetic agent was soon implicated. Much later it was shown that the effects of diethyl ether on leucocytes could be attributed to changes in hormone levels. It appears that anaesthetic agents may have both direct and hormonally mediated effects on immune mechanisms, and that alterations in hormone levels, whether related to anaesthetic agents themselves or to the nonspecific 'stress' response to anaesthesia and surgery, can affect many immune responses and resistance mechanisms.

High levels of circulating catecholamines are associated with increases in the number of neutrophils and lymphocytes, and alterations in their distribution and mobilization. The liberation of ACTH is also associated with neutrophilia, although a reduction in lymphocyte count may reflect toxic effects of steroids on these cells. In animals, steroids adversely affect protein synthesis, mitosis and thymus cell metabolism—although the doses used in such studies bear little relationship to the levels found clinically in the postoperative period. On the other hand, depression of phagocytosis *is* seen in patients on steroid therapy.

There are other minor factors which may affect perioperative immune status, including some antibiotics (for example, chloramphenicol), salicylates, blood transfusion (*see later*), and concurrent viral infections. Perioperative changes may also partly reflect normal cyclical variations in, for example, phagocytosis and lymphocyte reactivity.

Postoperative leucocytosis related to the hormonal effects of anaesthetic agents contrasts with reports that, in some circumstances, exposure may be associated with leucopenia. Transient reductions in leucocyte counts seen in some species following barbiturate, diethyl ether and chloroform anaesthesia may reflect direct toxicity or alterations in distribution. Prolonged exposure to, for example, nitrous oxide and halothane results in leucopenia attributable to adverse effects at several stages of the cell cycle as part of over all depression of cell metabolism.

Non-specific resistance mechanisms are depressed both during and after anaesthesia and surgery. Tracheal mucociliary flow decreases during anaesthesia (Forbes, 1976)—an effect exacerbated by atropine (Annis et al., 1976) and high inspired oxygen concentrations (Sachner et al., 1975). Pulmonary bactericidal activity is also depressed. The degree of depression of phagocytosis seems proportional to the degree of surgical stress—underlining the importance of the 'stress' component of anaesthesia and surgery. This presumably reflects adverse effects of steroids on phagocytic activity. The effects of anaesthesia on phagocytosis are both cellular (depression of mobilization, margination, chemotactic attraction etc.), and humoral (mediated by reductions in serum factors such as properdin seen following surgery). Volatile agents inhibit neutrophil function by decreasing calcium flux and superoxide production—both necessary for bactericidal activity. Calcium channel blockers such as verapamil and nifedipine have similar effects impairing the ability of neutrophils to kill common pathogens (Welch, 1986).

Both limbs of specific immunity are depressed postoperatively. The population of B lymphocytes is reduced, as is antibody production. Preformed antibodies are unaffected, and minor alterations in immunoglobulin levels are very variable. Reductions in antibody-producing cells following injury and burns supports the suggestion that the hormonal aspects of the stress response are very relevant. In support of the relatively minor role of anaesthesia in this respect is a study showing that halothane has no effect on the antibody response to immunization performed during anaesthesia (Salo et al., 1979).

The lymphocyte transformation and leucocyte migration inhibition tests have been used to demonstrate postoperative depression of T lymphocyte reactivity. The number of T lymphocytes falls and T lymphocyte responses in mixed lymphocyte culture and to tumour-derived antigens are diminished. Depression of T lymphocyte responsiveness has been seen following induction of anaesthesia but *before* the start of surgery (Espanol et al., 1974), but the degree and duration of postoperative depression seems, once again, to be related to the degree of surgical stress (Cullen and Van Belle, 1975). Hormone levels certainly affect T lymphocyte activity, as responsiveness is depressed by steroids, and, following various types of 'stress', prolonged skin graft survival and decreased skin reactivity clearly suggest impaired T lymphocyte function.

A recent study of postoperative immunocompetence in various age-groups (Linn and Jensen, 1983) suggests that although healthy young and old patients do not differ immunologically *before* surgery, following herniorrhaphy, depression of lymphocyte reactivity is more profound and prolonged in the latter group. It may be that the apparent increase in postoperative morbidity in the elderly may, in part, be due to decreased immunological resilience.

NK cell activity alters biphasically in the perioperative period. An increase is seen following premedication and there is *further* enhancement during anaesthesia and surgery (Tonnesen et al., 1983; Griffith et al., 1984). This apparent rapid, transient increase may be due to recruitment into the peripheral blood from the extravascular space, spleen or lymph nodes—possibly in response to the administration of premedicant and anaesthetic drugs. It is of interest that this enhancement is seen in patients with benign or *localized* malignancy, but not in those with disseminated disease—suggesting that, in the latter group, the vast majority of NK cells have *previously* been activated. Recent *in vitro* studies suggest that, at least at high concentrations, inhalational agents depress NK activity against tumour cells (Woods and Griffiths, 1986; Griffith and Kamath, 1986). However, the relevance of such a transient decrease in NK efficacy *clinically* is doubtful. On the other hand, NK activity *is* depressed postoperatively—possible due to release of suppressor monocytes (Uchida et al., 1982). As this is seen in patients operated on for malignancy but not in those with benign disease or in whom the tumour is not handled, it may be that the suppressor cells are released from the tumour itself during surgical manipulation. In addition, NK cell activity may be depressed by suppressor substances such as prostaglandins.

Practical Implications of Depression of Immune Status

Much postoperative morbidity relates to infections, and an increasing incidence of postoperative infections has been correlated with advancing age, poor nutritional status and, perhaps most significantly in this context, prolonged surgery and steroid therapy. No particular anaesthetic agent or technique has been associated with increased infection rates and, as susceptibility to infection in several species is increased following various types of trauma, it seems likely that the stress component of anaesthesia and surgery is yet again the most important factor. However, the effects of exposure to anaesthetic agents alone have been studied in this respect—with contradictory results. In some early studies, susceptibility to infections was increased, while in others, anaesthesia seemed to offer protection—with results varying with different species and infecting organisms. The beneficial effects of diethyl ether in some viral infections may reflect the *in vitro* ether sensitivity of some groups of viruses, and the drug has even been advocated for the treatment of canine distemper! More recently, it has been shown that exposure to halothane increases the morbidity and mortality among mice with various bacterial and viral infections. This is possibly of relevance to the poor prognosis among patients exposed to anaesthesia and surgery while developing coincidental acute viral hepatitis. Although potentially beneficial short-term inhibitory effects of anaesthetic agents on bacterial division rates have been reported, it seems that the overall depressant effects of anaesthesia and surgery on immune status may increase the likelihood of infections progressing in the postoperative period.

As discussed earlier, resistance to malignancy requires immunocompetence, and an increased incidence of malignant disease has been reported in immune deficiency states and in patients on immunosuppressant therapy. In animals, immunosuppression increases the oncogenic response to chemical agents and decreases tumour-directed cell mediated reactions. In seems possible, therefore, that depression of immune status in the perioperative period may favour the spread of malignant disease. Patients who have survived for years following removal of a primary tumour—without evidence of metastases, may succumb rapidly from metastatic spread following anaesthesia and minor unrelated surgery. This suggests that the balance between the malignant process and host immunosurveillance has been disturbed by exposure to the 'stress' of anaesthesia and even minor surgery—in favour of the malignancy. Postoperative *in vitro* lymphocyte responses to mitogens and antigens are reduced in patients with malignant disease, and it has been suggested that the degree and duration of postoperative lymphocyte depression may be even greater in such patients (Park et al., 1971). Some animal studies have shown that exposure to anaesthetic agents promotes the development of metastases and increases the 'success' rate of transplanted tumours, although other workers have reported unconvincing results. Cell mediated cytotoxic reactions are inhibited by halothane and nitrous oxide but short-lived effects of this nature are, once again, probably far less significant than the effects of surgical 'stress' in as much as the development of malignancy in animals is encouraged by surgery (without anaesthesia!) and the administration of steroids.

As patients with malignant disease are ill served by any therapy which unnecessarily depresses their immune responses, comparative studies of the depressant effects of various anaesthetic agents and techniques are of some interest. In general, it appears that a similar degree of postoperative depression is seen following comparable surgery under a wide variety of anaesthetic regimens. While, in some studies (Bruce et al., 1976; Ryhanen, 1977), no obvious differences emerged in this respect between various inhalational, intravenous and regional techniques, more recent reports have suggested that regional anaesthesia may offer some immunological advantages. Thus, following major orthopaedic procedures, postoperative monocyte and lymphocyte depression is far less in patients receiving epidural anaesthesia (Hole, 1984) and, following herniorraphy, leucocyte motility is relatively well preserved (Edwards et al., 1984). Further, it appears that postoperative depression of NK cell activity can be minimized by epidural anaesthesia—an effect once again related to diminution of the hormonal 'stress' response (Tonnesen and Wahlgreen, 1988). In general, the significance of apparent differences between agents or techniques immunologically speaking may be less than convincing in view of the normal diurnal variability in, for example, lymphocyte responsiveness. In other words, the 'signal to noise ratio' may be very poor! As has been repeatedly stated, the most important factors influencing the degree and duration of postoperative immunosuppression are the hormonal changes which form part of the stress response to anaesthesia and surgery. If epidural techniques, by reducing afferent stimuli, diminish this response, immunological benefits may accrue. Furthermore, it appears that psychological trauma may adversely affect several facets of the immune response (Editorial, 1987). It may be inferred, therefore, that a more aggressive approach to the perioperative relief of both physical *and psychological* 'stress' may have beneficial consequences—particularly for patients with malignancy. The author has seen apparent augmentation of lymphocyte responsiveness in some patients following premedication—suggesting that relief of pain and/or anxiety may, by reducing hormone levels, allow lymphocytes to react more effectively.

Evidence is accumulating that, following surgical removal of a primary tumour, recurrence rates are increased among patients who receive perioperative blood transfusions (Blumberg et al., 1986). As it appears that whole blood may be more harmful than red cells in this respect, it seems possible that homologous *plasma* contains factors that depress immune function in the recipient. Among patients receiving 'red cells', recurrence rates may be higher in those receiving four or more units. This suggests that 'plasma-reduced' blood contains enough plasma to produce the effect if sufficient units are administered. Thus, immunological considerations as well as the risk of infection and paucity of supply, should modify the attitudes of surgeons and anaesthetists to perioperative blood transfusion. At least in patients with malignancy, blood administration should be avoided unless really necessary and confined to 'red cells' whenever possible.

ADVERSE REACTIONS TO DRUGS

The terms 'allergy' and 'hypersensitivity' are very often loosely and erroneously applied to widely diverse, adverse reactions to drugs. In fact, these terms should only be used in patients in whom specific antibodies and/or sensitized lymphocytes can be demonstrated. In the absence of such evidence of either B or T lymphocyte involvement, reactions should more appropriately be described as 'intolerance' or 'idiosyncrasy', depending on whether the response is qualitatively normal or abnormal (Fig. 37.3). The term 'anaphylactoid' has been coined to describe adverse reactions which mimic true anaphylaxis in their clinical presentation but in which no evidence of immunological involvement can be found. Thus, if a drug releases histamine as part of its normal pharmacological activity, an adverse response in any patient related merely to excessive pharmacological histamine release would be labelled 'anaphylactoid'.

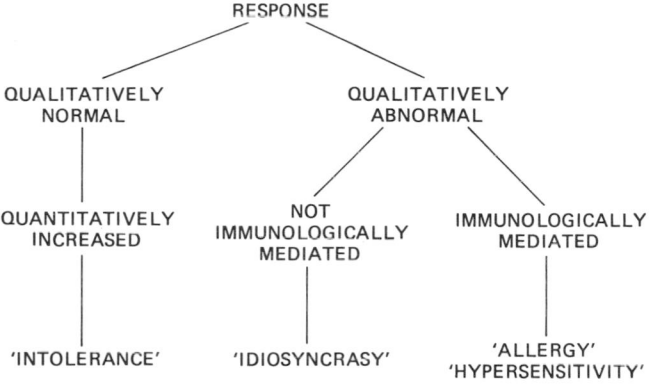

Fig. 37.3 Adverse drug reactions.

True allergic drug reactions include examples of all four main types of hypersensitivity reaction described earlier. Type I reactions (true anaphylaxis) include those to penicillin, procaine and iodine. Type II (cytotoxic) reactions, in which the drug (an antigen) binds to the surface of blood cells, include thrombocytopenia (sulphonamides), agranulocytosis (chloramphenicol) and haemolytic anaemia (para-amino salicylic acid). Penicillin and sulphonamides may be responsible for Type III (complex mediated) syndromes such as serum sickness, polyarthritis and glomerulonephritis. Finally, sulphonamides and local anaesthetics may evoke Type IV (cell mediated) reactions which present as contact dermatitis.

Intravenous Anaesthetic Agents

The reported incidences of adverse reactions to induction agents, muscle relaxants and plasma substitutes vary widely. Such reactions to propanidid (1 in 540 [Doenicke, 1974] to 1 in 1700 [Danneman and Lubke, 1970]) and althesin (1 in 900 [Fisher, 1975] to 1 in 11 000 [Clarke et al., 1975]) were considered by most authors to be more common than reactions to methohexitone (1 in 7000 [Driggs and O'Day, 1972]) and thiopentone (1 in 14 000 [Evans and Keogh, 1977]). On the other hand, reactions to barbiturates tend to be more severe. An overall incidence of 1 in 5000 for all induction agents and muscle relaxants has been suggested (Fisher, 1975), and it is at present thought that any of four mechanisms may be responsible (Watkins and Levy, 1988):

1. Type I hypersensitivity or true anaphylaxis, with IgE involvement, previous exposure necessary, and complement not usually activated until late.
2. Immune reactions involving other classes of immunoglobulins, with early complement involvement in histamine release.
3. Direct 'alternate' pathway activation of complement, with reactions possible on first exposure.
4. Pharmacological histamine release.

Although in all cases the cause of the clinical syndrome is histamine release, only (1.) and possibly (2.) can be called anaphylaxis, with the remainder being more accurately described as 'anaphylactoid'.

In contrast with barbiturate reactions, of which some 20% are thought to be true anaphylaxis and 65% pharmacological histamine release, althesin was thought to be responsible for true anaphylaxis only very rarely, with most cases falling into groups (3.) and (4.) above (Watkins et al., 1988). Concern that Althesin may have been responsible for adverse reactions more commonly than other induction agents lead to the suggestion that routine intradermal testing should be performed before exposing patients repeatedly to the drug (Jago and Restall, 1978). The impracticality of such advice and continuing concern about safety contributed to the withdrawal of both althesin and propanidid. Etomidate seems unique among induction agents in as much as it does not appear to cause histamine release. This correlates well with the extreme rarity of reports of adverse reactions (Watkins, 1983). Similarly, from the immunological point of view, ketamine seems very safe. Propofol, a new induction agent gaining popularity (particularly for out-patient procedures) has been implicated in several adverse reactions. Initially many of these were probably related to the vehicle, cremophor EL, but reformulation in fat emulsion has not eliminated completely such reports. Clinically severe anaphylactoid responses are being reported with increasing frequency as usage increases, although, in most cases, a concurrently administered neuromuscular blocker is thought to have been the culprit (Watkins, personal communication).

Identification of which of a number of injected drugs may be responsible for an 'anaphylactoid' reaction can be difficult. Clearly, intravenous challenge tests could have fatal consequences. *In vitro* methods, including leucocyte challenge and basophil degranulation tests, have been tried, although such tests are far from simple and are probably inappropriate for histamine releasing drugs. Successful results of intradermal tests have been reported and they appear relatively safe and easy to perform. Intradermal injections of 0.1 ml of suspected drugs in dilutions ranging from 1 in 100 (induction agents) to 1 in 100 000 (narcotics) were given, with a weal of 1 cm diameter lasting for 30 minutes being considered positive. Positive results were reported in 64% of patients studied (Fisher, 1979). However, concern about reliability of such tests remains and *in vitro* radio-labelled antibody sets are being developed. Such an approach may provide unequivocal specific evidence for sensitivity in patients exposed to polypharmacy as part of normal anaesthetic practice.

The reported incidences of reactions to plasma expanders also vary widely, between 1 in 1000 for gelatin derivatives and 1 in 10 000 for plasma protein preparations (Ring and Messmer, 1977). These reactions differ in some respects from those due to induction agents and muscle relaxants—possibly reflecting the ability of large molecules to be antigenic in their own right. Soluble immune complex aggregates have been reported (Richter et al., 1978) and dextrans may react specifically with antibodies [possibly produced previously in response to bacterial polysaccharides (Hedin et al., 1976)]. In severe reactions, complement activation has been noted, although such involvement may not be an important factor in the more common minor reactions. A recent study suggests that reactions to the polygelatin Haemaccel result from direct histamine release from mast cells, without complement activation (Lund, 1980).

There are several factors which apparently predispose some patients to adverse reactions to intravenous agents. These include a history of atopy or allergy to other drugs and underlying autoimmune disease associated with complement system instability. It may also be possible that the diverse alterations in immune status resulting from the hormonal aspects of the 'stress' response include an increased tendency to such reactions.

In patients thought to be 'at risk', a regimen involving etomidate, fentanyl and pancuronium has been recommended as being relatively 'safe', although regional and inhalational techniques may be more appropriate in such cases. For an up-to-date detailed analysis of adverse reactions to intravenous agents, readers are referred to Watkins and Levy, 1988.

Inhalational Anaesthetic Agents

In contrast with generalised adverse reactions to intravenous agents, some of which are clearly immunologically mediated, there is considerable doubt as to whether or not immunological mechanisms are responsible for the ostensibly rare organ specific adverse reactions reported in association with inhalational agents. Hepatic damage following exposure to chloroform and fluroxene and renal damage associated with methoxyflurane exposure are dose related phenomena attributable directly to toxicity of metabolic products. However, the feature of halothane-, enflurane-, and methoxyflurane- associated hepatitis, including apparent rarity, lack of dose-dependence, variable histology and latent period, suggest that, at least in some patients, an immunological mechanism may be more likely than direct hepatotoxicity.

The evidence advanced in favour of the hypersensitivity theory falls into three main categories:

1. Clinical Stigmata of Hypersensitivity. Many of the clinical features of hypersensitivity reactions reported in some patients with inhalational agent associated hepatitis are unconvincing. Reports of skin rash, arthralgia, bronchospasm, unexplained fever and leucocytosis have been considered useful 'evidence' for hypersensitivity (Doniach, 1970), although other authors have argued that such findings are more likely to be either uncommon chance associations or attributable to other non-anaesthetic causes (Dykes et al., 1972; Simpson et al., 1974). Much has been made of the significance of unexplained pyrexia following *previous* exposure to halothane, with the suggestion that such a history should preclude further exposure to the agent (Sharpstone et al., 1971; Moult and Sherlock, 1975).

Despite the fact that the value of such a common non-specific postoperative finding has been and *continues to be* questioned by several authors (Dykes, 1971; Walton et al., 1976; Spence, 1987), recent advice regarding halothane usage has, once again, stressed the importance of such a history (Editorial *Lancet*, 1986; Committee on Safety of Medicines, 1986).

On the other hand, some other clinical features *do* support the hypersensitivity theory more convincingly. These include multiple exposures (often rapidly repeated) to halothane (Inman and Mushin, 1978), methoxyflurane (Joshi and Conn, 1974), and enflurane (Lewis et al., 1983), eosinophilia, reduced latent period between exposure and onset of jaundice in patients with the 'syndrome' following multiple exposures, and ostensibly positive 'challenge' tests reported in the literature. However, several apparent clinical anomalies detract from the view that hypersensitivity is invariably involved—in as much as they are difficult to reconcile with accepted concepts of drug allergy. For example, it is difficult to explain why so many cases of alleged hypersensitivity occur after a single exposure. More than one third of patients with alleged halothane hepatitis recently reported to the Committee on Safety of Medicines had received halothane only once (C.S.M. Update, 1986). It is also odd that some patients with apparent halothane hepatitis have been subsequently re-exposed to halothane without problems and, even more peculiar, there are reports of patients receiving rapidly repeated exposures to halothane uneventfully and then, some years later, developing hepatitis following a further single exposure (Walton et al., 1976). Clearly, such anomalies lend weight to the generally held view that hypersensitivity may be a causative factor in some patients whereas, in others toxic reductive metabolites (formed particularly during periods of hepatic hypoxia) may *directly* damage the liver. Of course, such anomalies may merely illustrate the point that many patients labelled as anaesthetic agent associated hepatitis may actually be suffering from entirely unrelated syndromes—possibly co-incident viral hepatitis which, even now, cannot be excluded with *absolute* confidence.

2. Autoantibodies and Possible Predisposition. An early report of antimitochondrial antibodies (AMA) in some patients with halothane hepatitis was not confirmed by subsequent workers. However, the similar though distinct liver, kidney microsomal autoantibody (LKM) has been found in some patients—associated with persistent evidence for thyroid autoimmunity in the absence of overt thyroid disease (Walton et al., 1976). This latter finding suggested the possibility that patients with a predisposition to autoimmune disease may be more at risk although such an hypothesis has not been confirmed. It has been suggested that non-organ specific antibodies such as LKM may not be responsible for liver damage but may appear as a consequence. However, the concept that predisposition may be relevant in some cases is supported by the clear history in at least 20% of patients with halothane, methoxyflurane and enflurane associated hepatitis, and, in 15% of patients in the halothane group, a history of *drug* allergy can be elicited. Studies of halothane hepatitis susceptibility in guinea pigs (now thought by some to be a more relevant animal model than the arcane rat preparations popularized for years) suggest a genetic element (Lunan et al., 1986) and a recent study of the relatives of patients with halothane hepatitis has suggested a genetic predisposition to susceptibility to nucleophilic attack by drug metabolites. (Farrell et al., 1985). Of course, this latter report tends to support the direct hepatotoxicity theory rather than the hypersensitivity one but, in any event, the relevance of such familial studies to human halothane hepatitis seems in great doubt in view of the fact that throughout the world literature on this subject, only one single report has appeared of patients in the same family with the syndrome (Hoft et al., 1981).

3. Cell Mediated Immunity and Circulating Antibodies. Both the lymphocyte transformation and leucocyte migration inhibition tests have been used in attempts to demonstrate evidence for cell mediated immunity. Early studies, using halothane itself as the potential antigen, produced conflicting results and, in some respects, it would be surprising if halothane itself (a relatively small unreactive molecule) were capable of antigenicity in its own right. Much more likely is the concept that a metabolite of halothane might achieve antigenic status by combining with a protein. In animals, specific antibody responses and cellular hypersensitivity to metabolite-protein complexes have been produced, although they could not be correlated with hepatic lesions. However, positive migration inhibition (using halothane treated rabbit liver) and lymphocyte transformation (using halothane treated human plasma) results support the concept that metabolite-protein complexes may elicit cell mediated responses (Vergani et al., 1978; Saito and Kumagai, 1980). In addition, positive lymphocyte transformation results have been reported in one patient, using an unidentified metabolite of halothane as antigen, and this metabolite was shown to be bound to circulating antigen-antibody complexes (Williams et al., 1977).

In vitro cytotoxicity studies have demonstrated sensitization of leucocytes from patients with halothane hepatitis to human hepatocyte membrane lipoprotein coated target cells (Vogten et al., 1976), and halothane altered rabbit hepatocytes (Vergani et al., 1978). Subsequently, it has been shown that normal leucocytes can be induced to attack halothane altered rabbit hepatocytes (Vergani et al., 1980). As, in these studies, serum from a patient with halothane hepatitis was a prerequisite, it was postulated that such a patient has specific circulating antibodies which might prove of diagnostic value. More recently, these elegant tests have been developed further and specific antibodies to halothane altered rabbit liver microsomal fractions have been detected, using an enzyme-linked immunoabsorption assay, in about 70% of patients with relatively severe halothane hepatitis (Kenna et al., 1987).

In summary, in spite of the clear evidence that, in several animal species, the metabolism of halothane and other inhalational agents may, in some circumstances, produce highly reactive intermediate compounds and/or toxic metabolites, the relevance of animal models remains in some doubt. Many features of the syndrome in man suggest that, at least in some patients, direct hepatotoxicity is not the predominant mechanism involved. It seems likely that there are at least two distinct groups of patients presenting with postoperative hepatic dysfunction directly related to exposure to halothane or, indeed, methoxyflurane or enflurane. It is widely accepted that, in many patients, halothane and possibly enflurane may produce, by direct metabolite toxicity, variable degrees of hepatic damage. Several studies have compared the 'hepatotoxic' potential of repeated halothane and non-halothane anaesthetics, with conclusions based, in the main, on minor postoperative alterations in liver function test results. Two groups of workers (Trowell et al., 1975; Wright et al., 1975) reported that repeated halothane exposures were more likely to produce hepatic problems, although the results of other studies have not confirmed this (McEwan, 1976; Allen and Downing, 1977). As minor postoperative alterations in liver function test results may well reflect perioperative changes in hepatic blood flow and an element of hepatic hypoxia—unavoidable irrespective of the anaesthetic agents or technique used—the present author remains unconvinced that such minor alterations can necessarily be considered sinister evidence of low-grade hepatotoxicity. However, it is clear that, on rare occasions, severe hepatic damage may follow exposure to halothane or enflurane, and it is in these patients that immunological mechanisms may be involved. It seems likely that, in such cases, although the generation of toxic metabolites is not the main mechanism, metabolism remains a prerequisite. A reactive intermediate metabolite may combine with an intrahepatic protein to achieve antigenic status. Resultant antibody production may then trigger a toxic cellular response with ensuing liver damage. Whereas some 20% of halothane is metabolized in the liver, the figures for enflurane (2%) and isoflurane (0.2%) suggest that, whatever mechanism is involved, these 'replacement' agents may have less hepatotoxic potential. It remains to be seen whether, as halothane usage diminishes (for medicolegal, if not necessarily for scientifically satisfying reasons) in favour of the newer substitutes, the incidence of severe postoperative hepatitis diminishes also. It further remains to be seen, of course, whether such a trend is of benefit to *overall* patient safety.

REFERENCES

Allen P.J., Downing J.W. (1977). A prospective study of hepatocellular function after repeated exposure to halothane or enflurane in women undergoing radium therapy for cervical cancer. *Br. J. Anaesth.*, **49**, 1035.

Annis P., Landa J.F., Lichtiger M. (1976). Effects of atropine on velocity of tracheal mucus in anesthetised patients. *Anesthesiology*, **44**, 74.

Blumberg N., Heal J.M., Murphy P., et al. (1986). Association between transfusion of whole blood and recurrence of cancer. *Br. Med. J.*, **293**, 530.

Bruce D.L., Behbehani P., Land P.C. (1976). Lymphocyte reactivity of surgical patients. Paper read at International Anaesthetics Research Society (March).

Clarke R.S.J., Dundee J.W., Garrett R.T., et al. (1975). Adverse reactions to intravenous anaesthetics. *Br. J. Anaesth.*, **47**, 575.

Committee on Safety of Medicines, (1986). Halothane hepatotoxicity Current Problems, **18**, 1.

C.S.M. Update. (1986). *Br. Med. J.*, **29**, 949.

Cullen B.F., Duncan P.G., Ray-Keil L. (1976). Inhibition of cell mediated cytotoxicity by halothane and nitrous oxide. *Anesthesiology*, **44**, 386.

Cullen B.F., Van Belle G. (1975). Lymphocyte transformation and changes in leucocyte count: effects of anesthesia and operation. *Anesthesiology*, **43**, 563.

Danneman H., Lubke P. (1970). Complications during anaesthesia with epontol. *Prakt. Anaesth. Wiederbeleb.*, **5**, 237.

Doenicke A. (1974). Propanidid. In *Proc. IV Europ. Congr. Anesthesiology*, Madrid. p. 107. Amsterdam, Excerpta Medica.

Doniach D. (1970). Cell mediated immunity in halothane hypersensitivity. *New Engl. J. Med.*, **283**, 315.

Driggs R.L., O'Day R.A. (1972). Acute allergic reaction associated with methohexital anaesthesia: report of six cases. *J. Oral Surg.*, **30**, 906.

Dykes M.H.M. (1971). Unexplained postoperative fever. Its value as a sign of sensitisation. *JAMA*, **216**, 641.

Dykes M.H.M., Gilbert J.P., Schur P.H., et al. (1972). Halothane and the liver. *Canad. J. Surg.*, **15**, 217.

Editorial. (1986). Halothane-associated liver damage. *Lancet*, **1251**.

Editorial. (1987). Depression, stress and immunity. *Lancet*, **1467**.

Edwards A.E., Gemmell L.W., Mankin P.P., et al. (1984). The effects of three differing anaesthetics on the immune response. *Anaesthesia*, **39**, 1071.

Espanol T., Todd G.B., Soothill J.F. (1974). The effect of anaesthesia on the lymphocyte response to phytohaemagglutinism. *Clin. Exp. Immunol.*, **18**, 73.

Evans J.M., Keogh J.A.M. (1977). Adverse reactions to intravenous anaesthetic agents. *Br. Med. J.*, **2**, 735.

Farrell G., Prendergast D., Murray M. (1985). Halothane hepatitis. Detection of a constitutional susceptibility factor. *N. Engl. J. Med.*, **313**, 1310.

Fisher M. McD. (1975). Severe histamine-mediated reactions to intravenous drugs used in anaesthesia. *Anaesth. Intens. Care*, **3**, 180.

Fisher M. McD. (1979). Intradermal testing in the diagnosis of acute anaphylaxis during anaesthesia—results of five years' experience. *Anaesth. Intens. Care*, **7**, 58.

Forbes A.R. (1976). Halothane depresses mucociliary flow in the trachea. *Anesthesiology*, **45**, 59.

Gell P.G.H., Coombes R.R.A. (1975). In *Clinical Aspects of Immunology*, 3rd ed. (Gell P.G.H., Coombs R.R.A., Lachmann P.J. eds.). Oxford: Blackwell.

Griffith C.D., Rees R.C., Platts A., et al. (1984). The nature of enhanced natural killer lymphocyte cytotoxicity during anesthesia and surgery in patients with benign disease and cancer. *Ann. Surg.*, **200**, 753.

Griffith C.D.M., Kamath M.B. (1986). Effect of halothane and nitrous oxide anaesthesia on natural killer lymphocytes from patients with benign and malignant breast disease. *Br. J. Anaesth.*, **58**, 540.

Hedin H., Richter W., Ring J. (1976). Dextran-induced anaphylactoid reactions in man. Role of dextran reactive antibodies. *Int. Arch. Allerg. Immunol.*, **52**, 145.

Hoft R.H., Bunker J.P., Goodman H.I., et al. (1981). Halothane hepatitis in three pairs of closely related women. *N. Engl. J. Med.*, **304**, 1023.

Hole A. (1984). Pre and postoperative monocyte and lymphocyte functions: effects of—from patients operated under general or epidural anesthesia. *Acta Anaesth. Scand.*, **28**, 287.

Inman W.H.N., Mushin W.W. (1978). Jaundice after repeated exposure to halothane. A further analysis of reports to the committee on safety of medicines. *Br. Med. J.*, **2**, 1455.

Jago R.H., Restall J. (1978). Sensitivity testing for althesin. *Anaesthesia*, **33**, 644.

Joshi P.H., Conn H.O. (1974). The syndrome of methoxyflurane-associated hepatitis. *Ann. Int. Med.*, **80**, 395.

Kenna J.G., Neuberger J., Williams R. (1987). Specific antibodies to halothane induced liver antigens in halothane-associated hepatitis. *Br. J. Anaesth.*, **59**, 1286.

Lewis J.H., Zimmerman H.J., Ishak K.G., et al. (1983). Enflurane hepatotoxicity. A clinicopathological study of 24 cases. *Ann. Int. Med.*, **98**, 984.

Linn B.S., Jensen J. (1983). Age and immune response to a surgical distress. *Arch. Surg.*, **118**, 405.

Lunan C.A., Cousins M.J., Hall P. (1986). Genetic predisposition to liver damage in a guinea pig model of halothane hepatotoxicity. *Anesth. Analg.*, **65**, 1143.

Lund N. (1980). Anaphylactoid reaction to infusion of polygelatin (Haemaccel). A study in pregnant women. *Anaesthesia*, **35**, 655.

McEwen J. (1976). Liver function tests following anaesthesia. *Br. J. Anaesth.*, **48**, 1065.

Moult P.J.A., Sherlock S. (1975). Halothane-related hepatitis. *Quart. J. Med.*, **XLIV**, 99.

Park S.K., Brody J.C., Wallace H.A., et al. (1971). Immuno-suppressive effect of surgery. *Lancet*, **1**, 53.

Richter W., Messmer K., Hedin H., et al. (1978). Adverse reactions to plasma substitute: incidence and pathomechanisms. In *Adverse Responses to Intravenous Drugs*, p. 49 (Watkins J., Ward A.M. eds). London: Academic Press.

Ring J., Messmer K. (1977). Incidence and severity of anaphylactoid reactions to colloid volume substitutes. *Lancet*, **1**, 466.

Roitt I., Brostoff J., Male D. (1985). *Immunology*. London: Gower Medical Publishing.

Ryhanen P. (1977). Effects of anesthesia and operative surgery on the immune response of patients of different ages. *Ann. Clin. Res.*, **9**, (Suppl. 10).

Sachner M.A., Landa J.F., Hirsch J., et al. (1975). Pulmonary effects of oxygen breathing. A 6-hour study in normal men. *Ann. Int. Med.*, **82**, 40.

Saito K., Kumagai K. (1980). Postoperative hepatitis induced by halothane exposure and the lymphocyte transformation test. *Tohoku J. Exp. Med.*, **130**, 291.

Sulo M., Viljanen M., Kangas L. (1979). Effect of halothane anaesthesia on primary antibody response in the chicken. *Acta Anaesth. Scand.*, **23**, 344.

Sharpstone P., Medley D.R.K., Williams R. (1971). Halothane hepatitis— a preventable disease? *Br. Med. J.*, **1**, 448.

Simpson B.R., Strunin L., Walton B. (1974). Evidence for halothane hepatotoxicity is equivocal. In *Controversy in Internal Medicine II*, p. 580. (Ingelfinger J., Ebert R.V., Finland M. et al., eds.). Philadelphia: Saunders Co.

Spence A.A. (1987). Editorial: Halothane in the doldrums. *Br. J. Anaesth.*, **59**, 529.

Tonnesen E., Mickley H., Grunnet N. (1983). Natural killer cell activity during premedication, anaesthesia and surgery. *Acta. Anaesth. Scand.*, **27**, 238.

Tonnesen E., Wahlgreen C. (1988). Influence of extradural and general anaesthesia on natural killer cell activity and lymphocyte sub-populations in patients undergoing hysterectomy. *Br. J. Anaesth.*, **60**, 500.

Trowell J., Peto R., Crampton Smith A. (1975). Controlled trial of repeated halothane anaesthetics in patients with carcinoma of the uterine cervix treated with radium. *Lancet*, **1**, 821.

Uchida A., Kolb B., Micksche M. (1982). Generation of suppressor cells for natural killer activity in cancer patients after surgery. *J. Nat. Cancer Inst.*, **68**, 735.

Vergani D., Mieli-Vergani G., Alberti A., et al. (1980). Antibodies to the surface of halothane-altered rabbit hepatocytes in patients with severe halothane-associated hepatitis. *New Engl. J. Med.*, **303**, 66.

Vergani D., Tsantoulas D., Eddleston A.L.W.F. (1978). Sensitisation to halothane-altered liver compounds in severe hepatic necrosis after halothane anaesthesia. *Lancet*, **4**, 801.

Vogten A.J.M., Summerskill W.H.J., Shorter R.G. (1976). Cell mediated cytotoxicity against human hepatocyte membrane lipoprotein in halothane hepatitis: actuation by a serum factor? *Gastroenterology*, **71**, 934.

Walton B., Simpson B.R., Strunin L., et al. (1976). Unexplained hepatitis following halothane. *Br. Med. J.*, **1**, 1171.

Watkins J. (1983). Etomidate: an 'immunologically safe' anaesthetic agent? *Anaesthesia*, **38**, Suppl., 34.

Watkins J., Levy C.J. (1988). *Guide to immediate anaesthetic reactions*. London: Butterworths.

Welch W.D. (1986). Inhibition of neutrophil cidal activity by volatile anaesthetics. *Anesthesiology*, **64**, 1.

Williams B.D., White N., Amlot P.L., et al. (1977). Circulating immune complexes after repeated halothane anaesthesia. *Br. Med. J.*, **2**, 159.

Woods G.M., Griffiths D.M. (1986). Reversible inhibition of natural killer cell activity by volatile anaesthetic agents *in vitro. Br. J. Anaesth.*, **58**, 535.

Wright R., Eade O.E., Chisholm M. (1975). Controlled prospective study of the effect on liver function of multiple exposure to halothane. *Lancet*, **1**, 817.

E. BODY FLUIDS

38. Fluids and Electrolytes
K. Hillman

Traditionally, fluids and electrolytes have been considered together. There is some physiological basis for this. Fluid distribution within the body is largely determined by the distribution of sodium and potassium. The mechanisms responsible for renal control of electrolytes indirectly cause water loss or gain. However, other molecules, such as proteins also determine fluid distribution within the body and there are mechanisms such as antidiuretic hormone (ADH) secretion which directly control water intake and output independent of electrolytes. We will consider fluids and relevant aspects of electrolytes together in this chapter and emphasize their common features especially with respect to applied physiology.

FLUID COMPOSITION OF THE BODY

There are approximately 40 L of water in the average 70 kg adult male (Edelman and Leibman, 1959). The water is distributed in three compartments—the intravascular space (IVS), the interstitial space (ISS) and

intracellular fluid (ICF) (Fig. 38.1). Each of these three spaces has an unique composition and function. The IVS and ISS are considered together as extracellular fluid (ECF).

Body fluid compartments
(average for 70 kg male)

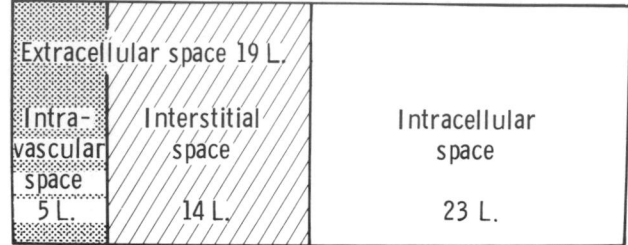

Fig. 38.1 Body fluid compartments. This represents the approximate proportion of body water in each of the three body compartments of a healthy 70 kg man. (Adapted with permission from Twigley and Hillman, 1985.)

The circulating fluid or IVS is a small but crucial component of the body fluid. Fluid in the ISS constitutes the matrix, or fluid in which the cells are bathed. It is the teleological remnant of sea water. Although the function of fluid in the IVS and ISS is distinct, the composition is similar and consists largely of salt and water. However, fluid in the IVS has a higher protein content, especially albumin, which generates a colloid osmotic pressure (COP). The COP confines the intravascular fluid to the circulating volume rather than the ISS. The composition of the cellular compartment consists largely of water, with the major cation being potassium.

FUNCTION OF FLUID COMPARTMENTS

Intravascular Fluid

The circulating fluid is responsible for the carriage and delivery of substrates, metabolites and gases needed for cellular function. The fluid is confined to the IVS by the nature of the endothelial cells which largely confine the circulating protein particles which in turn generate a COP.

Interstitial Fluid

While the vital role and function of fluid inside cells and in the circulating volume is largely self evident, the function of fluid in the interstitial fluid is less obvious. The interstitial fluid does not exist as a mobile liquid state—almost all of it is in the form of a gel filling the spaces between cells. The gel contains mucopolysaccharides, the most abundant of which is hyaluronic acid. However, the gel cannot move freely and the gel structure holds the interstitial fluid in place. This largely prevents free flow of fluid to dependent areas of the body. Apart from its structural properties the major function of the ISS is to facilitate transport between capillaries and cells. There is an ideal distance between the cell and capillary for optimum transport of substances. The maintenance of the right amount of interstitial fluid is therefore vital for cell nutrition.

The ISS cannot be discussed without considering the vital role of lymphatics. Lymph is interstitial fluid that flows into the lymphatic system. Valves at the terminal ends of lymphatics facilitate trapping of protein molecules which otherwise accumulate in the ISS. Lymph flow is further facilitated by the inherent pumping action of myo-endothelial fibres in conjunction with multiple valves along the length of the lymphatics. While most of the water is reabsorbed at the venous end of the capillaries almost none of the protein which leaks from the arterial ends of the capillaries is reabsorbed. The protein becomes concentrated in the interstitial fluid before it flows into the lymphatics.

The rapid removal of protein from the ISS by the lymphatics decreases the tissue fluid COP which allows the capillaries to reabsorb large quantities of fluid thus creating a negative pressure in the ISS (Guyton et al., 1971). The lymphatic pump also creates a slight degree of suction. The ISS pressure is approximately -6 mmHg. The significance of a negative ISS pressure cannot be overestimated in the understanding of body fluids. The negative pressure contributes to the integrity of cellular architecture. In oedematous states, the architecture is disrupted. Moreover, the negative pressure state of the ISS and the continual removal of fluid by lymphatics guarantees no excess fluid accumulation. Otherwise fluid would accumulate and diffusion distances would increase, interfering with cellular metabolism.

As long as the ISS pressure remains negative there is little change in the ISS volume. Any factor which increases ISS pressure such as elevated capillary pressure, decreased COP, increased ISS COP or increased permeability of the capillaries tends to increase lymphatic flow. The increase in lymphatic flow continues until it reaches approximately 10–50 times normal. Then the ISS pressure rises slightly above zero. Further flow is limited by distortion of the flap valves and collapse of lymph channels due to accumulation of surrounding fluid. Most of the compensation to prevent interstitial oedema occurs before the oedema actually appears.

There is a large increase in interstitial fluid volume when the interstitial fluid pressure becomes positive. The relationship between the pressure and volume is variable as each tissue has a different compliance. As soon as the ISS pressure becomes positive the compliance within that tissue markedly decreases. The same dynamics operate in the pulmonary circulation.

However, the pulmonary capillary pressure is lower, the pulmonary capillaries are relatively leaky to protein molecules, the rate of lymph flowing from the lungs is facilitated by their motion during breathing and the ISS's are very narrow (Meyer et al., 1968). As the alveolar epithelia can resist pressures no greater than approximately $+2$ mmHg, interstitial fluid can readily flow from the ISS into the alveoli causing overt pulmonary oedema. However, interstitial fluid does not normally accumulate because of the negativity of the ISS which pulls fluid away from the alveolar membrane, keeping the lungs dry.

Intracellular Fluid (ICF)

The ICF provides the milieu for cellular function to occur. Most enzymes are situated intracellularly and most metabolic reactions occur intracellularly. The maintenance of this fluid space is obviously vital for the life processes. The volume of the cell is critical for electrolyte concentrations and pH levels, which are in turn crucial for metabolic processes.

MAINTENANCE OF BODY FLUID SPACES

There are certain physical and physiological processes which maintain the composition and volume of body fluid spaces. These include basic physical laws such as diffusion created by chemical concentration gradients across the fluid compartments and the fact that lipophilic substances cross membranes at higher rates than hydrophilic substances. It is postulated that total volume flow across membranes occurs more rapidly than predicted by diffusion alone, because there are pores of varying size in the cell membrane.

The basic mechanisms of control of the ECF are through *osmolality* and *volume*. Although these mechanisms are directly sensed and operated through the ECF, the osmolality and volume of the ICF is then indirectly affected. Osmolality is largely adjusted by water retention or elimination and the volume is adjusted mainly by sodium retention or elimination. It can be seen that there is overlap between the two mechanisms. When water is retained or lost, volume and osmolality are affected. Moreover it is not only the volume of the ECF that is affected but also that of the ICF and total body water (TBW). Similarly sodium loss or retention affects osmolality and the volume of the ECF and ICF. A high serum sodium concentration for example, initially will cause water to move by osmosis from the ICF to the ECF, thus changing the volume of both fluid compartments in order to maintain isotonicity between the two spaces.

The ECF is divided into the ISS and the IVS by the capillary endothelial cells. These cells are relatively impermeable to protein molecules, particularly albumin, causing the oncotic pressure to be higher within the capillaries than in the ISS. The difference in oncotic pressure between the two spaces is facilitated by lymphatic drainage of protein from the ISS space.

Starling's forces define the oncotic and hydrostatic pressures in both fluid compartments. The oncotic pressure remains constant at both the arteriole and venule ends of the capillary bed, while the hydrostatic forces tend to result in fluid being forced out of the arterial end of the capillary and reabsorbed from the venous end. There is a net efflux of fluid out of the capillaries which is collected by the lymphatics. While the general concept of Starling's forces is probably valid it is variable between tissues. The filtration coefficient for each tissue is an expression of the permeability of the capillary systems and varies for each capillary bed. It is very small in both brain and muscle, larger in subcutaneous tissues and very large in the intestine and liver. Similarly, the concentration of protein in the ISS will increase as the filtration coefficient increases.

The intracellular and extracellular fluids are isotonic. This is largely because all cell membranes and capillary walls are freely permeable to water and therefore the principle of osmosis guarantees isotonicity between the fluid spaces. Osmosis is the movement of solvent molecules (usually water) across a membrane into a region where there is a higher concentration of solute to which the membrane is impermeable.

Sodium concentration is the prime determinant of ECF osmotic pressure and potassium of the ICF osmotic pressure. Sodium passes into the cells with difficulty and when it does it is continually extruded by the sodium-potassium pump. On the other hand, because of its small hydrated radius, potassium is more permeable across the cell membrane. Although potassium has a larger atomic weight than sodium, it has a smaller hydrated radius related to the number of water molecules surrounding it, and can diffuse across the membrane more readily.

Osmotic and electrical equality can only be satisfied by a relatively high concentration of mobile potassium within the cell together with a relatively low concentration of chloride and larger polyvalent anions. *While the volume and composition of the ECF is largely determined by the kidney, the volume and composition of the ICF largely depends on the efforts of each individual cell* (Leaf, 1970).

Osmolality

Osmolality of the ECF is sensed by 'osmoreceptor' cells in the anterior hypothalamus (Robertson et al., 1977). They in turn stimulate thirst and the synthesis of ADH from the neurones of the supraoptic nuclei which are part of the neurohypophyseal system (Schrier et al., 1979). Antidiuretic hormone then acts on the distal tubules and collecting ducts of the kidney causing reabsorption of water and the excretion of low volumes of urine with high osmolalities. This system is equisitively sensitive, keeping the serum osmolality normally within a range of 275–295

mosmol/L by varying the urine osmolalities between 15–1400 mosmol/L.

Volume

There is a paradox in the control of the ECF volume. While the receptors which determine volume of the ECF are mainly intravascular, the mechanism for volume regulation is based on retention of the sodium molecule which is distributed over the whole extracellular space—interstitial and intravascular. As the ISS is approximately three times larger than the IVS, sodium retention affects mainly the ISS and is an inefficient and long-term mechanism for controlling intravascular volume. As maintaining the circulating volume is crucial for life on a minute-to-minute basis, a more efficient and rapid response is needed to maintain it. This is achieved by the unique ability of the IVS, mediated by the sympathetic nervous system, to acutely constrict or dilate. The retention and excretion of water, although largely determined by ECF osmolality, is also affected by baroreceptors (Anderson et al., 1976) and affects the volume of TBW as well as individual body fluid compartments in a proportional manner.

SODIUM

Sodium is the major extracellular cation, maintained in a concentration range between 135–145 mmol/L. The total amount of body sodium is about 4000 mmol. The average dietary sodium intake is approximately 150 mmol/d with marked individual variations. Most ingested sodium is absorbed. To maintain the sodium balance, the amount absorbed from the gastrointestinal tract must equal that excreted in the kidneys. Like water, the kidneys have the ability to retain or excrete sodium over a wide range. The plasma osmolality and plasma sodium concentration are regulated by osmoreceptors in the hypothalamus that affect thirst and release of ADH. *Plasma sodium concentration is maintained mainly by changes in water content while the sodium balance is influenced mainly by intake and renal regulation of excretion.*

Renal Regulation of Sodium

Over the past 30 years there have been major developments in our knowledge of the factors which control sodium. However, there are still large gaps in our understanding. The mechanism of sodium control is closely linked to the mechanisms which control the size of the vascular bed i.e., vasoconstriction in response to hypovolaemia is usually accompanied by sodium retention and expansion of the ECF. Similarly, excessive intravascular pressures are associated with vasodilatation and sodium loss.

The three major determinants of sodium regulation

are the renin-angiotensin-aldosterone axis, intrarenal factors and atrial natriuretic factor (ANF).

Receptors

A change in sodium content of the body is reflected in extracellular volume. This in turn affects the intravascular volume where most of the receptors are. These are usually in the form of pressure receptors which detect either low-pressure capacitance areas (veins or atria), high-pressure resistance areas (arterial vascular tree) or juxtaglomerular apparatus intrarenal vascular pressures by the juxtaglomerular apparatus (Gauer and Henry, 1963; Smith, 1957). For example, the carotid sinus senses distending pressure in large arteries. This in turn stimulates acute changes in the tone of the vascular bed as well as the renin-angiotensin-aldosterone axis which help regulate sodium excretion.

Renin-angiotensin-aldosterone axis

This system simultaneously exerts the major control over sodium and potassium balance as well as playing a role in the regulation of arterial blood pressure (BP) (Laragh et al., 1972; Laragh and Sealey, 1973). The trigger for this system is renin release from the kidney, caused either by a fall in renal perfusion or a fall in sodium concentration in the distal tubule. Angiotensin II is then formed in the plasma and this is a powerful stimulant of aldosterone secretion. Aldosterone acts mainly on the distal renal tubules to increase sodium reabsorption and to promote potassium secretion. Decreased aldosterone excretion in response to a large sodium load may cause severe potassium loss. However, potassium remains stable in the face of a large sodium load and *vice versa*. This coregulation is accomplished by the renin system in conjunction with intrarenal compensation.

Intrarenal Factors

Sodium loading causes both the glomerular filtration rate (GFR) and peritubular interstitial pressure to increase resulting in decreased reabsorption of sodium from the proximal tubule (Beeuwkes et al., 1981). Sodium excretion is increased by factors which increase GFR or peritubular interstitial pressure. Similar factors which decrease GFR cause a net reabsorption of sodium from the proximal tubule (Beeuwkes et al., 1981; Mueller et al., 1951). Thus the intrarenal factors cause changes in distal tubular sodium concentration, which in turn contribute to sodium and potassium excretion as well as influencing the release of renin.

Atrial Natriuretic Factor (ANF)

Anomalies in renal sodium control previously unexplained by either intrarenal factors or the renin-angiotensin-aldosterone axis were ascribed to the so-called 'Third factor' (de Wardener et al., 1961). It has since become clearer that the atrial tissue contains peptides, at least one of which is secreted as a hormone regulating sodium excretion (de Bold et al., 1981). The peptides are collectively referred to as atrial natriuretic factor (ANF). Powerful diuretic, natriuretic and vasodilatory effects of the atrial peptides have been described (Laragh, 1985; Ballermann and Brenner, 1986; de Bold, 1986). It is suspected that the peptides are released in response to atrial distension which acts as a guide to the 'fullness' of the circulation. When released, ANF can cause an increase in GFR without increasing renal blood flow, there is relaxation of many vascular beds and a reduction in arterial BP. Moreover, the atrial peptides can inhibit renal renin secretion and adrenal cortical secretion of aldosterone, as well as opposing the vasoconstrictive action of angiotensin II. Thus ANF may play a major role in sodium balance as well as long-term regulation of arterial BP. However, there is still much to learn about the regulation of ANF release and its clinical significance in health and disease.

MEASUREMENT OF THE BODY SPACES

Fluid in the body can be measured either in a laboratory or in the clinical context. It is difficult to apply laboratory measurements to the clinical situation because they rely mainly on tracer dilutional techniques. These techniques are time consuming, complicated and rely on steady state or equilibrium conditions for accuracy.

It is uncommon to be able to achieve equilibrium conditions in clinical practice and when it is achieved in a normal and stable person the information cannot be extrapolated to unstable patients. We therefore use other methods such as intravascular pressure measurements and fluid balance charts as guidelines for the assessment of a patient's fluid status and their replacement needs.

Even in the normal population, body water distribution cannot be precisely estimated because of significant individual variations in body water content with age, sex and weight. Furthermore, there are wide differences in the relative amounts of ECF, ICF, plasma, interstitial fluid and transcellular fluid in normal individuals (Table 38.1) and even greater differences between normal and sick individuals.

LABORATORY MEASUREMENT OF BODY SPACES

Tracer-Dilutional Techniques

The volume of fluid distributed in a body compartment can be determined by injecting a substance which is largely confined to that space. The concentration of the substance must be capable of being measured and the amount excreted or metabolized

TABLE 38.1

REPRESENTATIVE NORMAL VALUES FOR TBW, ECF AND ICF AS %
OF TOTAL BODY WEIGHT

Age in years unless otherwise stated		% Total of body weight			
		TBW	ECF	ICF	ECF/ICF
Premature		80	—	—	—
Birth		75	42	33	1.27
1 month		70	32	38	0.84
1		65	26	39	0.67
10		62	26	36	0.72
Males	25	60	27	33	0.82
	45	53	24	29	0.83
	65	54	26	28	0.93
	85	51	26	25	1.04
Females	25	51	23	28	0.82
	45	48	23	25	0.92
	65	44	22	22	1.00
	85	43	22	21	1.05

Adapted from Pain R.W., 1977; Edelman and Leibman, 1959;
Moore et al., 1963.

known. Total body water (TBW), ECF, plasma
volume and red cell volume can be determined by
tracer-dilutional techniques. Intracellular fluid is
estimated as the difference between TBW and ECF.
Interstitial fluid is estimated as the difference between
ECF and plasma volume. The major disadvantage in
clinical practice is that the technique assumes that the
subject is in a steady metabolic state during the experimental period and this is rarely the case in the perioperative or seriously ill patient.

Total Body Water (TBW)

The most accurate and direct method for measuring
TBW is by desiccation of cadavers. The results
obtained by this technique and tissue sampling studies
have correlated well and with tracer-dilutional techniques.

The isotopes of water—deuterium oxide (D_2O) and
tritium oxide (THO) are frequently used for TBW
determination. Antipyrene and urea have also been
used (Pain, 1977). Both D_2O and THO are small
molecules which rapidly equilibrate within body water
and are not significantly metabolized over the 3–4
hour equilibration period. D_2O is non-radioactive
and being heavier than water, it is measured by densi-
metric or mass spectrometric methods.

Tritium is a weak β emitter and because it is technically easier to detect has become the method of
choice. Equilibration occurs within 4 hours and reproducibility is $\pm 2\%$ (Prentice et al., 1952). Total body
water accounts for approximately 75% of total body
weight at birth. It then gradually decreases to 50% at
age 85 in males and 40% in similarly aged females

(Edelman et al., 1959). We dry out and wrinkle as we
become older. This is important to remember when
prescribing intravenous fluids. Another important
variation occurs within the relationship between body
water and body fat content. Obese patients have proportionately less water for their body weight because
adipose tissue contains little water. This has led to the
concept of 'lean body mass' based on estimates of fat
free body weight (Hume, 1966). Seriously ill catabolic
patients lose muscle and fat tissue and the percentage
of their TBW falls as bone and dense connective
tissue accounts for an increasing proportion of body
weight.

Extracellular Fluid (ECF)

The ECF consists of all fluid external to cells. It consists of approximately 45% of TBW and 27% of total
body weight (Edelman et al., 1959). The ECF is
divided into the ISS and IVS. The ISS can be further
divided into functional or physiological water compartments some of which are more 'accessible' than
others (Table 38.2). The intravascular water is con-

TABLE 38.2

BODY FLUID COMPARTMENTS
(FOR A 70 KG YOUNG ADULT MALE)

Compartment	Percent body weight	Percent TBW	Volume in litres	ml/kg wt
Plasma	4.5	7.5	3.2	45
Interstitial-lymph	12.0	20.0	8.4	120
Dense connective tissue	4.5	7.5	3.2	45
Bone	4.5	7.5	3.2	45
Transcellular	1.5	2.5	1.0	15
ECF (Total)	27	45	19	270
Red cells	2.3	3.8	1.6	23
ICF (Total)	33	55	23	330
TBW	60	100	42	600

Note

The interstitial-lymph compartment includes 25% of connective tissue water and 10% of bone water. The dense connective tissue compartment is 'inaccessible'. It comprises
75% of connective tissue water and 90% of bone water.
Adapted from Pain R.W., 1977; Edelman and Leibman,
1959.

sidered as part of the plasma volume. However, the
water contained in red blood cells is not strictly ICF as
extracellular tracers equilibrate readily with the fluid
of red blood cells (Swan and Nelson, 1973).

The so-called normal values vary with illness.
Chronic disease and acute illnesses are often associated with an expansion of the ECF so that it may

even exceed the volume of the ICF. In stressed states, such as the perioperative period and in the acutely ill, catabolism of fat occurs with generation of 600–1000 ml of 'free' water a day (Moore, 1959). This is in association with other neuroendocrine mechanisms which promote sodium and water retention. Thus, the extrapolation of 'normal' values for fluid spaces to the clinical situation becomes even more precarious.

The volume of the ECF cannot be estimated with the same accuracy as TBW. The tracers used all have shortcomings and none are entirely confined to the ECF. They can be divided into two groups—crystalloids or non-electrolytes of medium molecular weight (e.g. inulin, sucrose and mannitol) or ionic substances (e.g. ^{82}Br, ^{36}Cl and ^{35}S. The crystalloids being of larger molecular weight only slowly penetrate the ECF with little leakage into cells, therefore tending to underestimate the total ECF. They are also rapidly excreted by the kidneys at a clearance rate approximately equal to the GFR. The ions are easier to measure but overestimate the ECF because they tend to leak into cells. Isotopes of chloride have half-lives which are either too short (37 minutes) or too long (400 000 years), whereas ^{82}Br has a more appropriate half-life of 36 hours and is not metabolized and only slowly excreted. It is currently the most widely accepted tracer for measuring the ECF. However, because of its tendency to penetrate cells it is more correct to talk in terms of a 'bromide space' rather than ECF. As the equilibration time is 20 hours, it is referred to as the '20 hour bromide space'. The tracer and the equilibration time should always be stated when referring to measurements of the ECF. Exponential regression of plasma levels to zero time allows for losses in the urine and elsewhere.

The rate of disappearance of ^{82}Br from the plasma occurs at two levels (Pain, 1977)—there is a rapidly equilibrating pool (20 minutes) referred to as the 'functional ECF'. It is approximately 8.4 L in volume and 20% of the TBW and represents that part of the ISS in constant and rapid equilibrium with the plasma. This pool includes 25% of the dense connective tissue and 10% of bone water. The second slowly equilibrating pool is the part of the ISS consisting of the remainder of dense connective tissue (e.g. cartilage, ligaments, tendons and bone). It comprises 15% of TBW and is 6.4 L in volume.

Although sodium is predominantly an extracellular cation, its space is larger than the ECF because a certain percentage is intracellular. The sodium space can be measured with Na-24 values obtained at 24 hours.

Red Cell Volume

The most accurate technique for determining red blood cell volume is by labelling red cells with radioactive chromium (^{51}Cr), reinjecting them and using the principles of tracer dilution. Alternatively, it can be determined from the plasma volume and haemato-crit. However, whole body haematocrit is greater than large vein haematocrit, resulting in errors of up to 7%. Red cell volume is approximately 2.0 L (29 ml/kg) in adult males and 1.5 L (25 ml/kg) in adult females and gradually decreases with age.

Plasma Volume

Plasma volume can be measured by two different types of tracer that bind to plasma albumin–dyes such as Evans blue or radioactive tracers such as radio-iodine labelled serum albumin (RISA). Albumin escapes at a rate of approximately 7–10% per hour from the IVS into the ISS causing an overestimation of plasma volume which is even greater in patients with nephrotic syndrome, sepsis, burns, trauma, ascites and cardiopulmonary disorders (Valeri and Cooper, 1973). To reduce errors in determining volume and distribution, equilibration time has to be short (approximately 10–15 min) or more accurately, extrapolated to zero time from multiple readings. The plasma volume is approximately 3.3 L (47 ml/kg body weight) in young adult males and 2.7 L (44 ml/kg body weight) in females (Edelman et al., 1959). These values decrease with age.

CLINICAL ASSESSMENT

Bedside assessment of TBW, ICF and ISS relies on crude estimates. The only fluid space we have reliable information about is the relatively small circulating volume or IVS (Hillman, 1986).

Intravascular Volume

Isotopic blood volume measurements have been attempted in clinical practice. Apart from being technically difficult and not able to be repeated at frequent intervals, there are the problems previously mentioned of unpredictable protein leakage and failure to achieve the equilibrium conditions necessary for these estimations.

We therefore mainly rely on indirect measurements of intravascular volume (see Table 38.3). Some of these rely on intravascular pressure measurements—central venous pressure (CVP), pulmonary artery wedge pressure (PAWP), systemic BP. Others involve flow—central flow is measured by cardiac output (CO) and peripheral flow is estimated by core versus peripheral temperature, peripheral filling time, partial pressure of oxygen measured transcutaneously (Ptc_{O_2}).

Peripheral blood flow in the skin can also be estimated using the Doppler principle.

An increase in heart rate is one of the first responses of the body to hypovolaemia. The haematocrit decreases gradually as interstitial fluid moves into the circulating volume in response to a decreased hydrostatic pressure. Organs manifest signs of decreased flow during hypovolaemia, e.g. decreased level of con-

TABLE 38.3
ASSESSMENT OF INTRAVASCULAR VOLUME

Indirect measurement isotopic dilution technique.

Measurement	Technique
Direct	Measurement by isotopic dilution
Indirect	
Vascular pressure	Central venous pressure (CVP)
	Pulmonary artery wedge pressure (PAWP)
	Arterial BP (BP)
	Dynamic mean systemic filling pressure
Blood flow	Cardiac output
Heart rate	
Haematocrit	
Organ blood flow	Brain—decreased level of consciousness
	Kidney—oliguria
	Skin—decreased peripheral temperature
	—Doppler
	—transcutaneous partial pressure of oxygen (Ptc_{O2})

sciousness and oliguria. Other organs may also suffer reversible damage during hypovolaemia and ischaemia e.g. liver dysfunction, decreased immunity, ileus or diarrhoea. These manifestations may not be immediately as obvious as, for example, oliguria with renal hypoperfusion and may not become clinically evident until hours or days after the initial ischaemia.

Systemic Blood Pressure
Changes in blood volume not only produce hydraulic changes within the cardiovascular system but also initiate many neural, endocrine and autoregulatory responses (Cowley et al., 1986). As blood volume is acutely decreased, the pressure receptors respond through the sympathetic nervous system and maintain BP by increasing stroke volume, heart rate and systemic vascular resistance. This reflex becomes less active in the elderly. Once hypotension, as a result of hypovolaemia, supervenes in young patients, the blood loss is usually severe. Blood volume can be increased markedly with no change in BP. Paradoxically, patients with a brittle cardiovascular system, such as hypertensives or patients with autonomic dysfunction such as in tetanus or Guillain Barré syndrome, can develop hypertension in response to hypovolaemia. This is corrected by fluid replacement.

Central Venous Pressure (CVP)
Central venous pressure measures the ability of the right heart to cope with venous return at the moment of measurement. As well as blood volume, right vent-

ricular function and the tone of the capacitance vessels have a large influence on CVP. It is possible to have a normal or even raised CVP as a result of intense vasoconstriction in the presence of hypovolaemia. Sykes (1963) noted that there could be variations of up to 10% of blood volume without changes in CVP. Any losses or gains in TBW or ISS fluid would have to be proportionately much greater than changes in the IVS to affect the CVP. Similarly, fluids which are distributed to the IVS such as blood or colloid would affect CVP readings much more than fluids such as crystalloid or 5% dextrose which are proportionately distributed mainly to other spaces.

Most acute pulmonary pathology causes a significant increase in pulmonary artery pressure which in turn causes an increase in right ventricular pressure and right atrial pressure. Thus the CVP reading may be a reflection of raised pulmonary artery pressure as a result of acute respiratory disease rather than an increase in intravascular volume. Interpretation is further complicated by intrathoracic pressures applied with artificial ventilation and positive end-expiratory pressure (PEEP) which unpredictably increase CVP. It is not surprising that since CVP readings were first used in the early 1950's, its accuracy in reflecting blood volume has been disputed (Prout, 1968; Baek et al., 1975; Shippy et al., 1984).

The measurement of CVP is most useful when there is simple uncomplicated haemorrhage with no associated organ failure and when used as part of the dynamic assessment of intravascular fluid replacement in conjunction with as many other intravascular measurements as possible. Even in these circumstances CVP is of little value in the acute resuscitation of severe haemorrhage.

Pulmonary Artery Wedge Pressure (PAWP)
The PAWP under certain conditions is a reflection of left atrial pressure which measures the ability of the left side of the heart to cope with venous return from the lungs. The PAWP is indirectly related to blood volume. There are, however, many physiological assumptions in this relationship. The assumption that PAWP always reflects left atrial pressure, left ventricular end diastolic pressure or left ventricular end diastolic volume has recently been challenged (Robin, 1985; Raper and Sibbald, 1986). Left atrial pressure itself reflects cardiac function as well as intravascular volume. In the clinical situation there has been a poor correlation between changes in blood volume and PAWP (Baek et al., 1975; Shippy et al., 1984). There is little place for PAWP in the management of acute haemorrhage. It may be of more benefit in fine tuning intravascular volume replacement and preventing pulmonary oedema. Even in these circumstances it should be used in conjunction with fluid challenges, looking at trends rather than being obsessed with single so-called normal values.

Heart Rate

Increased heart rate is part of a neuroendocrine response, mediated mainly through the sympathetic nervous system in response to hypovolaemia. It is best seen in simple haemorrhage, especially in young patients. Heart rate can also be influenced by concurrent drugs (e.g. anaesthetic agents, β-blockers and inotropes), underlying disease (e.g. bradyarrythmias or tachyarrhythmias associated with sepsis) and other factors such as pain and anxiety. Nevertheless, it can be a simple, albeit limited, guide to intravascular volume.

Urine Output

The hourly urine output is a good guide to intravascular volume. During fluid resuscitation, a urine output of more than 0.5 ml/(Kg·h) is desirable. Like other guidelines to intravascular volume, the urine output is an indirect assessment and subject to many other factors. These include drugs (e.g. diuretic inotropes, low or renal dose dopamine), underlying renal disease, concurrent acute renal failure, increased intrathoracic pressure which decrease renal blood flow and increased intra-abdominal pressure (e.g. abdominal tamponade) which decreases ureteric flow and renal blood flow.

Urine/plasma (U/P) osmolality ratio can help to differentiate prerenal renal insufficiency (inadequate volume replacement) from 'renal' renal failure. A U/P ratio of more than 2.0:1 is in favour of prerenal failure and < 1.5:1 is in favour of 'renal' renal failure.

Peripheral Perfusion

A simple and reliable guide to the adequacy of intravascular volume is peripheral perfusion of the skin. This is empirically detected by feeling the extremities or measuring peripheral (e.g. big toe) temperature. Like BP, the peripheral perfusion is a reflection of an active sympathetic nervous system in response to hypovolaemia rather than hypovolaemia itself. This is reinforced by the fact that cardiogenic shock is also associated with poor peripheral perfusion. In both cases there is a crude relationship between the degree of coldness in the periphery and the degree of shock. This can be quantified more accurately by directly measuring skin blood flow by the Doppler technique (Nilsson, et al., 1980; Waxman et al., 1987). The $P\text{tc}_{O_2}$ measured by a transcutaneous electrode on the skin is also a reflection of skin blood flow and the degree of hypovolaemia (Beran, et al., 1981; Tremper and Shoemaker, 1981). The $P\text{tc}_{O_2}$ tracks skin blood flow in shock when oxygenation is normal and tracks oxygenation when cardiovascular function is normal.

Cardiac Output

Cardiac output is significantly reduced during acute intravascular volume depletion. This is related to the decreased filling pressure as well as the increased afterload needed to maintain systemic arterial pressure. The reduction in CO is only an indirect guide to the assessment of intravascular volume and not accurately correlated with it (Shippy et al., 1984). While the place of CO monitoring for clinical estimation of blood volume is yet to be determined, its use in acute resuscitation is limited. It may have a place in the fine tuning of the circulation in conjunction with other measurements and as part of a fluid challenge.

Haematocrit

The changes in the haematocrit as a result of losses of intravascular fluid depend on many factors (Baek et al., 1975; Shippy et al., 1984). If the haematocrit is measured during active bleeding it will, of course, be normal. In response to bleeding and decreased hydrostatic pressure within the vascular space, salt and water will move from the ISS into the IVS. The kidneys simultaneously retain salt and water as a neuroendocrinological response to stress. Thus the IVS becomes diluted by salt and water and the haematocrit falls. However, this adaption occurs slowly. As well as the physiological changes resulting in the decreased haematocrit, simultaneous resuscitation with blood and other fluid would blunt the stress response and change the hydrostatic/oncotic pressure relationship between plasma and interstitial fluid. In the face of these dynamics, a haematocrit is at best a crude guideline to intravascular volume replacement, but a very useful measurement of red blood cell requirements.

Dynamic Mean Systemic Filling Pressure

Even if the blood volume could be accurately measured, the influence of that volume upon cardiovascular dynamics is not known unless the compliance of the vessel walls is also known. The mean circulatory filling pressure is a description of the relationship between the blood volume and the circulatory compliance (Guyton et al., 1954). The pressure is independent of cardiac function and vascular resistances and related only to compliance and the blood volume in excess of that required to fill the circulation to zero pressure. As it is measured after the heart is stopped and the circulation has been allowed to come to static equilibrium its place in clinical practice is limited. Using mathematic modelling, readily available cardiovascular measurements (CO, mean BP and right atrial pressure) as well as height, weight and age, the concept of dynamic mean systemic filling pressure has been developed and used in the clinical situation to predict intravascular volume requirements (Leaning et al., 1983; Parkin, 1986).

Interstitial and Intracellular Space

Most of our clinical information on fluid status concerns the relatively small IVS. However, assessment of the majority of the body's fluid is clinically inaccessible except by the crudest of techniques (Twigley and Hillman, 1985).

Fluid Balance Charts

Despite the considerable time invested in recording and interpreting fluid balance charts they provide scant information on the status of the body fluid compartments and therefore the nature and amount of fluid replacement.

When recording fluid input in a normal adult in a basal metabolic state there are more 'unseen' gains from the oxidation of food and water than 'seen' gains from fluid (Gruber and Allgower 1970). Approximately one litre of water is gained from the tissue breakdown and oxidation of 1 kg of tissue. This would provide a considerable source of 'unseen' water gains, especially in the critically ill and the perioperative hypercatabolic patient when excessive tissue breakdown is occurring.

Similarly, there are more 'unseen' than 'seen' losses in a normal basal metabolic adult. The insensible losses from the skin and lungs are approximately 900 ml compared to an average of 700 ml in urine. There are also small losses from faeces of about 150 ml. The 'unseen' losses from the critically ill and perioperative patients can be considerable, e.g. diarrhoea, intestinal sequestration and wound drainage.

Fluid balance charts must be looked at in the light of these shortcomings and the patient's clinical state. For example, it would be oversimplistic and illogical for example to replace what comes out with a similar volume. Apart from disregarding the composition of the fluid this approach ignores the inherent inaccuracies of fluid balance charts. Similarly it is futile to attempt to computerize fluid balance charts because of the fundamental inaccuracy of the figures. At best they provide a rough estimate of the source of major losses and gains.

History

A history can give an indication of the composition and to a lesser extent the volume of fluid loss. The composition of body fluids is variable. Pancreatic fluid and bile approach the composition of interstitial fluid whereas sweat and gastric contents have a higher water content and lower sodium content (Table 38.4). Depending on the site of the loss, the electrolyte composition can be estimated and the fluid compartments affected can then be determined, e.g. pancreatic fluid has an electrolyte composition similar to serum and therefore the loss is mainly from the ECF. Whereas the sodium concentration in gastric juice is lower and so would represent fluid from the ICF as well as the ECF. In both cases only a relatively small percentage would be from the intravascular volume.

Thirst is another common symptom associated with fluid disorders. Both osmotic and non-osmotic factors affect thirst (Phillips, 1977). The major effects are through the osmoreceptors and reflect either a change in body water or extracellular solute load (e.g. sodium). However, the symptom of thirst is also associated with acute intravascular depletion. Thirst is a non-specific finding, indicating total water depletion, osmolar load or intravascular volume depletion.

Chest X-ray

Extravascular lung water (EVLW) or pulmonary oedema may be an indication of expansion of the ISS in the lung (Shoemaker et al., 1981). However, it may also be related to other, often concurrent factors such as left ventricular dysfunction, overexpansion of the IVS and all of the many proposed aetiologies, including generalized capillary leak, of adult respiratory distress syndrome (ARDS). While the chest X-ray appearance correlates very well with the extent of EVLW (Halperin et al., 1985), the origin of EVLW cannot be ascertained.

TABLE 38.4
BODY FLUID COMPOSITION AND VOLUME

	Volume/24 h	Sodium mmol/L	Potassium mmol/L	pH
Sweat	500–1000 ml	50	10	—
CSF	100–160 ml	150	3	7.32–7.40
Saliva	1000–2000 ml	60	20	6.0–7.0
Bile	500–750 ml	145	5	7.8
Pancreatic	1000 ml	141	4	8.0–8.3
Gastric	2500 ml	60	9	1.0–3.5
Upper small bowel	2000–3000 ml	105	5	7.8–8.0
Ileum	1000 ml	117	5	6.5–8.0
Large intestine	150 ml	50		
Diarrhoea	500 + ml	75	30	—

(Adapted from Randall, 1976; and Fisher, 1977).

Serum Sodium

When blood glucose is normal, the variables which determine the serum sodium (Na_s) are the exchangeable stores of sodium (Na_e), the exchangeable stores of potassium (K_e) and the TBW (Edelman et al., 1958).

$$Na_s \propto \frac{Na_e + K_e}{TBW}$$

The most clinically significant effect of these variables, especially in the short-term, is the TBW. Thus hyponatraemia usually indicates excessive TBW and hypernatraemia indicates insufficient TBW. This general rule is one of the few clinical guidelines for TBW estimation and has important practical and therapeutic implications. *Serum sodium is the most important clinical indication of TBW status.*

Skin Turgor and Dry Mucous Membrane

Dry mucous membranes are a non-specific physical finding which may indicate TBW deficit (Dorrington, 1981). However, this is difficult to quantify especially in the presence of hyperventilation and oxygen face masks where gas flow can cause mucosal drying even in conditions of normal fluid balance.

Decreased skin turgor supposedly correlates with the degree of dehydration, where as dehydration may loosely mean a decrease in TBW or ISS. Firstly, it is impossible to state whether cells or the ISS is dehydrated by pinching a fold between the finger and thumb. Secondly, the TBW content of skin varies greatly with age (*see* Table 38.1). A newborn's skin is elastic compared to the elderly. Within these limitations skin turgor may be a crude indication of TBW or the ISS.

Measurement of Interstitial Space Pressure

Just as intravascular compartment pressure measurements such as BP, CVP and PAWP are a guide to the intravascular volume, measurement of ISS pressure is an indication of interstitial volume.

One of the difficulties has been that tissue pressure, which can be measured by a fluid filled needle in the ISS, includes both cellular and interstitial pressure (Guyton et al., 1971). This can be overcome by using an implantable capsule which has been allowed to equilibrate with the ISS (Guyton, 1963) or by using a wick directly implanted in the ISS (Fadnes et al., 1977). Although used experimentally in animals, it is not yet used widely in clinical practice.

In summary, although most of the fluids used in clinical practice are distributed mainly to the interstitial (crystalloids) or intracellular space (dextrose and water) our clinical measurements of those spaces are almost non-existent.

CLINICAL ASPECTS OF FLUID AND ELECTROLYTE THERAPY

Fluids and electrolytes are administered to replace or maintain the body's own requirements. We have already examined clinical methods for determining fluid status—each has its limitations. Even so, much of our current fluid therapy is illogical and irrational (Twigley et al., 1985)—often reduced to 2–3 L of a salt containing solution each day and a little more if there is excess drainage or a little less if the patient is small.

Intravenous Fluids

Intravenous fluids are commonly divided into blood, blood products, colloids, crystalloids as well as isotonic solutions with dextrose and varying amounts of sodium. Colloids are solutions containing colloid particles which are large molecules generally confined to the IVS. Just how much of the colloid solution remains in the IVS depends on the COP generated by these molecules and their half-life within the IVS. Examples include blood derivatives based on human albumin and other plasma proteins, dextrans, modified gelatins and hydroxethyl starch. Crystalloids are isotonic solutions with a similar fluid and electrolyte composition to the ECF but no colloid particles. These fluids are confined to the extracellular space—both the intravascular and ISS in a ratio of approximately 1:3. They include Ringer's lactate or Hartmanns solution and isotonic saline. The remaining isotonic fluids are largely based on dextrose. The dextrose is metabolized leaving either free water (5% dextrose) or a hypotonic solution containing varying amounts of sodium. Depending on the sodium concentration, these solutions are distributed to a greater or lesser extent over the TBW. A solution with no sodium is distributed equally to all three fluid spaces. Clearly there will only be a small amount distributed to the intravascular compartment—if there are 40 L of water in the average body, approximately 5/40 or $\frac{1}{8}$ will be distributed to the IVS. Similarly, because the ICS is the largest space, most of the water will be distributed to that space. Thus 5% dextrose would be an inappropriate and inefficient fluid to resuscitate the intravascular compartment for shock. Because a crystalloid is distributed equally in the ECF, at least $\frac{2}{3}$ will be to the interstitial fluid and $\frac{1}{3}$ to the intravascular compartment. Thus if a crystalloid is used for resuscitation in hypovolaemia, for each litre given, approximately 300 ml will remain in the intravascular compartment and the remainder will expand the ISS (Fig. 38.2). Crystalloids are therefore more efficient than 5% dextrose for hypovolaemia but not as efficient as colloid or blood. In this context the so-called crystalloid versus colloid controversy begs the wrong question. Crystalloids are excellent for expanding the whole ECF, the ISS more than the IVS, while colloids are more suitable for expanding the IVS.

Resuscitation of the correct body space

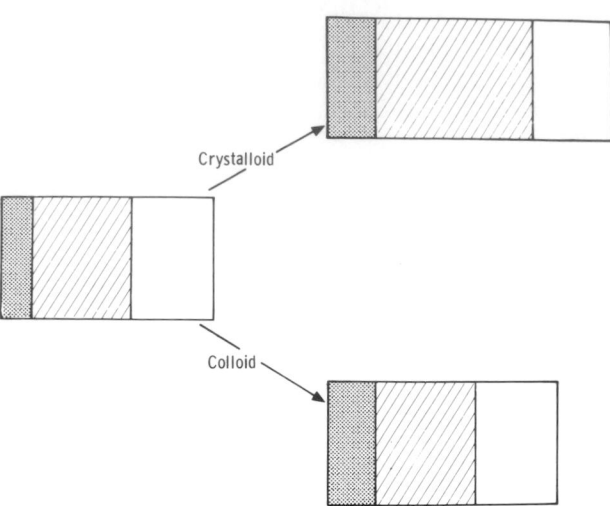

Fig. 38.2 The dotted area represents the intravascular compartment, the striped area the interstitial space (ISS), the unmarked area the intracellular space (ICS). Resuscitating a hypovolaemic patient with crystalloid will eventually restore the circulatory volume at the expense of an overexposed ISS, whereas whereas colloids are mainly confined to the intravascular compartment. (Adapted with permission from Twigley and Hillman, 1985).

Clinical Basis for Fluid Administration

When we administer an intravenous fluid we have to ask ourselves to which body fluid compartment the administered fluid will be distributed and on what basis do we estimate those compartments in order to give the correct amount.

The intravascular compartment is the most accessible. We are provided with many relatively 'hard' end-points about this small but crucial space—for example, pulse rate, BP, urine output, peripheral perfusion as well as right and left atrial pressures. However, most of these measurements owe as much to the performance of the heart and vascular resistance as to the volume status of the patient (Parkin, 1986). Even if blood volume could be conveniently measured it does not indicate the influence of that volume on cardiovascular dynamics. A 'normal' blood volume of 5 L may be inadequate for the vasodilated IVS associated with septicaemia. Intravascular pressure is therefore a more important indication of the adequacy of the blood volume for a particular IVS. If the heart could be stopped the distending pressure within all parts of the circulation would be equal and this pressure would depend on the blood volume and vascular compliances (Guyton et al., 1954). This pressure is called the mean circulatory filling pressure and is approximately 7 mmHg.

In practical terms to test the volume status of the circulation a fluid challenge is given. As many intravascular measurements as possible are made, then 200–300 ml of fluid is rapidly given and the measurements repeated. This manoeuvre is repeated until the normal circulating intravascular volume is restored.

Currently, there is very little information on the two largest body fluid compartments—the interstitial and intracellular spaces. 'Soft' end-points such as thirst, dry mucosa, tissue turgor and fluid balance charts offer empirical guidelines at best. Thus administration of a crystalloid solution which is largely distributed to the ISS is titrated against almost non-existent end points. The best that can be hoped for, if we assume that the body fluid compartments are intact, is that intravascular measurements will tell us the crystalloid solution is proportionately being distributed to the ISS at a rate of approximately 1:3. Water in the form of isotonic 5% dextrose will be distributed mainly to the ICF with proportionately less to the ISS and a small amount to the IVS. As we cannot measure the volume of ICS, the best clinical guide to body water needs is serum sodium. In the absence of factitious hyponatraemia or hyperglycaemia, the serum sodium concentration reciprocally reflects TBW (Edelman et al., 1958; Parkin, 1986). The gain or loss of body fluid with isotonic saline does not affect the plasma sodium concentration, rather it affects the volume of ECF. The major source of ion free water loss is from the urine or as insensible losses from the lungs and skin. Similarly, hypotonic losses will effect plasma sodium concentrations as well as ECF volume.

Water in the form of 5% dextrose can be titrated against plasma sodium concentration if it is high and alternatively water should be restricted if the serum sodium is low (Rose, 1986).

The principles of fluid and electrolyte management are the same whether it is for multi-trauma, sepsis, diabetic ketoacidosis or the perioperative period. The priorities are to urgently correct hypovolaemia and shock, then the serum potassium and finally to electively correct the water and other electrolyte abnormalities including sodium, phosphate, magnesium and calcium (Hillman, 1987a; b). For example, the major fluid and electrolyte problem in shock is hypovolaemia, not salt and water loss (Kaufman et al., 1984). Apart from hypovolaemia, the urgency and rate of correction of the other abnormalities depends on the rapidity with which they developed. For example, a serum sodium of 115 mmol/L should be slowly corrected (e.g. over 48–72 h) if it occurred over days to weeks; alternatively it should be rapidly corrected if it occurred over minutes to hours (Rose, 1986). Similarly, water losses should be replaced slowly if they occurred over days or weeks such as in diabetic ketoacidosis (Rose, 1986; Hillman, 1987b).

The Effects of Stress on Fluid and Electrolyte Balance.

There is a generalized metabolic response to stress, where stress includes insults such as surgery, trauma and other conditions associated with the critically ill. Moore and Ball (1952), in their classic studies demonstrated four phases associated with stress. Firstly, the phase of injury, characterized by adrenergic and adrenocortical hormone release resulting in salt and water retention, potassium loss and protein catabolism. To a greater or lesser extent this phase is prolonged by sepsis, shock and tissue necrosis. The other three phases are associated with recovery. The corticoid withdrawal phase occurs during the third to seventh uncomplicated postoperative day and is associated with a diuresis. The next phase results in regaining muscular strength and lasts two to five weeks. The final phase involves replacement of adipose tissue.

While Moore and Ball (1952), demonstrated salt and water retention in the early postoperative period, Shires et al., (1961) postulated that the extracellular volume decreased during major surgery due to internal redistribution of fluid, possibly as a result of wound oedema or ileus. While some studies have supported Shires's work others have failed to demonstrate a decrease in ECF and have criticized the experimental technique used by Shires (Twigley et al., 1985). The problem is largely related to the technical difficulties involved in measuring the ECF volume.

The practical conclusions are therefore difficult to summarize. Salt and water retention does occur in response to stress. Furthermore, up to 600–1000 ml of sodium free water is generated per day from catabolism in the postoperative period (Moore, 1959). Antidiuretic hormone (Sinnatamby et al., 1974) and aldosterone (Casey et al., 1957) are released in response to the stress of surgery. Whether the response is obligatory or not is as yet unknown. If it is obligatory, giving salt and water in the presence of salt and water retention would seem illogical (Fisher, 1977). However, it has been suggested that the stress response can be modified by adequate fluid replacement (Candell, 1968; Hayes et al., 1959; Irvin et al., 1972). Others suggest that despite adequate fluid replacement, ADH (Sinnatamby et al., 1974) and aldosterone (Hayes et al., 1957) increase in the perioperative period. If intravascular volume reduction is the major determinant of the salt and water retention associated with stress, then rapid correction with the appropriate fluid would seem logical. However, both Moore and Shires have urged moderation (Moore and Shires, 1967) in perioperative fluid regimes following excessive perioperative use of fluid after Shires et al. (1961) publication. Nevertheless, our fluid prescribing habits in the postoperative period are probably still on the generous side.

Complications of Expansion of the Interstitial Space

One of the complications of administering salt and water in the presence of salt and water retention is overexpansion of the ISS. If measurements of the IVS are used to administer fluids such as crystalloids which are mainly distributed to the ISS, they will inevitably cause an overexpansion of that space if adequate intravascular volume is to be achieved.

While as little as 1 litre of isotonic saline can adversely affect pulmonary function (Collins et al., 1973) moderate expansion of the ISS is probably not clinically significant. However, with major surgery or in the critically ill, large volumes of crystalloids are often needed to maintain the intravascular volume. This can cause overt hypoxia and pulmonary oedema (Boutros et al., 1979; Rackow et al., 1983; Shoemaker, 1976; Skillman et al., 1975). Moreover the cell architecture and integrity is disrupted and there is less efficient reabsorption of protein by lymphatics (Guyton et al., 1971).

Recently it has been demonstrated that expansion of the ISS in the periphery, resulting in peripheral oedema significantly impedes oxygen exchange (Hauser et al., 1980). This may be due to decreased diffusion between the capillaries and cells because of the increased distance or even occlusion of the capillaries by increased ISS pressure.

While small increases in the ISS may not be clinically important, doubling the ISS decreases tissue oxygen tension by such an extent that a twenty-fold increase in capillary flow is needed to re-establish the oxygen tension levels (Knisely et al., 1969) and these levels of tissue hypoxia are associated with delayed wound healing (Mangalore and Hunt, 1972).

In the critically ill, overexpansion of the ISS is potentiated by factors apart from administration of excessive salt and water and its retention as a result of neuroendocrine mechanisms. Positive intrathoracic pressure as a result of artificial ventilation reduces lymphatic return and increases extrathoracic venous pressure. Immobility and decreased COP can also contribute to oedema formation. Because of the extent of expansion of the ISS in these patients severe complications can result.

Overexpanded ISS in the lungs causes pulmonary oedema and hypoxaemia (Heughan et al., 1972; Shoemaker et al., 1981; Kaufman et al., 1984) resulting in decreased oxygen delivery. Over expansion of the ISS in the peripheral tissues causes decreased oxygen consumption (Hauser et al., 1980; Kaufman et al., 1984).

Manipulation of the Body Fluids
(Fig. 38.5)

Initial access to the body fluids is traditionally by venous cannulation of the IVS. The other spaces are not directly accessible. Each fluid's distribution can be largely predicted. Colloid or blood goes mainly into the IVS, crystalloid solutions are distributed mainly to the ISS and 5% dextrose to the intracellular space. Each body fluid space is, of course, in equilibrium with each other and the distribution of each fluid can be estimated by its COP and sodium content.

Apart from the IVS, elimination of fluid is more difficult. The IVS is uniquely amenable to drug manipulation, either by vasodilatation or vasoconstriction. Elimination of fluid from the interstitial and intracellular spaces can be achieved with drugs such as

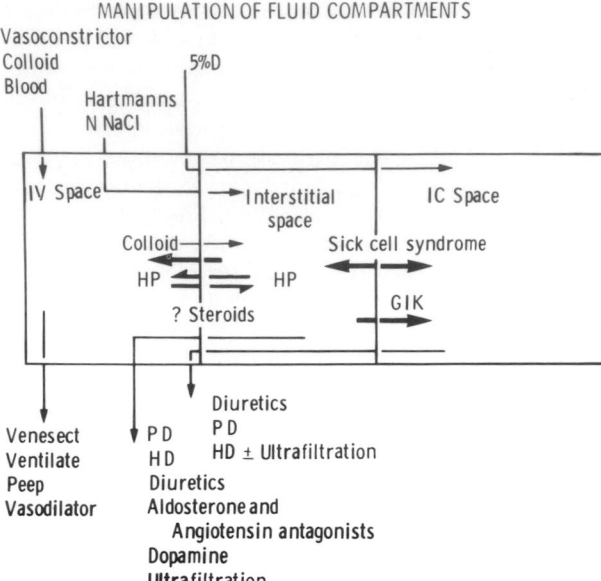

MANIPULATION OF FLUID COMPARTMENTS

Fig. 38.3 The different fluid compartments and how they may be manipulated are represented. By access through vascular cannulation the various fluids are mainly distributed to one compartment or another. Similarly, using various drugs or techniques fluid can be removed from the fluid compartments. Fluid can also be encouraged to move from one compartment to another. The following key is used:
PD–peritoneal dialysis,
HD–haemodialysis,
GIK–glucose insulin and potassium,
HP–hydrostatic pressure,
PEEP–positive end expiratory pressure,
IV–intravascular.

diuretics, aldosterone and angiotensin antagonists or by techniques such as dialysis or ultrafiltration.

Fluids can be encouraged to move from one compartment to another by a combination of strategies.

For example, a patient with peripheral oedema in the face of hypovolaemia and hypotension can be given a solution containing colloid to correct the hypovolaemia and increase the COP while simultaneously a diuretic or ultrafiltration decreases the ISS. Similarly glucose, insulin and potassium can be given to move water intracellularly.

Practical Guidelines to Fluid and Electrolyte Therapy

Perioperative fluid balance remains largely empirical. For example, a bottle of Ringer's lactate titrated against the BP intraoperatively and 2–3 L/d of salt containing solutions postoperatively. Whether this is logical or illogical and whether it has influenced perioperative morbidity and mortality in an adverse or beneficial way remains unanswered. For most uncomplicated procedures it is probably not clinically significant. Large errors in the administration of fluids and electrolytes are corrected by the body's own homeostatic mechanisms. These depend on the thirst mechanism to control intake, normal kidneys to control output and an intact gastrointestinal tract for absorption of both the fluids and electrolytes.

It is when these mechanisms are compromised that more precise knowledge and skills are needed. The medical staff must assume the role of the body's near-perfect system. In perioperative patients with large intraoperative fluid losses, where postoperative unconsciousness or compromised renal function is anticipated, a more meticulous approach is needed. Similarly, in the Intensive Care Unit, the patient is often unconscious with compromised renal function requiring large volumes of fluid, for example, in septic shock. We must be clear about which fluids are distributed to which spaces, how to assess those spaces clinically and what are the short-comings of that assessment. Moreover we must be familiar with drugs and techniques used to manipulate the fluid within those spaces, the physiological principles of move-

TABLE 38.5
COMPOSITION OF COMMONLY USED IV SOLUTIONS
(mmol/L)

	Na	K	Ca	Mg	Cl	Lactate	Dextrose g/100 ml	pH	Osmolality
0.9% NaCl	154	—	—	—	154	—	—	5.0	308
0.4% Saline (N/2)	77	—	—	—	77	—	—	5.2	154
Hartmanns Solution (Ringer's lactate)	131	5	1	1	112	29	—	6.5	280
4.3% Dextrose in fifth normal saline (0.18% NaCl)	31	—	—	—	31	—	43	4.0	300
5.0% Dextrose	—	—	—	—	—	—	50	4.0	278
2.5% Dextrose in 0.45 Saline (N/2)	75	—	—	—	75	—	25	4.0	280
3.75% Dextrose in 0.225% NaCl (N/4)	37.5	—	—	—	37.5	—	37.5	4.0	280

ment of fluid between the spaces and the danger of overfilling (e.g. interstitial oedema) or underfilling (e.g. hypovolaemia) the body's fluid spaces.

REFERENCES

Anderson R.J., Cronin R.E., McDonald K.M., et al. (1976). Mechanism of portal hypertension induces alterations in renal hemodynamics, renal water excretion, and renin secretion. *J. Clin. Invest.*, **58**, 964.

Baek S.M., Makabali G.G., Bryan-Brown C.W., et al. (1975). Plasma expansion in surgical patients with high central venous pressure (CVP); the relationship of blood volume to hematocrit, CVP, pulmonary wedge pressure and cardiorespiratory changes. *Surgery*, **78**, 304.

Ballerman B.J., Brenner B.M. (1986). Role of atrial peptides in body fluid homeostasis, *Circ. Res.*, **58**, 619.

Beeuwkes R. III., Ichikawa I., Brenner B.M. (1981). The renal circulations. In *The Kidney*, 2nd edn., p. 249. (Brenner B.M., Rector F.C. Jr. eds.). Philadelphia: W.B. Saunders.

Beran A.V., Tolle C.D., Huxtable R.F. (1981). Cutaneous blood flow and its relationship to transcutaneous O_2/CO_2 measurements. *Crit. Care Med.*, **9**, 736.

Boutros A.R., Ruess R., Olsen L., et al. (1979). Comparison of hemodynamic, pulmonary, and renal effects of use of three types of fluids after major surgical procedures on the abdominal aorta. *Crit. Care Med.*, **7**, 9.

Candell W.B. (1968). Parenteral Fluid Therapy. *Surg. Clin. N. Amer.*, **48**, 707.

Casey J.H., Bickel E.Y., Zimmerman B. (1957). The pattern and significance of aldosterone excretion by the post-operative surgical patient. *Surg. Gynecol. Obstet.*, **105**, 179.

Collins J.V., Cockrane G.M., Davis J., et al. (1973). Some aspects of pulmonary function after rapid saline infusion in healthy subjects. *Clin. Sci. Molec. Med.*, **45**, 407.

Cowley A.W. Jr., Barber W.J., Lombard J.H., et al. (1986). Relationship between body fluid volumes and arterial pressure. *Fed. Proc.*, **45**, 2864.

de Bold A.J. (1986). Atrial natriuretic factor: an overview. *Fed. Proc.*, **45**, 2081.

de Bold A.J., Borenstein H.B., Veress A.T., et al. (1981). A rapid and potent natriuretic response to intravenous injection of atrial myocardial extract in rats. *Life Sci.*, **28**, 89.

de Wardener H.E., Millis I.H., Clapham N.F., et al. (1961). Studies on efferent mechanism of sodium diuresis which follows administration of intravenous saline in dogs., *Clin. Sci.*, **21**, 249.

Dorrington K.L. (1981). Skin Turgor: do we understand the clinical sign? *Lancet*, **i**, 264.

Edelman I.S., Leibman J. (1959). Anatomy of body water and electrolytes. *Am. J. Med.*, **27**, 256.

Edelman I.S., Leibman J., O'Meara M.P. (1958). Interrelations between serum sodium concentration, serum osmolity and total exchangeable potassium and total body water. *J. Clin. Invest.*, **37**, 1236.

Fadnes H.O., Reed R.K., Aukland K. (1977). Interstitial fluid pressure in rats measured with a modified wick technique. *Microvasc. Res.*, **14**, 27.

Fisher M. McD. (1977). Postoperative intravenous therapy. *Anaesth. Intens. Care*, **5**, 339.

Gauer O.H., Henry J.P. (1963). Circulating basis of fluid volume control. *Physiol. Rev.*, **43**, 423.

Gruber V.F., Allgower M. (1970). Water and electrolyte balance. In *Scientific Tables*, (Diem K., Lentner C. eds.). Basle: Ciba-Geigy.

Guyton A.C. (1963). A concept of negative interstitial pressure based on pressures in implanted perforated capsules. *Circ. Res.*, **12**, 399.

Guyton A.C., Polizo D., Armstrong G.G. (1954). Mean circulatory filling pressure measured immediately after cessation of heart pumping. *Am. J. Physiol.*, **179**, 261.

Guyton A.C., Taylor A.E., Granger H.J., et al. (1971). Interstitial fluid pressure. *Physiol. Rev.*, **51**, 527.

Halperin B.D., Feeley T.W., Mihm F.G., et al. (1985). Evaluation of the portable chest roentgenogram for quantitating extravascular lung water in critically ill adults. *Chest*, **88**, 649.

Hauser C.J., Shoemaker W.C., Turpin I., et al. (1980). Oxygen transport responses to colloids and crystalloids in critically ill surgical patients. *Surg. Gynecol. Obstet.*, **150**, 811.

Hayes M.A., Brynes W.P., Goldenberg I.S., et al. (1959). Water and electrolyte exchanges during operation and convalescence. *Surgery*, **46**, 123.

Hayes M.A., Williamson R.J., Heidenreich W.F. (1957). Endocrine mechanisms involved in water and sodium metabolism during operation and convalescence. *Surgery*, **41**, 353.

Heughan C., Niinikoski J., Hunt E. (1972). Effect of excessive infusion of saline solution on tissue oxygen transport. *Surg. Gynecol. Obstet.*, **135**, 257.

Hillman K. (1986). Crystalloid or colloid. *Br. J. Hosp. Med.*, **35**, 217.

Hillman K. (1987a). Fluid replacement in the critically ill. *Med. Int.*, **2**, 1567.

Hillman K. (1987b). Fluid resuscitation in diabetic emergencies—a reappraisal. *Intens. Care Med.*, **13**, 4.

Hume R. (1966). Prediction of lean body mass from height and weight. *J. Clin. Pathol.*, **19**, 389.

Irvin T.T., Modgill V.K., Hyter C.J., et al. (1972). Plasma volume deficits and salt and water excretion after surgery. *Lancet*, **ii**, 1159.

Kaufman B.S., Rackow E.C., Falk J.L. (1984). The relationship between oxygen delivery and consumption during fluid resuscitation of hypovolemic and septic shock. *Chest*, **85**, 336.

Knisely M.H., Reneau D.D., Binely D.F. (1969). The development and use of equations for predicting limits on the rates of oxygen supply to the cells of tissues and organs. *Angiology*, **20**, 61.

Laragh J.H. (1985). Atrial natriuretic hormone, the renin-aldosterone axis, and blood pressure-electrolyte homeostasies. *N. Engl. J. Med.*, **313**, 1330.

Laragh J.H., Scaley J.E. (1973). The renin-angiotension-aldosterone hormonal system and regulation of sodium, potassium, and blood pressure homeostasis. In *Handbook of Physiology*, Section 8, p. 831. (Orloff J., Berliner R.W. eds.). Washington D.C.: American Physiological Society.

Laragh J.H., Sealey J.E., Brunner H.R. (1972). The control of aldosterone secretion in normal and hypertensive man: abnormal renin-aldosterone patterns in low renin hypertension. *Am. J. Med.*, **53**, 649.

Leaf A. (1970). Regulation of intracellular fluid volume and disease. *Am. J. Med.*, **49**, 291.

Leaning M.S., Pullen H.E., Carson E.R., et al. (1983). Modelling a complex biological system: the human cardiovascular system. 1. Methodology and model description. *Trans. Inst. Meas. Ctrl.*, **5**, 71.

Mangalore P.P., Hunt T.K. (1972). Effect of varying oxygen tensions on healing of open wounds. *Surg. Gynecol. Obstet.*, **135**, 756.

Meyer B.J., Meyer A., Guyton A.C. (1968). Interstitial fluid pressure. V. negative pressure in the lungs. *Circ. Res.*, **22**, 263.

Moore F. (1959). *Metabolic Care of the Surgical Patient*. p. 284 Philadelphia: W.B. Saunders.

Moore F., Olesen K., McMurrey J., et al. (1963). *The Body Cell Mass and its Supporting Environment. Body Composition in Health and Disease*. Philadelphia: W.B. Saunders.

Moore F.D., Ball M.R. (1952). *The Metabolic Response to Surgery*, 1st edn, Philadelphia: W.B. Saunders.

Moore F.D., Shires T. (1967). Moderation, *Ann. Surg.*, **166**, 300.

Mueller C.B., Surtshin A., Carlin M.R. (1951). Glomerular and tubular influences on sodium and water excretion. *Am. J. Physiol.*, **165**, 411.

Nilsson G.E., Tenland T., Oberg P.A. (1980). Evaluation of laser Doppler flowmeter for measurement of tissue blood flow. *IEEE Trans. Biomed. Eng.*, **27**, 597.

Pain R.W. (1977). Body Fluid Compartments. *Anaesth. Intens. Care*, **5**, 284.

Parkin G. (1986). Circulatory disorders: intervention and control. In *The Measurement in Medicine Series*. (Vol. 1), p. 313, (Cramp D.G., Carson E.R. eds.). London: Croom Helm.

Phillips P.J. (1977). Water metabolism. *Anaesth. Intens. Care*, **5**, 295.

Prentice T.C., Siri W., Berlin N.I., et al. (1952). Studies of total-body water with tritium. *J. Clin. Invest.*, **31**, 412.

Prout W.G. (1968). Relative value of central-venous-pressure monitoring and blood-volume measurement in the management of shock. *Lancet*, **i**, 1108.

Rackow E.C., Falk J.L., Fein I.A., et al. (1983). Fluid resuscitation in circulatory shock: a comparison of the cardiorespiratory effects of albumin, hetastarch, and saline solutions in patients with hypovolemic and septic shock. *Crit. Care Med.*, **11**, 839.

Randall M.T. (1976). Fluid electrolyte and acid-base balance. *Surg. Clin. North Am.*, **56**, 1019.

Raper R., Sibbald W.J. (1986). Misled by the wedge? *Chest*, **89**, 427.

Robertson G.L., Athar S., Shelton R.L. (1977). Osmotic control of vasopressin function. In *Disturbances in Body Fluid Osmolality*, p. 115. (Andreoli T.E., Grantham J.J., Rector F.C. Jr. eds.). Baltimore: Williams and Wilkins.

Robin E.D. (1985). The cult of the Swan-Ganz catheter. *Ann. Intern. Med.*, **103**, 445.

Rose B.D. (1986). New approach to disturbances in the plasma sodium concentration. *Am. J. Med.*, **81**, 1033.

Schrier R.W., Berl T., Anderson R.J. (1979). Osmotic and nonosmotic control of vasopressin release. *Am. J. Physiol.*, **236**, F321.

Shippy C.R., Appel P.L., Shoemaker W.C. (1984). Reliability of clinical monitoring to assess blood volume in critically ill patients. *Crit. Care Med.*, **12**, 107.

Shires T., Williams J., Brown F. (1961). Acute changes in extracellular fluids associated with major surgical procedures. *Ann. Surg.*, **154**, 803.

Shoemaker W.C. (1976). Comparison of the relative effectiveness of whole blood transfusions and various types of fluid therapy in resuscitation. *Crit. Care Med.*, **4**, 71.

Shoemaker W.C., Schluchter M., Hopkins J.A., et al. (1981). Fluid therapy in emergency resuscitation: clinical evaluation of colloid and crystalloid regimens. *Crit. Care Med.*, **9**, 367.

Sinnatamby D., Edwards C.R.W., Kitau M., et al. (1974). Antidiuretic hormone response to high and conservative fluid regimens in patients undergoing operation. *Surg. Gynecol. Obstet.*, **139**, 715.

Skillman J.J., Restall D.S., Salzman E.W. (1975). Randomized trial of albumin *vs* electrolyte solutions during abdominal aortic operations. *Surgery*, **78**, 291.

Smith H.W. (1957). Salt and water volume receptors: an exercise in physiologic apologetics. *Am. J. Med.*, **23**, 623.

Swan H., Nelson A. (1973). The chemical anatomy of extracellular water: contribution of erythrocyte water. *J. Cardiovasc. Surg.*, **14**, 515.

Sykes M.K. (1963). Venous pressure as clinical indication of adequacy of transfusion. *Ann. R. Coll. Surg.*, **33**, 185.

Tremper K.K., Shoemaker W.C. (1981). Transcutaneous oxygen monitoring of critically ill adults, with and without low flow shock. *Crit. Care Med.*, **9**, 706.

Twigley A.J., Hillman K.M. (1985). The end of the crystalloid era? *Anaesthesia*, **40**, 861.

Valeri C., Cooper A. (1973). Limitations of measuring blood volume with iodinated I^{125} serum albumin. *Arch. Intern. Med.*, **132**, 534.

Waxman K., Formosa P., Soliman H., et al. (1987). Laser doppler velocimetry in critically ill patients. *Crit. Care Med.*, **15**, 780.

39. Blood Transfusion and Notes on Related Aspects of Blood Clotting

D. James

Historical introduction
Blood groups
    The ABO blood group system
    The rhesus (Rh) blood group system
    Other blood group systems
Blood transfusion
Coagulation problems in relation to blood
    transfusion
    The coagulation mechanism
    Blood coagulation disturbances after
    massive blood transfusion

Historical Introduction

References in ancient Egyptian texts, Greek writings and medieval European records reflect the importance attached through the ages to the life giving properties of blood.

Initial attempts in the 17th century (e.g. by Lower in England and Denys in France) to effect transfusion of blood from one animal to another led eventually to transfusions from animals to humans, with disastrous consequences resulting in legal sanctions against the practice for about two centuries. Eventually, Blundell (1818) and others obtained occasional, though unpredictable successes using humans for both donors and recipients and thereby restored interest in the possibilities of blood transfusion therapy.

The key event in further progress was the work of Karl Landsteiner, whose researches into the differences between individuals of the same species led to the discovery of human blood groups. He described the blood groups, A, B and O (1900) and two of his co-workers described the fourth and rarest group (AB) of this system. Using animals immunized with human red cells, Landsteiner and Levine discovered the M, N and P groups and again using rabbits and guinea pigs immunized with erythrocytes of the monkey, *Macaca rhesus*, Landsteiner and Wiener discovered the Rhesus groups in 1939, a finding of paramount clinical importance.

In spite of the discovery of the ABO blood group system in the early 1900s, another major transfusion problem remained, namely the lack of a safe anticoagulant. In 1914–15 it was shown that non-toxic amounts of citrate could be used for this purpose and this led eventually to the development in 1943 by Loutit and Mollison of an acid-dextrose solution which has been in use in Britain since that time as ACD solution. This has the following composition:

Disodium citrate (monohydric)	2 g
Dextrose (anhydrous)	3 g
Water	120 ml

to be mixed with 420 ml of blood.

However, whole blood is now almost invariably supplied in plastic packs containing about 520 ml of citrated blood consisting of 450 ml of donor blood and 63 ml of citrate phosphate dextrose (CPD) anticoagulant solution or more recently CPD with added adenine (CPD-A). The adenine has improved red cell preservation and allowed extension of the expiry date to 35 days (previously only 21 days), the blood being stored at $4°–6°C$.

The development of techniques for freezing red blood cells (RBCs) under controlled conditions using added cryo-biological agents now allows almost indefinite preservation of the cells apparently with little loss of cell viability. Not only can blood of rare groups be stored and preserved but, where facilities and finances allow, the fear of sudden blood shortages due to strikes, storms etc can be virtually eliminated in the short term by hospitals able to maintain a stockpile of frozen blood.

The advent of an acceptable 'artificial blood' or non-cellular blood substitute still eludes discovery. Its potential value is immediately apparent. Not only could such an agent be used for military and civilian emergencies but also for patients needing long-term transfusions and less often for the patient refusing transfusion for religious reasons. The primary function of blood substitutes is the intravascular transport of oxygen but secondarily they could also act as short-term plasma expanders. Of those so far tested, only stroma-free haemoglobin and perfluorochemicals (PFCs) have shown much promise. However, free haemoglobin is too rapidly excreted while various PFCs may give rise to adverse reactions or require additional manipulations which make their use impractical. Thus some PFCs have a capacity for oxygen greater than that of erythrocytes but at normal P_{O_2} their ability to deliver oxygen is only 25–33% that of blood. To be used effectively, a 100% oxygen environment is necessary to maintain the normal arterial-venous oxygen difference. Another PFC (Fluosol-DA 20%) must be stored frozen to maintain its stability and while the initial results were promising, pulmonary complications and haemopoietic depression etc. have delayed its acceptance. Nevertheless, in view of the current AIDS epidemic and the danger of transmitting viruses to patients by transfusion, the urgent need for safe cell-free blood substitutes is obvious and the ongoing search for a satisfactory 'artificial blood' must be encouraged.

BLOOD GROUPS

Human blood groups are important clinically since

they are systems of antigens which may react with corresponding antibodies *in vivo* to produce harmful or even fatal results—(*see* Hazards of Blood Transfusion). Antigenic characteristics (or determinants) which represent the immunological differences between the red cells, etc. are under genetic control (*see* Inheritance of Blood Groups).

To date, a total of about eleven distinct blood group systems have been demonstrated, one of which (Xgᵃ) is unique in being sex linked. However, of the many blood group systems known, ABO and Rhesus are by far the most important in routine clinical work although from time to time tranfusion reactions and haemolytic disease of the newborn (HDN) occur due to less common blood group antigens.

White cells and platelets carry some of the antigens found on red cells, e.g. those of ABO, MN and P systems but apparently not others, e.g. the Rhesus system. Until recently, both white cells and platelets were thought to carry other (HLA) antigens not found on mature red cells and which were of particular importance in organ transplantation and rejection phenomena. Using automated techniques with increased sensitivity it has been shown, however, that some red cell antigens, e.g. Bgᵃ do have partial if not complete identity with certain HLA antigens (Morton et al., 1969, 1971). These leucocyte antigens are the subject of the rapidly developing field of 'tissue' or more correctly lymphocyte typing in relation to organ transplantation, etc. and will be considered later (*see* Hazards of Blood Transfusion).

Antigen is taken to mean any substance that has the ability to evoke an *in vivo* immune response upon parenteral injection into an immunologically competent animal. A most important requirement, especially for its detection, is that the antigen can react with the products of such a response, i.e. the corresponding antibody, both *in vivo* and *in vitro*.

Antibodies are specific serum proteins produced in the lymphoid tissue as a result of stimulation with an antigen and can react with the latter *in vivo* and *in vitro*.

Alleles in this context are taken to mean alternative forms of the genes (and hence the blood group antigens) concerned at a single locus on a chromosome.

Inheritance of Blood Group Antigens

A set of 23 chromosomes inherited from each parent resulting in a total of 46 chromosomes is found in the human somatic cell. The male is distinguished by the replacement of one of the two X chromosomes of the female by the smaller Y chromosome.

The genes controlling antigenic structure of a particular blood group system occupy specific loci on corresponding chromosomes. Such genes may be identical (homozygous, e.g. *BB*) or different (heterozygous, e.g. *BO*). Unless the gene is modified or suppressed then it can be demonstrated *in vitro* as a

particular blood group antigen, e.g. A or B; however, some genes do not produce demonstrable effects, e.g. the gene for group O. Hence an individual's genotype (i.e. the sum of the genetic blood group characteristics obtained from both parents) may not be the same as his phenotype (the demonstrable genes present), thus a phenotype of B may be of genotype *BB* or *BO* (Table 39.1).

TABLE 39.1
ABO GROUPS AND CORRESPONDING GENOTYPES

Blood group (phenotype)	Possible genotypes
A	*AA*
	AO
B	*BB*
	BO
O	*OO*
AB	*AB*

The fact that gene inheritance is Mendelian allows the prediction of the possible blood group of an unborn child. In practice this often permits the selection of blood of suitable group for exchange transfusion prior to its delivery. It may play an essential part in medico-legal cases involving paternity issues. An example is shown in Fig. 39.1.

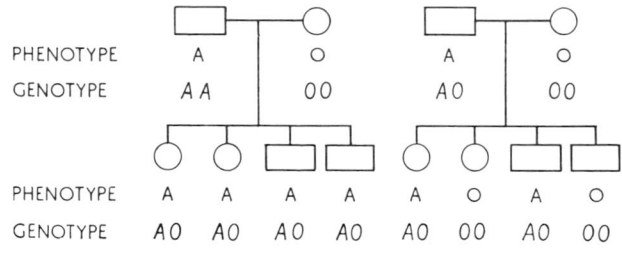

Fig. 39.1

To illustrate the mode of inheritance—a particular type of mating, as that in which a group A male mates with a group O female can be considered. The group A male may be of genotype *AA* or *AO* and the female will be of genotype *OO*, therefore within this mating subdivisions exist, namely (a) *AA* with *OO* and (b) *AO* with *OO*. The outcome of the two matings is shown in Fig. 39.1, namely, that the children of such a mating would be group (phenotype) A or O. Blood of group A and group O would be selected in advance for this case, should an exchange transfusion be under consideration.

Chemistry of the Blood Group Antigens

The studies of Morgan and Watkins, Kabat and others have shown that A, B, H and Lewis substances are glycoproteins combined with carbohydrates and appear to be closely related in structure and composition. They are thought to consist of a number of relatively short oligosaccharide chains attached at intervals to a peptide basis. The same five sugars and fifteen amino acids are found in pure A, B, H and Le^a substance. Differences in specificity depend partly on which sugar occupies the terminal position or side chains of the molecule and partly on the nature of the linkages between one sugar and the next.

Recent work has shown that the I antigen is a very complex system of antigens derived from a precursor glycoprotein devoid of A, B, H Le^a and Le^b activity. Similarly, the M and N antigens are now yielding to biochemical analysis. Desite its clinical importance the complex structure of the Rhesus antigens has not yet been fully resolved.

Blood Group Antibodies

Antibody activity is mostly confined to the gamma globulin fraction of plasma, forming the general group known as Immunoglobulins (Ig) which consists of five distinct classes called IgM, IgG, IgA, IgD and IgE based on physicochemical and serological properties. The blood group antibodies are associated with the IgM, IgG and IgA classes. The chemistry of IgG but not IgM and IgA has been well worked out and the structure of a typical IgG molecule is shown in Fig. 39.2.

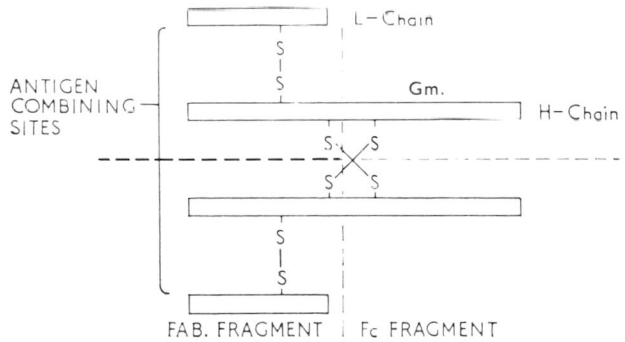

Fig. 39.2

In general, IgG represents the immune 'warm' acquired 7S antibodies with molecular weight of about 160 000 and which can cross the placenta, e.g. immune anti-D. IgM represents mainly naturally-occurring cold antibodies having a high molecular weight of about 900 000 which cannot cross the placenta, e.g. anti-A and anti-B. IgA antibodies form an intermediate group which also cannot cross the placenta (Table 39.2).

TABLE 39.2
GENERAL COMPARISON OF BLOOD GROUP ANTIBODY
TERMINOLOGIES AND PROPERTIES

	'Naturally occurring' antibodies	'Immune' antibodies
Synonyms	Complete	Incomplete*
	Saline agglutinating	Albumin agglutinating
	'Cold' (20°C and below)	37°C
Recent term	yM, β_2M	yG
Present name	IgM	IgG*
Molecular weight	900 000	c. 160 000
Sedimentation	19S	7S
Placental transmission	No	Yes

* Occasionally IgG antibodies occur as incomplete and/or complete antibodies.

The ABO Blood Group System

Following Landsteiner's discovery of the ABO blood group system, von Dungern and Hirszfeld (1911) not only first described subgroups of A but also showed that ABO genes were inherited. However, the exact mode of inheritance was determined by Bernstein (1924). The relationship of the gene O (recognized as Blood Group O) to the antigens H, A and B, has been explained by Morgan and Watkins. Thus beginning with a precursor mucopolysaccharide substance which is moulded by the gene *H* into H substance, the H in turn is partly converted by the independent genes *A* or *B* into A or B antigens. *O* is an amorphous gene which effects no conversion hence group O cells contain only H substance. The H antigen is of considerable importance then since it appears to be the basic ground substance from which the A and B antigens are derived. Occasionally anti-H, a 'cold' antibody, may achieve clinical significance if of high titre and if the individual has to undergo operation under hypothermic conditions.

Secretors

The antigens of the ABO system are found as glycolipid, alcohol-soluble components of all body tissue except perhaps brain and spinal cord. However, approximately 78% of individuals have the same antigens (corresponding to their ABO group) in a water-soluble form in their body secretions, e.g. saliva, urine, sweat, but not in CSF. Such individuals are termed 'secretors' and this hereditary characteristic has been used in genetic studies.

The Subgroups of A

Von Dungern et al., 1911, showed that there were two types of group A antigen A_1 and A_2, also that serum from group B individuals contains two types of anti-A antibodies. One reacted with all group A and group AB red cells, the other is an anti-A$_1$ which only reacts with A$_1$ or A$_1$B cells. The difference between A$_1$ and A$_2$ appears to be qualitative since a number of A$_2$ individuals and almost 26% of A$_2$B individuals have anti-A$_1$ in their serum, i.e. A$_1$ has some component which is missing in A$_2$. A$_1$ can also be identified using an anti-A$_1$ lectin prepared from the seeds of *Dolichos biflorus*. Other subgroups of A exist all of which are weaker than A$_2$ (which is weaker than A$_1$) and have been designated A$_3$, A$_4$, A$_5$, A$_x$, etc. The A subgroups are sometimes clinically significant because:

1. Anti-A$_1$, although usually an unimportant cold antibody not active over 30°C occasionally has a higher thermal range and can then cause a transfusion reaction.
2. Weak subgroups of A including A$_2$ can only be detected with high potency testing sera and failure to detect them may result in grouping the individual incorrectly as group O instead of A$_2$ or group B instead of A$_2$B. Subsequent transfusion with group O blood may lead to a reaction or accelerated destruction of the patient's A cells.

Weak subgroups of the B antigen exist but are extremely rare.

The ABO Isoantibodies

Anti-A and anti-B occur with such precise regularity in the plasma serum that Landsteiner formulated his 'Rule' that their presence or absence must be ascertained for the definitive establishment of the blood groups (Table 39.3). In addition 2% of A$_2$ individuals

TABLE 39.3
ANTIGEN AND ANTIBODY CONTENT OF THE RED CELLS AND
SERUM OF THE ABO BLOOD GROUP SYSTEM

Group	Antigen on red cells	Antibodies in serum	Frequency in English population (%)
O	NONE	anti-A, anti-B	47
A	A	anti-B	42
B	B	anti-A	8
AB	A and B	NONE	3

and 26% of A$_2$B contain anti-A$_1$. Because of the predictable occurrence of these antibodies in all individuals without apparent antigenic stimulation they are referred to as 'naturally occurring'. They are detectable by routine tests in the serum three to six months after birth—remaining throughout life. Their absence in infants of less than three months demands care in determination of the blood group, especially since at that age the A antigen is immature and may be only weakly reactive. The mechanism by which

anti-A and anti-B are produced is still disputed. Experimental evidence supports the theory that A and B antigens are ubiquitous in nature, e.g. in the bacterial flora of the intestinal canal, hence while a group A individual would not produce anti-A against a bacterial A antigen he would produce anti-B and vice versa.

Immune anti-A and anti-B may be found in individuals lacking the antigen and who have received it via transfusions, pregnancies or various vaccines such as tetanus and diphtheria toxoids (all of which may contain traces of A or B antigens). These immune antibodies differ in important respects from their naturally occurring counterparts in that they bind complement and are haemolytic both *in vivo* and *in vitro*, further they are most active at 37°C. Their possible and unsuspected presence in group O donor blood, the so called 'universal donor' should be noted since on many occasions the transfusion of group O to blood group A or B recipients has produced a brisk haemolytic reaction. Since the immune antibody is in the donor plasma, its potential danger will not be demonstrated on the major cross-match which tests only donor cells against recipient serum. Its presence must be suspected and excluded if, during the blood grouping of the donor, haemolysis is noticed in the tube containing incubated donor serum and control group A cells. A haemolytic titre of one in four or less is within normal limits; higher titres may make the donor a 'dangerous universal donor' and the blood should only be given to the group O recipient.

Basic blood grouping techniques have continued almost unchanged since the Landsteiner era, but more recently automation has been used in this field and most Blood Transfusion Centres as well as larger hospitals, now use automatic equipment for carrying out this exacting but monotonous routine work. Human anti-A, B, D and anti-IgG/Complement (Coombs) typing sera have now been replaced by monoclonal antibodies.

The Rhesus (Rh) Blood Group System

When the Rhesus blood group system was discovered in 1940 by Landsteiner and Wiener it was thought that only one antigen was involved—tests having shown that 85% of white individuals reacted with sera from rabbits immunized against *Macaca rhesus* red cells. Such individuals were termed Rhesus positive and the remaining 15% Rhesus negative. This antirhesus antibody appeared to be identical with that described by Levine and Stetson (1939) as the cause of haemolytic disease of the newborn in their patient and thus the human antibody was also named anti-Rh. Later work showed that these antibodies were, in fact, not identical.

With more refined techniques the Rhesus system was shown to contain at least five important antigens (of which the D antigen remains by far the most important from the clinical viewpoint) and two main terminologies are in current use, that of Fisher and Race

(1944) (used in this review) and that of Wiener (USA). Fisher (1943) postulated the existence of three pairs of allelomorphic genes occupying three separate but closely linked loci on each of a pair of chromosomes. The genes and the antigens they controlled were called C and its allele c, E and e and D and d. Rhesus 'negative' is taken to imply the absence of the D antigen (D negative) when applied to recipients but blood donors *must* be cde/cde. It should be noted that the genes for C and c and E and e are co-dominant and that the antigen c is, after D, the most potent and common cause of haemolytic disease of the newborn. Anti-d has not yet been found and this fact not only has theoretical implications but it means that the presence or absence of that antigen cannot be verified *in vitro*. Thus the decision whether an individual is homozygous or heterozygous for the D antigen can only be a statistical one, based on the frequency with which D occurs in relation to the antigens C, c, E and e, all of which can be demonstrated *in vitro* using the corresponding antibody. The genotype report therefore always refers to the 'probable genotype' except in the case of cde/cde. A knowledge of the father's genotype (especially in respect of D) is of paramount importance in families where severe haemolytic disease of the newborn has been encountered (Fig. 39.3). An individual who is homozygous for D would pass on the D antigen to all his offspring while in the heterozygous case there would be a 50% chance of one half of the offspring being D negative.

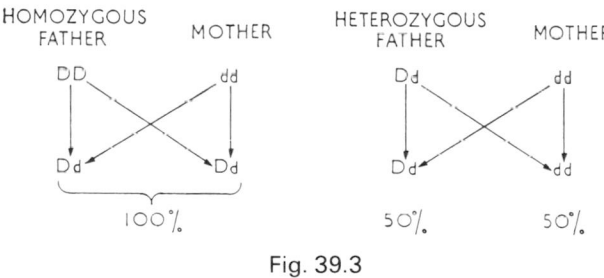

Fig. 39.3

Antigenic Variants

The D antigen is thought to be a mosaic composed of many factors called Rh^A Rh^B Rh^C Rh^D, etc. Where one or more components is missing the antigen is called a D^u. D^u individuals are usually detected because their cells will react with some anti-D sera but not with others. One variety of D^u is hereditary and here the D antigen may react so weakly *in vitro* that an antiglobulin test must be used to detect it. Another variety (non-hereditary) is due to the transposition of the C antigen in relation to the D. It can depress the D expression and is an example of 'gene interaction'. Rare individuals occur who are lacking in some Rh antigens, e.g. the variety —D— has the D antigen but

not C or E while the Rh null variety or ---/--- has no Rhesus antigen at all.

Rh Antibodies

Anti-Rh antibodies are most commonly found as incomplete agglutinins and require the addition of colloids such as albumin to the suspending media or the use of the antiglobulin technique of Coombs or enzymes for their detection. Naturally-occurring Rh antibodies are uncommon and in general D negative individuals never have anti-D antibodies unless they have received an antigenic stimulus through blood transfusion or pregnancy. Antibody production is dependent upon antigenicity and the frequency of occurrence of Rh antibodies suggests that the order of potency is D > c > C > E > e. Rh antibodies do not bind complement and are therefore not haemolytic.

Rh Groups and Haemolytic Disease of the Newborn (HDN)

Haemolytic disease of the newborn may be considered as an acquired haemolytic anaemia of the newborn of varying degree. The anaemia may be severe or very mild and it can cause intrauterine death. After delivery and without adequate treatment the associated hyperbilirubinaemia may cause bilirubin encephalopathy (kernicterus) and result in permanent brain damage.

Haemolytic disease of the newborn occurs when the mother lacks some blood group antigen and is immunized by fetal red blood cells, especially at delivery. In the event of subsequent pregnancies the resulting isoantibodies cross the placental barrier and react with the fetal erythrocytes leading to their destruction. Anti-D is by far the most important antibody in this respect. Paradoxically, the same immune anti-D given prophylactically after delivery of the first D-positive child to a D-negative mother has been shown conclusively to inhibit the sensitizing effect of the fetal cells on the mother. This treatment promises to end haemolytic disease of the newborn, due to the D antigen (which causes about 92 to 95% of all cases). The remainder of cases of haemolytic disease of the newborn due to anti-A or anti-B which are severe enough to require treatment are rare (about one in 3000 or less of all newborn infants): other blood group antibodies concerned include anti-c, anti-K, anti-k, anti-E and anti-Fy[a].

Other Blood Group Systems

Since the discovery of the ABO groups in 1900 many other blood group factors have been discovered. The discovery has usually resulted from the finding of an atypical antibody in the serum of a recipient of several transfusions or in that of a pregnant woman. In view of their lesser clinical significance only a very brief outline of them is considered here.

In the main the M, N, S and P groups are 'cold' agglutinins, i.e. giving strong reactions at about 20°C with little or no reactivity at 37°C. The significance of the corresponding antibodies in patients subjected to operation under hypothermic conditions remains unanswered but they are otherwise of little clinical importance unless their thermal range exceeds 30° above which they may be able to effect a reduced red cell survival time. Some have been known to cause tranfusion reactions, others have been associated with haemolytic disease of the newborn. It is doubtful if the P_1 and Lewis antigens have a role in histocompatibility and organ graft survival as was previously thought.

Kell (K), Cellano (k), Duffy (Fy^a and Fy^b), Kidd (Jk^a) and their related antigens are usually only detected by the antiglobulin (Coombs) reaction. They are often associated with transfusion reactions and occasionally cause haemolytic disease of the newborn, especially K and k which are exceptionally potent antigens, being second in strength only to D of the Rh system.

The I blood group system differs from others in many respects especially with regard to its slow maturation, its almost universal occurrence and the quantitative difference only existing between I positives and negatives. Anti-I and anti-i are cold agglutinins and may be found especially in the sera of patients suffering from primary atypical pneumonia and in autoimmune acquired haemolytic anaemia of the 'cold' antibody type. There is also a suspected inter-relationship between the I-i, ABO and P blood group systems.

Until the early 1960s all known red cell antigens were thought to be controlled by autosomal genes. The discovery of Xg as a sex linked blood group, i.e. occurring on the X chromosome, may assist considerably in chromosome mapping.

The Antiglobulin (Coombs) Test

The antiglobulin test, since its rediscovery and application by Coombs et al. (1945), resulted in the discovery of the Kell blood group system and has proved to be the outstanding serological finding in recent years.

The principle of the test was relatively simple and depended on the reasoning that since antibodies are globulins, then the injection of human sera or purified globulin into a susceptible animal would produce anti-human globulin antibodies. This reagent, suitably diluted, could be used to detect antibodies (globulins) on human red cells by allowing it to react with the antibody on the cell surface under controlled conditions, resulting in agglutination of the cells. The red cell itself simply becomes an indicator for the reaction.

Coombs and co-workers outlined two applications of the test—one to be performed on serum, referred to as the *indirect* test, and one to be used on red cells, known as the *direct* test. The *indirect* test is most frequently used to detect antibodies in the sera of pregnant women, or to learn whether antibodies are present in the recipient of a transfusion, as for example, in the crossmatch or compatibility test. The *direct* test is used to detect antibodies already absorbed or coated on the red cell surface. This may occur in haemolytic disease of the newborn in which case coating takes place *in utero* so that testing of cord blood will indicate whether the infant will be affected. Also, in cases of auto-immunization, e.g. acquired haemolytic anaemia, the test may be positive.

As in the case of blood grouping reagents, monoclonal rather than human antibodies are now used for this test.

Leucocyte (Lymphocyte) Agglutinins

The advent of 'tissue typing' for organ transplantation has accelerated the growth of knowledge regarding leucocyte antigens and antibodies. An extensive literature on white cell histocompatibility (HLA) antigens is now available. The significance of lymphocyte (HLA) antigens as a cause of graft *versus* host disease and HLA antibodies as a cause of febrile reactions is discussed under Hazards of Blood Transfusion.

BLOOD TRANSFUSION

A basic knowledge of human blood groups and antibodies is essential for those concerned with requesting or supervising blood transfusion procedures since otherwise they may be unaware of the many advantages and important hazards of this life saving procedure. The emphasis of this section is on the practical aspects of blood transfusion. For more detailed discussions the reader should refer to Mollison's textbook *Blood Transfusion in Clinical Medicine* (1988).

Blood Donors

Blood for transfusion is obtained in the UK from volunteer donors: in most other countries either all donors are paid or both systems operate. Donor protection includes restricting the frequency of donation to two or three times per year, the use of plasmapheresis wherever possible and insistence on a minimum haemoglobin level of 12.5 g per cent for females and 13.5 g per cent for males. Recipient protection depends mainly on accurate history taking from the donor to exclude maladies thought or known to be undesirable. Venereal diseases are excluded serologically. Patients who give a history of malaria or brucellosis should be excluded since these diseases are known to be transmissible by blood transfusion.

Very important advances have been made recently in detecting carriers of serum hepatitis (Hepatitis B). All blood donations issued by the British Blood Transfusion Centres are tested for the Hepatitis B surface antigen (HBsAg) and post-transfusion hepatitis B is claimed to have decreased significantly in the US since the advent of HBsAg testing. According to Barbara and Contreras (1986), 90% of cases are not now caused by the hepatitis A or B virus (non-A non-B hepatitis).

Transfusion-associated AIDS (acquired immune deficiency syndrome) has caused much concern in the general population regarding the safety of blood transfusions. AIDS is caused by a retrovirus, Human Immunodeficiency Virus (HIV), at first called Human T-cell Lymphotropic Virus (HTLV-111) or Lymph-adenopathy Associated Virus (LAV). Apart from exclusion of 'high risk' donors such as homosexuals and drug addicts, all blood donations are routinely tested for HIV antibodies.

Haemophiliacs who receive large amounts of clotting factor concentrates are particularly vulnerable and should only receive heat-treated clotting factor concentrates.

Care of Blood
Blood should not be issued for transfusion if it shows any evidence of haemolysis or is time expired.

The correct temperature for storage is from 4°–6°C (38°–42°F) and the refrigerator should have an automatic temperature recording device and battery operated alarm system. The temperature limits must be rigidly observed to preserve the red cells and minimize the multiplication of chance bacterial contaminants. Blood must never be allowed to freeze unless in a suitable medium such as glycerol, as used in long term preservation processes, since transfusion of blood which has been frozen and thawed may cause death. Food and pathological specimens must never be stored in the blood refrigerator. Blood for transfusion should not be out of the refrigerator for more than 30 minutes before transfusion, otherwise it should be discarded. Similarly, packed red cells, unless concentrated in a sterile closed system, e.g. plastic transfer pack, must be used within twelve hours and reconstituted plasma, fibrinogen or albumin within three hours. Packs of blood which have been partly used or entered in any way should always be discarded. No medicaments should be introduced into a blood pack prior to use.

Volume and Rate of Transfusion
The following factors must be considered:

1. The age of the patient.
2. The general condition.
3. The state of the circulation.
4. The indication for the transfusion.

The young adult with a normal myocardium will tolerate the rapid infusion of large volumes of colloid. On the other hand the chronically anaemic patient with an enfeebled myocardium or patients with respiratory or cardiac disorders or infective and toxic conditions should be transfused cautiously. The availability of potent diuretics, if correctly used, has significantly reduced the risk of circulatory overloading from over-transfusion. Severe injury with blood loss exceeding 20% of the circulating blood volume requires rapid and adequate restoration of the volume as the immediate aim.

In the treatment of anaemia it may be assumed that one unit of whole blood will raise the haemoglobin level about 1.0 g per cent. If, in the absence of continu-

ing blood loss the volume of whole blood required to raise the haemoglobin to the required level exceeds one third of the calculated blood volume, the transfusion should be given in two parts, separated by two days and the use of packed red cells should be considered.

The rate of administration should not normally exceed 20–40 ml per minute. In chronic anaemia with haemoglobin below 3.7 g per cent, cachexia, cardiac or respiratory disease, this rate may be halved and the venous pressure should be monitored for indication of overtransfusion. Patients with a septic condition or toxaemia should be treated with similar caution. Large volumes of fluid even if administered slowly over a long period should not be given as a single continuous transfusion in such conditions: it should be divided and given slowly as a number of small transfusions. It is usually recommended that no major surgical procedure should be carried out unless the haemoglobin is at least 10.4 g per cent. Where preoperative transfusions are necessary these should be completed at least twenty-four hours prior to the operation, partly to avoid the possibility of a reaction occurring at a time when the subjective signs would be masked by anaesthesia, but also because the oxygen dissociation curve of red cells stored in citrate is shifted to the left (storage lesion of red blood cells). For about twenty-four hours after transfusion such cells are incapable of releasing as much oxygen to the tissue as normal red cells, hence by diluting the patient's own blood in this way, there exists a temporary phase when the net effect is a decrease of oxygen availability for the tissues (Valtis and Kennedy, 1954).

Choice of Replacement Fluids
Transfusion should only be undertaken after careful assessment of the patient's clinical condition to determine the nature and volume of fluid to be transfused and the rate of administration. The patient may require whole blood, packed red cells, washed red cells, whole plasma or a specific blood component.

A transfusion should never be given without a definite indication in view of the element of risk involved (*see* Hazards of Blood Transfusion). It should never be used to correct moderate or slight degrees of anaemia. Emergency transfusions carry greater risks than well planned elective transfusions. Likewise the risk involved in giving single unit transfusions to adults often exceeds the possible benefits therefrom and these should be actively discouraged.

With continuing experience of blood transfusion therapy and important changes in emphasis in the mode of its application—the use of the standard product, i.e. stored whole blood, is rapidly giving way to a more sophisticated usage and range of blood products. Replacement fluids may be classified under:

A. Blood and cellular components.
B. Plasma and specific plasma components.
C. Plasma substitutes.
D. Electrolyte solutions.

A. Blood. Blood is still the most important therapeutic agent for the treatment of severe blood loss. The various forms in which it may be obtained are shown in Table 39.4.

B. Plasma and Specific Plasma Components. Since the shelf life of stored blood was only three weeks for ACD blood and was only five weeks for CPD-A blood now in current use, it is not surprising that there has been a ceaseless search for methods of producing longer term stable blood fractions. Table 39.5 shows some current stable plasma preparations and plasma components.

C. Plasma Substitutes (otherwise called plasma expanders, blood substitutes, etc.).

Natural plasma products or derivatives still form the best replacement fluids and some, e.g. Plasma Protein Fraction and Albumin have been heat treated during processing and therefore should be free from the AIDS and hepatitis viruses. However, the supply of these products is unlikely to meet the increasing demand for them—hence the need for infusion solutions containing artificial colloids. The requirements for a satisfactory artificial colloidal infusion solution include:

1. Should be capable of being administered at such

TABLE 39.4

A. BLOOD. SOME FORMS IN WHICH CELLULAR BLOOD PRODUCTS MAY BE AVAILABLE FOR TRANSFUSION

Form	Indication	Expiry	Comments
1. Stored whole blood: (a) Blood 450 ml CPD 63 ml	1. Haemorrhage—acute or chronic 2. Anaemia—acute or chronic 3. Oligaemic shock 4. Blood dyscrasias	35 days	CPD is the anticoagulant of choice for routine purposes
(b) Blood 450 ml Heparin 30 ml (2250 US units)	Where dilution of transfused blood is not desirable, e.g. cardiac surgery on infants	1–2 days	Heparinized blood deteriorates rapidly
2. Concentrated (plasma reduced) blood	Chronic refractory anaemias where increased haemoglobin is required but not blood volume	28 days	Increased viscosity may make transfusion more difficult
3. 'Almost fresh' whole blood	Transfusions in neonates	2 days	Used when minimal plasma potassium content and maximum survival of transfused red cells required
4. 'Washed' red cells (leucocyte reduced)	1. Paroxysmal nocturnal haemoglobinuria 2. Patients with known HLA or platelet antibodies 3. Transfusion reaction unrelated to red cell antigen systems (plasma reactors) 4. All pre and post organ transplantation patients 5. Patients with known immune deficiences, on massive irradiation or heavy immunosuppression therapy	Depends on preparation method About 6 h	Complete removal of leucocytes unlikely in practice
5. SAG–M (plasma reduced)	As for Form (1)	35 days	Plasma replaced with saline, adenine, glucose and mannitol solutions and viscosity problems should be avoided
6. Frozen red cells	As for Forms (1) and (4)	6 h after reconstitution	More expensive product but always available when required
7. Platelet rich plasma or concentrate	1. Thrombocytopenia with bleeding 2. Less than 40 000/mm³ before major surgery 3. During or after massive transfusion	72 h (store at 22°C)	One 50 ml (10^{10}) concentrate pack per 10 kg
8. Granulocyte transfusions	1. Myelosuppression and leucopenia in patients on cytotoxic therapy 2. Primary granulocytopenia 3. Severe overwhelming infection	24 h	May require irradiation to avoid danger of graft *v* host reaction

TABLE 39.5
B. PLASMA. SOME FORMS IN WHICH HUMAN PLASMA OR ITS COMPONENTS MAY BE AVAILABLE

Form	Indication	Expiry	Comments
1. Fresh frozen plasma	Replacement of all plasma clotting factors	1 year	Stored at − 25°C
2. Cryoprecipitate	1. Haemophilia 2. Von Willebrand's disease 3. Hypofibrinogenaemia	1 year	Stored at − 25°C. Moderate AHF content (80 IU) plus fibrinogen
3. Factor VIII (AHF) concentrate	Treatment of Haemophilia A	Freeze-dried Date on container	Contains 220 IU/ampoule Dosage based on 10–20 IU/kg
4. Plasma Protein Fraction (PPF)	1. Burns 2. Plasma expander for severe blood loss with oligaemic shock	Two years	Does not contain fibrinogen or gamma globulin. Preparation includes heat treatment—viruses inactivated
5. Albumin (salt poor)	1. Hypoalbuminaemia 2. Protein enteropathy 3. Nephrotic syndrome	2 years	20% solution Given to any blood group
6. Fibrinogen (3–4 g per bottle)	Afibrinogenaemia following severe bleeding, fibrinolytic therapy, defibrination	3 hours after preparation	Restricted supply

a concentration that its colloidal osmotic pressure is equivalent to that of normal blood plasma.

2. When employed to increase plasma volume after blood loss, there should be at least 50% retention for at least six and preferably for 12 hours.
3. The viscosity should not cause added work to the heart.
4. It should not interfere with haemostasis or blood coagulation at levels normally employed.
5. It should not interfere seriously with blood grouping.
6. It should be metabolized or eliminated from the body without causing delayed interference with the function of any organ, even after repeated administration.

The advantage of a satisfactory artificial colloidal solution would be:

1. It would help to save blood.
2. The risk of virus and other infections would be eliminated.
3. Such solutions could be kept available at places where emergency administration may be necessary, e.g. in ambulances.
4. Blood serology could be ignored and the solutions could be given irrespective of blood group.
5. Incidence of pyrogenic reactions, etc. would be reduced.
6. Long term storage would not present a problem.
7. The product would be available in unlimited quantities.

The plasma substitutes which are available are shown in Table 39.6.

Changes in Stored Blood
Certain changes occurring in stored blood are shown in Table 39.7.

Effects of Storage on Blood and Plasma Clotting Factors

Red Cells. In general, red cells in stored blood die at the rate of 1% for each day of storage and when stored under optimal conditions at 4°–6°C for 21 days should have a survival rate of not less than 70% for the first 24 hours after transfusion. The changes *in vitro* leading to loss of viability are still poorly understood.

Influence of Storage Medium
Red cells stored with trisodium citrate alone deteriorate rapidly with increased loss of potassium compared with storage in ACD. Storage with heparin alone results in clotting of stored blood after about 48 h.

Dextrose has a very favourable effect on preservation and probably provides energy for the synthesis of organic phosphate compounds particularly diphosphoglycerate and adenosine triphosphate (ATP) (Maizels, 1941).

Acidification is also beneficial hence the superiority of ACD over trisodium citrate alone. The ATP content of red cells falls more slowly in ACD solution which contains disodium hydrogen citrate-dextrose and there is good correlation between ATP content of stored red cells and their post-transfusion survival. Further improvement in prolongation of the expiry date has resulted from the addition of phosphate (CPD) and adenine (CPD-A) to the anticoagulant solution. Finally, replacement of the plasma with saline containing adenine, glucose and mannitol (SAG-M) also results in better red cell preservation permitting extension of the expiry time to 35 days (from the previous 21 days).

Influence of Storage Temperatures

Red Blood Cells. The accepted range of 4°–6°C repres-

TABLE 39.6
C. PLASMA. SUBSTITUTES

Form	Indication	Expiry	Comments
1. Dextran	1. Intitial treatment of haemorrhagic shock until compatible blood available 2. Shock conditions in burns, crash injuries, sepsis 3. Conditions where capillary circulation impaired (thrombosis, vascular insufficiency)	10 years	6% Dextran 70 (Macrodex) and 10% dextran 40 (Rheomacrodex) are most often used today. An extensive literature exists as to their respective merits. Blood for grouping and cross-matching should be taken before dextran is infused
2. Gelatin preparations: (a) Oxypolygelatin (b) Modified fluid gelatin (c) Crosslinked gelatin	Shock due to haemorrhage, burns, etc.		Crosslinked gelatin (Haemacel) is the best documented but in general there is insufficient data at present to recommend the use of gelatin preparations without reservations.
3. Polyvinyl pyrolidone (PVP)	Use discontinued		PVP cannot be metabolized in the body
4. Hydroxyethyl starch (HES) 6%	Volume expander		Undergoing clinical trials—insufficient data for full evaluation but initial results are optimistic

ents a temperature giving good preservation and one which is safely above the freezing point of blood. Red cell survival is significantly reduced if blood is stored at 25°C and deterioration is rapid at 37°C. Low temperatures also inhibit chance bacterial contaminants although some Gram negative bacilli can proliferate at blood bank temperatures.

Plasma Clotting Factors. Factor I (Fibrinogen) is stable in stored bank blood and fresh frozen plasma and can be successfully concentrated, permitting the administration of large amounts of fibrinogen in relatively small volumes of fluid.

Factor II (Prothrombin) is stable in bank blood under normal conditions of storage.

Factor V (Labile factor, Ac globulin) deteriorates

TABLE 39.7
CHANGES IN STORED CITRATED BLOOD (4° to 6°C)

According to Strumia and others					
Days	0	7	14	21	28
pH	7.1	6.85	6.75	6.68	6.65
Glucose mg%	350	300	245	210	190
Plasma Haemoglobin mg%	0–10	25	50	100	150
Potassium mmol/L	3–4	12	24	32	40
Ammonia µg%	50	260	470	680	—
Lactic acid mg%	20	70	120	140	150

during storage but the data is conflicting regarding its rate of disappearance *in vitro*.

Factor VII (Stable factor) is stable in bank blood under the usual conditions of storage.

Factor VIII (Antihaemophilic factor) deteriorates rapidly during storage of bank blood—as much as 50% may be lost after one or two weeks. It is best stored as fresh frozen plasma or as cryoprecipitate at $-20°C$ to $-30°C$.

Factor VIII concentrate is prepared freeze dried and can be stored at 4°C.

Factor IX is stable in bank blood.

Factor XI storage properties are not well documented.

Platelets. Platelets are transfused either as platelet rich plasma (PRP) or platelet concentrate (containing about 50% of the original platelets in 50 ml of plasma). Usually a pool of six ABO compatible platelet concentrates is used for an adult and repeated if necessary after two days, since the half-life of platelets is only about four days.

Unlike any other blood product, platelets are stored for up to five days at 22°C, preferably in modified plastic containers to allow optimal gaseous exchange and pH maintenance (Smith, 1987).

Leucocytes. Leucocyte transfusions are indicated essentially for neutropenic patients with severe infections not responding adequately to antibiotics. There are conflicting reports of the value of prophylactic granulocyte transfusions in severely neutropenic patients (Ford et al., 1980; Sutton et al., 1982).

The granulocytes may be prepared as buffy coats

from fresh blood donations (4–8 units being required for one adult treatment) or as concentrates obtained from single normal donors using a cell separator. The preparation must be transfused as soon as possible and well within 24 hours of collection. To avoid the danger of graft *versus* host reaction in immuno-suppressed patients, the leucocytes are irradiated (1500–2000 rad) without impairing their phagocytic properties.

Hazards of Blood Transfusion

Avoidance of transfusion hazards is the responsibility of the clinician and again it is stressed that every transfusion carries an element of risk and should never be given without a definite indication.

It is often forgotten that the donor also has to be protected against certain hazards. Thus a donor should not be bled (1) more often than 2–3 times yearly or (2) if pregnant and for one year following pregnancy or (3) if the haemoglobin in a female is less than 12.5 g per cent, in a male less than 13.5 g per cent—thus avoiding adverse effects on the iron balance. Additionally the donor is always at risk of vasovagal attacks, tetany due to hyperventilation, air embolism especially when blood is taken into glass bottles and sepsis at the point of insertion of the taking needle. A brief review of the main hazards to the patient is listed below:

1. Mortality. Mortality as a result of transfusion is about 0.1–1% and is thought to be comparable with that of appendicitis. Three thousand persons die annually in the USA due to transfusion; comparable figures are not available in the UK.

2. Transmission of Disease. The more important transfusion-transmitted diseases include (a) viral infections causing AIDS (acquired immune deficiency syndrome), hepatitis and cytomegalovirus (CMV) syndrome as well as (b) infections of non-viral origin such as syphilis, malaria and brucellosis. Screening tests of increasing sensitivity and specificity are used for all UK blood donations in respect of antibodies to the AIDS virus and for the hepatitis surface antigen (HBsAg). Syphilis is excluded serologically but exclusion of malaria and brucellosis depends initially on the donor's medical history.

Since at present there is no known cure for AIDS and its prevalence is increasing, the most careful selection of donors and restriction of blood transfusion only to patients for whom it is essential needs no emphasis. The most sensitive tests do not guarantee absence either of AIDS antibodies or the hepatitis viruses (Barbara et al., 1986).

3. Bacterial Contamination. Even with strict protocol for the arm-scrub procedure, a small degree (perhaps 2%) of bacterial contamination of stored blood can be expected from skin or air. The maintenance of optimal storage conditions (4°–6°C) is thus essential and

blood left out for more than 30 min at room temperature or higher at any one time and not used for immediate transfusion should be discarded. The greatest danger is caused by Gram negative bacteria, some cryophilic varieties being able to grow optimally at cold room temperatures. Less often, the contaminants may be Gram positive diphtheroids. Other points of entry for contaminants may be fine cracks in glass containers or tiny holes or faulty seals in the walls of plastic packs.

4. Pyrogenic Reactions. These may be due to pyrogens—polysaccharide products of bacterial metabolism—in the container or anticoagulant fluid. Tests for pyrogens in equipment and anticoagulant solutions are therefore essential before use. The incidence of pyrogenic reactions has decreased significantly following the use of disposable transfusion giving sets.

5. Incompatibility. A compatible blood transfusion is one in which transfused cells survive as long as the host red cells as well as *vice versa*. Incompatibility is where the survival time of transfused cells is reduced; this is not identical with haemolytic reactions which occur less frequently. Although the half-life of transfused cells is about 32 days, it has been shown that in 30% of all transfusions, especially in multi-transfused patients, the red cells only survive 14–16 days and then disappear from the vascular system, suggesting that the routine crossmatch by no means detects all patient–donor incompatibilities. The risk of iso-immunization is additive and is about 1% per blood transfusion.

6. Haemolytic Reactions. Haemolytic reactions refer to transfusion-associated events in which free haemoglobin is noted in the patient's post–transfusion serum, and often urine, or when an unexplained fall of the post–transfusion haemoglobin or haematocrit occurs. Haemolytic reactions initiated immunologically fall into two categories namely intravascular and extravascular transfusion reactions. The former are mediated by complement and may be fatal, the latter are invariably milder and often not detected except by chance. The majority are usually due to blood group incompatibility and may have a frequency of 0.2–0.3% or higher. Non-immunologic haemolytic reactions may be caused by blood incorrectly stored or time expired or already haemolysed, e.g. by overheating or freezing.

7. Allergic Reactions. These are relatively rare (1–1.5% of all transfusions) and range from urticarial reactions recognized by the distinctive urticarial rash (sometimes with pruritus) to the most severe form as anaphylactic shock with marked hypotension and requiring cessation of the transfusion and subcutaneous or intramuscular injection of adrenaline etc. Most allergic reactions allow continuation of the transfusion under antihistamine cover.

8. Citrate Toxicity. Stored blood contains citrate (as ACD or CPD) in solution and rapid transfusion of large volumes may cause tremors and cardiac arrhythmias due to metabolic acidosis. This is most likely to occur in severe shock, liver disease, in neonates or under hypothermic conditions. Plasma potassium elevation accompanies the decrease in pH. Normally the sodium citrate is rapidly metabolized to sodium bicarbonate in the liver and two litres of citrated blood can be transfused in about 20 minutes without danger of citrate intoxication. While 1 g of calcium gluconate is usually given per litre of citrated blood, Boyan and Howland (1969) suggest that calcium is not necessary and can sometimes be dangerous.

9. Acidity of Preserved Blood. ACD blood has a pH of about 7.1 decreasing to 6.6 with storage. Massive transfusion may cause a metabolic acidosis unless the blood is warmed under controlled conditions, and 3.75 g sodium bicarbonate given intravenously per 5 litres of blood is recommended by some workers to neutralize the acidosis. The more recent use of citrate phosphate dextrose (CPD) introduces two major differences from ACD, (1) the pH of stored whole blood is raised from about 6.6 to 7.3 and (2) the added phosphate with the raised pH together give better preservation of 2,3 diphosphoglycerate allowing more efficient unloading of stored oxygen especially in the first week of blood storage. The addition of adenine to the CPD (CPD-A) has extended red cell survival in stored blood from 21 to 35 days, thus allowing increased usage of available blood supplies.

10. Dangers of Cold Blood. Anaesthetized patients have impaired temperature regulation and if transfused rapidly with large volumes of cold blood suffer a fall in heart and body temperature. Oxygen consumption also increases. Children in particular are unable to compensate quickly for the fall in temperature and are prone to ventricular fibrillation and cardiac arrest (as in exchange transfusions). The value of using warm blood exclusively for massive transfusion, i.e. over 5 litres or so has been amply demonstrated. However, the blood must never be warmed over 40°C and warming devices must be thermostatically controlled.

11. Potassium Intoxication. Fresh stored blood contains about 4–5 mmol/L of plasma potassium—this may rise to 30 mmol/L or more by the expiry date, due to membrane leak of potassium out (and sodium into the cell) during storage. However, these changes are reversed on transfusion of the blood. For these reasons blood over 10 days old should not be given in large volumes to patients with impaired renal function, e.g. in shock or to neonates.

Hypokalaemia may be a greater problem than hyperkalaemia in the transfusion of blood products. The potassium leaked from the red cells will be lost in the case of washed red blood cells particularly, leaving potassium-depleted red cells for transfusion. These cells will replete the deficient potassium from their *in vivo* extracellular environment, i.e. the transfused patient. Hypokalaemia should be considered when large volumes of washed or frozen red cells are transfused.

12. Circulatory Overloading. At one time this was the commonest cause of death due to pulmonary oedema or cardiac arrhythmias following transfusion but this has now greatly diminished with the use of potent diuretics such as frusemide. However, lengthy operations involving both continuous blood loss and transfusions often result in an overtransfused patient. Knowledge of the central venous pressure and use of dyes or isotopes for measuring plasma volume (PV) and hence total blood volume (TBV) has reduced the hazards. However the haemodynamic fluid shifts due to shock etc. must always be allowed for when interpreting haematocrit and PV results in such patients. It is also good practice to auscultate the lung bases when giving large volumes of blood or when transfusing the elderly patient.

13. Effects of Anaesthetics and Drugs. In patients under the influence of anaesthetics or heavy sedation during transfusion the only two signs suggesting that incompatible blood may have been transfused are (1) hypotension despite apparently adequate blood replacement and (2) abnormal bleeding.

14. Graft versus Host (GVH) Reactions. These reactions are now recognized with increasing frequency in human patients; in all known cases they have been caused by administration of blood containing HLA incompatible immuno-competent lymphocytes to patients with severe disorders of the thymus-dependent immune system (e.g. lymphopenic hypogammaglobulinemia) or those previously exposed to massive irradiation or heavy immunosuppression and therefore unable to reject foreign cells. GVH disease in man is fatal unless the recipient has some remaining immuno-competence or the donor cells are compatible (Mewissen et al., 1969).

To prevent this possibly fatal complication of blood transfusion in patients susceptible to GVH disease, special precautions should be taken to remove or inactivate the lymphocytes by irradiation before transfusion.

Where the patient already has preformed anti-leucocyte (anti-HLA) antibodies, he may on transfusion suffer a febrile non-haemolytic (FNH) transfusion reaction which may range in intensity and pyrexia from mild to very severe. If no red cell incompatibility or bacterial contamination is found, the patient's plasma should be screened against a panel of HLA antigens using a two-stage microcytotoxicity or other technique. Up to 50% of such reactions are probably due to HLA antibodies. In these cases the patient should be transfused with plasma-reduced or washed or frozen red blood cells.

15. Rhesus (D) Positive Blood. Apart from the random immunization dangers of blood transfusion—a specific risk is attached to the transfusion of Rhesus (D) positive blood to D negative individuals. Thus, except as a life saving procedure, Rhesus (D) positive blood should never be given to a female below menopausal age since it could be the cause of haemolytic disease of the newborn. Younger D negative males should also not be transfused with D positive blood since they are more likely to produce anti-D than older males.

The Transfusion Reaction

The hazards of blood transfusion have already been discussed and it is again emphasized that the greatest risk of these is a *clerical* error. Technical mistakes account for a very small proportion of all reactions.

Allergic or febrile reactions unless very severe are treated with antihistamines but the transfusion is continued cautiously.

Where a haemolytic or severe febrile reaction is suspected or detected, the transfusion is stopped and the remainder of the transfused blood and the giving set are returned to the Blood Transfusion laboratory accompanied by a fresh blood specimen from the patient.

The basic scheme of investigating a blood transfusion reaction is shown in Fig. 39.4. Should a positive result be obtained, more detailed tests, e.g. antibody titres, cell survival studies, etc. will normally be carried out at the discretion of the Pathologist.

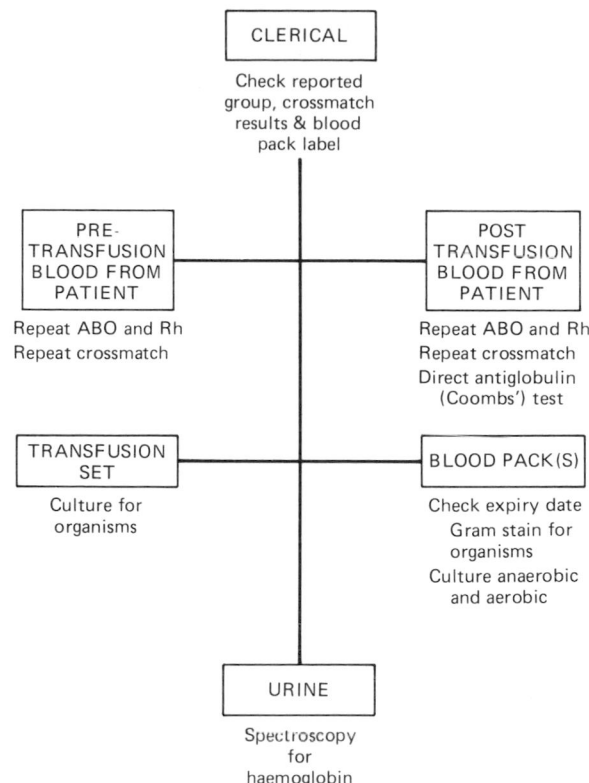

Fig. 39.4 Basic scheme of investigation of a blood transfusion reaction

COAGULATION PROBLEMS IN RELATION TO BLOOD TRANSFUSION

The Coagulation Mechanism

The importance of blood coagulation has been recognized since earliest recorded history and eventually led up to the Morowitz classical theory of coagulation (1905) which may be shown as:

$$\begin{array}{cc} \text{BLOOD} & \text{TISSUE} \\ \diagdown & \diagup \\ \text{THROMBOKINASE} \\ | \\ \text{Ca}^{++} \\ | \\ \text{PROTHROMBIN} \rightarrow \text{THROMBIN} \\ | \\ \text{FIBRINOGEN} \rightarrow \text{FIBRIN} \end{array}$$

He thus appears to have recognized the importance of the extrinsic and intrinsic systems even at this early date.

In the 1930s the one stage prothrombin determination of Quick and the two stage prothrombin procedure of Warner and co-workers brought coagulation studies into the routine clinical laboratory. Using these techniques, the cause of sweet clover disease of cattle as a bleeding disorder, was traced to decreased prothrombin after consumption of spoiled sweet clover. This led to the isolation of a dicoumarin derivative from spoiled clover and to the eventual inclusion of this and allied drugs in the modern range of conventional anticoagulants.

The rapid increase in knowledge of the coagulation mechanism led to several often unrelated names for each factor recognized. An International Committee now designates a number to each new factor which it recognizes (Table 39.8).

Although certain reactions in blood coagulation have long been considered to be enzymatic, recently there has developed a concept which holds that nearly all plasma coagulation factors circulate as pro-enzymes and are converted to enzymes during the process of clotting. The function of each enzyme derived from the pro-enzyme appears to be the activator of the pro-enzyme which succeeds it in the coagulation sequence. Thus blood coagulation may be considered as the result of a series of reactions in which the product of reaction 1 is the enzyme which catalyzes reaction 2 and the product of 2 is the enzyme which catalyzes reaction 3 and so on to the formation of fibrin. This concept has been called the 'enzyme cascade', 1964 of blood coagulation which is outlined in Fig. 39.5.

TABLE 39.8
INTERNATIONAL NOMENCLATURE FOR BLOOD COAGULATION

Factor	Synonym
I	Fibrinogen
II	Prothrombin
III	Tissue factor, tissue thromboplastin
IV	Calcium
V	Pro-accelerin, labile factor
VI	—
VII	Proconvertin, stable factor
VIII	Antihaemophilic globulin (AHG) or factor (AHF)
IX	Christmas factor, plasma thromboplastin component (PTC)
X	Stuart-Prower factor
XI	Plasma thromboplastic antecedent (PTA)
XII	Hageman factor
XIII	Fibrin Stabilizing Factor

The 'intrinsic system' represents reactions leading to coagulation of blood without addition of exogenous substances. 'Extrinsic system' involves the participation of exogenous tissue factor. Reference to Fig. 39.5 shows that in the intrinsic system activated factor VIII (i.e. factor VIIIa) activates factor X while in the extrinsic system tissue factor, factor VII and calcium are all involved in this reaction. The cascade concept has not displaced the much older notion of intrinsic and extrinsic systems since these differ in their speed of reaction; thus via the intrinsic system thrombin formation may take as long as 4–5 min to completion compared with 10–15 s when the extrinsic system (i.e. including tissue factor) is operative. It is not intended to study each step in detail but some points need special emphasis.

Factor XII. The intrinsic system begins with the activation of factor XII to XIIa by contact with any foreign surface, e.g. collagen, fibre, skin, etc.

The mechanism of activation is not understood and may involve removal of an inhibitor. The activated factor XII (XIIa) then appears to act as an enzyme in activating factor XI.

Factor X appears to be the beginning of the final common pathway of blood coagulation since it is the first factor involved in both intrinsic and extrinsic systems.

The 'extrinsic' system describes coagulation resulting from the addition of tissue extracts to whole blood. Tissue factor activity may be extracted from many organs including fresh lung, placenta and brain tissue. The role of this system in haemostasis and in inflammatory processes is not clear but is likely to be more important in the latter. Only extremely small amounts of tissue factor are necessary and the clotting reactions occur very rapidly. It may be that every wound causes the release of some tissue factor into the damaged vessels where it may induce rapid fibrin formation although this does not explain the mechanism of bleeding, e.g. in haemophilia. It is however clear that the extrinsic system does play an important part in pathological processes such as disseminated intravascular coagulation.

Implications of the Enzyme Cascade Concept
Macfarlane stresses the potential of the system for amplification since the enzymes are catalysts and a small quantity of enzyme would be expected to convert a large quantity of substrate to product. Since the product is also an enzyme each step leads to rapidly increasing enzymatic activity. The concept is a very acceptable one although it does not fully explain all known facts about coagulation and especially the function of platelets in the coagulation mechanism.

Blood Coagulation Disturbances after Massive Blood Transfusion

The most important disturbances in the coagulation mechanism of patients who require massive transfusions during surgery are (1) a marked reduction in the number of platelets, (2) a decrease in factors V and VIII, both effects being due to dilution. Such disturbances are often seen when the patient receives more than 5 L of blood in 24 h. Fresh blood is indicated for (1) while fresh blood or fresh frozen plasma can be used for (2).

Investigation of Abnormal Bleeding at Operation
The possible causes of abnormal bleeding at operation have been very adequately reviewed elsewhere (Ulin et al., 1964). However, in such an event, and especially

THE 'CASCADE' THEORY OF COAGULATION

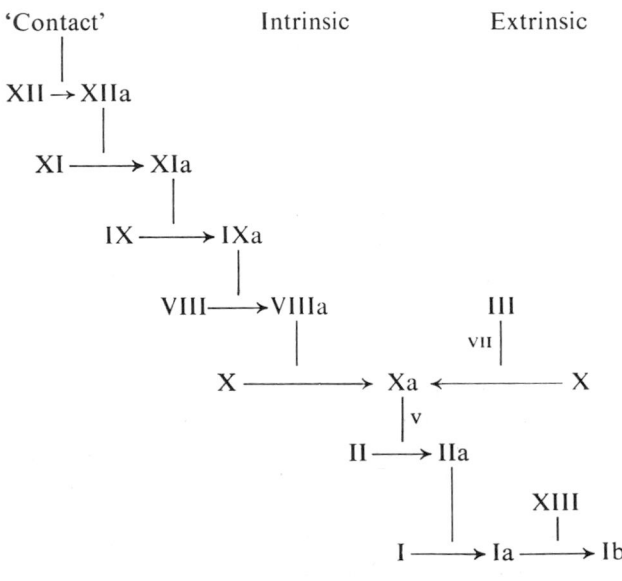

Fig. 39.5

where previous haematological investigations have not been carried out—a routine screening for possible haematological causes of bleeding should include:

1. Kaolin Cephalin Clotting Time and/or Hicks and Pitney screen test.
2. A total platelet count.
3. A plasma fibrinogen estimation measuring clottable protein.
4. A test for abnormal blood fibrinolytic activity.

The above are adequate as initial tests to exclude significant clotting abnormalities. It should be noted that the list does not include bleeding and clotting times since these are insensitive and reveal only gross abnormalities. Of the two alternatives in 1 above the Kaolin Cephalin Clotting Time is quicker and easier to perform.

The plasma fibrinogen *must* be estimated using a clotting technique. Chemical and immunological methods measure both fibrinogen and fibrin degradation products (formed during abnormal fibrinolysis and Arvin therapy) and may sometimes give grossly misleading high results.

Abnormal fibrinolysis is demonstrated by incubating a clotted blood sample in a water bath at 37°C for one hour with inspection at quarter hourly intervals—if present, the clot will have become smaller or will totally disappear. A more sensitive method involves the measurement of the euglobulin lysis time which provides a quantitative assessment of fibrinolytic activity.

Finally, it is important that blood samples for clotting tests be taken by a clean venepuncture and placed in containers with the correct anticoagulant. Thus:

Test	*Anticoagulant to be used*
Kaolin Cephalin test	— Disodium citrate
Hicks and Pitney	— Disodium citrate
Platelet count	— EDTA
Fibrinogen	— Disodium citrate
Fibrinolytic activity	— Disodium citrate (*and a* clotted blood specimen)

The Significance of Disseminated Intravascular Coagulation in Blood Transfusion Reactions and in the Shocked Patient

Disseminated intravascular coagulation (DIC) is a relatively new concept in the detection of disease. It is defined as acute, transient coagulation occurring in the blood flowing throughout the vascular tree and which may obstruct the microcirculation. It may or may not result in an accumulation of fibrin but does involve the transformation of fibrinogen into fibrin (Hardaway, 1966).

Briefly it is postulated that coagulation and fibrinolytic activity are two processes which go on continuously and normally in the vascular tree. They are in fact thought to be in dynamic equilibrium, with con-

stant removal of this fibrin mainly by the body's fibrinolytic system. Thus:

$$COAGULATION \rightleftharpoons FIBRINOLYSIS$$

However, certain factors may accelerate intravascular clotting so that fibrin accumulates. Such shifts in the equilibrium result in disseminated coagulation (DIC).

Typical findings in an episode of DIC are:

1. Sudden appearance of unexplained hypotensive shock with possible cyanosis and death.
2. Appearance of a clinical bleeding tendency which may be dramatic and can cause death.

The bleeding tendency may be due to:

(a) Partial or complete afibrinogenaemia and often deficiency of other clotting factors.
(b) Platelet deficiency.
(c) Presence of fibrin degradation products which act as circulating anticoagulants.
(d) Activation of the fibrinolytic system.

It is often difficult to decide whether intravascular coagulation or fibrinolysis have occurred either singly, together or in sequence. Although each case must be considered as a separate entity, it is a general finding that when fibrinolytic activation is *secondary* to intravascular coagulation then the number of circulating platelets is characteristically decreased, whereas in *primary* fibrinolytic activation (hyperplasminaemia) the plasminogen level is low but the platelet count is seldom decreased.

Plasminogen levels do not fall in uncomplicated fibrin formation and hence may serve to exclude intravascular clotting.

3. Finding of capillary thrombi at autopsy (particularly if epsilon amino-caproic acid (EACA) has been given).
4. Focal haemorrhagic necrosis in the liver, kidneys, etc., due to capillary obstruction by fibrin. The necrosis may cause death in renal failure.

Some Syndromes of Disseminated Intravascular Coagulation (DIC)

Many clinical syndromes are undoubtedly associated with DIC. Of immediate interest are the following:

1. Shock (inadequate capillary perfusion) due to:
   (a) Haemorrhage.
   (b) Trauma.
   (c) Burns.
2. Haemolytic syndromes including haemolytic blood transfusion reactions.
3. Obstetric syndromes:
   (a) Concealed accidental ante-partum haemorrhage with premature separation of the placenta.
   (b) Abortion.
   (c) Amniotic fluid embolism.
   (d) Retained dead fetus.
4. Extracorporeal circulation.

It is essential to note that the two immediate effects of DIC are inadequate capillary perfusion (shock) and an acute clotting defect. Although all shock (inadequate capillary perfusion) does not result from DIC, DIC invariably results in shock. Likewise all clotting defects do not result from DIC but DIC always results in a clotting effect.

Shock Following Incompatible Blood Transfusion
An incompatible blood transfusion may result in a haemolytic transfusion reaction with release of thromboplastin-like substance from the red cells. The syndrome that often results is without doubt due to DIC—the shock being caused by widespread obstruction of the microcirculation by micro-fibrin clots formed from the circulating fibrinogen. Chest pain, although partly due to bronchiolar constriction due to histamine-like substances, may also be due to the blocking of pulmonary blood vessels by agglutinates; likewise renal failure (and pain) may well be due to the obstruction of the renal microcirculation by fibrin, which undoubtedly occurs.

Principles of Treatment
If DIC is assumed to be the cause of abnormal bleeding (as indicated by laboratory tests), here a low platelet count and afibrinogenaemia are sensitive indicators, then immediate treatment is essential. If the afibrinogenaemia is associated with fibrinolytic activation then an acute life-threatening haemorrhagic state may develop.

Treatment must therefore include administration of fibrinogen until plasma level exceeds 100 mg per cent, with fresh whole blood or platelet concentrate to replace the platelets and additional fresh frozen plasma, if necessary, to supply other clotting factors.

Where DIC is thought to be still occurring then immediate *heparin* therapy is indicated to inhibit the clotting process and prevent further fibrin formation. The use of epsilon amino-caproic acid (EACA) to inhibit secondary fibrinolytic activity should only be considered as a last resort since the fibrinolysis is protecting the patient from the complications of intravascular coagulation. Further, any fibrin formed in the presence of EACA is incapable of being lysed later by the body's fibrinolytic system and so can only organize with resultant complications of fibrous tissue formation. EACA should never be used unless (a) violent fibrinolytic activation can be demonstrated, (b) life threatening bleeding is present, (c) blood clot formed after the drug becomes effective can be removed.

Occasionally DIC may result from transfusion, in which case anticoagulation with heparin should precede replacement therapy.

REFERENCES

Barbara J., Contreras M. (1986). Bacterial and parasitic diseases transmitted by blood transfusion. *Hosp. Update*, **12**, 629; and Viral diseases transmitted by blood transfusion. *Hosp. Update*, **12**, 697.

Bernstein F. (1924). Ergebnisse einer biostatischen zusammenfassenden Betrachtung über die erblichen Blutstrukturen des Menschen. *Klin. Wschr.*, **3**, 1495.

Boyan C.P., Howland W.S. (1969). Immediate and delayed mortality associated with massive blood transfusions. *Surg. Clin. N. Amer.*, **49**, 217.

Coombs R.R.A., Mourant A.E., Race R.R. (1945). Detection of weak and 'incomplete' Rh agglutinins: a new test. *Lancet*, **ii**, 15.

von Dungern E.V., Hirszfeld L. (1911). Über gruppenspezifische Strukturen des Blutes 111. *Z. Immun. Forsch.*, **8.**, 526.

Fisher R.A., cited by Race R.R. (1944). An 'incomplete' antibody in human serum. *Nature*, **153**, 771.

Ford J.M., Cullen M.H., Oliver R.T.D., et al. (1980). Possible prolongation of remission in acute myeloid leukemia by granulocyte transfusions. *N. Engl. J. Med.* **302**, 583.

Hardaway R.M. (1966). *Syndromes of Disseminated Intravascular Coagulation*. Springfield, Ill.: Charles C. Thomas.

Loutit J.F., Mollison P.L. (1943). Advantages of a disodium–citrate–glucose mixture as a blood preservative. *Br. Med. J.* **ii**, 744.

Maizels M. (1941). Preservation of organic phosphorus compounds in stored blood by glucose. *Lancet*, **1**, 722.

Mewissen H.J., Stutman O., Good R.A. (1969). Functions of the lymphocytes. *Seminars in Haem.*, **6**, 28.

Mollison P.L. (1988). *Blood Transfusion in Clinical Medicine*. Oxford: Blackwell Scientific Publications.

Morton J.A., Pickles M.M., Sutton L., (1969). The correlation of the Bg^a blood group with the HL-A7 leucocyte group: demonstration of antigenic sites on red cells and leucocytes. *Vox Sang.*, **17**, 536.

Morton J.A., Pickles M.M., Sutton L., et al. (1971). Identification of further antigens on red cells and lymphocytes. *Vox Sang.* **21**, 141.

Smith D.S. (1987). *The Appropriate Use of Diagnostic Services; (xv) A Guide to Blood Transfusion Practice*, pp. 12–16. Health Trends. London: DHSS.

Sutton, D.M.C., Shumak, K.H., Baker M.A. (1982). Prophylactic granulocyte transfusions in acute leukemia. *Plasma Ther. Transfu. Tech.* **3**, 45.

Ulin A.W., (1964). Bleeding in the surgical patient. *Ann. N.Y. Acad. Sci.*, **115**, 1.

Valtis D.J., Kennedy A.C. (1954). Defective gas–transport function of stored red blood cells. *Lancet*, **1**, 119.

40. Molecular Disorders of the Red Cell: Haemoglobino- pathies, Enzymopathies and Membrane Defects

J. Isbister

Anaesthetists are made constantly aware of the integrated nature of oxygen uptake, transport and delivery to the tissues. The red cell with its contained haemoglobin plays a pivotal role in this integrated process. Quantitative abnormalities seen in anaemia and polycythaemia are well accepted as impairing oxygen transport, but qualitative defects in red cell and haemoglobin may also impair oxygen transport to the tissues by several mechanisms. Disorders of the red cell provide us with prototypes of molecular disease and it was Linus Pauling in his studies of sickle cell disease who laid the foundations of molecular biology of disease. Haemoglobin has been the most studied molecule in biology and the one in which the greatest number of molecular defects has been identified. It has been possible to correlate genetics and structure with function in a manner that is only now becoming possible with other biological molecules.

The central dogma since Watson and Crick described the genetic code has been DNA → RNA → protein → function, seen as the unchangeable 'blueprint of life' transmitted in a one way fashion. Recent developments in molecular biology have clearly exposed a much more complex process and our initially simplistic theories on the mechanisms of molecular disease are being revolutionized and it would be far beyond the scope of this chapter to address the new concepts. However, the practitioner of medicine must have a working framework in which to understand and care for patients who may have these relatively common diseases causing specific clinical problems or problems in association with other disorders.

Figures 40.1 and 40.2 summarize the molecular defects of haemoglobin and the red cell. In the thalassaemias there is defective haemoglobin production with varying degrees of haemolysis. In other haemoglobinopathies where there is an abnormal amino acid substitution in the α or β chain of the haemoglobin molecule, a wide range of disorders may be observed including, an unstable haemoglobin molecule, a high or low oxygen affinity molecule, poor solubility of the haemoglobin molecule (sickle cell disease) and the methaemoglobinaemias. Various red cell enzyme deficiencies may also have effects on haemoglobin function, this is particularly the case in defects associated with the hexose monophosphate shunt, such as G6PD deficiency. There are also various disorders of the red cell membrane cytoskeleton, the commonest of which is hereditary spherocytosis, in which the red cell may be rigid, have a shortened life span and altered haemoglobin affinity. The aim of this chapter will be to review the various disorders in which there is a primary or secondary alteration in haemoglobin structure or function, which may impair oxygen transport or lead to various syndromes of clinical significance. Attention will concentrate on primary abnormalities in the production of the haemoglobin molecule and the clinical disorders which may result from a structurally abnormal haemoglobin molecule. However, for completeness, mention will be made of disorders where the haemoglobin molecule may be altered or denatured, secondary to enzyme deficiencies in the red cell or from excessive oxidant stress from toxins or drugs. Primary membrane disorders are briefly mentioned for completeness.

STRUCTURE OF THE HAEMOGLOBIN MOLECULE

Adult haemoglobin (Hb-A) is a tetramer in which each monomer is made up of a haem ring and a globin chain. Two of the monomers are α globin chains and the other two β globin chains. These pairs of α and β chains have their origin from maternal and paternal genes on chromosomes 16 and 11 respectively, with

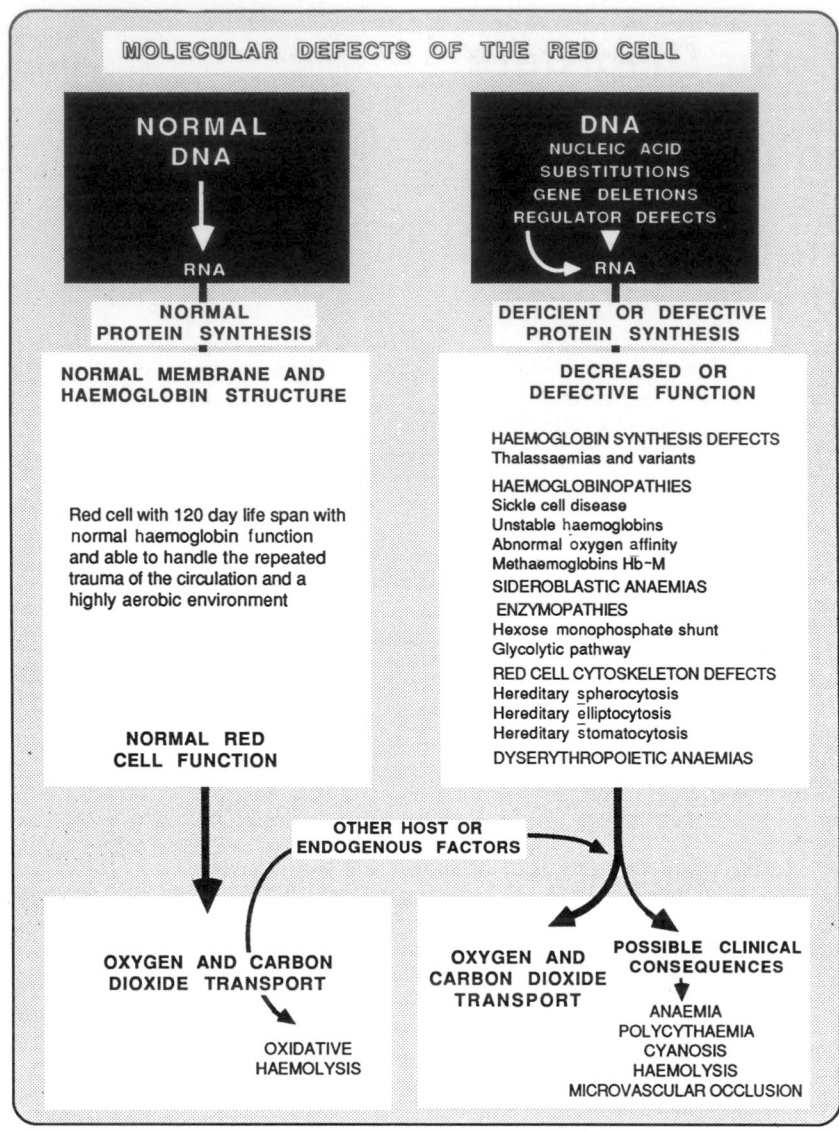

Fig. 40.1   A summary of the genetics of molecular defects of the red cell and haemoglobin.

two gene loci controlling α globin chain production and one controlling β globin chain synthesis. During binding for transport, elemental oxygen interacts with ferrous iron in the haem ring exchanging an electron thus converting the iron to its ferric state (Fig. 40.3). The reactive oxygen molecule is protected within the hydrophobic haem pocket. In the deoxygenated state the electron returns to the iron, reducing it to its original ferrous state. However, during the interchange between the oxygenated and deoxygenated form a small percentage becomes oxidized with the production of methaemoglobin (*see* below).

THE PATHOPHYSIOLOGY AND CLINICAL FEATURES

Figure 40.4 summarizes the molecular biology and pathophysiology of disorders of the red cell and haemoglobin. It should be emphasized that the majority of abnormal haemoglobins are not of clinical significance and physiological function is not significantly altered as a consequence of the molecular defect.

The haemoglobinopathies, enzymopathies and red cell membrane defects may result in a wide spectrum of clinical disorders depending on the nature of the defect. These clinical features may include:

1. Anaemia
Anaemia may occur on the basis of decreased haemoglobin production secondary to ineffective erythropoiesis or haemolysis secondary to precipitation and denaturing of the haemoglobin molecule with secondary red cell membrane damage. Anaemia primarily due to the haemoglobinopathy may also be complicated by other factors such as an aplastic crisis, folate deficiency or marrow suppression secondary to infec-

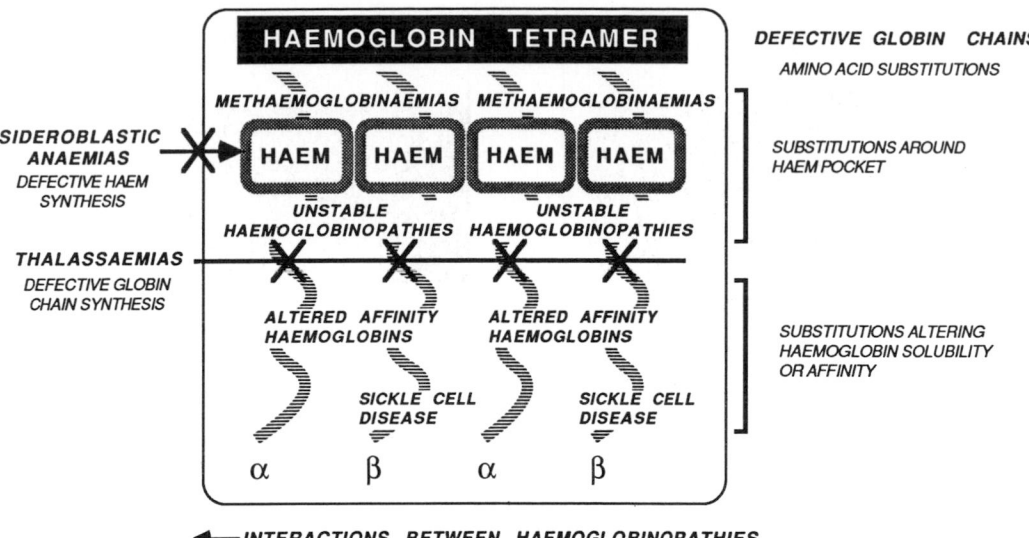

Fig. 40.2   Molecular defects of the haemoglobin molecule.

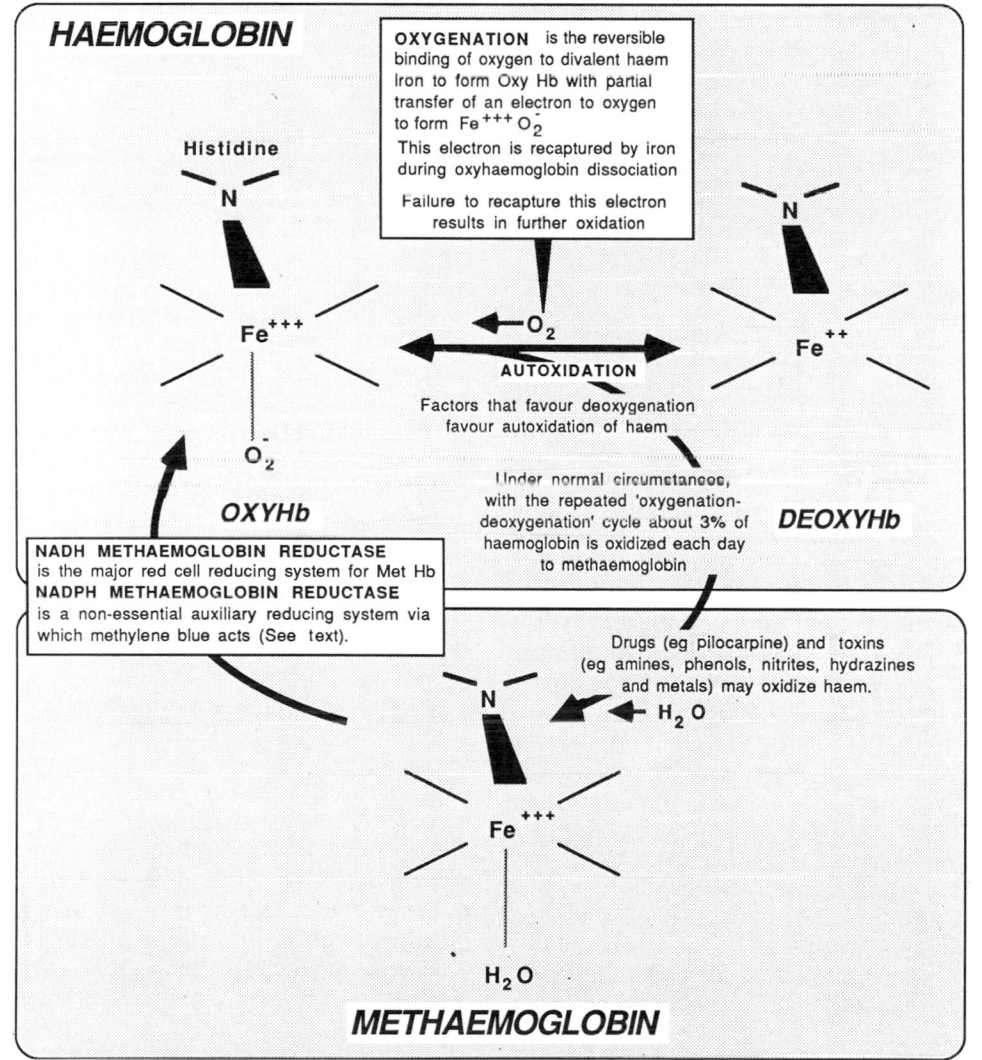

Fig. 40.3   The biochemistry of haemoglobin oxygenation and deoxygenation and formation and reduction of methaemoglobin.

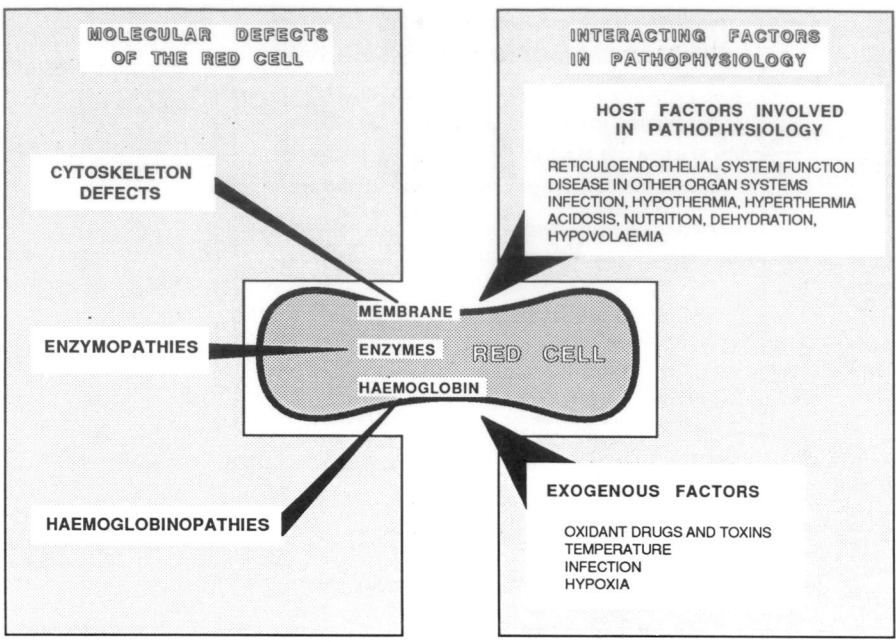

Fig. 40.4 The overall pathophysiology of molecular defects of the red cell, illustrating the various interacting host and environmental factors.

tion. Haemoglobin disorders in which there is a red cell production problem (e.g. thalassaemia, sideroblastosis, dyserythropoiesis) respond poorly to blood loss.

2. Haemolysis and its Associated Clinical Problems

Increased bilirubin production occurs as a result of shortened red cell survival resulting from chronic or acute haemolysis. It may also be the result of intramedullary death of developing red cell precursors as seen in congenital sideroblastic anaemia, thalassaemia and congenital dyserythropoietic anaemia.

An unconjugated hyperbilirubinaemia is usually indicative of haemolysis and conjugated hyperbilirubinaemia of cholestasis. Although this is generally true, it should be emphasized that a conjugated hyperbilirubinaemia does not exclude the presence of haemolysis. The transport of conjugated bilirubin from the hepatocyte to the biliary canaliculus is an energy requiring process and is susceptible to hypoxia and sepsis. In these circumstances, or others in which there is associated biliary obstruction, haemolysis may lead to a sudden load of bilirubin which may be rapidly conjugated, but delayed in its subsequent excretion. Any sudden rise in bilirubin, irrespective of its conjugation status, should alert one to the possibility of haemolysis. Another clue is an isolated rise in the bilirubin level in the absence of significant abnormalities in the hepatic enzymes (bilirubin/enzyme dissociated).

3. Polycythaemia

Haemoglobinopathies with increased oxygen affinity may cause tissue hypoxia with resultant increased red cell production and secondary polycythaemia.

4. Cyanosis

Methaemoglobinaemia and low affinity haemoglobins may cause cyanosis.

5. Microcirculatory Failure

Microvascular obstruction and tissue infarction is classically seen in sickle cell syndromes, but also may occur less dramatically in hereditary spherocytosis causing leg ulcers.

6. Iron Overload

Iron overload may occur as part of the red cell disorder if chronic haemolysis or ineffective erythropoiesis are a feature of the disease. This is commonly the case in thalassaemia, sideroblastic anaemia and hereditary spherocytosis. The degree of iron overload and tissue damage is variable and is possibly related in some patients to the coexistence of the haemochromatosis gene, which has a population frequency of approximately 1:20, in the heterozygous state. Repeated blood transfusion therapy may lead to iron overload. The effects of iron overload which warrant specific attention in acute medicine and anaesthesia are the tissue damaging effects on the heart (cardiomyopathy), the liver (dysfunction and cirrhosis) and host defences (infection).

7. Bone Abnormalities

These may be secondary to hyperplastic marrow and

occasionally present technical problems for the anaesthetist due to craniofacial abnormalities.

THE THALASSAEMIC SYNDROMES

Failure to synthesize one or more of the globin chains of the haemoglobin molecule results in defective haemoglobin formation, inadequate red cell haemoglobinization and hypochromic microcytic red cells. This group of haemoglobinopathies is becoming increasingly heterogeneous with complex molecular biological abnormalities. Although they are of great interest to the geneticist and the molecular biologist their importance to clinical medicine is essentially three-fold. Firstly, the homozygous form of thalassaemia (thalassaemia major) is a severe clinical disorder requiring constant medical attention. Secondly, the heterozygous states and the interaction of the thalassaemia genes with other haemoglobinopathies may produce a wide, and sometimes bizzare, spectrum of haematological abnormalities. Their correct recognition and diagnosis is essential if inappropriate therapy is to be avoided and acute crises minimized. Thirdly, with increasing understanding of these disorders, accurate genetic counselling and intrauterine diagnosis are becoming increasingly possible and it is likely that with the spectacular advances we are currently witnessing in genetic engineering, exciting new therapeutic interventions are likely. Table 40.1 briefly summarizes the laboratory findings in the clinically important thalassaemic syndromes. α thalassaemia is usually due to a structural gene deletion and is asymptomatic unless three or four of the gene loci on chromosome 16 are affected. With three genes affected Hb-H disease occurs which has a clinical picture of thalassaemia intermedia with an abnormal unstable haemoglobin present (Hb-His, a tetramer of β chains). These patients are susceptible to Heinz body haemolytic crises (*see* below). If four genes are deleted hydrops fetalis results which is incompatible with life.

In β thalassaemia the story has greater complexity with a more heterogeneous genetic picture with several different mechanisms responsible for the wide range of thalassaemic syndromes. Structural gene deletion is uncommon, in most patients the β globin gene is translated normally, but subsequent processing of the messenger RNA transcript is faulty. Many different regulatory mutations underlie the defective β chain synthesis. In the most common form $β^+$ thalassaemia, small amounts of β chains are synthesized and the reduced synthesis is due to a defect in the processing and transport of messenger RNA from the nucleus. In $β^0$ thalassaemia β globin chain synthesis is absent due to a variety of defects which results in defective messenger RNA processing.

Anaesthetic Implications of Thalassaemia

The anaesthetic importance of thalassaemia in any individual patient will depend on the specific defect. In patients with thalassaemia major anaemia may require preoperative transfusion. It should be emphasized that as with sickle cell disease thalassaemia major may be a multisystem disease and patients need to be carefully assessed. Iron overload may have led to extensive organ damage, especially cardiac and hepatic. Patients with thalassaemia major are also at increased risk of infection. Patients with lesser degrees or mild thalassaemic trait do not present any particular problems for the anaesthetist.

Diagnosis of Thalassaemia

Most patients with thalassaemia come to clinical attention during investigation of a hypochromic microcytic anaemia unless the patient is being investigated due to a positive family history. Correct diagnosis is probably more important than the anaesthetic significance of thalassaemia *per se* (Table 40.1).

TABLE 40.1

THE LABORATORY ABNORMALITIES IN THE THALASSAEMIAS

	Haemoglobin electrophoresis				Hb-H bodies	Globin chain synthesis
	Hb-F	Hb-A	Hb-A$_2$	Other Hb		
β *Thalassaemia*		Absence of				β Absent or
Major	↑↑	↓↓	↑	Various combinations	−	$β↓↓↓$
Intermedia		Variable levels		with other globin chain	−	β ↓
Minor		depending on severity		disorders: Hb-S, D, E,	−	β ↓
Trait	↑	N or ↓	↑	C, Lepore	−	β ↓
α *Thalassaemia*						
Barts Hydrops	Absent	Absent	Absent	Hb Barts	−	α Absent
Hb–H Disease	N	↓	N or ↓	Hb-H	+ + +	α ↓↓
Trait	N	N or ↓	N	Hb Barts at birth	+	α ↓

ABNORMAL HAEMOGLOBINS

Almost 400 structural variants of haemoglobin have been identified. In most cases there is a single abnormal nucleic acid resulting in a single amino acid substitution. Initially, letters of the alphabet were used for identification, but this was subsequently changed to using the name of the city or town of origin of the first reported case. As β globin chains are coded by two genes compared with four coding α globin chains, substitution in the β chain are of greater clinical importance. To produce a major clinical disease, expression in the homozygous state is usually necessary (e.g. sickle cell disease). However, unstable haemoglobins and abnormal oxygen affinity haemoglobins cause symptomatic disease in the heterozygous state.

Sickle Cell Syndromes

The particular racial groups in which the defect is common come from West Central Africa, Gabon and Zaire, Saudi Arabia and Central India. In America and other countries where immigration has occurred the gene frequency follows the migration patterns. The protective effect of the heterozygote state against falciparum malaria is used to explain the sustained high frequency of the sickle gene.

Classical sickle cell disease results from the homozygous inheritance of an abnormal haemoglobin in which a glutamic acid in the β chain is replaced by valine in the 6th amino acid position from the N terminus. This was one of the first molecular diseases to be recognized and is the most prevalent abnormal haemoglobin. The solubility of haemoglobin is defective with precipitation occurring when the cell is exposed to an hypoxic or acidic environment. The Hb-SS forms a gel in the red cell due to polymerization of deoxyHb-S, forming long crystals, tactoids, which distort the cells into the typical sickle shape, rendering the cell rigid (Fig. 40.5). Initially this sickling is reversible by reoxygenation, but the process can 'snowball' and eventually becomes irreversible, precipitating the patient into the 'viscous vicious cycle' and eventual haemolysis. Sickle cell disease is a classical example of a disorder in which the pathophysiology is attributable to abnormal rheological properties of blood.

Sickle cell trait in which the patient is heterozygous for the sickle cell gene is rarely symptomatic. The main importance of their identification has been for genetic counselling purposes. However, these patients may have impaired survival or increased susceptibility to certain diseases or environmental hazards. From the anaesthetic and intensive care point of view acute and severe hypoxia, acidosis and sepsis are the main risks.

Patients may be double heterozygous for the sickle and thalassaemia genes or another haemoglobinopathy (S/α thal, S/HPFH, SC, SD, S/O-Arab, S/Lepore, S/β thal). In these circumstances intermediate degrees of clinical severity may be seen and expert laboratory assistance is needed for correct diagnosis. However, all may be associated with the sickling phenomenon outlined above.

Clinical Features of Sickle Cell Syndromes

Symptoms of sickle cell disease appear after six months when β globin chain persistence of increased synthesis (Hb-S) are in full production. This tends to protect the patient against sickle cell crisis. The natural history of Hb-SS is one of chronic haemolytic anaemia, vaso-occlusive crises and progressive compromise of most organ systems, infection and failure to thrive.

1. Anaemia
Chronic haemolytic anaemia, haemolytic crisis, megaloblastic crisis, aplastic crisis and splenic sequestration.

2. Sickle Cell Vaso-occlusive Crisis
Acute or chronic microvascular occlusive disease may lead to microinfarction in many vascular beds, including splenic, bone marrow, gut, retinal (retinopathy, glaucoma), cutaneous (leg ulcers), renal (haematuria, papillary necrosis, renal failure, nephrotic syndrome) and pulmonary circulations. Bone and joint disease are particular features with aseptic necrosis of the femoral head, and osteomyelitis. Recognition of the crisis and its pathophysiology is of central importance. Although many precipitants are known in the majority of patients the attacks are unpredictable and unexplained. It should however be remembered that patients with sickle cell disease may suffer other unrelated disease and one should always be on guard against the 'double bluff'.

3. Susceptibility to Infection

Diagnosis of Sickle Cell Syndromes

Patients usually have a normocytic, normochromic anaemia with the typical diagnostic sickle cells in the peripheral blood. The sickle cell screening test gives a positive result with more definitive identification of Hb-S being made on haemoglobin electrophoresis. In homozygous disease the majority of the circulating haemoglobin is Hb-S with varying amounts of Hb-F.

Anaesthetic Management of Sickle Cell Syndromes

It is only patients with homozygous sickle cell disease (Hb-SS) and Hb-S associated with other haemoglobinopathies that present a practical anaesthetic and surgical problem. For a long time there has been a marked emphasis on the dangers of anaesthesia in patients who are heterozygous for sickle cell disease. Although these patients may have a sickle crisis precipitated by severe hypoxia or acidosis one would

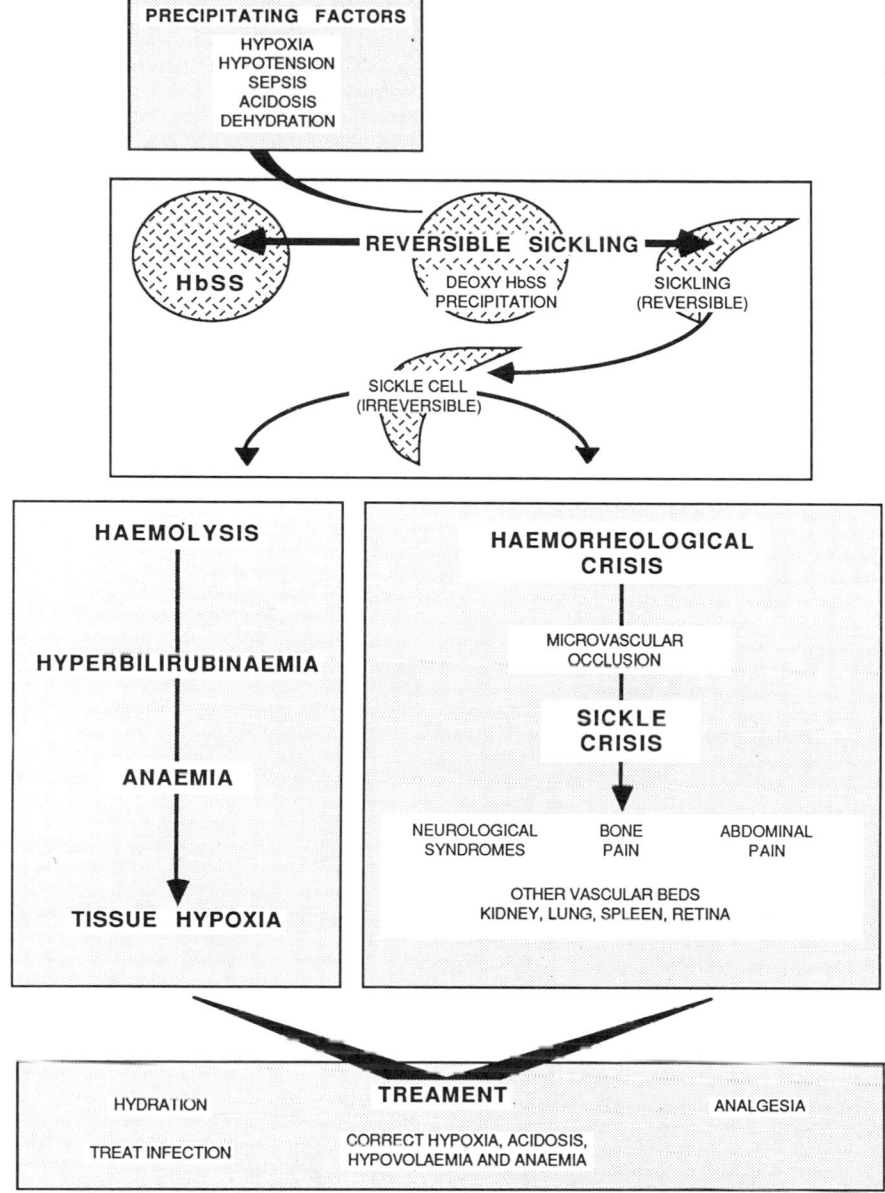

Fig. 40.5 The pathophysiology of sickle cell disease.

assume that such events would be uncommon these days with good anaesthetic practice. Most recent studies would confirm that with good anaesthetic technique there is no greater risk from anaesthesia in patients with sickle cell trait.

The following perioperative considerations are important when anaesthetizing patients with sickle cell disease:

● Adequate preoperative haemoglobin level— blood transfusion may be necessary, firstly to elevate the haemoglobin level to 11–12 g/dl and secondly to dilute the Hb-SS with normal Hb-A.
● Avoid—hypoxia, acidosis, hypovolaemia, dehydration, hypothermia. Supplemental oxygen and intravenous fluids are indicated.

● Prevent and/or diagnose sepsis early—prophylactic antibiotics may be indicated, and also chest physiotherapy.
● Correctly recognize sickle crisis during the course of other disease.
● Careful identification and treatment of complicating diseases (especially respiratory, cardiac, infectious)

HEINZ BODY HAEMOLYTIC ANAEMIAS

In the Heinz body haemolytic anaemias, the haemoglobin molecule tends to be oxidized and 'falls apart' within the red cell. A final product of this oxidation process is the precipitation of insoluble aggregates of denatured haemoglobin (Heinz bodies), followed by lysis of the red cell. These refractile particles attach to and rigidify the red cell membrane. On subsequent passage through the spleen, the Heinz bodies are removed producing 'moth eaten' spherocytes. The resultant cells have a limited life span. The haemoglobin molecule and cell membrane may become oxidized as a result of defects in aerobic glycolysis, an abnormal unstable haemoglobin molecule or overwhelming oxidant stress on a normal red cell (Fig. 40.6).

ENZYME DEFECTS IN HEXOSE MONOPHOSPHATE SHUNT

Faulty reductive capacity of the red cell due to enzyme deficiency in the hexose monophosphate (HMP) shunt or the glutathione pathways impairs the red cell's ability to handle normal and abnormal oxidant stresses and exposes the red cell membrane to free oxygen radical damage. The red cell is constantly exposed to stresses which oxidize haemoglobin and vital sulphydryl groups in the membrane. The HMP provides the major reductive capacity of the normal red cell. Defects in this system will expose the red cell and the haemoglobin molecule to intolerable oxidative influences. The red cell has several mechanisms for dealing with superoxides and hydrogen peroxide, which have the potential to lyse the red cell, such as superoxide dismutase, and catalase, but the main antioxidant mechanism is the glutathione system. Reduced glutathione (GSH) is oxidized to the disul-

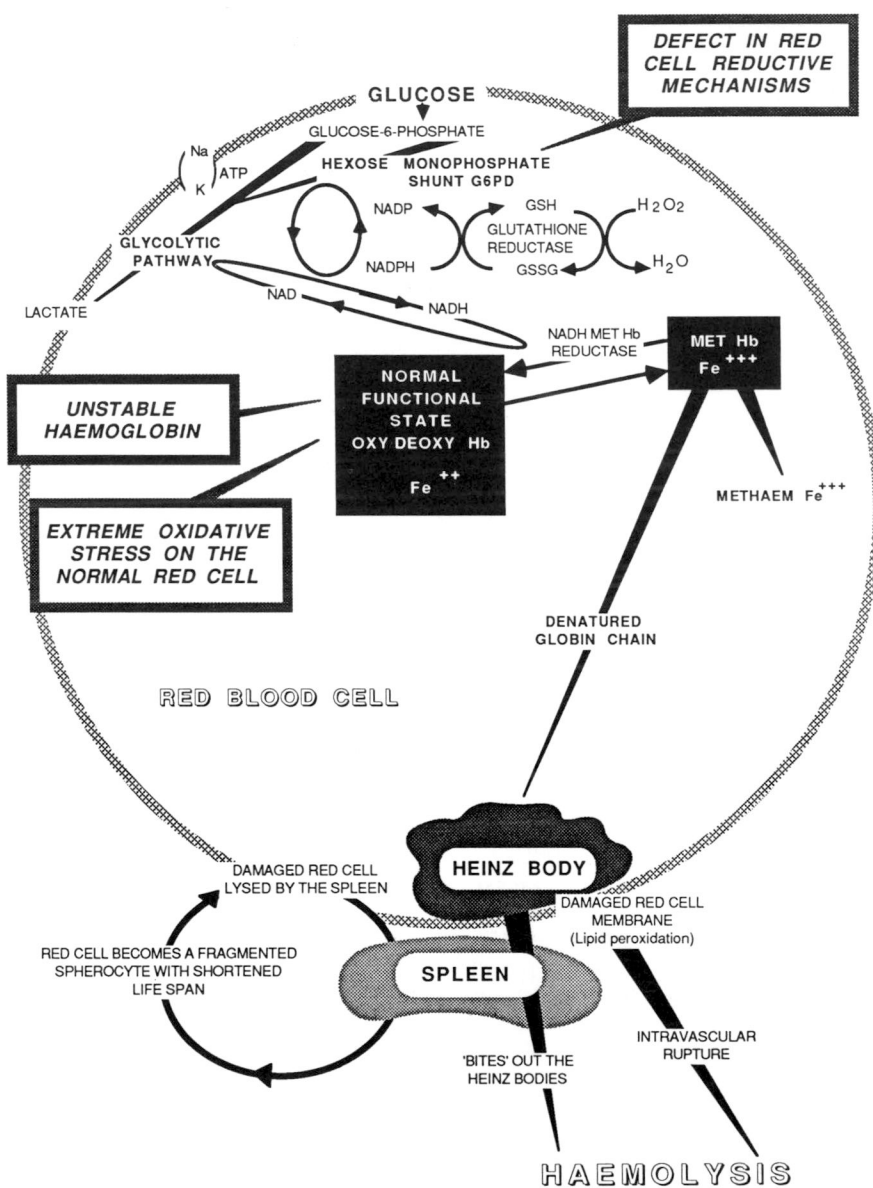

Fig. 40.6 The pathophysiology of the Heinz body haemolytic anaemias.

phide form (GSSH) in the process of converting hydrogen peroxide to water. NADPH is necessary for the reduction of GSSH back to GSH for the process to continue. Glucose-6-phosphate dehydrogenase (G6PD) catalyses the first step in the HMP shunt resulting in the reduction of NADP to NADPH to produce the only NADPH in the red cell. Deficiency of this enzyme is the most frequent cause of Heinz body haemolysis and is also the commonest known red cell enzyme deficiency.

G6PD Deficiency

This is a heterogenous group of disorders with as many as 250 variants known. There are two forms of G6PD which are regarded as normal, the commonest, the B form is found in the majority of people and the A form in some Africans. The clinical severity is usually classified on the basis of enzyme activity.

- Class I < 10% enzyme activity: life-long haemolysis.
- Class II < 10% enzyme activity: acute episodes of haemolysis.
- Class III 10–60% enzyme activity: episodic haemolysis on exposure.
- Class IV Normal enzyme activity.
- Class V Increased enzyme activity.

Any of the variants are susceptible to varying degrees of acute intravascular haemolysis in association with oxidant chemicals or drugs, infectious episodes or acidosis. Most patients with G6PD deficiency are asymptomatic until stressed. The Mediterranean variant, classically seen in favism in children exposed to broad beans, may be associated with severe clinical problems and the enzyme levels are usually lower. The African type, referred to as A − is more likely to give a chronic type of Heinz body haemolysis.

Unstable Haemoglobin Molecule

There are hereditary disorders in which the haemoglobin tetramer is inherently unstable due to substitution of amino acids in the α or β chains, introducing hydrophilic amino acids into the interior, modifying the haem pocket, affecting the helical structure or modifying the interface between the α_1 and β_1 subunits. The molecule thus has a constant tendency to 'fall apart' spontaneously or following exposure to the slightest oxidant stress. The same unstable state occurs in Hb-H disease, a variant of α thalassaemia in which the tetramer of β globin (Hb-H) is unstable.

Drug or Toxin Oxidation of an Otherwise Normal Red Cell

There is a limit to the oxidant stress a red cell can tolerate and a total breakdown is seen in such conditions as moth ball poisoning and in relation to cer-

tain drugs. The sulphonamides have a particularly bad name in this respect especially sulphasalazine and dapsone. The reason for this probably relates to the slow metabolic acetylator status of some patients.

Management of Heinz Body Haemolytic Anaemias

Identify precipitants and avoid their use in future, this especially applies to drugs (e.g. antimetabolites and sulphonamides). In patients commencing drugs which have a high association with Heinz body haemolysis, such as sulphasalazine or dapsone, the blood count should be checked one week after commencing therapy. Infections should be identified early and treated expeditiously, control of fever is probably important. G6PD deficiency is not specifically a risk factor in general anaesthesia, but in the analysis of any postoperative clinical events one must consider G6PD deficiency as possibly playing an interactive role or an unexpected event being a direct manifestation of the deficiency. As long as oxidant drugs are avoided and infection recognized and treated G6PD deficiency should not be an anaesthetic problem.

ENZYME DEFECTS IN ANAEROBIC GLYCOLYSIS: EMBDEN MEYERHOF PATHWAY

Pyruvate Kinase (PK) Deficiency

Pyruvate kinase deficiency is the commonest red cell enzyme defect after G6PD deficiency, but deficiency of hexokinase, triose phosphate isomerase and 3-glycerophosphoglycerate kinase may rarely occur. PK deficiency is an autosomal recessive disorder which may be due to a heterogeneous variety of defects in qualitative or quantitative enzyme function. The deficiency causes a nonspherocytic haemolytic anaemia but occasional 'spikey' spherocytic red cells may be seen on the blood film. The 2,3-DPG level is elevated secondary to the metabolic block, resulting in a right shift in the oxygen dissociation curve. The patient has less symptoms of anaemia than would normally be expected for the degree of anaemia. The haemolysis shows considerable variation in severity. Unless the typical cells are seen in the peripheral blood there are no diagnostic clinical or laboratory features. In the postsplenectomy state the abnormal cells are greatly increased in number and are easily identifiable. The patients usually have a chronic compensated haemolysis. The autohaemolysis test is abnormal, with no correction with added glucose, but correction with ATP. Screening tests and quantitative enzyme assays are available.

METHAEMOGLOBINAEMIA

Methaemoglobin is the oxidized form of haemoglobin in which the iron in haem is in the ferric state and the molecule is unable to carry oxygen. Less than 1% of haemoglobin is methaemoglobin and a balance is maintained between methaemoglobin formation and reduction by the NADH methaemoglobin reductase pathway (*see* Fig. 40.3). Similar to the Heinz body haemolytic anaemias, methaemoglobinaemia may result from abnormalities in the reducing capacity of the NADH methaemoglobin reductase pathway, variant haemoglobins (Hb-M) and from the oxidant effects of various toxins and drugs (aniline dyes, nitrates and nitrites) (Fig. 40.7). A chocolate coloured cyanosis occurs with methaemoglobinaemia which is not correctable by the administration of oxygen. Progressive tissue hypoxia develops as the level rises above 30%, being more severe if anaemia is also present. The affected haemoglobin cannot interact with oxygen and the unaffected haemoglobin has increased oxygen affinity, with a left shift in the oxygen dissociation curve.

Methaemoglobin should be treated by first identifying and then removing the cause or precipitating factor/s, except for oxygen, other therapy is not usually necessary. To those in which a variant Hb-M is not involved, methylene blue (1–2 mg/kg) can be administered intravenously. Methylene blue in its oxidized form (blue) is converted to leukomethylene blue (clear) by accepting electrons from NADPH in the presence of NADPH methaemoglobin reductase. The leukomethylene blue acts as an electron donor and non-enzymatically reduces methaemoglobin to haemoglobin. Methylene blue should not be used in patients with G6PD deficiency. In severe and resistant cases of methaemoglobinaemia blood transfusion, red cell exchange or hyperbaric oxygen may be indicated.

ALTERED AFFINITY HAEMOGLOBINS

There are now over 60 haemoglobin variants with altered affinity for oxygen. Polycythaemia may result from an increase in haemoglobin affinity secondary to an amino acid substitution disturbing haem/haem interaction or 2,3-DPG interaction with the haemoglobin molecule. Mild anaemia and/or cyanosis may result from amino acid substitutions which reduce haemoglobin affinity. The altered affinity haemoglobins are of minor clinical significance except in relation to diagnostic alarm and/or dilemma they may cause.

RED CELL MEMBRANE DISORDERS

Hereditary Spherocytosis (HS)

Any pathological process leading to red cell membrane loss will result in the red cell discocyte being transformed into a spherocyte. Figure 40.8 illustrates several interacting pathologies and host factors which may lead to spherocytosis and ultimate red cell lysis. In general there is either an intrinsic defect in the red cell (as discussed above) or an extrinsic attack. Secondary to these defects the reticuloendothelial system, especially the spleen, plays an important role in filtering and free radical attack on the damaged red cell and ultimate haemolysis.

Hereditary spherocytosis is an autosomal dominantly transmitted haemolytic anaemia with a heterogeneity of the molecular defect from variable expression of the responsible gene abnormalities. It is usually suspected after examination of the blood film in the appropriate clinical setting. There is a red cell membrane defect with progressive oxidation and loss of membrane during the life span of the cell, resulting from repeated passage through the spleen. The nature of the membrane defect remains *sub judice*, but involves the membrane cytoskeleton (spectrin in particular) and it is likely that there will be heterogeneity in relation to the specific molecular causes. The spleen

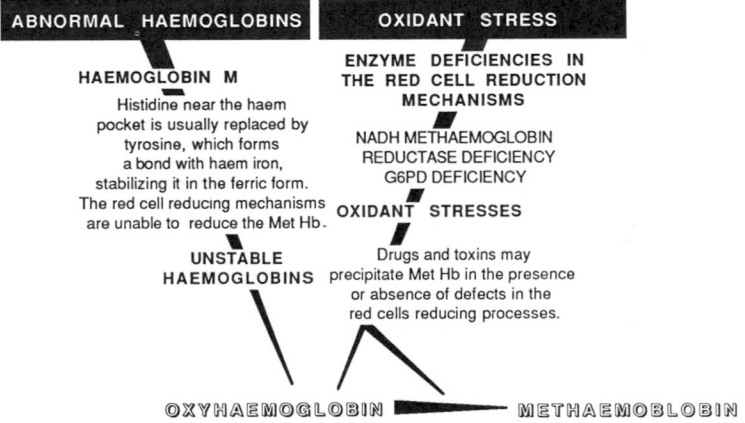

Fig. 40.7   The pathophysiology of methaemoglobinaemia.

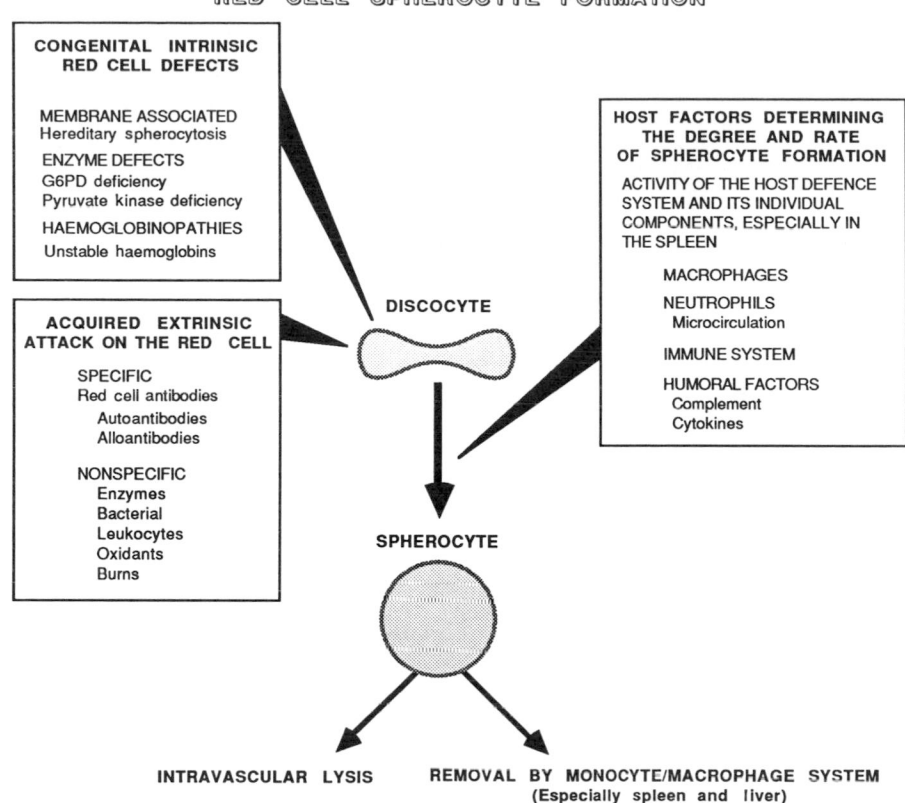

Fig. 40.8   The pathophysiology of red cell spherocyte formation.

is the main site for this 'eating away' at the membrane until the cells are no longer able to survive.

Clinical Features of Hereditary Spherocytosis

Patients with HS are commonly asymptomatic and are detected incidentally, as a result of a blood count. Clinical presentations include: neonatal jaundice, episodes of jaundice with infections, leg ulcers, poor exercise tolerance, biliary colic, splenomegaly or investigation as a part of a family study. Due to the rigidity of the spherocytic red cells and a low 2,3-DPG the patient's symptoms of impaired exercise tolerance tend to be greater than the level of haemoglobin would suggest. This has resulted in the misapprehension that HS is a well compensated haemolytic anaemia. Osmotic fragility and autohaemolysis studies are used for diagnosis, but they are not definitive diagnostic tests for hereditary spherocytosis as they may be positive in any spherocytic haemolytic anaemia. It may not be long before definitive identification of the molecular membrane defect in the individual patients with the disease is possible.

Although splenectomy provides a definitive form of therapy, returning the red cell life span towards normal, it should not be performed without due consideration. Chronic anaemia, repeated haemolytic episodes, pigment gall stones and leg ulcers would be accepted as indications for splenectomy in any patient over the age of seven years. Constant lethargy and poor exercise tolerance may also be accepted and the beneficial effects reported through the family by members who have had their spleen removed may encourage others to do likewise.

HEREDITARY ELLIPTOCYTOSIS AND HEREDITARY STOMATOCYTOSIS

Hereditary elliptocytosis and hereditary stomatocytosis are membrane disorders which are less frequently encountered than hereditary spherocytosis. Unless they represent severe disease they are not usually of major clinical significance, but may cause some concern due to their impressively abnormal blood films.

CONCLUSION

Molecular defects of the red cell are relatively common and, on the one hand, may be responsible for life threatening pathology, whereas in other people they may be of no pathological significance. Diagnosis is of paramount importance, particularly to assist in the identification, removal and avoidance of precipitants and aggravators of crises. Figure 40.9 outlines an approach for the clinician when caring for patients with molecular defects of the red cell in conjunction with other disorders.

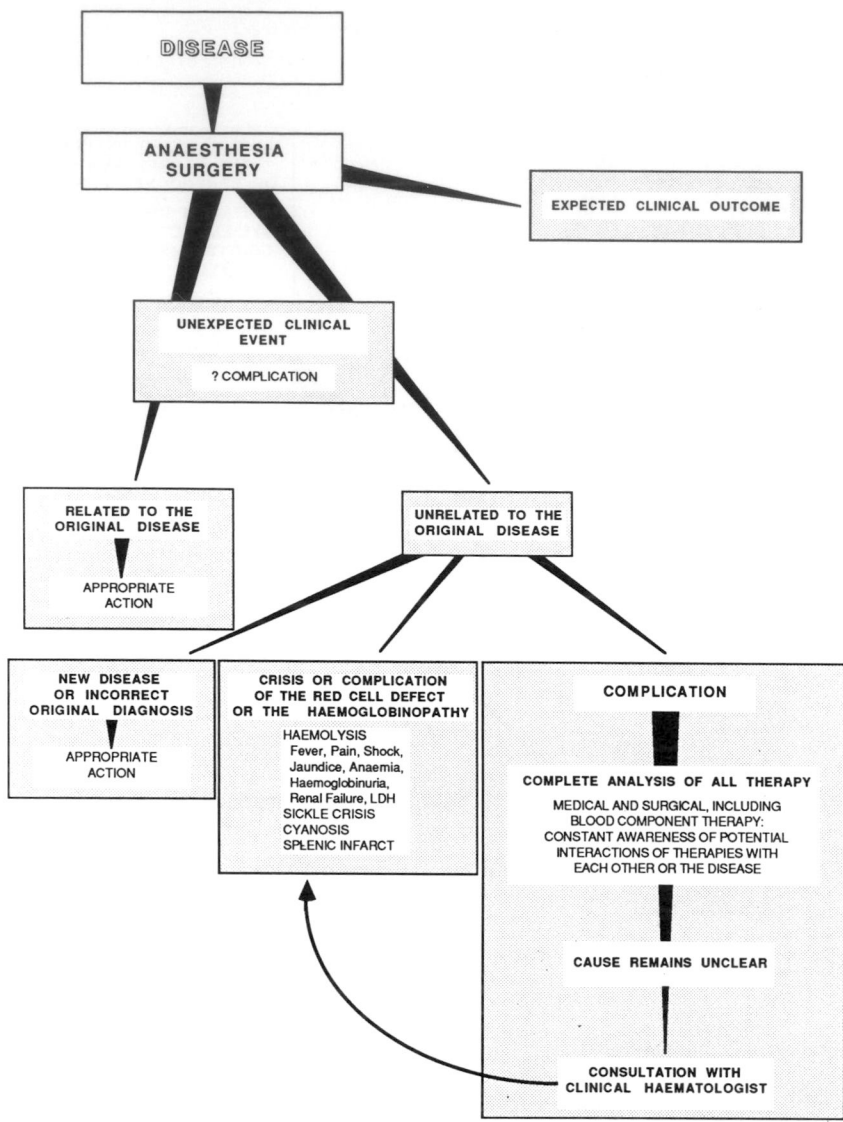

Fig. 40.9 An approach to the management of patients who have an associated molecular defect of the red cell.

41. Oxygen Delivery by Haemoglobin

R. Macdonald

Tissue oxygenation is a function of blood flow, oxygen transport by the blood and the unloading of oxygen at cellular level.

The Oxygen Cascade

The partial pressure of oxygen in dry air or at sea-level is 21.2 kPa. It falls in a stepwise fashion as it traverses the respiratory tract and is carried by the systemic circulation to the mitochondria where the P_{O_2} may be as low as 0.5–3 kPa. This stepwise decrease in the P_{O_2} is called the oxygen cascade. If any step in the cascade is increased this will result in hypoxia in the mitochondria and a change from aerobic to anaerobic metabolism. Factors affecting each step in the cascade are well described by Nunn (1977).

Oxygen Transport

The quantity of oxygen transferred in the blood in 1 min is called the oxygen flux (Nunn and Freeman, 1964) and is equal to:

cardiac output
    × arterial oxygen saturation
    × haemoglobin concentration
    × 1.39 (volume of oxygen in ml combining with
      1 g of haemoglobin).

The oxygen flux is the product of 3 variables and 1 constant (ignoring oxygen in solution). Decreases in any of these variables requires compensatory changes by the other two or hypoxia will occur. The oxygen flux has an inbuilt 'reserve' of oxygen since the value of the oxygen flux is 1000 ml/min and the conscious resting subject utilizes 250 ml/min. Therefore mixed venous blood is approximately 75% saturated and the first sign of increased oxygen requirements will be venous desaturation (as occurs in exercise).

The three different types of hypoxia occur as a result of failure of any of these variables, e.g.

1. cardiac output → stagnant hypoxia
2. arterial oxygen saturation → hypoxic hypoxia
3. haemoglobin concentration → anaemic hypoxia.

Prevention of hypoxia requires intact and functioning cardiovascular and respiratory systems with adequate gas exchange taking place in the lungs. An adequate functional haemoglobin concentration with the ability to vary its oxygen affinity is also necessary.

The oxygen affinity of haemoglobin governs oxygen unloading at the tissue or mitochondrial end of the oxygen cascade. Oxygen affinity is also affected by inter-related factors which may permit adequate tissue oxygenation in many potentially hypoxic conditions.

THE OXYHAEMOGLOBIN DISSOCIATION CURVE

Oxygen affinity may be graphically illustrated by reference to the oxyhaemoglobin dissociation curve (ODC) (Fig. 41.1).

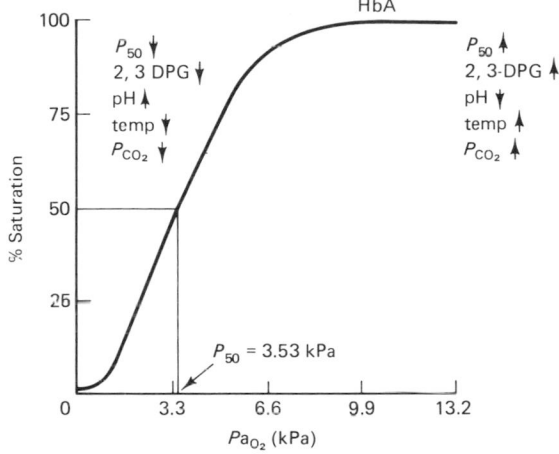

Fig. 41.1 Factors controlling the position of the oxyhaemoglobin dissociation curve.

The position of the curve is usually denoted by the P_{50}, i.e. the partial pressure of oxygen when haemoglobin is 50% saturated at pH 7.4 and a temperature of 37°C. The normal value is approximately 3.5 kPa.

A *decrease* in oxygen affinity shifts the curve to the right and *increases* the P_{50} whereas an *increase* in affinity shifts the curve to the left and *decreases* the P_{50}.

The normal sigmoid shape of the oxygen dissociation curve, due to the haem–haem interaction means that large shifts have little effect at the upper end of the curve, i.e. oxygen loading, but at the low P_{O_2} encountered in the tissues, i.e. oxygen unloading, a small change in P_{O_2} is associated with a large change in oxygen saturation. This is why an appreciation of the P_{50} and shape of the ODC is useful in clinical interpretation of changes in oxygen saturation and P_{O_2} in various disease processes. In general it may be assumed that a right shifted curve will facilitate oxygenation whereas a left shifted curve will impair it.

In 1904, Bohr elucidated the effects of hydrogen ion concentration (pH), partial pressure of carbon dioxide (P_{CO_2}) and temperature on the position of the oxyhaemoglobin dissociation curve, and in 1967 it was shown that the functional capability of haemoglobin was controlled by red cell 2,3-diphosphoglycerate (2,3-DPG) (Benesch and Benesch, 1967; Chanutin and Curnish, 1967). Increases in red cell 2,3-DPG concentration effect a significant reduction in haemoglobin oxygen affinity and permit the red cell to act as an oxygen donor under physiological conditions. Although all phosphates exert an effect on oxygen affinity, the di and triphosphates are the most potent. Only 2,3-DPG and adenosine triphosphate (ATP) are present in substantial concentrations in the erythrocyte, and 2,3-DPG is the most important since the intraerythrocytic molar concentration is about 4 times that of ATP and approximately equal to that of haemoglobin (Benesch and Benesch, 1969). This chapter discusses the role of 2,3-DPG as a mediator of oxygen delivery and its interaction with other factors affecting oxyhaemoglobin dissociation. The clinical implications of changes in oxygen affinity in some pathophysiological conditions will be discussed.

Biochemistry of 2,3-DPG

The synthesis and breakdown of 2,3-DPG is controlled in the phosphoglycerate cycle of Rapoport and Luebering (Fig. 41.2), a side shuttle off the main Embden–Meyerof pathway (Fig. 41.3). Approximately 80% of the glycolytic flux is via this shuttle. Factors controlling the concentration of 2,3-DPG are:

1. The concentration of 2,3-DPG itself. A negative

feedback mechanism inhibits the activity of 2,3-DPG phosphatase (*see* Fig. 41.1).

2. Inorganic phosphate concentration. In hypophosphataemia 2,3-DPG concentration is low and in hyperphosphataemia it is high.

3. Hydrogen ion concentration. Phosphofructokinase is pH sensitive and appears to be the pacemaker of the Embden–Meyerof pathway. In alkalosis the rate of glycolysis is increased, and the conversion of glyceraldehyde-3-phosphate to 1,3-diphosphoglycerate is favoured resulting in an increased concentration of 2,3-DPG. Decreased red cell pH inhibits phosphofructokinase, slows the rate of glycolysis and activates 2,3-DPG phosphatase which accelerates 2,3-DPG catabolism.

However, 2,3-DPG is a non-penetrating anion. As the concentration increases and especially when the 2,3-DPG/haemoglobin ratio becomes greater than 1, there is a fall in intraerythrocytic pH via the Donnan membrane equilibrium effect. This drop in pH limits further increase in 2,3-DPG concentration. Therefore the magnitude of any increase in 2,3-DPG is limited both by product inhibition and by its effect on intraerythrocytic pH (Duhm, 1971).

Binding of 2,3-DPG to Haemoglobin

Haemoglobin exists between two quaternary conformations: the deoxygenated or T-tense state with a very low oxygen affinity and an oxygenated or R-related state with a high oxygen affinity. These two forms are the extremes. The transition of one to the other leads to the smooth relationship between the partial pressure of oxygen and saturation of haemoglobin (the oxyhaemoglobin dissociation curve ODC).

X-ray crystallographic studies (Arnone, 1972) have shown that 2,3-DPG binds specifically to deoxyhaemoglobin in the central cavity where it acts as a

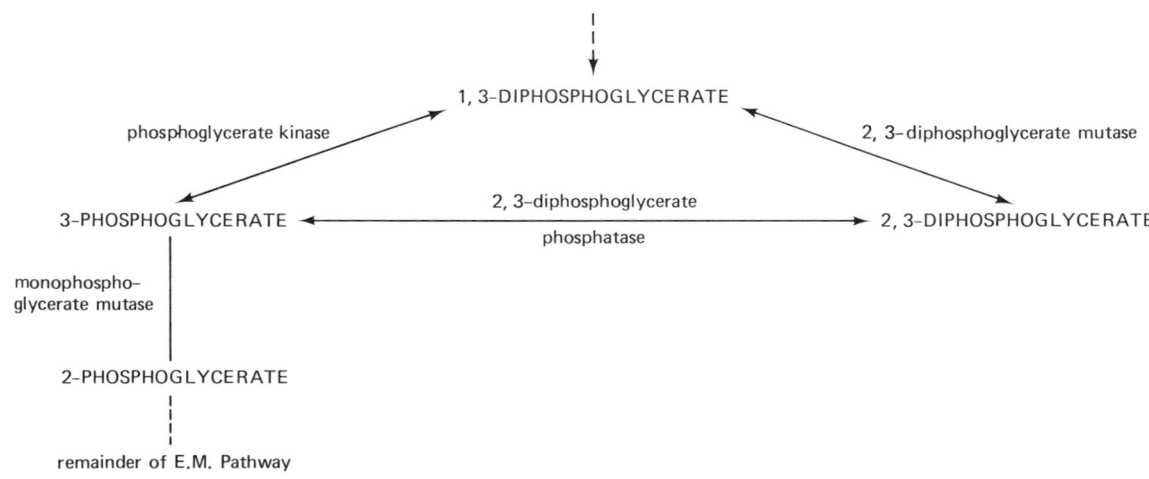

Fig. 41.2   The phosphoglycerate cycle of Rapoport and Luebering.

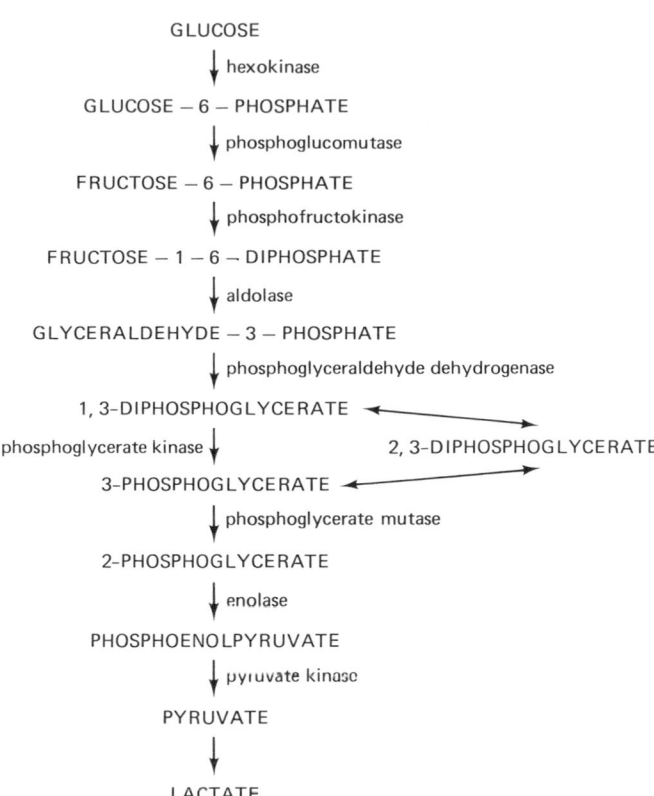

GLUCOSE

↓ hexokinase

GLUCOSE − 6 − PHOSPHATE

↓ phosphoglucomutase

FRUCTOSE − 6 − PHOSPHATE

↓ phosphofructokinase

FRUCTOSE − 1 − 6 − DIPHOSPHATE

↓ aldolase

GLYCERALDEHYDE − 3 − PHOSPHATE

↓ phosphoglyceraldehyde dehydrogenase

1, 3-DIPHOSPHOGLYCERATE

phosphoglycerate kinase ↓   2, 3-DIPHOSPHOGLYCERATE

3-PHOSPHOGLYCERATE

↓ phosphoglycerate mutase

2-PHOSPHOGLYCERATE

↓ enolase

PHOSPHOENOLPYRUVATE

↓ pyruvate kinase

PYRUVATE

↓

LACTATE

Fig. 41.3   The Embden–Meyerof pathway.

'clamp' maintaining the T state of the molecule and reducing oxygen affinity. The central cavity of relaxed, 'crumpled' oxyhaemoglobin is smaller and unable to accommodate 2,3-DPG.

2,3-DPG, hydrogen ions and carbon dioxide are all 'allosteric effectors' since they produce a change in the equilibrium between deoxy and oxyhaemoglobin.

2,3-DPG also binds non-specifically to the N-terminal amino groups of the β chains of both oxy and deoxyhaemoglobin. This is important since otherwise high concentrations of 2,3-DPG would fix haemoglobin in the deoxy or T state and uptake of oxygen in the lungs might be impaired. Many haemoglobinopathies exhibit changes in oxygen affinity which can be explained by altered binding of 2,3-DPG, secondary to genetically produced changes in the amino acid sequence.

Factors Influencing Haemoglobin–Oxygen Affinity

Intraerythrocytic 2,3-DPG, pH, P_{CO_2} and temperature all affect oxygen affinity and all these factors are inter-related. The effects of pH on the oxygen dissociation curve are difficult to dissociate physiologically from the effects of pH on 2,3-DPG concentration and the direct effect of 2,3-DPG on intraerythrocytic pH, e.g. a decrease in pH *increases* the P_{50} but also decreases

2,3-DPG concentration which results in a *decrease* in the P_{50}. Conversely an increase in pH, which *decreases* the P_{50} also increases 2,3-DPG concentration which not only *increases* the P_{50} but ultimately will produce a fall in intraerythrocytic pH which will also affect the position of the oxygen dissociation curve. In fact about 35% of the effect of 2,3-DPG on oxygygen affinity is due to its effect on intra-erythrocytic pH (Bellingham et al., 1971). pH is the major physiological factor producing instantaneous changes in the P_{50} whereas the 2,3-DPG effect takes several hours to develop. This is important in some clinical situations.

When the 2,3-DPG haemoglobin ratio is less than one its effect on oxygen affinity would appear to be due to its role as an allosteric effector stabilizing the deoxy configuration. When the ratio exceeds one, its main effect is to reduce intracellular pH which affects oxygen affinity via the Bohr effect. (Samaja and Winslow, 1979). It was originally thought that CO_2 exerted its effect on the curve solely via pH but it is now known that CO_2 produces a pH independent effect by binding to the N-terminal amino acid residues of haemoglobin. The Bohr effect is increased by about 25% when pH is changed by varying P_{CO_2}. CO_2 and 2,3-DPG compete for binding sites at N-terminal amino groups of the β chains. However at a low pH 2,3-DPG binding is stronger, thus increasing the CO_2 component of the Bohr effect whereas a high pH reduces it.

The effect of temperature on oxygen affinity is also important—an increase in temperature producing a shift towards the right and making oxygen more available when an increase in oxygen demand is accompanied by a rise in temperature. It has been suggested that the effect of 2,3-DPG on P_{50} decreases with increasing temperature. Mean corpuscular haemoglobin concentration (MCHC) also affects oxygen affinity. Increases in the MCHC, as occurs in acidosis, increase the P_{50} and decreases in the MCHC decrease the P_{50}. When a pH change occurs the MCHC changes rapidly to ensure that the P_{50} remains relatively unchanged as 2,3-DPG concentration alters.

Benesch et al. (1969) have shown that sufficiently high concentrations of anions, e.g. sodium chloride have the same effect on oxygen affinity as 2,3-DPG but when haemoglobin is saturated with 2,3-DPG, i.e. fixed in the deoxy T-tense form the position of the curve becomes independent of the salt concentration. 2,3-DPG can be considered as 'super-salt' because it achieves its physiological effect at a concentration compatible with *osmotic equilibrium* within the erythrocyte. It is the making and breaking of salt bridges, the subsequent binding and unbinding of 2,3-DPG which leads to the coexisting conformational and physicochemical equilibrium resulting in the smooth ever changing *dynamic* relationship between P_{O_2} and CO_2. The varying effects of these factors on oxygen affinity and their inter-relationship are summarized in Fig. 41.4.

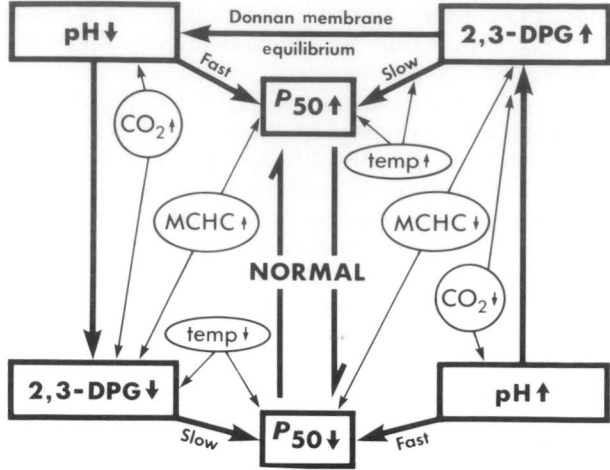

Fig. 41.4 Physiological parameters controlling the P_{50}. 2,3-DPG, exerts primary control. MCHC, P_{CO_2} and temperature exert secondary control. Any change in one parameter produces compensatory changes in the others. The system is geared to maintain a normal or increased P_{50}.

Measurement of Oxygen Affinity

Accurate construction of the oxyhaemoglobin dissociation curve requires classical tonometry. Arterial blood is equilibrated with mixtures of varying oxygen concentrations at a constant pH, P_{CO_2} and temperature. The saturation and temperature are measured and the curve is plotted. Tonometry is extremely difficult to master and its usefulness in the clinical situation is limited.

However, Severinghaus developed a slide rule for the approximation of P_{50} from a single venous sample and measuring P_{O_2}, CO_2, pH and temperature. This is based on the observation that the ratio of the P_{O_2} of blood from a shifted curve to that of a normal curve at any given saturation between 20% and 80% is constant.

Thus:

$$\text{Estimated } P_{50} = \frac{3.5 \, P_{O_2} \text{ sample}}{P_{O_2} \text{ standard}}$$

where 3.5 kPa is the normal P_{50}. The saturation of the sample must be measured to derive the standard P_{O_2}. The Severinghaus slide rule allows simultaneous correction for temperature, pH, and base excess. It would not seem unreasonable to derive the P_{50} in the clinical situation. Most intensive care units have an automatic blood gas analyser and the saturation of the sample could be measured photoelectrically (Taylor and Whitwam, 1986). In the Intensive Care Unit, a computer programme is being developed. Blood gas analyses and saturation are performed on venous and arterial bloods. The results are entered and the computer displays the patient's ODC on the VDU. The programme enables theoretical manipulation of the curve before therapeutic intervention is instituted (Bamber, 1989). This has prompted much thought about patient management and subtle changes of therapy. The work continues and hopefully heralds developments in better management of cellular oxygenation.

CHANGES IN OXYGEN AFFINITY

Oxygen affinity is the result of the interplay of many physiological parameters, e.g. following myocardial infarction 2,3-DPG concentration has been found to be raised secondary to the increased deoxyhaemoglobin:haemoglobin ratio and metabolic alkalosis (Lichtman et al., 1974). However, although the *in vitro* P_{50} was increased it was modified by the high pH. Consequently, changes in oxygen affinity secondary to an increased or decreased 2,3-DPG concentration will be discussed *only* where results have been consistent.

1. Hypoxia
a. **Hypoxic Hypoxaemia.** This is due to low inspired oxygen tension. Although an increased 2,3-DPG concentration is part of the physiological adaptation to altitude, above 12 000 feet the right shifted ODC offers little advantage as it impairs oxygen loading in the lungs. This has been elegantly verified for specific altitudes by Samaja et al. (1986) who showed that at altitudes above 5400 m an increase in the 2,3-DPG:Hb ratio is detrimental, irrespective of the state of exercise since larger blood flows are required for a given oxygen uptake. This rise in 2,3-DPG concentration appears to be less important than ventilatory compensation since people with a high affinity haemoglobinopathy can still adapt to altitude (Hebbel et al., 1978). The increase in 2,3-DPG concentration at altitude is thought to be due initially to alkalosis secondary to hypoxia induced hyperventilation. Once the pH has returned to normal by increased renal excretion of bicarbonate, 2,3-DPG concentration still remains high. This is secondary to the increased deoxygenation of haemoglobin which is associated with an intraerythrocytic alkalosis continuing to stimulate 2,3-DPG production.

b. **Anaemic Hypoxaemia.** In anaemia displacements of the oxygen dissociation curve to the right are produced by increased concentrations of 2,3-DPG, thus making normal oxygen delivery possible without such a large rise in cardiac output. This explains the exercise tolerance and lack of symptoms experienced by patients with mild anaemia.

The importance of this decreased oxygen affinity can be illustrated by reference to the anaemias associated with hexokinase and pyruvate kinase deficiency. In pyruvate kinase deficiency (2,3-DPG↑ P_{50}↑) exercise tolerance is much greater than in hexokinase deficiency (2,3-DPG↓ P_{50}↓). However, the magnitude of the increase in 2,3-DPG varies with different types of anaemia at the same haemoglobin concentration due to variation in MCHC and cell size.

2. Hypophosphataemia
Parenteral feeding, with solutions lacking added inorganic phosphorus (e.g. aminosol) leads to hypophosphataemia, low 2,3-DPG concentration and an increased oxygen affinity which can be accompanied by symptoms suggestive of hypoxia. Use of non-phosphate containing i.v. fluids following surgery also leads to hypophosphataemia, and although 2,3-DPG concentration is not significantly lowered there may be serious implications in patients in whom oxygen affinity is already disordered (Macdonald et al., 1979).

In children before puberty, increased inorganic phosphate leads to an increased 2,3-DPG concentration. The subsequent decrease in oxygen affinity and increased oxygen delivery results in a lower erythropoietin drive from the kidney and hence a reduction in red cell mass and haemoglobin concentration, thus explaining the physiological 'anaemia' of childhood (Card and Brain, 1973).

Chronic renal failure is a metabolic disease encompassing changes in electrolyte, phosphate and acid–base balance. In general 2,3-DPG concentration is elevated in patients on regular haemodialysis. The resulting reduction in haemoglobin–oxygen affinity enables these patients to function with such low haemoglobin concentrations. Therefore acidosis or hypophosphataemia should be avoided.

3. Hormonal Disorders
Aldosterone, growth hormone, androgens and adequate pituitary function are all required to maintain normal 2,3-DPG concentration and metabolism. The results of investigations in thyroid hormone dysfunction are conflicting.

In diabetes there is altered oxygen affinity. In uncontrolled diabetic ketoacidosis the low pH leads to a low 2,3-DPG concentration which will reduce the Bohr effect. If the pH is corrected too quickly with i.v. bicarbonate then this low 2,3-DPG concentration manifests itself on the position of the ODC and leads to a low P_{50}.

2,3-DPG concentration is increased in stable diabetics (Madsen and Ditzel, 1984) although the P_{50} is normal. Diabetics have an increased concentration of haemoglobin A_{1c} which has a high affinity for oxygen. The increased 2,3-DPG by lowering the affinity of the remaining HbA balances this, the overall effect being a normal P_{50}. The effects of intermittent ketoacidosis on oxygen affinity may account for the higher incidence of retinopathy and peripheral vascular disease in unstable or badly controlled diabetics.

4. Exercise and Temperature
The results of studies on the effects of acute exercise and physical training on oxygen affinity remain contradictory. Katz et al. (1984), concluded that the de-crease in oxygen affinity during strenuous exercise depended mainly on the degree of lactacidosis and temperature regulation.

5. Anaesthesia and Oxygen Affinity
Anaesthesia may alter oxygen affinity by affecting pH, electrolyte balance etc. Since halothane and methoxyflurane are capable of localized and specific interactions with haemoglobin resulting in a conformational change in its structure altered oxygen affinity might be expected.

OXYGEN AFFINITY AND STORED BLOOD

In 1954 Valtis and Kennedy observed that the ODC of blood stored in acid citrate dextrose solution (ACD) is shifted to the left. This effect can be explained by the decrease in 2,3-DPG concentration during storage. When blood is stored in citrate–phosphate–dextrose solution (CPD) 2,3-DPG concentration is maintained for longer.

If ACD or CPD blood is deep frozen within 24 h of collection 2,3-DPG concentration can be maintained and many blood transfusion centres offer this for special cases.

Depletion of 2,3-DPG does not rob the red cells of all their value because they regenerate 2,3-DPG—about one half being restored in 4 h and synthesis is almost complete after 1 day. It must be remembered that many patients survive massive blood transfusion. Nevertheless there will still be a transient increase in oxygen affinity. Its return to normal will depend not only on the volume of blood transfused but the physical condition of the patient, e.g. acid–base status, the availability of phosphate, the preoperative position of the ODC, the ability to increase the cardiac output. The implications for patients with preexisting cardiac or cerebrovascular disease are obvious. Blood transfusion with 2,3-DPG depleted blood in patients who have an adaptive increase in 2,3-DPG, e.g. anaemia, renal failure, old age, pregnancy may lead to an increase in oxygen affinity sufficient to cause symptoms of hypoxia.

Smoking and Oxygen Affinity

In people who smoke up to 15% of available oxygen binding sites may be occupied by carbon monoxide which results in a 25% reduction of available oxygen (Jones et al., 1987). Smokers compensate for this by increasing their haemoglobin and/or 2,3-DPG concentrations.

Anaemic or pregnant patients who smoke will suffer a *further* reduction of their functional haemoglobin concentration. Since these patients already have an increased 2,3-DPG concentration they may be unable to effect an even greater increase because of product inhibition and the effects of 2,3-DPG on intraerythrocytic pH.

CLINICAL RELEVANCE OF OXYGEN AFFINITY

Oxygen affinity is primarily controlled by erythrocytic 2,3-DPG and pH, with P_{CO_2}, temperature, MCHC and inorganic phosphorus exerting secondary control. This constitutes an elegant physiological mechanism but what is the clinical relevance?

Inadequate concentration of 2,3-DPG will assume greater importance in pathophysiological conditions in which it would be normally elevated, e.g. anaemia, old age, renal failure, pregnancy etc. Thus, acidosis, hypophosphataemia and blood transfusion, all of which reduce 2,3-DPG concentration should, if possible be avoided, e.g. not infrequently patients are hurriedly transfused the evening prior to theatre to obtain a haemoglobin concentration acceptable to the anaesthetist. If preoperative transfusions are deemed necessary in elderly or anaemic patients this should be carried out at least 48 h prior to surgery. It is not the *absolute* haemoglobin concentration which must be considered but the *functional* haemoglobin concentration.

In pregnancy, 2,3-DPG concentration is increased by about 20%. It follows that transfusion of the anaemic pregnant patient near term is hazardous since the reduction in maternal 2,3-DPG concentration may lead to fetal hypoxia. This explains why blood transfusions near term may result in premature labour. If blood transfusion is absolutely necessary then fresh blood should be used and continuous fetal heart monitoring should be carried out during the transfusion.

Tissue, i.e. fetal, oxygenation in pregnant patients who smoke is precarious. The may explain why patients who continue to smoke during pregnancy have smaller babies.

The relatively short half-life of carboxy-haemoglobin means that the cessation of smoking for as short a time as 12 h (Jones et al., 1987) is beneficial. While smoking should positively be discouraged it might profitably be *prohibited* prior to anaesthesia in patients with disordered oxygen affinity, e.g. anaemia, old age, diabetes, renal failure, etc. Therapeutic intervention and treatment of oxygen affinity in the clinical situation has been hampered by the difficulty of measuring the P_{50}. The assessment of oxygenation has depended on invasive intermittent blood gas analyses. It is not enough to measure the P_{CO_2} as the saturation of haemoglobin with oxygen is important. Continuous noninvasive oxygen saturation monitoring is now possible and several machines are available to do this (Taylor et al., 1986). The ease with which the haemoglobin is going to part with the oxygen must also be considered with reference to the pH and general metabolic state.

The oxyhaemoglobin dissociation curve is *dynamic*. Oxygen affinity may be only one link in the chain of oxygen transport from the lungs to the tissues. Strengthening that will compensate for weakness in others and ultimately benefit cellular oxygenation and prevent hypoxia.

REFERENCES

Arnone A. (1972). X-ray diffraction study of binding of 2,3-diphosphoglycerate to human deoxyhaemoglobin. *Nature*, **237**, 146.

Bamber P. (1989). Personal communication about a computer programme for display and theoretical manipulation of the oxyhaemoglobin dissociation curve.

Bellingham A.J., Detter J.C., Lenfant C. (1971). Regulatory mechanisms of haemoglobin oxygen affinity in acidosis and alkalosis. *J. Clin. Invest.*, **50**, 700.

Benesch R., Benesch R.E. (1967). The effect of organic phosphates from the human erythrocyte on the allosteric properties of haemoglobin. *Biochem. Biophys. Res. Commun.*, **26**, 162.

Benesch R., Benesch R.E. (1969). Intracellular organic phosphates as regulators of oxygen release by haemoglobin. *Nature*, **221**, 618.

Card R.T., Brain M.C. (1973). The 'anaemia' of childhood. Evidence for a physiological response to hyperphosphataemia. *New Engl. J. Med.*, **288**, 388.

Chanutin A., Curnish R.R. (1967). Effect of organic and inorganic phosphates on the oxygen equilibrium of human erythrocytes. *Arch. Biochem. Biophys.*, **121**, 96.

Duhm J. (1971). Effects of 2,3-diphosphoglycerate and other organic phosphate compounds on oxygen affinity and intracellular pH of human erythrocytes. *Pfluegers Archive: Eur. J. Physiol.*, **326**, 341.

Hebbel R.P., Eaton J.W., Kroneuberg R.S., et al. (1978). Human llamas: adaptation to altitude in subjects with high haemoglobin oxygen affinity. *J. Clin. Invest.*, **62**, 593.

Jones R.M., Rosen M., Seymour L. (1987). Smoking and anaesthesia. *Anaesthesia*, **42**, 1.

Katz A., Sharp R., King D.S., et al. (1984). Effect of high intensity interval training on 2,3-diphosphoglycerate at rest and after manual exercise. *Eur. J. Appl. Physiol.*, **52**, 331.

Lichtman M.A., Cohen J., Young J.A., et al. (1974). The relationships between arterial oxygen flow rate, oxygen binding by haemoglobin and oxygen utilization after myocardial infarction. *J. Clin. Invest.*, **54**, 501.

Macdonald R., Guillou P.J., Kester R.C. (1979). Plasma phosphate and red cell 2,3-diphosphoglycerate following abdominal surgery. *Anaesthesia*, **35**, 339.

Madsen H., Ditzel J. (1984). Red cell 2,3-diphosphoglycerate and haemoglobin oxygen affinity during normal pregnancy. *Acta Obstet. Gynecol. Scand.*, **63**, 399.

Nunn J.F. (1977). Oxygen, in '*Applied Respiratory Physiology*'. London: Butterworths.

Nunn J.F., Freeman J. (1964). Problems of oxygenation and oxygen transport during haemorrhage. *Anaesthesia*, **19**, 206.

Samaja M., Di Prampero P.E., Cerretelli P. (1986). The role of 2,3-DPG in oxygen transport at altitude. *Resp. Physiol.*, **64**, 191.

Samaja M., Winslow, R.M. (1979). The separate effects of H^+ and 2,3-DPG on the oxygen equilibrium curve of human blood. *Br. J. Haematol.*, **41**, 373.

Taylor M.B., Whitwam J.G. (1986). The current status of pulse oximetry. *Anaesthesia*, **41**, 943.

Valtis D.J., Kennedy A.C. (1954). Defective gas transport function of stored red blood cells. *Lancet*, **226**, 119.

FURTHER READING

For a more complete list of references to original work on oxygen affinity and erythrocytic 2,3-diphosphoglycerate readers are referred to the following review articles:

Harken A.H. (1977). The surgical significance of the oxy-haemoglobin dissociation curve. *Surg. Gynaecol. Obstet.*, **144**, 935.

Macdonald R. (1977). Red cell 2,3-diphosphoglycerate and oxygen affinity. *Anaesthesia*, **32**, 544.

Meldon J.H. (1986). Blood gas transport and 2,3-DPG. *Adv. Exp. Med. Biol.*, **191**, 63.

International forum. (1978). What is the clinical importance of alterations of the haemoglobin oxygen affinity in preserved blood—especially as produced by variations of red cell 2,3-DPG content? *Vox Sanguinis*, **34**, 111.

F. SPECIAL PHYSIOLOGY

42. Neuromuscular Transmission and Block

S. A. Feldman

Neuromuscular transmission
 Anatomy of the neuromuscular junction
 Neuromuscular transmission
 Postjunctional membrane potential
 Depolarization of the postsynaptic membrane
 Formation and release of acetylcholine
 Margin of safety of neuromuscular transmission
Neuromuscular block
 Depolarization block (agonist block)
 Non-depolarization block (antagonist or competitive block)
 Other conduction blocks
 Desensitization block
 Channel block ('in use' block)
 Gate block
Tests and measurement of neuromuscular block
 Summary

NEUROMUSCULAR TRANSMISSION

In the chain of events that starts with the stimulation of a motor nerve and ends with the contraction of muscle, the most vulnerable link is the synapse between the nerve and muscle—the neuromuscular junction. It is here that the neuromuscular blocking agents exert their action and that many physical and chemical factors have their effect.

Anatomy of the Neuromuscular Junction

The motor end plate is a specialized part of the post-junctional region of the muscle and it is separated from the motor nerve ending by the synaptic cleft. The cleft is enclosed by a membrane, the Schwann cell membrane, which anatomically separates it from the ECF. This membrane fuses with the perimysium of the muscle postjunctionally and is believed to be an extension of the Schwann cell covering the myelinated part of motor nerve proximal to the neuromuscular junction. The fundamental anatomy of the neuro-muscular junction was elucidated by Birks et al. in 1960 (Fig. 42.1). Modern techniques have demonstrated refinements of histological detail which, in turn, have given us greater insight into the way the synapse functions. Details of the presynaptic membrane have shown it to be traversed by an apparent grid between the lines of which acetylcholine vesicles discharge their contents by exocytosis into the synaptic cleft. The postsynaptic membrane is folded into longitudinal gutters (Fig. 42.2). Along the ridges of these gutters lie the openings to the secondary clefts. This area is rich in cholinesterase and stains with gold

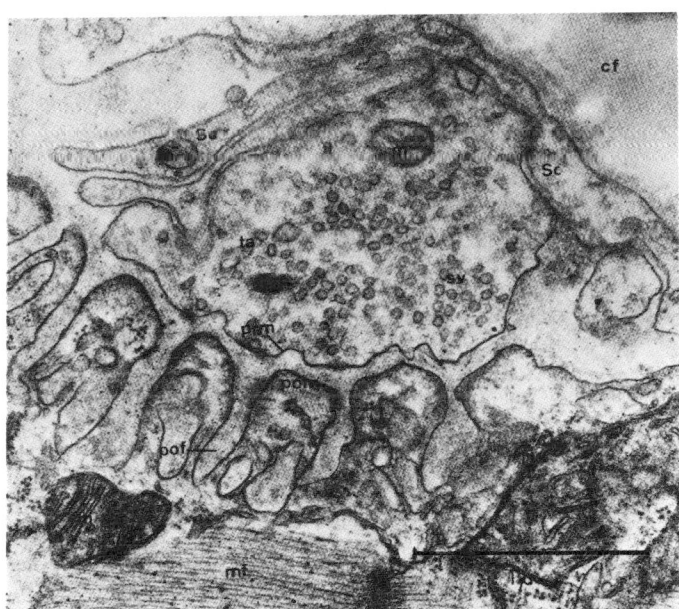

Fig. 42.1 Electron microscopy of a neuromuscular junction. prm = presynaptic membrane; pom = postsynaptic membrane; pof = secondary synaptic cleft; mf = muscle fibre. The acetylcholine vesicles and the mitochondria (m) (ta) are contained in the motor nerve terminal. (With permission from Birks et al., 1960, and the Editor of *J. Physiol., Lond.*)

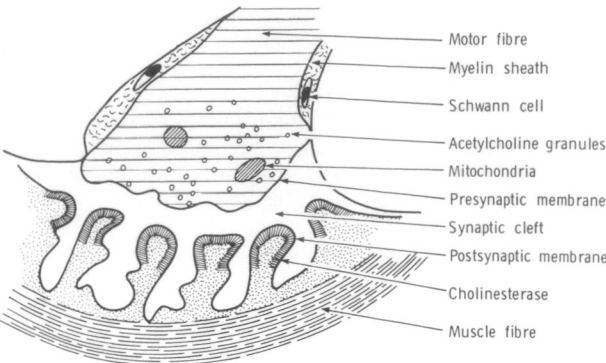

Motor fibre
Myelin sheath
Schwann cell
Acetylcholine granules
Mitochondria
Presynaptic membrane
Synaptic cleft
Postsynaptic membrane
Cholinesterase
Muscle fibre

Fig. 42.2 Schematic representation of the neuromuscular junction. The postsynaptic membrane is folded into longitudinal gutters.

thioacetate (Nickel and Waser, 1968). This area corresponds to the site of binding of labelled toxiferine and α bungarotoxin (Waser, 1972). Freeze etch imaging allows the visualization of clusters of tiny protrusions in this area between 7–9 nm diameter each of which surrounds a sodium channel. It is on these minute surface mounds that the receptors for acetylcholine and non-depolarizing neuromuscular blockers are found.

Freeze etched images of frog muscle endplate by Hirokawa and Heuser (1982) have shown that the synaptic cleft, which measures about 50–70 nm in width is filled with sheets of a mucopolysacchride material folded upon themselves in a manner that causes them to appear on tranverse section like a disorganized lattice. Further elucidation of the ultrastructure of this important region has revealed that it contains a high density of 'long tailed' cholinesterase molecules trapped in the interstices of this lattice. It is through this minute space that the acetylcholine molecules, released presynaptically, must travel in order to produce depolarization of the postsynaptic membrane and trigger off an action potential.

It has been postulated that there may be channels between the presynaptic membrane and the crests of the secondary clefts on the postsynaptic membrane where the highest density of receptors are found. In this manner acetylcholine, when released as a transmitter, would rapidly reach the receptors without contact with cholinesterase, but when it is displaced from the receptor, it would diffuse into the cleft where it would be rapidly destroyed.

Neuromuscular Transmission

A motor nerve containing many hundreds of nerve fibres serves many thousands of muscle fibres. The relationship between the number of muscle fibres innervated by one nerve fibre is an index of the refinement of control of motor function that is possible in that motor unit. Muscles capable of fine movements, such

as those of the eye and the hand, have fewer muscle fibres related to each motor nerve while the postural muscles have many hundreds of muscle fibres innervated by one nerve fibre. The stimulation of each motor nerve fibre has to be of threshold strength to produce a propagated action potential. If the motor nerve stimulation causes the release of sufficient transmitter substance to cause a suprathreshold change in the resting membrane potential of the motor end plate, then muscle contraction will ensue. This 'all or none' phenomenon controls excitation of each muscle unit. It therefore follows that the only way of producing a reduction in the strength of muscle contraction is by activating a smaller number of motor units. Because of this phenomenon, when quantitative comparisons of muscle activity are to be made, it is necessary to ensure all the muscle fibres that can contract are activated, by using a supramaximal stimulation of either the motor nerve (indirect stimulation) or muscle (direct stimulation). Even when this is achieved, changes in contractility of the muscle due to physical factors, such as the initial stretch of the muscle fibres, may occur. To minimize this effect, a standard preload is applied to the muscle whose contraction is to be measured. Under conditions of supramaximal stimulation and standard preload, the difference in the twitch response occurring when the motor nerve is stimulated from that produced when the muscle is stimulated indicates changes at the neuromuscular junction. (For true direct stimulation the muscle should be stimulated in the presence of a non-depolarizing muscle relaxant to prevent retrograde conduction of the impulse along the muscle to the motor end plate causing postsynaptic stimulation of the muscle.)

Acetylcholine, the transmitter substance released at the motor nerve terminals was shown by Dale and Feldberg (1934) to cause contraction of the muscle if applied to the sensitive area of the muscle, at the motor end plate. In 1936 Dale et al. demonstrated that curare did not inhibit the release of acetylcholine in doses that produced neuromuscular block. Electrophysiological studies have demonstrated that the action of acetycholine at the postsynaptic membrane is associated with a change in the resting membrane potential producing depolarization. If the voltage change is adequate and conditions are suitable, the depolarization produces a propagated action potential resulting in muscle contraction.

Postjunctional Membrane Potential

The electromagnetic potential across the postjunctional membrane of the receptor area of the neuromuscular junction is controlled by the sodium channels. The membrane potential is a reflection of the uneven distribution of ions across the surface membrane (*see* Chapter 26). In the resting state with the sodium channels closed, the end plate membrane is far more permeable to K^+ ions than Na^+ ions. As a result K^+ ions pass out of the cell along their concentration gradient until the accumulation of positively charged ions on the outside of the membrane produces an electromagnetic force which opposes further migration of the positively charged potassium ions. This point of equilibrium determines the resting membrane potential. If one regards the end plate membrane as being semipermeable, the resting EMF can be expressed in accordance with the Gibbs–Donnan rule as being proportional to the ratio of the concentrations of the most permeable ion (potassium) on the two sides of the membrane (Hodgkin and Horrowicz, 1959). This is expressed in the Nernst equation.

$$\text{EMF} = \frac{RT}{F} \ln \frac{[\text{K}^+]_o}{[\text{K}^+]_i}$$

$[\text{K}^+]_i$ = potassium ion concentration inside cell; $[\text{K}^+]_o$ = potassium ion concentration outside cell membrane; R = universal gas constant; T = absolute temp; F = Faraday constant. In mammalian muscle this resting potential is about -90 mV.

As the magnitude of this resting membrane potential will determine the relative ease by which it is depolarized, it is evident that alterations in the ratio of potassium ions between those inside the cell (normally about 150 mmol) and those in the extracellular fluid (normally about 5 mmol) will have a profound effect on neuromuscular conduction. If this ratio is raised (i.e. by decreasing the extracellular potassium concentration relative to that inside the cell), then hyperpolarization of the membrane occurs and will result in resistance to depolarization by acetylcholine. This causes an increased sensitivity to non-depolarizing relaxants (Feldman, 1963). It has been recognized since the work of Jennerick and Gerard in 1953 that if the end plate potential falls from its normal resting value of -90 mV to below -57 mV, then further depolarization produces an insufficient energy flux to trigger off an action potential. Depolarizing neuromuscular blocking agents produce their effect by lowering the resting membrane potential causing it to become insensitive and neuromuscular block to be established. Depolarization of the membrane increases the speed of closing of the sodium channel following depolarization making further ionic flux more difficult while hyperpolarization delays the closure of the sodium channels making it easier for drugs to enter the ionophore producing 'channel block' (Bowman, 1986).

Depolarization of the Postsynaptic Membrane

Acetylcholine produces depolarization of the postsynaptic membrane by opening sodium channels causing an increase in its permeability to Na$^+$ ions. As a result, the membrane becomes more permeable to sodium than potassium, and the transmembrane potential changes from the resting value (-90 mV) that reflected the concentration ratio for potassium to one that is determined by the ionic gradient for

sodium. The opening of the sodium barrier causes a change in the EMF across the membrane, and the immediate entry of sodium ions into the cell. The extent of this depolarization is determined by the pressure head of sodium trying to enter the cell along a positive concentration and electrostatic gradient, and by the number of sodium channels that are opened. The actual extent of the movement of sodium ions is limited and influenced not only by the number of open sodium channels that are available, but also by the duration for which they are kept open. Thus drugs that retard the closing of sodium channels (like germine diacetate, veratrum alkaloids and 4 aminopyridine) prolong the duration of the action potential enhancing the action of acetycholine. At the receptor, acetylcholine reacts with specific sites on the α subunits of the five-unit structure that forms the cholinoceptor protein (Fig. 42.3) (*see* Chapter 52). These

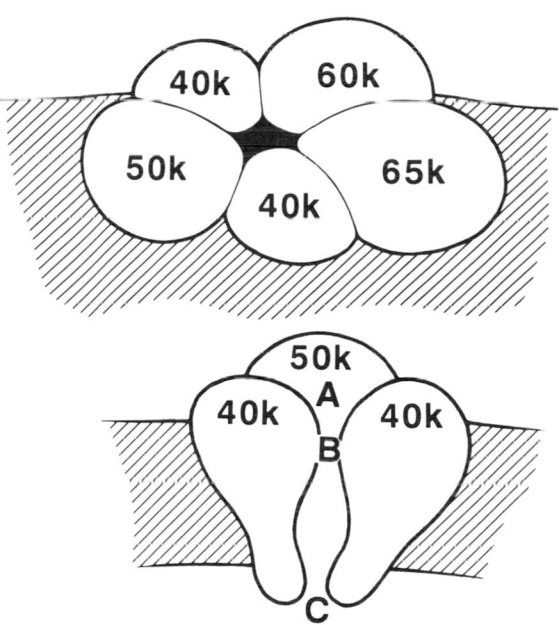

Fig. 42.3 The five-unit structure penetrating the postsynaptic membrane that constitutes the cholinoceptor. 40 K units = α units; sites A, B and C are potential sites of neuromuscular blocking. A, postsynaptic receptor site; B, channel block site; C, cytoplasmic block site.

units penetrate the surface membrane and surround the central pore which, in its open state, allows passage of sodium ions along their concentration gradient into the cell. In order to open this channel, pairs of acetylcholine specific recognition sites on the two α subunits must be simultaneously activated. The receptors are in the region of the disulphide bonds in the chain of amino acids that make up the α units (Changeax et al., 1984; Sheridan and Lester, 1982). Changes induced by acetylcholine produce a contraction of both α units. Due to the asymmetry caused by the uneven number of units, a rotational effect is produced along with contraction of the subunits resulting in an increased diameter of the central channel. In order to prevent this acetylcholine induced response, non-depolarizing muscle relaxants have to occupy a certain critical number of receptor sites or act to bridge the ionophore imposing a rigidity on the structure that prevents deformation.

Formation and Release of Acetylcholine

Acetylcholine is formed from the acetylation of choline under the influence of choline-o-acetyltransferase (cholineacetylase). The enzyme is associated with large mitochondria in the axoplasm of the nerve. In normal circumstances its ability to synthesize acetylcholine does not appear to be a rate limiting factor in neuromuscular transmission.

Choline is present in the ECF and blood as a result of hepatic synthesis and dietary intake (its concentration falls in starvation). However, about half the choline taken into the nerve for acetylcholine synthesis is recycled choline from hydrolyzed acetylcholine. Choline is positively charged and is transported by an active, highly specific carrier mechanism across the axonal membrane. The choline carrier may be blocked either by chemically similar substances, such as hemicholinium, or by substances that act as alternative substitutes for choline leading to the formation of false transmitter (Potter, 1968). Once in the axoplasm, acetylation of choline takes place and the newly formed acetylcholine is then loaded against its concentration gradient into densely packed vesicles. This is achieved by a specific energy dependent carrier which depends upon calcium and ATPase. The mechanism underlying this process has been extensively studied by Marshall and Parsons (1987) using phenylpiperidino cyclohexanol (vescimicol) which blocks the loading process.

Acetylcholine is present in the vesicles (quantal store) and axoplasm (non-quantal). In the quantal form, it is either in a reserve store (R.ACh), or as part of an immediate available source (IAS ACh) (Fig. 42.4). It is the size of the pool of immediately available acetylcholine that determines the amount of quantal transmitter release following stimulation of the motor nerve. The discharge of vesicles is a random process, the greater the concentration of vesicles, the more will be discharged per unit time following nerve stimulation (Fig. 42.5). If vesicles are lost from the IAS, then the rate of acetylcholine release per nerve stimulus will fall until the rate of discharge equals the rate of replenishment of IAS. This is believed to be the mechanism underlying the train of 4 fade when stimulation is at a rate of 2 Hz. The reduced acetylcholine release only becomes apparent in the partially curarized or myasthenic patient. However, if the rate of stimulation is greater, i.e. 50–100 Hz, tetanic stimulation, then fade is minimized by a positive feedback resulting from the acetylcholine liberated during the

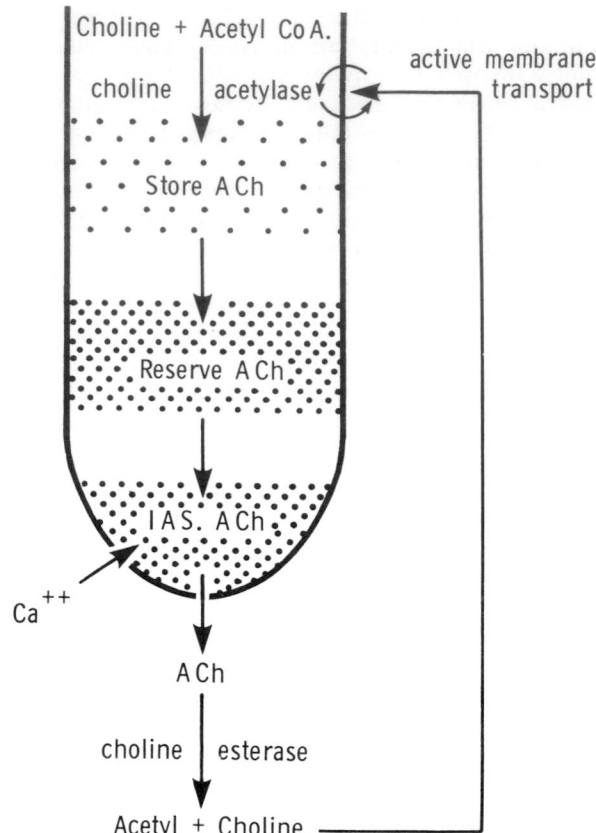

Fig. 42.4 Formation and release of acetylcholine. (From S. A. Feldman, 1979. *Muscle Relaxants; Major Problems in Anaesthesia*, I. (2nd edn.) Philadelphia: Saunders.)

tetanic stimulation, acting upon presynaptic cholinoceptors on the motor nerve. The effect of this feedback is to stimulate the transfer of acetylcholine into the IAS at a rate that keeps pace with the loss into the synaptic cleft, thus effectively limiting the fade. In the presence of presynaptic block produced by some neuromuscular blocking agents, the prejunctional feedback is reduced and fade is exaggerated (Bowman et al., 1984). This has been used by Bowman and Webb (1976; Bowman, 1985) to study the presynaptic site of activity of neuromuscular blocking agents. Following the cessation of tetanic stimulation and increased transmitter mobilization, there is a short

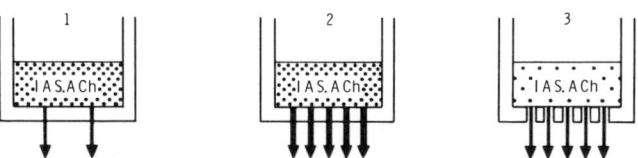

Fig. 42.5 The size of the immediately available store of acetylcholine (IAS) determines the number of quanta of transmitter released when the motor nerve is stimulated. 1, resting state; 2, active state; 3, active state with depleted IAS causes less quanta to be released.

period of overshoot during which time a single nerve stimulus will produce an unusually large release of acetylcholine. This is seen in partially curarized patients where it produces post-tetanic potentiation. The duration of this effect is measured in the post-tetanic count which provides an index of recovery from neuromuscular block.

There is a constant leak of acetylcholine from the presynaptic region. This is both quantal and non-quantal. The quantal leak, representing the discharge of 1 or 2 vesicles at a rate of about 2 Hz at normal temperature gives rise to postsynaptic voltage changes of 0.5–1 mV termed mini end plate potentials (mepps). The non-quantal leak of acetylcholine produces insignificant postsynaptic voltage changes. The acetylcholine is thought to originate both in the motor nerve and also in the Schwann cells.

Following stimulation of a motor nerve, the potassium channels on the prejunctional membrane open. These channels also permit the inward passage of calcium ions. The rate of entry of calcium depends upon the external concentration and the duration of the open state of the channel. Thus a small fall in extracellular calcium or a prolonged open channel state will cause a profound effect upon this process. Drugs such as tetraethylammonium and 4 aminopyridine which delay closure of the potassium channels increase the calcium influx, as does a fall in body temperature. Calcium influx activates calmodulin and ATPase and leads to a large synchronous quantal discharge of acetylcholine into the synaptic cleft. One nerve impulse causes the simultaneous discharge of some 200–300 quantal vesicles. The prejunctional simultaneous release of some 10 000 molecules of acetylcholine usually results in a postjunctional action potential of sufficient magnitude to trigger off a propagated muscle action potential. This will cause excitation of the sarcolemma, activating the T tubules of the sarcoplasmic reticulum which, in turn, leads to muscle contraction (*see* Chapter 43). It has been proposed by Long et al. (1983) that the production of antibodies to this calcium transport involving the calmodulin system may be responsible for the neuromuscular weakness of the Eaton–Lambert syndrome (myasthenic syndrome).

In addition to the quantal release of acetylcholine, Thesleff and Molgo (1983) have described a release of acetylcholine which is not calcium dependent. It has been suggested that this non-quantal acetylcholine may have a trophic effect upon the end plate. It is possible that acetylcholine produced in Schwann cells also determine the anatomical integrity of normally innervated neuromuscular junctions. The loss of this trophic influence following denervation may be the cause of the dispersion of receptor material away from the specific receptor area. The spread of sodium channel protein containing the receptors to acetylcholine over the surface of the muscle is the cause of the large potassium flux that occurs when denervated muscles are exposed to depolarizing agents.

Margin of Safety of Neuromuscular Transmission

The concept of the margin of safety of neuromuscular transmission was introduced by Paton and Waud (1967). They demonstrated that unless more than 75% of the receptors were occupied by d-tubocurarine, it was not possible to detect a reduction in the indirectly elicited twitch response (Fig. 42.6). This extent of receptor occupancy is necessary to reduce

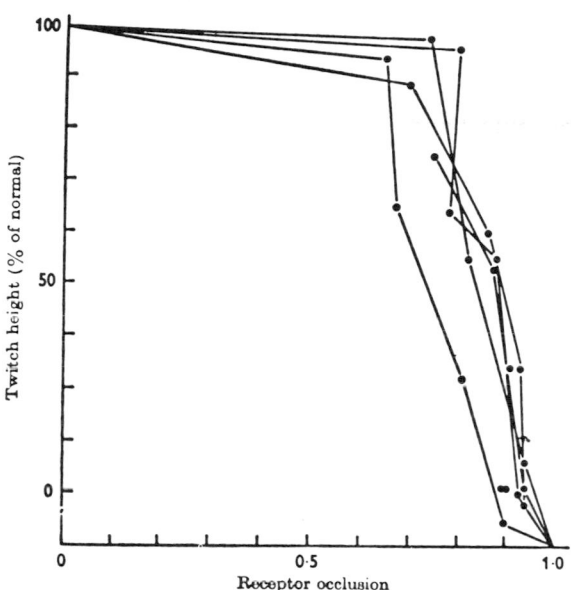

Fig. 42.6 Margin of safety of neuromuscular transmission. No depression of twitch response can be detected until over 75% of the receptors are occluded. (With permission from W.D.M. Paton and D. Waud, 1967, and the Editor of *J. Physiol., Lond.*)

the random probability of adequate acetylcholine-receptor interaction taking place to cause a change in membrane potential of sufficient magnitude to trigger off a propagated action potential. The concept was developed by Waud and Waud (1971), who demonstrated that the margin of safety was reduced if tetanic rather than twitch rates of stimulation were used. However, even at fast physiological rates of stimulation, at least 50% of the receptors have to be occupied by curare before the muscle twitch response is lost. As the reaction between receptor and transmitter is random, the margin of safety reflects the normal superfluous production of acetylcholine and excessive number of receptor sites available. If less transmitter is released, then a minor reduction in receptor availability, which would normally be without any physiological effect, may cause neuromuscular block.

One consequence of the high margin of safety of neuromuscular transmission is that in order to effect neuromuscular block over 75% of receptors must be occupied by non-depolarizing drugs whilst depolarization can occur if over 25% of receptors are activated. This might explain the slowness of the onset of postsynaptic receptor block by non-depolarizing drugs compared to the rapid action associated with depolarizing agents.

The basis of the priming principle in which a small dose of a non-depolarizing relaxant is administered 3 min before the full dose in order to increase the rate of onset of paralysis can be explained on the basis of the large safety margin of neuromuscular transmission. It has been demonstrated that irrespective of agent used, a priming dose that just produces diplopia and difficulty in controlling the muscles of the tongue must be administered if onset of total block is to be achieved in 60 s following injection of the paralytic dose. This strongly suggests that a critical receptor occupancy must be obtained by the priming dose requiring only a further 10–20% receptor occupancy to be achieved in order to obtain complete neuromuscular block (Harrop-Griffiths et al., 1986; Jones, 1989).

NEUROMUSCULAR BLOCK

Various ways have been proposed in which a block of the nervous transmission to the muscle may be effected. Some of these are undoubtedly important in pharmacologically induced neuromuscular block whilst the role of others in clinical practice is more uncertain.

The two most important clinical components of neuromuscular block by muscle relaxant drugs are depolarizing, agonist block and non-depolarizing, antagonist (competitive) block of the postsynaptic membrane. With the advent of the new drug ORG 9426 interest has been stimulated in the characteristics of non-depolarizing presynaptic blocks in clinical practice.

Depolarization Block (Agonist Block)

Depolarization of the postsynaptic membrane to 57 mV or less results in unresponsiveness of that membrane to acetylcholine and causes neuromuscular block (Burns and Paton, 1951; del Castillo and Katz, 1956). Gissen and Nastuk (1970) confirmed that decamethonium produced this degree of depolarization. Although suxamethonium was demonstrated to produce a slightly lesser depolarization, it still produced conduction block. It is proposed that the continuing association and dissociation of agonist drug molecules with receptors on the postsynaptic membrane produce continuing depolarization and block. The duration of the action will therefore depend upon the maintenance of a critical concentration of drug in the synaptic cleft. It is a characteristic of this type of block that it is rapid in onset and recovery, does not exhibit tetanic fade nor post-tetanic potentiation. It is not reversed by anticholinesterase drugs. It is also found that all agonists studied are capable of causing a phase II block when the end plate is exposed to a high concen-

tration of drug for a prolonged period. This may be the result from a failure of hydrolysis of suxamethonium, following excessive neostigmine administration in the absence of residual non-depolarizing block, or following prolonged or excessive administration of suxamethonium or decamethonium.

Non-Depolarization Block (Antagonist or Competitive Block)

Non-depolarizing, antagonist or competitive block follows the use of drugs such as d-tubocurarine, alcuronium, pancuronium, vecuronium and atracurium. The classical concept of the mechanism of this block is that molecules of the drug compete with molecules of acetylcholine for postsynaptic receptor sites. If there is a relative preponderance of drug relative to acetylcholine it will occupy sufficient receptor sites to achieve neuromuscular block. The characteristics of such a block have been established by Gaddum and by Schild and others. They are:

1. The inhibitory effect of the drug can be overcome by increasing the dose of agonist or lowering the dose of antagonist.
2. That increasing the concentration of competitive antagonists in discrete steps displaces the *log* dose response for the agonist to the right in a parallel fashion in a manner described by the Schild plot.

Unfortunately although the predications of the second of these pre-requisites are fulfilled in laboratory experiments using the isolated phrenic nerve diaphragm preparation of the rat, neither they nor the first characteristic can be reconciled readily with clinical observations or with findings in intact animals. Thus:

1. It is a common experience that is well documented that in the presence of even sub-paralytic plasma concentrations of some non-depolarizing drugs it is impossible to reverse the action by neostigmine (Baraka, 1977). However, once the plasma concentration is lowered reversal is easily achieved by anticholinesterases. (Feldman and Levi, 1963).
2. Rapidly lowering the plasma concentration of drug in the isolated arm of volunteers from an ED_{95} concentration to a sub-paretic level does not cause a rapid reversal of drug action. Indeed the rate of reversal appears not to depend on the plasma concentration, the blood flow or the physical properties of the drug, but upon its electrochemical structure (Feldman and Tyrrell, 1970).
3. Mixing various doses of neostigmine, from 0.5 mg to 2.5 mg with 2 mg of d-tubocurarine and administering the mixture into the blood of arms isolated from the general circulation by a tourniquet does not prevent the onset of neuro-

muscular block or alter its effectiveness (Feldman and Agoston, 1980). This is the in vivo equivalent of the agonist-antagonist experiments used to construct the Schild plot in vitro experiments.

This has led to an alternative hypothesis to the simple competitive concept of non-depolarizing block. Feldman and Tyrell (1970) proposed a theory of action based upon Paton's Rate Theory (1961). This envisages the antagonist molecules reacting with the receptor sites to cause a receptor occupancy whose duration is determined by physio-chemical properties of the specific drug-receptor association. Whilst the drug occupies the receptor it denies it access to the biological transmitter and so produces neuromuscular block. The block is reversed by acetylcholine disrupting the drug-receptor association.

The relatively slow dissociation of non-depolarizing drugs from the receptor when compared to the rate of association was demonstrated by Armstrong and Lester (1979) who found a ratio of onset/offset times of 1/20 for d-tubocurarine. They explained this on the basis of 'buffered diffusion'. Buffered diffusion proposes that the microenvironment within the synaptic cleft is strongly influenced by the high density of receptors with their affinity for the positively charged onium heads of the acetylcholine and muscle relaxant drug molecules. As a result, although competition between acetylcholine and drugs may exist within this environment, drug molecules not associated with receptors are still concentrated within the barrier of the Schwann cell membrane. Factors that reduce receptor density or destroy the Schwann cell membrane hasten recovery from neuromuscular block in vitro in isolated nerve-muscular preparations.

An alternative suggestion is that the high density of mucopolysaccharide in the synaptic cleft may act in a similar manner by acting as a local depot (acceptor) of high affinity for drug molecules with a strong positive charge. As a result reversal of the non-depolarizing block by anticholinesterase drugs would only have a temporary effect as the displaced drug would be held in the synaptic cleft ready to reassociate with the receptor once the concentration of acetylcholine was reduced.

It has been demonstrated that two steps are essential before non-depolarizing neuromuscular block can be reversed.

1. Drug must be displaced from the receptor by acetylcholine.
2. Drug plasma level must be sufficiently low for displaced drug to leave the synaptic cleft along its concentration gradient.

Agoston et al. (1979) demonstrated that the rate of spontaneous recovery following pancuronium block was strongly influenced by the circulating plasma concentration of drug (Fig. 42.7).

Non-depolarizing block is characteristically slow in

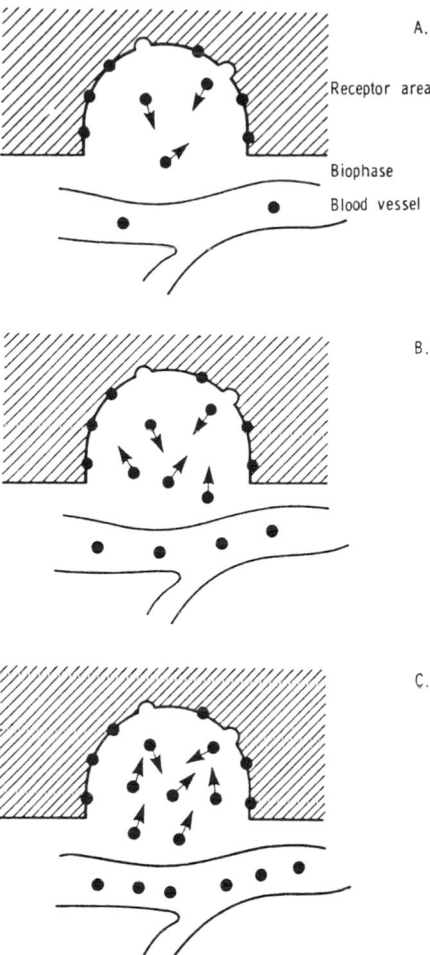

Fig. 42.7 The effect of increasing blood concentration of drug is to reduce the rate at which drug displaced from the receptor site can leave the neuromuscular junction. Low blood concentration of drug (A) allows rapid reversal of block. High blood concentration of drug (C) prevents reversal of block.

onset, reversed by neostigmine or other anticholinesterase drugs, shows fade on a train of 4 stimulation (2 Hz) or tetanic stimulation and demonstrates post-tetanic potentiation.

Other Conduction Blocks

Presynaptic Block
Just as acetylcholine released during tetanic stimulation reacts with presynaptic cholinoceptors to mobilize acetylcholine, so it is possible for non-depolarizing agents to block this process. This property is well demonstrated with d-tubocurarine and with ORG9426 (Gibb and Marshall, 1984; Bowman, 1984; Muir et al., 1989). Tetanic fade occurs as a result of presynaptic block and is less obvious in drugs with little or no presynaptic activity. Its importance in clinical practice is uncertain but interest in the properties

of this block have been aroused by the introduction of ORG9426. Presynaptic activity of depolarizing agents has also been proposed (Riker, 1965; Galindo, 1971).

Desensitization Block

This term was used by Thesleff (1955) to explain the prolongation of block following exposure to depolarizing agents after the membrane potential has been restored. At this time the muscle appeared totally unresponsive to indirect stimulation and to acetylcholine. It is now thought unlikely that true desensitization occurs except in laboratory conditions where it may represent a chronic ion depletion.

Channel Block ('*In Use*' Block) (Site B, Fig. 42.3)

It has been proposed that some drugs exert their action by blocking ionic pores either at the narrow neck of the channel within the cell membrane (site B, Fig. 42.3) or at the intracellular surface on the cytoplasmic side of the membrane (site C, Fig. 42.3) (i.e., local anaesthetics). The possibility that neuromuscular blocking drugs may enter the channel has been suggested (Rang, 1981) although the significance of this has been questioned (Bowman, 1985). For channel block to occur the sodium channels must be open, hence the term 'in use' block or 'use dependent' block. The membrane may be electrically hyperpolarized to achieve open channels or else subjected to rapid repetitive stimulation to provide ideal conditions for the block to occur. In these circumstances smaller drug molecules, such as gallamine may enter the channels contributing to the resultant neuromuscular block. It is characteristic of this block that it occurs with molecules small enough in the hydrated form to enter the channel, it is encouraged by anticholinesterases and it is relatively short lived. It has only been convincingly demonstrated to occur with gallamine in a concentration relevant to clinical practice.

Gate Block

The gating concept envisages an opening and closing of an electrical and chemical gate mechanism to modulate the ease of propagation of excitatory influence from the end plate to the muscle. It is proposed as one of the possible sites of action of those volatile anaesthetics that potentiate the action of the neuromuscular blocking drugs (*see* Chapter 43).

TESTS AND MEASUREMENT OF NEUROMUSCULAR BLOCK

The principal methods for quantitative evaluation of neuromuscular conduction are:

1. Measurement of strength of muscle contraction following indirect stimulation.
2. Measurement of the compound electromyograph, following indirect stimulation.

Of the two methods, recording electrical activity from the muscle belly has the advantage of being less influenced by physical factors affecting contractility and also of recording activity in the train of events that occurs during muscle contraction. It is therefore closer to any changes in neuromuscular transmission than is a record produced by muscle contraction itself. EMG methods are especially suitable for use in small animals and neonates as they require less cumbersome apparatus attached to the subject.

The disadvantage of electromyographic recordings is that it is difficult to obtain good records during clinical conditions in the operating theatre and that it is less directly related to the actual end product of neuromuscular conduction—the muscle contraction—that determines that patient's ability to make an active effort and which ultimately determines his ability to survive.

The simplest device for recording the evoked muscle response is a form of ergometer constructed from a 20 ml syringe with the plunger attached to the thumb. If this is filled with fluid connected to a CVP manometer the strength of adduction of the pollucis muscles can be usefully quantified.

More elaborate monitors such as the Statham UC3 force displacement transducer and the Grass strain gauge can be used (Fig. 42.8), together with a suitable amplifier and recording system.

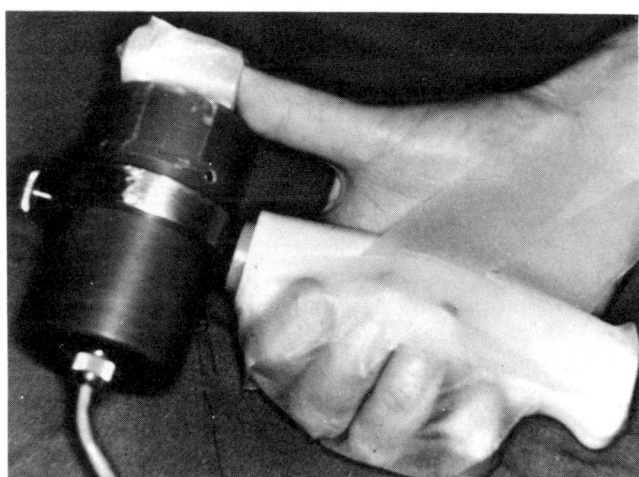

Fig. 42.8 A Statham UC3 load cell mounted in a bicycle handle grip can be used to measure the force of adduction of the thumb produced by stimulation of the ulnar nerve.

A development of the force transducer is the Accelograph (Biometer). This simple apparatus utilizes a strain gauge strapped to the thumb to record change in acceleration of the thumb following stimulation of the ulnar nerve.

As force = mass × acceleration, acceleration is a

first derivative of force and hence its measurement should parallel that of applied force. This instrument offers potential advantages because of its simplicity and ease of use.

Nerve stimulation should be supramaximal and of less than 0.5 ms duration to avoid stimulation on 'make and break' (0.2 ms is usually used) if quantative comparisons are to be made with other patients. Submaximal stimulation will give valid indication of the recovery of neuromuscular transmission in one particular patient being studied, but if these results are to be compared with those of another patient, or with a subsequent experience with that patient, it is essential that all the nerve fibres capable of conducting are stimulated. Needle electrodes (EEG needles are ideal for this purpose) placed subcutaneously parallel to the nerve are preferable to surface electrodes, as they are not affected by variations in skin resistance. However, care must be taken to ensure that the needle is not impinging on the nerve or that its point, and hence its highest current density, is not directed at the nerve lest it causes thermal trauma to the nerve.

The rate of twitch stimulation should be as slow as is consistent with useful recording, rates—0.1 Hz to 0.5 Hz are usual. Tetanic stimulation starts at 15–20 Hz and provides useful information up to rates of 50 Hz. Stimulation rates greater than 100 Hz are unphysiological, as the interval between stimuli is shorter than the refractory period of the synapse and it may cause thermal injury to the nerve.

Test of Residual Curarization

The most satisfactory test of adequate neuromuscular conduction is the ability of the patient to lift his head from the pillow for more than 5 seconds. This has been shown to correlate well with a return of normal respiratory function parameters.

If the patient is unconscious or uncooperative, the occurrence of post-tetanic potentiation of the twitch response or of more than 30% reduction in the height of the fourth to first stimulus with the train of 4 stimuli, indicates significant neuromuscular block with significant depression of respiratory function, due to occupancy of over 80% of the receptors by the antagonist drug (Ali et al., 1975).

Post-tetanic potentiation must be distinguished from the normal physiological post-tetanic facilitation of muscle contraction which can be especially well demonstrated in patients receiving halothane or enflurane. Post-tetanic facilitation reflects enhancement of muscle contractility and is seldom greater than 25% more than the pre-tetanic twitch height. True post-tetanic potentiation should be at least 50% greater than the pre-tetanic twitch response. The cause of this response is believed to be an increased rate of mobilization of immediately available acetylcholine from the reserve pool. When tetanic stimulation stops there is an overshoot of production and hence the next few twitch stimuli will liberate more

acetylcholine than usual. The train of 4 stimuli was based on an observation of Berry (1966) that 2 stimuli applied in rapid (1–1.8 ms) succession showed fade in the presence of neuromuscular block. Ali et al. (1970) introduced it as a test for residual curarization. It consists of resting the nerve for 2 seconds followed by the administration of 4 or more stimuli at 2 Hz. If the fourth twitch response is less than 70% of the first, then residual curarization is present. The reason for this effect is believed to be the 'running down' of the store of immediately available acetylcholine by stimulation at this slow rate. By the 3rd–5th stimulation the rate of mobilization of transmitter from the reserve is sufficient to replace that being lost at each stimulation and the twitch response is maintained at its new lower level.

Summary

Neuromuscular conduction can be chemically blocked at several levels. It can be depressed by interference at the level of choline transport across the axoplasm, in the synthesis and vesicular packaging of acetycholine and in the mobilization of reserve acetylcholine. These produce a slow onset of muscle weakness and often incomplete paralysis. Depression of acetylcholine release or the ability of transmitter to activate the receptor can cause a rapid and complete neuromuscular block. Finally, the process by which an endplate action potential triggers off a propagated muscle action potential producing muscle contraction can be chemically depressed causing neuromuscular block. Of these processes, it is only those blocking receptor activation that have found favour in anaesthesia, but it is important to appreciate that the neuromuscular synapse is vulnerable to block at various stages in the complex process of neuromuscular conduction.

REFERENCES

Agoston S., Feldman S.A., Miller R.D. (1979). Plasma concentrations of pancuronium and neuromuscular block after injection into the isolated arm, bolus injection and continuous infusion. *Anesthesiology*, **51**, 119.

Ali H.H., Utting J.E., Gray T.C. (1970). Stimulus frequency in the detection of neuromuscular block in humans. *Br. J. Anaesth.*, **42**, 967.

Ali H.H., Wilson R.S., Savarese J.J., et al. (1975). The effect of tubocurarine on indirectly elicited train-of-four muscle response and respiratory measurements in humans. *Br. J. Anaesth.*, **47**, 570.

Armstrong D.L., Lester H.A. (1979). The kinetics of tubocurarine action and restricted diffusion within the synaptic cleft. *J. Physiol.*, **294**, 365.

Baraka A. (1977). Irreversible curarization. *Anaesthesia and Intensive Care*, **5**, 244.

Birks R., Huxley H.E., Katz B. (1960). The fine structure of the neuromuscular junction of the dog. *J. Physiol. (Lond.)*, **150**, 134.

Berry F.R. (1966). Detection neuromuscular block in man. *Br. J. Anaesth.*, **38**, 929.

Bowman W.C. (1985) The neuromuscular junction. Recent developments. *Eur. J. Anaesthesiol.*, **2**, 59.

Bowman W.C. (1986). Physiology and basic pharmacology of the neuromuscular junction. *Anesth. Reanin.*, **3**, 18.

Bowman W.C., Marshall I.G., Gibb A.I. (1984). Is there feedback control of transmitter release at the neuromuscular junction? *Sem. Anaesth.*, **4**, 275.

Bowman W.C., Webb S.W. (1976). Tetanic fade during partial transmission failure produced by non-depolarizing neuromuscular blocking drugs in the cat. *Clin. Exp. Pharmacol. Physiol.* **3**, 545.

Burns B.D., Paton W.D.M. (1951). Depolarization of the motor end plate by decamethonium and acetylcholine. *J. Physiol. (Lond.)*, **115**, 41.

del Castillo J., Katz B. (1956). Interaction at end plate receptors between different choline derivatives. *Proc. R. Soc. Lond. (Biol.)*, **146**, 369.

Changeaux, J.P., DeVilliers-Thiery A., Chemonilli P. (1984). Acetylcholine receptor. An allosteric protein. *Science*, **225**, 1335.

Dale H.H., Feldberg W. (1934). Chemical transmission at motor nerve endings in voluntary muscle. *J. Physiol. (Lond.)*, **81**, 39.

Dale H.H., Feldberg W., Vogt M. (1936). Release of acetylcholine at voluntary motor nerve endings. *J. Physiol. (Lond.)*, **86**, 353.

Feldman S.A. (1963). Effects of changes in electrolytes hydration and pH upon the reactions to muscle relaxants. *Br. J. Anaesth.* **35**, 546.

Feldman S.A., Agoston S. (1980). Failure of neostigmine to prevent d-tubocurarine neuromuscular block in the isolated arm. *Br. J. Anaesth.*, **52**, 1199.

Feldman S.A., Tyrrell M.F. (1970). A new theory of the termination of action of muscle relaxants. *Proc. Royal Society of Medicine*, **63**, 692.

Galindo A. (1971). Depolarizing neuromuscular block. *J. of Pharmacology Exp. Therapy*, **178**, 339.

Gibb A.J., Marshall I.G. (1984). Pre- and postjunctional effects of d-tubocurarine and other nicotinic antagonists. *J. Physiol.*, **351**, 275.

Gissen A.J., Nastuk W.L. (1970). Succinylcholine and decamethonium; comparison of depolarization and desensitization. *Anesthesiology*, **33**, 611.

Harrop-Griffiths A.H., Grounds R.M., Moor M. (1986). Intubating conditions following pre-induction priming with alcuronium. *Anaesthesia*, **41**, 2, 87.

Hirokawa N., Heuser J.E. (1982). Internal and external differentiation of the postsynaptic membrane at the neuromuscular junction. *J. Neurocytol.*, **11**, 487.

Hodgkin A.F., Horrowicz P. (1959). The influence of potassium and chloride ions on the membrane potential of the single muscle fibres. *J. Physiol. (Lond.)*, **148**, 127.

Jennerick H.P., Gerard R.W. (1953). Membrane potential and threshold of single muscle fibres. *J. Cell. Congs. Physiol.*, **42**, 79.

Jones R.M. (1989). (Editorial). The priming principle. *Br. J. Anaesth.*, **63**, 1.

Long B., Newsom Davies J., Prior C., et al. (1983). Antibodies to motor nerve terminals in electrophysiological studies of human myasthenic syndrome transferred to mouse. *J. Physiol. (Lond.)*, **344**, 335.

Marshall I.G., Parsons S.M. (1987). Novel methods of blocking neuromuscular transmission. In *Clinical Neuromuscular Pharmacology. An International Symposium.* Publ. UCLA Educational Foundation.

Muir A.W., Houston J., Green L., et al. (1989). Effects of a new neuromuscular blocking agent (ORG 9426) in anaesthetised cats and pigs and in isolated nerve muscle preparation. *Br. J. Anaesth.*, **63**, 400.

Nickel E., Waser P.G. (1968). Electronemikrostopiche Unterschungen am Diaghragma der Maus nach Einsterteger Phrenikotomie. *Z. Zelliforsch.*, **88**, 278.

Paton W.D.M. (1961). A theory of drug action based on the rate of drug-receptor combination. *Proc. Royal Society and (biol.)*, **154**, 21.

Paton W.D.M., Waud, D.R. (1967). The margin of safety of neuromuscular transmission. *J. Physiol. (Lond.)*, **191**, 59.

Potter L.T. (1968). Uptake of choline by nerve endings isolated from the rat cerebral cortex. In *The Interactions of Drugs and Subcellular Components of Animal Cells.* London: Churchill Livingstone.

Riker W.F. (1965). Prejunctional effects of neuromuscular blocking and facilitatory drugs. In *Muscle Relaxants* (Katz R.L., ed.) Amsterdam Exerpta Medica, p. 59.

Sheridan R.E., Lester H.A. (1982). Functional stoichiometry at the nicotinic receptor. *J. Gen. Physiol.*, **80**, 499.

Thesleff S., Molgo J.A. (1983). A new type of transmitter release at the neuromuscular junction. *Neuroscience*, **9**, 1.

Waud D.R., Waud B.E. (1971). The relation between tetanic fade and receptor occlusion in the presence of competitive neuromuscular block. *Anesthesiology*, **35**, 456

Waser P.G. (1972). Affinity labelling of cholinergic receptors with curarizing and depolarizing drugs. Pharmacology Congress, San Francisco, 1972. Basel: Karger.

43. The Mechanism of Skeletal Muscle Contraction
I. Neering and T. A. Torda

STRUCTURE OF SKELETAL MUSCLE

Microscopic Structure

Skeletal muscle consists of muscle fibres, connective tissue elements, blood and lymphatic vessels and nerves. The muscle fibres, which are multinucleated cells of $10–100\,\mu m$ diameter of up to 40 mm length, are arranged in regular bundles, surrounded by connective tissue elements. The external, dense, sheath (epimysium) extends thin septa into the muscle (perimysia) which segregate groups of fibres into fascicles. Within the fascicles, each fibre is surrounded by a delicate connective tissue layer, the endomysium. This connective tissue structure serves to bind loosely together the component fibres of a muscle. It carries the vasculature and nerves, and also binds the muscle to its origin and insertion where it may condense into tendons. The individual fibres rarely run the whole length of a muscle and thus must rely on the connective tissue to transmit the force generated by muscle

contraction. The connective tissue makes a significant contribution to the elastic properties of muscle.

The sarcoplasm of each muscle fibre contains from a few dozen up to about 10 000 myofibrils, which are longitudinal bundles of the muscle's contractile subunits, $1–2\,\mu m$ in diameter. As a consequence of the regular arrangement of these elements the muscle fibre presents a characteristic pattern of transverse striations. These consist of alternate light *I bands* and dark *A bands*. Each I band bears in its middle a dark, transverse *Z line* and in the centre of the A band is a lighter zone, the *H band*. The repetitive subunit of the contractile mechanism, the *sarcomere*, extends from Z line to Z line, and is about $2.5\,\mu m$ long (Fig. 43.1).

Electron Microscopy

With electron microscopy further detail can be distinguished. In the A band lie 'thick' myosin filaments, about 10 nm thick, parallel to the long axis of the fibre and about 45 nm apart. The 'thin' actin filaments which alternate with them have a diameter of about 5 nm and have one end attached to the Z line. In the sarcomere, which is the 'unit' of contraction, the H band is that portion which consists of thick filaments only. For most of the A band, the thick and thin filaments overlap. During contraction or stretch, the width of the A band remains unchanged but the H band narrows, corresponding to the change in the length of the sarcomere (the distance between the Z lines). In cross section the arrangement of the filaments is hexagonal, each thick filament surrounded by 6 thin filaments.

At the junction of the A and I bands in mammals (in frogs and toads at the Z lines), openings exist in the sarcolemma (caveolae) through which a complex system of tubules which invades the muscle fibre, the *transverse tubular system* (*TTS*), opens to the interstitial space. This system brings the deeper myofibrils into close association with the extracellular fluid and the sarcolemma. Finally, an extensive membrane system which overlies more than 40% of the surface of the myofibrils, the *sarcoplasmic reticulum* (*SR*), can be demonstrated. Portions of this, the *terminal cisternae*, are closely associated with the TTS at each A–I band junction. The association of two cisternae and the tubule form the *triad*. Large and prominent mitochondria lie between the myofibrils, especially in red muscle fibres.

Function of Muscle Elements

The Bands and their Molecular Components
The microscopically visible bands which have been described correspond to known molecular entities. The A band is formed by the 'thick' *myosin* filaments which are bundles of characteristically shaped protein molecules. They are usually described as 'golf club' like, 150 nm long and 2–4 nm in diameter. The 'shaft' is the *light meromyosin* (*LMM*) component, a strand

about 100 nm long, 2 nm in diameter and 150 000 dalton molecular weight. The head of the club is the *heavy meromyosin* (*HMM*), 30 nm long, 4 nm in diameter and 350 000 dalton molecular weight. The function of LMM appears to be structural only. HMM, however, has two functions at least. It contains the ATP hydrolysis site for energy production and binds to actin, which is the basis of contractile function (Fig. 43.1).

Actin filaments are attached to the Z membrane. G (globular) actin consists of 5.5 nm globules of 60 000 dalton molecular weight. Each molecule binds one molecule of ATP. F (fibrous) actin is a double helical strand formed by polymerization of the G-actin. *Tropomyosin* is also a thin polar molecule of about 40 nm in length. It contains two polypeptide chains in the form of a coiled helix which lies along the actin strands. Each tropomyosin molecule is related to seven G-actin globules. At a specific site on each tropomyosin molecule, a troponin (Tn) molecule is attached. This is a complex of three subunits, the TnT

subunit, which is attached to the tropomyosin, the TnC which has a Ca^{2+} binding site and the TnI which serves to inhibit the actin–myosin interaction. If the Ca^{2+} binding site becomes occupied, a binding site on the actin becomes exposed to the HMM of the myosin filament and the contraction process is initiated. Actin and myosin represent about 55% of the protein of striated muscle. Other contractile proteins exist, such as actinin and β-actinin but their function is not understood.

Transverse Tubules

The TT system communicates with the extracellular environment and brings the extracellular fluid with its high Na^+ and Ca^{2+} concentration into extensive contiguity with the terminal cisternae of the SR. The flattened tubes of the TT system are 25–80 nm in diameter and increase the sarcolemmal surface by about 70%. The membrane of the TT system not only contains Na^+, K^+ and Cl^- channels, but also Ca^{2+} channels which are discussed below.

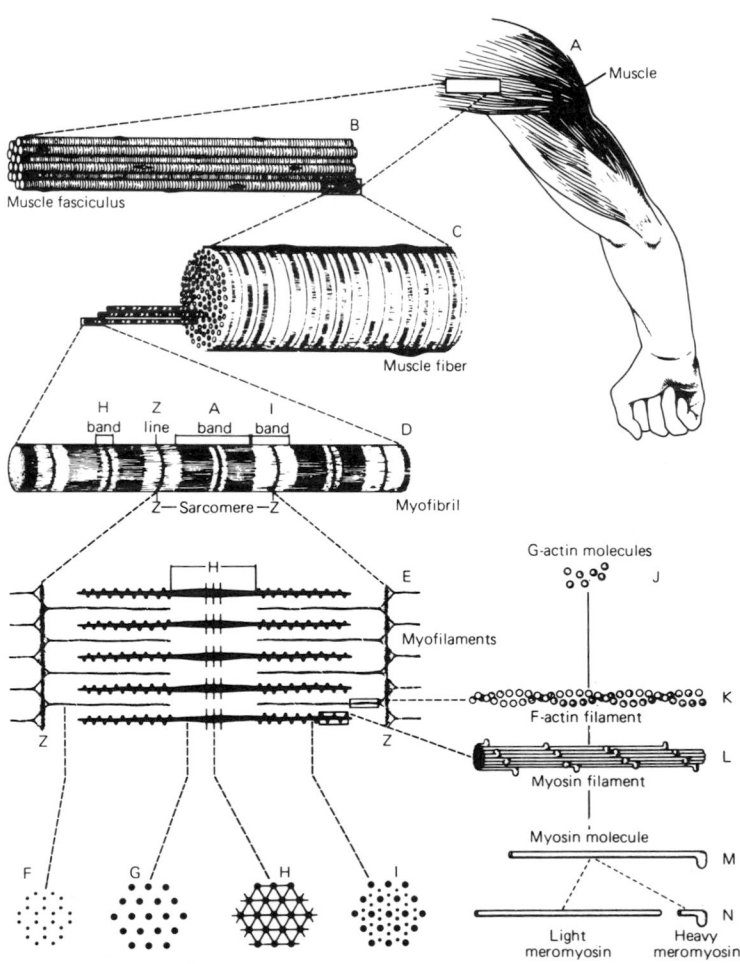

Fig. 43.1 The structure of muscle. Reproduced with permission from W. Bloom and D.W. Fawcett, 1968. *A Textbook of Histology*, 9th edn. Drawing by Sylvia Collard Keene, Philadelphia: W.B. Saunders.

Sarcoplasmic Reticulum

The SR forms a second tubular system enveloping each myofibril. It consists of three elements, the terminal cisternae which adjoin and cover the TT system, the intermediate cisternae and the lateral SR, or fenestrated collar which overlies much of the myofibril surface. The SR acts as a source and sink for Ca^{2+} facilitating the initiation and termination of the contractile process (Fig. 43.2).

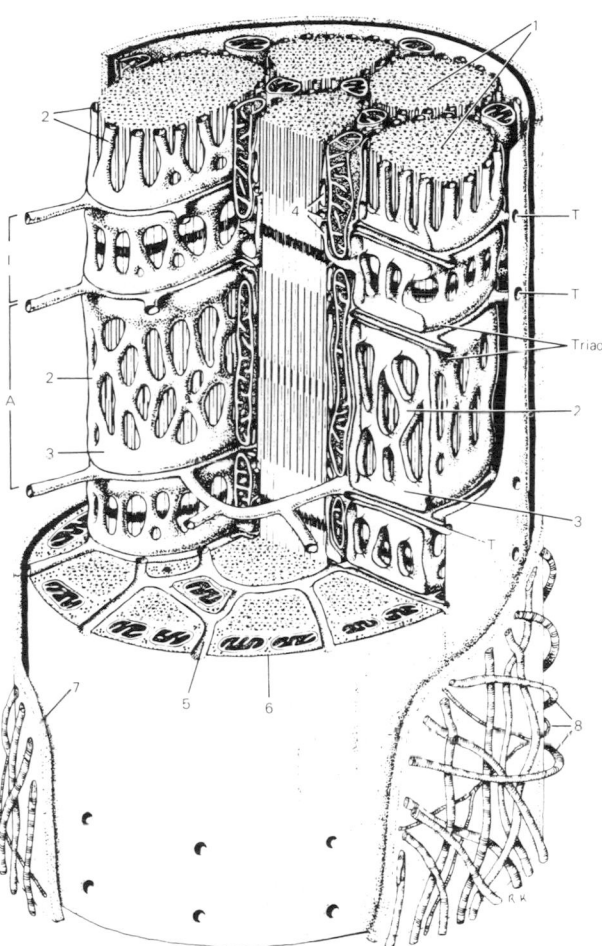

Fig. 43.2 Diagram of the ultrastructure of a mammalian muscle segment. 1, muscle fibres; 2, sarcoplasmic reticulum; 3, terminal cisterna; 4, mitochondria; 5, T openings of the transverse tubular system (caveolae); 6, sarcolemma; 7, basal lamina; 8, collagen fibres, which form the epimysium with the basal lamina. (Reproduced with permission from Kistic R.V. (1979). *Ultrastructure of the Mammalian Cell*, Heidelberg: Springer-Verlag.

Triads

Where the TT and two terminal cisternae of the SR systems come into apposition, the three structures form the so called triads. About 60–80% of the surface of the TT system is surrounded by the SR and a gap of only 12–14 nm exists between the two. This space is occupied by feet, evenly spaced structures, disposed in a regular tetragonal arrangement. The lumina of the two systems do not appear to communicate and contain fluid of differing composition.

FILAMENT INTERACTION

The process of contraction is initiated by an elevation of the intracellular Ca^{2+} concentration (*see below*). Calcium binds to TnC and the resultant conformational change moves tropomyosin deeper into the groove separating the actin chains. This exposes myosin recognition sites on the actin molecules.

In addition to binding sites for actin, the myosin heads have a separate site for the binding and subsequent hydrolysis of ATP. ATP is bound and split to ADP and phosphate, (which remains bound to the myosin) with the consequent release of energy before the myosin molecule attaches to actin to form a cross bridge. The energy released by the hydrolysis of ATP is transferred to the myosin, producing an activated form. The subsequent binding of this activated myosin to actin, triggers the discharge of the energy stored in the myosin. The myosin heads then bend or rotate through an angle of about 45°, presumably as the result of the attraction between adjacent charged sites on the surface of the globular actin molecules and the myosin heads. This rotation produces a translational movement of thin filament over thick filament. Following rotation of the myosin head, the cross bridge must be broken and this is achieved when a new molecule of ATP is bound but not split by the myosin head. ADP and phosphate are released at this time. This process constitutes a single cross bridge cycle.

Cross bridge formation is asynchronous. Rather like the 'hand over hand' motion of a number of workers hauling on a rope. Since rotation of a single myosin head results in a movement of no more than 5–10 nm, it follows that at least 10^{10} cross bridges in parallel would need to be activated to account for the force characteristics of a single muscle fibre.

ELECTROPHYSIOLOGY

Ionic Channels

Ion movements which generate the potentials across the muscle membrane take place through aqueous pores in the lipid bilayer of the cell membrane. It is convenient to divide these channels into two basic types, the agonist or chemically activated (or gated) channels, confined mostly to the region of the neuromuscular junction in normal muscle, and the electrically activated (or voltage gated) channels elsewhere on the cell membrane and the TT system.

Agonist Activated Channels

The motor end-plate contains agonist activated channels only. They serve an amplifying function, rendered necessary by the high impedance of the gap between the motor nerve and the muscle membrane. Other chemically gated channels, which differ from those of the end-plate in some of their kinetic characteristics are found in a 500 μm region about the junctions. The function of these extra junctional channels is unknown. Unlike channels elsewhere on muscle membrane (voltage activated channels), these channels are not greatly cation selective, although relatively impermeable to Cl⁻. All currents which contribute to the end-plate potential and its termination are generated in these channels.

In denervated muscle agonist activated channels proliferate and spread along the cell membrane beyond the bounds of the neuromuscular junction. When activated by suxamethonium, these channels appear to be responsible for a massive K^+ leak from muscle cells.

Voltage Activated Channels

These channels do not require a chemical trigger, but are activated by membrane depolarization. Among the voltage gated channels on the muscle cell membrane there is a high degree of ion specificity. Separate types of channels exist for each major cation, Na^+, K^+ (three or four distinct types) and Ca^{2+} as well as for Cl⁻. These channels are responsible for the dominant conductance at rest and for the generation of action potentials.

Membrane Potential

In the resting state the muscle cell membrane is mainly permeable to K^+ and Cl⁻ ions and only slightly to Na^+. Considering K^+, the high intracellular concentration of this ion is electrically balanced mainly by nonpermeable anions. Therefore if the membrane were permeable to K^+ alone, the transmembrane potential difference would be equal to the equilibrium potential of a K^+ electrode, as defined by the Nernst equation:

$$E_K = \frac{RT}{nF} \cdot \ln \frac{[K]_0}{[K]_i}$$

where E_K is the potassium equilibrium potential in mV, R the universal gas constant, T the absolute temperature, n the valency of the ion and F the Faraday number. Similarly, the potentials due to Cl⁻ and Na^+ can be calculated. Allowing for the different permeabilities of the membrane for the three ions, the Goldman equation for the membrane potential can be set up:

$$E_m = \frac{RT}{nF} \cdot \ln \frac{P_1[K]_0 + P_2 \cdot [Na]_0 + P_3 \cdot [Cl]_i}{P_1 \cdot [K]_i + P_2 \cdot [Na]_i + P_3 \cdot [Cl]_0}$$

where E_m is the membrane potential in mV, and P_1, P_2 and P_3 constants representing the permeability of the membrane to each ion. The normal E_m in mammalian muscle is about -85 mV. The gradients in concentrations of K^+ and Na^+ across the cell membrane are maintained by a pump mechanism using ATP as its energy source. Because of the relatively low permeability for Na^+, K^+ is the principal ion responsible for the E_m and because the cell membrane is relatively impermeable to them, other ions (Ca^{2+}, Mg^{2+} etc.) play no significant role in its establishment. The Cl⁻ gradient is essentially passive and results from the presence of nonpermeable anions within the cell and the concentration gradients of the cations.

End-plate Potential

The postjunctional membrane of the motor end-plate has high concentrations ($7500 \ \mu m^{-2}$) of agonist activated channels, located principally at the crests of the junctional folds. When the motor nerve action potential releases about 200 quanta of transmitter, (a quantum is the content of a single vesicle in which the transmitter, acetylcholine, ACh, is stored) each containing about 2000–10 000 transmitter molecules, it is estimated that of a total 10^7 channels at an end-plate, about 250 000 are opened. By the technique of patch clamping the current generated by each individual channel opening can now be recorded. The mean open channel life time is about 1 ms in mammalian muscle at room temperature and about 0.3 ms at 37°C. The conductance of the individual channel is 18–30 pS. It is estimated that during 1 ms about 10 000 Na^+ and K^+ ions cross the same channel and the current generated is about 2 pA. The conductance of the single channel shows little temperature dependence. As the channels open and current flows, there is some depolarization of the membrane and reduction in the driving force of the current. Thus summation of these single currents is not linear and the total end-plate current generated is about -400 nA (the negativity indicates inward current by convention). The distribution of transmitter after its release is not uniform along the whole end-plate and only 50–75% of the channels in the area of distribution of the transmitter are opened following a single evoked transmitter release.

The actions of ACh are terminated mainly by acetylcholinesterases (AChE) which tend to be aggregated in the depths of the synaptic clefts as well as on the presynaptic membrane. This anatomical arrangement enables the clefts to function as sinks for the transmitter. After release, the reduction of free transmitter concentration in the cleft is very rapid as is dissociation from the recognition sites. It is estimated that within 10–100 μs there is little free transmitter left and the duration of channel opening is much longer than the transmitter–receptor association. So the events leading to channel activation are best described by two steps, with independent rate constants:

$$2A + R \underset{k_2}{\overset{k_1}{\rightleftharpoons}} A_2 R \underset{b}{\overset{a}{\rightleftharpoons}} A_2 R^*$$

where k_1 and k_2 are the association and dissociation constants for the reaction between two molecules of the transmitter, A and the receptor R and a and b are the rate constants for opening and closure of the channel $A_2 R^*$ represents the open channel.

The EPC causes depolarization of the surrounding membrane. If the depolarization is sufficient, the voltage gated channels are activated and an action potential (AP) is generated in the surrounding membrane. The ratio of the end-plate potential (EPP) to the minimum EPP required to initiate the AP is the safety factor of the neuromuscular junction and usually has a value of about 4.

Action Potential

Once the end-plate potential has activated the voltage gated channels of the muscle membrane, the upstroke of the action potential is caused by a regenerative increase in Na^+ conductance, including the overshoot beyond zero potential (reversal potential) which results from the Na^+ equilibrium potential of about $+50\,mV$. Repolarization results from inactivation of the Na^+ conductance and activation of the delayed rectifier type K^+ channels. These channels have an equilibrium potential of -70 to $-80\,mV$ and bring the membrane potential back to this value relatively rapidly. The negative afterpotential reflects the slow time course of recovery from this potential to the resting potential, which depends on the inward rectifier channels, another K^+ type of channel whose equilibrium potential is about $-100\,mV$. In slow twitch fibres, there may be a significant contribution to a positive afterpotential by the slow K^+ channels. Using isotopes, a net Na^+ entry of 15.6 and a net K^+ exit of $9.6\,pmol\,cm^{-2}$ per impulse have been measured. These lead to negligible alterations in the electrolyte composition of the cell and its environment following short bursts of tetanic stimulation. After more prolonged stimulation a late afterdepolarization can develop, due to accumulation of K^+ in the TT system.

Asymmetrical Charge Movement

Slow asymmetrical charge movements can be recorded with contractions from muscles, under appropriate conditions. These currents or charge movements show particular properties expected of gating charges:

1. On depolarization (ON charge) the charge moves outwards and on repolarization (OFF charge) inwards.
2. At any membrane potential the ON and OFF currents are equal, as would be expected if the currents were due to the movement of the same charges.
3. With large depolarizations the current saturates as if there were only a finite number of charges to move.

It is believed that these charge movements reflect at least in part, the gating currents of the T system Ca^{2+} channels, and play a part, as yet undefined, in the excitation–contraction coupling process.

EXCITATION–CONTRACTION COUPLING

Contraction of skeletal muscle is triggered by an increase in intracellular Ca^{2+} concentration. As contractility is maintained for some time in the absence of extracellular Ca^{2+}, the source of Ca^{2+} must be intracellular. This source is the sarcoplasmic reticulum (SR). The process of excitation–contraction coupling (ECC) is thus concerned with the regulation of intracellular Ca^{2+} concentration. Three important steps govern this process.

Transmission of Membrane AP to Site of Ca^{2+} Release

The AP propagates from the cell surface along the transverse tubular (TT) system to the terminal cisternae (TC) of the SR, the site of Ca^{2+} storage and release. The manner of transmission of the impulse from the TT system to the SR is still a matter of debate and several hypotheses have been advanced of which three will be discussed briefly.

Calcium-Induced Release of Calcium (CROC)

In cardiac muscle the movement of Ca^{2+} during the slow inward current is believed to trigger the release of Ca^{2+} from the SR. In vertebrate skeletal muscle, however, while a Ca^{2+} current can be recorded at the level of the TT system, calcium channel blocking drugs do not alter the ability of the muscle to contract under normal conditions. Thus while Ca^{2+} influx during TT activation may modify the EC coupling mechanism, it does not trigger the process of Ca^{2+} release.

Charge Movement

It has been previously suggested that asymmetric charge movement associated with the gating of Ca^{2+} channels may be located at the TT. If this is the case, then Ca^{2+} release by the SR may be initiated by a long molecule, extending between the gating molecule in the TT system and the adjacent TC. Analogy can be drawn to a cam (the gating molecule) attached by a rod to a plug in the SR. Rotation of the cam would open the plug and allow Ca^{2+} to flow from the SR.

Alternatively, a second messenger might be involved; released from the electrically activated TT system to diffuse across to the SR and initiate Ca^{2+} release. Inositol trisphosphate (IP_3) which has been shown to have just this effect on Ca^{2+} stores of smooth muscle and nerve cells has been suggested as a possible candidate for this role in skeletal muscle as well. This suggestion remains to be confirmed.

Channels Between the TT System and the SR

Electron microscopic studies of the triad region of vertebrate skeletal muscle have revealed pillars of electron dense material (feet) which appear to connect the TT system to the SR. It has been suggested that these feet contain ionic channels which open upon depolarization of the TT system and directly transmit the current to the lateral sacs of the SR. Proponents of this theory explain the asymmetric charge movement previously discussed as arising from a membrane with linear capacitance (TT system) coupled in series with a non-linear conductance, the electron dense pillars or feet.

Calcium Release from the SR

The concentration of free Ca^{2+} in the sarcoplasm of resting skeletal muscle is less than 10^{-7} mol L^{-1}. In the resting state most of the intracellular calcium (1–2 mmol kg^{-1} muscle fibre) is contained in the SR which constitutes 9–13% of fibre volume. The calcium concentration in TC is about 50 mmol L^{-1} and that in the longitudinal SR about 5 mmol L^{-1}. This unequal distribution of calcium may be related to selective pumping from the longitudinal SR into the TC, or to differences between the calcium binding protein of the TC (calsequestrin) and that of the longitudinal SR. Most of the calcium in the SR is thought to be bound either to these proteins or to other calcium binding sites such as phospholipids or the Ca–ATPase system which line the internal surface of the SR membrane. The actual amount of calcium in the SR in free but non-ionized form is likely to be quite small. The large concentration gradient of Ca^{2+} ions between the SR and the myoplasm provides the driving force for a purely passive Ca^{2+} outflux when the Ca^{2+} permeability of the membranes of the TC increases as a result of activation.

During contraction the peak free Ca^{2+} concentration rises to about 2–3 μmol L^{-1}. This figure may, however, be misleading as higher concentrations would be reached but for buffering by troponin and other soluble or structural proteins. The relation between the Ca^{2+} transient, as measured by the intra-cellular Ca^{2+} indicator, aequorin, and force in fast and slow twitch muscles of the rat are shown in Fig. 43.3. During these isometric twitches, the Ca^{2+} transients peak well before the force and the maximum rate of rise of force and cross bridge cycling correlates with the amplitude of the Ca^{2+} transient which in turn declines more rapidly than the tension. The duration of the Ca^{2+} transient thus recorded is a good indicator of the active state of the muscle, that is, the period during which cross bridge cycling is taking place.

Calcium Re-Uptake by the SR

As discussed previously, cross bridge cycling in mammalian skeletal muscle will occur as long as calcium remains bound to TnC. It follows that muscle relaxation occurs as calcium becomes unbound from TnC when the free Ca^{2+} concentration declines. The most

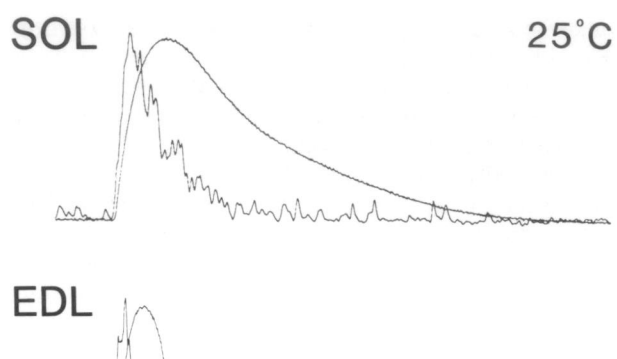

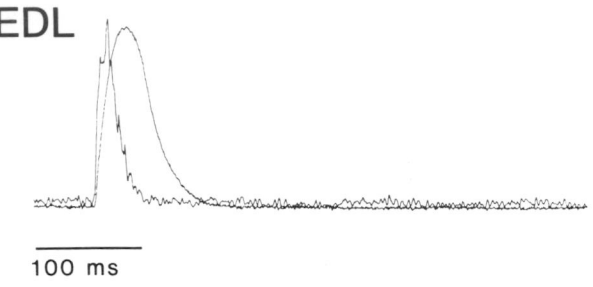

100 ms

Fig. 43.3   Recordings of force and intracellular free calcium concentration (measured with the photoprotein aequorin) during contractions of the soleus and extensor digitorum longus muscles of the rat. (EDL) (Unpublished data by Fryer M.W. and Neering I.R.)

important calcium sequestration system is the SR itself. Calcium uptake is achieved by a translocator molecule in the membrane of the SR. This molecule is a magnesium requiring ATPase, which, by hydrolyzing one molecule of ATP, moves two molecules of calcium against a concentration gradient of several orders of magnitude. The equilibrium constant of the translocator–calcium complex is about 10^6 per mole, which indicates that even at resting intracellular Ca^{2+} concentration of 10^{-7} mol L^{-1}, calcium pumping by the SR is still taking place. The movement of calcium ions into the SR is essentially electroneutral since there are compensating movements of H^+, K^+ and Cl^-. Nevertheless, there is a small potential difference of about 10 mV (inside positive) across the SR membrane.

The rate of calcium pumping by the SR ATPase and thus the capacity of the SR to accumulate calcium is regulated by the calcium concentration of the myoplasm. As mentioned above, the calcium pump is active at a basal level below the resting Ca^{2+} concentration of 10^{-7} mol L^{-1}. It reaches maximal activity at about 10^{-6} mol L^{-1} free Ca^{2+}, but decreases with time as the SR becomes filled with calcium. Thus, the presence of calcium in the myoplasm, following release, stimulates its reuptake.

From the preceding discussion which describes the relationship between calcium uptake by the SR and relaxation, one would expect the calcium uptake of slow twitch muscles to be slower than that of fast twitch muscles. This can be seen in Fig. 43.3. Such differences in calcium uptake by the SR have been explained on the basis of differing ATPase activities of the SR as well as a greater number of pump sites in the SR of fast twitch muscles.

Recently, it has been suggested that soluble calcium binding proteins in the myoplasm such as parvalbumins may play a role in the relaxation process. In the muscles where such proteins are found, they may sequestrate calcium in parallel with the SR at high Ca^{2+} concentration and then unload their calcium to the SR when the intracellular Ca^{2+} approaches its resting level.

ENERGY METABOLISM

The machinery of muscle requires a continuous supply of energy, which is derived from the hydrolysis of ATP. By far the greatest consumption of energy occurs during contraction, when the development of force is the consequence of the cycling of large numbers of cross bridges; here, formation of a single cross bridge consumes one molecule of ATP. During relaxation ATP is required to fuel the Ca–ATPase pumping system of the sarcoplasmic reticulum and to repay energy debts incurred during activity. There is also a relatively small basal consumption of ATP in the resting state associated with the maintenance of ion gradients and catabolism of cellular constituents. Resting muscle concentration of ATP is about 3 mmol L^{-1}, which is only enough to support about 10 twitches of a fast twitch (type IIB) muscle. Obviously this is insufficient to support physiological muscle activity and the means whereby this limitation is overcome in various muscles is discussed below. For details of the biochemistry of energy generation in muscle the reader is referred to appropriate biochemical texts.

Energy Production

Glycolysis

The substrate for glycolytic energy production is either glucose, or its branched polymer, glycogen which forms granules in the cytoplasm of muscle fibres, large enough to be visible in electron micrographs. The glycolytic breakdown of glucose to pyruvate or lactate yields 2 moles of ATP for each mole of glucose. Where glycogen rather than glucose is the initial substrate, glucose residues are split off as glucose 1-phosphate and do not require phosphorylation to enter the glycolytic path, increasing the energy yield to 3 moles of ATP. If oxygen is available, further oxidation of pyruvate to acetyl CoA and CO_2 increases the net yield of ATP to 6 moles. The glycolytic process is very rapid in its rate of energy production and is activated by calcium release from the SR, the same process which initiates contraction. Calcium activates phosphorylase kinase, which in turn activates phosphorylase, one of the enzymes which splits off glucose 1-phosphate from glycogen. Fast twitch fibres contain sufficient glycogen to sustain between 600–700 contractions, if the glycogen stores were the sole energy substrate available.

Oxidative Phosphorylation

This process is the main source of energy in muscles which have the capacity for sustained activity. In contrast to glycolysis it is relatively slow but much more efficient, yielding 30 moles of ATP for each mole of glucose. It takes place in mitochondria, rather than the cytosol, which is the location of the glycolytic process. The tricarboxylic acid (citric acid, Krebs) cycle takes acetyl CoA as its initial substrate, thus linking carbohydrate, fat and amino acid metabolism to the oxidative energy producing mechanism. Thus under optimal circumstances, the metabolism of a molecule of glucose from glycogen can yield 6 molecules of ATP during glycolysis and a further 30 molecules of ATP during oxidative breakdown, for a total of 36 molecules of ATP. Thus the same glycogen store which was sufficient for 600 twitches under anaerobic conditions would provide sufficient energy for about 12 000 twitches.

Direct Phosphorylation

When the glycolytic and the oxidative paths are both blocked (e.g. by iodoacetate and cyanide, respectively) muscles can still contract many times. The source of this alternative energy is creatine phosphate, whose phosphoryl group can be transferred to ADP by creatine kinase to form ATP. In fast twitch muscle the concentration of creatine phosphate is about 20 mmol L^{-1}, sufficient for about 70 twitches. There is one more mechanism of direct phosphorylation in muscle, the transfer of a phosphoryl group between molecules of ADP by adenylate kinase (myokinase), yielding one molecule each of ATP and AMP. This reaction appears to play a regulatory role in glycolysis, but its contribution to muscle energy is probably minimal (Fig. 43.4).

Muscle Fibre Types

Mammalian muscle fibres differ not only in the way in which limitations of energy storage are overcome, but also in several other characteristics. The speed of contraction of muscle fibres is related to the rate at which myosin ATPase is able to hydrolyze ATP and thus regulate the rate of cross bridge cycling. Two main types of myosin can be distinguished by histochemical techniques. *Fast myosin*, mainly found in *fast twitch fibres*, has a rate of ATP hydrolysis about three times as fast as *slow myosin*, which is predominantly contained in *slow twitch* (type I) fibres. There are also fibres intermediate in type between the two, sometimes called oxidative fast twitch (type IIA) fibres. The characteristics and differences between the three types of twitch fibres are summarized in Table 43.1. Some true slow fibres (as distinct from 'slow twitch' fibres) are also found in mammals, in the intrinsic muscles of the oesophagus and the ear and in some extraocular

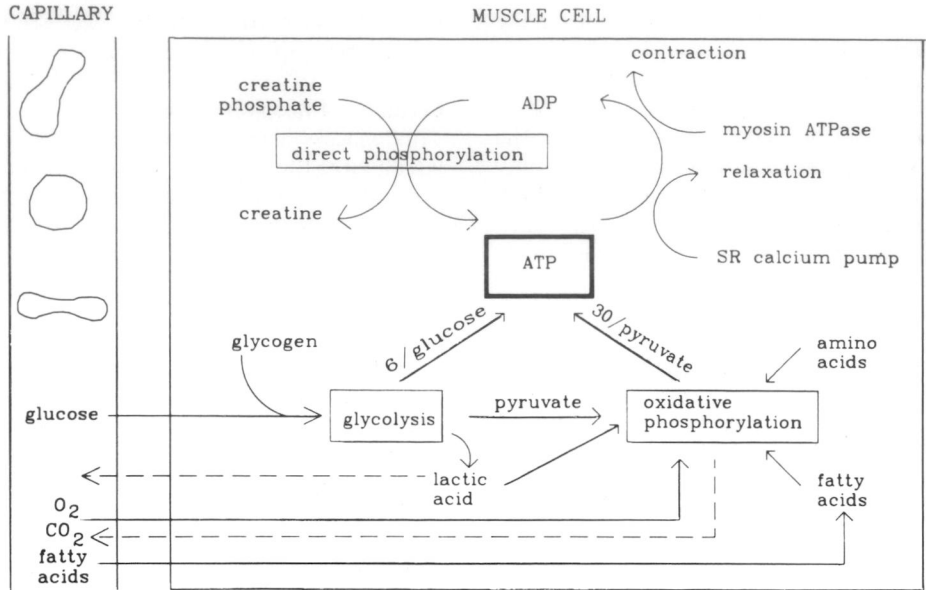

Fig. 43.4 Summary of the metabolic processes of skeletal muscles. The numbers 6 and 30 indicate the relative amounts of ATP produced.

muscles. The slow fibres resemble the slow muscle fibres of invertebrates, they have multiple innervation and do not respond by a twitch to a single nerve impulse but require nerve volleys to produce contraction. Their importance and function is uncertain.

Motor Units

Most muscles contain all three types of twitch fibre, fast, slow and intermediate, although one type may predominate. A group of muscle fibres innervated by branches of the same lower motor neurone is a motor unit. A motor unit is always composed of muscle fibres of the same histochemical type. There is strong evidence to indicate that the motor nerve plays a major role in determining the fibre type. Figure 43.3

shows the force responses and changes in intracellular calcium concentration associated with contraction from two muscles from the rat in which the motor unit composition is relatively homogeneous; the slow twitch soleus muscle and the fast twitch extensor digitorum longus.

Oxidative Slow Twitch (Type I, Red) Fibres

These fibres are characterized by low myosin ATPase activity and high oxidative capacity. They contain numerous mitochondria, in close proximity to a rich capillary network which permits a high rate of oxygen delivery to them. The diameter of these fibres is small and they contain large amounts of myoglobin which facilitates oxygen diffusion into the cells and serves as

TABLE 43.1

PROPERTIES OF MAMMALIAN MUSCLE FIBRE TYPES

	Slow twitch	*Intermediate*	*Fast twitch*
Alternative names	Type I oxidative	Type IIA oxidative–glycolytic	Type IIB glycolytic
	red	red	white
Colour	red	red/pale	pale
Diameter	small	intermediate	large
Capillary network	profuse	intermediate	sparse
Mitochondria	many	intermediate	few
Myosin ATPase activity	high	intermediate	low
Ca^{2+} uptake by SR	slow	intermediate	fast
Fatigability	low	intermediate	high
Contraction speed	slow	fast	fast
Force developed	low	intermediate	high

a small oxygen reservoir. In addition, the myoglobin imparts to these fibres their characteristic red colour. These fibres thus have a high capacity for sustained oxidative phosphorylation and a rate of energy utilization limited by the low myosin ATPase activity. They are well adapted to sustained activity and they are relatively resistant to fatigue. Slow twitch fibres are usually predominant in those muscles which are continuously active for prolonged periods, such as the postural antigravity muscles.

Glycolytic Fast Twitch (Type IIB, White) Fibres

Fast twitch fibres are characterized by high myosin ATPase activity and a high capacity for glycolysis. Although mitochondria are few and their capillary network is less well developed than that of red fibres, they contain high concentrations of glycolytic enzymes and large stores of glycogen. These fibres contain little or no myoglobin and accordingly, muscles containing predominantly this type of fibre are called white. Their SR is much more extensive than that of the slow twitch fibres, well adapted for rapid activation and inactivation of the contractile mechanism. Since the glycolytic process is able to produce ATP at a rapid rate, it is suited to the provision of energy for brief bursts of high force output. The process is however relatively inefficient in its energy yield and glycogen stores are soon exhausted. For this reason, fast muscles are much less resistant to fatigue than muscles containing predominantly slow twitch fibres. They tend to subserve rapid phasic movements as in the extraocular muscles and the small muscles of the hand.

Oxidative Fast Twitch (Type IIA, Intermediate) Fibres

These fibres have a mixed metabolic pattern with high myosin ATPase activity and intermediate oxidative and glycolytic capacity. Their force kinetics resemble those of the fast glycolytic fibres, and their ability to withstand fatigue is intermediate between the oxidative and glycolytic fibres.

MECHANICS

Recording Contraction

Two different systems exist for recording contraction of muscle, isotonic—constant tension and isometric—constant length systems. The former is typified by attachment of the muscle to a weight, over a pulley. When the muscle is stimulated, it contracts against a constant load and the change in length is recorded. In the isometric system the muscle is attached to a fixed transducer which measures the force developed when the stimulated muscle contracts at a fixed length. The recording systems are never perfect. Friction adds a variation to the load of isotonic systems while there is usually some movement in the transducer of an isometric system. Physiological movement is generally neither isotonic nor isometric, but somewhere in

between, with variation in both load and length. Sometimes this is called *auxotonic* contraction. Electromyography (EMG) records the electrical activity of contracting muscle. The amplitude of the compound EMG (electrical activity of the whole muscle, recorded with electrodes outside the muscle) or the integrated EMG (time integral of the EMG) correlates closely with isometric force measurements.

Length–Tension Relation

From the previous discussion of filament interaction it should be clear that force development is dependent upon the number of cross bridges formed between thin and thick filaments. The initial degree of overlap between filaments has a crucial effect on the ability to generate force. At low sarcomere lengths, where there is much overlap of the thin filaments, and at long sarcomere lengths, where there is little or no overlap, force development is limited. Muscles produce their greatest force at about their normal resting length (Fig. 43.5).

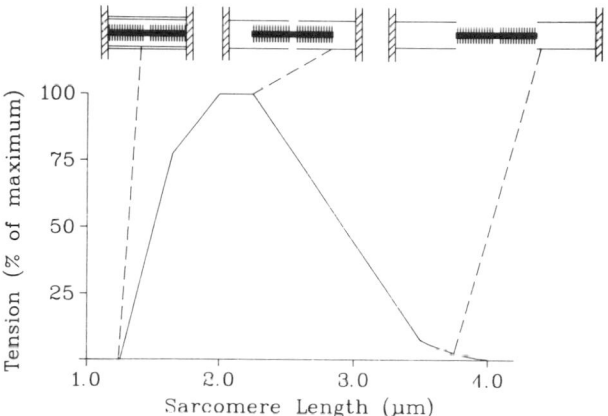

Fig. 43.5 The relationship between sarcomere length (degree of filament overlap) and the force developed by skeletal muscle. (Data from A.M. Gordon et al. (1966). *J. Physiol.*, **184**, 170.)

Summation, Tetanus and Modulation of Contraction

A muscle fibre can be modelled as elastic components both in series and in parallel with the active contractile mechanism. For greater accuracy, a viscous element (damping forces) can be added in series with the contractile component. The parallel elastic components include the sarcolemma, the SR and the collagen of the basement membrane. The series elastic components are the cross bridges, the Z disks and the tendons. The filaments have little resistance to stretch and act as viscous elements principally. This model can be used to explain many of the mechanical properties of muscle (Fig. 43.6).

The duration of electrical refractoriness of muscle

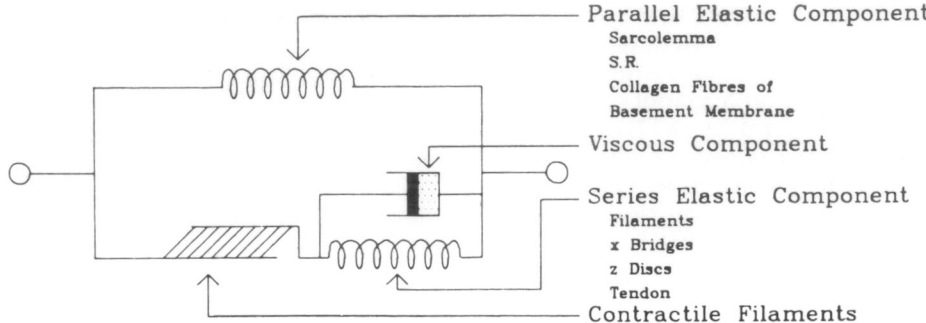

Fig. 43.6 Mechanical model of a muscle fibre, relating cellular entities to the components of the model.

membrane is short relative to the duration of a twitch. After a contraction is initiated the fibre is ready to contract again, well before the force of the previous contraction has waned. So when two stimuli are delivered in rapid succession, the contractile responses will sum. Although the first twitch does not fully stretch the series elastic components of the muscle fibre, the contraction induced by the second stimulus acts on a partly stretched elastic element. Less energy is expended on overcoming internal elasticity and more is available for external work. At low stimulation frequencies (< 30 Hz) individual contractions may be discerned—this is *partial tetanus*. As the frequency of stimulation increases, so does the force developed until a smooth, sustained, and maximal contraction results—*fused tetanus*. Fused tetanus represents the maximal amount of work which a muscle can perform and the force generated is usually about four times that achieved in a twitch.

The modulation of the force of contraction of muscles depends on two mechanisms. The force developed by the individual fibre depends on the initial fibre length, as discussed above. The total force then depends on the number of fibres contracting (recruitment), which is under neural control. The control of complex movements of course involves co-ordination of agonist and antagonist muscle groups simultaneously.

PHARMACOLOGY

A number of compounds have been shown to have effects on muscle activity. Some of these are briefly discussed below.

Antibiotics

Four groups of antibiotics have been implicated in reports of muscle paralysis:

Aminoglycosides

The principal paralytic action of the aminoglycosides is reduction of the evoked acetylcholine release (Mg^{2+} like). They also have a slight postjunctional blocking action. Direct action on muscle has not been demonstrated.

Lincosamides

Both clindamycin and lincomycin have been reported to be associated with paralysis in postoperative patients. In isolated nerve–muscle preparations clindamycin induced paralysis is preceded by marked increase in both directly and indirectly evoked twitch tension. Clindamycin has postjunctional receptor and open-channel blocking activity as well as direct depressant action on muscle. Lincomycin appears to have similar receptor and channel blocking actions, but does not appear to act on muscle directly.

Polymyxins

Polymyxins depress muscle contractility both directly and through the neuromuscular junction. Neuromuscular block involves both pre and postjunctional actions but like the direct action on muscle, they are poorly understood. Washing of experimental preparations reverses the indirect but not the direct action.

Tetracyclines

Both oxytetracycline and tetracycline reduce the quantal content of the EPP and also the amplitude of the MEPP, demonstrating both pre and postjunctional action at the motor end-plate. In the mouse hemidiaphragm preparation the directly elicited twitch is also blocked and contracture occurs. The mechanisms are not known.

Volatile Anaesthetics

The 'relaxant' effects of the volatile anaesthetics are principally manifestations of their effects on the CNS. Their augmentation of the non-depolarizing neuromuscular blockers is probably due to reduction of the mean open-channel life time. Their direct action on muscle appears to be facilitation of the evoked contraction at concentrations up to about 5 MAC and depression of the response at higher concentrations. As the augmentation of caffeine-induced contracture by halothane is not abolished by disruption of the TT system, it is thought that their action is on Ca^{2+} release by the SR.

Other Drugs

Dantrolene Sodium

This drug inhibits the depolarization-induced passive movement of calcium from the SR during normal activation. Interestingly, it is more effective at inhibiting calcium release from terminal cisternae than from the longitudinal SR. This is of particular value in the treatment of malignant hyperthermia where it significantly reduces muscle tone. Its effect on SR calcium release of muscles thus affected is much greater than on normal muscles, which are minimally affected by therapeutic concentrations.

Caffeine

This drug has a dual effect on the SR. It stimulates calcium release from the SR and slows its reuptake. Thus at low concentrations it potentiates muscle contraction by increasing the time–$[Ca^{2+}]$ integral. At high concentrations, caffeine directly causes calcium release from the SR, contraction occurring without depolarization of the muscle membrane. An addtional effect of caffeine is to sensitize the contractile apparatus to calcium.

Ryanodine

This compound causes paralysis of muscle by inhibition of calcium release from the SR. Its clinical use, however, is limited by the fact that its actions are irreversible.

Butanedione monoxime

This compound has two main actions. It inhibits calcium release from the SR. In addition, it interferes with the interaction of the contractile proteins with each other and with calcium. The paralysis thus produced is readily reversible *in vitro*.

FURTHER READING

Blines J.R., Wier W.G., Hess P., et al. (1982). Measurement of Ca^{2+} concentration in living cells. *Prog. Biophys. Molec. Biol.*, **40**, 1.

Dulhunty A.F., Gage, P.W. (1983). Asymmetrical charge movement in slow- and fast-twitch mammalian muscle fibres in normal and paraplegic rats. *J. Physiol.*, **341**, 213

Ebashi S. (1980). Regulation of muscle contracton. *Proc. R. Soc.*, **207**, 259

Franzini-Armstrong C., Peachey L.D. (1981). Striated muscle—contractile and control mechanisms., *J. Cell. Biol.*, **91**, 166S.

Luttgau H.C., Stephenson G.D. (1986). Ion movements in skeletal muscle in relation to the activation of contraction. In *Physiology of Membrane Disorders*, (Andreoli, T.E., Hoffman J.F., Fanestil D.D., Schultz S.G., eds.). New York: Plenum Publishing Corp.

Morgan D.L., Proske U. (1984). Vertebrate slow muscle: its structure, pattern of innervation, and mechanical properties. *Physiol. Rev.*, **64**, 103.

Peper K., Bradley, R.J., Dreyer, F. (1982). The acetylcholine receptor at the neuromuscular junction. *Physiol. Rev.*, **62**, 1271.

Ruegg J.C. (1986). Calcium in muscle activation. In *Zoophysiology*, Vol. 19. Berlin: Springer-Verlag.

Stefani E., Chiarandini D.J. (1982). Ionic channels in skeletal muscle. *Ann. Rev. Physiol.*, **44**, 357.

44. Neonatal Physiology
W. J. Glover

Many physiological differences exist between the newborn infant and the adult. This chapter deals with those differences which are most relevant to the anaesthetist.

Infant mortality has fallen considerably, especially in preterm infants. The neonatal period is defined as the first 28 days after birth and in normal circumstances refers to an infant born at 40 weeks gestation. In view of the increasing numbers of preterm infants surviving it is sometimes practical to think in terms of postconceptual age.

Compared with infants of normal gestation, preterm infants are more likely to suffer from conditions such as intraventricular haemorrhage, necrotizing enterocolitis, patent ductus arteriosus, inguinal hernia and respiratory distress syndrome. They are therefore more likely to present to the anaesthetist.

THE PRETERM INFANT

An estimate of gestational age is important as it indicates the degree of maturity of various organs. The mother's menstrual history may be unreliable and body weight is a poor guide to gestational age. Clinical examination will reveal increasing muscle tone and increasing flexion of upper and lower limbs with increasing gestational age.

Accurate assessment of fetal maturity can be made by measuring biochemical substances in the amniotic fluid. The sphingomyelin remains constant throughout pregnancy, while lecithin (which indicates surfactant production) begins to appear at about 28 weeks. By 35 weeks the lecithin/sphingomyelin ratio is normally greater than 2.0 and it is then almost certain that respiratory distress syndrome will not develop (see p. 520). Differences, affecting many organs, arise between the preterm and fullterm baby. Most of the differences will be dealt with under the appropriate headings in the remainder of the chapter but two are so specific to the preterm that they are dealt with here.

Cerebral Circulation and Intraventricular Haemorrhage

Neonatologists are increasingly successful in achieving survival even at 23–28 weeks gestational age. In one large series 7% survival at 23 weeks rising to 75% survival at 28 weeks gestation has been reported (Yu et al., 1986). However, the major concern is the high incidence of neurological handicap in the survivors and this is associated with intraventricular haemorrhage which affects approximately 40–50% of all preterm infants under 35 weeks gestation and is the major cause of death or handicap (Volpe, 1981).

The aetiology of intraventricular haemorrhage is not clear but may be related to the state of the vascular system. The periventricular capillary bed is an immature vascular plexus (Pape and Wigglesworth, 1979). The vessels consist only of a layer of endothelium without smooth muscle, collagen or fibrin (Haruda and Blanc, 1981) and there is only loose connective tissue surrounding these vessels over the basal ganglia. Rapid changes in arterial or venous pressure will predispose to rupture of these thin-walled vessels.

Intraventricular haemorrhage is associated with prematurity, respiratory distress of all types, mechanical ventilation, metabolic acidosis, hypoxia and hypercapnia. Surges in arterial pressure or in venous pressure should be avoided. Therefore rapid transfusion or the administration of hyperosmolar solutions of glucose or sodium bicarbonate may be harmful. Hypoxia causes venous congestion and even the safety of awake intubation in sick preterm infants has been questioned (Sumner and James, 1987). Attempts should be made to keep the systolic blood pressure within normal limits of 5.3–9.3 kPa (40–70 mmHg). The major risk period is the first week of life and prognosis may be helped by the use of ultrasound (Yu et al., 1986; Stewart et al., 1987).

Retinal Vasculature

Vascularization of the retina takes place until about the 44th week of gestation and progresses from the nasal to the temporal side. It has been known for many years that high retinal arterial oxygen tensions can cause retinal arterial vasoconstriction in immature babies. This causes retinal fibrosis. New vessels proliferate through the vitreous causing retinal detachment which is described as retrolental fibroplasia (RLF). However the control of inspired oxygen to preterm babies has not eliminated RLF. With the increased survival rate of infants under 1500 g more cases of RLF have occurred. There is some evidence that relative hypoxia after hyperoxia leads to RLF (Phelps and Rosenbaum, 1982). It seems possible that fluctuations in blood flow causing a rise in transluminal pressure may be a factor. A recent review of the role of oxygen in RLF suggests a multifactorial origin in which oxygen is but one factor (Lucey and Dangman, 1984). They point out that the retinal circulation is subject to the same wide fluctuations as the cerebral circulation in newborn infants. It seems prudent therefore to take the same precautions to avoid wide variations in inspired oxygen and fluctuations in pressure as is advisable in avoiding intraventricular haemorrhage.

RLF should not be considered an avoidable iatrogenic disease in very low birth weight infants because the cause in these infants is not known (Lucey et al., 1984). The precise safe level of Pa_{O_2} is unknown. It has been suggested that a reasonable level is 9.3–10.7 kPa (70–80 mmHg) (Hatch and Sumner, 1986). The recent introduction of pulse oximeters facilitates the achievement of a steady state for these infants.

CONTROL OF BODY TEMPERATURE

Mortality rises considerably if small babies are nursed in surroundings more than a degree or so below the optimum range. The cause of the increased mortality is uncertain. The basal metabolic rate of the newborn is higher than that of the adult per unit of body weight but it is considerably less per unit of surface area. Resting heat production per unit of surface area is particularly low in preterm babies of low birth weight.

Heat Loss

The average newborn has about twice the surface for heat loss per kilogram of tissue compared with the adult. Although thermoregulatory control over skin blood flow is well developed even in very small babies, heat is readily lost because tissue insulation in the newborn is much less than in adults and is even less in babies of low birth weight (Hey et al., 1970). Under ideal environmental conditions for the newborn, about one quarter of basal heat production is lost by evaporation of water from the skin and respiratory tract. The remainder is lost by radiation and convection. In warm surroundings the evaporative heat loss may increase considerably due to sweating and in cold surroundings the heat loss by radiation and convection will increase.

Response to Cold

Most newborn mammals respond to cold exposure by a large increase in oxygen consumption and heat production. In several species and in the human infant this is largely achieved without shivering. The main source of this additional heat production is the oxidation of fat within the brown adipose tissue (Hull, 1966). Brown adipose tissue is widely distributed in the neonate, between the muscles of the neck and back, in the axillae and groins and especially around the kidney and adrenal glands.

Oxygen is required for oxidation of the fat and the infant's increased oxygen consumption as a result of cold stress may be up to 60%. Consequently an infant who is in respiratory distress will deteriorate if nursed in a cool environment. Anaesthesia suppresses this metabolic response to cold, therefore the temperature of an infant will fall considerably in the operating theatre if steps are not taken to minimize heat loss. A baby's ability to respond to cold stress is impaired by severe hypoxia. This is important in respiratory distress syndrome.

Response to Warmth

Skin blood flow increases sufficiently in warm surroundings to reduce tissue insulation to one-third of its amount in the cold. In addition the infant can sweat efficiently at 36–37 weeks gestation and therefore evaporative water loss can increase three-fold (Roberton, 1979). If vasodilatation and sweating fail to prevent body temperature rising, oxygen consumption will increase.

Neutral Thermal Environment

Between the extremes of environment which cause either the metabolic response to cold or sweating there is a narrow neutral zone. In this zone, body temperature can be controlled by changes in posture and blood flow alone and oxygen consumption is minimal. This neutral zone cannot be defined in terms of temperature alone because heat loss is determined by many factors, e.g. radiation, ambient humidity, presence or absence of draughts and, most important, whether the infant is clothed or naked.

Under standard conditions, free from thermal stress, the main factors determining the neutral environmental temperature are age and weight. The low basal heat production (per unit of surface area) and low tissue insulation make it necessary to maintain a high environmental temperature to provide neutral conditions for a *naked* infant in the neonatal period. For example 32°C for a fullterm baby of more than 2 days old and 35°C for a 1 kg infant in the first few days of life (Hey, 1972).

It has become common practice, when babies require constant observation, to keep them naked in incubators or under radiant heat canopies. In the operating theatre the infant can be placed on a thermostatically controlled heating pad, hot air mattress or water blanket and the limbs wrapped in foil or cotton wool.

RESPIRATORY SYSTEM

Transition from Fetal to Neonatal State

The lungs are filled with fluid before birth. This fluid differs in composition from amniotic fluid and plasma and it appears to be an ultrafiltrate of plasma with selective reabsorption or secretion. A variable amount of this fluid is squeezed out from the air passages in the final stages of delivery and as the compressed chest emerges some air is drawn in to replace the fluid previously present. Most of the fluid still remains in the lungs at this stage. This residual fluid is absorbed mainly by the lymphatics and to a lesser extent by the capillaries during the first 24 hours after birth.

During the first breath considerable force is required to overcome the viscosity of the fluid in the lungs, the surface tension of the air/fluid interface and the tissue resistive forces. Pressures measured in the oesophagus during the first breath are of the order of -1 to -7 kPa (-10 to -70 cmH$_2$O) on inspiration maintained for 0.5–1.0 s, and 2–3 kPa (20–30 cmH$_2$O) on expiration. Much of the inspired air remains in the lungs as residual volume. After the first few breaths the lungs are almost completely and evenly expanded and the functional residual capacity reaches about 75% of its ultimate volume within a few minutes. Once respiration is established the arterial P_{O_2} reaches the neonatal level in 5 min, the hypercapnia is corrected by 20 min and the acidosis by 24 h.

The lungs must be mature before they are capable of sustaining life. The alveoli must form by flattening of the cuboidal epithelium at the terminal air sacs and the pulmonary vasculature must develop until the pulmonary capillaries are sufficient for gaseous exchange. In the human this stage is reached at about 28 weeks gestation. In parallel with this anatomical development biochemical development of the lungs must also occur. The normal alveolar lining layer produces surface active phospholipids and adequate amounts of these substances are required to maintain lung stability and avoid atelectasis. In the normal infant some degree of biochemical development is reached at about 28 weeks gestation.

These phospholipids (known collectively as pulmonary surfactant) have been identified as a number of saturated lecithins and are synthesized in the lung tissue by the type II alveolar cells and excreted into the air space to form surface active lining layers. The enzymes for lecithin synthesis are sensitive to cold, hypoxia and acidaemia. Postnatal exposure to temperatures of less than 35°C and a pH of less than 7.25 causes a rapid fall in the amount of surfactant in pharyngeal aspirates.

It has been noted that in very preterm infants, boys have a significantly lower survival than girls (Yu et al., 1986). Boys have slower lung maturation than girls of similar gestation and this probably explains their higher mortality (Khoury et al., 1985).

Certain conditions cause acceleration or delay of maturation of the fetal lung independent of maturation of other organs, e.g. chronic retroplacental bleeding, renal or cardiac hypertension and steroids injected into the mother stimulate early lung maturation. Premature rupture of the membranes may cause a particularly rapid rise in the lecithin/sphingomyelin (L/S) ratio in the course of 72 hours. In some types of diabetes mellitus delay in lung maturation to the 37th week of gestation may occur.

The most widely used indicator of fetal lung maturity is the L/S ratio. L/S ratios greater than 2.0 have predicted the absence of respiratory distress syndrome (RDS) with 98% accuracy in over 2000 patients (Kulovich et al., 1979). The remaining 2% who developed RDS had diabetic mothers, a history of asphyxia *in utero* or hydrops fetalis.

In early gestation with L/S ratios of less than 2.0 the predictability of RDS is much less certain. It is considerably improved by measuring the percentage of another phospholipid in surfactant, phosphatidyl glycerol (PG). PG normally appears at 35 weeks gestation and increases until term but will appear earlier when fetal lung maturation is accelerated. If the percentage of PG in total phospholipid is 3% or more than even when the L/S ratio is less than 2.0, RDS is unlikely to occur. An accuracy of 93% has been reported (Kulovich et al., 1979). The presence of PG is an important step in the biochemical maturation of surfactant.

The relationship between the pressure (P), surface tension (T) and radius (r) of a sphere is expressed by the Laplace equation $P = 2T/r$. This means that the smaller the sphere the higher the pressure within that sphere. One would therefore expect the pressure in the smaller alveoli of the lung to be relatively high with a tendency to empty into adjacent larger alveoli at lower pressure. This would cause an unstable situation with extensive atelectasis. It does not occur because extracts of normal lungs have the remarkable property of altering surface tension, the smaller the surface area, the lower the surface tension (Clements et al., 1958). This explains the phenomenon that the smaller air spaces in the lung remain expanded instead of becoming atelectatic and is based on an assumption that the alveolus is lined with a continuous layer of fluid thereby resembling a bubble.

Recently this concept of a continuous layer of liquid in the normal physiological state has been challenged (Hills, 1987). Hills suggests that the continuous layer of liquid is present only in pathological states and that in the normal lung the gas transfer surface of the alveolus is dry as a result of water repellancy induced by a monolayer of surfactant absorbed onto the epithelial surface. Any fluid present in the alveolus is repelled by the surfactant to form droplets at the corners of the alveolus.

Surfactant is very much reduced or absent in infants

dying from respiratory distress syndrome and this accounts for the generalized atelectasis in this condition. This disease occurs in 30% of all premature births and there have been recent encouraging reports of the efficacy of instillation of bovine or artificial surfactant into the lungs of very preterm infants with respiratory distress syndrome (Raju et al., 1987; Ten Centre Study Group, 1987).

Neonatal Lung

The respiratory region of the lung continues to differentiate during the last three months of gestation. Additional respiratory bronchioles develop with terminal saccules which are capable of gas exchange. New alveoli grow until 8 years of age.

A fairly stable functional residual capacity is established by 8–10 min after birth. Continuing ventilation is associated with decreasing pulmonary vascular resistance leading to a great increase in pulmonary blood flow (*see below*). The absorptive process of the fluid in the lungs by the lymphatics and pulmonary capillaries takes several hours and the increase in the specific compliance of the lung is near its maximum at 24 hours, $6\,ml\cdot cmH_2O^{-1}$. Airway resistance decreases during the same period from about $9\,kPa/(L/s)$, i.e. $90\,cmH_2O/(L/s)$, in the first minute to about $2.5\,kPa/(L/s)$, i.e. $25\,cmH_2O/(L/s)$. This means that normal breathing then requires only about $0.5\,kPa$ ($5\,cmH_2O$) pressure change.

Whereas the specific compliance of the infant's lung at one week of age is similar to that of the adult, the neonatal chest wall is about five times as compliant as that of the adult. As a result there is very little work due to breathing in the normal fullterm infant once ventilation is properly established. There are however disadvantages due to the compliant chest wall. It does not adequately oppose the inward recoil force of the lung which leads to:

1. A low resting functional residual capacity which in turn predisposes to hypoxia.
2. An intrapleural pressure which is less negative than in adults causing a tendency to closure of small airways. This can lead to increased intrapulmonary shunting and hypoxia.

The degree of venous admixture in the normal neonate is about 20% compared with about 5% in the adult. In the normal neonate the arterial P_{O_2} is 10–10.7 kPa (75–80 mmHg) and the arterial P_{CO_2} is low, 4.7 kPa (35 mmHg). The preterm infant is more prone to respiratory difficulties. The respiratory problems resulting from lack of surfactant have already been described. Even when respiratory distress syndrome is not present there is further reduction in lung volume and an increase in small airway closure compared with the fullterm infant. This leads to an increase in venous admixture and a lowering of arterial oxygen tension.

The tendency to apnoea in preterm infants is in-

creased after general anaesthesia and this has implications for postoperative analgesia (*see below*). It is generally recommended that infants below 44 weeks postconceptual age should not be treated as day cases following general anaesthesia.

In the normal fullterm infant the resting oxygen consumption per unit of body weight is twice that of the adult, $7\,ml/(kg\cdot min)$ compared with $3.5\,ml/(kg\cdot min)$. This leads to a higher alveolar ventilation per unit of lung volume than in the adult and accounts for the lower arterial P_{CO_2} in the neonate. The minimum oxygen requirements exist when the neonate is nursed in a neutral thermal environment. As there is normally a greater demand placed on the lung of an infant, there is less respiratory reserve in the infant than in older individuals.

Calculations based on normal data for compliance and resistance indicate that the work of breathing is at its minimum at a rate of 35–40 per min in a healthy neonate. This may explain the higher rate of the infant compared with an older individual. Respiratory work uses about 1% of a fullterm neonate's energy consumption but in preterm infants it may require a great deal more. Any respiratory disease which increases the mechanical work of breathing can cause very great physical energy expenditure in a baby.

The ratio of dead space to tidal volume is the same in infants as in adults.

The preference for nose breathing is a very serious factor in infants with bilateral choanal atresia as the infant will not breathe through its mouth and asphyxia may ensue. The situation is immediately relieved by inserting an oropharyngeal airway which is well tolerated by a neonate.

CARDIOVASCULAR SYSTEM

Fetal Circulation

In utero the placenta provides a means of gaseous exchange and nutrition for the fetus. Most of the blood in the descending aorta passes via the hypogastric arteries and their continuation the umbilical arteries, to the placenta and returns to the fetus via the umbilical vein. From the umbilical vein the blood passes via the ductus venosus, thereby by-passing the liver, to the right atrium. From the right atrium the blood goes through the foramen ovale to the left atrium and thus to the left ventricle and ascending aorta. The superior vena caval blood returning to the right atrium enters the right ventricle and then the pulmonary artery from which it passes through the ductus arteriosus to enter the descending aorta.

Circulatory Changes at Birth

After birth the lungs and liver must serve the functions of the placenta and therefore the circulation must adjust accordingly. The circulation via the umbilical arteries ceases and the ductus venosus should close. The patent ductus arteriosus and foramen ovale should close so that the blood flows through the pulmonary circulation before reaching the left heart and aorta.

The main mechanism which causes an increase in blood flow through the pulmonary circulation is ventilation of the lungs with air thereby exposing the pulmonary vessels to a higher oxygen tension. This causes a decrease in the pulmonary vascular resistance probably by a direct local effect rather than by a reflex via the aortic and carotid chemoreceptors. The first breath therefore causes an increase in pulmonary blood flow which raises the left atrial pressure above that of the inferior vena cava and right atrium. Consequently the foramen ovale closes functionally by a valve-like action of the membrane which is on the left atrial side.

The blood from both inferior vena cava and superior vena cava now enters the pulmonary artery from the right side of the heart. As the resistance in the pulmonary vessels falls so the blood flow through the pulmonary vascular bed increases rapidly with a consequent diminution in the flow through the ductus arteriosus. In the first hour after birth there may be left-to-right and right-to-left shunts via the ductus in normal infants. The right-to-left shunt decreases rapidly within the first hour and after this time is unusual in the resting normal infant. If the ductus remains open a left-to-right shunt will develop. The pulmonary vascular resistance does not fall to adult levels immediately, otherwise a large shunt would develop from left-to-right through the still patent ductus leading to an overwhelming pulmonary blood flow. As the left ventricular output is increased after birth and the systemic vascular resistance rises, a large left-to-right shunt causing an additional output from the left ventricle might precipitate failure.

Oxygenation of the systemic arterial blood causes constriction of the ductus and functional closure occurs within a few hours but histological closure may take 2–3 weeks. A significant reduction in arterial oxygen tension may reopen a constricted ductus in the first few days. This is of considerable importance to the anaesthetist because the lowered oxygen tension will cause an increase in pulmonary vascular resistance leading to a right-to-left shunt through the ductus. This could cause a considerable degree of desaturation in the systemic circulation.

In certain types of congenital heart disease the ductus arteriosus may be the only means by which a significant amount of blood can reach the pulmonary vasculature, e.g. severe pulmonary stenosis, or by which communication between the pulmonary and systemic circulations can occur, e.g. transposition of the great arteries. Early spontaneous closure of the ductus can cause a fatal deterioration in the patient's condition in such lesions (Glover, 1977).

Prostaglandin E_1 is known to dilate the ductus arteriosus of the neonate. Clinically it has been used as a short-term palliative in the above conditions to enable the patient's hypoxic and metabolic state to be improved before surgical correction of the defect.

In some infants a high pulmonary artery pressure persists with a right-to-left shunt through a patent ductus arteriosus or patent foramen ovale. This is called 'persistent fetal circulation'. It occurs in respiratory distress syndrome, in some cases of diaphragmatic hernia and there are instances of unknown aetiology. Ventilation and a high inspired oxygen mixture are valuable in lowering the pulmonary vascular resistance. If there is a poor response tolazoline may be used; if it is ineffective then epoprostenol (prostacyclin) may be effective (Lock et al., 1979).

Cardiac Output

The average cardiac output of the human infant is about 180 ml/(kg·min) and is double the adult value per kg. The heart rate and cardiac output in both fetus and newborn are so high that there is not much room for further increase (Dawes, 1971). In the adult 60% of cardiac muscle is contractile mass but in the neonate it may be as low as 30% (Smith and Smith, 1982). The infant therefore has less capacity to increase its stroke volume.

Sympathetic and parasympathetic reflexes to the heart are active from birth and anything which reduces cardiac rate will lower cardiac output. Hypoxia is the best example but inhalational anaesthetic agents where infants have not been given atropine will often produce slowing of the rate with considerable reduction in cardiac output.

BODY FLUIDS

Total Body Water

Approximately 80% of the total body weight in the newborn is fluid. This proportion drops to 75% in the young child and 55–60% in the adult. There are wide variations in body composition between individual newborn infants due to differences in the size of the skeleton and thus in the proportions of bone and soft tissue as well as in fat content.

Distribution of Water

The extracellular volume (plasma plus interstitial fluid) in the neonate is relatively increased and constitutes about 40% of the body weight at birth. It falls to 32–35% at weights of 5–20 kg and 25% in adults. The intracellular fluid in the newborn amounts to only 30% body weight compared with over 40% in adults.

The blood volume represents about 10% of the total fluid volume throughout life. Consequently, because of the high proportion of fluid in the newborn the blood volume is about 80 ml/kg body weight whereas in adult males it is about 65–70 ml/kg and in females about 55–65 ml/kg varying inversely with the amount of body fat present.

Water Balance

In the first few days of life there is normally a large loss of weight, approximately 10%. This is related to the duration of the restriction of water intake and can be reduced by starting a water intake soon after birth. Of this 10% loss, less than one-third can be accounted for by the urine passed. Apart from some of the remainder which is used for metabolic processes, most of the weight loss is due to insensible loss via the expired air and skin. Once feeding begins, fluid metabolism rapidly increases reaching a peak at two years of age. Consequently the infant and young child will become depleted much more rapidly than the adult.

Water Requirements

For parenteral replacement in fullterm neonates (provided there are no abnormal losses) it is suggested that little or no fluid is essential during the first 36–48 h after birth. The normal intravenous requirement is met by 30 ml/(kg · 24 h) on the first day of life increasing by approximately 20 ml/(kg · 24 h) until it reaches 120 ml/(kg · 24 h) near the end of the first week. However, abnormal losses almost always occur in preterm infants mainly by insensible loss through the skin, e.g. in newborn infants weighing over 2 kg the insensible fluid loss is between 0.7 and 1 ml/(kg · h) whereas in infants weighing less than 1 kg it has been measured at 2.5–3 ml/(kg · h). Insensible water loss will increase considerably when radiant heat canopies are used and unless absorption by the oral route is adequate, intravenous fluid therapy will be required.

Due to the metabolic response to *major* surgery the normal maintenance requirements should be reduced by approximately 30% in the first 24 h postoperatively but infants with abnormal kidneys may not show this antidiuretic response.

Renal Function

The neonatal kidney has a remarkable capacity to conserve sodium and potassium in the first week of life. If given a water load, infants excrete it well but they can not excrete a given water load within 4 h. Adults can achieve this.

The urine of infants is hypotonic compared with that of older children and their renal clearances of urea, sodium, potassium and chloride are always low even when the plasma concentrations are raised. Nevertheless the range of function of infantile kidneys is adequate for the infant's needs in neonatal life. If large quantities of glucose solution or saline are given, especially intravenously, the limited capacity to excrete a water load and the low renal clearances of sodium and potassium may lead to retention of large quantities of fluids.

Metabolic Aspects

One week after birth the normal neonate taking breast milk will retain in the body 65% of its intake of protein, sodium and potassium and incorporate it in new tissue. Growth therefore relieves the kidney of much of its excretory load but it is important that there is an adequate calorie intake to enable this anabolic mechanism to function properly. Therefore on a diet of breast milk under normal circumstances the neonate kidney is amply fitted for the functions it has to perform. Cow's milk, however, has a renal solute load nearly three times as high as breast milk. If it is administered to an infant who is unable to concentrate his urine (due to water losing disease) he will be in negative water balance even on an apparently adequate intake. Under these circumstances a dangerously hyperosmolar state may occur.

Unlike adults, surgical trauma in neonates does not seem to produce the well-defined metabolic response to surgery (protein breakdown, release of antidiuretic and adrenal cortical hormones causing water and salt retention) unless the surgery is extensive or the baby's general state poor.

The brain accounts for two-thirds of the basal metabolism in infancy whereas in adult life it only accounts for a quarter (Holliday, 1971). It is, therefore, particularly important to ensure that the metabolic sources of energy are adequate. Glucose is of special importance and hypoglycaemia has been recognized as a major cause of preventable mental subnormality. The lower limit of normal in fullterm infants in the first week is 30 mg%. In low birth weight babies it may be 20 mg%. Clinically at these levels the infants appear normal. Symptoms of hypoglycaemia occur if the blood glucose falls below 20 mg% for some time and apnoea and fits may occur. Very preterm infants born before fat and glycogen deposits have been laid down may become hypoglycaemic at any time during the first week or two of life especially if their caloric intake is inadequate.

Newborns have deficient stores of vitamin K and clotting deficiencies therefore exist in the neonate due to an inadequate amount of vitamin K dependent factors. This may be partly prevented by the administration of 1 mg vitamin K parenterally and this is normal practice.

RESPONSE TO RELAXANTS

Stead reported that when assessed by respiratory function, infants under one month of age showed a marked sensitivity to d-tubocurarine and an increased tolerance to succinylcholine compared with older patients (Stead, 1955). Other workers have confirmed Stead's findings on succinylcholine and it is generally accepted that this is due to the infant's proportionately large extracellular volume throughout which the drug is distributed resulting in a lower plasma concentration.

The pharmacokinetics and dynamics of d-tubocurarine in neonates, infants, children and adults have been studied by Fisher et al. (1982). They showed that compared to adults, neonates are sensitive to d-tubocurarine when its effect is determined by the plasma level at which 50% depression of the electromyograph twitch occurs. However as the drug is distributed in a larger volume, due to the high percentage of extracellular fluid in the neonate, leading to a lower plasma concentration for equivalent doses, the dose requirement does not differ with age. Thus the age related changes in volume distribution and neuromuscular junction sensitivity are counter-balancing.

Fisher et al. (1982) also found that in neonates the elimination half-life is longer than in older patients because the larger volume of distribution results in lower plasma concentration at any given time. The drug is therefore less accessible for clearance by glomerular filtration which in turn is also reduced in the neonate. An important consequence of this finding is that second and subsequent doses will be required at less frequent intervals than in older children.

Many workers have found a marked variation response to doses of d-tubocurarine in the neonate. Consequently it is advisable to give small incremental doses until the desired clinical effect is achieved (Bush, 1985; Hatch et al., 1986). It is suggested that fullterm infants should be given an initial dose of 0.5 mg followed by incremental doses of 0.25 mg while these amounts should be reduced to 0.25 mg and 0.125 mg respectively in the preterm infant.

The newer relaxant vecuronium seems to behave in the same way in the neonate as d-tubocurarine whereas atracurium, subject to work still in progress, differs in that the dose interval is similar for neonates and older patients. This is presumably due to its elimination in tissue as well as plasma (Fisher, 1986; Nightingale, 1986).

RESPONSE TO PAIN

A functioning cerebral cortex is necessary for sensation and perception and there is some evidence that this is so. Torres and Anderson (1985) have shown that auditory, olfactory and tactile stimuli cause cortical electroencephalographic activity in preterm neonates. In neonatal convulsions cortical potentials occur with peripheral muscle contractions. We must therefore consider the possibility that the neonate can perceive pain at cortical level (Booker, 1987).

On the other hand myelination of nerve fibres is incomplete at birth and reflexes which depend on cutaneous stimuli are more widespread in the preterm. The increased sensitivity to opiates and general anaesthetics is due to incomplete myelination in the CNS. There are theoretical reasons to suspect that neonatal perception of pain is reduced in proportion to the degree of myelination of the CNS (Hatch, 1987).

Newborns have a higher circulating level of β-endorphins than adults and the immature blood–brain barrier may allow them to cross to the CNS (Sanner and Woods, 1965). This may explain the reduced need for analgesics in this age group (Hatch et al., 1986). It is remarkable how neonates can settle down to sleep after surgery provided they can be fed orally.

For many years most doctors have withheld powerful analgesics from neonates postoperatively. Recently this attitude has been challenged. However even if it is clearly established that the neonate can perceive pain the consequences of using powerful analgesics intra or postoperatively may be serious for the following reasons:

1. An increasing number of neonates requiring surgery are preterm.
2. Apnoeic periods (by definition lasting 20 s or more) occur frequently in preterm infants. This is increased after general anaesthesia and will be greatly aggravated by opioid analgesia intra or postoperatively.
3. Enzyme activity involved in the metabolism of opioids is poor in the neonate and therefore their action will be prolonged.

Apnoea in the neonate is extremely serious and the cumulative effects of repeated attacks can be disastrous neurologically. If opioids are to be used it must be done with great care and only in robust fullterm neonates. Alternatively, it may be more reasonable to institute intubation and ventilation when they are given (Hatch, 1987).

REFERENCES

Booker P.D. (1987). Editorial: postoperative analgesia for neonates. *Anaesthesia*, **42**, 343.

Bush, G.H. (1985). Neuromuscular blockade: use in paediatric surgery and intensive care. In *Clinics in Anaesthesiology*, **3**, 405. (Norman J. ed.). London, Philadelphia, Toronto: W.B. Saunders.

Clements J.A., Brown E.S., Johnson R.P. (1958). Pulmonary surface tension and mucus lining of the lungs: some theoretical considerations. *J. Appl. Physiol.*, **12**, 262.

Dawes G.S. (1971). Fetal and neonatal respiration. In *Recent Advances in Paediatrics* 4th edn (Gairdner D., Hull D. eds). London: Churchill.

Fisher D. (1986). The use of muscle relaxants in children. In *1986 ASA Annual Refresher Course Lectures*, Lecture 256.

Fisher D.M., O'Keeffe C., Stanski D.R., et al. (1982). Pharmacokinetics and pharmacodynamics of d-tubocurarine in infants, children and adults. *Anesthesiology*, **57**, 203.

Glover W.J. (1977). Management of cardiac surgery in the neonate. *Br. J. Anaesth.*, **49**, 59.

Haruda F., Blanc W.A. (1981). The structure of intracerebral arteries in premature infants and the autoregulation of cerebral blood flow. *Ann. Neurol.*, **10**, 303.

Hatch D.J. (1987). Editorial: analgesia in the neonate. *Br. Med. J.*, **1**, 920.

Hatch D.J., Sumner E. (1986). *Neonatal Anaesthesia and Peri-Operative Care*, 2nd Edn. London: Edward Arnold.

Hey E.N. (1972). Thermal regulation in the newborn., *Br. J. Hosp. Med.*, **8**, 51.

Hey E.N., Katz G., O'Connell B. (1970). The total thermal insulation of the newborn baby. *J. Physiol.*, **207**, 683.

Hills B.A. (1987). Editorial: bursting the alveolar bubble. *Anaesthesia*, **42**, 467.

Holliday M.A. (1971). Metabolic rate and organ size during growth from infancy to maturity and during late gestation and early infancy. *Pediatrics*, **47**, 169.

Hull D. (1966). The structure and function of brown adipose tissue. *Br. Med. Bull.*, **22**, 92.

Khoury M.J., Mark J.S., McCarthy B.J., et al. (1985) Factors affecting the sex differential in neonatal mortality; the role of respiratory distress syndrome. *Am. J. Obstet. Gynecol.*, **151**, 777.

Kulovich M.V., Hallman M.B., Gluck L. (1979). The lung profile. I. Normal pregnancy. *Am. J. Obstet. Gynecol.*, **135**, 57.

Lock J.E., Olley P.M., Cocani F., et al. (1979). Use of prostacyclin in persistent fetal circulation. *Lancet*, **1**, 1343.

Lucey J.F., Dangman B. (1984). A reexamination of the role of oxygen in retrolental fibroplasia. *Pediatrics*, **73**, 82.

Nightingale D.A. (1986). Use of atracurium in neonatal anaesthesia. *Brit. J. Anaesth.*, **58**, Suppl. 1, 32S.

Pape K.W., Wigglesworth J.S. (1979). Haemorrhage, ischaemia and the perinatal brain. In *Clinics in Developmental Medicine*, Nos. 69/70. Spastics International Medical Publications, Oxford: Heinemann Medical.

Phelps D.L., Rosenbaum A.L. (1982). The effect of marginal hypoxaemia during the recovery period in oxygen-induced retinopathy in the kitten. *Clin. Res.*, **30**, 146A.

Raju T.N., Vidyasagar D., Bhat R., et al. (1987). Double-blind controlled trial of single-dose treatment with bovine surfactant in severe hyaline membrane disease. *Lancet*, **1**, 651

Roberton N.R.C. (1979). Perinatal physiology. In *Clinical Paediatric Physiology*, p. 134 (Godfrey S., Baum J.D. eds.). Oxford, London, Edinburgh, Melbourne: Blackwell.

Sanner J.H., Woods L.A. (1965). Comparative distribution of tritium labelled dihydromorphine between maternal and fetal rats. *J. Pharmacol. Exp. Ther.*, **148**, 176.

Smith P.C., Smith N.T. (1982). The special considerations of the premature infant. In *Some Aspects of Paediatric Anaesthesia*. (Steward D.J. ed.). Amsterdam: Elsevier.

Stead A.L. (1955). The response of the newborn infant to muscle relaxants. *Br. J. Anaesth.*, **27**, 124.

Stewart A.L., Reynolds E.O.R., Hope P.L., et al. (1987). Probability of neurodevelopmental disorders estimated from ultrasound appearance of brains of very preterm infants. *Dev. Med. Child Neurol.*, **29**, 3.

Sumner E., James I. (1987). Paediatric anaesthesia and intensive care. In *Anaesthesia Review*, **4**, p. 125 (Kaufman L. ed.). Edinburgh, London, Melbourne and New York: Churchill-Livingstone.

Ten Centre Study Group (1987). Ten centre trial of artificial surfactant (A.L.E.C.: artificial lung expanding compound) in very premature babies. *Br. Med. J.*, **1**, 991.

Torres F., Anderson C. (1985). The normal EEG of the newborn. *J. Clin., Neurophysiol.*, **2**, 89.

Volpe J.J. (1981). Neonatal intraventricular haemorrhage. *New Engl. J. Med.*, **304**, 886.

Yu V.Y.H., Loke H.L., Bajuk B., et al. (1986). Prognosis for infants born at 23 to 28 weeks gestation. *Br. Med. J.*, **1**, 1200.

SECTION 3
PHARMACOLOGICAL BASIS OF THE SCIENCE OF ANAESTHESIA

45. Factors Affecting The Action of Drugs
A. Lant

Drug disposition
Passage of drugs across cell membranes
  Membrane structure
  Transport mechanisms
  Pinocytosis and phagocytosis
Drug transfer across specialized membranes
  Blood–brain barrier (BBB)
  Placenta
Binding of drugs and molecular mechanisms
  of drug action
  Plasma–protein binding
  Cellular binding
  Drug action not mediated by receptor
    interaction
  Excretion of drugs
  Renal excretion
  Pulmonary excretion
  Biliary excretion
  Kinetics of drug elimination

With the increased complexity and sophistication of modern drug therapy, it is becoming virtually impossible for any one individual to acquire complete knowledge of the actions and potential hazards of all available therapeutic agents. This poses a particularly difficult problem for the anaesthetist, since the drugs employed in anaesthetic practice cover an unusually wide spectrum of compounds of diverse structure, physical and pharmacological properties. Although the mechanisms of action of few are explicable in molecular terms, advances made in the sphere of biochemical pharmacology in recent years have shown that the pharmacodynamics of drug action in general are governed and often determined by certain common physicochemical principles. In this chapter, attention has been focused on some of these fundamental principles with the aim of providing the requisite background for understanding the actions of drugs and the basis for their rational use in clinical practice. So as to retain the historical perspective of the advances in knowledge, references to several of the older, and now classic, papers in the literature, have been included.

DRUG DISPOSITION

The ultimate purpose in administering any drug is to achieve an adequate concentration at its site or locus of action sufficient to trigger the desired pharmacological effect. After administration by whichever route, the medium of drug transfer is the plasma water, and it is through this medium that the drug arrives at its site of action or tissue receptor. Only a small proportion of the total number of drug molecules in the circulation reaches and reacts with the receptor, the absolute number depending on the relative activities of various processes which influence the concentration of free drug in the plasma.

After a drug enters the circulation, a number of fates await it. A variable proportion becomes bound to *plasma protein* and is no longer diffusable. Part is bound to *tissue structures* which have nothing to do with the specific drug effect. A small fraction reaches the site of action and reacts with the *specific receptors* (*see* p. 538). Circulation free drug is in a state of dynamic equilibrium with these three processes. The equilibrium state is, however, constantly being disturbed by loss of free drug either by excretion of the unchanged molecule or as metabolites formed by processes of metabolic transformation and conjugation.

It is clear that from the time of administration until its ultimate elimination from the body, the state of distribution of a drug at any given time is dependent on the relative activities of the processes of plasma and tissue binding, metabolism and excretion depicted in Fig. 45.1.

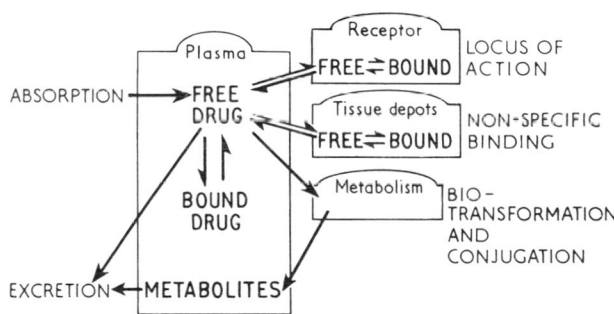

Fig. 45.1 Schematic representation of the factors which influence the plasma concentration of a drug.

Furthermore, participation in these various processes involves either directly or indirectly the crossing of a succession of membrane barriers. These barriers range from rather simple membranes like the blood capillary and red cell to the complex multicellular barriers of the gastric mucosa, intestinal and renal tubular epithelia. It is, therefore, important to consider the mechanisms whereby drugs traverse body membranes and the physicochemical properties of molecules and membranes that characterize these transport processes.

PASSAGE OF DRUGS ACROSS CELL MEMBRANES

Membrane Structure

(Second International Conference on Carriers and Channels in Biological Systems—Transport Proteins, 1980; Hoffmann and Simonsen, 1989)

Natural membranes can be broadly classified into two groups: those which surround individual cells (plasma membranes) and those which surround subcellular structures (cytoplasmic membranes such as the endoplasmic reticulum and the envelopes enclosing intracellular organelles). Although there may be considerable individual variations in structural detail, the general picture which has emerged from chemical, X-ray diffraction and electron microscopic studies is of a basically similar architecture for all cell membranes. This consists of a bimolecular layer of lipid molecules covered with an adsorbed monolayer of protein on both sides, the long axes of the lipids being perpendicularly orientated in relation to the membrane surface. The thickness of the membrane is of the order of 8–10 nm. The question of whether body membranes consist of a continuous lipid barrier or a discontinuous lipid mosaic interspersed with aqueous channels or 'pores' remains a controversial issue. The presence of 'pores' seems necessary to account for the ready passage of water and small lipid insoluble molecules and ions across the membrane. This is particularly so for the blood capillary membrane which behaves as a typical 'lipid-pore' barrier; lipid-soluble substances penetrate readily at a rate determined by their lipid/water partition coefficients, whilst water-soluble substances penetrate less readily at rates determined by molecular size and electrical charge. However, whereas lipid-soluble substances appear to traverse the entire capillary surface, even the smallest hydrophilic molecules (including water) behave as though only a small fraction (about 0.2%) of the total cross-sectional area of the capillary surface was available for transfer. Such behaviour is consistent with the belief that membrane structure incorporates a system of pores, and studies of comparative permeability to various substances have allowed measurements to be derived of equivalent pore radii of different natural membranes. Matrix proteins, as for example, porin or spectrin have been isolated and appear to play an important role in the function of membrane pores and their transport characteristics (Benz et al., 1980; Gardner and Bennett, 1989).

Transport Mechanisms
(Schafer and Barfuss, 1986)

There are two general mechanisms whereby drugs cross membranes: (1) passive transfer, in which the membrane behaves as an inert system through which the drug passes; (2) specialized transport, in which the membrane plays an active role in the process of transferring the drug through it.

Passive Transfer

Simple Diffusion and Filtration. Most drugs cross membranes by *simple diffusion* where the rate of transfer is proportional to the concentration gradient across the membrane, and the driving force is thermal agitation of the molecules in accordance with Fick's law. As well as being related to surface area and thickness of the membrane, the speed of transfer is also determined by inherent properties of the drug, such as its molecular size, spatial configuration and degree of ionization if it is an electrolyte and lipid solubility. In general, substances of low molecular weight diffuse readily, but as size increases, the lipid solubility of the molecule becomes more important. The significance of lipid solubility was first emphasized by Overton (1899) who showed that the permeability of membranes to lipid-soluble molecules increased as the molecule became more soluble in non-polar solvents. The subsequent finding that the potency of various inhalational anaesthetics correlated with their oil/water partition coefficients formed the basis of the 'lipid solubility' theory of anaesthesia (Meyer-Overton). However, correspondence between lipid solubility and anaesthetic potency does not necessarily imply a cause and effect relationship and may represent a phenomenon quite distinct from the fundamental mechanism of action of general anaesthetics at a cellular or molecular level. There is no doubt, however, that in the case of most drugs, lipid solubility is a major determinant in the ability to penetrate the cell membrane. It is of particular importance in relation to those drugs which undergo partial ionization at body pH, for membrane permeability to the non-ionized form of a weak electrolyte is very much greater than to the ionic form. Indeed, the membrane can be regarded as virtually impermeable to the latter. The amount of drug present in the lipid-soluble unionized form is a function of the dissociation constant of the native molecule and the pH of the fluid in which it is dissolved (*see below*).

On the other hand, a number of lipid insoluble substances cross a membrane as if it were a fine sieve, smaller molecules and ions crossing faster than larger ones to an extent not affected by pH. Presence of a system of 'pores' or polar discontinuities in the lipoprotein barrier offers a means whereby such hydrophilic substances can cross the membrane. Although 'pores' have not been visualized with certainty even with the electron microscope, their presence has been inferred from studies of comparative membrane permeability to various substances and their average size can be expressed mathematically in the form of an 'equivalent pore radius'. Small lipid-insoluble molecules may diffuse directly through aqueous-filled pores, or, when a hydrostatic or osmotic pressure difference exists across the membrane, the flow of water in bulk through the 'pores' may drag with it any solute molecules whose dimensions are small enough to penetrate the 'pores'. This process has been called 'solvent drag'. A figure of about 0.4 nm is representative of the equivalent pore radius of the plasma membrane of most cells and thus penetration by pore filtration is restricted to substances, whose molecular radius in at least one dimension is less than 0.4 nm. Thus urea (MW 60), with an equivalent radius of 0.2 nm, passes readily across cell membranes. Most drug molecules have radii considerably larger than this and filtration by pores is, therefore, of minor importance as a route of cell entry for drugs. Attempts to correlate molecular and pore sizes may be misleading, for example in the case of penetration of membranes by ions. The volume of an ion may be much larger than indicated by molecular weight on account of hydration. Furthermore, with some ions transfer may be more dependent on charge than size. For example, although the size of the hydrated ions of K^+ and Cl^- is about the same, the permeability of the red cell membrane to Cl^- is very much greater than to K^+.

The situation is different in the case of certain body membranes such as the sheet-like structures formed by the epithelial cells of blood glomerular capillaries. Although these membranes possess the lipoidal characteristics of the membranes of their constituent cells, the sheets of cells do not fit together tightly with the result that the effective pore size may be as high as 3 nm in radius. The result is that these membranes are highly 'porous' and most drugs pass from one side to the other with relative ease. Plasma albumin (MW 69 000) is borderline in size and tends to be restrained by the normal capillary and glomerular membranes, as are molecules of drug which are albumin-bound.

Diffusion and Drug Ionization. The majority of drugs are weak electrolytes capable of undergoing ionization in aqueous solution. The cell membrane is preferentially permeable to the lipid-soluble non-ionized form, but resists penetration of the water-soluble ionized form. The extent of ionization of a drug is a function of its dissociation constant and the pH of the surrounding solution. By international convention, the dissociation constants for both acids and bases are expressed on the same scale in the form of K_a. Because these constants are small, it is more convenient to use the expression pK_a, which represents the negative logarithm of the dissociation constant. The pK_a scale is analogous to pH notation and provides a useful way of comparing the strengths of acids and bases. The stronger an acid, the lower its pK_a; the stronger a base, the higher its pK_a (Fig. 45.2).

The relationship between pK_a and the proportion of total drug which has undergone ionization can be represented by the Henderson–Hasselbalch equation which results from application of the law of mass action.

$$\text{For a weak acid, } pH - pK_a = \log_{10} \frac{(\text{ionized form})}{(\text{unionized form})}$$

$$\text{For a weak base, } pH - pK_a = \log_{10} \frac{(\text{unionized form})}{(\text{ionized form})}$$

At 50% ionization, the logarithmic fraction equals unity and $pH = pK_a$. If C_I and C_{II} are the concentrations of total drug on sides I and II of a biomembrane, the ratio $R = C_I/C_{II}$, can be expressed in the following form:

$$\text{For a weak acid, } R = \frac{1 + \text{antilog}_{10}(pH_I - pK_a)}{1 + \text{antilog}_{10}(pH_{II} - pK_a)}$$

$$\text{For a weak base, } R = \frac{1 + \text{antilog}_{10}(pK_a - pH_I)}{1 + \text{antilog}_{10}(pK_a - pH_{II})}$$

From these relationships, it is clear that a small change in pH can make a large change in the extent of ionization, particularly if the values of pK_a and pH lie close together. The pH partition hypothesis can be employed to calculate the theoretical distribution of drugs across various body membranes where distinct pH differences are known to exist in the media bathing either side of the membrane. Thus, there is an unequal distribution of weak acids and bases between the highly acid gastric juice and plasma with its pH close to neutral. In the stomach, strong acids with pK_a less than 1 are largely in an ionized form and are not absorbed. Drugs of weaker acidity such as salicylates (pK_a 3.0–3.5) or barbiturates (pK_a 7.5–7.9) exist as unionized molecules which, being lipid soluble, are readily absorbed. Alkalinization of the stomach contents by addition of $NaHCO_3$ decreases the absorption of salicylate through conversion of a large part of the drug to the ionized form, whereas a drug like thiopentone (pK_a 7.6) is but little affected by increase in pH, since even at pH 8 it is largely in non-ionized form. On the other hand, absorption of weak bases can be markedly increased when stomach contents are neutralized. Absorption from the intestine resembles that from the stomach in that there is rapid penetration by lipid-soluble non-ionized molecules. Passage of drugs across the mucosa is dictated to a considerable extent by the pK_a and the differential pH gradient. It is the gradient between the pH at the absorbing (membrane) surface and plasma rather than that existing between plasma and the bulk contents within the lumen which determines the degree to which ionization affects absorption. Experimental work has shown that the pH in the immediate environment of the intestinal mucosa is about 5.3, a value somewhat more acidic than that usually associated with intestinal contents. Strong acids and bases are present in both intestine and plasma, mainly in ionized form, and are poorly absorbed.

In general, there is negligible intestinal absorption of acids with $pK_a < 2.5$ and of bases with $pK_a > 8.5$. Within these limits there is good absorption of both acids and bases, though the extent in individual cases may differ aaccording to the lipid solubility of the non-ionic form of the drug. Other factors which may make the pattern of gastrointestinal absorption devi-

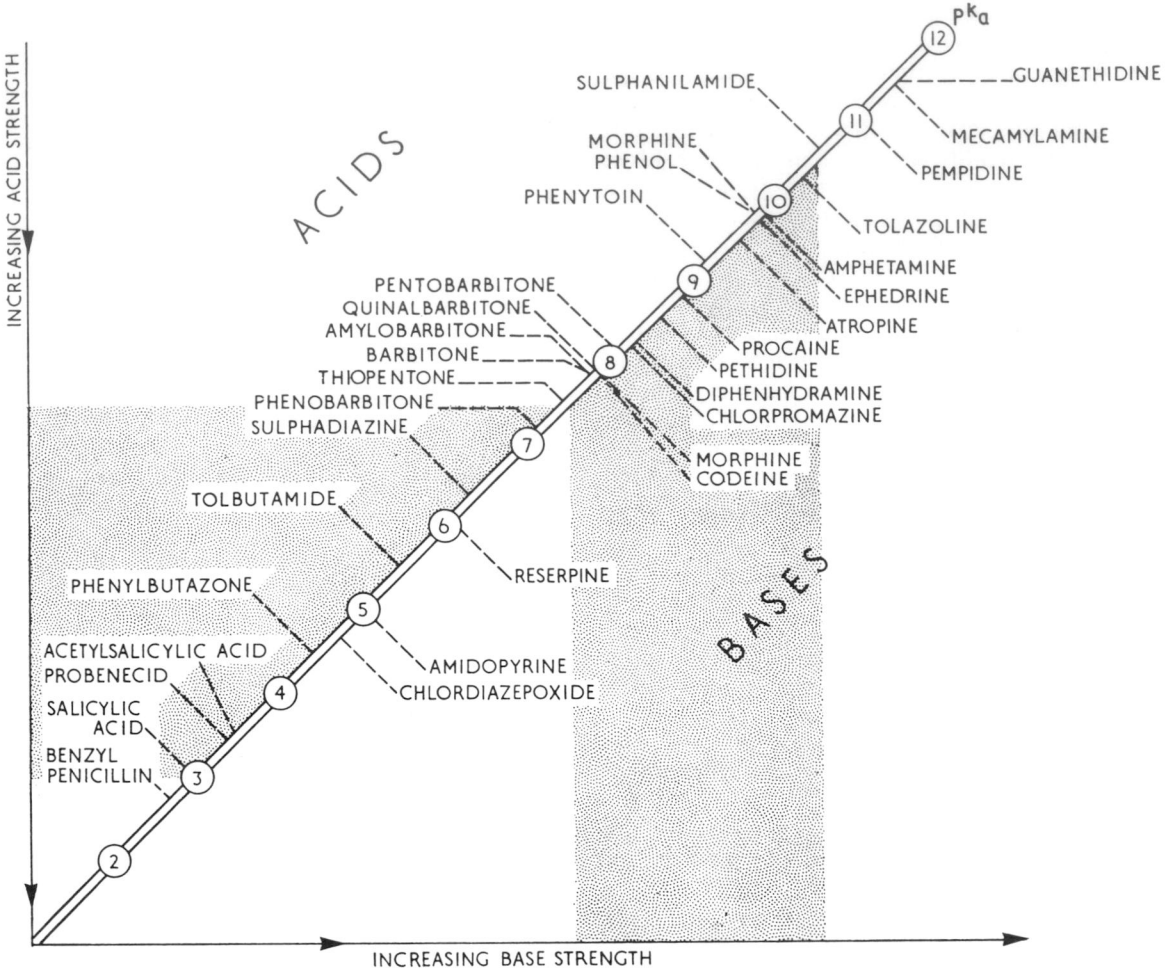

Fig. 45.2 pK$_a$ values of some commonly used drugs. The shaded areas represent the ranges of pK$_a$ for weak acids (3.0–7.5) and weak bases (7.5–10.5) whose urinary excretion displays the phenomenon of pH-dependence.

ate from that predicted by theory include variations in blood supply and motility of the gut, viscosity and pH of secretions, as well as drug formulation.

Degree of ionization and the lipid-solubility of the unionized drug moiety play a major role in determining the rate at which many drugs penetrate into the CSF and brain. The blood-brain and blood-CSF boundaries which comprise the 'blood-brain barrier' behave basically like other lipid biomembranes. Drugs with very high lipid solubility such as the anaesthetic gases diffuse across freely to an extent limited not by lipid solubility, but almost entirely by rates of blood flow. In the case of more polar compounds, however, the role of ionization becomes increasingly important. Because there is only a very small pH gradient between plasma and CSF (the pH of the latter normally being 0.1 unit less than plasma), distribution of drugs between the two components is largely a function of pK$_a$ and the lipid solubility of the undissociated molecules present. The degree of binding of drug to plasma protein is also critical because the rate of diffusion across a membrane is proportional to the

unbound and not *total* concentration of drug in the plasma.

Realization of the important roles of lipid solubility and extent of ionization which underlie the pH-partition hypothesis have provided much insight into the mechanisms whereby drugs penetrate cell boundaries. It has become clear that alterations in extracellular pH, whether of respiratory or metabolic origin, can have far-reaching consequences on the biological efficacy of any drug which undergoes ionization in body fluids, for distribution of drug, ability to attain equilibrium at the tissue site of action, metabolism and elimination may all be profoundly affected.

The special role of the renal tubular epithelium in relation to drug elimination will be considered later.

Specialized Transport

A number of naturally-occurring non-electrolytes are readily transported across cell membranes under physiological conditions, although they are too large to traverse 'pores' and too polar to dissolve in the lipid biophase. In some cases, a remarkable degree of stereospecificity of the membrane exists, as for example in the selective intestinal absorption of l-amino acids as compared to their d-enantiomorphs. Such lipid-insoluble materials are believed to traverse the membrane by a specialized transport system, which involves the formation of a complex with a 'carrier' in the membrane. 'Carriers' are pictured as membrane components which combine with substrate at one surface of the membrane; the complex then moves across the membrane under its own diffusion gradient, substrate is released and the carrier returns to the original surface for another trip. The analogy of the ferry boat has been suggested. A considerable literature has developed on the subject of carrier-mediated transport, which has been extended also to explain the transmembrane movements of certain inorganic and organic ions. Isolation with certainty of membrane carriers has proved difficult. The behaviour of a number of ion transporting systems suggests that ion channels may function by virtue of conformational changes in specific binding sites occupied by a mobile carrier protein.

At least three types of carrier-mediated transport are recognized.

(a) Active Transport. If the substrate molecule is moved against a concentration gradient or, in the case of an ion, against an electrochemical gradient, chemical energy is needed and the process is called 'active transport'. The maximum rate of carrier-mediated transport is limited by the concentration of carrier molecules in the membrane. The transport system can become saturated with substrate if the concentration of substrate molecules is high enough and then formation and breakdown of the carrier-substrate complex within the membrane will follow Michaelis-Menten kinetics (*see* p. 540). In many cases the system displays a high degree of structural and stereo-specificity for chemical configuration. If two substances of similar chemical structure are transported, one will competitively inhibit the other. Because active transport is 'uphill transport', and requires the expenditure of cellular energy, it can be blocked by metabolic inhibitors. The details of how the chemical reactions of cellular metabolism are coupled to the transport mechanism are not fully understood. Active transport systems are widely distributed in living tissues. An example of an active transport system of considerable significance is the 'sodium pump' found within cell membranes. It uses energy from the hydrolysis of adenosine triphosphate (ATP) to expel Na and accumulate K and is responsible for maintaining the low concentration of Na and high concentration of K found in most body cells (Fig. 45.3). At least two separate transport systems have been discovered in renal tubular epithelium which are energy-dependent and fulfil the criteria for processes of active transport. However, judging from the wide heterogeneity of chemical substances which can be handled,

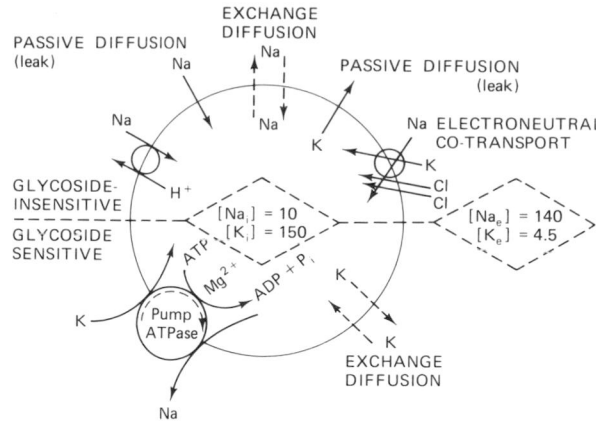

Fig. 45.3 Diagrammatic representation of the interrelationships between active and passive cation movements in cells and the sensitivity of ion fluxes to the inhibitory effects of cardiac glycosides. Cell volume and cation content are kept constant by the balance which normally exists between the downhill movement of passive diffusion (leak) and the active transport of Na and K via the sodium pump in the membrane. The curved arrows connected by the circle represent the active ion fluxes which oppose the attainment of diffusion equilibrium. The outward pumping of Na is linked to the inward pumping of K. The glycoside-sensitive Mg^{2+}, Na^+, K^+—ATPase, located in the cell membrane either constitutes the pump or is a major component of its mechanism. ATP = adenosine triphosphate; ADP = adenosine diphosphate; P_i = inorganic phosphate; $[Na_i]$, $[K_i]$ = intracellular Na and K concentrations (mmol/kg intracellular water); $[Na_e]$, $[K_e]$ = extracellular Na and K concentrations (mmol/L).

these systems appear to lack any clear structural requirements as to substrate configuration.

A few synthetic drugs are absorbed from the intestine by an active transport mechanism, because they closely resemble natural substrates. An example is the anti-hypertensive agent, α-methyldopa, which is structurally related to phenylalanine.

Transfer of biologically important peptides may pass from the circulation via the blood-brain barrier (BBB) to enter brain interstitial space by binding to specific peptide carriers. This receptor-mediated transport process is referred to as transcytosis (*see* BBB, p. 533).

(b) Facilitated Diffusion. This term is applied to carrier-mediated transport in which the substrate moves down a concentration gradient just as in the case of simple diffusion, but considerably faster than by the latter process alone. Thus, for example, glucose readily traverses the red cell membrane attaining the same concentration inside as on the outside, by a process which displays specificity, saturability and sensitivity to certain metabolic inhibitors. A number of volatile anaesthetics compete with monosaccharides for the carrier within the red cell membrane and it is possible that these agents may, therefore, traverse the membrane both by simple and facilitated diffusion.

(c) Exchange Diffusion. This term describes the transport system in which the carrier complex moves the substrate from one surface of the membrane to the opposite and, after releasing the substrate, reacts with another molecule of substrate which it then returns to the original surface. No net movements of substrate occur by this route. An example would be the rapid exchange between substrate and its isotope placed on either side of a membrane.

Pinocytosis and Phagocytosis

This is the process by which cells engulf small drops of the external medium and occurs classically in amoebae and mammalian macrophages. The mammalian intestinal mucosa may engulf fat droplets and perhaps other large molecules in this way. The absorption of cyanocobalamin-intrinsic factor complex in the ileum may involve pinocytosis, but whether such a process affects drug absorption in general to any significant extent is unknown.

DRUG TRANSFER ACROSS SPECIALIZED MEMBRANES

Blood-brain Barrier (BBB)
(Pardridge, 1988)

The resistance of the brain and CSF to penetration by various substances led to the formulation of the concept of a 'blood-brain barrier' (BBB). In recent years, it has become clear that the boundaries between blood and brain and blood and CSF, though differing

anatomically, behave in an analogous manner to other lipoidal plasma membranes with regard to their permeability to drugs. The blood-brain barrier consists essentially of the blood capillary wall and a surrounding layer of glial cells closely applied to the basement membrane of capillary endothelium. Because of this investment of the brain capillaries by a cellular sheath, their permeability characteristics are closer to those of the plasma membranes of cells rather than the more porous structure of capillary endothelium. The blood-CSF boundary consists mainly of the epithelium of the choroid plexus. The blood-brain and blood-CSF boundaries resist the entrance of highly ionized compounds such as quaternary ammonium derivatives like *d*-tubocurarine or gallamine. With drugs that undergo only partial ionization at plasma pH, penetration rates are proportional to the lipid/water partition coefficient of the unionized molecules, allowing for variations in the individual degrees of binding to plasma protein. Highly lipid soluble drugs such as the inhalation anaesthetics enter the brain so rapidly that barriers to diffusion are not demonstrable and blood flow becomes the main rate-limiting factor. A less obvious example of high lipid solubility affecting the onset and duration of drug action is the behaviour of thiopentone as an intravenous anaesthetic agent. Thiopentone is largely non-ionic at plasma pH and has a very high partition coefficient. Its oxygen homologue, pentobarbitone, is even less ionized at pH 7.4 and is much less protein-bound, but because of the low partition coefficient of the non-ionized form, its penetration is very slow. The low lipid solubility of barbitone is also responsible for its slow penetration despite a negligible degree of protein binding and similar degree of ionization to thiopentone (Table 45.1). Thus, for any weak electro-

TABLE 45.1

COMPARISON OF THE STRUCTURES AND PHYSICOCHEMICAL PROPERTIES OF THREE BARBITURATE DERIVATIVES

Drug	X	Y	Z	pK_a	Fraction non-ionized at pH 7.4	Fraction bound to plasma protein at pH 7.4	Partition coefficient (n-heptane/water) of non-ionized form
Thiopentone	$-CH_2-CH_3$	$-CH-(CH_2)_2-CH_3$ $\quad\vert$ $\quad CH_3$	$=S$	7.6	0.61	0.75	3.30
Pentobarbitone	$-CH_2-CH_3$	$-CH-(CH_2)_2-CH_3$ $\quad\vert$ $\quad CH_3$	$=O$	8.1	0.83	0.40	0.05
Barbitone	$-CH_2-CH_3$	$-CH_2-CH_3$	$=O$	7.5	0.56	<0.02	<0.002

[Data based on Morgan et al., 1981a]

lyte to act upon the central nervous system, it should have a suitable combination of the following properties which will allow ready penetration of the blood-brain barrier: low ionization at plasma pH; low binding to plasma protein and a fairly high lipid water partition coefficient. Increase in the degree of ionization by deliberate molecular modification may hinder passage of drugs across the blood-brain barrier. For example, atropine and physostigmine (eserine) are tertiary amines which penetrate brain tissue readily, whilst their quaternarized derivatives, atropine methyl sulphate and neostigmine, are more highly ionized and are effectively excluded from the central nervous system. The latter drugs have the advantage of evoking the same autonomic effects in the periphery as the parent molecules from which they are derived, but their parenteral use is free from the complications of central effects. The boundary, consisting of ependyma and pia which separates brain and CSF, has a high degree of permeability, so that diffusion of most molecules, including lipid insoluble compounds, is essentially unrestricted. Recent studies have used isolated brain capillaries as an *in vitro* model of the BBB and have led to the discovery of a number of specific peptide receptors. These receptors appear to play a major role as transport systems as well as in altering BBB permeability to circulating plasma proteins, nutrients and drugs (Hawkins, 1986).

Unlike entry of drugs into the central nervous system, passage of drugs out of the CSF is less dependent on lipid solubility and extent of ionization. There are two possible routes whereby lipid-insoluble compounds may leave the CSF. First, they may be swept out via the valve-like structures of the arachnoid villi, as CSF drains in bulk from the subarachnoid space to the dural blood sinuses. The porosity of these villi is so great that a small molecule like mannitol and a large molecule like albumin flow out at similar rates. Second, the epithelium of the choroid plexuses offers an alternative exit route. Available evidence indicates the presence in the choroidal cells of two distinct active transport mechanisms, one pumping out organic anions and the other cations. These specialized transport mechanisms appear to function separately, a situation analogous to that occurring in the renal tubular epithelium (*see later*).

Placenta
(Nation, 1980)

Although there has been a considerable interest in recent years in the potential teratogenicity of drug therapy in pregnancy, surprisingly little is known of the mechanisms governing transplacental passage of drugs. It has become clear that it is an oversimplification to regard the placenta as a homogeneous semi-permeable barrier, although the features of drug transfer do, in many cases, parallel those of other lipid biomembranes. The situation is, however, complicated by the extensive anatomical and physiological changes which the placenta undergoes in the course of development. The mature placenta is a remarkably active organ, which is not only capable of transporting many substances of physiological importance, but also possesses organized enzyme systems capable of synthesizing hormones such as gonadotrophins, oestrogens and progesterone. Because of the understandable technical difficulties involved, there is extremely little quantitative information on the kinetics of drug penetration of the placenta at different stages of pregnancy. Nevertheless, the concept of the blood-placenta barrier as a modified lipid membrane has gained ground from the behaviour of drugs with differing degrees of ionization and lipid solubility. Drugs with high degrees of ionization and low lipid solubility such as the quaternary ammonium neuromuscular blocking drugs, apparently penetrate poorly, whilst drugs that are fat soluble at physiological pH penetrate almost simultaneously. Thus, for example, thiopentone attains lipid equilibrium with fetal blood as do the inhalational anaesthetics (Morgan et al., 1981b). Other drugs known to traverse the placental barrier include narcotic analgesics of the opiate group, phenothiazine derivatives, and sulphonamides. Local anaesthetics such as lignocaine, bupivacaine or mepivacaine, whether given in labour by the epidural, caudal or paracervical routes, cross the placenta without difficulty and may cause dose-related bradycardia in the fetus. Various antibiotics including penicillins, cephalosporins, tetracyclines, the aminoglycoside and macrolide derivatives, cross the placenta, but rather slowly and at varying rates. The gradient of drug achieved across the placenta is primarily a function of the amount administered to the mother. However, other factors such as distribution in the maternal and fetal extracellular spaces, metabolism and excretion in the mother, infant and placenta and also maternal and fetal blood flow rates are of importance. The speed of maternal–fetal equilibration is also influenced by the degree of binding to plasma proteins, because binding can clearly occur on either side of the placenta. The fetal plasma proteins act as a reservoir for drug molecules after they cross the placenta in free form and the speed of equilibration can be retarded particularly in cases where the process of diffusion is rate-limiting. The inhalational anaesthetics diffuse and equilibrate very rapidly, the rate of equilibration being limited more by variations in placental blood flow than by protein-binding.

Pathological changes in the placenta secondary to hypoxia, hypertension, dehydration, etc., can all affect the selectivity of the membrane barriers and alter the efficacy of the protective mechanism which nature has provided for the fetus. This is especially important in the newborn, since it is placed in a vulnerable state by having immature and inefficent drug-metabolizing and detoxifying systems (*see below*). More systematic studies of drug transfer kinetics across the placenta are needed before firm conclusions can be drawn and predictions made as to the safety of drugs administered during various stages of gestation, during labour and at delivery.

BINDING OF DRUGS AND MOLECULAR MECHANISMS OF DRUG ACTION

Plasma-protein Binding
(Tozer, 1984)

Within the vascular compartment, a variable proportion of the drug is reversibly bound to plasma proteins. Only the free or unbound drug is diffusible and pharmacologically active. For this reason, to speak of the 'plasma level' of a drug has only limited meaning. The value of functional significance is the *unbound* component. The protein most generally involved in drug-binding is albumin, a single chain peptide structure with a non-specific reactivity for binding a variety of drugs. The muscle relaxant *d*-tubocurarine is somewhat of an exception in that it appears to bind predominantly to gamma globulin.

Nature of Binding Forces
Although the subject of much study, the detailed mechanisms responsible for holding drugs in combination with protein remain obscure. The major physicochemical forces which may be involved in binding are as follows:

1. Attractive forces
(a) *Covalent Bonding.* This is the familiar strong bond which holds together the carbon atoms of organic molecules. It is formed by the sharing of a pair of electrons by two atoms and has a bond energy of about 40–200 kcal/mol. Such bonding is usually irreversible at ordinary temperatures unless enzymatic cleavage is involved. Because of its high stability, the covalent bond plays little part in the readily reversible binding of drugs to protein. It may have an important role in reaction mechanisms, which involve the formation of unusually stable complexes such as, for example, the inactivation of cholinesterase by organophosphate insecticides.

(b) *Electrostatic or Ionic Bonding.* This arises from electrostatic attraction between oppositely charged particles. Electrons of one atom are transferred to a different atom. The bond strength is of the order of 4–6 kcal/mol. Combination of acidic or basic drugs which undergo ionization at plasma pH may bind in this way to oppositely charged sites on the protein molecule.

(c) *Hydrogen Bonding.* The hydrogen nucleus, a proton, has a strong electropositive nature. It is able to accept readily an electron pair in part from each of two electron donor atoms such as oxygen, nitrogen or fluorine and forms a bridge approximately 3 Å long between them. The bond strength ranges between 2 and 7 kcal/mol. Water, by its chemical nature, can readily form hydrogen bonds both by its constituent H and O atoms.

(d) *Hydrophobic Bonding.* This type of bonding represents an interaction between non-polar molecules or groups and the aqueous environment. Formation of hydrophobic bonds is associated with a decrease in entropy implying that some more ordered structure has been formed. It is believed that a layer of 'structured' or 'icelike' water forms either round the drug molecule or in the immediate proximity of the binding protein. Dissolution of this 'iceberg' when drug and binding-protein meet may contribute to the free energy of hydrophobic binding. A characteristic of this type of binding is its lack of high structural specificity on the part of the involved molecules. There has been considerable interest in the role which changes in water structure in the vicinity of non-polar binding-sites in protein or other tissue macromolecules may play in the molecular mechanism of anaesthesia.

(e) *Van der Waals Forces.* These represent short-range attractive forces which develop whenever two atoms approach each other closely. They are in essence the result of slight distortions in the electron clouds surrounding each nucleus. The bond energy is only 0.5–2.0 kcal/mol, but in the case of close-fitting groups of atoms or molecules, such forces may become sizeable and cause the groups to cling together. At least three different types, named Keesom, Debye and London forces respectively, have been distinguished as components of this group.

2. Repulsive forces
(a) *Ionic and Dipole Repulsions.* Clearly, where similarly charged chemical groups come close together, a decrease in drug-protein binding interaction is to be expected. The repulsive Born force comes into this category.

(b) *Steric Hindrance.* This refers to certain three-dimensional characteristics of chemical structure such as the orientation of certain radicals or the inflexibility of certain bonds to distortion, which influence the overall reactivity of a drug molecule. Certain variations in molecular architecture may thus hinder the ability of substances to bind with protein or other macromolecules.

Extent of Protein-binding
It is evident that for binding to be reversible, the tertiary structure of the binding protein must remain intact. The overall extent of drug-protein binding

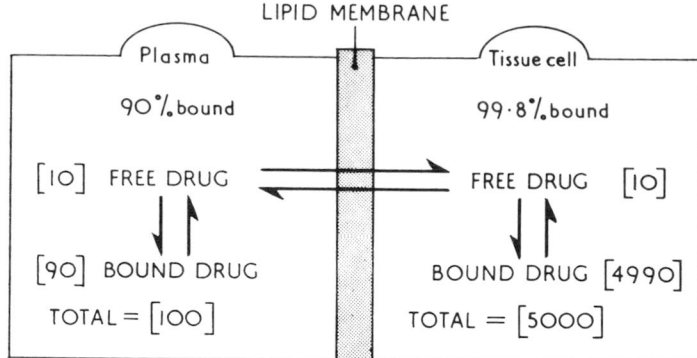

Fig. 45.4 Theoreticl steady-state distribution between a tissue cell and plasma of a drug such as chlorpromazine which has a higher binding affinity for intracellular protein than for plasma albumin. Only the unbound moiety equlibrates across the membrane.

depends on the concentration of drug, the capacity and number of sites for interaction and the affinity of the drug for them (Fig. 45.4). Although the detailed mechanisms involved in binding are not fully understood, it is probable that several of the binding forces considered above are involved together in the process. In some cases, the degree of binding is considerable as, for example, has been found with iodinated derivatives of β-phenylpropionic acid ($C_6H_5 \cdot CH_2 \cdot CH_2 \cdot COOH$); the compound hydroxy-triiodo-ethyl-cinnamic acid was used at one time as a contrast medium in diagnostic cholecystography. The half-life of the albumin complex of this drug is about 2.5 years. In other instances, hardly any protein-binding occurs as, for example, in the case of the pyrazolone analgesic, antipyrine or the non-depolarizing muscle relaxant, pancuronium. Protein-binding of drugs may be impaired in certain disease states; thus, for example, the binding of phenytoin and other acidic drugs to plasma albumin is decreased in uraemia.

Protein-binding and Volatile Anaesthetics

Volatile anaesthetics have a greater solubility in plasma and whole blood than can be accounted for by their lipid or water solubility alone. This has directed attention to possible interactions with circulating proteins such as albumin and haemoglobin. Binding to fixed protein or other macromolecular components of tissue cells may also play an important role in the mechanisms of anaesthesia at a molecular level. Experimental work on the association of volatile anaesthetics with various protein molecules including haemoglobin and myoglobin has shown that this interaction occurs without the anaesthetic undergoing any chemical change and that under physiological conditions, ionic or covalent bonds are not involved. Available evidence points to this being a triple association involving anaesthetic, water and protein

molecules. These appear to be held together by the concerted effects of hydrogen bonding, hydrophobic bonding and Van der Waals forces, though the precise details of the binding mechanism have not been worked out yet.

Kinetics of Binding

The interaction of a drug D with the unoccupied binding sites of a protein P can be considered as a reversible reaction obeying the law of mass action:

$$[D] + [P] \underset{k_2}{\overset{k_1}{\rightleftharpoons}} [DP]$$

$$\text{drug} \qquad \text{protein} \qquad \text{drug-protein} \atop \text{complex}$$

where k_1 and k_2 are the rates of forward and reverse reactions respectively and DP is the drug-protein complex.

At equilibrium, the forward and reverse reactions are equal and

$$\frac{[D].[P]}{[DP]} = K_D \tag{1}$$

where K_D equals the dissociation constant.

If the drug is able to combine with a certain number of binding sites, n, on each protein molecule, the total number of these sites equals $n[P_T]$ where $[P_T]$ equals the total concentration of protein.

It follows that $n[P_T] = [P] + [DP]$

$$\therefore \quad \frac{[D]\{n[P_T] - [DP]\}}{[DP]} = K_D$$

$$[D].n[P_T] - [D].[P] = K_D.[DP]$$

and

$$\frac{[DP]}{n[P_T]} = \frac{[D]}{[D] + K_D} \tag{2}$$

If F equals the fraction, ratio of bound drug to total

number of drug molecules, then by definition

$$F = \frac{[DP]}{[DP] + [D]} = \frac{1}{1 + \dfrac{[D]}{[DP]}}$$

However, it has been shown above that

$$[DP] = \frac{n[P_T] \cdot [D]}{[D] + K_D}$$

$$\therefore \quad F = \frac{1}{1 + \dfrac{K_D}{n[P_T]} + \dfrac{[D]}{n[P_T]}} = \frac{[P_T]}{[P_T] + \dfrac{K_D}{n} + \dfrac{[D]}{n}} \quad (3)$$

From this equation, it is evident that since in plasma, P_T is fixed, and n and K_D are determined by the particular drug under consideration, the fraction of bound drug becomes inversely related to the concentration of drug $[D]$, the terms $K_D/n[P_T]$ and $n[P_T]$ being invariant. At sufficiently high concentrations, all drugs saturate the binding sites; if the concentration is increased further, additional drug is free, and F decreases toward zero. Although at such concentration levels the maximum amount of drug is bound, this still represents only a very small fraction of total drug. As the drug concentration $[D]$ declines, for example through processes of elimination from the body, F tends to increase. If the binding affinity is very high (K_D very low) and provided the number of binding sites is high enough, practically all the drug present will be bound and F approaches unity.

Structural Requirements for Binding

There appears to be no correlation between chemical structure and the extent and stability of binding to plasma protein such as albumin. Binding occurs with a diversity of drugs ranging from single anions and cations to complex aromatic and heterocyclic compounds. It also occurs with hydrophilic as well as lipid-solule substances. Increase in lipid solubility, however, is associated with increase in degree of protein binding, and this suggests that hydrophobic forces may be of importance. Thus, thiopentone is more lipid soluble than its oxygen analogue pentobarbitone and is also more highly bound to plasma albumin (*see* Table 45.1). Thiopentone binding to plasma albumin displays characteristics of concentration dependence and may range from a fraction of 0.97 at a drug concentration of 0.2 μg/ml to 0.60 at 150 μg/ml (Morgan et al., 1981a).

The lowered polarity resulting from ethyl and allyl quaternarization of the nitrogen atoms in the molecules of gallamine and alcuronium may account for the higher binding affinity of these muscle relaxants for plasma albumin as compared with *d*-tubocurarine. The latter compound binds preferentially to globulin and this behaviour has been ascribed to greater hydrophilic nature associated with presence in the molecule of *d*-tubocurarine of two free phenolic hydroxyl groups.

Significance of Binding

Except for the very small fraction of drug bound to specific receptors in the tissues, protein-bound drug molecules are pharmacologically inert and are hindered from gaining access to the sites of metabolism and excretion. Yet, binding to protein is not as disadvantageous as it might seem at first sight. Provision of a 'reservoir' from which free drug is liberated slowly prolongs biological activity and tends to prevent the wide fluctuations in plasma concentration of unbound drug which might otherwise occur. The reversibility of the drug-plasma protein interaction may be likened to the stabilizing behaviour of a buffer ystem. Although at true equilibrium, the rate at which DP would be formed (k_1) and the rate at which it is dissociated (k_2) equal one another, this is rarely the situation *in vivo*. The plasma levels of unbound drug tend naturally to decline through occurrence of processes of metabolism and elimination. Because of the ready reversibility of the drug protein complex, there is a continuous dissociation of bound to unbound drug and provided the total amount of bound drug, DP, is sufficient, this buffering effect tends to replenish and maintain the circulating level of unbound drug. If the processes of excretion and metabolic inactivation occur at sufficiently rapid rates at, for example, active transport sites in the kidney or enzymatic sites in hepatic tissue, the concentration of free drug molecules may be lowered locally to infinitesimal levels. As a result, the equilibrium of the plasma protein-drug interaction is shifted to the left with rapid conversion of bound to unbound drug to an extent dependent on the rate constant for dissociation, k_2. This explains why drugs such as penicillins, which are highly bound to plasma protein, may nevertheless be virtually cleared from plasma in a single passage through the kidney.

Drug Displacement from Binding Sites

Analysis of the binding characteristics of various drugs to plasma albumin has shown that whereas, at physiological pH, several binding sites exist for basic compounds, acidic drugs attach to no more than two primary binding sites and often to only one. Where only a single binding site is available as, for example, with sulphonamides, the carrying capacity of plasma is limited to one molar equivalent of its albumin content. This is about 7×10^{-4} M, which at an average molecular weight for sulphonamides of 300, is equivalent to a plasma concentration of drug of about 0.2 g/L. Beyond this concentration, the fraction of unbound drug increases rapidly and it becomes available for diffusion to tissue sites of metabolism and excretion. A maximum plasma concentration of drug may eventually he reached regardless of dosage, because the processes of metabolism and elimination have kept pace with the increased availability of unbound drug. A number of acidic drugs with high affinity for binding may compete for and may displace each other from the same protein binding sites. Thus, for example, phenylbutazone, coumarin anticoagulants, sulphinpyrazole and salicylic acid are all capable of displacing 'long-acting' sulphonamides from plasma albumin. Since these sulphonamides are not rapidly metabolized, the displaced molecules diffuse from the plasma to the tissues where their antibacterial action is continued despite the fact that the total plasma concentration of sulphonamide is decreased. Similar competitive displacement from plasma albumin may increase the effective antibacterial activity of acidic antibiotics such as the semi-synthetic penicillins. Thus a reduction of only 5% in the plasma protein-binding of oxacillin by administration of sulpha-methoxy-pyridazine almost doubles the plasma concentrations of unbound oxacillin in the circulation. Displacement of plasma bound drug by another chemical may have dangerous results, especially where the binding to plasma albumin is extensive and the free drug normally represents only a very small fraction of the total. Thus, the potentiating effect of certain sulphonamides on the hypoglycaemic action of tolbutamide or the increase in anticoagulant efficacy of coumarin and indancdiane compounds by co-administration of clofibrate, phenylbutazone, or tolbutamide can be explained on the basis of this same mechanism. The non-diuretic benzothiadazine derivative, diazoxide, binds firmly to one major site on plasma albumin. As well as being markedly diabetogenic, diazoxide is an effective antihypertensive agent when administered by rapid intravenous injection. It is not metabolized to any significant extent and hence any appreciable displacement from its binding site by other more strongly bound drugs such as, for example, warfarin, could result in sustained and serious hypotension.

Drugs may displace endogenous substances such as bilirubin that are bound to plasma albumin. Premature infants have relatively low levels of albumin and the acidic binding sites are readily saturated with bilirubin. After administration of certain sulphonamides to such infants, bilirubin may be displaced from its albumin complex and the resultant increase in circulating unbound bilirubin may lead to the development of kernicterus. The premature infant is in a particularly vulnerable position, because the glucuronyl transferase system in the liver is not properly developed and hence elimination of bilirubin as its glucuronide is retarded. It follows that neonates should not be given acidic drugs such as sulphonamides, salicylates, phenylbutazone or indomethacin, which are highly bound to albumin and can readily uncouple bilirubin from its binding site. The reverse situation may also occur in that a number of naturally occurring substances may compete with exogenous drugs for the same limited number of protein-binding sites. Thus, for example, fatty acids are transported in plasma bound to albumin. Release of free fatty acids into the blood as a result of physiological stimuli as in major surgery may serve to displace drug bound to albumin. Similarly, impaired protein-binding of acidic drugs in renal disease is due in part to accumulation of endogenous metabolites such as fatty acids strongly bound to plasma albumin.

Few drugs have a primary affinity for plasma globulins, but a number of endogenous hormones including thyroxine and cortisol bind to α-globulins, and d-tubocurarine binds to γ-globulins. It has been suggested that the mechanism of action of certain antirheumatic drugs such as phenylbutazone and indomethacin may be linked to their ability to displace endogenous corticosteroids from their binding to the globulin, transcortin, thereby increasing the tissue concentrations of free corticosteroid. Subsequent work did not support this hypothesis.

Cellular Binding

Non-specific Storage Depots

A number of molecular structures besides the plasma proteins may bind drugs. Many tissues serve as storage depots because drugs combine with cellular constituents and as a result accumulate in higher concentrations than in extracellular fluid. The major part of this tissue binding is 'non-specific' in the sense that it is not involved in the process whereby the drug interacts with a cell component or receptor to evoke a specific pharmacological effect. Such secondary binding is, nevertheless, of considerable importance in providing extensive pools for drug storage in the body. Without these, many drugs would be metabolically inactivated and excreted so quickly that their effects would be too transient to be of therapeutic value. Non-specific binding is generally a reversible process. The stored drug remains in dynamic equilibrium with unbound drug which is then free to diffuse into the circulation and replenish drug eliminated by processes of metabolism and excretion (*see* Fig. 45.4). Some drugs are stored in connective tissue because they are bound to the strongly anionic radicals of mucopolysaccharides. Gallamine has a strong affinity for mucopolysaccharide which is shared by suxamethonium, but not by other muscle relaxants (Fig. 45.5). Bones, teeth and nails may serve as reservoirs for drugs such as heavy metals and tetracyclines. Other drugs such as the antimalarials, mepacrine and chloroquine, have a special affinity for binding to tissue nucleoprotein; in the case of chloroquine, significant amounts have been detected in blood and urine of patients for as long as five years after the last administration of the drug.

By contrast, there are a few drugs which have no significant binding affinities for tissue constituents, and for them body water may serve as a storage reservoir. Thus barbitone and amidopyrine are examples of drugs which remain confined to body water as unbound molecules until they are excreted from the body.

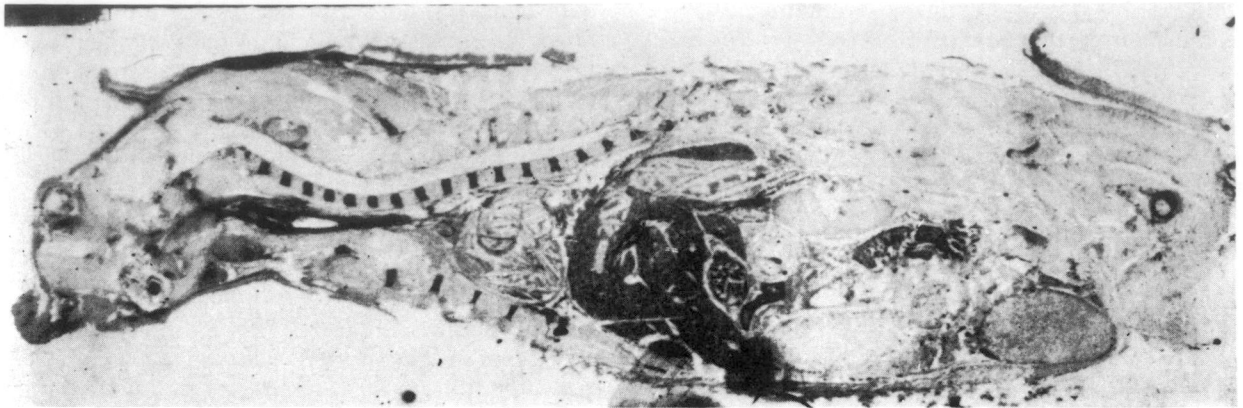

Fig. 45.5 Autoradiograph showing the localization of ^{3}H-gallamine in cartilaginous tissues of the rat in the intervertebral discs, sternal cartilage etc. (*Reproduction by courtesy of Dr S. A. Feldman*)

Adipose Tissue. Drugs with high lipid/plasma partition ratios tend, understandably, to accumulate in adipose tissue. The significance of fat as a storage depot for lipid-soluble drugs is emphasized by the fact that in obesity, fat content may amount to over 35% of the body weight, whilst even in starvation, the level does not fall much below 10%. Body fat behaves as a relatively homogeneous substance attracting lipophilic drugs in quite an indiscriminate manner. Binding is mainly by the close-range intermolecular attraction of Van der Waals forces. A good illustration of the role of lipid storage in determining drug pharmacodynamics is the behaviour of thiobarbituates. At one time, the ultra-short activation of thiopentone was attributed to rapid metabolic inactivation. This view is now known to be incorrect, since the barbiturate is metabolized and excreted slowly. After a single dose, most tissues well supplied with blood, including brain and muscle, rapidly take up considerable amounts of thiopentone in proportion to their bulk and the plasma level falls abruptly; thereafter the tissue levels decline slowly in parallel with plasma level. On the other hand, the level of drug in fat is low at first and then raises rapidly to a peak level of about ten times that in plasma in about 3 h. At this time, about 70% of the drug remaining in the body is localized to adipose tissue. The main clinical implication of this high lipid localization coupled with a slow rate of metabolism is that the duration of anaesthesia after a large dose of thiopentone may be prolonged out of all proportion to the dosage needed for induction of anaesthesia. Although not thiobarbiturates, hexobarbitone and other N-methylated derivatives of barbituric acid are also localized extensively in fat. There are two main reasons for this: first, presence of the N-methyl group at position 3 renders them such weak acids that they are essentially unionized at pH 7.4; second, the methyl group also increases lipid solubility by eliminating the hydrogen bonding between the adjacent nitrogen and oxygen atoms at positions 3 and 4 of the barbiturate ring. The compound N-methyl thiopentone is both a thiobarbiturate *and* possesses a methyl substituent at position 3. It is characterized by a very high degree of lipid solubility coupled with a relatively slow rate of metabolism.

Further examples of lipid-soluble drugs which accumulate preferentially in body fat are α-receptor blocking drugs, phenoxybenzamine and dibenamine.

Specific Tissue Binding
Concept of Drug Receptors. It is self-evident that any drug must achieve adequate concentrations at its site of action if it is to produce its desired effects. Although obviously a function of the amount given, the amount ultimately reaching the site of action is necessarily dependent on the relative avidities of other processes such as non-specific binding, metabolism and excretion, which are all competing for disposal of the active form of the drug (*see* Fig. 45.1). Most drugs display a degree of specificity of action and correlation of pharmacological activity with chemical structure which leads to the presumption that the biological response is the consequence of an interaction with a specific tissue element called the *drug receptor*. The theory that drugs produce their effects through discrete cellular sites had its origins in the pioneer work of Ehrlich and Langley in the late nineteenth century. However, identification and characterization of drug receptors has proved extremely difficult. With the vast majority of drugs, the nature of the receptor is still unknown and has to be discussed in the abstract. Although this vagueness is but a reflection of ignorance, the *concept* of the receptor has, nevertheless, proved most valuable, since it has allowed the application of thermodynamic principles in seeking to explain the fundamental action of drugs at a molecular level. Such theoretical analyses of the mechanisms of drug-receptor interaction have been undertaken by many pharmocologists following on the classical studies of

Clark (1926). A useful discussion of the various experimental approaches that have been used in studying drug-receptor interaction is to be found in Lamble (1981).

A receptor can be considered as the functional component of a cell with which a drug combines reversibly to initiate a response. There has been considerable lack of agreement between biochemists, physiologists and pharmacologists as to what exactly is meant by the term 'receptor'. In the present state of knowledge, it seems best to avoid the confusion of semantic arguments and equate 'drug receptor' with 'site of action'. Two of the most important mediators of molecular specificity in biological systems—enzymes and antibodies—are proteins, and it has, therefore, been reasonable to assume that the receptor, too, is a specialized section of a protein or related macromolecule. When a specific macromolecule affected by a drug 'does something' which is readily measurable, attempts to isolate and purify the receptor substance may be fruitful. Thus, for example, the elucidation of the molecular mechanisms of action of drugs which inhibit specific enzymes, e.g. anticholinesterases or folic acid reductase inhibitors (*see below*), has been possible because the sophisticated techniques of enzymology could be utilized and readily applied. However, when it comes to investigating possible receptor proteins without enzymic or other readily measured activity, the problem is much more difficult, the approaches become indirect and results often highly speculative.

If a working hypothesis is accepted that a receptor is part of a protein molecule, drug-receptor interaction can be looked upon as a special case of reversible protein-binding involving the combined operation of the various binding forces considered above (p. 534). The essential difference between this type of binding and non-specific binding is that only drug-receptor interaction is followed by the drug response.

The secondary and tertiary structures of protein are unstable systems held together by interaction of a considerable number of these same relatively weak binding forces. The structure of the whole depends on the structural integrity of the constituent subunits. When a foreign molecule interacts with part of the chemical grouping of a cellular macromolecule, the development of new forces at the binding site or sites may lead to a general alteration in tertiary structure and influence the stability of the protein as a whole. Many of the ideas on mechanisms of drug-receptor interaction have developed directly from knowledge of substrate-enzyme combination. Thus, the receptor for drug molecules may be looked upon as analogous to the active site or centre of an enzyme. Since changes in enzyme conformation have been shown to accompany formation of enzyme-substrate complexes, it may be inferred that similar conformational changes occur secondary to drug-receptor interaction. One important difference lies in the consequences. In the case of the enzyme, the induced structural change in the

protein leads to a change in the substrate. In the case of the receptor, molecular disturbances occur in the matrix of the protein of which the receptor is a constituent part; these changes of conformation then initiate a chain of biochemical and physiological events which characterize the pharmacological response to the drug.

Consequences of Drug-receptor Interaction

The major part of an administered dose of drug is either directed to non-specific binding sites, metabolized or excreted, without ever reaching the selected receptor. Interaction of the minute fraction of drug which does combine with its receptor can manifest itself in a number of ways.

Drugs which combine with the receptor and generate a response are called *agonists*. They must possess two important properties. First, they just have *affinity* for the receptor and second, *intrinsic activity* or *efficacy*, the power to initiate the subsequent response.

The quantitative analyses of drug-receptor interaction developed by Clark (1926) and Gaddum (1937) have emphasized that pharmacological response is proportional to the number of receptors occupied (*occupation theory of drug action*). Paton (1961) suggested a different interpretation based on the proposal that the response to a drug is not a function of the number of receptors occupied, but of the rate of drug-receptor combination (*rate theory of drug action*). These two theories may not be mutually exclusive and it is conceivable that the occupation theory may be valid for certain receptors, whilst the rate theory is valid for others.

Agonists that produce a smaller maximal effect than other agonists with the same receptor are said to have intermediate efficacy and are called *partial agonists*. If a partial agonist and full agonist act on the same receptor simultaneously, the effects may be additive or the partial agonist may competitively antagonize the full agonist, depending on the relative concentrations of the two drugs. In certain situations, a substance may react with the same receptor as a 'full agonist' but, because it lacks intrinsic activity, its action becomes that of a *competitive antagonist*.

Kinetics of Drug-receptor Interaction

The reaction between a drug and its receptor is a reversible process governed by the law of mass action. It can be expressed mathematically in a manner analogous to the reaction of non-specific protein-binding considered on p. 535. Thus, if an agonist D reacts with a receptor R:

$$[D] + [R] \underset{k_2}{\overset{k_1}{\rightleftharpoons}} [DR] \qquad (4)$$

Drug   Receptor   Drug-receptor complex

However, unlike non-specific binding, drug receptor interaction is characterized by a second event in which the drug-receptor complex acts further to evoke a pharmacological effect, Q_D. The complex mechanisms involved in this second event are largely obscure at the present time. The reasonable assumption may, however, be made that during this phase of response the receptor reappears, otherwise drug action would imply destruction of the receptor, which is in general known not to be the case. The complete scheme of events may be described as follows:

$$[D] + [R] \underset{k_2}{\overset{k_1}{\rightleftharpoons}} [DR] \overset{k_3}{\to} Q_D + [R]$$

where k_1, k_2 and k_3 = the rate constants for each partial reaction.

At equilibrium $\quad K_D = \dfrac{k_2}{k_1} = \dfrac{[D][R]}{[DR]} \qquad (5)$

(cf. equation 1, p. 535), where K_D = the dissociation constant of the drug-receptor complex.

If the total receptor concentration equals $[R_T]$, it follows that $[R_T] = [R] + [DR]$. On substituting in the above equations, we obtain:

$$K_D = \frac{[D]\{[R_T] - [DR]\}}{[DR]} \text{ or } \frac{[DR]}{[R_T]} = \frac{[D]}{K_D + [D]} \quad (6)$$

Now, $Q_D = k_3[DR]$, indicating that the response is proportional to the concentration of DR.

If $Q_{\max}$ equals the maximal response which the system is capable of, then, $Q_{\max} = k_3[R_T]$.

$$\frac{Q_D}{Q_{\max}} = \frac{[DR]}{[R_T]} = \frac{[D]}{K_D + [D]} \qquad (7a)$$

$$Q_D = \frac{Q_{\max} \cdot [D]}{K_D + [D]} = \frac{Q_{\max}}{\dfrac{K_D}{[D]} + 1} \qquad (7b)$$

The derivation of these last equations is identical to that of the well-known *Michaelis-Menten equation* which expresses the velocity V of an enzyme reaction as a function of the concentration of substrate, S, the enzyme-substrate dissociation constant, K_s and the maximal velocity when the enzyme is saturated with substrate, $V_{\max}$:

$$v = \frac{V_{\max}}{\dfrac{K_s}{S} + 1} \qquad (8)$$

When $v = V_{\max}/2$, S is equal to K_s. The value of S which is experimentally found to give half the maximum velocity is written as Km, *the Michaelis constant*, so that under these conditions $Km = K_s$. With the drug-receptor interaction, the parallel situation arises when $Q_D = Q_{\max}/2$, whereupon $[D]$ becomes equal to K_D.

If the phamacological activity of a drug is assumed to be proportional to the magnitude of the response, Q_D, then the ratio $Q_D/Q_{\max}$ of equation (7a) will be a constant for each particular drug. This ratio of

maximum effect is given the symbol α^E, and expresses the *efficacy* or *intrinsic activity*. α^E is usually expressed as a constant relative to a standard drug which evokes maximum effect in the particular biological system under consideration. The reciprocal of the dissociation constant, K_D, gives a measure of the *affinity* of a drug for its receptor. It may conveniently be expressed as pK_D, by analogy with pH, where $pK_D = -\log_{10} K_D$; thus the higher the value of pK_D, the greater the affinity of a drug.

Equation (7b) may be transformed to its reciprocal form just as Lineweaver and Burk transformed the Michaelis-Menten equation.

$$\frac{1}{Q_D} = \frac{K_D}{Q_{\max}} \cdot \frac{1}{[D]} + \frac{1}{Q_{\max}} \qquad (9)$$

The advantage of this manoeuvre is that when the variables $1/Q_D$ and $1/[D]$ are plotted against one another, a straight line is obtained whose slope equals $K_D/Q_{\max}$, whilst the intercept of the $1/[D]$ axis, i.e. when $1/Q_D = 0$, equals $-1/K_D$ and thus gives a direct measure of affinity. This double-reciprocal plot has been widely applied to the analysis of the kinetics of enzyme inhibition; it has also provided considerable theoretical insight into the mechanisms of drug antagonism.

Chemical Identity of Receptors. The best way to gain information about the chemical nature of a receptor would be to identify and isolate it. Unfortunately, this direct approach is beset with pitfalls and difficulties, but considerable progress has been made in recent years in this direction. The study of structure-activity relationship (SAR) has offered a most valuable way of gaining indirect data on receptor structure. This approach is based on the fundamental premise that the interaction of an agonist molecule with its receptor involves the mutual attraction of chemically reactive groups which are spatially orientated in a pattern complimentary to one another. Many of the inferences regarding the chemical structure of receptors have been drawn from SAR studies undertaken particularly amongst autonomic neurotransmitters and narcotic analgesics.

Study of SAR data on members of the polymethylene bis-methonium compounds has indicated that the receptors for the cholinergic transmitter at autonomic ganglia and the skeletal neuromuscular junction have different structures. The prototype structure for this series is a symmetrical molecule containing two cationic groups separated by a simple aliphatic chain:

$$_3(CH_3)N^+ - (CH_2)_n - N^+(CH_3)_3$$

When the biological activity of derivatives with differing chain length was investigated, the ganglionic site was found to interact most strongly with C_5 (pentamethonium) or C_6 (hexamethonium) compounds. These drugs cause ganglion blockade by preventing the receptor from responding to acetylcholine. On the other hand, compounds with longer chain length such as C_{10} (decamethonium) and succinylcholine show great selectivity for the neuromuscular end plate, suggesting that the anionic sites on the latter receptor are spaced further apart.

On the basis of detailed SAR studies of sympathomimetic drugs, it appears that the grouping

$$C_6H_5-\overset{|}{\underset{|}{C}}-\overset{|}{\underset{|}{C}}-N\diagdown$$

is the one that fits the essential sites of attachment of the adrenergic or adrenoceptor receptor. A model can be constructed which defines the relationship between catecholamine structure and the hypothetical α and β sites of a single adrenergic or 'adrenoceptive' receptor. Three essential chemical features appear to be: (1) a flat surface to which the benzene ring can be closely applied; (2) a cationic site where ion pairing can occur; (3) a chelation site which may involve a metallic ion like Mg^{2+} in the formation of hydrophobic bonding with aqueous layers in the vicinity of the receptor surface. These are depicted diagrammatically in Fig. 45.6. Substitution on the N atom especially of bulky

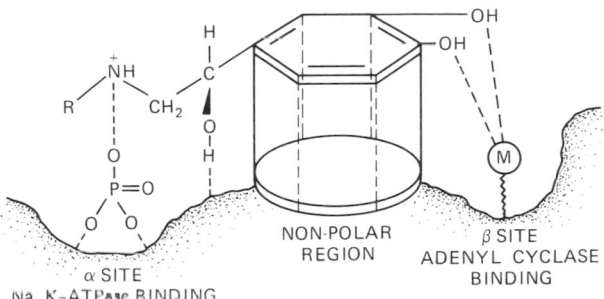

NON-POLAR REGION

β SITE ADENYL CYCLASE BINDING

α SITE Na, K-ATPase BINDING

Fig. 45.6 Diagram of a catecholamine and the concept of its fit with a receptor model containing an α site which forms an ionic bond and a β site at which chelation with a metal, M (possibly magnesium), occurs. At the α site, binding may occur to membrane-bound ATPase with catalysis of ATP hydrolysis: the β site is located on the enzyme adenylcyclase and thus binding involves formation of cyclic AMP.

alkyl groups like isopropyl (as in isoprenaline or propranolol) increases the affinity of a compound for the β site, probably by steric hindrance of the ion-pairing necessary for α site attachment. The phenolic-OH groups attached to the benzene nucleus contribute to intrinsic activity at the β site. The alcoholic-OH at the β carbon atom on the side-chain appears to serve mainly to strengthen attachment to the α site of the receptor (i.e. causing an increase in affinity); its presence gives rise to an asymmetrical carbon in the molecule and optically active stereoisomers. For both agonists and antagonists pharmacological activity is much greater in the (−)isomer.

SAR amongst stereoisomers has been particularly valuable in allowing certain inferences to be drawn

about the three-dimensional structure of receptor surfaces. This has been done extensively with narcotic analgesics and has allowed the construction of a model of a hypothetical receptor surface for morphine and its congeners. In this case only the D (−)-isomers can fit the surface features of the receptor and in both the natural and synthetic compounds, only D (−)-molecules have analgesic activity.

Although construction of models of receptor structure is a highly speculative undertaking, it has the particular merit of seeking to explain the molecular action of drugs in physicochemical terms. Thus, for example, the benzodiazepine receptor in the central nervous system has been purified, its cDNA has been cloned and functional receptors have been expressed in oocyte preparations (Schofield et al., 1987). This receptor emerges as a macromolecular complex which includes a binding site for the inhibitory neurotransmitter GABA; the receptor also includes recognition sites for barbiturates and even ethanol. Further work in this direction should not only provide an answer to the fundamental problem of how drug interaction with the cell receptor is translated into pharmacological response, but should make it feasible to design new drugs with even greater specificity of action.

Recent studies have confirmed that most synapses within the central nervous system employ excitatory amino-acids (EAA) as their neurotransmitters. At least four different receptor types have been defined besides the N-methyl-D-aspartate (NMDA) receptor (Fagg et al., 1986). Excitatory transmission appears to involve actions mediated by one or more combinations of actions at these receptors (Monaghan et al., 1989) [see also Chapter 53].

Enzyme Receptor Sites. A number of drugs appear to act through known specific enzymatic mechanisms. The mechanism of action may involve direct inhibition of an enzyme. Alternatively, the ininhibition may be indirect; if the drug has close chemical similarities with the normal substrate, it may serve as a substrate substitute for the enzyme and thereby block a key reaction in a vital metabolic sequence. In either event, the subunit of the enzyme macromolecule which contains the functional three-dimensional region for binding the specific substrate, i.e. the active or catalytic centre, may be regarded as the drug receptor. An important difference between binding of drugs to receptor sites of macromolecules in general and the active sites of enzymes in particular is that, in the former case, initiation of the pharmacological response does not usually involve making or breaking of covalent bonds in the agonist, whereas this can readily occur in reactions of enzymatic catalysts.

Inhibition of Cholinesterase. Anticholinesterases are classic examples of drugs whose pharmacological effects are mediated by inhibition of a specific enzyme. There are two types of mammalian cholinesterase with different specificities and affinities for both substrates and inhibitors. These are true or acetylcholinesterase (AChE) and pseudo or butyryl cholinesterase (BuChE); the latter enzyme is considered in detail below. The clinical effects of anticholinesterase drugs are almost entirely due to inhibition of AChE whose physiological substrate is acetylcholine.

Acetylcholine has in its molecule only two functional groups, an ester and quaternary ammonium group, which it can offer for attachment to an enzyme receptor site. The active centre of cholinesterase is believed to consist of two sites approximately 7 Å apart, an *anionic site* that forms an ionic bond with the cationic 'onium' head of acetylcholine and an *esteratic site* at which the ester bond is actually split (Fig. 45.7).

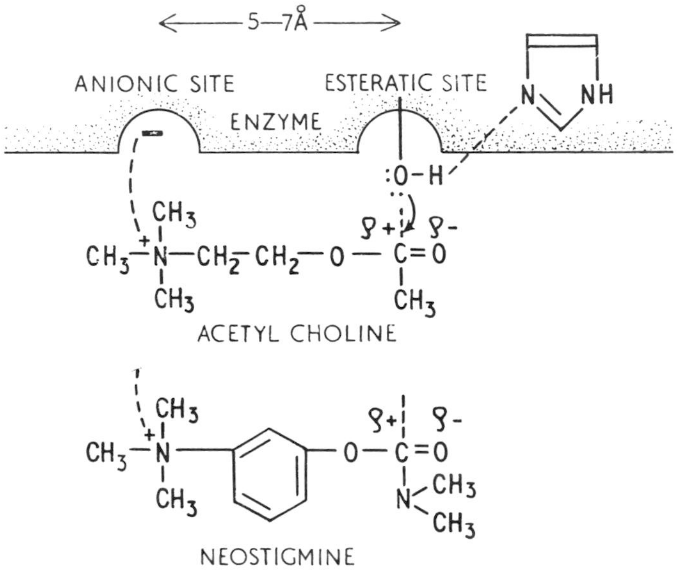

ACETYL CHOLINE

NEOSTIGMINE

Fig. 45.7 Substrate and inhibitor interactions with the active centre of AChE. :O—H represents the essential electron-rich group at the esteratic site which makes a nucleophilic attack on the substrate by donating electrons to the electrophilic $\diagdown$C = O radical of the ester. The nucleophilic group to the enzyme is made more nucleophilic by formation of H-bonding with the imidazole N atom of a neighbouring histidine residue. Attachment of the carbon atom to the serine oxygen leads to formation of the acyl-enzyme complex (acetylated enzyme, if the substrate is acetyl choline).

The anionic site is composed of ionized carboxyl groups whose main function is to anchor the cationic head of the substrate and keep it there for the few microseconds needed for hydrolysis to occur. The esteratic site represents an electron-rich centre which includes an essential serine residue. The initial interaction at the esteratic site is thought to be electron donation to the electrophilic carboxyl C atom. This carbon is then linked to a serine OH group and choline is split off, leaving an acetylated esteratic site. The acetylated enzyme has only a very transient existence and is rapidly hydrolysed in about 100 μs to

yield acetic acid and the regenerated free enzyme. This may be represented as follows:

$$\textcircled{E}\text{-H} + S \underset{k_{-1}}{\overset{k_1}{\rightleftharpoons}} [\textcircled{E}\text{-H}\ldots S] \overset{k_2}{\rightarrow} \textcircled{E}\text{-acyl} + \text{choline}$$

$$\downarrow k_3$$

$$\textcircled{E}\text{-H} + \text{acetic acid}$$

where $\textcircled{E}$-H represents AChE and S equals substrate, acetylcholine in this case; $\textcircled{E}$-acyl is the unstable acylated enzyme which rapidly decomposes to regenerate the original enzyme.

Anticholinesterases may compete with acetylcholine for the active sites of the enzyme and interfere with hydrolysis of the natural substrate. They may do this in two ways:

(a) *Rapidly reversible inhibitions* by combining only with the anionic site, e.g. edrophonium, which is a *bis*-quaternary ammonium compound not containing an ester radical.

(b) *Acylation*, namely formation of an acylated enzyme which is considerably more stable than the acetylated enzyme formed by reaction with acetylcholine. Anticholinesterases acting via an acylation mechanism are the carbamates and organophosphates. The carbamates, e.g. the quaternary amine, neostigmine, form a carbamylated AChE which reacts with water at less than one-millionth the rate of the corresponding acetylated form (*see* Fig. 45.7). The organophosphates react at the esteratic site to form a phosphorylated AChE which is extremely stable. If the alkyl groups attached to the organophosphates are — CH_3 or — C_2H_5, significant regeneration of the enzyme occurs spontaneously in several hours. With isopropyl groups as in DFP, however, the phosphoryl-enzyme bond undergoes negligible spontaneous hydrolysis; recovery of AChE activity depends on synthesis of new enzyme protein, a process that may take months. Reactivation of the phosphorylated enzyme can be achieved much more rapidly by employing certain nucleophilic agents such as hydroxylamine (Fig. 45.8). Unfortunately, high doses of hydroxylamine are needed and these are not tolerated *in vivo*. It was reasoned that if a hydroxylamine derivative could be synthesized, which also possessed a cationic head that would fit simultaneously into the anionic site of the enzyme (i.e. at a distance of approximately 7 Å from the N-OH radical, reactivation potency might be enhanced further. A number of quaternary pyridine aldoximes, such as pralidoxime and TMB-4, fulfil this requirement and are rapid and less toxic reactivators.

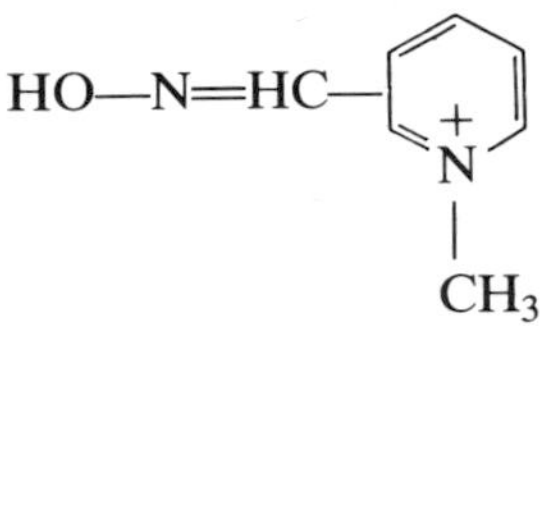

$HO-N=HC-$ pralidoxime

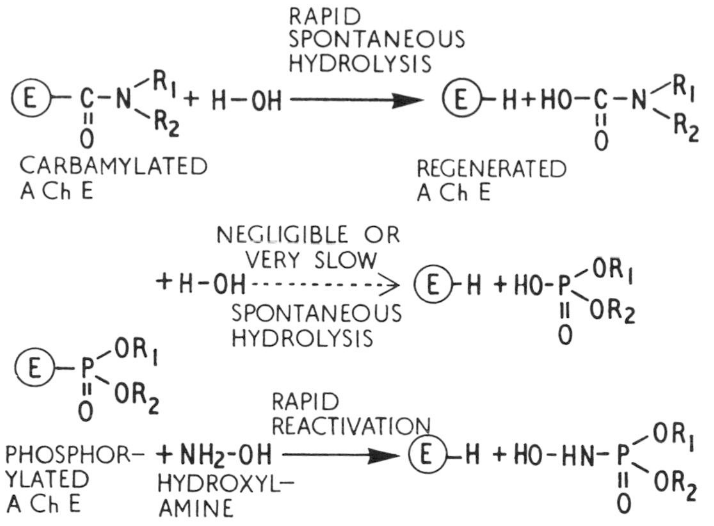

Fig. 45.8 Spontaneous and stimulated reactivation of carbamylated (a) and phosphorylated (b) forms of AChE. The native enzyme is represented as E—H.

They are of considerable value as antidotes in the treatment of poisoning by organophosphate insecticides.

Evidence gleaned from a number of experimental approaches including thermodynamic studies and investigation of structure-activity relationships, raises the possibility that, rather than there being different cholinergic receptors, the active centre of AChE may represent the fundamental cholinergic or cholinoceptive receptor. It is conceivable, though not proven, that the so-called muscarinic and nicotinic 'receptors' may merely represent altered conformations of the same enzyme protein being a standard active centre as receptor site for the neurotransmitter.

Inhibition of Other Enzymes. Examples of other drugs whose pharmacological activity is a direct expression of enzyme inhibition include inhibitors of carbonic anhydrase (e.g. acetazolamide); of xanthine oxidase (e.g. allopurinol); of aldehyde oxidase (e.g. disulfiram and of angiotensin converting enzyme (e.g. captopril).

Antimetabolites. The antibacterial sulphonamides are representative of a class of drugs which exert their biological effects by acting as antimetabolites. There is a close chemical similarity between sulphonamides and p-aminobenzoic acid (PABA), an essential growth factor and biosynthetic intermediate in the metabolism of many bacteria. PABA is normally condensed enzymatically with a glutamylpteridine compound to form dihydropteroic acid, a precursor of folic acid. Sulphonamides, because of their close structural likeness to PABA can also act as substrate for the condensing enzyme and thereby inhibit competitively the normal entry of PABA into the folic acid pathway.

The ultimate consequence is bacterial folic acid deficiency manifested as a reversible inhibition of bacterial growth.

Antimetabolites have also been developed for use in cancer chemotherapy. Some of these act by the mechanism of counterfeit incorporation into biosynthetic pathways. The pyrimidine antagonist, 5-flurouracil, differs from uracil merely by substitution of F for H at position 5 in the ring. Fluorouracil is handled metabolically like uracil forming a riboside and riboside phosphate.

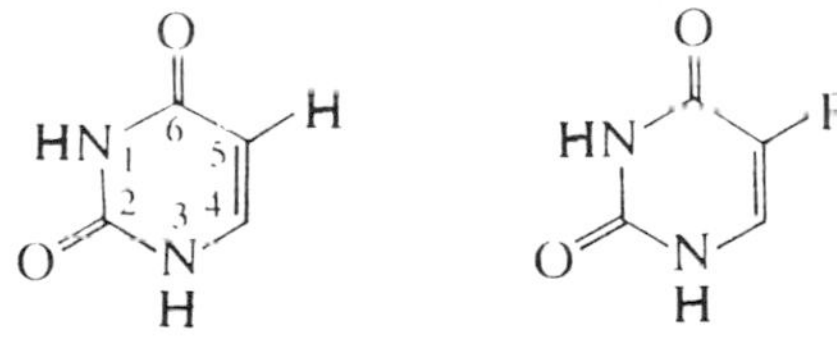

uracil   5-fluorouracil

The enzyme thymidine synthetase which normally methylates uracil to thymidine is inhibited. In addition, fluorouracil is converted to the corresponding nucleoside triphosphate and then incorporated into messenger-RNA in place of uracil (Diasio and Harris, 1989). Miscoding may result through misinterpretation of codons containing fluorouracil during the assembly of amino acids into polypeptide chains.

Drug Action not Mediated by Receptor Interaction

The pharmacological effects of a variety of drugs do not appear to involve attachment to receptors possessing a high degree of structural specificity. Substances as unrelated chemically as diethyl ether, nitrous oxide, halothane or xenon all produce very similar effects of depression of the central nervous system. As a group, the volatile anaesthetics are remarkable for the lack of any obvious correlation between chemical structure and pharmacological activity. The term 'chemically inert' which has frequently been applied to this class of drugs is somewhat misleading. First, there is now good evidence that many of these compounds undergo significant metabolism in the body (Chapter 56, p. 649).

Second, under certain conditions, hydrophobic associations may develop with other substances including water as in clathrate formation or bonding to tissue or circulating macromolecules. However, because the volatile anaesthetics do not enter into a reaction of distinct chemical specificity with the organism, most approaches aimed at defining the molecular environment in which these drugs act have focused attention on correlations between potency and certain physical properties. Many such correlations have been noted as for example with vapour pressure, polarizability, molecular size and shape of free energy of drug-membrane adsorption. Detailed discussion of the cellular and subcellular mechanisms involved in the action of general anaesthetics is given in Chapter 27.

Excretion of Drugs

The unbound diffusible fraction of a drug may be eliminated from the body either unchanged or in forms modified by metabolism or as a mixture of both native drug and biotransformed products. The basic mechanisms operating in excretion are applicable to both the unaltered or metabolized molecule.

Drugs may be excreted through the lung, kidneys, biliary system, intestine, salivary and sweat glands. By far the major route for most drugs is the kidney, with the exception of the inhalation anaesthetics which are eliminated predominantly via the lungs.

Renal Excretion
(Lant, 1979; Brater and Chennavasin, 1984)

Excretion of drugs by the kidney involves the triple processes of glomerular filtration (passive), proximal tubular secretion (active), tubular diffusion (passive).

Plasma is filtered at the glomerular capillaries whose porous membranes permit the passage of most solutes. Unbound drug diffuses into the glomerulus in an amount proportional to the transfer of plasma water and hence filtration does not disturb the plasma equilibrium between bound and unbound drug. Meaningful values for clearance of drug from the plasma are only obtainable if the degree of protein-binding is known at the relevant drug concentration. Factors such as hypertension or dehydration which reduce glomerular filtration rate (GFR) reduce the filtered load, whilst correction of such abnormalities or infusion of mannitol may increase GFR and filtered load. The plasma ultrafiltrate then flows down the nephron, the subsequent fate of filtered drug molecules depending on their physicochemical properties. The lining of the tubules consists of a continuum of closely-packed epithelial cells with characteristics similar to other biomembranes. The principles which govern passage of drug back from the filtrate across the tubular epithelium are the familiar ones relating to transfer of solute across other lipid boundaries. Polar compounds including ions are not lipid-soluble and do not diffuse back, unless they are of small enough size to traverse the pores or are undergoing reabsorption by a carrier-mediated transport system. Drugs with high lipid/water partition coefficients will undergo ready tubular reabsorption.

Active Secretion in the Proximal Tubule. The tubular epithelium closely resembles that in the biliary tract and choroid plexus in having a dual character with regard to transfer of drugs. It functions as a lipid boundary in permitting ready passage of unionized lipid-soluble molecules and, in addition, also possesses two carrier-mediated mechanisms for transporting many organic acids and bases from plasma to urine. Unlike glomerular filtration, both the protein bound and free drug forms are available for active tubular secretion. As free drug is removed by the tubular cells, there is rapid dissociation of the drug-protein complex to maintain the equilibrium with plasma water. Very strong protein-binding may, however, limit the rate of tubular secretion because uptake of drug by the cells, the first step of active transport, is dependent on the initial content of free drug in plasma water.

Results of competitive experiments have shown that the secretory pathways for organic acids and bases are quite separate. Although the characteristics of secretion by both pathways fulfil the criteria for active transport, neither mechanism is as selective as those for naturally occurring substances. The tubules are able to secrete a large number of acids and bases of diverse chemical structure, molecular size and ionic strength. The acid-secreting mechanism transports the ionized forms of a variety of acidic drugs ranging from sulphonic acids to amino acid conjugates, ester and ether glucuronides, ethereal sulphate, acetylated sulphonamides, benzothiadiazines, heterocyclic carboxylic acids such as the penicillins and cephalosporins, aliphatic organic acids such as acylglycine and oxalic acid, and enolic compounds such as phenylbutazone. The competition displayed between these various anionic compounds for the secretory mechanisms has been taken advantage of in the clinical use of probenecid (Dixey et al., 1988). Probenecid also blocks the rapid renal secretion of penicillin and prolongs the duration of action of the antibiotic. This is of particular value in septicaemic infections and also where use of a particularly expensive derivative, such as carbenicillin, is indicated and dosage can be thereby kept to a minimum without decreasing clinical efficacy.

Secreted organic bases vary from the weakly basic

primary (e.g. histamine), secondary (e.g. mecamylamine) and tertiary (e.g. N-methyl nicotinamide) amines to the highly ionized quaternary ammonium compounds such as choline and hexamethonium.

An interesting parallel can be drawn between the non-specific functions of the renal secretory mechanisms which handle organic acids and bases and the microsomal enzyme systems which metabolize drugs in the liver. In discussing the evolutionary significance of the hepatic enzyme system, which functions essentially to convert non-polar to polar substances, Brodie and Hogben (1957) speculated that this development was necessary for the 'emancipation of life from the sea'. It is conceivable that the proximal tubule system has evolved in an attempt to enhance the elimination of polar and non-polar compounds and thereby keep the plasma content of potential toxins at lower levels than would otherwise obtain by glomerular filtration alone.

Diffusion and pH-dependent Excretion. In addition to the non-specific transport systems considered above, elimination of drugs occurs also by passive diffusion across the tubular epithelium. Drugs which are water soluble and of moderate molecular size as, for example, the polymeric carbohydrate, inulin (MW 5500) or cyanocobalamin (MW 1355) do not diffuse across the tubular cells. Such substances are filtered at the glomerulus and are neither reabsorbed nor secreted by the tubules. They can, therefore, be used for measuring GFR. Other water-soluble compounds of small molecular size such as urea may diffuse readily across the tubular epithelium. The clearance of such substances is less than the glomerular filtration rate, is unaffected by pH, but is sensitive to changes in urine flow. Thus renal clearance is increased when high flow rates are induced with an osmotic diuretic like mannitol, for with high urinary flow rate, there is insufficient time for significant back-diffusion to occur. Processes of diffusion are potentially bidirectional, but as water is progressively abstracted from the tubular fluid on its passage down the nephron, intraluminal concentrations of dissolved drug increase and back-diffusion occurs.

The majority of non-volatile drugs are weak electrolytes and the relative proportions of unionized and ionized components on either side of the tubular epithelium will conform to the tenets of the pH-partition hypothesis and, therefore, depend on pH and pK_a as shown by the Henderson–Hasselbalch equation. Weak acids tend to be excreted more rapidly in alkaline urine, weak bases in acid urine. Variations in drug clearance with altered primary urinary pH, which are achieved in practice, are usually lower than the theoretical maxima for a number of reasons. These include the following factors: the tubular epithelium does not usually display an absolute impermeability to the ionized forms of weak acids or bases; when urine flow rate is high, there may be incomplete equilibration in the time available; back-diffusion in

the distal nephron may be restricted on account of the relatively low rate of blood flow in the renal medulla.

Although atypical in a number of respects, output of ammonia by the kidney is probably one of the most important examples of pH-dependent excretion. In this instance, the main direction of diffusion is from its site of production in the tubular cells into the lumen. Diffusion of ammonia into highly acid urine and its combination with secreted H^+ to form NH_4^+ constitutes a major mechanism for eliminating the acid products of metabolism and thereby maintaining acid-base homeostasis. In general, excretion of acidic or basic drugs is pH-dependent if the unionized fraction is lipid soluble and if the pK_a is within the range of 3.0–7.5 for weak acids and 7.5–10.5 for weak bases (*see* Fig. 45.2). This, therefore, includes the weak acids, salicyclic, phenobarbitone, nitrofurantoin, certain sulphonamides, nalidixic acid and phenylbutazone; the weak bases, mepacrine, procaine, amphetamine, pethidine, imipramine and amitriptyline.

The phenomenon of pH-dependent excretion has found an important application in the clinical management of acute poisoning. Appropriate manipulation of urinary pH may expedite the elimination of a drug present in the plasma in toxic concentrations. Rapid alkalinization of the urine by intravenous administration of sodium bicarbonate or lactate has been found useful in treating aspirin (pK_a 3.5) and phenobarbitone (pK_a 7.2) over-dosage (Fig. 45.9). Most other barbiturates have higher pK_a values and their urinary excretion is virtually unaffected by changes in urinary pH. Rapid acidification of the urine is more difficult to attain in practice. There is a slow drop in urinary pH after oral administration of ammonium chloride, and intravenous use of this salt

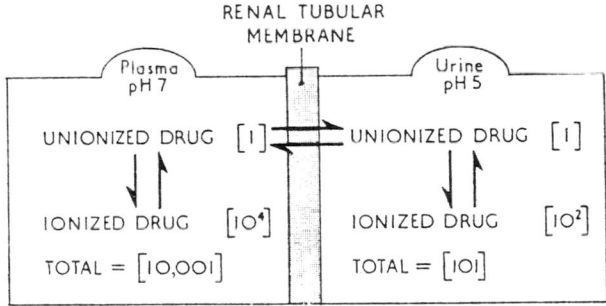

Fig. 45.9 Theoretical steady-state distribution of salicylate ($pK_a = 3.0$) between urine and plasma. The concentrations of unionized and ionized forms of the drug in the two compartments have been calculated from the Henderson-Hasselbalch equations. pH values have been rounded off for simplicity. Only the unionized moiety equilibrates across the tubular epithelium. At physiological pH, most of plasma salicylate is in the ionized form and is reversibly bound to albumin. Increases in urinary pH from 5 to 8 increases the fraction of drug in unionized form from [10^2] to [10^5] and therefore aids elimination from the body.

may be hazardous. Intravenous administration of the hydrochlorides of arginine or lysine is safer and usually efficacious. Urinary acidification may be valuable in treating overdosages, with pethidine, amphetamine or its analogue fenfluramine, especially where there is impairment of hepatic function and the normal metabolism of these compounds is disturbed.

Clinical Role of Renal Excretion

Removal of unchanged drug by the kidney is a less common means of terminating drug action *in vivo* than metabolic degradation. However, for those drugs whose elimination is primarily renal, the state of renal function is very important in relation to possible accumulation and toxic effects. From the anaesthetist's point of view, the main drugs to be borne in mind in this respect are the non-depolarizing muscle relaxants, ganglion blockers, various antibacterial agents and cardiac glycosides. Table 45.2 lists

TABLE 45.2

ELIMINATION RATE CONSTANT FOR VARIOUS ANTIMICROBIAL AGENTS

| Drug | Overall rate constant of elimination | |
	Normal renal function	Anuria
Penicillins		
Benzylpenicillin	1.40	0.02
Ampicillin	0.80	0.12
Cephalosporins		
Cephaloridine	0.40	0.08
Cephalexin	0.70	0.04
Tetracyclines		
Chlortetracycline	0.12	0.08
Doxycycline	0.03	0.03
Macrolides and related agents		
Erythromycin	0.50	0.25
Lincomycin	0.15	0.40
Polymyxins		
Colistin	0.31	0.07
Aminoglycosides		
Streptomycin	0.27	0.04
Kanamycin	0.35	0.03
Gentamicin	0.30	0.02
Tobramycin	0.35	0.02

the elimination rate constants for a number of antibiotics whose main route of elimination is the kidney. The aminoglycosides, polymyxins and oxytetracycline, potentiate the actions of non-depolarizing muscle relaxants in man and are particularly liable to do so when there is accumulation in the presence of renal insufficiency.

Pulmonary Excretion

Inhalation anaesthetics are metabolized to a small extent in the body (*see below*); they are, however, mainly eliminated in unchanged form through the lungs, their site of absorption. The healthy alveolar-capillary membrane allows free diffusion of anaesthetic gases in both directions and poses no significant barrier to their transfer. The factors which govern the elimination of volatile anaesthetics are in effect the same ones that are concerned in the uptake of these agents. In essence, three factors are of special importance. First, the *solubility of the agent in blood* expressed as the blood/gas partition coefficient (λ) representing the ratio of anaesthetic concentration in blood to anaesthetic concentration in the gas phase when the two are in equilibrium. The coefficient varies from as high as 12.10 in the case of diethyl ether to 2.30 for halothane. Second, *cardiac output* as reflected in pulmonary blood flow, since this will influence the rate at which efficient elimination of gases can occur from the blood traversing the alveoli. Third, the *tension gradient* of anaesthetic existing between the mixed venous blood and alveoli.

Elimination of the anaesthetic takes place as a reversed image of the uptake phase. When a low-solubility agent such as nitrous oxide or cyclopropane ($\lambda = 0.47$) is discontinued the arterial blood concentration falls very quickly as venous blood is almost cleared completely of anaesthetic in the lungs. A steep concentration gradient is thus provided which, with the high blood flow/mass ratio of brain tissue (a vessel rich group-VRG body tissue), favours rapid transfer of anaesthetic from brain to cerebral capillary blood and consciousness is rapidly regained. Conversely, after discontinuing a high solubility agent, once equilibration of body water has occurred, the arterial tension falls slowly and desaturation of brain tissue tends to be limited by the rate of elimination of anaesthetic from the whole of body water. Recovery is therefore slow.

The factors influencing uptake distribution and elimination of inhalational anaesthetics are considered in detail in Chapter 48.

Biliary Excretion
(Rollins, 1984)

The excretion of drugs via the liver cells into bile has not been studied extensively. Available evidence indicates that the endothelium of the hepatic sinusoids behaves as an extremely porous barrier, which allows ready equilibration between plasma and bile of virtually all compounds whose molecular size is less than that of albumin. The membrane of the hepatic parenchymal cell has a porosity which is less than that of the sinusoidal epithelium, but greater than that of many other cells. Quite a number of relatively hydrophilic compounds are thus able to traverse the liver cells. Although many drugs diffuse in small quantity into bile in the unchanged state, the majority undergo metabolic transformation in the liver and appear in bile as conjugates such as glucuronides, glycine or glutamine conjugates, ethereal sulphates, etc. Experimental studies in animals have shown that drugs of low molecular weight (< 200) only appear in bile to the extent of less than 5% of the dose, including the conjugates. Their main route of excretion is via the kidney. Compounds of higher molecular weight, particularly if they contain a suitably placed polar grououp such as —OH or —OCH_3 in the molecule, are more likely to be excreted in bile provided they can be metabolized and conjugated. Thus, for example, excretion in bile is the major route of elimination of the drug carbenoxolone following glucuronide conjugation in the liver. Many conjugates are polar acidic compounds which, being highly ionized, are not readily reabsorbed from the intestine. They may be excreted unchanged in the faeces or may be split by enzyme activity emanating from intestinal cells or the bacterial microflora to yield other compounds which can be absorbed. An enterohepatic circulation of the compound and its metabolites may, therefore, arise which rather than assist in drug elimination, has the opposite effect of prolonging drug action. Such continuous recirculation of foreign compounds and metabolites could have toxicological significance.

In addition, there is evidence for at least two carrier-mediated systems for transporting organic acids and bases from blood to bile analogous to the secretory mechanisms of the renal tubule. Like the kidney, the biliary systems have the features of active transport mechanisms of low structural specificity.

Kinetics of Drug Elimination
(Gambertoglio, 1984)

After a dose of any drug is administered by whatever route, its ultimate fate will be its elimination from the body. The term 'elimination' is used here to include all the processes which operate to reduce the effective drug concentration in body fluids. Most elimination mechanisms are approximately *first order*, that is, the rate of elimination is proportional to the concentration of drug in the body at any given time. Thus, a plot of concentration of drug in plasma versus time gives a typical exponential curve. If D equals the total drug in the body at time t, D_0 is the drug present at zero time and K equals the rate contant for elimination (in this case the sum of rate constants for metabolism, urinary excretion or other drug disposing process), then

$$D = D_0 e^{-Kt}$$

and
$$\log_{10} D = \log_{10} D_0 - \frac{K}{2.303} \cdot t$$

If $t_{\frac{1}{2}}$ equals the time for D_0 to decrease to one-half the initial concentration, i.e. $D = D_0/2$, it follows that

$$t_{\frac{1}{2}} = \frac{2.303 \log_{10} 2}{K} = 0.693/K$$

$t_{\frac{1}{2}}$, the half time for elimination is often termed the *biological half-life*; from this equation, it is clearly independent of D_0.

When a drug is mainly excreted via the kidney, the plasma half-life is determined by the volume of distribution (V_d) and by the renal clearance of the drug (Cl_r). Thus:

$$t_{\frac{1}{2}} = 2.303 \ \log_{10} 2 \cdot \frac{V_d}{Cl_r}$$

The volumes of distribution and renal clearance tend to be inversely related because a major influence on their respective magnitude is the inherent diffusibility of drugs across lipid biomembranes. Thus, for example, a highly lipid-soluble drug might possess an apparent V_d much greater than total body water; its renal clearance would be low because of substantial back diffusion from the tubular fluid, possibly by a pH-dependent mechanism. The biological half-life would be long provided rapid metabolic inactivation in the liver was not occurring at the same time. The formula for $t_{\frac{1}{2}}$ is not affected by protein-binding of the drug provided the same measurement of drug concentration (i.e. either total concentration or protein-free component) is used for calculating V_d and Cl_r. In practice, $t_{\frac{1}{2}}$ values vary widely. For example, the half-life of a drug like PAH will be very short because V_d is small (localization of drug to the extracellular fluid) and Cl_r is at the level of renal blood flow. In the case of the antimalarial mepacrine, because of its high affinity for intracellular binding sites and low excretion rate, $t_{\frac{1}{2}}$ is unusually long and significant amounts of drug may be found in the body for as long as two months after a single dose.

If the major elimination mechanisms of a drug can become saturated, and the concentration of drug rises above saturation level, then elimination will follow *zero order kinetics* (constant rate). Examples of this are the renal and biliary transport systems for drug secretion for which there is always a maximum transport capacity or *Tm*. If the plasma level of a drug is so high that *Tm* is exceeded, zero order kinetics will be obeyed until the concentration falls below the saturation level; subsequent elimination will be exponential and follow first order kinetics. The elimination of ethanol is an example where zero order kinetics apply. Ethanol is very slowly excreted through the kidneys and lungs, its chief route of elimination being oxidation by liver alcohol dehydrogenase via an NAD-coupled reaction:

$$C_2H_5OH + NAD^+ \rightleftharpoons CH_3CHO + NADH + H^+ \rightarrow$$
$$CH_3CO \cdot CoA$$
acetyl coenzyme A

The rate of metabolism in man is essentially constant at about 10 ml/h regardless of the concentration of alcohol, and zero order kinetics arise mainly because NAD^+ cannot be made available at a sufficient rate. Using the same notation as for first order kinetics, a zero order reaction obeys the following equation:

$$D = D_0 - Kt$$

If $t_{\frac{1}{2}}$ equals the time taken for D to decrease to a value of $D_0/2$, then by substitution, $t_{\frac{1}{2}} = D_0/2K$, indicating that in this instance, the half-life is directly related to the initial concentration of drug. It is only as the circulating concentration of ethanol falls to low levels at which NAD^+ supply is no longer the limiting factor, that elimination kinetics become exponential.

REFERENCES

Benz R., Janko K., Läuger P. (1980). Pore formation by the matrix protein (porin) of *Escherischia coli* in planar bilayer membranes. *Ann. N. Y. Acad. Sci.*, **358**, 13.

Brodie B.B., Hogben A.M. (1957). Some physico-chemical factors in drug action. *J. Pharmacol.*, **9**, 345.

Brater D.C., Chennavasin P. (1984). Effects of renal disease. In *Pharmacokinetic Basis for Drug Treatment*, pp. 119–147. (Benet L. Z., Massoud N., Gambertoglio J.G., eds.) New York: Raven Press.

Clark A.J. (1926). The reaction between acetyl choline and muscle cells. *J. Physiol.*, **61**, 530.

Diasio R.B., Harris B.E. (1989). Clinical pharmacology of 5-fluorouracil. *Clin. Pharmacokinet.*, **16**, 215.

Dixey J.J., Noormohamed F.H., Pawa J.S., et al. (1988). The influence of nonsteroidal anti-inflammatory drugs and probenecid on the renal response to and the kinetics of piretanide in man. *Clin. Pharmacol. Ther.*, **44**, 531.

Fagg G.E., Foster A.C., Ganong A.H. (1986). Excitatory amino acid synaptic mechanisms and neurological function. *Trends in Pharmacol. Sci.*, **7**, 357.

Gaddum J.H. (1937). Discussion on the chemical and physicial bases of pharmacological action. *Proc. R. Soc.*, B, **121**, 598.

Gambertoglio J.G. (1984). Effects of renal disease: altered phamacokinetics. In *Pharmacokinetic Basis for Drug Treatment*, pp. 149–171. (Benet L.Z., Massoud N., Gambertoglio J.G., eds.) New York: Raven Press.

Gardner K., Bennett G.V. (1989). Recently identified erythrocyte membrane-skeletal proteins and interactions. In *Red Cell Membranes*, pp. 1–29. (Agre P., Parker J.C., eds.) New York: Marcel Dekker.

Hawkins R.A. (1986). Transport of essential nutrients across the blood-brain barrier of individual structures. *Fed. Proc.*, **42**, 2055.

Hoffmann E.K., Simonsen L.O. (1989). Membrane mechanisms in volume and pH regulation in vertebrate cells. *Physiol. Rev.*, **69**, 315.

Lamble J.W., ed. (1981). *Towards Understanding Receptors. Current Reviews in Biomedicine*. Amsterdam: Elsevier.

Lant A.F. (1979). Renal excretion and toxicity of drugs. In *Renal Disease*, pp. 617–639. (Black D.A.K., Jones N.F., eds.) Oxford: Blackwell.

Monaghan D.T., Bridges R.J., Cotman C.W. (1989). The excitatory aminoacid receptors: their classes, pharmacology, and distinct properties in the function of the central nervous system. *Ann. Rev. Pharmacol.*, **29**, 365.

Morgan D.J., Blackman G.L., Paull J.D., et al. (1981a). Pharmacokinetics and plasma binding of Thiopental, II: studies at Caesarian section. *Anaesthesiology*, **54**, 474.

Morgan D. J., Blackman G.L., Paull J.D., et al. (1981b). Pharmacokinetics and plasma binding of Thiopental, I: studies in surgical patients. *Anesthesiology*, **54**, 468.

Nation R.L. (1980). Drug kinetics in childbirth. *Clin. Pharmacokinet.*, **5**, 340.

Overton E. (1899). Uber die allgemeinen osmotischen Eigenschaften der Zelle; ihre vermutlichen ursachen und ihre bedeutung fur die Physiologie. *Vertljschr. naturforsch. Ges.*, **44**, 88.

Pardridge W.M. (1988). Recent advances in blood-brain barrier transport. *Ann. Rev. Pharmacol.*, **28**, 25.

Pauling L. (1961). A molecular theory of anesthesia. *Science*, **134**, 15.

Rollins D.E. (1984). Pharmacokinetics and drug excretion in bile. In *Pharmacokinetic Basis for Drug Treatment*, pp. 77–88. (Benet L.Z., Massoud N., Gambertoglio J.G., eds.) New York: Raven Press.

Schafer J.A., Barfuss D.W. (1986). Mechanisms of transmembrane transport in isolated cells and their experimental study. In *Membrane Transport of Antineoplastic Agents*, pp. 1–37. (Goldman I.D., ed.) Oxford: Pergamon Press.

Schofield, P.R., Darlison M.G., Fujita N., et al. (1987). Sequence and functional expression of the GABA receptor shows a ligand-gated super-family. *Nature*, **328**, 221.

Second International Conference on Carriers and Channels in Biological Systems—Transport Proteins (1980). Shamoo A.E., ed. *New York Acad. Sci.*, **358**, 1.

Tozer T.N. (1984). Implications of altered plasma protein binding in disease states. In *Pharmacokinetic Basis for Drug Treatment*, pp. 173–193. (Benet L.Z., Massoud N., Gambertoglio J.G., eds.), New York: Raven Press.

46. An Introduction to the Mechanisms of Drug Action

D. H. Jenkinson

DRUG ACTION IN GENERAL

This chapter addresses the general question of how drugs produce their effects on cells and tissues, a topic often summarized as pharmacodynamics. The first step in drug action is almost always the combination of the drug molecule with specific sites on or in the cells. There are only a few exceptions to this (e.g. the osmotic diuretics). These aside, Paul Ehrlich's famous generalization that substances must bind in order to act (*corpora non agunt nisi fixata*) remains a good starting point for an account of pharmacodynamics.

The site of attachment is often a receptor, though it is increasingly clear that many useful drugs act on other structures. Some examples follow, to illustrate the range of possibilities. The 'calcium antagonists' such as verapamil and nifedipine reduce the movement of calcium into cells through ion channels of a subtype that is particularly important in cardiac and smooth muscle, and that normally opens in response to a fall in membrane potential. Some antidepressant drugs (e.g. imipramine, amitriptyline) block a mechanism for the transport of monoamines (e.g. noradrenaline and serotonin) into nerve endings. The antihypertensive drugs captopril and enalapril inhibit a specific enzyme responsible for the conversion of angiotensin I to the much more active angiotensin II. The diuretic amiloride blocks sodium channels in the distal tubules of the nephron. The antibiotics represent another major class of drugs that do not act through receptors; some (e.g. the penicillins) interfere with the action of enzymes concerned in the synthesis of bacterial cell walls; others (e.g. streptomycin) inhibit protein synthesis by binding to a non-enzymic site on bacterial ribosomes.

In each of these examples, the drug in question combines with a specific structure, be it an ion channel, a transport protein, or the substrate binding region of an enzyme. While such a structure may in a sense be described as a receptor, the term is probably better reserved for those binding sites that are concerned in the physiological control of cell activities by neurotransmitters and by local and systemic hormones. Such substances (e.g. acetylcholine, histamine, hydrocortisone) are able to activate their corresponding receptor (i.e., they are agonists) in a way that has no close parallel with a transport protein, or an ion channel.

Even this restricted definition of a receptor needs a little further qualification, for the term can be used to denote either the whole macromolecule through which the agonist acts or the particular region of the macromolecule to which it binds. Though both usages are current, it will generally be clear which is intended.

An intriguing and instructive problem in this context is posed by the general anaesthetics; can these diverse agents be regarded as acting through receptors, in the sense already discussed? If so, the following criteria might be expected to be met.

1. The binding site or sites would be expected to display some degree of selectivity, in terms of the size, shape and electron distribution of the molecules of the anaesthetic
2. Binding of the anaesthetic to its site of action should be saturable
3. Much more speculatively, the anaesthetic molecules might compete with a naturally occurring ligand for its binding sites

A good deal of evidence to support the first two of these predictions has been presented, though some of it is still quite circumstantial. Articles by Franks and Lieb (1984, 1987) provide a succinct introduction to the 'specific site' hypotheses of general anaesthetic action, and a more general account can be found in the review by Miller (1987), and in Chapter 27 of this volume.

AGONISTS AND ANTAGONISTS

Full and Partial Agonists

As already noted, substances that combine with receptors and thereby initiate a cellular response are described as agonists. If there is combination, but no response, then the agent is a competitive antagonist (because it will reduce the response to an agonist, by occupying receptors). Partial agonists have intermediate properties, that is, though they are able to initiate a response, it is never as great as that produced by a large concentration of a full agonist of the same pharmacological class. The maximum response to a partial agonist, expressed as a proportion of that to the full agonist, is termed the intrinsic activity. Another measure of the ability of a partial agonist to elicit a response is efficacy (Stephenson, 1956). According to the convention introduced by Stephenson, a partial agonist which can produce, at most, a half-maximal response has an efficacy of unity. (The term efficacy is, of course, being used in a specifically pharmacological sense). The distinction between efficacy and intrinsic activity is subtle, and outside the scope of this article (*see* the reviews by Kenakin, 1984, 1985).

Returning to practicalities, some β-adrenoceptor blocking drugs are weak partial agonists, and hence are said to possess sympathomimetic activity. This may be clinically important as discussed, for example, by Northcote (1987). Other examples of drugs that are partial agonists include ergotamine (acting at α_1-adrenoceptors), prenalterol (at β-adrenoceptors) and nalorphine (at opioid receptors).

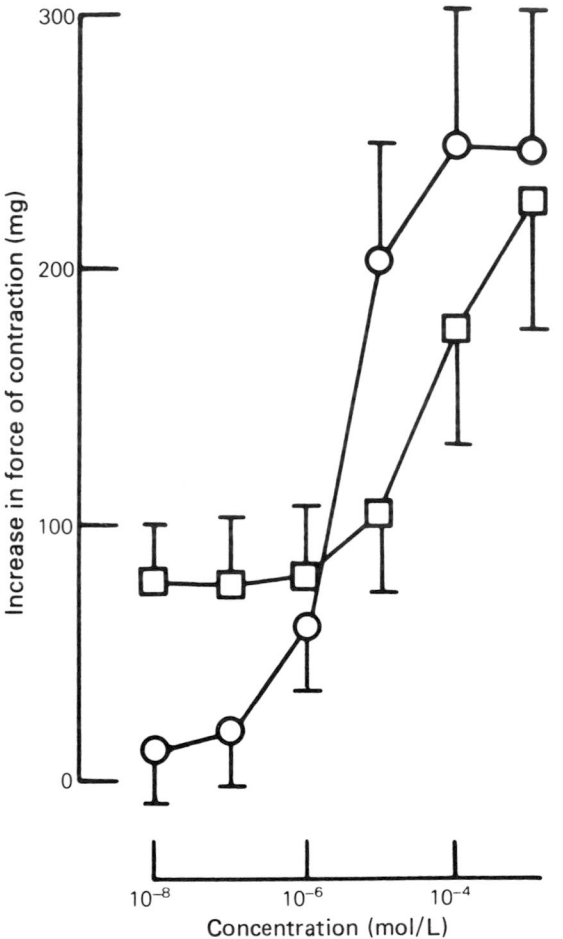

Fig. 46.1 The influence of a partial agonist (impromidine) on the effect of histamine in increasing the force of contraction of an isolated, electrically driven, human left ventricular papillary muscle preparation. *Circles:* response to histamine alone, at the concentrations shown on the abscissa. *Squares:* response to histamine in the presence of a fixed concentration (10^{-5} mol/L) of impromidine. (Reproduced with permission from English et al., 1986.)

What will happen when a tissue is exposed to a full and a partial agonist together? As Fig. 46.1 illustrates, the outcome depends on the relative concentrations. At large concentrations of the full agonist (histamine in this instance), the partial agonist reduces the response. The simplest explanation is that the presence of the partial agonist diminishes the numbers of receptors available to histamine. At low concentratons, many free receptors are available, and the occupation of some of them by the partial agonist, and of others by the full agonist, results in a greater response than would be seen were only one or the other present.

Competitive Antagonists

This important class of drug (e.g. propranolol, tubocurarine, cimetidine) acts by competing with agonists for their binding sites. If the combination between the antagonist and the receptor is freely reversible, as it often is, the effect of the antagonist can be overcome by a large enough increase in the concentration of agonist, so that the tissue response is restored. Such an antagonist causes the curve which relates the equilibrium response to the log of the agonist concentration to shift to the right in a parallel fashion (Fig. 46.2, *left*). The extent of the shift is expressed by the *dose ratio*, that is, the factor by which the concentration of agonist has to be increased in order to restore a given submaximal response in the presence of the antagonist. Competitive antagonists can be remarkably active; an atropine concentration of only 1 nmol/L is needed for a dose ratio of 2 at the muscarinic receptors in e.g. the pacemaker region of the heart, or in bronchial smooth muscle.

Application of the law of mass action leads to the prediction that the following simple relation should hold between the dose ratio, r, and the concentration, [B], of a competitive antagonist:

$$ r - 1 = \frac{[B]}{K_B} $$

Here K_B is the equilibrium constant (i.e., the reciprocal of the affinity constant) for the combination between the antagonist and the receptor. This relationship (the Schild equation—*see* Jenkinson, 1987, for an historical account, and Kenakin, 1982, 1984 for reviews) holds for a wide range of tissues, competitive antagonists and concentrations. Its applicability is generally tested by plotting $(r - 1)$ against [B] on logarithmic scales. This is the Schild plot, and is illustrated in Fig. 46.2, *right*. A straight line should be obtained, with a slope of unity, and an intercept of log K_B. Returning to the previous example (the action of atropine on muscarinic receptors), K_B has the value of 1 nmol/L. It is no coincidence that this is the same as the concentration of atropine giving a dose ratio of 2; the Schild equation implies that they should be identical if the antagonism is competitive and reversible.

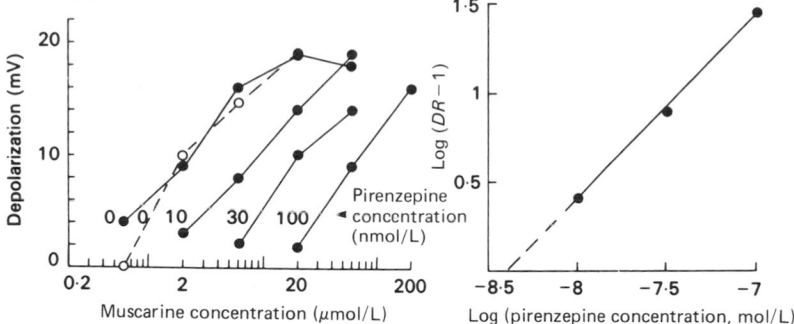

Fig. 46.2 Competitive antagonism. *Left:* The effect of three concentrations of the muscarinic antagonist pirenzepine on the action of muscarine. The response measured was depolarization of a single neurone in the submucous plexus of the guinea-pig small intestine. The open circles show the recovery of the response after removing the antagonist. *Right:* Schild plot (*see* text) based on these results. (Reproduced with permission from North et al., 1985.)

(The negative logarithm of the concentration of antagonist for which the dose ratio is 2 is sometimes written as the pA_2 value for the antagonist in question: for atropine on the muscarinic receptors it is 9.0.)

The quantitative approach to drug antagonism just outlined has important practical applications. Three will be mentioned. First, it is widely employed in the development of new competitive antagonists (since the value of K_B for a novel compound is a direct indication of its affinity for the receptors). Second, it is invaluable for receptor classification, because the K_B value for the combination between a receptor and a well characterized antagonist (or, better, a series of such antagonists) can provide an 'autograph' for that receptor. Third (and perhaps rather surprisingly) it can be applied to the classification of agonists (since if a novel agonist acts through the same receptors as a known one, it should be antagonized to the same degree by a competitive antagonist acting at that receptor).

Quantitative methods are of course equally applicable to the study of drugs acting by enzyme inhibition, though the procedures used are rather different. One approach is to plot the reciprocal of the initial velocity of the enzyme reaction against the reciprocal of the substrate concentration. If a straight line is obtained by this procedure (the Lineweaver–Burk plot), the nature of the changes in its slope and intercept observed when the enzyme inhibitor is also present can provide information about the character of the inhibition, and about the equilibrium constant for the combination of the inhibitor with the enzyme (*see* Fersht, 1985, for an account of this and other more recent approaches to the study of enzyme inhibitors). The Lineweaver Burk procedure is rarely applicable to the study of drugs active on receptors in whole cells, tissues and organisms. This is because it is quite unlikely that the measured response is directly proportional to the occupancy of the receptors by the agonist

(whereas the velocity of an enzyme reaction, for simple enzymes at least, bears a direct relationship to the concentration of the enzyme–substrate complex). When intact tissues are to be examined, the dose ratio method for studying the actions of antagonists is preferable, because it avoids the need to know the exact relation between receptor occupancy and tissue response.

Two other complications in the study of competitive antagonism deserve mention. Both can be illustrated in relation to skeletal muscle relaxants such as tubocurarine. Though the Schild equation applies to the blockade of acetylcholine by tubocurarine (for references *see* Colquhoun, 1986a), the interpretation of the 'equilibrium constant' obtained is complicated by the fact that the nicotinic receptor macromolecule has two binding sites for acetylcholine. If these have different affinities for tubocurarine (for a discussion of the evidence on this, again *see* Colquhoun, 1986a), the apparent equilibrium constant is a function of the individual affinities of the two sites (Sine and Taylor, 1981; Colquhoun, 1986a).

The other complication arises when one comes to consider the effect of tubocurarine on neuromuscular transmission rather than on the response to uniformly applied acetylcholine. In the former instance, the acetylcholine released by the nerve endings is present for only a millisecond or so following each nerve impulse, and its concentration is far from uniform. Indeed the transmitter lasts for so short a time that few of the antagonist molecules are likely to dissociate from the receptors while it is present. Quantitative methods are still applicable (*see* e.g. Paton and Waud, 1967; Armstrong and Lester, 1979), and the antagonism is still competitive in the sense that the presence of tubocurarine reduces the number of binding sites available to acetylcholine. (For a discussion of the usage of 'competitive' in this context, *see* Ginsborg and Jenkinson, 1976).

A more complete account of the action of neuromuscular blocking agents can be found in Bowman (1980) and in the book edited by Kharkevich (1986)—*see* also Chapter 42 in the present volume.

Irreversible Antagonists

Some antagonists (including a few used in therapeutics) combine irreversibly with the binding site for the agonist. There are also a number of drugs that react irreversibly with the active site of enzymes (e.g., the organophosphorus anticholinesterases; some monoamine oxidase inhibitors). Usually the irreversibility arises because the drug forms a covalent bond with some component of the binding site. Such bonds are much stronger, and hence longer lasting (hours or even days for some drug molecules), than the other kinds of forces (ionic, hydrophobic, Van der Waals) involved in the reversible binding of small molecules to receptors, enzymes and transport proteins. However, irreversibility on a similar time scale can sometimes be seen when the small molecule (the ligand) fits the binding site so closely that the cumulative contribution of these other forces (which increase steeply with proximity, over a certain range) becomes comparable to that of a covalent bond. This degree of complementarity is rarely achieved in the laboratory, despite the best efforts of medicinal chemists, but is encountered in animal toxins. A good example is α-bungarotoxin, a small protein found only in the venom of certain snakes. This toxin can form an effectively irreversible bond with the nicotinic receptor at the neuromuscular junction (resulting in paralysis of the prey of the snake). α-bungarotoxin has proved a most valuable tool for the study of the control of these receptors in health and disease (*see later*, and Chapter 52).

NATURE, SYNTHESIS AND CONTROL OF RECEPTORS

Receptors are usually glycoproteins, with relative molecular masses in the broad range 50 000–500 000. Most are located in the cell membrane, which they span. Exceptions include the receptors for steroidal and thyroid hormones, and retinoic acid, which are found in the nucleus and cytosol. In membrane-spanning receptors, the glycosylation sites are on the outer (i.e. extracellular) surface, as are the agonist binding regions for 'fast' (e.g. nicotinic) receptors (*see later*).

Cells make receptors by the usual protein synthetic pathways. These can now be studied directly by an ingenious method in which messenger RNA (from a tissue which expresses the receptor of interest) is injected into the cytosol of another cell that does not. Amphibian oocytes are often used for the latter purpose, because of their size and synthetic capabilities. For example, following the injection of messenger RNA from a tissue that displays nicotinic receptors, the oocytes begin to synthesize these receptors which, moreover, become inserted into the plasma membrane, where they are functional, i.e., the oocyte now responds to nicotinic agonists (Barnard et al., 1982). For another example of the application of the technique (in this instance, to serotonin receptors) *see* Lübbert et al. (1987).

The rate at which a cell *in situ* makes and degrades receptors is influenced by several factors. When a skeletal muscle is chronically denervated, the total number of acetylcholine receptors increases greatly (by up to 30-fold), and they are now found along the whole length of the muscle fibres, rather than almost exclusively at the endplate region. There is a concomitant rise in the corresponding messenger RNA and a change in its spatial distribution (Merlie and Sanes, 1985). The nature of the signal that initiates the increase in receptor synthesis which follows denervation is not yet fully understood, though the reduction in muscle activity is known to be an important factor.

Other receptors are under hormonal control. For example, progesterone receptors increase in number in response to oestrogen secretion during the menstrual cycle. Receptor numbers may also change in the course of physical training (Butler et al., 1982) and during drug administration. This has been studied in some detail for the β-adrenoceptors. Here, agonists (e.g. terbutaline) cause the number of β-receptors on circulating lympocytes to fall, whereas the reverse is seen with β-adrenoceptor blockers (e.g. Hedberg et al., 1986). These changes occur in other tissues and are described as *down-* and *up-regulation* respectively. They can have clinical implications during both the administration and the withdrawal of drugs (*see* Hollenberg, 1985). The phenomenon is not unique to receptors, and is seen, for example, with ion channel blockers such as the calcium antagonists which can cause the numbers of calcium channels to increase.

The number of receptors may also alter as a consequence of immune reactions. A striking example is the reduction in functional acetylcholine receptors in the neuromuscular junction of patients with the autoimmune disease myasthenia gravis (*see* the review by Lindstrom, 1985).

The importance of methods for assessing the numbers of receptors will be clear from the foregoing. In the case of the acetylcholine receptors at the muscle endplate, this can be done with radio- or fluorescently-labelled α-bungarotoxin. More commonly, labelled drugs which form reversible rather than irreversible bonds with the receptors are now used, and many are commercially available. The procedure employed (the radioligand binding technique) provides information not only on the numbers of receptors but also on the value of the equilibrium constant for their combination with the ligand. The measurements may be made with biopsy samples, or with the formed elements of blood. A general problem is how to distinguish binding to the receptor of interest from that to other sites. This can often be clarified by studying the binding both in the presence and in the absence of a suitable unlabelled displacing agent, that is, a substance which binds mainly (ideally, solely) to the receptor in question. The difference between the binding with and without the displacing agent provides an estimate of the binding to the receptor. The procedure is illustrated in Fig. 46.3 and a full account can be found in the book edited by Yamamura et al. (1985). It has also now become possible to study receptors *in vivo* using the technique of positron emission tomography (*see* Kuhar, 1987).

Receptor Isolation and Sequencing

Knowledge of the structure and function of receptors has been transformed by recent successes in receptor isolation, and by the determination of the complete amino acid sequences of several of the receptors so isolated. These advances have been made possible by two main techniques. The first is that of affinity chromatography. A column is prepared in which beads of an inert material are 'baited' by the covalent attachment of a molecule to which only the receptors can be

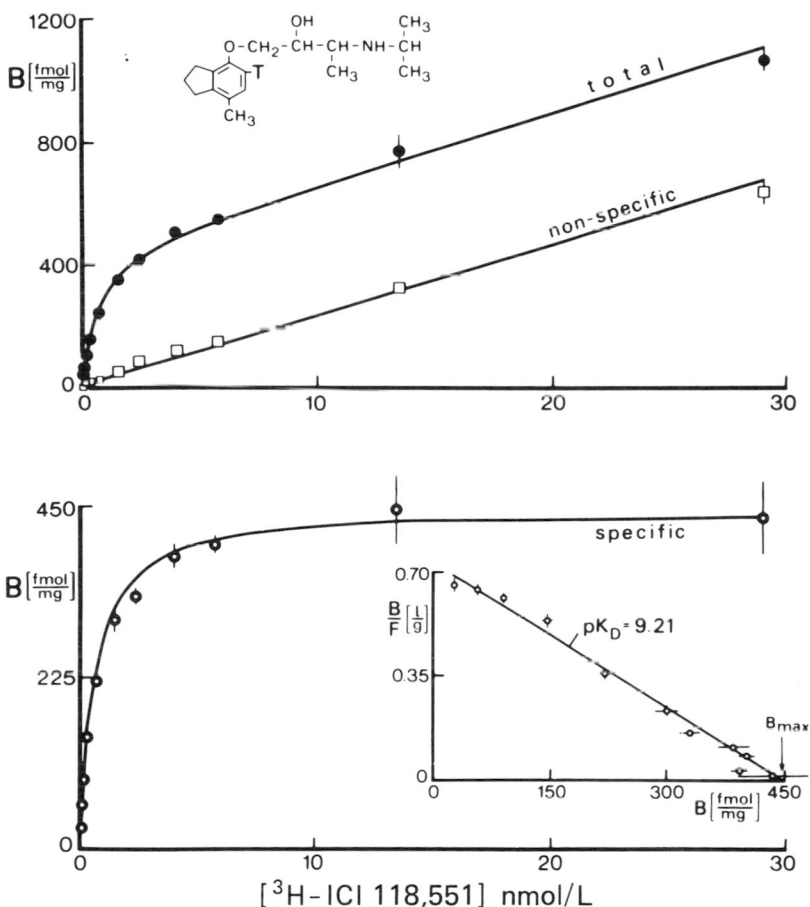

Fig. 46.3 The radiolabelled ligand binding technique. In this example, the ligand is a tritiated β_2-adrenoceptor antagonist, ICI 118,551 (for structure see top: T indicates the position of the label). The tissue being studied is guinea-pig lung, and the upper graph shows the amounts of the ligand binding to membrane particles at various ligand concentrations. 'Total' and 'non-specific' refer to the binding (B) observed in the absence and presence respectively of 0.2 mmol/L (−)-isoprenaline which was used to determine what proportion of the binding is non-specific, i.e. not to the receptors (*see* text). The lower graph plots the specific binding, again as a function of the free (i.e. unbound) concentration (F) of [^{3}H]-ICI 118,551. The inset illustrates a means of analysing the binding data in order to obtain estimates of the affinity constant for binding, and of the maximum binding capacity (B_{max}). For further details, and an account of the exacting statistical analysis which was applied (the lines show the theoretical fit), *see* Lemoine et al. (1985) from which this illustration is taken, with permission.

expected to bind with high affinity. Animal toxins have been invaluable for this purpose, and the first successful isolation of a receptor (the nicotinic subtype of the acetylcholine receptor) was made possible by the availability of the snake venom neurotoxins already mentioned. Cobra toxin has been particularly useful, since the bonds it forms with nicotinic receptors are somewhat less irreversible than those with α-bungarotoxin. Solubilized membrane macromolecules are then applied to the column, and only those (ideally the receptors alone) with a high affinity for the 'bait' become trapped by attachment to the material of the column. The receptor is then eluted using a high concentraton of a small ligand (e.g. carbachol or gallamine) for which the receptor has an adequate affinity.

Once the receptor macromolecule has been isolated, its amino acid sequence can be determined. This would be a formidable task were direct chemical methods to be used, since there may be many hundreds of amino acids. Sequencing is invariably done indirectly using the procedures of molecular biology, and in particular, gene cloning. This is the second of the techniques mentioned above. Though a detailed account would be beyond the scope of this article, the important breakthrough has been the ability to obtain large amounts of a particular DNA by inserting a 'foreign' gene (e.g. one coding for a specific receptor) into the DNA of another cell (often *E. coli*) which can be grown in bulk. The DNA of interest (normally a cDNA) can then be isolated in quantity and decoded to provide the amino-acid sequence of the receptor. For an example of this approach, and references to earlier work, *see* Kobilka et al. (1987) and also the later section on slow acting receptors. It hardly needs pointing out that knowledge of the sequences provides a new and powerful tool for receptor classification. This has already led to the identification of additional subtypes of the muscarinic receptors for acetylcholine (*see* Bonner, 1989).

At the time of writing, the sequences of more than ten receptors have been determined, and we can expect that by the next edition of this volume, the primary structures of all the major receptors will be known. What has already become clear is that receptors can be placed into several distinct classes on the basis of their structures. Not surprisingly, these classes correspond to different mechanisms of action. This is the final topic to be discussed.

HOW RECEPTORS INFLUENCE CELL ACTIVITY

Fast Acting Receptors

These are exemplified by the nicotinic receptors for acetylcholine, and are so named because their action develops within microseconds of exposure to agonist. Others in this category are the receptors for glycine and glutamate, and the A subtype of the GABA

receptor. In each instance the receptor spans the cell membrane and projects on either side, as illustrated for the nicotinic receptor in Fig. 46.4 (upper). Binding of an agonist molecule to each of the two binding sites possessed by the nicotinic receptor macromolecule allows the receptor to change shape in such a way as

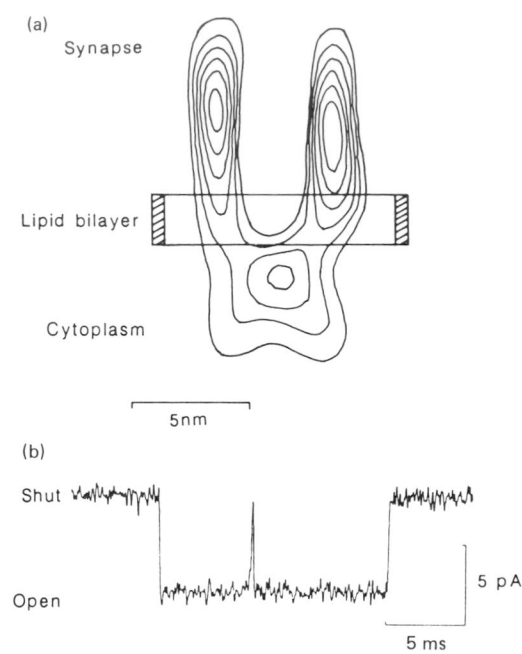

Fig. 46.4   Structure and function of the nicotinic acetylcholine receptor. (a) Electron image map of a cross section of the receptor macromolecule, perpendicular to the plane of the membrane. The wide mouth of the ion channel in the centre of the structure is clearly seen. (b) A record of the electrical current which flows into a muscle cell when a single acetylcholine receptor ion channel opens. The opening lasts for about 14 ms, but for a brief closure of about 100 μs. (Reproduced with permission from Colquhoun (1986b).)

to create a channel for the movement of cations across the cell membrane, hence causing depolarization (*see* Chapter 52). With the receptors for glycine and GABA, the channel is anion rather than cation selective, in keeping with the inhibitory actions of these neurotransmitters. Remarkable advances in electrophysiology have enabled the current flow associated with the opening and shutting of a single channel to be observed. As Fig. 46.4 (lower) shows, the transition from the closed to the open channel, and back again, occurs very rapidly. The average duration of the opening of a mammalian nicotinic receptor channel is about 0.3 ms.

Experiments of this kind have also shown that the amplitude of the current flow does not vary when different agonists are tested; it is the *duration* of the channel opening that differs. The most likely explanation is that receptor activation is 'all or none', as represented in the following scheme.

$$A + R \rightleftharpoons AR \rightleftharpoons AR^* \rightleftharpoons AR_D$$

On this model, the receptor, R, when combined with agonist, A, isomerizes spontaneously between an inactive (AR) and an active (i.e. channel open) form (AR*). The position of the equilibrium between AR and AR* determines the efficacy of the agonist (for a critical discussion of the concept of efficacy in this context, *see* Colquhoun, 1987). AR* may also convert to a second, inactive ('desensitized') state, AR_D. An additional possibility, now well documented, is that the agonist (and some antagonists) may also block the open ion channel (*see* Ogden and Colquhoun, 1985). Receptor desensitization of this kind may contribute to the change with time in the nature of the neuro-muscular block caused by suxamethonium (for discussions of this still rather controversial issue *see* Zaimis, 1976, and Colquhoun, 1986a).

Desensitization also occurs with many other kinds of receptor, though the mechanism varies. β-adrenoceptor desensitization has been studied in great detail and at least three factors have been shown to contribute (*see* Sibley and Lefkowitz, 1985; Sibley et al., 1987; Mahan et al., 1987). One is a reduction in the ability of the receptor to activate a guanine nucleotide binding protein which has a key role in the

initiation of the response (*see* the next section). Another is sequestration of the receptors, which enter the cells. Indeed, receptor endocytosis has a more general role in that it is important in the control of the numbers, and in some instances, the actions, of certain receptors (e.g., for insulin). A third factor in β-adrenoceptor desensitization is *down-regulation*, whereby the total number of receptors (membrane bound and internalized) declines over a much longer time scale (several hours or days).

Receptors with an Intermediate Speed of Response

Examples here include the α and β-adrenoceptors, the H_1 and H_2 receptors for histamine, muscarinic receptors, the receptors for opioids and for many other neuropeptides. The response to the agonist develops after a delay which may be as little as some tens of milliseconds for some receptors, and as great as a second or two for others. The delay is thought to reflect the complexity of the underlying events. Each of the receptors in this class, when activated by the binding of an agonist molecule, becomes capable of influencing a second membrane protein which carries a binding site for a guanine nucleotide, guanosine di or triphosphate (hence the abbreviation G, or sometimes N, protein). The outcome is that the G protein is now able to activate specific membrane enzymes

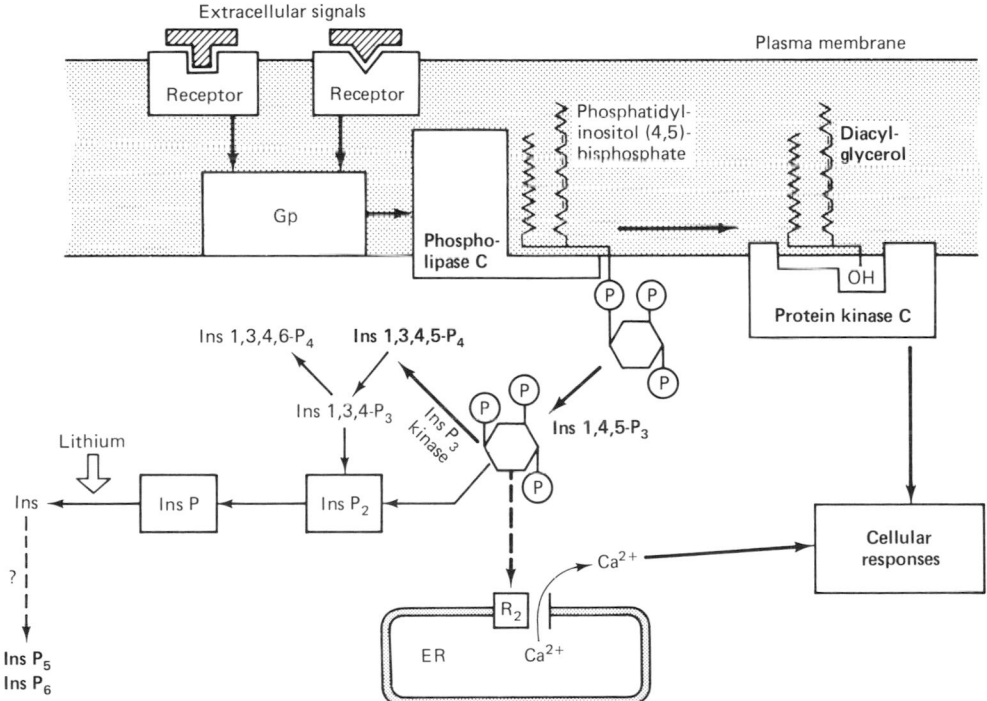

Fig. 46.5   Mechanism of action of receptors (e.g., α_1-adrenoceptors, histamine H_1, muscarinic) that activate, via a G protein (G_p), the enzyme phospholipase C, which operates on a specific membrane phospholipid. The outcome is the formation of inositol polyphosphates and diacylglycerol, both of which alter cell function in a variety of ways (*see* text). (Reproduced with permission from Altman, 1988.)

HUMAN β₂AR

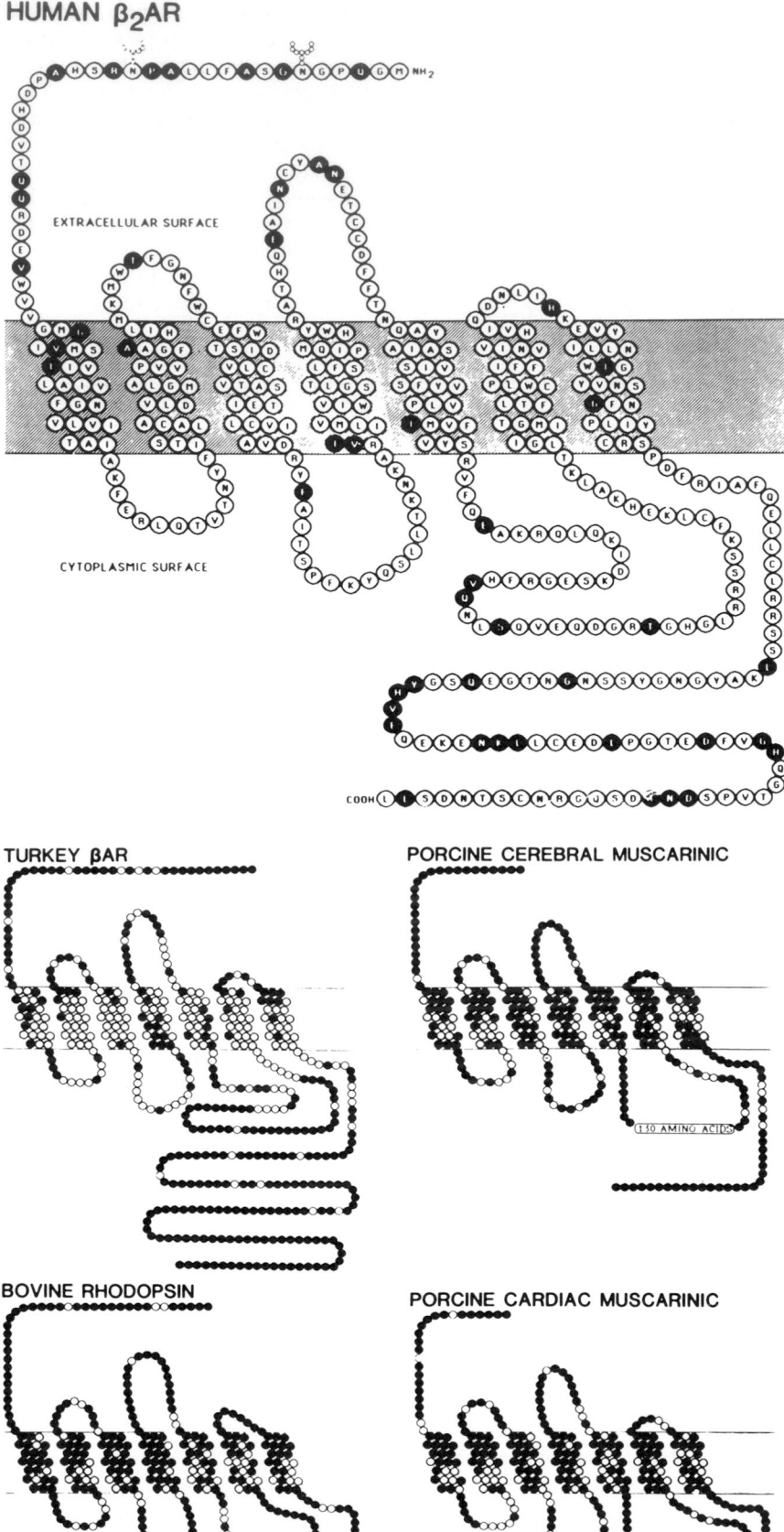

Fig. 46.6 Structures of the human β_2-adrenoceptor, the turkey β-adrenoceptor, porcine muscarinic receptors (cerebral and cardiac) and bovine rhodopsin, as they may be organized within the membrane. The open circles represent amino acids that are identical with those of the hamster β_2-adrenoceptor. (Reproduced with permission from Dohlman et al., 1987.)

which catalyse the formation of molecules that alter events at the membrane, and within the cell (*see* Gilman, 1987, for a review). A well characterized example of such a 'signalling' enzyme is adenylate cyclase, which converts ATP to the second messenger, cyclic AMP. The activity of this enzyme can be altered in either direction by two distinct G proteins. One (G_s) stimulates the enzyme, and the other (G_i) inhibits it (*see* Casperson and Bourne, 1987).

Yet other G proteins (G_p, G_o) when activated by, for example, an α_1-adrenoceptor will in turn increase the activity of a second signalling enzyme, a phospholipase C (*see* Berridge, 1987; Stahl et al., 1988), which can hydrolyse a specific membrane phospholipid (phosphatidylinositol bisphosphate). The outcome is the formation of inositol polyphosphates, and diacylglycerol (Fig. 46.5). These substances initiate a variety of cellular responses (Berridge, 1987). For example, inositol 1,4,5-trisphosphate causes the release of calcium from storage sites within the cell, leading to, for example, the contraction of vascular smooth muscle, and glycogenolysis in liver cells (Exton, 1988). Diacylglycerol, the other product, increases the activity of an enzyme (protein kinase C) which catalyses the phosphorylation of ion channels, receptors and other enzymes, with widespread consequences for cell function.

The elucidation of the amino acid sequences of several of the receptors in this class has revealed remarkable and previously unsuspected similarities. The peptide chain of each receptor has seven stretches which are mainly hydrophobic. These are thought to lie within the membrane, and span it (Fig. 46.6). A surprising feature is that the agonist binding site is located within one of the hydrophobic regions (Dixon et al., 1987; Wheatley et al., 1988).

Slow Acting Receptors

These are exemplified by the receptors for the steroid and thyroid hormones. The physiological response to these substances develops only after some minutes or more often hours. This again reflects the mechanism of action which in this instance involves receptors in the nucleus and perhaps also the cytosol. The locus of action is the DNA transcription mechanism in the nucleus; changes in transcription lead to alterations in protein synthesis, resulting in the modifications in cell function finally observed (*see* Ringold, 1985). Specific proteins may be involved. An example is the formation of lipocortin in response to the action of glucocorticoids. This protein and its proteolytic fragments (Huang et al., 1987) inhibit the generation, via phospholipase A_2, of prostaglandins, platelet activating factor and leukotrienes. The reduction in these substances, all of which are concerned in inflammation (*see* Vane and Botting, 1987), can account for part at least of the anti-inflammatory action of the glucocorticoid steroids.

Though the above classification in terms of the rapidity of response is useful, certain receptors are not easily accommodated within it. Examples are those for insulin and epidermal growth factor (EGF). Though many of the actions of these substances develop slowly, the earliest steps may occur within a minute. These steps are not fully understood, though it is known that the insulin and EGF receptors are initially membrane bound, and that they are also enzymes which are able to phosphorylate not only other proteins, but also regions of their own peptide chains (*see* Sibley et al., 1987). An additional factor is that combination with insulin or EGF causes the corresponding receptors to aggregate into clusters which are then internalized by endocytosis. This internalization is thought to be important for some of the actions of both insulin (Kahn, 1985) and EGF (Carpenter, 1987).

Evidently, there is a hierarchy of complexity on passing from the (relatively) simple fast receptors, with their intrinsic ion channels, through receptors acting via second messengers, to those for steroids, insulin and EGF. Establishing how the latter act is one of the major remaining challenges.

REFERENCES

Altman J. (1988). Ins and outs of cell signalling. *Nature*, **331**, 119.

Armstrong D.L., Lester H.A. (1979). The kinetics of tubocurarine action and restricted diffusion within the synaptic cleft. *J. Physiol.*, **294**, 365.

Barnard E.A., Miledi R., Sumikawa K. (1982). Translation of exogenous messenger RNA coding for nicotinic acetylcholine receptors produces functional receptors in *Xenopus* oocytes. *Proc. R. Soc. (Biol.)*, **215**, 241.

Berridge M.J. (1987). Inositol trisphosphate and diacylglycerol: two interacting second messengers. *Ann. Rev. Biochem.*, **56**, 159.

Bonner T.I. (1989). The molecular basis of muscarinic receptor diversity. *Trends Neurosci.*, **12**, 148.

Bowman W.C. (1980). *Pharmacology of Neuromuscular Function*. Bristol: John Wright.

Butler J., O'Brien M., O'Malley K., et al. (1982). Relationship of β-adrenoceptor density to fitness in athletes. *Nature*, **298**, 60

Carpenter G. (1987). Receptors for epidermal growth factor and other polypeptide mitogens. *Ann. Rev Biochem.*, **56**, 881.

Casperson G.F., Bourne H.R. (1987). Biochemical and molecular genetic analysis of hormone-sensitive adenylyl cyclase. *Ann. Rev. Pharmacol. Toxicol.*, **27**, 371.

Colquhoun D. (1986a). On the principles of postsynaptic action of neuromuscular blocking agents. In *New Neuromuscular Blocking Agents, Handbook of Experimental Pharmacology*, Vol. 79, pp. 59–113 (Kharkevich D.A., ed.). Berlin: Springer-Verlag.

Colquhoun D. (1986b). Structure and function of acetylcholine-receptor ion channels. *Nature*, **321**, 382.

Colquhoun D. (1987). Affinity, efficacy and receptor classification: Is the classical theory still useful? In *Perspectives on Receptor Classification*, pp. 103–114 (Black J.W., Jenkinson D.H., Gerskowitch V.P., eds.). New York: Liss.

Dixon R.A.F., Segal I.S., Rands E., et al. (1987). Ligand binding to the β-adrenergic receptor involves its rhodopsin-like core. *Nature*, **326**, 73.

Dohlman H.G., Caron M.G., Lefkowitz R.J. (1987). A family of receptors coupled to guanine nucleotide regulatory proteins. *Biochemistry*, **26**, 2657.

English T.A.H., Gristwood R.W., Owen D.A.A., et al. (1986). Impromidine is a partial H$_2$-receptor agonist on human ventricular myocardium. *Br. J. Pharmacol.*, **89**, 335.

Exton J.H. (1988). The roles of calcium and phosphoinositides in the mechanisms of α$_1$-adrenergic and other agonists. *Rev. Physiol. Biochem. Pharmacol.*, **111**, 117.

Fersht A. (1985). *Enzyme Structure and Mechanism*. New York: Freeman.

Franks N.P., Lieb W.R. (1984). Do general anaesthetics act by competitive binding to specific receptors? *Nature*, **310**, 599.

Franks N.P., Lieb W.R. (1987). Anaesthetics on the mind. *Nature*, **328**, 113.

Gilman A.G. (1987). G Proteins: transducers of receptor generated signals. *Ann. Rev. Biochem.*, **56**, 615.

Ginsborg B.L., Jenkinson D.H. (1976). Transmission of impulses from nerve to muscle. In *Neuromuscular Junction, Handbook of Experimental Pharmacology*, Vol. 42, pp. 229–364 (Zaimis E., ed.). Berlin: Springer-Verlag.

Hedberg A., Gerber J.G., Nies A.S., et al. (1986). Effects of pindolol and propranolol on beta adrenergic receptors on human lymphocytes. *J. Pharmacol. Exp. Ther.*, **239**, 117.

Hollenberg M.D. (1985). Pathophysiological and therapeutic implications of receptor regulation. *Trends Pharmacol. Sci.*, **6**, 334.

Huang K.S., McGray P., Mattalians R.J., et al. (1987). Purification and characterization of proteolytic fragments of lipocortin I that inhibit phospholipase A2. *J. Biol. Chem.*, **262**, 7639.

Jenkinson D.H. (1987). Heinz Schild's contribution to receptor classification. In *Perspectives on Receptor Classification*, pp. 1–10, (Black J.W., Jenkinson D.H., Gerskowitch V.P., eds.). New York: Liss.

Kahn C.R. (1985). The molecular mechanism of insulin action. *Ann. Rev. Med.*, **36**, 429.

Kenakin T.P. (1982). The Schild regression in the process of receptor classification. *Can. J. Physiol. Pharmacol.*, **60**, 249.

Kenakin T.P. (1984). The classification of drugs and drug receptors in isolated tissues. *Pharmacol. Rev.*, **36**, 165.

Kenakin T.P. (1985). The quantification of relative efficacy of agonists. *J. Pharmacol. Methods*, **13**, 281.

Kharkevich D.A. (1986). (ed.) *New Neuromuscular Blocking Agents. Handbook of Experimental Pharmacology*, vol. 79. Berlin: Springer Verlag.

Kobilka, B.K., Dixon R.A.F., Frielle T., et al. (1987). cDNA for the human beta-2 adrenergic receptor: a protein with multiple membrane spanning domains and encoded by a gene whose chromosomal location is shared with that of the receptor for platelet-derived growth factor. *Proc. Nat. Acad. Sci., USA*, **84**, 46.

Kuhar M.J. (1987). Imaging receptors for drugs in neural tissue. *Neuropharmacology*, **26**, 911.

Lemoine H., Ehle B., Kaumann A.J. (1985). Direct labelling of β$_2$-adrenoceptors. Comparison of binding potency of ^{3}H-ICI 118,551 and blocking potency of ICI 118,551. *Naunyn-Schmiedeberg's Archives of Pharmacology*, **331**, 40.

Lindstrom J. (1985). Immunobiology of myasthenia gravis,

experimental autoimmune myasthenia gravis and Lambert–Eaton syndrome. *Ann. Rev. Immunol.*, **3**, 109.

Lübbert H., Hoffman B.J., Snutch T.P., et al. (1987). cDNA cloning of a serotonin 5-HTIC receptor by electrophysiological assays of mRNA-injected Xenopus oocytes. *Proc. Nat. Acad. Sci., USA*, **84**, 4332.

Mahan L.C., McKernan R.M., Insel P.A. (1987). Metabolism of alpha and beta-adrenergic receptors *in vitro* and *in vivo*. *Ann. Rev. Pharmacol. Toxicol.*, **27**, 215.

Merlie J.P., Sanes J.R. (1985). Concentration of acetylcholine receptor mRNA in synaptic regions of adult muscle fibres. *Nature*, **317**, 66.

Miller K.W. (1987). General anaesthetics. In. *Drugs in Anaesthesia: Mechanisms of Action*, pp. 133–159. (Feldman S.A., Scurr C.F., Paton W.D.M., eds.). London: Arnold.

North R.A., Slack B.E., Surprenant A. (1985). Muscarinic M$_1$ and M$_2$ receptors mediate depolarization and presynaptic inhibition in guinea-pig enteric nervous system. *J. Physiol.*, **369**, 435.

Northcote R.J. (1987). The clinical significance of intrinsic sympathomimetic activity. *Int. J. Cardiol.*, **15**, 133.

Ogden D.C., Colquhoun D. (1985). Ion channel block by acetylcholine, carbachol and suberyldicholine at the frog neuromuscular junction. *Proc. R. Soc. [Biol]*, **225**, 329.

Paton W.D.M., Waud D.R. (1967). The margin of safety of neuromuscular transmission. *J. Physiol.*, **191**, 59.

Ringold G.M. (1985). Steroid hormone regulation of gene expression. *Ann. Rev. Pharmacol. Toxicol.*, **25**, 529.

Sibley D.R., Benovic J.L., Caron M.G., et al. (1987). Regulation of transmembrane signalling by receptor phosphorylation. *Cell*, **48**, 913.

Sibley D.R., Lefkowitz R.J. (1985). Molecular mechanisms of receptor desensitization using the β-adrenergic receptor-coupled adenylate cyclase system as a model. *Nature*, **317**, 124.

Sine S.M., Taylor P. (1981). Relationship between reversible antagonist occupancy and the functional capacity of the acetylcholine receptor. *J. Biol. Chem.*, **256**, 6692.

Stahl M.L., Ferenz C.R., Kelleher K.L., et al. (1988). Sequence similarity of phospholipase C with the non-catalytic region of src. *Nature*, **332**, 269.

Stephenson R.P. (1956). A modification of receptor theory. *Br. J. Pharmacol.*, **11**, 379.

Vane J., Botting R. (1987). Inflammation and the mechanism of action of anti-inflammatory drugs. *FASEB J.*, **1**, 89.

Wheatley M., Hulme, E.C., Birdsall N.J.M., et al. (1988). Peptide mapping studies on muscarinic receptors: receptor structure and location of the ligand binding site. *Trends Pharmacol. Sci.*, **9**, Supplement on Subtypes of Muscarinic Receptors III, 19.

Yamamura H.I., Enna S.J., Kuhar M.J. (Eds.). (1985). *Neurotransmitter Receptor Binding*. New York: Raven.

Zaimis E. (1976). The neuromuscular junction: areas of uncertainty. In *Neuromuscular Junction, Handbook of Experimental Pharmacology*, Vol. 42, pp. 1–21. Zaimis E. (Ed.). Berlin: Springer-Verlag.

FURTHER READING

Ariëns E.J., Soudijn W., Timmermans P.B.M.W.M. (eds.). (1983). *Stereochemistry and Biological Activity of Drugs*. Oxford: Blackwell.

Black J.W., Jenkinson D.H., Gerskowitch V.P. (eds.). (1987). *Perspectives on Receptor Classification*. New York: Liss.

Dean P.M. (1987). *Molecular Foundations of Drug Receptor Interaction*. Cambridge: Cambridge University Press.

Kenakin T.P. (1987). *Pharmacologic Analysis of Drug Receptor Interaction*. New York: Raven.

Limbird L.E. (1986). *Cell Surface Receptors: A Short Course on Theory and Methods*. Boston: Martinus Nijhoff.

Wallach D.F.H. (1987). *Fundamentals of Receptor Molecular Biology*. New York: Dekker.

47. Pharmacokinetics of Drugs Administered Intravenously
M. Ghoneim and K. Pearson

Distribution
  Tissue size, blood flow, and partition
    coefficient
  Ionization
  Plasma protein binding
  Molecular size and active transport
Elimination
  The liver
  The kidney
Pharmacokinetic models
  First-order processes
  Half-life ($t_{\frac{1}{2}}$)
  The volume of distribution
  Clearance
  Relation between elimination half-life,
    volume of distribution, and clearance
  Relation between distribution, elimination,
    and duration of drug action
  The plasma concentration-time curves and
    the compartment models
  Non-linear pharmacokinetics
Clinical applications
  Plasma target concentration strategy
  Rational dosage regimens
Summary

Pharmacokinetics is the quantitative study of the processes of drug absorption, distribution, biotransformation and elimination. It is carried out by the use of mathematical models to describe and predict drug concentrations in the body as a function of time after treatment. This study of the dose-concentration relationship under various physiological and pathological states can help the physician to prescribe dosing regimes that result in optimal concentration profiles in the body. The drug blood levels would be associated with maximum therapeutic effectiveness and minimum toxicity. First we plan to review the physiologic principles governing drug distribution

and elimination followed by a discussion of the concepts of pharmacokinetic analysis. The chapter ends with a brief discussion of the clinical applications of pharmacokinetic data.

DISTRIBUTION

When a drug is injected intravenously, it passes first through the lungs where some part may be metabolized and/or stored before reaching the general circulation. Once in the latter, it is distributed to various organs and tissues of the body regardless of its site of therapeutic action. The important factors affecting the distribution of many drugs are: (1) blood flow to the tissues; (2) the mass of tissues into which the drug distributes; (3) the partition coefficient of drug between the tissues and blood; (4) the extent of ionization of the drug; (5) the magnitude of protein binding of the drug in plasma and tissues; (6) molecular size; and (7) active transport or facilitated diffusion processes.

Tissue Size, Blood Flow, and Partition Coefficient

The Body's Three Physiologic Compartments

For the sake of simplicity, the tissues of the body other than the vascular system can be assigned, according to their perfusion, to three groups (Table 47.1).

1. Vessel-rich group (VRG) which comprises the brain, heart, liver, kidneys, glands, and gastrointestinal tract. These tissues represent only 9% of body weight, but are perfused by 75% of cardiac output.
2. Muscle group (MG) has a larger mass than the preceding group, but is supplied with less blood.
3. Fat group (FG) which is the least perfused.

For individual characterization of different regions of the body the reader is referred to articles by Mapleson (1963) and Dedrick and Bischoff (1968).

Influence on Rate and Mass of Distribution

The magnitude of the blood flow to the tissues as seen in Table 47.1 determines how *fast* a drug can be delivered to a certain region of the body. For example, thiopentone reaches the brain very quickly following injection to produce rapid loss of consciousness

TABLE 47.1
PHARMACOKINETIC COMPARTMENTS*

Compartment	% Body mass	% Cardiac output	Blood flow/weight (L/(kg tissue · min))
VRG‡	9	75	0.75
MG	50	18	0.033
FG	19	5.4	0.022

Note
*Figures are for a standard man of 70 kg body weight, 1.83 m² surface area and 30–39 years old.
‡VRG is the vessel rich group, e.g. brain, heart, viscera, MG is the skeletal muscle group, and FG is fat.

because of the rich blood supply to the brain; however, it accumulates in fat slowly because of its poor blood supply. The *amount* of drug which is distributed to, or stored in, a tissue will depend on the mass of the tissue and the ability of the drug to concentrate there. The latter is known as the tissue/blood partition coefficient and is defined as the ratio of drug in tissue to that in blood when equilibrium has been achieved, i.e. no further movement of drug between blood and tissue. For example, the fat/blood partition coefficient of thiopentone is eleven. This means that thiopentone will move from blood to accumulate in fat as long as the thiopentone concentration in fat is less than eleven times that in blood (Saidman, 1974).

Drug Transfer Between Tissues
Taking thiopentone as an example, very rapid equilibrium occurs between the VRG and blood after administration of the drug because of the high perfusion of these tissues, their relatively small mass and their modest partition coefficients. As the plasma concentration falls due to continued distribution to other tissues, the drug leaves the VRG and returns into the blood where it will be redistributed to other tissues which have not yet achieved equilibrium. In the first five minutes following injection, most of the drug will go to the muscle mass (Price, 1960), thus accounting for the rapid initial recovery following administration of the drug (Fig. 47.1).

Effects of Changes in Tissue Blood Flow on Volume of Distribution
Changes in the perfusion of tissues influence significantly the distribution of drugs. Decreased cardiac output due to heart failure or haemorrhage impairs tissue perfusion, often decreases the volume of distribution of the drug, and results in an increase in the plasma concentration (Wilkinson, 1976). Since physiological compensation in such conditions tries to maintain perfusion to essential organs like the brain and heart at the expense of other tissues like muscle and fat where vasoconstriction takes place, toxic levels of the drug may occur in adequately perfused tissues. Distribution of the drug to other tissues will

not lower these high drug concentrations because perfusion of these tissues is impaired.

Drugs affecting the cardiovascular system can alter their own distribution as well as the distribution of another drug administered concomitantly. For example, the cardiovascular depressant effect of halothane slows its own distribution (Smith et al., 1972) and the distribution and redistribution of another concomitantly administered drug like ketamine (White et al., 1976).

Ionization
Many drugs are either weak acids or weak bases (Table 47.2) which may ionize in solution depending on the pH of their fluid or tissue environment. Weak acids tend to dissociate in an alkaline medium and the opposite occurs with weak bases (Table 47.3). The tendency of any given acid or base to dissociate is

TABLE 47.2
EXAMPLES OF ACIDIC AND BASIC DRUGS

Acid	Base
Anticoagulants (Heparin is a strong acid)	Antihistamines (Diphenhydramine, pK_a 9.1)
Barbiturates (Pentobarbitone, pK_a 8.1*; Secobarbitone, pK_a 7.9; Thiopentone, pK_a 7.6)	Benzodiazepines (Chlordiazepoxide, pK_a 4.8; Diazepam, pK_a 3.3)
Penicillins (Penicillin G, pK_a 2.8)	Local anaesthetics (Bupivacaine, pK_a 8.1; Lignocaine, pK_a 7.9; Mepivacaine, pK_a 7.6)
Salicylates (Acetylsalicyclic acid, pK_a 3.5)	Opioids (Codeine, pK_a 8.1; Pethidine, pK_a 8.5; Morphine, pK_a 7.9)
Sulfon amides (Sulfacetamide, pKa 5.4; Sulfathiazole, pKa 7.1)	Vasopressors (Ephedrine, pK_a 9.6)

Note that an acid cannot be distinguished from a base by the value o pK_a. For example, pentobarbital and bupivacaine have the same pK_a.

Immediately After Injection:

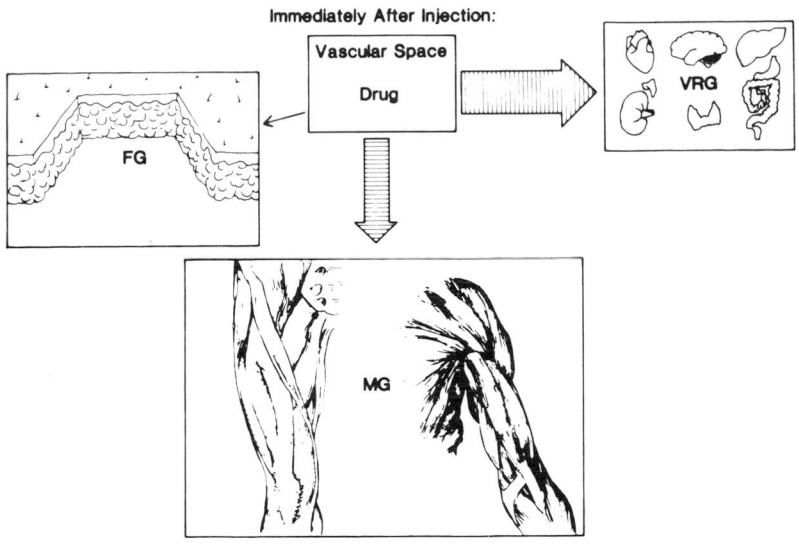

5 Minutes After Injection:

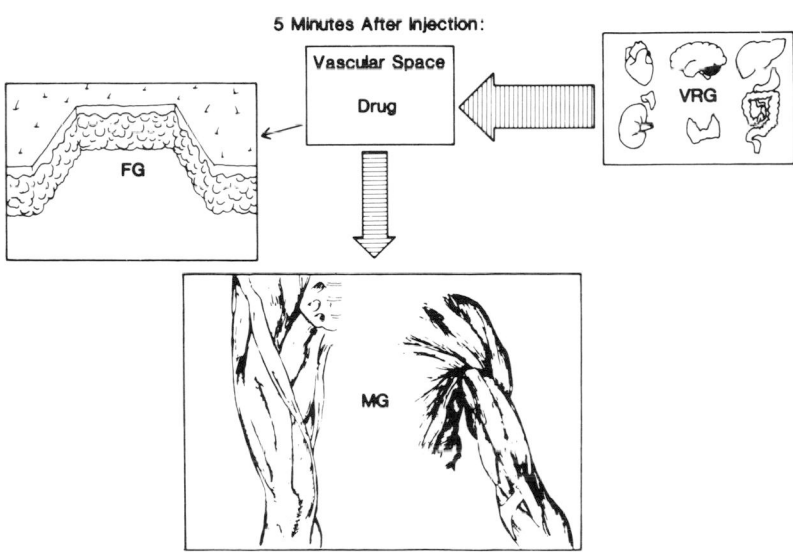

Fig. 47.1 Early distribution of thiopentone. VRG is the vessel rich group. MG is the muscle group and FG is fat. The size of the arrows is schematically proportional to the amount of drug reaching the tissues and the direction of the arrows represents the direction of movement of drug. (The idea of the figure is credited to Dr. L. J. Saidman, San Diego, California.)

given by its dissociation constant, K (pKa is the negative logarithm of K).

The degree of ionization can be calculated from the Henderson–Hasselbalch equation. Thus for a weak acid

$$pH = pK_a + \lg \frac{[\text{ionized weak acid}]}{[\text{unionized weak acid}]}$$

and for a weak base

$$pH = pK_a + \lg \frac{[\text{unionized weak base}]}{[\text{ionized weak base}]}$$

TABLE 47.3

INFLUENCE OF pH ON IONIZATION OF WEAK ACID AND BASE DRUGS*

Drug type	Acid (Low pH) medium	Alkaline (High pH) medium
Weak acid	R-COOH	R-COO⁻ + H⁺
Weak base	R-NH₃⁺	R-NH₂

*(Reprinted with permission from Robinson D.S. (1975). Pharmacokinetic mechanisms of drug interactions. *Postgrad. Med.*, **57**, 55.)

Relation of pKa to pH

When pH equals pK_a the drug will be 50% ionized. The change in degree of ionization will be large if the pH is close to the pK_a value of the drug and will be small if the pH is far removed from the pK_a. As an example, consider Fig. 47.2 which shows the degree of ionization of thiopentone (pK_a 7.6) with changes in pH.

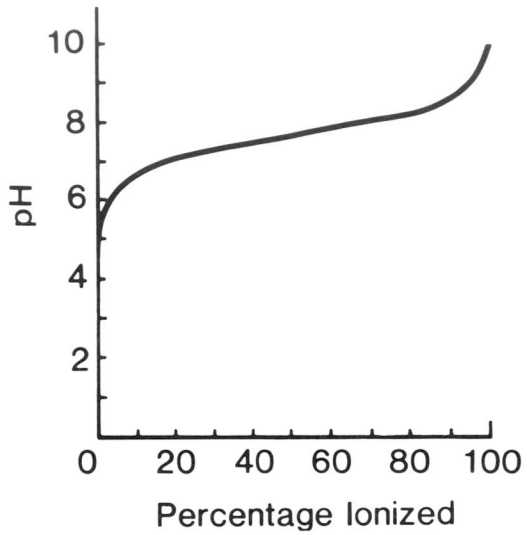

Fig. 47.2 Relationship between pH and degree of ionization of thiopentone (pKa 7.6).

Pharmacological Significance

Cellular membranes resist the penetration of the ionized form of a drug because of its poor lipid solubility and the electric charge on the drug molecule. The latter may cause the drug to be repelled from similarly charged portions of a membrane or attracted and bound by oppositely charged membrane components. A concentration gradient can occur across membranes separating fluids of different pH (Fig. 47.3). At equilibrium the concentrations of unionized drug will be the same on both sides of the membrane, but the total amount of the drug may be considerably different. For a weakly acidic drug like thiopentone, a high pH in the plasma will favor its ionization with the result that less drug will cross cellular barriers. The opposite will occur with acidosis (Brodie et al., 1950; Waddell and Butler, 1957). Weak basic drugs like opioids and local anaesthetics will be sequestrated in low pH areas like the stomach or an acidotic fetus (Stoeckel et al., 1979; Biehl et al., 1978; Kennedy et al., 1979). The reader should note that analytical techniques measure total drug concentrations and do not differentiate between ionized and unionized forms.

Plasma Protein Binding

The great majority of drugs are partially bound to plasma proteins during their stay in the blood. The

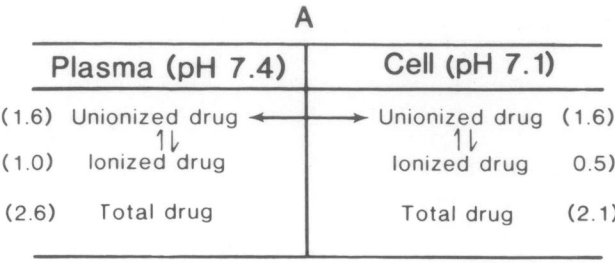

A	
Plasma (pH 7.4)	**Cell (pH 7.1)**
(1.6) Unionized drug ⟷	⟶ Unionized drug (1.6)
⇅	⇅
(1.0) Ionized drug	Ionized drug 0.5)
(2.6) Total drug	Total drug (2.1)

B	
Plasma (pH 8.1)	**Cell (pH 7.1)**
(1) Unionized drug ⟷	⟶ Unionized drug (1)
⇅	⇅
(3.1) Ionized drug	Ionized drug (0.3)
(4.1) Total drug	Total drug (1.3)

Fig. 47.3 The distribution of thiopentone (pKa 7.6) in plasma and cells under (A) physiological state and (B) a rise in plasma pH. The total intracellular drug content in (B) is decreased and the plasma content is increased although the concentration of unionized drug is the same. (pH gradients exist between extra and intracellular fluids. Waddell and Bates, 1969; and Roth, 1983.)

association is usually reversible and can be explained by the law of mass action:

$$\text{Free Drug} + \text{Protein} \underset{K_2}{\overset{K_1}{\rightleftharpoons}} \text{Drug–Protein Complex} \tag{1}$$

K_1 and K_2 are the rate constants of the association and dissociation reactions.

The extent of binding of a drug depends on: the number of binding sites available, the affinity of the drug for those sites, and the concentration of the drug itself (Fig. 47.4).

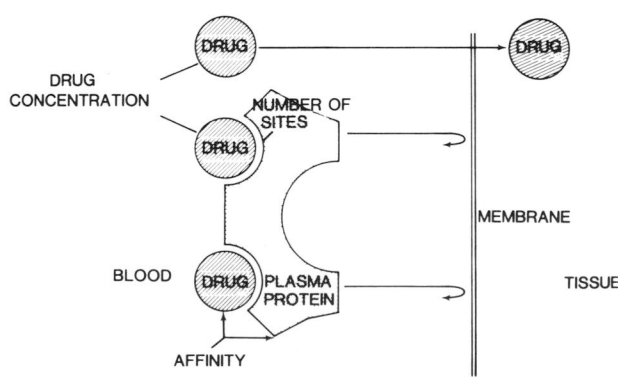

Fig. 47.4 Factors that influence the binding of drugs to plasma proteins

Pharmacological Significance

Generally it is the unbound, or free, fraction of the drug which is pharmacologically active because it can diffuse through capillary walls and reach the site of action. A decrease in the magnitude of binding of a drug as, for example, due to displacement by another drug may temporarily increase the concentration of the drug in the tissues. This may enhance the intensity of the drug action and alter its duration of action (Ghoneim et al., 1976). Decreased binding of an extensively bound drug may also complicate the interpretation of its blood level measured by its total (bound plus free) concentration. For example, a total plasma phenytoin level of 20 µg/ml in a uremic patient with decreased drug binding may be associated with signs of drug toxicity which would be absent in a patient with normal binding. Calculations of pharmacokinetic parameters (e.g. clearance, *defined later*) based on total drug assays will also underestimate their actual values.

Rate of Injection and Binding

The rate of intravenous injection of highly protein bound drugs can influence the intensity of their actions. During rapid intravenous injection of such drugs, the binding capacity of the proteins in the limited blood volume with which the drug initially mixes may be exceeded resulting in a high level of free drug. This will result in turn, in a high drug concentration in the richly perfused tissues (Ghoneim et al., 1976). During a slow intravenous injection, the drug is allowed to mix with the entire blood volume containing a large number of protein receptor sites. Mixing is complete in two or three circulations and will result in lower free drug levels. A more intense and prolonged pharmacologic action after rapid rather than after slow intravenous injection has been demonstrated for thiopentone and diazoxide (Koch-Weser and Sellers, 1976). It is also prudent to inject highly protein bound drugs which act on the richly perfused tissues at a slower rate than normal in patients with decreased binding.

Factors that Affect Binding

For the great majority of drugs, particularly the acidic ones, binding to plasma albumin is quantitatively the most important. The α_1-acid glycoprotein contributes significantly to binding of basic drugs (Piafsky and Borga, 1977). Drugs vary markedly in the extent of their binding to plasma proteins. Unfortunately, it is not possible to predict the plasma binding of a drug from its chemical structure or physical properties. Various physiological and pathological states may affect the magnitude of binding. Age may be one variable, with binding relatively low in neonates and perhaps old age (Wood and Wood, 1981; Wallace and Verbeeck, 1987). Binding may be less in females than in males, and it may also be decreased in pregnancy (Song et al., 1970; Yoshikawa et al., 1984). Temperature and pH can affect the number of binding sites and their dissociation constants, particularly *in vitro*. Competition for the plasma protein binding sites by endogenous substances such as free fatty acids may be important. Competition between drugs for the same binding sites may produce clinically important interactions by decreasing the magnitude of binding of one or both drugs. The binding of many drugs is decreased in renal disease, liver disease, and hypoalbuminaemic states in general (Vallner, 1977). The concentration of α_1-acid glycoprotein is increased in obesity, trauma, burns, after surgery, after myocardial infarction, malignancy, and various inflammatory diseases (Routledge, 1986).

Molecular Size and Active Transport

In general, large molecular weight water-soluble substances and drugs pass through cellular membranes less readily than smaller molecules (Bradbury, 1979). Some molecules (e.g. penicillin) are transported in the body by active or carrier mediated transport processes (Lorenzo and Spector, 1976). These processes profoundly affect distribution (and excretion) of these drugs. In the case of penicillin, pretreatment of animals and man with probenecid (which blocks the active transport of penicillin in liver, kidney, and choroid plexus) decreases significantly the volume of distribution of the drug (Gibaldi et al., 1970).

ELIMINATION

This occurs mainly through the liver and kidney, usually by hepatic biotransformation followed by renal excretion.

The Liver

Biotransformation. Most drugs are lipophilic substances that cannot be excreted unchanged in the aqueous urine. These drugs must undergo chemical changes to transform them into water-soluble (polar) compounds. The chemical changes usually are 'Phase I or preparatory reactions' like oxidation, reduction, or hydrolysis, and 'Phase II or synthetic reactions' like glucuronide conjugation or acetylation. Drug metabolism may involve only one phase or more commonly a sequence of both phases.

Relation between hepatic extraction ratio, perfusion, enzyme activity, and drug protein binding. The elimination of drugs that are readily extracted from the blood passing through the liver (e.g. lidocaine, morphine, methohexitone) is very sensitive to changes in this organ's blood flow, but is relatively insensitive to changes in either its enzyme activity or protein binding of the drug and/or its partitioning into red blood cells (Wilkinson and Shand, 1975). On the other hand, the elimination of drugs that are poorly extracted by the liver (e.g. thiopentone) is very sensitive to changes in the organ's enzyme activity and plasma protein binding, but is insensitive to changes in hepatic perfusion. Drugs with an intermediate hepatic extraction ratio (e.g. midazolam) are partially dependent on all the above factors.

The rate of drug elimination is generally inversely proportional to its magnitude of plasma protein binding due to inaccessibility of the drug to the biotransformation sites. The exception will be drugs that are concentrated in the hepatic cells by active transport mechanisms. Free drug molecules withdrawn from the plasma will be immediately replaced by more free drug resulting from dissociation of the protein–drug complex (Koch-Weser et al., 1976).

The Kidney

Mechanisms. Some drugs are excreted principally by passage into the glomerular filtrate whereas other drugs are also secreted by active transport processes (for example, penicillin). Part of the excreted drug may be reabsorbed from the tubular lumen back into the blood stream.

Renal Perfusion, Drug Ionization, and Protein Binding. Both the clearance of drugs by glomerular filtration and its secretion by the renal tubules are dependent on renal blood flow. It is important to remember that renal blood flow is decreased by many general anesthetics (Deutsch, 1975). This would prolong the action of another drug which is largely excreted in the unchanged form. Tubular reabsorption of drugs involves passive diffusion of nonionized molecules. It may, therefore, be affected by the urine pH if the drug is a weak acid or base (*see* the section on ionization, and Goldstein et al., 1974). The relation between the rate of elimination and plasma protein binding is analogous to that of the liver. The magnitude of binding will affect the rate of glomerular filtration of a drug in an inverse proportion, but will not generally limit the rate of its active tubular secretion (Koch-Weser et al., 1976).

PHARMACOKINETIC MODELS

In the previous sections, we described the distribution and elimination of drugs in anatomical and physiological terms. Because it is not possible to measure tissue drug concentrations in human subjects, construction of physiological models to characterize drug disposition in individuals, as has been done schematically in Fig. 47.1, is not feasible. Sampling of blood, urine and saliva is, however, relatively easy. Recent interest in clinical pharmacokinetics evolved because of the development of sensitive analytical methods for measuring drug concentrations in these fluids and the formulation of relatively simple mathematical terms (helped by the wide use of computers) to describe the processes of drug absorption, distribution, and elimination. This is the basis of the compartment pharmacokinetic models, conceiving the body to consist of

distinct compartments interconnected by first-order (*see below*) mass transfer constants.

The body may be conceived to consist of one, two, or three compartments (Fig. 47.5). The reader will

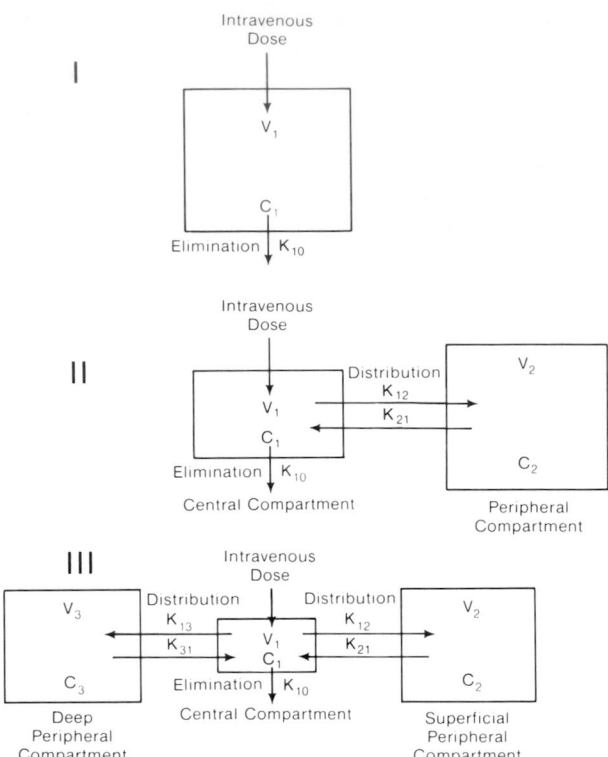

Fig. 47.5 One, two and three open compartment models. V represents the apparent volume of the compartment and C the drug concentration in it. K represents the first-order rate constants of drug transfer between compartments (K_{12}, etc.) and elimination (K_{10}). It is assumed that drugs are administered into and irreversibly eliminated only from the central compartment. The terms central, peripheral, superficial, and deep have no anatomical implications.

note that these compartments are depicted as empty boxes, unlike those in Fig. 47.1, to emphasize the fact that these are mathematical spaces whose precise anatomical contents are unknown. Three parameters are necessary for designing appropriate drug dosage regimens: half-life, volume of distribution, and clearance. These will now be discussed.

First-order Processes

The kinetic behavior of a large number of drugs follows a relatively simple law, the first-order model. The rate of change of drug concentrations over time varies in proportion to the concentration at any given moment. This may be illustrated by the following example from Gladtke and von Hattingberg (1979).

A man is standing in an enclosed space with butterflies flying around (Fig. 47.6). The man has a net and,

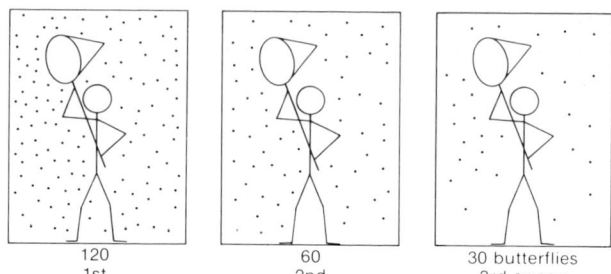

120
1st

60
2nd

30 butterflies
3rd sweep

Fig. 47.6 First-order process. A constant *fraction* (half) of the butterflies are eliminated at every sweep. The numbers remaining are illustrated. Please read the text for explanation. (After Gladtke and von Hattingberg, 1979.)

at each sweep with it, he catches a certain percentage of the insects. Suppose that before the first sweep there are 120 butterflies. The man catches half of them with his first sweep, leaving 60 with him in the space. These 60 butterflies are soon uniformly distributed again. He now makes another sweep and again removes half the butterflies, that is, of 60 butterflies he catches 30. With the next sweep he catches 15, followed by 7.5. Each time, half the butterflies are eliminated.

If we plot a graph of the number of butterflies on the ordinate and the sequence of sweeps of the net expressed as time on the abscissa, we get the curve shown in Fig. 47.7, which is a plot of an exponential

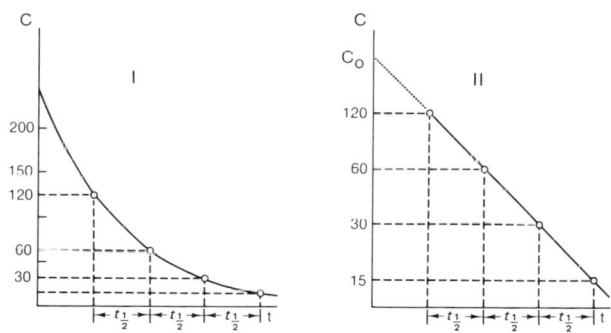

Fig. 47.7 I. The model from Fig. 47.6 is expressed as a linear plot where the ordinate = number of butterflies and the abscissa = number of catches = time. $t_{\frac{1}{2}}$ is the elimination half-life. II. The same curve is ploted with a logarithmic ordinate (Reproduced with permission from Gladtke and von Hattingberg, 1979.)

function, that is, a function of the first-order. At high concentrations, the rate of decline is rapid, while at low concentrations the decline rate is slow. The ordinate of the graph can be changed from a number of butterflies to drug concentration to describe a kinetic drug behavior.

In mathematical terms, the change [usually a decline, (d)] in drug concentration (C) over time (t):

$$\frac{dC}{dt} = -kC \tag{2}$$

K is a proportionality constant that defines the fraction of the amount of drug in the body that will be eliminated in unit time. For example, if $k = 0.01 \text{ min}^{-1}$, the concentration will decrease by 1% each minute. The minus sign indicates decline of drug concentration with time.

When the curve in Fig. 47.7 is replotted with a logarithmic ordinate, a straight line is produced.

Half-Life ($t_{\frac{1}{2}}$)

This characteristic of first-order processes, defines the time necessary for the drug concentration to fall by one-half (Fig. 47.7). The figure also shows that after four half-life intervals, first-order processes are more than 90% complete.

Equation (2) is a differential one which can be integrated:

$$C = C_0 e^{-kt} \tag{3}$$

where C_0 is the theoretical initial concentration at time t = 0 and e the base of the natural logarithm.

Substituting C by $C_0/2$ which is half of the initial drug concentration C_0':

$$\frac{C_0}{2} = C_0 e^{-kt_{\frac{1}{2}}} \tag{4}$$

Division of the equation by C_0 gives:

$$\tfrac{1}{2} = e^{-kt_{\frac{1}{2}}} \tag{5}$$

Substituting into logarithms:

$$\ln \tfrac{1}{2} = -kt_{\frac{1}{2}} \tag{6}$$

Reversing the signs,

$$-\ln \tfrac{1}{2} = kt_{\frac{1}{2}} \tag{7}$$

Since $-\ln \tfrac{1}{2} = \ln 2$, we obtain

$$\ln 2 = kt_{\frac{1}{2}} \tag{8}$$

$$t_{\frac{1}{2}} = \frac{\ln 2}{k} \tag{9}$$

$$t_{\frac{1}{2}} = \frac{0.693}{k} \tag{10}$$

The number 0.693 is an approximation of the natural logarithm of 2.

The most frequently cited pharmacokinetic half-life is that which describes the process of drug removal from the body, 'the elimination half-life' ($t_{\frac{1}{2}}\beta$). It indicates the rate of drug disappearance from the body after treatment and the rate of its accumulation after repeated dosing to reach a plateau or 'steady state.'

The Volume of Distribution

The volumes of compartments in the pharmacokinetic models are as fictitious as the compartments themselves (hence the often used term 'apparent'), but they are nevertheless important characteristics of drugs

(Klotz, 1976). They are calculated by relating the dose and concentration together.

By definition:

$$\text{Concentration} = \frac{\text{Dose}}{\text{Volume}} \qquad (11)$$

$$\text{Volume} = \frac{\text{Dose}}{\text{Concentration}} \qquad (12)$$

In the one compartment model, the volume of distribution (V_d) is calculated as follows:

$$V_d = \frac{\text{Dose}}{C_0} \qquad (13)$$

where dose = amount of drug administered. C_0 = initial plasma concentration at time zero after instantaneous distribution, but before the start of elimination.

Drugs that are represented by a two compartment model (see Fig. 47.5) have at least two separate volumes of distribution; the initial or 'central' volume of distribution (V_{d1}) and the volume of distribution at steady state (V_{dss}). A logarithmic plot of the drug's concentration in plasma, versus time, yields a curve with two separate linear components, as shown in Fig. 47.8.

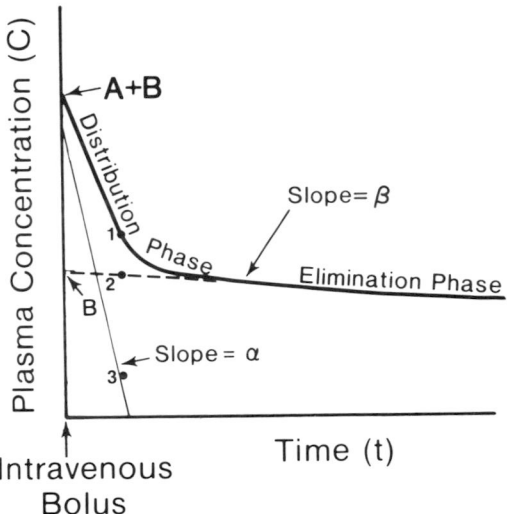

Fig. 47.8 Semilogarithmic plot of plasma concentration of drug (C) *versus* time after a single intravenous bolus. The biphasic graph relates to the two compartment open model.

The initial distribution volume equals the amount of drug in the body following injection and instantaneous mixing divided by the initial concentration in the blood:

$$V_{d1} = \frac{\text{Dose}}{A + B} \qquad (14)$$

where A = intercept at time zero of distribution phase line B = intercept at time zero of elimination phase line. The magnitude of this volume depends on several factors that affect the drug concentration measured within the first few minutes after injection and which were discussed under the physiologic principles governing drug distribution. One may speculate that the initial distribution space for many drugs is composed mainly of the blood volume and the vessel rich group of tissues (see Fig. 47.1).

The volume of distribution at steady state (V_{dss}) is the overall volume achieved when a constant serum concentration of drug has been reached and distribution equilibrium has been attained between the compartments. It can be calculated from the following equation:

$$V_{dss} = V_{d1}\left(1 + \frac{K_{12}}{K_{21}}\right) \qquad (15)$$

where K_{12} and K_{21} = intercompartment rate constants. Lipid solubility affects the magnitude of this volume, in addition to the other factors previously discussed. While the initial distribution volume would be of particular importance during induction of anesthesia, the volume of distribution at steady state would be of more importance hours later.

Volumes of distribution indicate the extent of extravascular tissue uptake of drugs. Highly lipid-soluble drugs are extensively distributed with large apparent volumes of distribution that exceed the size of the body, e.g. two or more L/kg. Because drug concentration is measured only in blood, it is assumed that the drug is distributed homogeneously throughout the other tissues, when calculation is made. Obviously this is an over-simplification because many drugs accumulate in various tissues at concentrations exceeding those in blood.

In the first section, the effects of changes in tissue blood flow on the volume of distribution have been described. Renal and hepatic disease can also cause an increase in the volume of distribution due to a decrease in plasma binding (Klotz, 1976).

Clearance

This is the volume of blood or plasma from which the drug is removed in unit of time. It can be calculated from the slope of the elimination phase of the blood concentration-time curve, β (see Fig. 47.8) and the volume of distribution:

$$\begin{aligned} Cl &= \beta \times V_d \\ &= k \times V_d \end{aligned} \qquad (16)$$

where Cl = clearance
k = first-order rate constant of drug elimination which was defined before with equation (2).

This important kinetic parameter indicates the efficiency of drug elimination from the body and is the main determinant of the extent of drug accumulation during multiple-dose treatment.

Relation between elimination half-life, volume of distribution and clearance

The equation for the elimination half-life:

$$t_{\frac{1}{2}\beta} = \frac{0.693}{k} \qquad (10)$$

Substituting the equation of clearance:

$$t_{\frac{1}{2}\beta} = \frac{0693 \times V_d}{Cl} \qquad (17)$$

It is apparent that the magnitude of the elimination half-life is dependent on both the volume of distribution and clearance. The $t_{\frac{1}{2}\beta}$ would become longer or shorter in direct proportion to V_d if Cl remains the same. By the same token, $t_{\frac{1}{2}\beta}$ would change inversely with Cl if V_d remains fixed. Simultaneous proportional changes in both V_d and Cl would leave $t_{\frac{1}{2}\beta}$ unchanged. It may, therefore, be misleading to use $t_{\frac{1}{2}}$ as an index of drug metabolism or excretion. Cl is the proper parameter. Although Cl can be calculated mathematically from V_d, the two parameters are physiologically independent, unlike the hybrid quality of $t_{\frac{1}{2}}$. (There is no reason why a change in a drug's affinities for tissues would affect the efficiency of its metabolism or excretion.)

Relation between Distribution, Elimination, and Duration of Drug Action

It is commonly assumed that the administration of a drug with a long half-life will result in a long duration of action and the opposite for a drug with a short half-life. This is often erroneous; because as was illustrated with thiopentone, the rate of distribution is a more important determinant of the duration of drug action after *single* doses than is the elimination half-life (Burch and Stanski, 1983). Another example is the case of benzodiazepines; a single dose of diazepam (0.2 or 0.3 mg/kg) will produce effects of about 4 h duration, despite a $t_{\frac{1}{2}}$ of about 30 h (Ghoneim et al., 1984), while lorazepam in an equi-potent dose will produce effects of about double that duration, despite a $t_{\frac{1}{2}}$ of only 10 h (Shader et al., 1986).

There may be two exceptions to the generalization about the importance of the distribution phase to a drug's duration of action after single doses. First, if the drug has a high clearance in addition to a rapid rate of distribution, then elimination will contribute to the termination of its action. Second, residual effects of a drug may relate to its elimination. For example, the minimal effective concentration of thiopentone required for anesthesia will fall on the steep distribution phase of the drug decay curve (Fig. 47.8) while concentrations relating to physical and mental sedation following initial recovery of consciousness may fall on the terminal elimination part (Korttila et al., 1975). However, the development of acute tolerance to CNS-active drugs (Ghoneim et al., 1986) complicates the correlation between effects of the drug and its late plasma concentrations.

The Plasma Concentration-Time Curves and the Compartment Models

In the one-compartment model, distribution of a drug is instantaneous and the decline of plasma concentration with time due to elimination follows a straight line on a semilog arithmetic plot (*see* Figs. 47.5 and 47.7). For most drugs, however, the one-compartment model does not describe the entire course of the plasma concentration because distribution to all tissues does not occur at the same rate (*see* Fig. 47.1). The drug concentration appears to decay in two or three phases. For drugs that follow the two-compartment model (*see* Fig. 47.5), distribution of the drug into tissues, i.e. movement from the central to the peripheral compartments, results in the initial rapid decline (Fig. 47.8) and elimination from the body, i.e. irreversible movement out of the central compartment, causing the second slower decline. (Distribution and elimination occur simultaneously, from the moment the drug enters into the blood stream to the time when the last molecule leaves the body, however, one process dominates the other because distribution occurs more rapidly than elimination.)

The two processes can be plotted separately by 'feathering away' the contribution that the elimination phase makes to the distribution curve (Fig. 47.8). The elimination phase line is extrapolated back to intercept the Y axis. The intercept at time zero gives the value B and the slope β. By subtracting point 1 (the plasma concentration during the distribution phase) from point 2 (the corresponding plasma concentration on the extrapolated elimination phase line) the difference can be plotted as point 3. This is done at several time intervals of the distribution phase and the 'difference' points constitute a line with an intercept at time zero A and a slope α. Mathematically, the plasma concentration-time relationship can be expressed by the equation:

$$C = Ae^{-\alpha t} + Be^{-\beta t} \qquad (18)$$

where C is the drug concentration in plasma at time t.

For some drugs, the plasma curve shows two distribution phases which are best satisfied by a three-compartment model (*see* Fig. 47.5) and characterized by a triexponential equation. The decision about the number of exponentials in the equation which best describes the concentration-time data and, therefore, the number of compartments is usually done by a statistical test. There is no pharmacological significance to the particular model for which the drug conforms. More frequent and intensive sampling immediately after drug administration tends to yield data that must be described by equations containing more exponential terms than would be required by less frequent and intensive sampling.

Non-Linear Pharmacokinetics

At usual therapeutic concentrations, first-order or linear processes describe the pharmacokinetic behavior of most drugs. For a few drugs, however, one or more processes governing drug disposition may deviate from such behavior. There are at least three reasons for this. The most common is saturable metabolism in the liver. At high plasma concentrations of drugs like thiopentone (Stanski et al., 1980), phenytoin and salicylates, the enzyme systems for their biotransformation become saturated and their elimination proceeds at a fixed rate (zero-order or Michaelis–Menten model). A second cause is that plasma protein binding may not be constant in the concentration range studied. As the concentration of the drug increases in plasma, the amount of unbound drug will increase as binding sites become saturated. For example, the unbound fraction of salicylate is approximately twice as great at a concentration of 1 mmol/L as compared to 0.1 mmol/L. A third cause of non-linearity is the presence of carrier-mediated active transport process for the drug which is saturable. As an example, the clearance of penicillin by the kidney depends on active carrier-mediated secretory processes as well as first-order processes. The important implication of non-linear kinetics is that half-life is no longer a constant but changes as a function of drug concentration. During multiple-dose or continuous infusion therapy, the steady-state plasma concentration will not be proportional to the dose. Instead, a given increase in dosage will result in a rapidly increasing excessively high concentration.

CLINICAL APPLICATIONS

Plasma Target Concentration Strategy

The plasma target concentration strategy is one in which a steady state mean plasma concentration of a drug is chosen as a therapeutic objective, rather than some physiological end-point. This is particularly useful for drugs where there is a wide individual variability in pharmacokinetics and/or a small therapeutic index. Also, for some drugs the pharmacological response is not easily quantifiable particularly when the drug is given for prophylactic purposes. (Examples include lignocaine, lithium, phenytoin, theophylline, etc.) Three criteria must be met for monitoring plasma drug concentrations: the intensity of drug action must be proportional to its concentration at the receptor site, the latter must be proportional to the free concentration in the plasma and the effect–time curve must parallel that of concentration (Greenblatt and Shader, 1985).

There have been some studies of the plasma concentrations needed to produce analgesia or unconsciousness with opioids (Hug, 1984; Ausems et al., 1986) and anesthesia with intravenous anesthetics (Becker, 1978; Hudson et al., 1983). However, the anesthetist needs on-line methods to measure drug concentrations during surgery if he is to use these data or others to adjust the dosage of anesthetic drugs.

Rational Dosage Regimens

The simplest kinetic model, the one compartment open model, allows us to adopt a sensible approach to the calculation of dosage regimens (Rowland, 1978).

Loading dose. The initial loading dose of a drug needed to achieve a certain plasma concentration depends only upon the volume of distribution, that is on the size of the single compartment to be filled.

$$\text{LD} = V_d \times C_p \qquad (19)$$

LD is the loading dose, V_d is the volume of distribution and C_p is the desired plasma concentration.

Repetitive dosing. With repeated administration of a drug, its concentration reaches a plateau or steady state. This state is reached because the rate at which the drug is removed becomes equal to the rate of its entry into the body. At steady state, the rate of elimination of the drug depends only upon the clearance times the plasma concentration.

$$\text{MD} = Cl \times C_p \qquad (20)$$

where MD is the maintenance dose.

Example: If we assume that a sufentanil plasma concentration of $0.2\,\mu g/L$ would be effective in supplementing nitrous oxide and oxygen anesthesia without causing excessive postoperative respiratory depression and knowing that the volume of distribution of the drug is approximately 3 L/kg and its clearance 12 ml/(kg·min); the loading and maintenance doses can be calculated approximately as follows:

$$\text{Loading Dose} = 0.2 \times 3 = 0.6\,\mu g/kg$$
$$\text{Maintenance Dose} = 0.2 \times 0.012 \times 60\,\text{min/h}$$
$$= 0.14\,\mu g/(kg \cdot h)$$

Dosing Interval. Usually a series of maintenance doses are required to keep the drug concentration at the therapeutic level. The frequency of dosing needs, therefore, to be determined. A rational dosing interval for most drugs approximates the elimination half-life. If the drug is administered at more frequent intervals, significant accumulation may occur, while at longer intervals, the drug may stay below the minimum effective concentration (i.e. becomes clinically ineffective) for a good part of the time (Fig. 47.9).

Continuous Infusion. The use of intermittent injections results in a peak and valley effect in drug concentrations (Fig. 47.9); some time the drug concentration is too low to be effective, and other times the drug concentration is too high leading to toxicity. The use of an infusion eliminates these fluctuations in plasma concentrations and results in decreased dosage requirements and a better therapeutic response (White, 1983).

There are several methods available to design infusion regimens (Fig. 47.10) and calculate the rates required to achieve a certain plasma concentration.

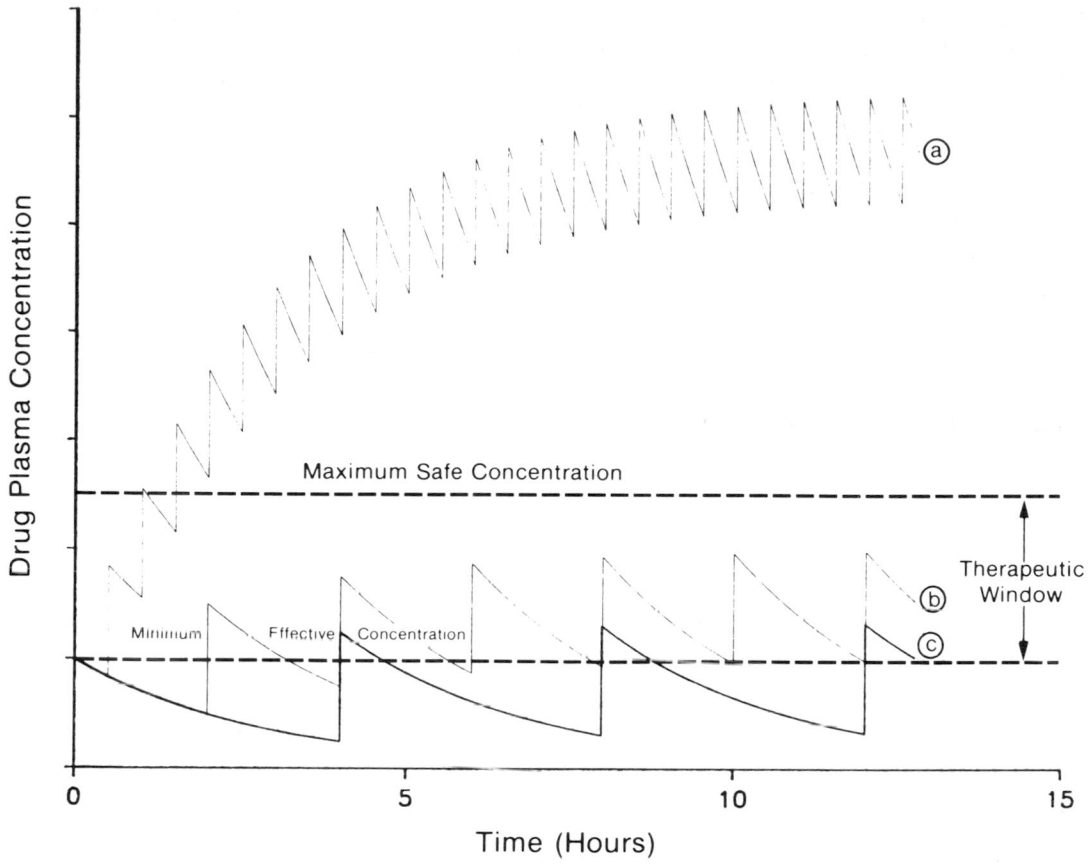

Fig. 47.9 Simulated plasma concentrations of a drug with an elimination half-life of 2 hours following administration of the same dose every 0.5 hour (curve a), every 2 hours (curve b), and every 4 hours (curve c).

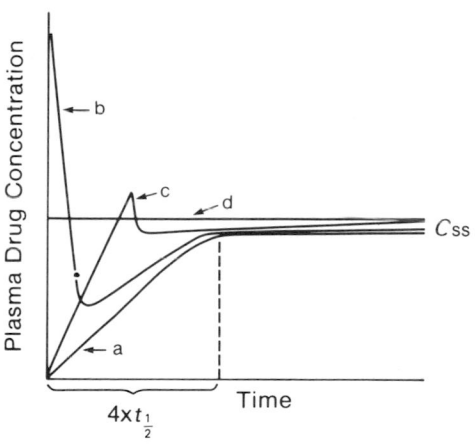

Fig. 47.10 Schematic plasma concentration curves following four infusion methods. (a) Constant rate infusion. (b) Loading dose followed by a constant rate infusion. The initial dose only fills the central compartment. (c) Two rate infusion. (d) Variable rate infusion after Vaughan and Tucker (1976). C_{ss} is the concentration at steady state which is also the target concentration. $t_{\frac{1}{2}}$ is the drug half life.

(1.) A constant rate infusion. At steady state the plasma concentration is dependent only on the clearance (equation 20), but the target concentration will not be approached for at least four half-lives. (2.) A loading dose followed by a constant rate infusion. If one starts with a loading dose, the target concentration will be reached more rapidly. The loading dose can be calculated according to equation 19. In the case of a multi-compartment model, if the bolus dose only 'loads' the central compartment at time zero, the plasma concentration will decrease rapidly as the drug is distributed to the other comparatment(s) before increasing gradually towards the target concentration due to the infusion. If the bolus is large enough to 'load' all compartments, the plasma concentration will not decrease below the target concentration. However, the initial plasma concentration will greatly exceed the target concentration which may lead to toxicity. (3.) A two-rate infusion. Wagner (1974) described two sequential infusions for a two compartment model; an initial rapid one to fill the central compartment followed by a slower one to fill the peripheral compartment. Variables needed for calculation are the clearance and half-life of a given drug. This type of infusion will not expose the patient to a large initial dose of the drug, but achievement of the steady state plasma concentration will be rather slow, particularly if the time of administration of the initial infusion is long (4.) Variable rate infusion. Vaughan and Tucker (1976) described a more complex regimen. Their method involves a bolus dose to fill the central compartment, followed by a maintenance infusion together with an exponentially declining infusion superimposed upon the maintenance rate, which would compensate for movement of drug into the peripheral compartment(s).

Clinical application of infusion schemes can be aided by computer-assisted infusion pumps. The user provides the computer with the appropriate pharmacokinetic data for the specific drug. The computer then drives an infusion pump to administer the drug to the desired plasma concentration. If the clinical response needs to be changed, the user increases or decreases the target plasma concentration (Schüttler et al., 1983; Ausems et al., 1985).

SUMMARY

Pharmacokinetics accounts quantitatively for the fate of drugs in the body and relates this information to their pharmacological responses. The knowledge assists the physician in establishing and maintaining therapeutic yet nontoxic amounts of drugs in the body and at the pharmacologic site of action. Once a drug reaches the blood stream, it is distributed to various tissues of the body. The rate and extent of distribution are determined by how well each tissue is perfused with blood, the binding of drug to plasma proteins and tissue components and the permeability of tissue membranes to the drug. Elimination of the drug becomes more important as distribution progresses in time. It occurs by metabolism and/or excretion. Mathematical models have been developed to explain the distribution and elimination processes, which conceive the body to consist of compartments. Three pharmacokinetic parameters are related and are of particular importance: half-life, the time it takes for the drug plasma concentration to be reduced by 50%; volume of distribution, a measure of the apparent space in the body available to contain the drug; and clearance, a measure of the body's ability to eliminate the drug. The initial loading dose depends only upon the volume of distribution. With repeated dosing, the time to achieve a steady state depends on the drug's half-life, whereas the actual drug level achieved depends only on clearance. There has been a recent interest by anesthetists in administration of drugs by continuous infusions. Pharmacokinetics is particularly useful in the design of these regimens. However, the mathematical precision provided may be counterbalanced by interpatient variability. The clinician should measure the drug effect whenever feasible (e.g.

by monitoring the muscle twitch in the case of muscle relaxants) and adjust the dose accordingly.

Acknowledgement
The authors thank R. Spector, M.D. for his contribution to the previous edition of this chapter.

REFERENCES

General

Rowland M., Tozer T.N. (1980). *Clinical Pharmacokinetics: Concepts and Applications*, Philadelphia: Lea & Febiger.
Stanski D.F., Watkins W.D. (1982). *Drug Disposition in Anesthesia*, New York: Grune & Stratton.

Specific

Ausems M.E., Stanski D.R., Hug C.C. Jr. (1985). An evaluation of the accuracy of pharmacokinetic data for the computer assisted infusion of alfentanil. *Br. J. Anaesth.*, **57**, 1217.
Ausems M.E., Hug C.C. Jr., Stanski D.R., et al. (1986). Plasma concentrations of alfentanil required to supplement nitrous oxide anesthesia for general surgery. *Anesthesiology*, **65**, 362.
Becker K.E. (1978). Plasma levels of thiopental necessary for anesthesia. *Anesthesiology*, **49**, 192.
Biehl D., Shnider S.M., Levinson G., et al. (1978). Placental transfer of lidocaine: effects of fetal acidosis. *Anesthesiology*, **48**, 409.
Bradbury M. (1979). *The Concept of a Blood–Brain Barrier*, pp. 84–115. New York: John Wiley & Sons.
Brodie B.B., Mark L.C., Papper E.M., et al. (1950). The fate of thiopental in man and a method for its estimation in biological material. *J. Pharmacol. Exp. Ther.*, **98**, 85.
Burch P.G., Stanski D.R. (1983). The role of metabolism and protein binding in thiopental anesthesia. *Anesthesiology*, **58**, 146.
Dedrick R.L., Bischoff K.B. (1968). Pharmacokinetics in applications of the artificial kidney. *Chem. Eng. Prog. Symp. Ser.*, **64**, 32.
Deutsch S. (1975). Effects of anesthetics on the kidney. *Surg. Clin. North Am.*, **55**, 775.
Ghoneim M.M., Pandya H.B., Kelley S.E., et al. (1976). Binding of thiopental to plasma proteins: effects on distribution in the brain and heart. *Anesthesiology*, **45**, 635.
Ghoneim M.M., Hinrichs J.V., Mewaldt S.P. (1984). Dose-response analysis of the behavioural effects of diazepam: I., Learning and memory. *Psychopharmacology*, **82**, 291.
Ghoneim M.M., Hinrichs J.V., Chiang C-K., et al. (1986). Pharmacokinetic and pharmacodynamic interactions between caffeine and diazepam. *Clin. Psychopharmacal.*, **6**, 75.
Gibaldi M., Davidson D., Plaut M.E., et al. (1970). Modification of penicillin distribution and elimination by probenecid. *Int. Z. Klin. Pharmakol. Ther. Toxicol.*, **3**, 182.
Gladtke E., von Hattingberg W. (1979). *Pharmacokinetics. An Introduction*, p. 10, New York: Springer-Verlag.
Goldstein A., Aronow L., Kalman S.M. (1974). Drug elimination: the major routes. In *Principles of Drug Action: The Basis of Pharmacology*, pp. 210–216, second edn., New York: John Wiley & Sons.

Greenblatt D.J., Shader R.I. (1985). *Pharmacokinetics in Clinical Practice*, p. 95, Philadelphia: W.B. Saunders.

Hudson R.J., Stanski D.R., Saidman L.J., et al. (1983). A model for studying depth of anesthesia and acute tolerance to thiopental. *Anesthesiology*, **59**, 301.

Hug C.C. Jr. (1984). Pharmacokinetics of new synthetic narcotic analgesics. In *Opioids in Anesthesia*, pp. 50–60. (Estafanous F.G., ed.), Boston: Butterworth.

Kennedy R.L., Erenberg A., Robillard J.E., et al. (1979). Effects of changes in maternal-fetal pH on the transplacental equilibrium of bupivacaine. *Anesthesiology*, **51**, 50.

Klotz U. (1976). Pathophysiological and disease-induced changes in drug distribution volume: pharmacokinetic implications. *Clin. Pharmacokin.*, **1**, 204.

Koch-Weser J., Sellers E.M. (1976). Binding of drugs to serum albumin. *N. Engl. J. Med.*, **294**, 311.

Korttila K., Linnoila M., Ertama P., et al. (1975). Recovery and simulated driving after intravenous anesthesia with thiopental, methohexital, propanidid, or alphadione. *Anesthesiology*, **43**, 291.

Lorenzo A.V., Spector R. (1976). The distribution of drugs in the central nervous system. In *Transport Phenomena in the Nervous System*, pp. 447–461. (Levi, Battistin and Lajtha, eds.) New York: Plenum Press.

Mapleson W.W. (1963). An electric analogue for uptake and exchange of inert gases and other agents. *J. Appl. Physiol.*, **18**, 197.

Piafsky K.M., Borga O. (1977). Plasma protein binding of basic drugs. II. Importance of α_1-acid glycoprotein for interindividual variation. *Clin. Pharmacol. Ther.*, **22**, 545.

Price H.L. (1960). A dynamic concept of the distribution of thiopental in the human body. *Anesthesiology*, **21**, 40.

Roth K.M. (1983). Regulation of intracellular acid–base equilibrium in rats. *Acta Anaesthesiol. Scand.*, **27**, 443.

Routledge P.A. (1986). The plasma protein binding of basic drugs. *Br. J. Clin. Pharmacal.*, **22**, 499.

Rowland M. (1978). Drug administration and regimens. In *Clinical Pharmacology. Basic Principles in Therapeutics*, pp. 25–70. (Melmon and Morrelli, eds.) New York: MacMillan.

Saidman L.J. (1974). Uptake, distribution and elemination of barbiturates. In *Anaesthetic Uptake and Action*, Chap. 17 (Eger E.I. II ed.) Baltimore: The Williams and Wilkins Company.

Schüttler J., Schwilden H., Stoekel H. (1983). Pharmacokinetics as applied to total intravenous anaesthesia. *Anaesthesia* (Suppl.), **38**, 53.

Shader R.I., Dreyfuss D., Gerrein J.R., et al. (1986). Sedative effects and impaired learning and recall after single oral doses of lorazepam. *Clin. Pharmacol. Ther.*, **39**, 526.

Smith N.T., Zwart A., Benchen J.E.W. (1972). Interaction between the circulatory effects and the uptake and distribution of halothane. *Anesthesiology*, **37**, 47.

Stanski D.R., Mihm F.G., Rosenthal M.H., et al. (1980). Pharmacokinetics of high-dose thiopental used in cerebral resuscitation. *Anesthesiology*, **53**, 169.

Stoeckel H., Hengstmann J.H., Schüttler J. (1979). Pharmacokinetics of fentanyl as a possible explanation for recurrence of respiratory depression. *Br. J. Anaesth.*, **51**, 741.

Song C.S., Merkatz I.R., Rifkind A.B., et al. (1970). The influence of pregnancy and oral contraceptive steroids on the concentration of plasma proteins. *Am. J. Obstet. Gynecol.*, **108**, 227.

Vallner J.J. (1977). Binding of drugs by albumin and plasma protein. *J. Pharm. Sci.*, **66**, 447.

Vaughan D.P., Tucker G.T. (1976). General derivation of the ideal intravenous drug input required to achieve and maintain a constant plasma drug concentration. Theoretical application to lignocaine therapy. *Eur. J. Clin. Pharmacol.*, **10**, 433.

Waddell W.J., Butler T.C. (1957). The distribution and excretion of phenobarbital. *J. Clin. Invest.*, **36**, 1217.

Waddell W.J., Bates R.G. (1969). Intracellular pH, *Physiol. Reviews*, **49**, 285.

Wagner J.G. (1974). A safe method for rapidly achieving plasma concentration plateaus. *Clin. Pharmacol. Ther.*, **16**, 691.

Wallace S.M., Verbeeck R.K. (1987). Plasma protein binding of drugs in the elderly. *Clin. Pharmacokin*, **12**, 41.

White P.F., Marietta M.P., Pudwill C.R., et al. (1976). Effects of halothane anaesthesia on the biodisposition of ketamine in rats. *J. Pharm. Exp. Ther.*, **196**, 545.

White P.F. (1983). Use of continuous infusion versus intermittent bolus administration of fentanyl or ketamine during outpatient anesthesia. *Anesthesiology*, **59**, 294.

Wilkinson G.R., Shand D.G. (1975). A physiological approach to hepatic drug clearance. *Clin. Pharmacol. Ther.*, **18**, 377.

Wilkinson G.R. (1976). Pharmacokinetics in disease states modifying body perfusion. In *The Effect of Disease States on Drug Pharmacokinetics*, pp. 13–32. (Benet L.Z. ed.), Washington, D.C.: American Pharmaceutical Association.

Wood M., Wood A.J.J. (1981). Changes in plasma drug binding and α_1-acid glycoprotein in mother and newborn infant. *Clin. Pharmacol. Ther.*, **29**, 522.

Yoshikawa T., Sugiyama Y., Sawada Y., et al. (1984). Effect of late pregnancy on salicylate, diazepam, warfarin, and propranolol binding: use of fluorescent probes. *Clin Pharmacol. Ther.*, **36**, 201.

48. The Pharmacokinetics of Inhalational Anaesthetic Agents

C. Hull

When an anaesthetic gas or vapour is inhaled, it mixes with gases already in the pulmonary alveoli, crosses into the arterial blood, and is distributed to all tissues of the body. That which enters the brain diffuses from capillary to the biophase, where it interacts directly with 'target structures'. To a great extent these are as yet undefined, but may be regarded here as hydrophobic sites on neuronal cell membranes, interaction with which induces the state we call anaesthesia. If this process were allowed to continue for a very long period an equilibrium would be reached at which the anaesthetic concentrations in the inspired gas, alveoli, arterial blood, brain interstitial fluid and biophase would be constant.

The *manner* in which this equilibrium is approached is of primary importance to the clinical anaesthetist since rarely, if ever, will a surgical procedure require anaesthesia so prolonged that steady state is actually achieved. It is not sufficient to *observe* that some anaesthetic agents seem to act more rapidly than others, and that some are more potent than others; we must know *why*. In the process of finding out we may also discover why the concentrations in gas, blood, brain, muscle, liver etc. are all different at equilibrium! The study of uptake distribution and elimination of drugs is called *pharmacokinetics*. Of course, there is an important step between the arrival of a drug at its site of action and the appearance of some pharmacolog-

ical effect. There may be many complex processes contributing to this step, and they are encompassed by the term *pharmacodynamics*. Holford expressed the distinction between the two processes very neatly. *Pharmacokinetics is what the body does to the drug, while pharmacodynamics is what the drug does to the body.*

This chapter considers the pharmacokinetics of inhaled vapours and gases in an essentially non-mathematical way, although some equations are, unfortunately, inevitable.

MOLECULES IN GASES AND SOLUTIONS

Before considering the complexities of gas uptake and distribution in the body, we must understand the physical laws governing the processes involved. Consider a closed system (Fig. 48.1) which contains some liquid L_1 above which is a mixture of two soluble gases A and B. The total pressure in the gas phase is 100 kPa (1 bar), which approximates to 1 atmosphere.

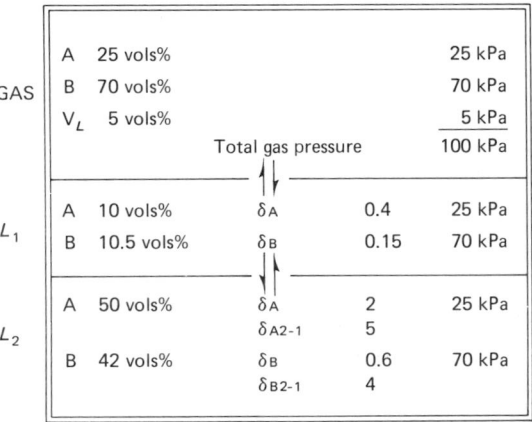

Fig. 48.1 Solubility of gases in liquids. A closed system at pressure 100 kPa contains two gases A and B, which dissolve in liquid L_1. The gas phase also contains vapour V_L from liquid L_1, which exerts a vapour pressure. A second liquid phase L_2 lies beneath L_1, into which dissolved gases may diffuse. The partial pressure of each gas remains constant in all phases, but the volumes of gases in the two liquids vary according to solubility. From the dissolved volumes it can be calculated that gas A has a partition coefficient between the two liquids (δ_{A2-1}) of 50/10 = 5. Similarly, δ_{B2-1} = 42/10.5 = 4. *See* following sections on solubility, partition coefficients and gas tension.

The system can be described in familiar terms. Each gas will exert a *partial pressure* as if it alone were present, and the sum of the partial pressures is the total pressure (Dalton's law of partial pressures). The partial pressures reflect the fractional concentrations of the three components by volume (remembering that the liquid evaporates to exert its own partial, or vapour pressure). Thus gas A exerts $0.25 \times 100 = 25$ kPa, and gas B, $0.7 \times 100 = 70$ kPa. The vapour

L_1 amounting to 5% of the gas phase (V_L), exerts $0.05 \times 100 = 5\,kPa$.

Each of the gases dissolves to some extent in the liquid. In each case the amount dissolved is proportional to the partial pressure in the gas phase (Henry's law). However, we find that at equilibrium the liquid contains more molecules of A than B, despite the greater partial pressure of B. This is because A is more soluble than B.

Solubility and Partition Coefficients

Solubility is usually expressed as the Ostwald coefficient, this being the volume of gas dissolving in unit volume of liquid at some stated temperature. It can also be expressed as a partition coefficient δ, which is the ratio of the amounts of gas in the two phases at some stated temperature. This more general definition can be compared directly with partition coefficients between other phases, and is, in fact, numerically identical to the Ostwald coefficient. Thus if the liquid contains 10 vol.% of gas A, the solubility coefficient is: $0.1 \div 0.25 = 0.4$. The liquid contains 10.5 vol.% of gas B, whose solubility coefficient is: $0.105 \div 0.7 = 0.15$.

What *determines* the pressure exerted by the two gases, and the concentrations they reach in the liquid at equilibrium?

Gas molecules can be seen as vibrationally energetic particles which occupy an infinitesimally small proportion of the space, travelling at random and colliding only with the boundaries, thus exerting a pressure. Interactions between gas molecules are insignificant. This pressure depends upon the number and energy of boundary collisions. In fact it is closely related to the temperature-dependent thermodynamic quantity known as *chemical potential*, which expresses the tendency by which a gas tends to escape through its boundaries; the higher the energy with which molecules strike the boundary, the greater the probability that some will escape. This determines the rate at which gas molecules enter the liquid phase of our system; i.e. dissolve.

When molecules enter the liquid they continue to move and exert forces upon their boundaries. However, interactions with liquid molecules are now very numerous, Van der Waal's attractive forces tending to reduce the energy with which gas molecules strike the boundaries, thereby reducing also the probability of escape into the gas phase. Thus equal *concentrations* of molecules in the two phases will be associated with very *unequal* numbers of boundary crossings in the two directions. Clearly, there will be a net transfer of molecules into solution until the rates of boundary crossings are equal. This will occur when the concentration of gas molecules in solution rises to a level where the greater number of collisions compensates for the lower probability of escape. A gas whose energy is reduced by interaction with the liquid must reach a higher concentration before equilibrium is

reached; in other words it is more soluble. At equilibrium the chemical potentials of the gas in the two phases are equal.

Chemical Potential and Tension

In the gas phase we can see the chemical potential expressed clearly as the *partial pressure* of the gas. In the liquid phase it is more difficult, but we use the word *tension* to express that quantity which makes gas molecules leave solution at the same rate as they enter at a given partial pressure. Tension is conveniently expressed in terms of the *pressure* which it can support in an adjacent gas phase, and therefore has the dimensions and units of pressure, such as mmHg or kPa.

Partition Coefficients with Other Liquid Phases

The argument can be extended to other liquid phases. If gas A in solution reaches a permeable membrane on the other side of which is a second liquid phase L_2, in which it is more soluble, concentration in that phase will increase until equilibrium is reached.

We can state confidently that since L_2 is in equilibrium with a liquid phase that supports $25\,kPa$ gas pressure, it also *would* support $25\,kPa$, and therefore can be stated to have a *tension* of $25\,kPa$. Thus the 'driving force' which brings dissolved gases to equilibrium is not *concentration* but *tension*, or more explicitly, chemical potential.

We have seen that the process by which a gas dissolves in the blood and then distributes to different tissues depends upon *tension*. At equilibrium, the gas *tensions* in the alveoli and all tissues will be very similar, the only exceptions being those tissues from which gas molecules are eliminated by metabolism or other means.

Lipid Solubility and Potency

At the hydrophobic site of action, we can safely retain the Meyer–Overton concept of a critical gas concentration in a lipid phase. While many new concepts struggle to explain *how* this leads to anaesthesia, it remains axiomatic that it *does*. The implication is that in this 'target' lipid phase it is concentration that matters; therefore in adjoining aqueous phases (such as interstitial fluid) the anaesthetic concentration is that which, when partitioned with the lipid target, will result in the critical concentration therein. Thus a certain level of anaesthesia will be attained at a much lower plasma concentration of a very lipid-soluble agent, such as trichloroethylene, than a poorly lipid-soluble gas such as nitrous oxide. As may be expected, there is a close relationship between lipid solubility and potency over several orders of magnitude.

Diffusion Through Membranes

So far we have considered only the transfer of gas

molecules between phases, and then only at equilibrium. In the body, phases are separated by membranes through which anaesthetic gas molecules must pass. Anaesthetic gases cross cell membranes by simple diffusion along tension gradients, and Graham's law states that the rate of diffusion is proportional to the square root of molecular size. For a simple membrane area A and thickness X the actual rate of drug transfer is

$$K \cdot A \cdot (\phi_1 - \phi_2)/X,$$

where $(\phi_1 - \phi_2)$ is the tension gradient and K the diffusion constant for the substance concerned.

However, red cell membranes are selectively permeable, so that small, lipid-soluble substances can pass more rapidly than those which are large, lipid-insoluble or worse still, highly ionized. All anaesthetic gas molecules are small (MW < 200) and relatively lipid-soluble. Nitrous oxide, the least lipid-soluble, is also the smallest (MW 44). In practice, all anaesthetic gas molecules cross cell membranes quite rapidly, so that diffusion is not a limiting step in the onset of anaesthesia.

PHYSICOCHEMICAL CHARACTERISTICS OF ANAESTHETIC AGENTS

It is evident that the rates of diffusion and partitioning of individual gases depend largely upon solubility coefficients. The most important are those which determine how the gas molecules distribute to various body tissues. Some important values are listed in Table 48.1.

The table is organized in descending order of blood/gas partition coefficient. Although there are some notable exceptions, this order applies also to the oil/gas coefficient. Brain/blood and muscle/blood coefficients are generally small, indicating that solubility in blood is a broad indicator of solubilities in other tissues.

THE DISPOSITION OF ANAESTHETIC GASES

Let us start by making some assumptions and definitions. We will assume that the gas is inert; that is, it exists in *simple solution* and does not bind selectively to proteins, cell membranes etc. Similarly, it is not *metabolized* to any significant degree (not true for agents such as halothane, but a reasonable simplification). *Pulmonary ventilation* can be seen as a simple process of equilibration between the partial pressures (gas tensions) of inspired and alveolar gases. Similarly, the *circulation* provides an equilibrating pathway between lung and each tissue of the body. Each major tissue group can be considered as a *compartment*. This can be defined as a homogeneous space into which a certain *volume* of gas distributes. We will deal in *volumes* of gas rather than masses, since all gases at the same temperature and pressure contain the same number of molecules (Avogadro's hypothesis), and therefore (ideally) behave identically. The use of mass requires correction for the molecular weight of each substance, and adds nothing to clarity.

Apparent Volume of a Compartment

The increase of gas tension following the addition of unit volume of gas depends upon the volume into which it *appears* to distribute; the *apparent volume*. If the compartment contains only gas (such as would be true for the lung), or has a solubility coefficient of 1, the apparent volume V_C will equate with the physical volume V_P, and the gas tension ϕ will continue to be the product of fractional concentration (by volume) and volume F_{GAS} and atmospheric pressure P_{ATM}. However, if the gas is more soluble in some compartment, the increase in tension following the addition of unit gas volume would be smaller than might be expected from the *physical* volume. Thus so far as *tension* is concerned, the apparent volume is larger than the physical volume. The mathematics are very simple: $V_C = V_P \cdot \delta$.

For a given gas volume V_{GAS} dissolved in a compartment of volume V_C, the tension can be calculated as the product of fractional concentration (by volume) and atmospheric pressure P_{ATM}. Thus: $\phi = F_{GAS} \cdot P_{ATM}$.

We will also assume that gas tensions in the various compartments will equilibrate with that in the lung in a *first-order* manner; that is, they will approach equi-

TABLE 48.1
DATA FROM EGER, 1980

	Blood/gas	Brain/blood	Muscle/blood	Fat/blood	Oil/gas
Nitrogen	0.015				
Nitrous oxide	0.47	1.1	1.2	2.3	1.4
Cyclopropane	0.5	0.76	1.2	13	12
Isoflurane	1.4	2.6	4.0	45	98
Enflurane	1.8	1.4	1.7	36	98
Halothane	2.3	2.3	3.5	60	224
Trichloroethylene	9	1.7	1.5	52	714
Diethyl ether	12	1.0	1.0	3.7	65
Methoxyflurane	12	1.7	1.3	49	970

librium at any time at a rate proportional to the tension gradient at that time.

The body may now be seen as a system of compartments, with the rates of equilibration between them determined by first-order rate constants. This could be characterized by a set of first-order differential equations, solution of which will predict the tension in any compartment at any time, following any stated initial conditions. To most clinicians such equations are decidedly unfriendly, and do nothing to improve our understanding of gas kinetics! This difficulty can be overcome by allowing a computer (Mapleson, 1978) to solve the equations, and then present the information in a more palatable form. Mapleson has derived an elegant analogue model based upon containers of water, which behaves mathematically in precisely the same manner as the compartmental model, and is a valuable aid to comprehension (Mapleson, 1984). The volume of water in each container (Fig. 48.2) represents the volume of gas in a compartment, and the water level represents gas tension.

The surface area of each container represents that container's capacity for water (or gas), since it determines how much the water level (tension) will rise for a given added volume of water (gas). On reflection, this must be the apparent volume of distribution V_C. The interconnecting pipes represent the transfer clearances, with high clearances represented by wide bores and *vice versa*. The inspired gas tension is seen as a source container with an appropriate water level

which remains constant despite gas uptake into the model. We can use the analogue model to understand the processes underlying the induction, maintenance and recovery phases of inhalational anaesthesia.

Gas Uptake from a Constant Inspired Concentration

As can be seen from the model (Fig. 48.2) inhaled gas passes through a cascade of compartments before reaching the site of action in the brain. We will consider these in turn.

Pulmonary Exchange

First consider the gas tension in the pulmonary alveoli. In model terms, fresh gas comes from a reservoir whose water level remains constant. When the tap is turned on, the water level in the 'lung' container rises rapidly, and as the patient breathes, each tidal volume brings the alveolar tension nearer to that in inspired air. If none were to pass on to other compartments equilibration would be attained rapidly. The rate of equilibration is clearly dependent upon alveolar ventilation, or, in the model, the diameter of the 'ventilation' pipe.

Uptake into the Bloodstream

In fact, the alveolar gas equilibrates even more rapidly with arterial blood, so that pulmonary venous blood has almost the same tension as that in the alveoli. As the alveolar tension rises, uptake into the bloodstream

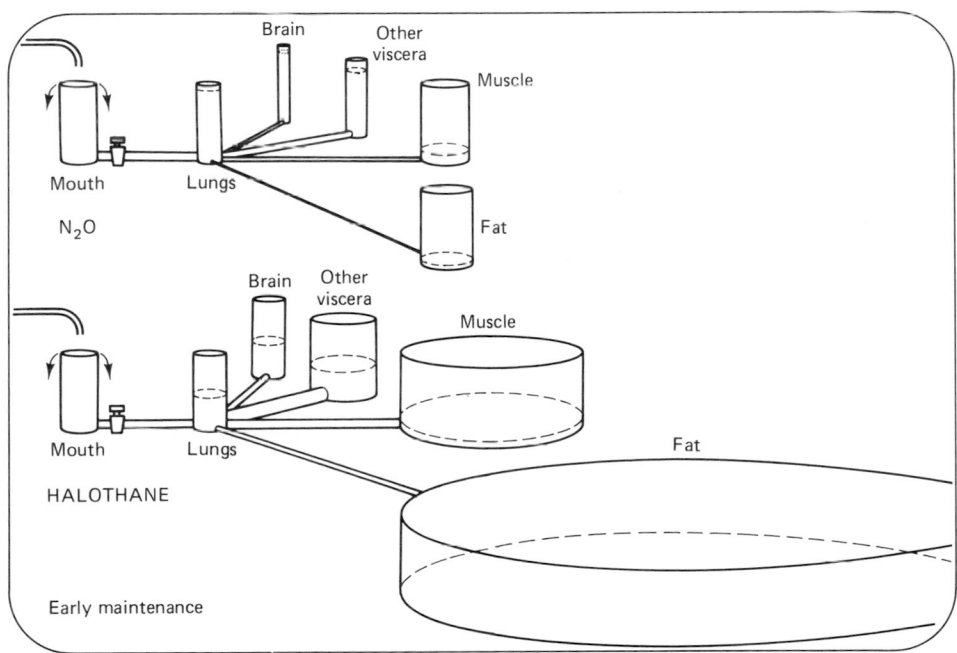

Fig. 48.2 Mapleson's water analogue models for the disposition of nitrous oxide and halothane. The water levels in this illustration correspond to the early maintenance phase. Note that this simple model for nitrous oxide does *not* account for the concentration effect. (Reproduced with permission from Mapleson, 1984. Pharmacokinetics of inhaled anaesthetics. In *Pharmacokinetics of Anaesthesia*, pp. 89–111. (Prys-Roberts C., Hug Jr. C.C., eds.). Oxford: Blackwell Scientific Publications.)

increases in direct proportion. Thus during the initial *mixing* phase alveolar tension rises very rapidly as successive tidal volumes mix with the FRC. This is followed quickly by an *uptake* phase, during which increasing quantities of alveolar gas are absorbed into the bloodstream and alveolar tension therefore rises more slowly. Since alveolar tension rises more slowly, so does arterial blood tension and finally brain tension. During this uptake phase, the tissue compartments fill with gas at rates determined by their respective volumes and clearances. Later, in an *equilibration* phase, the rate of increase diminishes further as the tension gradients between alveolar and tissue compartments become even smaller and the whole system approaches equilibrium. Eventually a steady state is achieved, at which alveolar tension is constant and uptake is limited to replacement of gas eliminated by non-pulmonary routes (*see later*).

During the early phases alveolar tension can be seen as the resultant of two opposing tendencies; ventilation causing an increase and uptake causing a decrease. If the gas is (like nitrogen) very blood-insoluble the fractional concentration of gas dissolved in blood (F_{GAS}) is also small, with uptake having very little effect upon alveolar concentration. Thus arterial tension rises at almost the same rate as alveolar tension. If the gas is also very insoluble in brain tissues, the tension in brain interstitial fluid and biophase follows suit, with the patient losing consciousness very rapidly indeed.

However, anaesthetic gases are all much more soluble than nitrogen ($\delta = 0.015$). Nitrous oxide is 30 times more soluble ($\delta = 0.47$), while methoxyflurane is 380 times more soluble than nitrogen ($\delta = 12$). Thus uptake into pulmonary capillary blood *does* have a significant effect upon alveolar tension, especially in the case of the more soluble gases.

Distribution to Tissues
Blood leaving the pulmonary circulation distributes the dissolved gas to all tissues of the body. Some, like brain and viscera are well-perfused, while others, such as resting muscle, are less so. Body fat is very poorly perfused. In the model these differences are apparent from the differing bores of the tubes connecting 'lung' to the tissues concerned. The apparent volumes of distribution for each compartment vary with both physical volume and solubility coefficient. Thus apparent muscle volume is larger than brain, but smaller than fat. When comparing agents of differing solubilities, the apparent volumes for halothane are seen to be much larger than those for nitrous oxide. The connecting pipes are also wider, reflecting the greater transport capacity of blood for a soluble agent.

Equilibration with Tissues
All the tissue compartments can be seen as equilibrating with gas tension in the lung. Body fat may take days to reach steady state, so that gas tensions in fat and pulmonary alveoli are likely to differ widely

throughout anaesthesia. Obviously, such a compartment has almost no influence upon the gas tension in lung and well-perfused tissues. By contrast, the visceral and muscle compartments have a profound effect if the agent is even moderately soluble, since their combined effect (Fig. 48.3) is to restrict severely the rate at which lung tension can rise towards the inspired value.

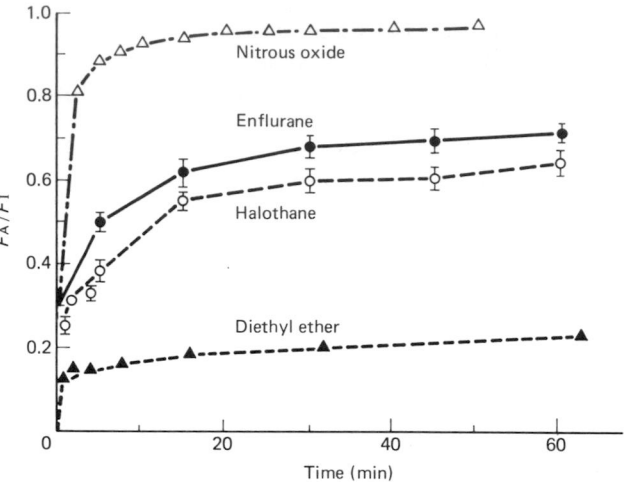

Fig. 48.3 The rate at which alveolar concentration F_A rises towards inspired concentration F_I when breathing a constant inspired gas mixture. If all gases behaved identically, then plots of F_A/F_I would all follow the same path, regardless of concentration. In most part, the *differences* are due to variations in blood-gas partition coefficient (δ). Thus N_2O ($\delta = 0.47$) rises very rapidly, while diethyl ether ($\delta = 12$) equilibrates very slowly. Halothane and enflurane have intermediate characteristics. (Reproduced with permission from Eger, 1980. Inhalational anaesthesia: pharmacokinetics. In *General Anaesthesia*, 4th edn., pp. 67–97. (Gray T.C., Nunn J.F., Utting J.E., eds.). London: Butterworths.)

Equilibration with Brain and Biophase
A small, well-perfused compartment, such as brain, will lag only slightly behind lung tension. This is very important, since onset of anaesthesia may be expected to follow rapidly upon attainment of an effective tension in the lung. For a relatively insoluble agent such as nitrous oxide the apparent volume of the brain is small and equilibration is very rapid indeed. However, halothane, and to an even greater extent trichloroethylene are soluble in brain tissue (Table 48.1). As a result, brain tension 'lags' significantly behind arterial tension.

Perfusion also plays an important role, and alterations in cerebral bloodflow have a significant effect on the rate of equilibration.

Halothane vs Nitrous Oxide
It might appear difficult to compare the uptake characteristics of two agents with such differing potency, which must be administered in very different concen-

trations. In fact they *can* be compared (Fig. 48.3) by plotting alveolar tension as a fraction of the inspired tension (F_A/F_I) against time, thereby normalizing the two gases for inspired concentration.

Using this construct, all gases with identical uptake and distribution kinetics should follow identical paths, regardless of potency. In fact, alveolar tension of a moderately blood-soluble agent such as halothane rises much more slowly than that of nitrous oxide. This is mainly because continuing equilibration with large compartments, such as muscle, has a marked braking effect upon the rate at which alveolar, and therefore brain tension rises. Inspection of Fig. 48.2 shows why as alveolar tension of halothane rises, outflow to muscle and viscera is almost as great as uptake into the lung, so that the rate of alveolar tension increase is slow. By contrast, the uptake of nitrous oxide is proportionately lower, since it has only one fifth the blood solubility of halothane. Furthermore, the 'compartmental' containers have much smaller surface area (or distribution volume) and therefore fill much more rapidly. As they fill, uptake diminishes and so alveolar tension also rises more rapidly.

The Concentration Effect

If Mapleson's basic model is used to predict gas uptake over a range of concentrations, we find that F_A/F_I for a gas rises along the same pathway, regardless of concentration. For many commonly used anaesthetic vapours, inhaled at concentrations below 10%, this is confirmed in practice. However, Eger showed many years ago (Eger, 1963a,b) that nitrous oxide does not behave as predicted; F_A/F_I for 70% nitrous oxide rises more rapidly than for 10% (Fig. 48.4). This phenomenon is known as the *concentration effect*. If widely differing nitrous oxide concentrations are compared, the effect can be seen to be quite large. For instance, it would take three times as long for alveolar tension to reach 80% of inspired tension with 1% nitrous oxide as with 80% (Mapleson, 1984). However, the comparison is rather academic since 1% nitrous oxide is not particularly effective. Nevertheless, in practice nitrous oxide reaches its effective alveolar tension much more quickly than would otherwise be predicted. Therefore it is important to understand *why*.

What Causes the Concentration Effect?

Consider in a rather crude analysis what happens when the patient makes a 500 ml alveolar inspiration (thus ignoring deadspace) from a 10% mixture of some gas in air. The 500 ml inspired volume containing 50 ml gas mixes with the Functional Residual Capacity (FRC) of, say 2500 ml, to yield an alveolar gas concentration of about 1.7%. Since the gas is freely diffusible across the alveolar membrane, we would expect the amount absorbed by the bloodstream to be proportional to concentration. Assume that 10% (5 ml) of the gas is absorbed during inspiration, and that about 16% of what remains will be lost

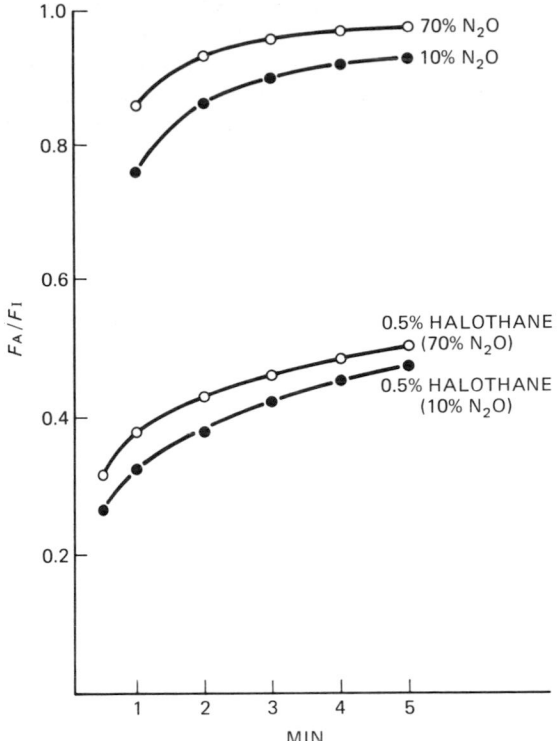

Fig. 48.4 Plots of F_A/F_I for N_2O and halothane measured during the first 5 min of inhalation (means of five studies). The upper curves for 10 and 70% N_2O demonstrate the *concentration effect*, while the lower curves for 0.5% halothane in the presence of 10 and 70% N_2O demonstrate the *second gas effect*. (Reproduced with permission from Epstein et al., 1964 and the Editor of *Anesthesiology*.)

as the patient exhales 500 ml of alveolar air. It follows that the end-tidal gas concentraton will be 1.5% and $F_A/F_I = 0.15$.

Were the patient to breathe 80% gas, all values would be correspondingly greater except F_A/F_I, which remains 0.15. Even if the patient breathes 100% gas, the numbers come out the same.

The important difference lies in the actual volumes of *gas absorbed into the bloodstream*. Whereas the single inspiration of 10% gas results in 5 ml absorption, 80% gas leads to 40 ml and 100% gas to 50 ml absorption. What happens to the lung volume previously occupied by that gas? There are several possibilities: the volume or pressure of the lung contents might diminish, some more fresh gas might replace that absorbed or alternatively the expired volume might diminish in order to maintain a constant FRC.

Since the alveoli are in direct communication with the fresh gas source, changes in lung volume are most unlikely. However, since gas uptake must continue during both inspiration and expiration, both accentuation of inspired volume and reduction in expired volume are inevitable. Gas absorbed during inspiration will simply draw more fresh gas down the trachea, whereas gas absorbed during expiration causes a reduction in expired volume and therefore a raised Pa_{CO_2}. This will quickly lead to a chemoreceptor-mediated rise in inspired minute volume. Thus uptake during both phases of respiration have the same end-result; increased inspiratory ventilation. This has a marked effect upon the rate at which FA/FI increases.

Following the above example, we can adjust the values of FA/FI for the estimated effects of expiratory uptake and enhanced inspiration; with 10% gas FA/FI becomes 0.14 and with 80% gas, 0.15. As breathing continues the difference becomes more marked, since the more rapidly rising FA/FI of the 80% gas causes more uptake and so more inspiratory augmentation, while expiratory uptake leads to increased respiratory drive and therefore greater minute ventilation. If our very simplified calculation is continued for 10 inspirations, we find that whereas FA/FI for 10% gas has risen to 0.47, that for 80% gas has risen to 0.71 despite almost 300 ml uptake into the bloodstream. The sequence of events is expressed diagrammatically in Fig. 48.5.

The effect is greatest in the unlikely event that 100% gas is administered. Here, uptake is followed by increased ventilation with 100% gas, such that uptake has no influence whatever upon the rate at which FA/FI rises. The nearer to 100% inspired gas, the more effective the mechanism becomes.

The Role of Nitrogen in the Concentration Effect
It might be expected that a patient breathing nitrous oxide in oxygen might not exhibit the concentration effect, since absorption of nitrous oxide should be balanced by washout of nitrogen. To a degree, it is, but nitrogen is 30 times less blood-soluble than nitrous oxide and therefore dissolved in much smaller volume. The small volume of nitrogen coming out does little to offset the large volume of nitrous oxide going in.

We have seen that the concentration effect is an entirely predictable consequence of gas uptake. Although a consequence of breathing *any* anaesthetic gas or vapour, it only reaches clinical significance if the gas is breathed in high concentration. Therefore all the vapours with MAC values less than 5% will be unaffected, and nitrous oxide is the only agent which need be considered.

The concentration effect is not easily reconciled with the water analogue because, quite clearly, during the early uptake phase inspired and expired volumes are not identical and cannot be simulated by such a simple first-order model (Mapleson, 1984).

The Second Gas Effect
If FA/FI for 1% halothane in 10% nitrous oxide is compared with that for the same halothane concentration in 80% nitrous oxide, we find that the latter mixture yields a steeper increase and a more rapid induction would be expected. This has been termed the *second gas effect* (Epstein et al., 1964). It is a

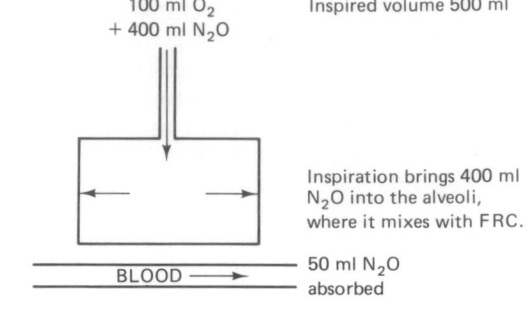

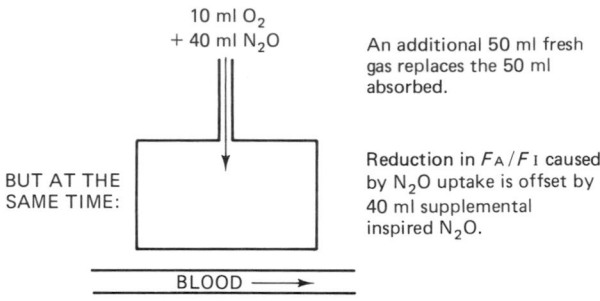

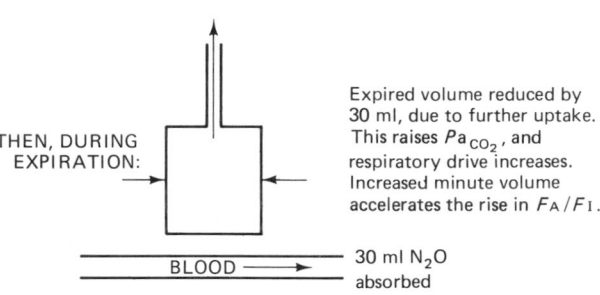

Fig. 48.5 The three diagrams show, in sequence, the events leading to the concentration effect.

natural consequence to the concentration effect, caused by the increased inspired volumes which follow the uptake of nitrous oxide. Since the minute inspired volume rises by the volume of nitrous oxide absorbed, the amount of halothane reaching the alveoli increases by proportion, causing a more rapid approach to the inspired concentration.

Uptake by Enclosed Gas Spaces
As a gas distributes to all tissues of the body, it will diffuse into any enclosed gas space. Such spaces are normally limited to the middle ear and the intestinal lumen, because blood leaving capillary beds has a total gas pressure averaging some 9 kPa below atmospheric. This ensures that gas 'pockets' do not *normally* develop in the pleural and peritoneal cavities.

However, in the unsteady state following administration of a gas such as nitrous oxide, this does not apply (Hunter, 1955). Consider a patient with a small, newly formed pneumothorax whose composition is still that of air. With the patient breathing air this will be slowly diminishing in size as the oxygen tension reduces to the mixed venous level. Now he breathes 79% nitrous oxide in oxygen for several minutes (Fig. 48.6).

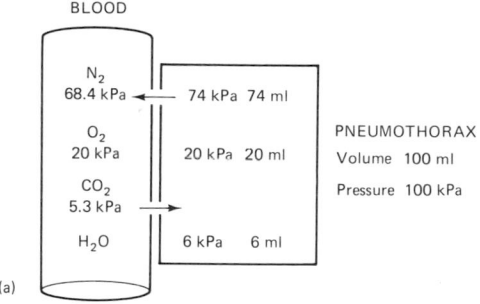

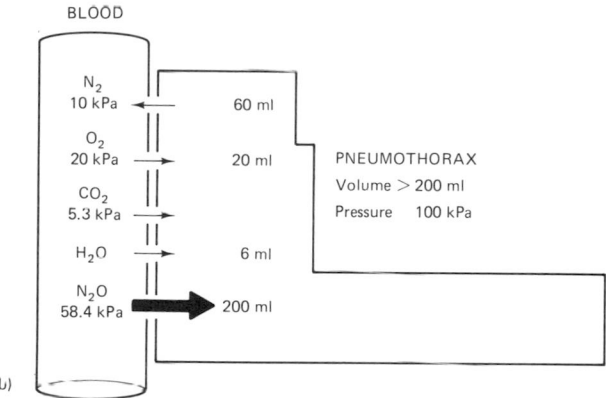

Fig. 48.6   (a) A fresh pneumothorax containing humidi-fied air equilibrates slowly with arterial blood. N_2 diffuses out, and a little CO_2 diffuses in. (b) Breathing 79% N_2O in O_2 for some minutes, the plasma P_{N_2} has fallen to 10 kPa, and P_{N_2O} has risen to 58.4 kPa. N_2 continues to diffuse *slowly* out of the cavity, but N_2O diffuses in much more rapidly, expanding the volume greatly. This dilutes the O_2, CO_2 and H_2O vapour to lower partial pressures, so these gases also, diffuse into the cavity.

During this period, the arterial nitrogen tension declines from 75 to 10 kPa, Pa_{O_2} remains unchanged and arterial nitrous oxide tension rises from zero to 60 kPa. This set of partial pressures equilibrate with the contents of any gas space in the body.

If nitrogen were to diffuse *out* of the space as rapidly as nitrous oxide diffuses *in*, the cavity volume and pressure would remain unchanged. However, due to its very poor plasma solubility it does not, and may take many hours to equilibrate. Consequently, the total gas volume in the cavity tends to increase until the partial pressures (and therefore the proportions) of gases are the same as in plasma (Eger and Saidman, 1965). Nitrous oxide now diffuses rapidly into the

cavity until the partial pressure reaches 60 kPa. If no nitrogen diffuses out at all, this will require that the cavity volume increases by 150%. Some while later the arterial nitrous oxide tension has risen to 70 kPa; now the space must increase to 230% of the original volume. A long-established pneumothorax, such as those induced during the management of pulmonary tuberculosis, may contain as much as 90% nitrogen. In such a case, the theoretical limit to expansion would be even greater.

Some gas-filled spaces, such as the middle-ear, cannot expand so readily. Now the total gas pressure rises with increasing nitrous oxide tension unless vented spontaneously through the Eustachian tube. The theoretical limiting pressure is the sum of atmospheric pressure and the nitrous oxide tension in plasma: 101 + 70 = 171 kPa. Perreault and his colleagues (Perreault et al., 1982) showed that in the presence of an occluded Eustachian tube middle ear pressure can increase by as much as 30 mmHg when breathing nitrous oxide.

The volumes and pressures of endotracheal tube cuffs initially filled with air will increase to a variable degree following exposure to nitrous oxide. For instance, Stanley found that the changes depended upon the type of cuff and the volume and pressue of initial inflation. In the most extreme instances he found volumes to be increased by 100% and pressures by as much as 80 mmHg (Stanley et al., 1974; Stanley, 1975).

In fact, the theoretical limits for volume or pressure are almost never reached, since some nitrogen *does* diffuse out of the space as nitrous oxide diffuses in. A possible exception is the air bubble accidentally injected into blood (Munson and Merrick, 1966). Here, diffusion of nitrous oxide can be very rapid and the bubble reach its theoretical size almost immediately. Therefore, nitrous oxide presents a significant hazard to a patient with, or likely to sustain, air embolism.

The Maintenance Phase; Approaching Steady-state

As inhalation continues, the body compartments approach equilibrium. In the case of a relatively insoluble agent such as nitrous oxide this process is 95% complete within 2 h. Using trichloroethylene it might take weeks.

The volume of halothane in the body approaches steady state very slowly once the well-perfused tissues are fully equilibrated and the only uptake is into a very 'slow' fat compartment. Under these conditions alveolar tension is very close indeed to inspired tension and the resulting depth of anaesthesia virtually constant. Trichloroethylene presents a more difficult case. It takes a very long time to equilibrate despite high blood solubility which provides an efficient means of carrying drug from lung to tissues. This is because the 'fat' compartment takes a long time to fill despite high delivery. As a result of this high tissue delivery, the rate of uptake from the lung remains high for an extended period. Alveolar and therefore brain tensions remain much lower than the inspired tension throughout any possible period of anaesthesia, and therefore require special administration techniques if of any clinical usefulness whatever.

Non-pulmonary Elimination

For many agents, achievement of steady state does not mean that uptake ceases, since any drug eliminated by non-pulmonary routes must be replaced. Thus nitrous oxide escapes through the skin in small quantities (Orcutt and Waters, 1933), while as much as 15% of halothane taken up by the body is metabolized.

The Pharmacokinetics of Recovery

When administration ceases, and the inspired gas becomes air, oxygen, or a mixture of both, the anaesthetic agent will be eliminated along a reciprocal pathway to that followed during induction. The alveolar tension will decline rapidly at first due to mixing with the new inspired gas. However, the declining alveolar tension leads to diffusion of anaesthetic gas from bloodstream to alveolus, such that the rate of fall of F_A/F_I is slowed appreciably (Stoelting and Eger, 1969). Now the effectiveness of this 'braking' action depends upon the tension of agent in mixed venous blood; depending in turn upon the tissue tension achieved during administration. Thus the rate of recovery is not only dependent upon the previous *depth* of anaesthesia, but also upon the *duration* of administration (Fig. 48.7).

Needless to say, the solubility of the agent has a profound effect upon the significance of these changes. Even after prolonged nitrous oxide anaesthesia recovery is rapid, because the rate at which the gas returns from tissue compartments declines very rapidly; there is simply not enough nitrous oxide in the body to do otherwise. By contrast, cessation of trichloroethylene administration is followed by a high rate of drug clearance from tissue compartments, so that alveolar tension may remain in the anaesthetic range long after administration has stopped. Prolongation of narcosis after such soluble agents depends strongly upon the duration of administration, since the effect depends upon there being a large reservoir of drug in the tissues. After only short administrations recovery may, in fact, be quite rapid.

Diffusion Hypoxia; the Fink Effect

If a patient breathes 70% nitrous oxide for, say, 30 min, and then switches abruptly to room air, a sequence of events follows which depends upon the same factors as the concentration effect, but in reverse (Fink, 1955). As nitrous oxide is flushed out of the lungs by the first few breaths, it is replaced by room air; 79% nitrogen and 21% oxygen. As the alveolar nitrous oxide tension falls abruptly, rapid equilibration with mixed pulmonary capillary blood releases some 1000 ml nitrous oxide per min into the alveoli, but only very little nitrogen diffuses in the opposite direction. Thus the alveoli are flooded with both nitrogen and nitrous oxide, and therefore the expired volume begins to exceed the inspired volume. Consequently, both oxygen and carbon dioxide are diluted and washed out of the alveoli, making the patient both hypocapnic and hypoxic. The ensuing reduction

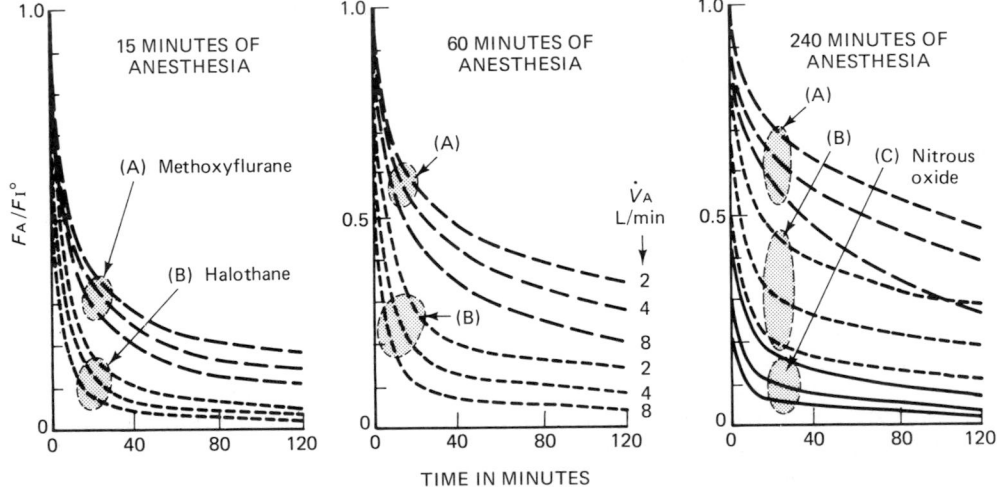

Fig. 48.7 Simulated plots of F_A/F_I^0 against time, during the recovery phase following different periods of anaesthesia. (F_I^0 is the alveolar fraction immediately before the inspired mixture is restored to air). Because recovery from short exposures is as much due to distribution as to elimination, the curves for different minute volumes are much closer together after 15 minutes anaesthesia than after 240 minutes. (Modified with permission from Stoelting and Eger, 1969 and the Editor of *Anesthesiology*.)

in inspired ventilation only serves to make things worse. This phenomenon, originally called 'diffusion anoxia', is more precisely described as 'diffusion hypoxia' (Sheffer et al. 1972). In recognition of the original description, the author favours 'the Fink effect'.

Arterial oxygen saturation may decline precipitously as a result, with considerable risk to the patient (Fig. 48.8). However, as every clinical anaesthetist is

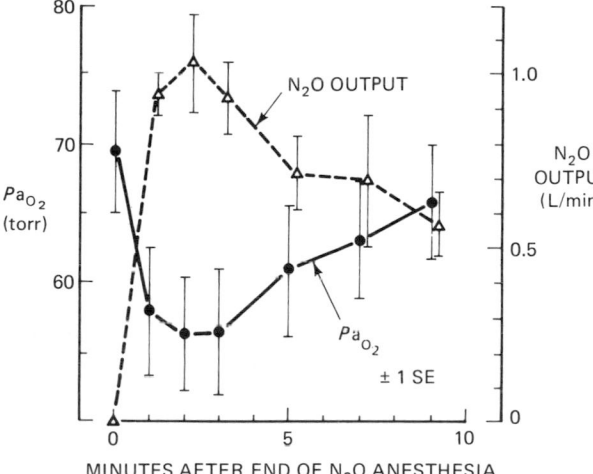

Fig. 48.8 Diffusion hypoxia. Eight young males breathed 79% nitrous oxide in oxygen with methoxyflurane for surgical procedures lasting 2–3 h. The diagram shows the changes in Pa_{O_2} after the inspired mixture was changed to air. N_2O output is also shown. (Adapted with permission from Sheffer et al., 1969. Nitrous oxide-induced diffusion hypoxia in patients breathing spontaneously, *Anesthesiology*, **37**, 439.)

aware, even a very short period of oxygen breathing following cessation of nitrous oxide administration prevents the phenomenon altogether; first by raising the alveolar oxygen tension itself, but also by providing a more exchangeable gas than nitrogen during the period of maximal nitrous oxide excretion.

THE INFLUENCE OF ALTERED ANATOMICAL AND PHYSIOLOGICAL STATES

The most important variations to consider are those in pulmonary ventilation and cardiac output.

Effect of Changing Pulmonary Ventilation

It is self-evident that the rate at which the alveolar and therefore brain tension of an anaesthetic gas rises must be strongly dependent upon pulmonary ventilation. As in previous sections we will compare halothane with nitrous oxide (Fig. 48.9).

The uptake curve for nitrous oxide is displaced upwards and to the left, but to a much less extent than that of halothane. Whereas doubled ventilation

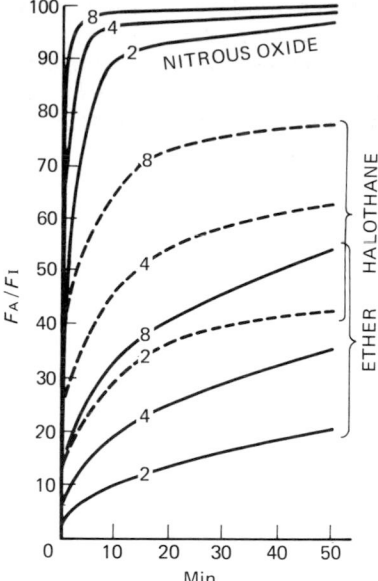

Fig. 48.9 The effect of changing pulmonary ventilation on the uptake of nitrous oxide, halothane and diethyl ether (computer simulations). The uptake characteristics at minute volumes of 2, 4, and 8 L/min are drawn for each agent. (Reproduced with permission of Eger, 1963b.)

during the induction phase results in a 4% increase in F_A/F_I for nitrous oxide at 5 min, the F_A/F_I value for halothane increases by 50% (Eger, 1963b).

Now this might be taken to indicate that induction with nitrous oxide is little affected by changing ventilation. This is by no means so; it depends simply upon how the data are expressed. So far as clinical practice is concerned, we are more interested in the time it takes to induce anaesthesia than in small differences in depth once it is achieved. In fact, the time taken to reach $F_A/F_I = 0.9$ is halved by doubled ventilation, and increased by a factor of 3 when ventilation is halved. The reasons are plainly demonstrated by Mapleson's model, viewed in conjunction with Fig. 48.9. Since the pipe between 'fresh gas' and 'lung' will always make the alveolar partial pressure lag behind that of inspired gas, it follows that a change in ventilation must always have some effect, however rapid the equilibrating process.

However, it should be noted that the greatest effect will occur in the very early phase when F_A/F_I is low. During this period the alveolar tension is finely balanced between the influences of ventilation, tending to increase F_A/F_I, and uptake, tending to lower F_A/F_I. Were it not so, the concentration effect would not occur.

In fact, were it not for the concentration effect, the effect of ventilation upon nitrous oxide and halothane could be said to be very similar; if allowance were made for the very different rates of equilibration of the two agents. By comparing the effect upon the nitrous oxide curve when $F_A/F_I = 0.9$ with the halothane curve when $F_A/F_I = 0.5$, we are not making a fair or even reasonable comparison. The effect of a reduction in ventilation upon the nitrous oxide curve makes this clear; by displacing F_A/F_I down towards the mid-zone, there is a much greater effect upon the curve than that caused by an increase in ventilation.

As might be expected, changing ventilation has no effect whatever upon disposition when the agent has reached equilibrium. However, during recovery the same factors apply as during induction; increased ventilation leads to faster recovery, and *vice versa*.

The Effects of Altered Pa_{CO_2}

Changes in Pa_{CO_2} may occur with or without alteration in minute volume. Thus if the patient hyperventilates in response to mask placement, accelerated onset of anaesthesia might be expected whichever agent is used. In fact, the reduction in cerebral bloodflow caused by the inevitable hypocapnia largely offsets the effect of hyperventilation. Munson and Bowers (1967) went so far as to suggest that because the onset of nitrous oxide anaesthesia is little affected by hyperventilation, the associated reduction in cerebral blood-flow might even cause induction to be prolonged. While hypercarbia causes widespread physiological changes, not least an increase in cardiac output, the most important is an *increase* in cerebral bloodflow. This leads to more rapid equilibration between alveolar and brain tensions and therefore more rapid induction or recovery.

The Effect of Changing Cardiac Output

From the above consideration of ventilation, cardiac output is obviously another key factor in determining the rate at which the vapour or gas tension in blood approaches that in 'fresh gas'. However, while increasing ventilation promotes F_A/F_I and therefore the rate of induction, rising cardiac output does the opposite. This may seem paradoxical, in that an increased cardiac output might be expected to carry drug to the brain more rapidly. Indeed it does, but at a lower tension which does nothing to hasten induction. The point is that increased cardiac output promotes the rate of equilibration with well-perfused viscera and muscle, manifested in Mapleson's model as an increase in the diameter of the pipes connecting 'lung' to these compartments. During the induction phase these wider pipes carry more water away from the 'lung', so that the F_A/F_I curves follow a lower path (Fig. 48.10) and so the biophase tension reaches the anaesthetic threshold more slowly. The effect is accentuated by the fact that cerebral bloodflow remains relatively unchanged over a wide range of cardiac outputs, so that the brain does not even gain benefit of more rapid equilibration with arterial gas tensions as cardiac output rises.

As with ventilation, the F_A/F_I curves for nitrous oxide and halothane behave differently. As before, those nearest the mid-zone are most affected. At 5 min, halving the cardiac output causes a 3% in-

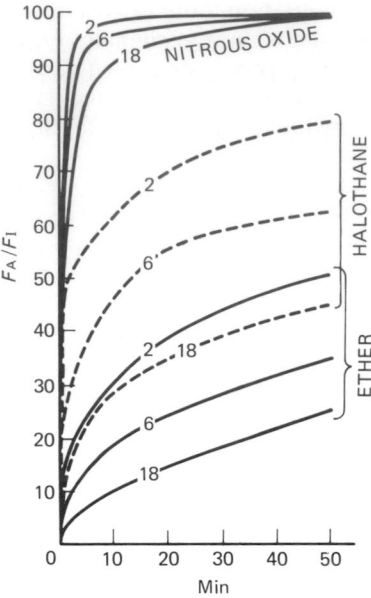

Fig. 48.10   The effect of changing cardiac output on the uptake of nitrous oxide, halothane and diethyl ether (computer simulations). The uptake characteristics at cardiac outputs of 2, 6, and 18 L/min are drawn for each agent. (Reproduced with permission from Eger, 1963b.)

crease in F_A/F_I for nitrous oxide, but a 50% increase in that for halothane. As before, the effects upon nitrous oxide are much greater than they seem because of the time-scale effect. In fact, doubled cardiac output causes the time taken to reach 90% to increase from 4 min to 10 min. To the practical anaesthetist, not an insignificant difference.

It should be noted that an increase in cardiac output does, in fact, accelerate the general process of equilibration. Because uptake is increased, all compartments must reach final equilibrium more quickly. This is of little practical importance to nitrous oxide, but has profound effects upon the total uptake of a more soluble agent such as halothane over, say, a 3h period. Thus if cardiac output remains high during the early phases of the procedure but later diminishes (not an unusual occurrence), recovery may be protracted as continuing outflow from the tissue compartments sustains the alveolar and therefore brain tension at a narcotic level.

The Effect of Body Size and Obesity

In general, cardiac output, ventilation and distribution volumes change in proportion to the patient's physical size. Therefore, large patients require the same concentrations, given for the same periods, as small patients.

Children have greater cardiac outputs and respiratory minute volumes in relation to their size, than adults. This means that the sequence of events proceeds exactly as in adults, but with a compressed time-scale. However, it should be noted that small children have been found to have higher MAC values for halothane (Gregory et al., 1969) and therefore require greater inspired concentrations if the same effects are to be achieved.

Moderately obese patients differ from normals only in respect of a greatly increased mass of adipose tissue. Although fat is poorly perfused, the total bloodflow to fat does constitute a greater proportion of the cardiac output than in normals. However, this has little influence on the time-course of alveolar tension at any phase of anaesthesia (Saraiva et al. 1977).

THE INFLUENCE OF ANAESTHETIC TECHNIQUE UPON DISPOSITION

A number of anaesthetic techniques have been devised whose aim is to achieve more rapid induction and recovery. For instance, if a patient is administered a gaseous agent only at a concentration sufficient to *maintain* anaesthesia, say 1% halothane, the induction process may be very protracted. By administering an initial concentration of 5%, followed by successive reductions as the patient loses consciousness, more rapid induction is achieved; the so-called 'over-pressure' technique. The rationale is obvious; a high inspired concentration raises the alveolar tension and therefore the brain tension much more rapidly. The skill lies in adjusting the inspired concentration so as to keep the blood tension at exactly the right level against a constantly changing background of pulmonary ventilation, cardiac output and tissue uptake. The recent development of end-tidal anaesthetic concentration monitoring instruments enables constant alveolar tensions to be both achieved and maintained with some precision.

In the days of ether anaesthesia, patients were often given high concentrations of CO_2 during induction with the dual objectives of increasing cerebral blood-flow and discouraging breath-holding.

For many years, anaesthetists have toyed with the idea that an artificially hyperventilated patient should recover consciousness more rapidly than if limited to a 'physiological' minute volume. The advent of routine capnography in the operating theatre has made this a practical proposition since it is now possible to add CO_2 to the inspired air such that the patient does not become hypocapnic. Unfortunately, patients anaesthetized with even moderately soluble agents such as halothane are at some risk from such procedures. Because hyperventilation washes halothane rapidly from plasma, brain, even some well-perfused tissues, the patient recovers consciousness rapidly. However, a short period of hyperventilation has removed but a small fraction of the halothane. It is more than likely that redistribution from other tissue compartments will restore the plasma halothane level to anaesthetic levels and the patient will be re-anaesthetized; possibly in a most dangerous location where skilled help is not at hand. However, the recent introduction of less soluble agents such as enflurane

and isoflurane may allow this technique to be used safely.

REFERENCES

Eger E.I., II (1986a). The effect of inspired concentration on the rate of rise of alveolar concentration. *Anesthesiology*, **24**, 679.

Eger E.I., II (1963b). Applications of a mathematical model of gas uptake. In *Uptake and Distribution of Anaesthetic Agents*, p. 96, (Papper E.M., Kitz R.J., eds.). New York: McGraw-Hill.

Eger E.I., II. (1980). The uptake and distribution of inhalational anaesthetic agents. In *General Anaesthesia*, 4th edn., (Gray T.C., Nunn J.F., Utting J.E., eds.). London: Butterworths.

Eger E.I., II, Saidman L.J. (1965). Hazards of nitrous oxide anaesthesia in bowel obstruction and pneumothorax. *Anesthesiology*, **26**, 61.

Epstein R.M., Rackow H., Salanaitre E., et al. (1964). Influence of the concentration effect on the uptake of anaesthetic mixtures: the second gas effect. *Anesthesiology*, **25**, 364.

Fink B.R. (1955). Diffusion anoxia. *Anesthesiology*, **16**, 511.

Gregory, G.A., Eger E.I., II and Munson E.S. (1969). The relationship between age and halothane requirement. *Anesthesiology*, **30**, 488.

Hunter A.R. (1955). Problems of anaesthesia in artifical pneumothorax. *Proc. R. Soc. Med.*, **48**, 765.

Mapleson W.W. (1978). Circulation-time models of the uptake of inhaled anaesthetics-nitrous-oxide-induced diffusion hypoxia in patients breathing spontaneously. *Anesthesiology*, **37**, 436.

Mapleson W.W. (1984). Pharmacokinetics of inhaled anaesthetics. In *Pharmacokinetics of Anaesthesia*, pp. 89–111, (Prys-Roberts C., Hug C.C. Jr., eds.), Oxford: Blackwell Scientific Publications.

Munson E.S., Bowers D.L. (1967). Effects of hyperventilation on the rate of cerebral anaesthetic equilibration. *Anesthesiology*, **28**, 377.

Munson E.S., Merrick H.C. (1966). Effect of nitrous oxide on venous air embolism. *Anesthesiology*, **27**, 783.

Orcutt F.S., Waters R.M. (1933). The diffusion of nitrous oxide, ethylene and carbon dioxide through human skin. *Anesth. Analg.*, **12**, 45.

Perrault L., Normondin N., Plamondon L., et al. (1982). Middle ear pressure variations during nitrous oxide and oxygen anaesthesia. *Can. Anaesth. Soc. J.*, **224**, 253.

Saraiva R.A., Lunn J.N., Mapleson W.W., et al. (1977). Adiposity and the pharmacokinetics of halothane. The effect of adiposity on the maintenance of and recovery from halothane anaesthesia. *Anaesthesia*, **32**, 240.

Sheffer L., Steffenson J.L., Birch A.A. (1972). Nitrous oxide induced diffusion hypoxia in patients breathing spontaneously. *Anesthesiology*, **37**, 436.

Stanley T.H. (1975). Nitrous oxide and pressures and volumes of high and low-pressure endotracheal tube cuffs in intubated patients. *Anesthesiology*, **42**, 637.

Stanley T.H., Kawamura R., Graves C. (1974). Effects of nitrous oxide on volume and pressure of endotracheal tube cuffs. *Anesthesiology*, **41**, 256.

Stoelting R.K., Eger E.I., II (1969). Influence of ventilation and solubility on recovery from anaesthesia: an *in vivo* and analog analysis before and after equilibrium. *Anesthesiology*, **30**, 290.

49. Passage Across Membranes
Felicity H. Hawker

Biological membranes play a crucial role in almost all cellular phenomena. The plasma membrane defines the cell boundary and has important functions in communication between cells, and in cell adhesion and immunogenicity (Houslay and Stanley, 1982). However, the most important function of the plasma membrane is its role as a continuous barrier around the cell which selectively limits or facilitates the passage of substances into and out of the cytoplasm. It therefore maintains essential differences between cell contents and the environment. Intracellular membranes both delineate and mediate various functions of cell organelles. Passage of substances across membranes is the subject of this chapter.

MEMBRANE COMPONENTS AND THEIR ORGANIZATION

Structure of Membranes

All biological membranes, both plasma membranes and the internal membranes of eucaryotic (nucleated) cells, have a common overall morphology. The basic structure is a continuous double layer of lipid molecules (Gorter and Grendell, 1925), which has fluid properties and acts as a relatively impermeable barrier to water and charged molecules. This bilayer is punctuated with a wide variety of embedded proteins which mediate the various functions of the membrane, and act as specific receptors, enzymes and transporters. This model of membrane structure is termed the *fluid mosaic model* (Singer and Nicolson, 1972; Fig. 49.1), and is developed from thermodynamic considerations of the various membrane components. Thermodynamic theory requires that the membrane

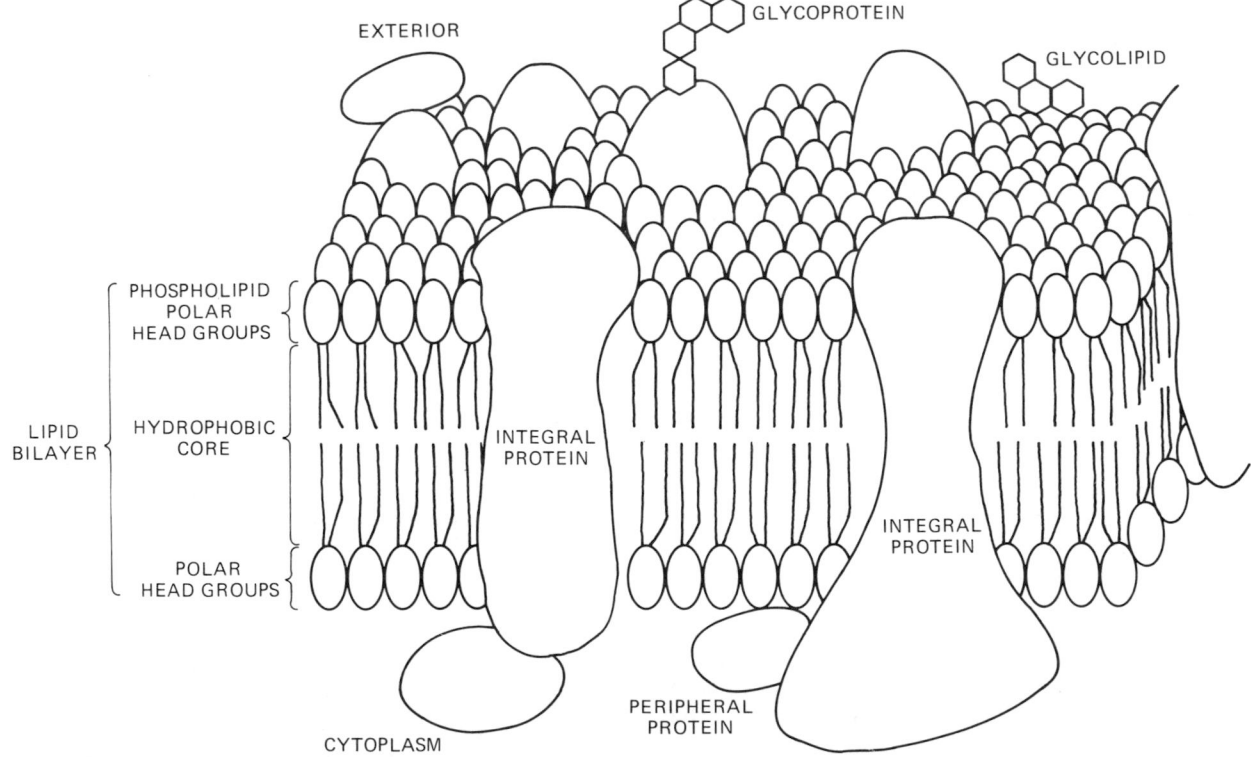

Fig. 49.1 Model of membrane structure. The continuous double layer of phospholipid molecules is arranged with polar headgroups at the membrane surfaces and the fatty acid chains meeting in the interior of the membrane. Integral proteins are embedded in the bilayer whereas peripheral proteins are loosely attached at the membrane surfaces. Carbohydrate groups are confined exclusively to the external or noncytoplasmic membrane surface.

adopts its lowest free energy state. In hydrophobic interactions, thermodynamic factors are responsible for the sequestering of nonpolar groups away from water. On the other hand, in hydrophilic interactions, thermodynamic factors dictate that ionic and polar groups prefer an aqueous rather than a nonpolar environment. Both membrane lipids and membrane proteins are amphipathic, that is, their molecules have both hydrophobic and hydrophilic domains. Hence nonpolar amino acid residues of membrane proteins, and the fatty acid chains of phospholipids are sequestered away from water in the membrane interior; while the ionic and polar groups of the proteins, lipids and oligopolysaccharides are in contact with the aqueous environment on the peripheral faces of the membrane.

With this conformation, the intact membrane achieves its lowest free energy state. Other noncovalent interactions such as hydrogen bonding and electrostatic interactions make a contribution to macromolecular structure. In this model, both lipids and proteins can both rotate and diffuse laterally in the plane of the membrane, although lateral movement of membrane proteins may be limited to some extent by the cell cytoskeleton (Schlessinger, 1983). Under usual circumstances, for the above thermodynamic reasons, neither lipids nor proteins transfer from one half of the bilayer to the other. The cell membrane is also asymmetrical (Rothman and Lenard, 1977). The lipid and protein components of the cytoplasmic and external faces differ in ways that reflect the different functions performed at the two surfaces. For example, the phosphatidylinositols, a specific class of membrane phospholipid involved in the arachidonic acid cascade and the calcium second messenger system, are located in the inner leaflet of the plasma membrane (Rasmussen, 1986). These phospholipids will be discussed later in this chapter.

Although aspects of this model have been criticized (Houslay et al., 1982), it provides a useful structural basis for understanding membrane transport phenomena.

Membrane Components

Lipids

Three major classes of lipids; phospholipids, cholesterol and glycolipids are present in animal cell membranes. In keeping with the fluid mosaic model, these lipid molecules are arranged with their polar headgroups towards the aqueous interfaces and their fatty acid chains meeting in the centre, so that the long axis of the lipid molecule is perpendicular to the plane of the membrane (Fig. 49.1). A typical phospholipid molecule has two hydrophobic hydrocarbon tails, which vary in length and normally consist of 14–24 carbon atoms. One chain is usually unsaturated and has one or more cis-double bonds resulting in a 'bend' in one tail; while the other is saturated. These differences in tail length and saturation influence the fluid-

ity of the membrane (Quinn and Chapman, 1980). The two hydrocarbon chains are esterified via a glycerol molecule and phosphate ester, to a hydrophilic base. In glycolipids, the glycerol is esterified directly to the carbohydrate units. Cholesterol molecules are orientated with their hydroxyl groups close to the polar head groups of the phospholipid molecules, and their steroid rings interact with, and partly immobilize those regions of the hydrocarbon tails closest to the headgroups (Alberts et al., 1983). The cholesterol content of the membrane also influences its fluidity. At 37°C, cholesterol tends to make the membrane less fluid. However, at low membrane temperatures, cholesterol conserves fluidity (Darnell et al., 1986).

Proteins

Specific membrane processes are carried out largely by membrane proteins. The amount and type of proteins reflect the functions of the membrane. For example, the protein content of myelin sheaths is approximately 18% of the dry weight of the membrane, whereas the internal membranes of mitochondria are approximately 76% protein. Most plasma membranes are approximately 50% protein (Table 49.1).

TABLE 49.1
CHEMICAL COMPOSITION OF SOME PURIFIED MEMBRANES (PER CENT OF TOTAL)

Membrane	Protein	Lipid	Carbohydrate
Myelin	18	49	3
Plasma membrane			
Human erythrocyte	49	43	8
Human platelets	33–42	58–51	7.5
Mouse liver cells	44	52	4
Mitochondrial			
Inner membrane	76	24	0
Sarcoplasmic reticulum	67	33	0

Adapted with permission from Guidotti, 1972.

Membrane proteins can be classified as 'peripheral' or 'integral' depending upon the ease with which they can be removed from the membrane (Fig. 49.1). Peripheral membrane proteins, such as the cytochrome C of mitochondrial membranes, can be washed off the membrane using buffers, whereas integral proteins require detergents or organic solvents for extraction. Approximately 70% of membrane proteins are integral proteins. Those that span the membrane and are exposed to an aqueous environment on both sides are termed transmembrane proteins. These may be fibrous or globular. Because water is excluded from the interior of the membrane, polar groups of polypeptide chains form hydrogen bonds with each other, and these chains are therefore arranged mainly as α-helices or β-sheets. Fibrous proteins usually have only a

TABLE 49.2
PROPERTIES OF TRANSPORT PROCESSES

Diffusion	*Diffusion through channels*	*Facilitated diffusion*	*Activated transport*
Mediated by membrane lipid	Mediated by membrane proteins	Mediated by membrane proteins	Mediated by membrane proteins
Net flux ceases at electro-chemical equilibrium	Net flux ceases at electro-chemical equilibrium	Net flux ceases at electro-chemical equilibrium	Achieves transport against electro-chemical gradient
No energy coupling	No energy coupling	May be indirectly coupled to electrochemical energy	Directly coupled energy supply
Low specificity	Variable specificity	High specificity	High specificity
Non-saturating	Non-saturating	Saturates at high substrate concentration	Saturates at high substrate concentration
No counter transport	No counter transport	Displays counter transport	Almost irreversible

single α-helical strand of polypeptide spanning the hydrophobic segment of the membrane and are often heavily glycosylated on the extracytoplasmic surface. Globular proteins have many loops of polypeptide chain spanning the membrane and a much higher percentage of hydrophobic surface. Most tend to have a dimeric structure (Klingenberg, 1981) and are probably transport proteins. The protein, band 3 of the erythrocyte membrane is a typical globular transmembrane protein that crosses the membrane at least 12 times (Kopito and Lodish, 1985). Other proteins do not span the bilayer and are exposed to an aqueous environment on only one side of the membrane. These are bound to specific integral membrane proteins by ionic or other weak interactions.

Carbohydrate

Most proteins exposed at the cell surface and some lipid molecules in the outer lipid monolayer are covalently bound to oligosaccharide chains forming glycoproteins and glycolipids respectively. The proportion of carbohydrate in plasma membranes varies between about 2 and 10% by weight (Alberts et al., 1983). These complex oligosaccharide side chains are located exclusively at the noncytoplasmic membrane surface, and together with additional proteins, such as fibronectin, make up the glycocalyx. Sialic acid residues are usually found at the ends of the carbohydrate side chains and are mainly responsible for the net negative charge that characterizes all eukaryotic cells. The functions of membrane carbohydrates are unclear. They may be responsible for orienting, anchoring and stabilizing glycoprotein molecules and some may play a part in cell-to-cell recognition processes (Luft, 1976).

MEMBRANE TRANSPORT PROCESSES

Passage of small molecules across membranes may occur by passive diffusion, which is chiefly a function of the lipid bilayer, by diffusion through channel proteins, or by the more complex processes of facilitated diffusion and active transport, also mediated by membrane proteins (Table 49.2). These transport processes are shown schematically in Fig. 49.2 and will be considered individually.

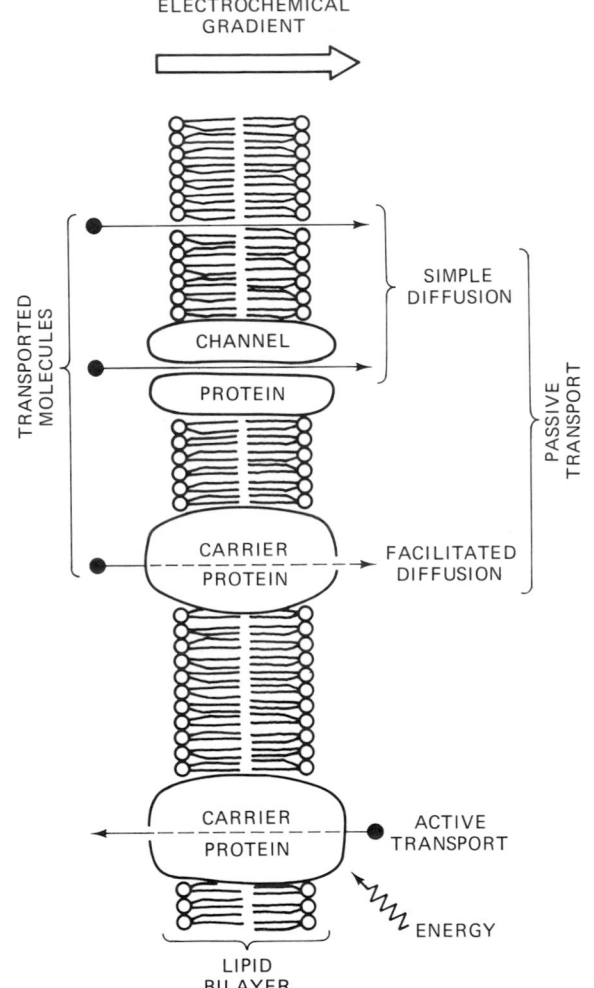

Fig. 49.2 Schematic representation of membrane transport processes. Some molecules may pass across membranes by several transport processes. For example, calcium ions enter cells by diffusion through channels (calcium channels) and are removed from cells by carrier proteins; by facilitated diffusion (sodium–calcium exchange) and by active transport (Calcium ATPase). (Adapted with permission from Alberts et al., 1983. *Molecular Biology of the Cell*, New York: Garland Publishing Inc.).

Passive Diffusion

Random movements of molecules in solution cause a solute to disperse from areas of high concentration until the solution is homogeneous. This process of diffusion can also occur between compartments separated by a biological membrane and is largely a property of the membrane lipid bilayer. Membranes represent a considerable barrier to the diffusion of all types of molecules as the close packing and hydrophobic nature of the hydrocarbon chains in the centre of the membrane limit the type of molecules that can diffuse into or out of cells. Discrete binding sites are not involved and hence passive diffusion does not saturate at high substrate concentrations.

Passive diffusion of uncharged molecules across a biological membrane depends only on the diffusion coefficient of the molecule under the given conditions, and its concentration gradient across the membrane. The diffusion coefficient depends largely on the size of the molecule and its relative solubility in oil. Thus, small, nonpolar molecules diffuse across lipid bilayers rapidly. Small uncharged, polar molecules may also diffuse across membranes. For example urea (molecular weight 60 daltons) crosses rapidly, but glucose (180 daltons) diffuses hardly at all (Alberts et al., 1983). Molecules that are charged or large are almost entirely excluded unless a specific transport system exists (Fig. 49.2).

The rate of penetration of nonelectrolytes across membranes of isolated cells shows marked temperature dependence, and increases if cholesterol is removed from the membrane. This suggests that solute molecules pass through the lipid hydrocarbon region of the membrane, whose fluidity increases both with temperature and with cholesterol removal (Houslay et al., 1982).

Diffusion Through Ion Channels

Many molecules have greater rates of penetration into cells than predicted by their size and oil–water partition coefficients. These substances are transported by membrane proteins. These proteins are either carrier proteins with characteristics of membrane-bound enzymes which will be discussed in the next section, or proteins that form transmembrane hydrophilic channels through which solutes of appropriate size and charge can pass by diffusion, without directly contacting the hydrophobic core of the lipid bilayer. Transport through channel proteins can occur at a very much faster rate than transport mediated by carrier proteins. If the molecule is uncharged, only the concentration gradient across the membrane determines the direction of transport. However, if the solute carries a net charge, then both the concentration gradient and the membrane potential (the electrochemical gradient) influence its transport through channel proteins (Fig. 49.3).

While some channels are continuously open, most

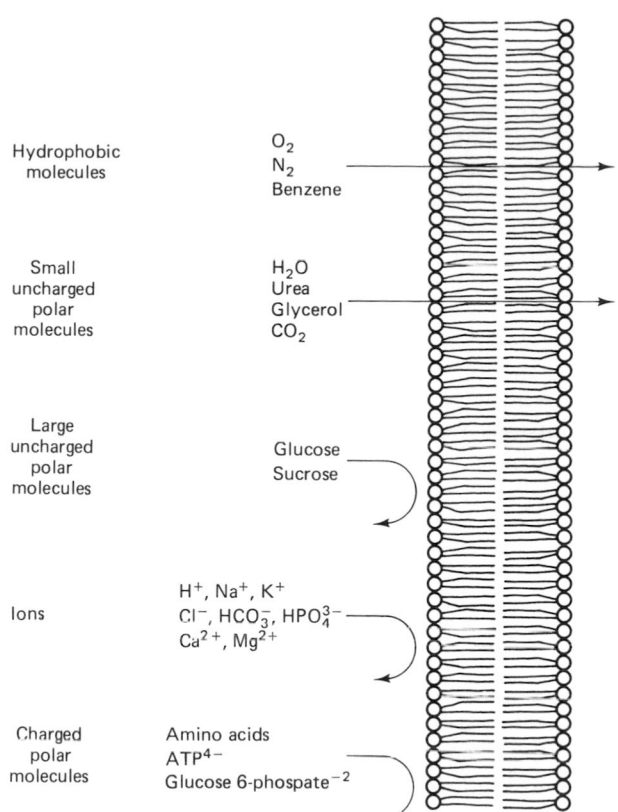

Fig. 49.3 The relative permeability of an artificial bilayer to different classes of molecules. (Adapted with permission from Molecular Cell Biology by James E. Darnell et al. Copyright © 1986 Scientific American Books, Inc.)

are open only transiently and are said to be gated. Some are voltage-gated, and open in response to a change in membrane potential (such as the sodium ion (Na^+) channel in electrically active cells), and others open in response to an extracellular ligand binding to a specific cell surface receptor. For example, the Na^+ and potassium ion (K^+) channels of muscle cell membranes open in response to the binding of acetylcholine. In the vertebrate brain, neuronal inhibition is mediated by ligand binding to the γ-aminobutyric acid (GABA)/benzodiazepine receptor which opens an integral chloride (Cl^-) channel (Schofield et al., 1987). Benzodiazepine and barbiturate drugs act at this receptor. These channels are said to be ligand-gated.

Ion Channels and Nerve Conduction (Hodgkin and Huxley, 1952)
All cells have gradients of Na^+ and K^+ across their membranes, which are maintained by Na^+-K^+ dependent adenosine triphosphatase (ATPase). This ion pump will be described in more detail under 'Active transport'. Sodium ions are pumped out of the cell while potassium ions are pumped in. These ions also leak back across the membrane through their respective ion channels. Since the resting plasma membrane

is about 100 times more permeable to K^+ than it is to Na^+ or anions, an electrical as well as a concentration gradient is established. In the neurone the resting membrane potential is approximately -70 mV. The membrane potential is largely determined by the K^+ gradient, which in turn is determined by the properties of specific proteins in the plasma membrane itself.

The depolarization and subsequent recovery of the membrane potential is achieved by Na^+ and K^+ channels in the membrane, which allow ions to leak down a steep concentration gradient. These ion channels are voltage-gated. Thus if an electrical impulse is applied to the membrane such that a certain threshold is achieved, the Na^+ channels in that vicinity open and sodium ions rush into the cell until the local membrane potential is abolished or even slightly reversed. This action is sufficient to trigger the opening of adjacent Na^+ channels so that a self propagating signal is produced. Na^+ permeability is then shut off and potassium ions moving in the opposite direction restore the membrane potential. While the Na^+ channel has closed but the K^+ channel is still open, the membrane potential achieves a higher value than the resting potential, thus giving a refractory period before the membrane can depolarize again and giving directionality to the impulse. The Na^+ and K^+ gradients are quickly restored by Na^+-K^+ ATPase. The rapid response of the Na^+ channels to changes in membrane potential govern the size, rate of rise and rate of transmission of the action potential.

Tetrodotoxin specifically inhibits sodium transport in electrically excitable tissues by binding to a site on the external surface of the sodium channel and physically occluding the pore (Keynes, 1979). Detergent solubilization of the tetrodotoxin-membrane complex has led to the isolation of a glycoprotein of molecular weight 260 000, believed to be the major component of the Na^+ channel. Two smaller polypeptides have also been identified which may be either components of the channel itself or regulatory molecules (Catterall, 1986). The amino acid sequence and tertiary structure of the sodium channel protein have been determined with four similar units surrounding a central transmembrane pore that serves as the ion conducting pathway. It is believed that voltage-dependent conformational changes occur in these subunits of the Na^+ channel, probably as a result of reorientation of charged and/or dipolar amino acid residues of the channel protein within the electric field. These conformational changes allow the channel to open and close in response to changes in membrane potential (Catterall, 1986). Less is known about the K^+ channel protein due to the absence of a high affinity ligand that would aid its isolation and purification.

Calcium Channels

Unlike the Na^+ channel which appears to be a unique molecular structure, Ca^{2+} channels are probably a family of channels of different structure in different membranes. When these Ca^{2+} channels open, calcium ions diffuse into the cell down their electrochemical gradient. In non-excitable cells calcium channels may be open permanently or may be ligand-gated. However, in excitable cells, Ca^{2+} channels, which normally are closed, are sensitive to the membrane potential. These channels begin to allow Ca^{2+} influx as the potential rises above -30 mV, and at $+30$ mV about 70% of the Ca^{2+} channels are open (Carafoli and Penniston, 1985). For example, depolarization of the cardiac muscle cell membrane results in opening of voltage-gated Ca^{2+} channels, often called 'slow channels'. Entry of Ca^{2+} into the cell stimulates further release of Ca^{2+} from the sarcoplasmic reticulum causing muscle contraction. At the neuromuscular junction, voltage-gated Ca^{2+} channels in the plasma membrane of the axon terminal open in response to the action potential. The resulting increase in free Ca^{2+} concentration inside the nerve terminal stimulates the release of acetylcholine, by activating an acetylcholine transporter in the nerve terminal membrane (Rasmussen, 1986). It is likely that electrical gating of Ca^{2+} channels is achieved by a conformational change of the protein induced by the alteration of the electric field across the membrane. Calcium channels that are opened by ligand binding may be regulated by phosphorylation of the channel protein itself (Carafoli et al., 1985).

Ligand-gated Ion Channels

Voltage-gated ion channels are usually named for the ion that passes through them, whereas ligand-gated ion channels are named by the ligand that regulates the channel. An example of this latter group is the acetylcholine receptor (AChR), which is a ligand-gated cation channel, permeable to Na^+ and K^+, that is transiently opened by binding of acetylcholine. The resultant flow of Na^+ into and K^+ out of the muscle cell results in a localized depolarization of the muscle membrane. This depolarization opens adjacent voltage-gated Na^+ channels causing a wave of depolarization of the whole membrane. Voltage-gated Ca^{2+} channels in the sarcoplasmic reticulum open in response to this action potential, initiating muscle contraction (Darnell et al., 1986).

Mediation of a physiological response by closure of ion channels occurs in the membranes of retinal rod cells. Rod cells are highly permeable to Na^+ in their resting state, in the dark. Light falling on rhodopsin closes these channels resulting in a transient hyperpolarization of the rod cell membrane which is transmitted to the visual cortex, mediating the visual response (Altman, 1985). The likely mechanism is that the photon activates rhodopsin by inducing isomerization of a component of rhodopsin, 11-cis retinal. Activated rhodopsin catalyzes the binding of guanosine triphosphate (GTP) to GTP-binding protein, sometimes called G protein or transducin. Activated G protein, in turn activates a cyclic guanosine monophosphate (cGMP) phosphodiesterase. Cyclic GMP is the ligand that maintains these Na^+ channels in the open state. Activation of phosphodiesterase results in breakdown of cGMP and the closure of membrane channels (Schnapf and Baylor, 1987).

Facilitated Diffusion

Unlike channel proteins, carrier proteins bind the specific molecule to be transported and transfer it across the membrane. If these specific molecules are metabolically utilized, they are translocated down a concentration gradient, and this can take place without a direct input of energy. This process is termed facilitated diffusion. On the other hand, the establishment and maintenance of concentration gradients of ions that are not consumed requires energy and it is termed active transport. This will be discussed in the next section.

In both these processes, the transport system saturates at high substrate concentrations, and in some cases, the carrier transports only one stereo-isomer. This is evident in the transport of glucose into erythrocytes, where the nonbiological L-isomer is hardly transported at all, but D-glucose is transferred readily (Darnell et al., 1986). These properties distinguish this process from passive diffusion.

Carrier proteins have similar characteristics to enzymes. Each protein has a specific binding site for its substrate. When the carrier is saturated, the rate of transport is maximum. This rate, referred to as V_{max}, is characteristic of the specific carrier. In addition, each carrier protein has a characteristic binding constant for its solute, K_m, equal to the concentration of solute when the transport rate is half its maximum value. Solute binding to carrier proteins can be blocked specifically by competitive or noncompetitive inhibitors. The transmembrane flux (J) may be described by the Michaelis–Menten equation for enzyme velocity:

$$J = \frac{SV_{max}}{K_m + S}$$

where S is the concentration of substrate.

Since, however, a flux can occur in both directions, the net flux is given by the equation

$$\text{Net flux} = J_{in} - J_{out}$$
$$= \frac{S_{in}V_{max}}{K_m + S_{in}} - \frac{S_{out}V_{max}}{K_m + S_{out}}$$

When there is no substrate inside the cell the flux is entirely unidirectional since $J_{out} = 0$. However, as the concentration inside the cell increases towards a chemical equilibrium, exchange of substrate will occur. Thus, the net flux is much slower than the rate of exchange. In some cases the net flux is so small that the system may be regarded simply as an exchange reaction. An example of this type of transport is the carnitine: acylcarnitine exchange transporter of the mitochondrial inner membrane. During fatty acid oxidation, fatty acyl groups are transported into mito-

chondria by exchange of cytoplasmic acylcarnitine with mitochondrial carnitine. This transport is energy independent and symmetrical, allowing bidirectional exchange of carnitine and acylcarnitine. The purpose of this transport system is the entry of fatty acyl groups into the mitochondrion for oxidation. However, when the proportion of acetylated carnitine in the mitochondrion increases, acylcarnitine is transported out of the mitochondrion and net influx of acyl groups slows or even ceases (Houslay et al., 1982).

Models of Membrane Transport Proteins

An early model of membrane transport suggested that carriers shuttled between the two membrane surfaces. However, direct evidence against moving carrier molecules comes from the consistent orientation of proteins in the membrane. Also the attachment of bulky antibodies to the surface of these proteins does not adversely affect their function.

The current model of a transport protein proposes that the substrate passes through hydrophilic pores between subunits of a multimeric membrane protein. The pore is not a fixed structure, and in this aspect differs from a membrane channel. This transport protein can exist in two states interconvertible by a conformational change. One of the properties of a multimeric protein is that a relatively low input of energy can give rise to a large rearrangement of the subunits. In facilitated diffusion, it is possible that the energy of substrate binding is sufficient to achieve this. In active transport the phosphorylation of subunits would be capable of inducing conformational change (Houslay et al., 1982).

Anion Exchange in Erythrocytes

The anion exchange protein of the erythrocyte membrane catalyzes a one-for-one exchange of chloride ions (Cl^-) for HCO_3^-. This protein has been identified as band 3 polypeptide (Steck, 1978). It is the predominant protein of the erythrocyte membrane which is about 100 000 times more permeable to Cl^- than other plasma membranes. In capillary blood, carbon dioxide (CO_2) diffuses into the erythrocyte and is converted to HCO_3^- by the action of carbonic anhydrase. Release of oxygen by haemoglobin allows binding of the H^+ derived from the reaction of CO_2 with water. The HCO_3^- produced is transported out of the cell by band 3 protein and exchanged for an entering Cl^- (Fig. 49.4). This exchange greatly increases the ability of blood to transport carbon dioxide. The process is reversed in the pulmonary capillaries (Fig. 49.4).

Co-transport and Energy Coupling

Facilitated diffusion of two substances can be coupled by a common transport protein and is then termed co-transport (Gunn, 1980). The transfer of one solute depends on the simultaneous or sequential transfer of a second solute, either in the same direction (symport) or in the opposite direction (antiport). When the co-substrate is an ion like Na^+ or K^+ it is possible to

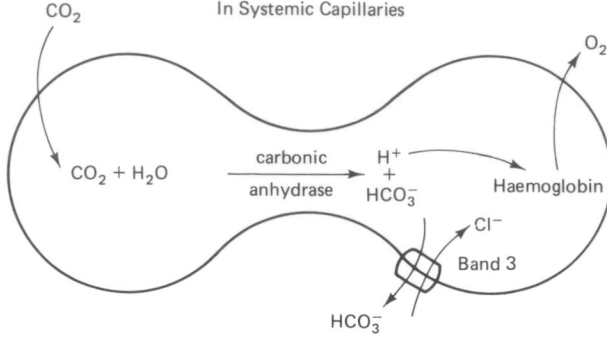

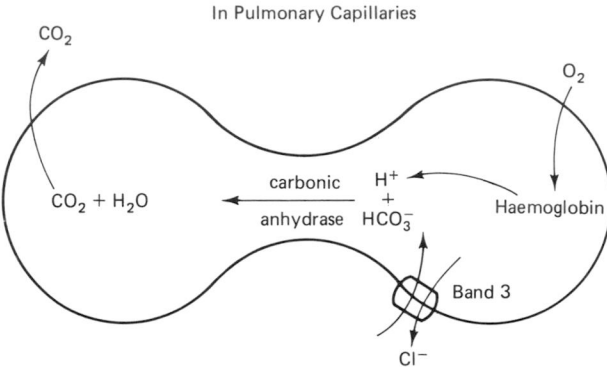

Fig. 49.4 Schematic representation of anion transport through the erythrocyte membrane by band 3 polypeptide. In the systemic capillaries, CO_2 diffuses into the cell and is converted into HCO_3^- which is exported from the cell in exchange for Cl^-. In pulmonary capillaries the process is reversed. HCO_3^- is transported into erythrocytes by band 3 polypeptide and then converted to CO_2 which diffuses out of the cell. (Adapted with permission from *Molecular Cell Biology* by James F. Darnell et al. Copyright © 1986 Scientific American Books, Inc.)

move substances across the membrane against a concentration gradient using the energy stored in ion gradients created by Na^+-K^+ ATPase. It is likely that both substrate binding sites on a co-transport protein must be occupied before the conformational change can occur.

Glucose uptake into intestinal cells is achieved by a symport system in which glucose and Na^+ bind to different sites on the glucose carrier protein; Na^+ moves into the cell down its electrochemical gradient and 'drags' glucose with it (Fig. 49.5). The rate of glucose entry is proportional to the Na^+ gradient, and if the Na^+ concentration in the extracellular fluid is markedly reduced, glucose transport stops. The Na^+ that enters the cell with glucose is pumped out by the Na^+-K^+ ATPase which therefore indirectly drives glucose transport. Insulin increases glucose uptake into cells, possibly by inducing rapid translocation of glucose carrier proteins from an intracellular pool to the plasma membrane (Mueckler et al., 1985). In adipocytes, it is likely that insulin increases the efficiency of

this transporter by decreasing its K_m for glucose (Mueckler et al., 1985). Most amino acids are transported into cells by similar symport sytems with Na^+ (Oxender, 1972).

Energy may also be coupled indirectly to facilitated diffusion by the active modification of the substrate transported into the cell. Glucose is rapidly phosphorylated by hexokinase thus removing it from the chemical equilibrium of glucose across the membrane.

An example of an antiport system is the export of Ca^{2+} from cells in exchange for an entry of Na^+ down the electrochemical gradient established by Na^+-K^+ ATPase. This so called sodium–calcium exchanger complements the activity of Ca^{2+} ATPase (*see below*). Three Na^+ ions move into the cell for every Ca^{2+} ions removed. Both chemical and electrical gradients drive this antiport system (Carafoli et al., 1985). The cardiac glycosides such as digoxin inhibit Na^+-K^+ ATPase and therefore result in a small increase in intracellular Na^+ concentration. Sodium–calcium exchange then causes Ca^{2+} to enter the cell in exchange for intracellular Na^+, and in cardiac muscle, the force of myocardial contraction is increased (Colucci et al., 1986). This is the likely mode of action of these drugs.

Recent observations suggest that co-transport systems may transport more than two substances. The (Na^+-K^+-Cl^-) co-transport system is coupled so that all three ions are carried across the cell membrane together, and all three are necessary for transport. This co-transport system is inhibited by loop diuretic drugs such as frusemide. (Na^+-$K^+$$Cl^-$) co-transport is involved in the epithelial absorption of NaCl, and has been implicated in secretion, cellular accumulation of Cl^- and, more controversially, in the aetiology of hypertension (Chipperfield, 1986).

Active Transport

Transport of specific solutes against their concentration gradients is termed active transport. Unlike passive transport (diffusion and facilitated diffusion), active transport must be tightly coupled to a source of energy. This energy may be supplied by light (in photosynthetic membranes), by oxidation (in mitochondrial membranes) or by metabolic processes, either via a proton gradient or by hydrolysis of ATP. Although many substrates are transported by co-transport systems with ions indirectly using stored energy, Na^+, K^+, Ca^{2+} and H^+ are the only known substances whose transport into and out of cells is *directly* coupled to ATP hydrolysis. These ion pumps will be considered in more detail.

Sodium–Potassium ATPase

The Na^+-K^+ pump is found in the plasma membrane of virtually all animal cells (Sweadner and Goldin, 1980). This pump operates as an antiport, actively pumping sodium ions out of the cell and potassium ions in against their concentration gradients; and in

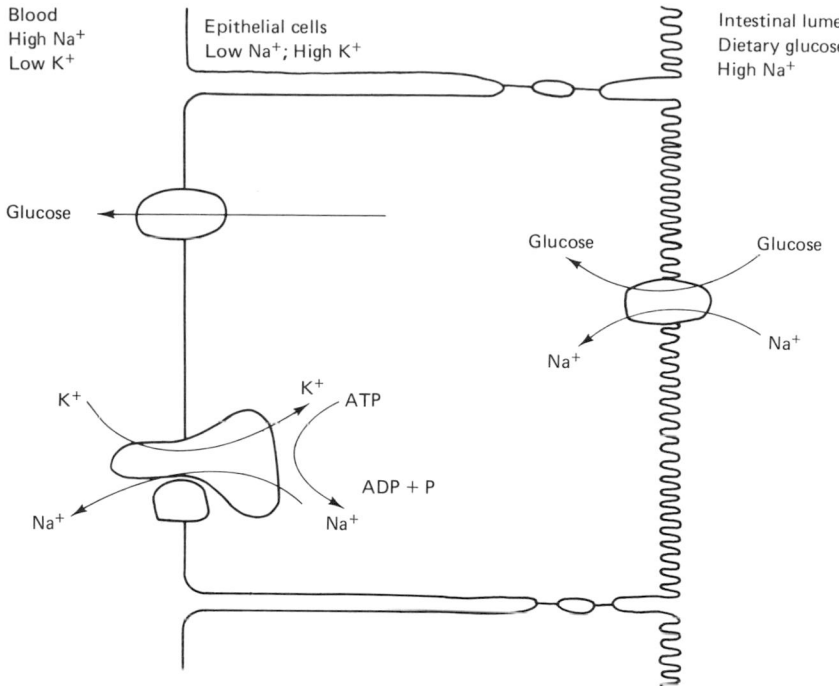

Fig. 49.5 Glucose transport into intestinal epithelial cells. Glucose is transported into the cell through the apical membrane by a symport system with Na^+. The Na^+ gradient driving the glucose symport is maintained by Na^+-K^+ ATPase. Glucose is transported out of the cell, down a concentration gradient by facilitated diffusion mediated by a different glucose carrier protein. (Adapted with permission from *Molecular Cell Biology* by James E. Darnell et al. Copyright © 1986 Scientific American Books, Inc.)

the case of Na^+, against an electrical gradient as well. These ion gradients are responsible not only for the cell's membrane potential, but also for controlling cell volume (Alberts et al., 1983) and for the transport of sugars and amino acids and other ions (as outlined in the previous section). It is estimated that approximately one third of an animal cell's energy requirement is consumed by the Na^+-K^+ pump; this figure approaches 70% of the total energy requirement of electrically active cells (Alberts et al., 1983).

The Na^+-K^+ pump is a membrane-bound ATPase that hydrolyzes ATP to ADP and phosphate and requires Na^+ and K^+ for optimum activity (Skou, 1957). Na^+-K^+ ATPase is shown schematically in Fig. 49.6. For every molecule of ATP hydrolyzed, $3Na^+$ are transported out, and $2K^+$ are transported into the cell (Post and Jolly, 1957). This tends to generate an electrical potential across the plasma membrane, with the inside negative relative to the outside (Thomas, 1969). The Na^+-K^+ pump therefore makes a small direct contribution to the membrane potential. Depending on the membrane studied, the potential is principally due either to the ion gradients maintained by the Na^+-K^+ ATPase or the greater permeability of the plasma membrane to K^+ than to Na^+ or anions. Active transport of Na^+ and K^+ in

red blood cell ghosts is inhibited by the cardiac glycoside ouabain (Glynn, 1968). K^+ and ouabain competes for the same site on the ATPase on the external surface of the membrane (Fig. 49.6). The binding sites for ATP and Na^+ are on the cytoplasmic surface (Glynn, 1968). ATP hydrolysis and ion transport are linked by transfer of the terminal phosphate group of the ATP to an aspartyl residue of the ATPase in the presence of Na^+ (Alberts et al., 1983). The binding of Na^+, and the subsequent phosphorylation on the cytoplasmic face of the ATPase induce the enzyme to change conformation so that Na^+ transfers across the membrane and is released on the external surface (Fig. 49.7). This reaction requires magnesium ions (Mg^{2+}). The binding of K^+ on the external surface and subsequent dephosphorylation of the protein return it to its original conformation which transfers K^+ across the membrane and releases it into the cytoplasm (Alberts et al., 1983). In red blood cell ghosts, sufficiently high concentrations of Na^+ on the outside and K^+ on the inside can drive the pump in the reverse direction and result in synthesis of ATP from ADP and inorganic phosphate (Garrahan and Glynn, 1967). Under physiological conditions, the pump is apparently asymmetric and drives active transport in only one direction (Sweadner et al., 1980).

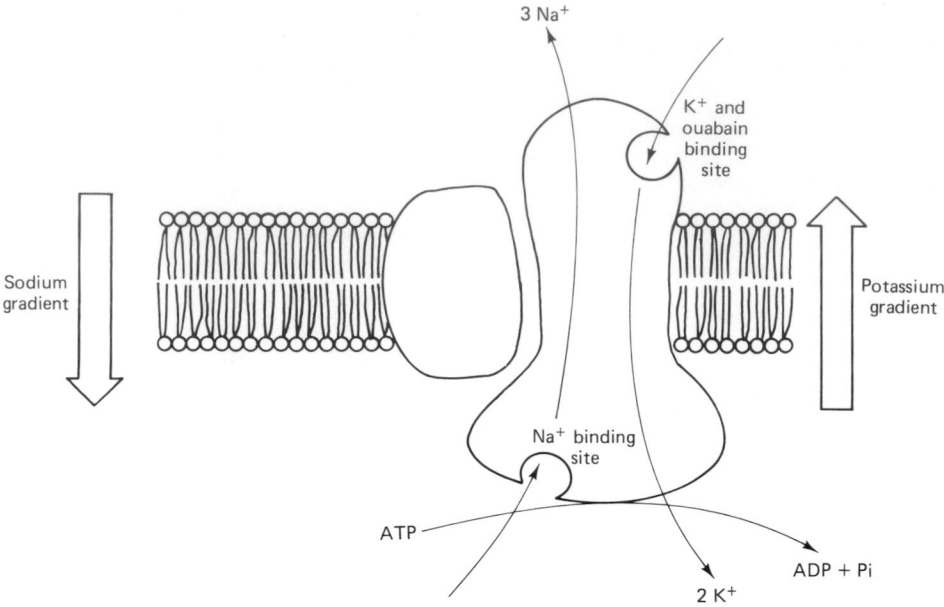

Fig. 49.6 Schematic diagram of Na^+-K^+ ATPase. Na^+ and ATP bind at the cytoplasmic surface. The K^+ and ouabain binding site is at the external surface. (Adapted with permission from Alberts et al., 1983. *Molecular Biology of the Cell*. New York: Garland Publishing Inc.)

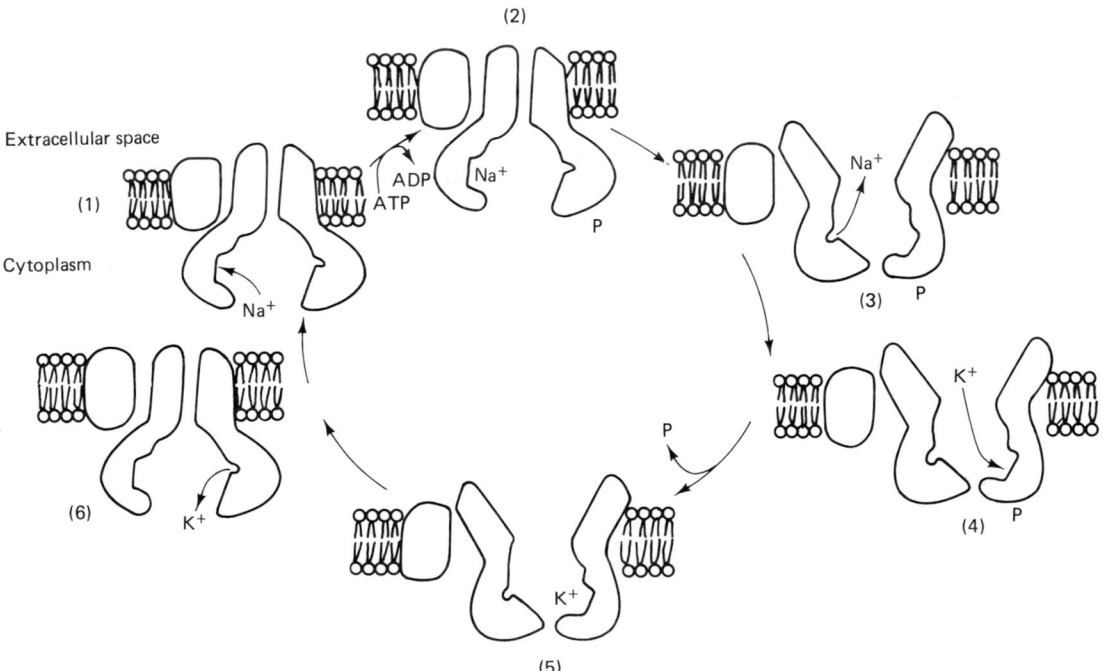

Fig. 49.7 Schematic model of Na^+-K^+ ATPase. Na^+ binds to the ATPase (1), the protein becomes phosphorylated (2) resulting in a conformational change which transfers Na^+ out of the cell (3). K^+ then binds to the ATPase (4) which becomes dephosphorylated (5). This returns the protein to its original conformation and K^+ is transferred into the cell (6). (Adapted with permission from Alberts et al., 1983. *Molecular Biology of the Cell*. New York: Garland Publishing Inc.)

The Na^+-K^+ ATPase probably exists as a dimer and each subunit consists of two polypeptide chains, a transmembrane catalytic subunit (approximately 110 000 daltons), called the α subunit; and an associated glycoprotein (approximately 55 000 daltons), the β subunit. The former has binding sites for Na^+ and ATP on its cytoplasmic surface and for K^+ and ouabain (or digoxin) on its external surface and is reversibly phosphorylated and dephosphorylated. The function of the glycoprotein is unknown (Shull et al., 1985).

Calcium ATPases

In a typical mammalian cell the concentration of free Ca^{2+} is 10^{-7} M, ten-thousand times less than its concentration in plasma. This Ca^{2+} gradient is maintained by the plasma membrane-bound Ca^{2+} ATPase, which is present in virtually every kind of mammalian tissue. It has been best characterized in erythrocytes (Carafoli et al., 1985), where for each Ca^{2+} transported out, $2H^+$ are transferred into the cell. The erythrocyte plasma membrane Ca^{2+} ATPase contains the Ca^{2+}-binding regulatory protein, calmodulin, as an essential subunit. A rise in intracellular Ca^{2+} concentration induces binding of Ca^{2+} to calmodulin. This both increases the maximum capacity of the ATPase (V_{max}) and increases its efficiency (lowers the K_m for Ca^{2+}), accelerating the removal of Ca^{2+} from the cell (Rasmussen, 1986). This Ca^{2+} ATPase 'fine-tunes' intracellular Ca^{2+} concentration and has been termed the high-affinity, low-capacity transporter. On the other hand, the Na^+-Ca^{2+} exchanger, the cotransport protein with no direct energy requirement described under 'Facilitative diffusion', is termed the low-affinity, high-capacity Ca^{2+} transporter. This latter protein removes ions from the cell when intracellular free Ca^{2+} concentration increases to about ten times its resting level due to repetitive stimulation or cell damage (Carafoli et al., 1985).

A similar membrane-bound Ca^{2+} ATPase is present in muscle cells, and this pump transports Ca^{2+} against a concentration gradient from the cytosol into the sarcoplasmic reticulum. The sarcoplasmic reticulum is responsible specifically for release of Ca^{2+} into the muscle cytosol causing muscle contraction. Rapid removal of Ca^{2+} by the ATPase contributes to relaxation. This ATPase constitutes more than 80% of the integral protein component of the sarcoplasmic reticulum. The ATP binding site is on the outside or cytoplasmic side of the membrane. The purified enzyme catalyzes Mg^{2+} and Ca^{2+}-dependent hydrolysis of ATP, and like the other ATPases it becomes reversibly phosphorylated. It pumps two Ca^{2+} ions into the sarcoplasmic reticulum for every molecule of ATP hydrolyzed, and it is likely that monovalent cations serve as counter ions (Racker, 1978). Within the sarcoplasmic reticulum, Ca^{2+} binds to two proteins, calsequestrin and the 'high-affinity calcium binding protein'. These proteins serve as an

intracellular store of Ca^{2+} and, by reducing the concentration of free Ca^{2+} within the organelle, decrease the energy required to pump Ca^{2+} (Darnell et al., 1985). These calcium pumps can also theoretically work in reverse and synthesize ATP (de Meis and Vianna, 1979).

ATP-dependent Proton Pumps

Hyrolysis of ATP is coupled to the transport of H^+ out of gastric parietal cells, resulting in hydrochloric acid secretion into the stomach (Forte et al., 1980) (Fig. 49.8). Active transport of H^+ from the cells into the lumen of the stomach is accompanied by passive transport of Cl^-. The H^+ secreted by the parietal cell is derived from the hydration of CO_2 by carbonic anhydrase within the cell. The HCO_3 produced by this reaction is exchanged for Cl^- by means of an anion exchanger in the basolateral membrane which is similar to the erythrocyte band 3 protein (Fig. 49.8). An ATP-dependent proton pump is also present in lysosomal membranes and is responsible for the acid environment inside lysosomes (Ohkuma et al., 1982).

MEMBRANE EVENTS IN HORMONE ACTION

Hormones initiate effects on target tissue by binding to receptors. They can be classified into those hormones that bind to cell surface receptors, such as adrenaline and insulin, and those that bind to intracellular receptors, such as steroid and thyroid hormones. Cell surface receptors are transmembrane proteins with specific binding sites on the external surface of the plasma membrane. Binding of a hormone to its specific receptor protein may either directly cause phosphorylation of cellular proteins (as in the case of epidermal growth factor (Carpenter and Cohen, 1979)) or activate a cytoplasmic 'second messenger' such as cAMP or Ca^{2+}.

Cyclic AMP

Cyclic AMP is a common intracellular mediator of peptide and protein hormones (including glucagon, ACTH, TSH and parathyroid hormone) and catecholamines (Pasten, 1972; Sutherland, 1972). It is generated from ATP by the action of adenylate cyclase, a membrane protein with its active site at the cytoplasmic surface of the plasma membrane (Ross and Gilman, 1980). Different receptors share a common pool of adenylate cyclase molecules which can move independently in the lateral plane of the membrane. Activation of adenylate cyclase first requires binding of a hormone to a unique receptor protein. The resulting change in conformation of the receptor activates guanosine triphosphate (GTP) binding protein or G protein, which is a membrane protein which binds GTP to its cytoplasmic surface when activated (Rodbell, 1980). The resulting conformational change in the G protein activates an adenylate cyclase molecule to synthesize cAMP (Fig. 49.9). The G protein is a

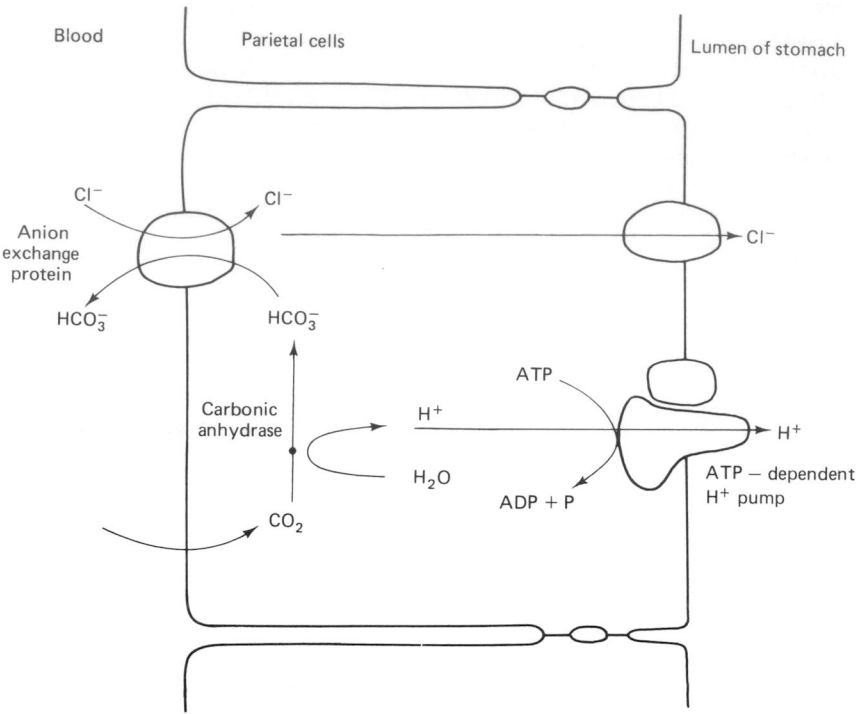

Fig. 49.8 Schematic representation of hydrochloric acid secretion by gastric parietal cells. Carbon dioxide diffuses into the cell and is converted to H^+ and HCO_3^- by carbonic anhydrase. The H^+ is transported into the lumen of the stomach against a concentration gradient by an ATP-dependent proton pump in the parietal cell membrane. HCO_3^- is exchanged for Cl^- by means of an anion exchange protein in the basolateral membrane. Chloride ions are then transported into the stomach down a concentration gradient. (Adapted with permission from *Molecular Cell Biology* by James E. Darnell et al. Copyright © 1986 Scientific American Books, Inc.)

GTPase that hydrolyzes its bound GTP to GDP and inorganic phosphate, which returns the cyclase to its original inactive state. Thus the function of hormone receptors, e.g. the adrenergic β-receptor, involves at least three different intrinsic proteins of the plasma membrane. Another specific GTP-binding protein (Gi protein) inhibits adenylate cyclase when ligands such as α-adrenergic agents and opiates bind at inhibitory receptors (Schramm and Selinger, 1984).

Cyclic AMP stimulates cAMP-dependent protein kinases to phosphorylate specific target proteins (Cohen, 1982), which serve as effectors or modulators of various cellular reactions. Each cell has characteristic sets of target proteins and responds in a specific way to a change in intracellular cAMP concentration. The role of G protein as a 'transducer' between the binding of a hormone and the production of cAMP allows both a rapid response to changes in hormone concentration and amplification of the original extracellular signal, since each activated receptor protein may activate many molecules of G protein.

Calcium Ions

In the case of hormones such as angiotensin II and

vasopressin, Ca^{2+} acts as the second messenger (Rasmussen, 1986). The intracellular concentration of Ca^{2+} is normally maintained at a low level by the action of plasma membrane-bound Ca^{2+} ATPase. Binding of these hormones induces opening of Ca^{2+} channels allowing Ca^{2+} to enter the cytosol, without depolarization of the plasma membrane. In this case the receptor-hormone interaction also activates a phospholipase C that catalyzes the hydrolysis of phosphatidylinositol 4,5, biphosphate (PIP2) to produce diacyglycerol (DG) and inositol triphosphate (IP3). IP3 induces Ca^{2+} release from the endoplasmic reticulum resulting in an increase in intracellular Ca^{2+} concentration. This free Ca^{2+} binds to and alters the conformation of calmodulin (Cheung, 1980), and the Ca^{2+}–calmodulin complex in turn activates many different target proteins, including Ca^{2+}-dependent protein kinases, allowing characteristic responses (Cohen, 1982). DG is a precursor of arachidonic acid.

In some circumstances the roles of cAMP and Ca^{2+} are related. Stimulation of hepatic glycogenolysis by glucagon is mediated by cAMP; when it is stimulated by vasopressin, Ca^{2+} is the second messenger (Rasmussen, 1986).

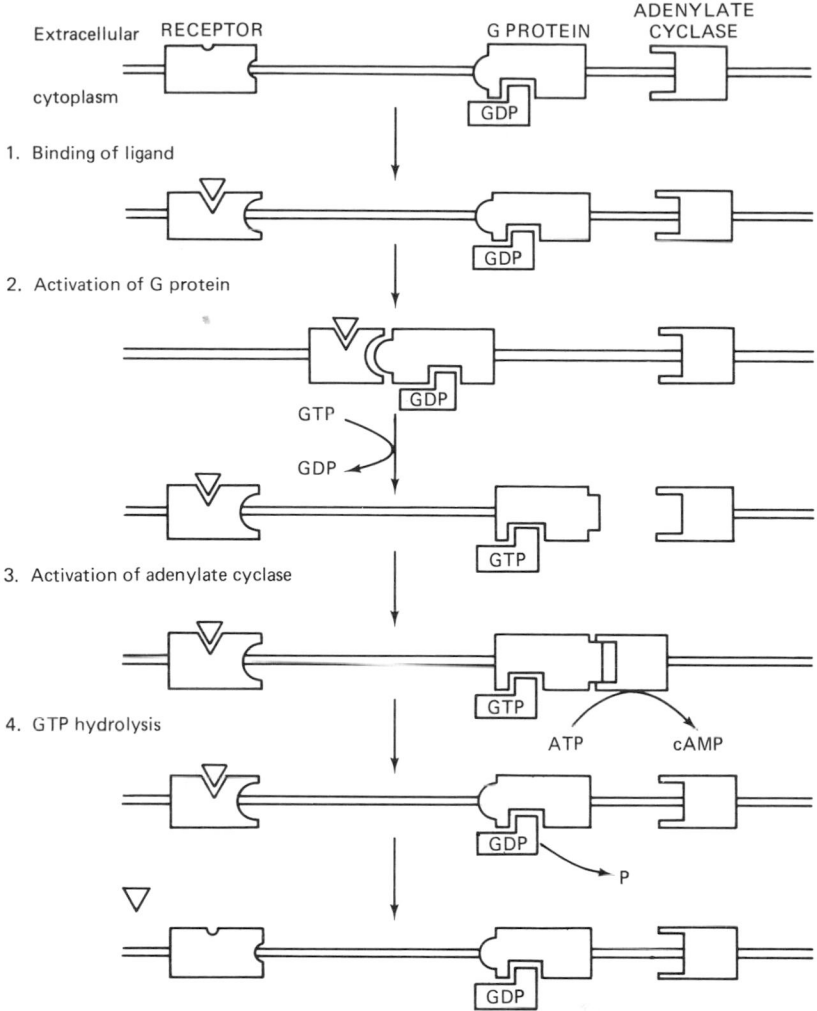

Fig. 49.9   The 'collision' model of adenylate cyclase activation. In this model the receptor protein, G protein and adenylate cyclase molecules are assumed to move independently in the membrane. Ligand binding results in a conformational change in the receptor protein (1) which activates G protein (2) so that it binds GTP and changes conformation. Activated G protein in turn activates adenylate cyclase to produce cAMP (3). Hydrolysis of GTP returns G protein to its original conformation (4). (Adapted with permission from Alberts et al., 1983. *Molecular Biology of the Cell*. New York: Garland Publishing Inc.)

For insulin, the molecular mechanisms of action are poorly understood, and the cytoplasmic 'second messenger', if it exists, remains to be elucidated (Houslay et al., 1986).

Hormones with intracellular receptor proteins are hydrophobic molecules that diffuse through the plasma membrane. Steroid hormones bind to specific receptor proteins in the cytosol and the hormone–receptor complex acquires an affinity for DNA and accumulates in the cell nucleus (Yamamoto and Alberts, 1976); whereas thyroid hormones probably bind in the nucleus (Narayan et al., 1984). In both cases the hormone–receptor complex affects gene transcription. Second messengers are not involved.

TRANSPORT OF MACROMOLECULES

Although membrane proteins transport many small polar molecules into and out of cells, they cannot transport macromolecules, such as proteins, polynucleotides and polysaccharides. These macromolecules are secreted and ingested by exocytosis and endocytosis respectively. In exocytosis, the contents of special intracellular vesicles are released to the outside by fusion with the plasma membrane. In endocytosis the process is reversed and localized regions of the plasma membrane pinch off to form small (pinocytotic) or large (phagocytotic) vesicles. Most cells continuously endocytose sections of their plasma membrane and thus ingest extracellular fluids and solutes, a process called fluid-phase endocytosis. Large extracellular particles, such as cell debris and micro-organisms are usually endocytosed by specific phagocytic cells. A specialized form of endocytosis, involving coated pits, will be described in more detail.

Receptor Mediated Endocytosis

A variety of macromolecules which bind to cell surface receptors are transported to the interior of the cell by receptor mediated endocytosis. These include low density lipoproteins (LDL), glycoproteins, transferrin, insulin and epidermal growth factor (Krogstad and Schlesinger, 1987). The ligand first binds to specific cell surface receptors which cluster in specialized regions on the cell surface called coated pits. These coated pits have submembrane protein coats consisting primarily of clathrin, a fibrous protein of mol. wt. 180 000. This forms a characteristic polygonal network on the pit surface (Ungewickell and Branton, 1981). Coated pits are rapidly internalized as coated vesicles by invagination of the plasma membrane into the cytoplasm, after which the submembrane coats begin to disassemble and the contents of the coated pit are deposited in a smooth endosome. This then fuses with an uncoupling vesicle called CURL (compartment of uncoupling of receptor and ligand), that is characterized by an internal pH of about 5.0. The acid environment causes the receptor–ligand complex to disassociate. Finally, the ligand enters a secondary lysosome with the acid hydrolases from a primary lysosome. The receptor and other membrane components may be recycled to the cell surface (Fig. 49.10).

Cholesterol bound to LDL is internalized by receptor mediated endocytosis and used for new membrane synthesis or stored as cholesterol ester. The LDL receptors are recycled. LDL receptors appear to be incorporated into coated pits in a process that is independent of LDL binding (Goldstein et al., 1979). On the other hand, insulin receptors do not associate with coated pits until after ligand binding (Dautry-Varsat and Lodish, 1984). In the case of insulin, many of the internalized insulin receptors are degraded in lysosomes along with the insulin, so that the concentration of insulin receptors on the cell surface is decreased. By this process, called downregulation, the concentration of hormone in the extra-cellular fluid can regulate the concentration of its receptors on the target cell surface. Exposure of cells to high concentrations of a number of hormones, including insulin, growth hormone, TRH and catecholamines reduces the number of receptors for these hormones (Raff, 1976). The acid vesicle system also has important functions in degradation of internalized macromolecules, intracytoplasmic entry of internalized viruses and some bacterial toxins, antigen processing and normal cell growth and differentiation (Krogstad et al., 1987).

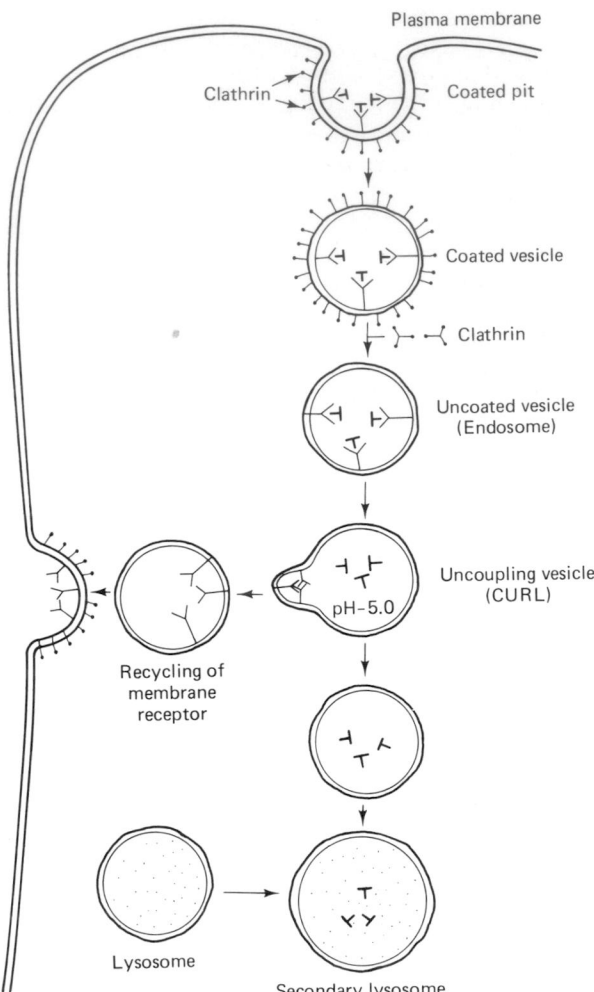

Fig. 49.10 Receptor mediated endocytosis. The ligand binds to its receptor protein and the receptor–ligand complex is internalized in a clathrin coated pit that pinches off to become a coated vesicle. The vesicle loses its coat and fuses with an uncoupling vesicle (CURL). In the case of LDL, the LDL receptors are recycled to the membrane surface and the LDL particles are degraded in secondary lysosomes. (Adapted with permission from *Molecular Cell Biology* by James E. Darnell et al. Copyright © 1986 Scientific American Books, Inc.)

The ability of cells to selectively regulate the passage of substances across both plasma membranes and internal membranes is necessary for their survival, and for the normal function of tissues and whole organs. Some commonly used drugs, such as digoxin which inhibits Na^+–K^+ ATPase, and the calcium channel antagonists, exert their therapeutic effects by influencing membrane transport processes. Many mediators of disease disrupt normal membrane function. For example, activated complement binds to cell membranes, forming a huge pore, which results in collapse of ion gradients across the membrane and osmotic disruption of the cell (Houslay et al., 1982). In oxygen toxicity, the hydroxyl radical exerts its major action against cell membrane lipids by converting polyunsaturated fatty acid side chains into lipid peroxides, a process called lipid peroxidation. This results in a gradual loss of membrane fluidity and membrane potential, increases membrane permeability to ions such as Ca^{2+}, and eventually causes loss of membrane integrity. Membrane-bound enzymes and receptors are also activated (Halliwell and Gutteridge, 1985).

An understanding of the principles of passage across membranes is a necessary basis for the understanding of normal cellular physiological and biochemical processes, the action of many therapeutic agents and the underlying mechanisms of many disease processes.

REFERENCES

Alberts B., Bray D., Lewis, J., et al. (1983). *Molecular Biology of the Cell*. New York: Garland Publishing.

Altman J. (1985). New visions in photoreception. *Nature*, **313**, 264.

Carafoli E., Penniston T. (1985). The calcium signal. *Sci. Am.*, **253**, 50.

Carpenter G., Cohen S. (1979). Epidermal growth factor. *Ann. Rev. Biochem.*, **48**, 193.

Catterall W.A. (1986). Voltage-dependent gating of sodium channels: correlating structure and function. *Trends NeuroSci.*, **9**, 7.

Cheung W.Y. (1980). Calmodulin plays a pivotal role in cellular regulation. *Science*, **207**, 19.

Chipperfield A.R. (1986). The (Na^+-K^+-Cl^-) co-transport system. *Clin. Sci.*, **71**, 465.

Cohen P. (1982). The role of protein phosphorylation in neural and hormonal control of cellular activity. *Nature*, **296**, 613.

Colucci W.S., Wright R.F., Braunwald E. (1986). New positive inotropes in the treatment of congestive heart failure. Mechanisms of action and recent clinical developments. (First of two parts). *N. Eng. J. Med.*, **314**, 290.

Darnell J., Lodish H., Baltimore D. (1986). *Molecular Cell Biology*. New York: Scientific American Books.

Dautry-Varsat A., Lodish H.F. (1984). How receptors bring proteins and particles into cells. *Sci. Am.*, **250**, 48.

Forte J.G., Machen T.E., Obrink K.J. (1980). Mechanism of gastric H^+ and Cl^- transport. *Ann. Rev. Physiol.*, **42**, 111.

Garrahan P.J., Glynn I.M. (1967). The incorporation of inorganic phosphate into adenosine triphosphate by reversal of the sodium pump. *J. Physiol.*, **201**, 495.

Glynn I.M. (1968). Membrane adenosine triphosphate and cation transport. *Br. Med. Bull.*, **24**, 165.

Gorter E., Grendell S. (1925). Bimolecular layers of lipoids on chromocytes of blood. *J. Exp. Med.*, **41**, 439.

Goldstein J.L., Anderson R.G.W., Brown M.S. (1979). Coated pits, coated vesicles, and receptor-mediated endocytosis. *Nature*, **279**, 679.

Guidotti G. (1972). Membrane Proteins. *Ann. Rev. Biochem.*, **41**, 731.

Gunn R.B. (1980). Co and counter-transport mechanisms in cell membranes. *Ann. Rev. Physiol.*, **42**, 249.

Halliwell B., Gutteridge J.M.C. (1985). Oxygen radicals and the nervous system. *Trends NeuroSci.*, **8**, 22.

Hodgkin A.L., Huxley A.F. (1952). A quantitative description of membrane current and its application to conduction and excitation in nerve. *J. Physiol.*, **117**, 500.

Houslay M.D., Stanley K.K. (1982). *Dynamics of Biological Membranes*, pp. 1–39 and 281–325. New York: John Wiley and Sons.

Houslay M.D., Wakelam M.J.O., Pyne N.J. (1986). The mediator is the message: is it part of the answer of insulin's action. *Trends Biochem. Sci.*, **11**, 393.

Keynes R.D. (1979). Ion channels in the nerve-cell membrane. *Sci. Am.*, **240**, 98.

Klingenberg M. (1981). Membrane protein oligomeric structure and transport function. *Nature*, **290**, 449.

Kopito R.R., Lodish H.F. (1985). Primary structure and transmembrane orientation of the murine anion exchange protein. *Nature*, **316**, 234.

Krogstad D.J., Schlesinger P.H. (1987). Acid-vesicle function, intracellular pathogens, and the action of chloroquine against plasmodium faciparum. *N. Engl. J. Med.*, **317**, 542.

Luft J.H. (1976). The structure and properties of the cell surface coat. *Int. Rev. Cytol.*, **45**, 291.

de Meis L., Vianna A.L. (1979). Energy interconversion by the Ca^{2+}-dependent ATPase of the sarcoplasmic reticulum. *Ann. Rev. Biochem.* **48**, 275.

Mueckler M., Caruso C., Baldwin S.A., et al. (1985). Sequence and structure of a human glucose transporter. *Science*, **229**, 941.

Narayan P., Liaw C.W., Towle H.C. (1984). Rapid induction of a specific nuclear mRNA precursor by thyroid hormone. *Proc. Natl. Acad. Sci. USA*, **81**, 4687.

Ohkuma S., Moriyami Y., Takano T. (1980). Identification and characterization of a proton pump on lysosomes by fluorescein isothiocyanate-dextran fluorescence. *Proc. Natl. Acad. Sci. USA*, **79**, 2758.

Oxender D.L. (1972). Membrane transport. *Ann. Rev. Biochem.*, **41**, 778.

Pasten I. (1972). Cyclic AMP. *Sci. Am.*, **227**, 97.

Post R.L., Jolly P.C. (1957). The linkage of sodium, potassium, and ammonium active transport across the human erythrocyte membrane. *Biochim. Biophys. Acta*, **25**, 118.

Quinn A.J., Chapman D. (1980). The dynamics of membrane structure. *Crit. Rev. Biochem.*, **8**, 1.

Racker E. (1978). Mechanisms of ion transport and ATP formation. in *Membrane Transport in Biology 1. Concepts and Models*. (Giebisch G., Tosteson D.C., Ussing H.H., eds.). Berlin: Springer-Verlag.

Raff M. (1976). Self regulation of membrane receptors. *Nature*, **259**, 265.

Rasmussen H. (1986). The calcium messenger system. (First of two parts). *N. Engl. J. Med.*, **314**, 1094.

Rodbell M. (1980). The role of hormone receptors and GTP-regulatory proteins in membrane transduction. *Nature*, **284**, 17.

Ross E.M., Gilman A.G. (1980). Biochemical properties of hormone-sensitive adenylate cyclase. *Ann. Rev. Biochem.*, **49**, 533.

Rothman J., Lenard J. (1977). Membrane asymmetry. *Science*, **195**, 743.

Schlessinger J. (1983). Mobilities of cell-membrane proteins: how are they modulated by the cytoskeleton? *Trends NeuroSci.*, **6**, 360.

Schofield P.R., Darlison M.G., Fujita M., et al. (1987).

Sequence and functional expression of the GABA receptor shows a ligand-gated receptor super-family. *Nature,* **328**, 221.

Schnapf J.L., Baylor D.A. (1987). How photoreceptor cells respond to light. *Sci. Am.,* **256**, 32.

Schramm M., Selinger Z. (1984). Message transmission: receptor controlled adenylate cyclase system. *Science,* **225**, 1350.

Shull G.E., Schwartz A., Lingrel J.B. (1985). Amino acid sequence of the catalytic subunit of the (Na⁺K⁺)ATPase deduced from complementary DNA. *Nature,* **316**, 691.

Singer S.J., Nicholson G.L. (1972). The fluid mosaic model of the structure of cell membranes. *Science,* **175**, 720.

Skou J.C. (1957). The influence of some cations on adenosine triphosphatase from peripheral nerves. *Biochim. Biophys. Acta,* **23**, 239.

Steck T.L. (1978). The band 3 protein of the human red cell membrane: a review. *J. Supramol. Struct.,* **8**, 311.

Sutherland E.W. (1972). Studies on the mechanism of hormone action. *Science,* **177**, 401.

Sweadner K.J., Goldin S.M. (1980). Active transport of sodium and potassium ions. *N. Engl. J. Med.,* **302**, 777.

Thomas R.C. (1969). Membrane current and intracellular sodium changes in a snail neurone during extrusion of injected sodium. *J. Physiol.,* **201**, 495.

Ungewickell E., Branton D. (1981). Assembly units of clathrin coats. *Nature,* **289**, 420.

Unwin P.N.T., Zampighi G. (1980). Structure of the junction between communicating cells. *Nature,* **283**, 545.

Yamamato K.R., Alberts B.M. (1976). Steroid receptors: elements for modulation of eukaryotic transcription. *Ann. Rev. Biochem.,* **45**, 721.

50. Endogenous Opioid Peptides

A. H. Dickenson

The discovery of endogenous opioid peptides has had two major impacts on concepts of sensory processing and modulation in the CNS. Firstly, the realization that peptides can function as transmitters or modulators in the brain and peripheral nervous system has added several dozen candidates to the list of centrally active neurotransmitters. Secondly and of great importance to anaesthesiology is the major step forward in understanding opiate analgesia produced by comprehension of opioid peptide systems in the brain and the possibility of novel therapeutic agents based on this knowledge.

SYNTHESIS OF OPIOID PEPTIDES

The three main biologically active classes of opioid peptides, the enkephalins (methionine and leucine), β endorphin and the dynorphins have, in common with other peptides, a slow synthesis pathway compared to the rapid synthesis and turnover of other transmitters such as acetylcholine or the catecholamines. The opioid peptides are released as cleavage products of a large precursor or parent molecule, which are produced in the cell body (Fig. 50.1). The propeptide (proopiocortin, proenkephalin and prodynorphin)

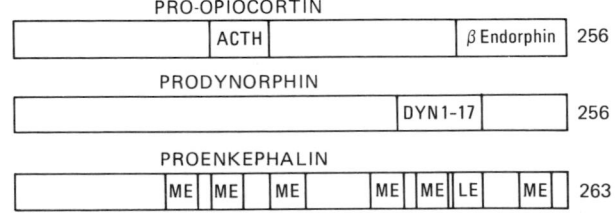

Fig. 50.1 The opioid propeptide precursors. Dyn = dynorphin, ME = methionine enkephalin., LE = leucine enkephalin. The numbers refer to the number of amino acids in the sequence.

consists of the neuropeptide plus signal segments and following synthesis is transferred from the genetic apparatus to the endoplasmic reticulum and thence the Golgi apparatus where it is formed into granules. En route to the terminal or in the terminal itself the parent propeptide is cleaved by specific enzymes to liberate the final peptides which are then released into the synapse. Of course, the classical transmitters (glutamate, noradrenaline, dopamine etc) are rapidly synthesized in the terminal from precursors so that the time span from synthesis to release can be short. An important consequence of the slower peptide synthesis is that large or sustained release of the peptide may lead to a depletion of the neuropeptide. However, the production of opioid peptides by this means allows genetic, enzymatic and post-translational influences to modulate the pool of opioids available for release.

Modification of Synthesis

In the case of proopiocortin single copies of the opioid peptide are produced whilst six copies of met-enkephalin are contained within the sequence of proenkephalin. Various products arise from pro-dynorphin. The relative size of fragments of β endorphin produced vary from tissue to tissue and alter with the stages of development of the animal. Hypothalamic β-endorphin fragments can be manipulated by interference with dopamine function, an example of gene expression being modulated by central transmitters.

Conclusions

The synthesis of peptides differs from all other transmitters since the biologically active peptide is formed from large precursor peptides. Complex post-translational modulation seems to occur.

RELEASE AND BREAKDOWN

The opioid peptides are released into the synapse by a calcium dependent process but unlike many central transmitters are not seemingly subject to reuptake by either neurones or glia. Thus, the situation at central opioid synapses is now akin to the neuromuscular junction where acetylcholine is broken down by cholinesterases. The opioids are broken down by a variety of peptidases and this process is exemplified by enkephalin for which the enzymatic metabolism is best characterized.

Enzymatic Breakdown

What then are the enzymes that degrade the enkephalins? Three membrane-bound peptidases seem to be involved; one, termed 'enkephalinase' cleaves between the amino acids glycine and phenylalanine. The two others are an aminopeptidase (probably aminopeptidase M) releasing tyrosine from the N-terminal part of the enkephalins and a third aminopeptidase, a dipeptidylaminopeptidase, which may also be involved in the hydrolysis of the Gly^2-Gly^3 bond (Fig. 50.2). These enzymes are ubiquitous (enkephalinase, is associated with aminopeptidase M in kidney and intestine) and a broad substrate spectrum of these enzymes may reflect multiple actions of the enzymes on many other non opioid peptides. Many *in vitro* studies have demonstrated the involvement of these enzymes in hydrolysis of the enkephalins. As a result of this enzymatic assault the effects of the enkephalins are very brief and in the case of the dynorphins the actions of this family on biological processes may be due to fragments as well as the original opioid.

Conclusions

Opioid peptides are broken down by many peptidases and in the case of the enkephalins the degradation is

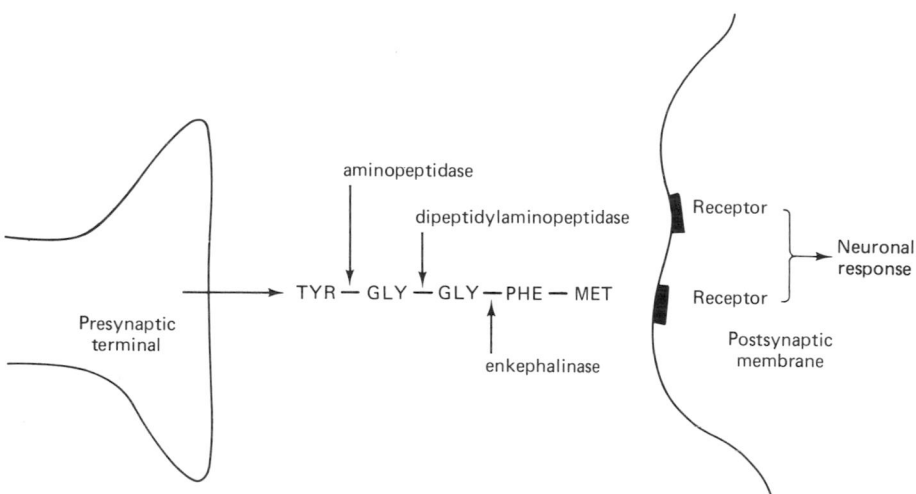

Fig. 50.2 The three enzymes demonstrated to degrade methionine enkephalin.

so rapid that physiological effects are difficult to observe.

OPIOID RECEPTORS

Five types of opioid receptor have been described, although only three, the mu (μ) delta (δ) and kappa (κ) (*see* Table 50.1) have been well characterized. The sigma (σ) subtype may be better described as an amino acid receptor rather than opioid. These three main subtypes of receptor are widely distributed in the CNS and PNS and certain peripheral tissues containing one type of receptor have been useful model systems in elaboration of the pharmacology of these receptors.

Mu Receptor

The mu receptor is the subtype through which morphine (and morphine like opiate drugs) produce its effects and the receptor for which naloxone, the opiate antagonist, has highest affinity. However the endogenous opioid ligand for this receptor is a point of dispute and somewhat puzzling since although β endorphin is a candidate the receptor is found in some tissue bereft of the opioid, and likewise although methionine enkephalin has affinity for the receptor it is very low. A possibility is metorphamide which is a cleavage product from proenkephalin. All the clinical effects of morphine like drugs are produced via this receptor which explains the ready reversal of these actions by naloxone, by competitive antagonism at this receptor. Activation of the receptor is always inhibitory, hyperpolarising neurones (via activation of potassium channels) inhibiting both transmitter release and adenyl cyclase.

Delta Receptor

The delta receptor like the mu receptor has been shown to be coupled to potassium channels and again mediates inhibitory influences on a variety of neural processes. The enkephalins have high affinity for this receptor and so are likely to be the endogenous ligands. Stable enkephalin analogues, protected from degration by chemical modification can be used as probes for this receptor. There is evidence both for and against coupling of the mu and delta receptors so this at present is an open question, but so far mu and delta receptors have not been found on the same neurone but their distribution in the CNS is rather similar. Naloxone has a much lower affinity for this receptor compared to the mu subtype.

Kappa Receptor

Kappa receptor activation is believed to close calcium channels leading to inhibition of neurones and transmitter release. Various fragments of dynorphin are likely to be the endogenous ligands at this receptor and some synthetic opiates such as pentazocine, ethylketocylclazocine and bremazocine have kappa affinity. However *in vitro* and *in vivo* studies indicate that some *kappa agonists* can act as *mu antagonists* which might explain precipitation of withdrawal from patients receiving morphine when pentazocine is administered. It may be that the mixed agonist-antagonist opioids may be explained by these opposite mu and kappa effects.

Conclusions

The opioid receptors can be subdivided into at least three main subtypes, the mu, delta and kappa for which morphine, the enkephalins and the dynorphins, respectively, have highest affinities. Activation of the receptors predominantly leads to neuronal inhibitions.

DISTRIBUTION OF OPIOIDS AND RECEPTORS

A variety of techniques have been used to localize the

TABLE 50.1
OPIOID RECEPTOR SUB TYPES

Receptor type	μ (*mu*)	δ (*delta*)	κ (*kappa*)
Endogenous agonist	*β endorphin met-enkephalin metorphamide	met-enkephalin leu-enkephalin	dynorphin peptides
Selective agonist	morphine dago	D PEN DPEN enkephalin	U50488h + ethylketocyte
Clinically used agonist	morphine × analogues	D ALA DLEU enkephalin	pentazocyte
Antagonist	naloxone kappa agonists	naloxone plus some experimental drugs	naloxone

Notes: * several CNS areas contain mu receptors buit no β ENDORPHIN.
    + non selective and possesses mu agonist activity

main three types of opioid receptors, the distribution of β endorphin, enkephalins and dynorphin (or propeptides) and to a more limited extent a cleavage enzyme for the propeptide (enkephalin catalase) and enkephalinase, a degradation peptidase. Although there is a degree of overlap there is an uneven distribution of the opioid receptors and their endogenous ligands. Neurones containing opioids are generally short interneurones although some far ranging connections have been observed. Cell bodies for β endorphin seem confined to the hypothalamus and the nucleus of the solitary tract although some long running projections from these areas may indicate actions on other CNS areas. β endorphin is known to be co-released with ACTH from the pituitary.

Enkephalins are formed in high levels in many areas of the CNS notably the superficial dorsal horn of the spinal cord and caudal trigeminal, periaqueductal and periventricular areas, amygdala, brainstem and hypothalamus, substantia nigra and peripherally in the adrenal medulla, autonomic ganglia and other tissues.

Dynorphin is found in the spinal cord where interestingly it may be present in sensory fibres as well as in interneurones, brainstem and hypothalamus. The distribution of the mu and delta receptors parallels that of the enkephalins in a general fashion and likewise the propeptide for enkephalin, enkephalin catalase and enkephalinase are concentrated in the areas containing the enkephalins. However exceptions can be mentioned—the periaqueductal grey matter contains enkephalins, dynorphin and some endorphin terminals but only mu receptors in any great number—by contrast the superficial dorsal horn of the spinal cord contains, as well as intrinsic opioid peptides, dynorphin from afferent fibres, enkephalin from descending fibres from the brainstem and high levels of mu, delta and kappa receptor binding sites as well as enkephalinase.

Conclusions

The endogenous opioids and their receptors have a discrete but wide distribution in the CNS reflecting their likely roles in many central functions.

FUNCTIONAL ASPECTS OF OPIOIDS

Two problems arise in this context. Firstly the rapid degradation of the enkephalins renders study of their actions frustratingly difficult and secondly, the use of naloxone as a probe for opioid effects is complicated by its relatively low affinity for the delta and kappa receptors as compared to the mu receptor. Despite these provisos I now wish to address the functional aspects of the opioids in processes relevent to anaesthesiology in the framework of the effects of morphine, exogenous ligand for the mu receptor. Morphine produces analgesia by actions at two main sites in the central nervous system. One is a direct action on the spinal cord and the second is an action

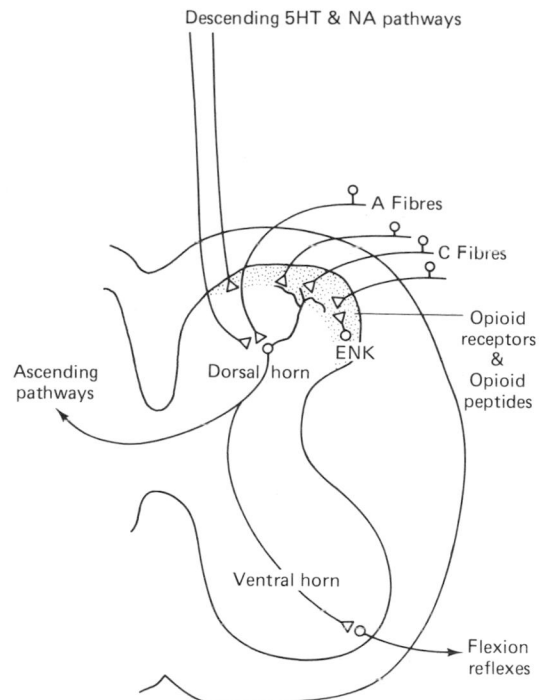

Fig. 50.3 Anatomical organization of the spinal cord and brain stem descending pathways involved in pain modulation.

on the spinal cord but via descending controls of brainstem origins (Fig. 50.3). Additional actions at thalamic and cortical levels may occur but since the ascending input to latter areas depends on spinal mechanisms the first two actions are likely to be of paramount importance.

Direct Depressive Action at the Spinal Level: Morphine

Over many years several groups have reported that systemic opiates can produce a differential depressive effect on spinal reflexes: polysynaptic reflexes are markedly reduced whilst monosynaptic reflexes are only influenced by higher doses. Since the reflexes can be reduced in animals with sections of the spinal cord at thoracic or cervical levels following systemic administration and since a peripheral effect of opiates can be excluded these findings are indicative of a spinal mechanism of action. These studies have been recently confirmed in chronic traumatic paraplegics considered as completely spinal by neurological criteria: the intravenous injection of morphine produced a long lasting marked depression of nociceptive reflexes without influencing monosynaptic reflexes. In intact man, a similar effect has been observed after epidural morphine. Following morphine (2 mg/kg i.v.) the spontaneous activity of convergent neurones in the cat spinal cord responding to A and C fibre inputs and so to tactile and noxious stimuli, is rapidly depressed; the depression lasts at least 50 min and can be considerably longer. The time course and degree of the effects on evoked activity is similar; for example responses to noxious pinch are reduced by about 50%. In the rat, 3 mg/kg i.v. of morphine strongly inhibits the responses of convergent neurones and also nociceptive specific cells to noxious radiant heat. However all neurones are not influenced in the same manner; the responses to low intensity stimuli are not altered whilst the responses of the same cells to nociceptive stimuli are greatly reduced. These effects are specific as demonstrated by their reversal by naloxone, the opiate receptor antagonist. These findings are similar to those of other groups studying the effects of systemic morphine. The ability of morphine to reduce this type of response has been gauged following recording of ascending axons, particularly those in the anterolateral quadrant; in the spinal animal, morphine, administered systematically, strongly depresses the discharges evoked in these axons by Aδ and C fibre strength stimulation of the sural nerve. Over the dose range 1–9 mg/kg i.v. morphine the mean curve reveals a highly significant dose-response relationship for the Aδ and above all, C fibre responses which was naloxone reversible. A weak and non specific effect was seen for the Aβ responses. This demonstration of a significant dose response relationship is an additional argument for the pharmacological nature of this cellular inhibition. A dose dependent depression of C fibre evoked activity, reversed by naloxone, of convergent neurones following intrathecal morphine in the rat has recently been described. Again this effect was selective with Aβ response being little altered.

In addition using more prolonged noxious stimuli to evoke dorsal horn neuronal activity the ability of a mu receptor peptide to inhibit the responses is greatly increased when pretreatment is used. Thus almost complete inhibition of the neuronal activity is caused by application of the opioid before the noxious stimulus is given whereas the opioid effects are reduced once the activity is allowed to build up. This may well have relevance to the effectiveness of opioid pretreatment in reducing postoperative pain in man.

Finally the clinical use of clonidine to potentiate morphine analgesia has a basis in animal studies where this has been observed but for a marked increase in the efficacy of morphine, particular doses of clonidine are needed.

The ability of epidural and intrathecal opioids, such as morphine and diamorphine which are used to relieve pain in humans, lends testimony to this spinal action of opioids.

Conclusions

A clear direct spinal action of morphine has been extensively documented in many animal studies and is manifest by a selective inhibition of activity transmitted into the cord by fine afferent nociceptive fibres, and forms the basis for the use of spinal opioids in man.

Site of Action of Opioids in the Spinal Cord

These results allow one to conclude as to a direct spinal action of morphine on the transmission of nociceptive messages. The differential effect on the responses of convergent neurones to the stimulation of various fibre types suggest that morphine does not act directly on the neuronal membrane but rather on elements presynaptic to the recorded cell. The hypothesis of additional mechanisms of action, including postsynaptic actions cannot however be totally excluded. At the spinal level opiate receptors are predominantly located in the most superficial laminae of the dorsal horn; the marginal zone of Waldeyer (lamina I) and the substantia gelatinosa (lamina II). The convergent neurones are mainly located in the dorsal horn, the most numerous being around lamina V. It seems from anatomical evidence that these cells send dendrites towards the superficial laminae of the dorsal horn. In addition, the majority of C fibre terminals and the dendrites of the convergent neurones are largely found in the superficial zones of the dorsal horn (Fig. 50.4).

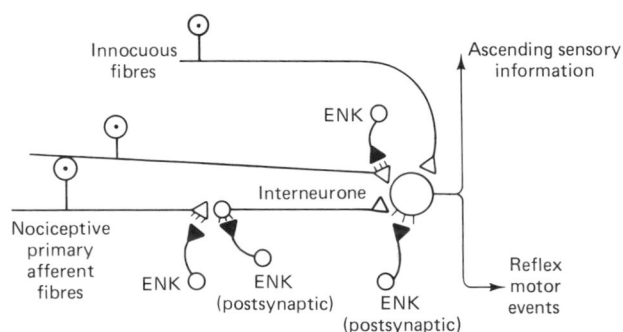

Fig. 50.4 The synaptic arrangements in the spinal cord by which opioid modulation of pain may occur. Presynaptic reduction in transmitter release and postsynaptic inhibition of interneurones would allow selective inhibition of noxious messages. Postsynaptic inhibition of the output neurones may also occur. ENK = enkephalin.

The work of Duggan and North (1984) has used microelectrophoresis to demonstrate the site of action of morphine as being situated in the superficial zones; following recording of convergent neurones they have observed that morphine injected near the cell body of the neurone has little effect but the injection into the substantia gelatinosa causes an inhibition of the neuronal responses to noxious stimuli without altering responses to innocuous stimuli. These inhibitions were long lasting and could be reversed by electrophoretic or low doses of intravenous naloxone. The overall importance of this type of effect is demonstrated by the reversal of the inhibitory effects of systemic morphine on C fibre responses by iontophoresis of naloxone into the substantia gelatinosa.

Endogenous Opioids and Spinal Analgesia

The effects of morphine have been compared to those of endogenous opioids. The iontophoresis of met-enkephalin into substantia gelatinosa produces an inhibition equally selective of the responses of convergent neurones to a noxious stimulus. However, the action of metenkephalin seems more widespread since injection close to the cell body is also effective. In this regard one should note that enkephalinergic terminals have been observed on the soma and dendrites of dorsal horn cells projecting in the spinothalamic tract. In this context although the superficial dorsal horn contains high levels of met and leuenkephalin, these opioids are also found in lamina V. The products of prodynorphin (dynorphins, α neoendorphin) are by contrast concentrated in lamina I.

Recent electrophysiological studies have compared the effects of intrathecal morphine with those of enkephalin analogues with varying affinities for the mu (morphine preferring) and delta (enkephalin preferring) opiate receptors (*see* Fig. 50.1). Morphine, methadone and DAGO, all with high selectivity for the mu receptor produce inhibitions of the C fibre evoked activity which can be complete with appropriate doses and the dose-response curve is steep. Delta agonists also produce selective effects but the dose-response curve is shallower. Both groups of ligands produce effects antagonized by intrathecal naloxone although, in keeping with the highest affinity of naloxone for the mu receptor, only the effects of delta ligands require higher doses. In contrast, dynorphin and stable synthetic analogues with kappa receptor selectivity produced both dose-dependent inhibitions and excitations of convergent neurones, the mean effect being little overall change in activity of the population of cells. Thus whereas morphine and enkephalin like compounds produce inhibitory effects which differ only quantitatively, kappa agonists produce more complex effects which have no clear relationship to analgesia.

Returning to morphine as already discussed, the selective effect on responses due to activation of fine fibres allows the ideas of a principal site of action being elsewhere than on the membrane of the neurone being recorded, most probably then an action in the substantia gelatinosa. Several mechanisms have been considered, with an action of morphine on the fine primary afferent fibres by a presynaptic mechanism attracting most attention. Biochemical studies support this hypothesis: the finding that a dorsal rhizotomy is accompanied by a drop in the number of specific binding sites for opiates in the dorsal horn suggests that a number of opiate receptors are situated on primary afferents.

Thus so far one can conclude that morphine and enkephalin like peptides can inhibit nociceptive responses of dorsal horn cells whereas dynorphin and related peptides seem to lack this spinal site of action. Confirmation of these conclusions arises from behavioural studies in rats and primates, mostly from the work of Yaksh and Noueihed (1985). Here intrathecal administration of morphine, delta ligands and other morphine like opiates produce marked antinociception in a variety of behavioural tests. However kappa agonists seem to produce little effects on cutaneous stimuli but may become effective when the test employed uses visceral stimulation. In this respect it is interesting to note that whereas the release of spinal substance P from afferent fibres produced by a cutaneous noxious stimulus is reduced by μ and δ agonists, kappa compounds do not share this action. A final problem is marked flaccidity elicited by dynorphin in rats after spinal administration.

Despite the clear potential of the delta receptor agonists, mostly modified protected enkephalins in producing analgesia at spinal levels, which has been reported very recently in man, albeit in, as yet, a small number of cases, the enkephalins themselves produce weak or no effect on either the behavioural thresholds or the neuronal responses. The reason for this would seem to be the rapid degradation of these peptides. Very recently peptidase inhibitors have been produced. Bestatin inhibits aminopeptidases, thiorphan blocks enkephalinase and kelatorphan is an inhibitor of both enzymes. Since the peptidases are metallo peptidases, the inhibitors are designed to chelate the Zn^{2+} and from *in vitro* and *in vivo* studies clearly protect the enkephalins from breakdown.

Conclusions

The effects of spinally applied mu receptor opioids such as morphine are shared by delta receptor agonists in both electrophysiological and behavioural studies, although quantitative differences may exist. Kappa opioids produce less obvious effects. The site of action of opioids is probably predominantly presynaptically on the terminals of nociceptive fibres.

MANIPULATION OF ENDOGENOUS OPIOIDS

So, do the peptidase inhibitors produce antinociception? The answer would seem to be yes, but with the proviso that the effects seem dependent on the test used and the circumstances. Thus animal tests which seem clearly amenable to naloxone, the opiate antagonist, such as vocalization, writhing and hot plate jumping illustrate the antinociceptive activity of bestatin and thiorphan which generally have similar magnitudes of effect. Furthermore, coadministration leads to additive effects equivalent to that of kelatorphan. By contrast, tail flick and hot plate licking tests are not sensitive to the inhibitors. Electrophysiological studies have demonstrated thiorphan-induced inhibitory effects on thalamic nociceptive neurones but no influence of the inhibitor on spinal cord neurones. However, in the spinal cord, neither thiorphan nor bestatin have much influence on spontaneous or depolarization-evoked release of enkephalin whereas kelatorphan and coadministration increase overflow *in vivo* and *in vitro*. These findings are reflected in recent observations on the ability of these agents to elicit inhibitions of nociceptive neurones in rat cord where kelatorphan produces inhibitions comparable to stable enkephalin analogues. Whereas the disparate results with thiorphan may reflect the relative importance of the various peptidases in degradation of the enkephalins at different CNS sites, the types of stimulus and the response of the animal or man may govern the release of enkephalins and/or the ability of available enkephalins to block the stimulus. In any case, inhibition of only one enzyme is probably insufficient. In many of these studies the positive effects of the inhibitions were naloxone reversible, indicating actions at opiate receptors. Nevertheless, the effects of kelatorphan antagonized by naloxone would indicate that both enkephalinase and aminopeptidase M (for which kelatorphan has a good selectivity, contrasting with the broad inhibition of all aminopeptidase by bestatin) are important in termination of the physiological effects of the enkephalins. In this regard, the use of labelled inhibitors will be a useful means to locate the three enzymes in the CNS. Using autoradiography, enkephalinase is found in areas high in both enkephalin levels and mu and also delta receptor binding sites, such as the striatum, periaqueductal grey matter, substantia nigra and spinal cord. Visualization of binding sites for the three inhibitors in discrete areas of the CNS should shed light on the relative importance of the degrading enzymes and the roles of enkaphalins in different areas and in various circumstances. Obviously, what these inhibitors do not tell you is whether the increased availability of the enkephalins results from either a pool of tonically released peptide or peptide released as a result of a particular stimulus.

The potential of this approach to the production of 'physiological analgesia' is high, especially since effects mediated by the delta (enkephalin-preferring) opiate receptor may produce less of the problematic side effects mediated by the mu-preferring agonist morphine. Furthermore, the results from animal studies discussed previously would indicate that the more integrated measures of nociception may be altered by the inhibition of enkephalin degradation whereas reflex tests seem, in general, insensitive.

Conclusions
As a result of their rapid breakdown by peptidases, inhibitors of these enzymes serve to protect the endogenous enkephalins, in a manner akin to monoamine oxidase inhibitors and anticholinesterases. Animal studies indicate that these enzyme inhibitors can elicit analgesia.

SUPRASPINAL ANALGESIA
Whereas the spinal actions of opioids are now reaching a reasonable level of understanding so that consensus would be that μ and δ but not κ opioids are effective, the supraspinal sites are much less well documented.

Sites of Action: Morphine
It is clear however that morphine by actions within the periaqueductal grey matter of the midbrain and further caudally within the medial brainstem can elicit behavioural analgesia. There may also be actions within the thalamic areas and at cortical levels. The latter has not been directly studied, mostly due to our ignorance of cortical pain mechanisms but there is a differential distribution of μ, δ and κ receptors within the laminae of the sensory cortex. Thus the ability of intraventricular morphine to relieve pain in man and to elicit analgesia in animals is presumed to be due to actions at one or more of these sites.

It is generally held that opioid receptors in the periaqueductal grey matter, particularly in ventral zones and more caudally within the raphé nuclei of the brainstem are involved in these supraspinal effects of morphine. Thus microinjection of opioids into these zones produces a naloxone reversible analgesia and conversely, systemic morphine analgesia is reduced by either destruction of or naloxone injection into these areas.

The periaqueductal grey projects to the raphé magnus of the brainstem which in turn sends massive descending projections, mainly using 5-hydroxytryptamine as transmitter, onto the spinal cord. Interference with 5HT alters morphine analgesia and animal studies have illustrated that 5HT agents can modulate the nociceptive threshold. A second descending system is a noradrenergic pathway which may also be involved in opioid analgesia.

The action of morphine on these areas is apparent with low doses of systemic opioids and it is likely that the opioid reduces these descending inhibitions from the brainstem which themselves are triggered by noxious inputs. The descending control of the spinal transmission of pain is thus probably reduced by morphine and since these controls may act to filter and integrate sensory messages the analgesia would be in keeping with the loss of the unpleasant aspect of pain reported clinically with low doses of opioids. Higher doses would elicit the spinal action as well so producing profound analgesia.

Conclusions
Although these zones where microinjection of morphine produces analgesia are reasonably well mapped the final mechanisms underlying these effects are less well understood. However an interaction between opiates and descending inhibitory controls, probably serotoninergic and noradrenergic projections onto the spinal cord is likely as are effects on the forebrain processing of painful messages.

Endogenous Opioids

What then is the situation regarding endogenous opioids? Enkephalins produce an analgesia when administered into the nucleus raphé magnus and also adjacent zones and a transient effect is also seen on (intra cerebro ventricular) i.c.v. injection. These relatively weak effects, as previously described at spinal levels are probably due to rapid degradation since i.v. thiorphan and kelatorphan alone produce analgesia in mice and rats. However it is interesting to note that the behavioural tests used are differentially sensitive to the enzyme inhibitor. Thus the tail flick and hot plate licking are not altered whereas more complex and integrated nonreflex tests of nociception such as the vocalization threshold to electrical stimulation, writhing and hot plate jump test are amenable to the treatment. Similarly these latter tests are sensitive to naloxone whereas reflex activity, at least in intact animals, is not. Thus the nonmotor tests seem sensitive to protected enkephalins indicating that these supraspinal actions of the enkephalins depend on particular neural events.

Dynorphin 1–13 and synthetic kappa agonists, by contrast to spinal administration produce behavioural analgesia without other overt effects following i.v. injection.

Although the above may indicate that the delta and kappa receptors mediate supraspinal analgesia as well as the mu receptor, the involement of the delta receptor is not yet confirmed. The ability of a variety of opioids to elicit analgesia following i.v. injection correlates in a linear fashion with their affinity for the mu receptor and within the periaqueductal grey matter there are mu and kappa binding sites but very few delta sites. It may therefore be that the enkephalins produce their supraspinal actions by interactions with the mu receptor, for which they have low but appreciable affinity, and this contrasts with the clear role of the delta receptor at spinal levels.

Conclusions

Whereas morphine and other agonists at the mu receptor have clear supraspinal sites of action in producing analgesia, particularly at midbrain and brainstem sites the influence of other opioids is as yet unclear.

CIRCUMSTANCES BEHIND RELEASE OF ENDOGENOUS OPIOIDS

This field of study has been fraught with many difficulties, mostly technical problems related to the measurement of authentic peptide and not fragments and the difficulty in separating peptides with similar or common amino acid sequences.

The Problems Involved

However there is evidence that circulating β endorphin and ACTH levels increase following stress or noxious stimuli although it is clearly difficult to separate the two possible causal stimuli. It is, however, unlikely that the β endorphin can cross the blood brain barrier to produce central actions from the systemic circulation. Deep brain stimulation of periaqueductal areas causing pain relief has been claimed to elevate cerebrospinal fluid (csf) β endorphin levels but other studies find no correlation between these levels and pain relief. The contrast medium used in these studies has been reported to interfere with the endorphin assay, another problem added to the confusion. Human and animal studies are likewise unclear as to whether naloxone reduces stimulation induced analgesia. The literature on the affects of naloxone on pain levels in man and nociceptive and reflex behaviours in animals is sufficiently polarized for no conclusions to be reached. However use of naloxone as a tool to probe endogenous opioids is problematic for several reasons. Firstly, it is not a good antagonist at the delta or kappa receptors so that enkephalins and dynorphins acting at these receptors may not be antagonized. Secondly rapid breakdown of the enkephalins makes study of their physiological actions difficult and thirdly, due to the complexities of pain transmission and modulation a clear role in setting the pain threshold is likely to be wishful thinking. An illustration is the dose dependent biphasic effect of naloxone on nociceptive thresholds and pain levels reported by several studies. However despite these points there is evidence for an involvement of enkephalins and dynorphins in certain pain related phenenoma.

Endogenous Opioids and Pain Relieving Procedures

Noxious cutaneous stimuli elevate enkephalin levels in superfused spinal cord as does tooth pulp stimulation, alogenic chemical stimulation and nerve stimulation. There may also be a release from midbrain areas. Enzyme inhibitors markedly enhance the levels of metenkephalins released in the cord. Dynorphin levels are likewise increased by noxious stimuli at spinal levels. However the spinal release of enkephalin is only segmental to a minor extent and much of the release depends on an intact spinal cord. Thus the conclusion would be that a noxious stimulus in addition to eliciting a segmental excitation also activates descending pathways that produce an extrasegmental spinal release of enkephalin. There is clear electrophysiological and behavioural evidence for this premise in that distant noxious stimuli can inhibit neuronal activity and behavioural nociception in a naloxone reversible manner. This has been shown to occur in man with experimental pain and may be the basis for acupuncture-like and counterirritant-produced analgesia. In fact high intensity transcutaneous nerve stimulation and extrasegmental acupuncture analgesia have been reported to be opioid in nature whereas dorsal column stimulation and segmental low intensity stimuli are generally held to be nonopioid. Here then is evidence that noxious or high intensity stimuli can activate opioid systems. Possibly pertinent here are reports of opioids elevating mood and pain thresholds following prolonged exercise—'runners high'.

Persistent Pain and Opioids

Studies using more prolonged noxious stimuli, likely to approach chronic or persistent pain in man have been largely based on studies on arthritic rats. Here akin to studies using other prolonged stimuli the opioid systems seem to alter or adapt to the stimulus. In arthritic rats synthesis of β endorphin increases but whether this is stress or pain induced is not known. Enkephalin and dynorphin levels increase in the cord, the latter in concert with the development of the arthritis, but kappa receptor binding density diminshes (mu and delta remain unchanged). Dynorphin staining and synthesis increase, and in line with the kappa receptor changes the effects of kappa agonists are reduced in these animals.

Conclusions

Despite technical difficulties, there is good evidence that opioids can be released by a variety of noxious or stressful stimuli which may be the basis for acupuncture-like analgesia and various other environmentally elicited analgesiae.

SIDE EFFECTS OF OPIOIDS

Dependence

Dependence and withdrawal can be elicited in animals following long-term endogenous opioid administration using either isolated tissues or gross behaviour as criteria. However despite an abundance of studies on endogenous opioid systems and dependence on morphine and related drugs, there is no evidence which suggests that opiate dependence results from alterations in endogenous opioids. However the protection of enkephalins by peptidase inhibition seems to produce little dependence and kappa ligands appear to be aversive rather than rewarding like μ agents and so do not support self administration in animals.

Endocrine Systems

Where studied, the direction of change in hormone levels produced by single dose enkephalin opioids acting on the hypothalamic-pituitary axis is the same as morphine, despite the receptors being different (δ and μ), and there is probably some resting activity in the opioid systems since naloxone alone has opposing effects. Thus growth hormone and prolactin levels increase (the latter via an inhibition of dopamine) whereas LH and TSH levels fall. Other hormones and the effects of longer dosage regimes are not clearly consistent.

Respiratory Depression

The reduced sensitivity of the brainstem centres to increased P_{CO_2} produced by morphine is likely to occur following application of exogenous opioid peptides since metenkephalin depresses tidal volume and respiratory rate when applied locally to the medulla. However many other studies have used nonselective opioids to gauge respiratory depression so are difficult to interpret. It may be that kappa opioids produce little respiratory depression whilst the primary effect of mu receptors is decreased tidal volume, while rate is controlled more by delta receptors.

Gastrointestinal Function

The constipation produced by morphine has both central and peripheral components since it can be produced by spinal application as well as systemic. High levels of enkephalins and dynorphin are found in the myenteric plexus and likewise opiate receptors. Again studies are difficult to interrelate but it seems likely that both the central and local effects of opioids on propulsion are predominantly mu receptor mediated with delta receptors producing lesser effects and kappa receptors unlikely to be significant.

To redress the balance back to kappa mediation of certain neural events, the suppression of appetite and diuresis (produced via ADH inhibition and direct renal actions) seems exclusively kappa mediated. All three subtypes of receptor can reduce epileptic activity. The cardiovascular effects of endogenous opioids are poorly understood and complicated by use of nonselective or unproven agents. However it is clear that the baroreceptor inhibition and bradycardia seen with morphine results from an interaction with the μ receptor. Holaday has extensively studied the role of opioids in conditions of spinal injury and circulatory shock. The general conclusions are that naloxone increases recovery following spinal shock in animals, an effect which seems to result from increased local vascular perfusion. Recent evidence indicates that the opioid producing the detrimental effects may be a dynorphin peptide. In recovery from stroke the findings are less clear which may relate to the value of animal models of stroke and also the circumstances of the stroke.

ENDOGENOUS ANTI-OPIOID SYSTEMS

There is now accumulating evidence that in addition to the effects mediated by the mu, delta and kappa opioid receptors, other transmitters or indeed other opioids can antagonize each other. Thus, cholecystokinin (CCK) has been reported to antagonize analgesia and neuronal depressions whereas proglumide, a possible CCK antagonist, enhances morphine effects. A kappa opioid by contrast seems to act as a CCK antagonist, but as yet it is not clear as to whether these are receptor mediated effects on parallel systems with a common target site. However it does seem clear that a variety of kappa receptor agonists can act as antagonists at the mu receptor, and that complex interrelations exist between opioid and other CNS transmitter systems.

FINAL CONCLUSIONS

The evidence for the existence of multiple endogenous opioids and their receptors, together with the rapid increase in our understanding of their pharmacology, physiological effects and functional roles in little over a decade since their discovery lends testament to the interest in their field.

It is now clear that the three types of opioid receptor, the mu, delta and kappa together with the three families of opioid peptides arising from pro-opiocortin, proenkephalin and prodynorphin mediate different CNS events and have different distributions within the brain. Thus by comparison to the effects of morphine acting at the mu receptor, delta and kappa agonists may be useful agents with differing spectra of effects. Finally our ability to manipulate endogenous opioids may hold novel therapeutic potential.

GLOSSARY

Opioid: Synonymous with opiate in this chapter, any substance, synthetic or endogenous with actions attributable to activation of the opioid receptors. The criterion that the effects of the opioid should be antagonized by naloxone is useful (*see* Fig. 50.3).

Peptide: A chemical made up from amino acid chains.

Propeptide: A precursor or large parent molecule which is cleaved to produce the biologically active peptide.

Peptidases: The enzymes which degrade the peptides. Enkephalinase, aminopeptidase, dipeptidylcarboxypeptidase.

Ligand: A chemical that binds to a receptor.

Substantia gelatinosa: The translucent zone of the dorsal horn where most opioid peptides and receptors are found at this level and where C fibres terminate. (laminae II & III).

Periaqueductal grey matter: Zone in the midbrain surrounding aqueduct.

$A\alpha\beta$ fibres: Peripherally afferent fibres conveying mainly tactile ($A\alpha\beta$) messages, mainly noxious (C) and mixed ($A\delta$).

$A\delta$ fibres:
C fibres: Divided on the basis of conduction velocity with C fibres transmitting slowly (0.5 m/s).

Laminae of the spinal cord: The Rexed classification, divided into laminae I-V for the dorsal horn.

Convergent neurone: Neurones responding to both innocuous and noxious stimuli from skin, muscle and viscera.

Iontophoresis: The injection of small quantities of drugs or transmitters from a micropipette by the passage of current.

FURTHER READING

Books and General Reviews

Besson J.M., Chaouch A. (1987). Peripheral and spinal nociception. *Physiol. Rev.*, **67**.

Besson J.M., Lazorthes Y. (eds.). (1985). Spinal opioids and the relief of pain. *INSERM* (Paris).

Dubner R., Bennett G.J. (1983). Spinal and trigeminal mechanisms of nociception. *Ann. Rev. Neurosci.*, **6**, 381.

Jessel T. (1982). Pain, *Lancet*, **Nov**, 1084.

Yaksh T.L. (ed.). (1986). *Spinal Afferent Processing*. New York: Plenum Press.

Opioid Peptide and Receptor Pharmacology

Akil H. et al. (1984). Endogenous opioids. Biology and Function. *Ann. Rev. Neurosci.*, **7**, 223.

Hollt V. et al. (1985). Multiple opioid ligands and receptors in the control of nociception. *Phil. Trans. R. Soc. Lond.* **B. 308**, 299.

Kosterlitz H. (1985). Opioids peptides and their receptors. *Proc. R. Soc. Lond.* **B225**, 27.

Martin W.R. (1984). Pharmacology of Opioids. *Pharm. Rev.*, **35**, 285.

Spinal Opioids

Cousins M.J., Mather L. (1984). Intrathecal and epidural administration of opioids. *Anesthesiology*, **61**, 276.

Dickenson A.H., Sullivan A.F. (1986). Electrophysiological studies on the effects of intrathecal morphine on nociceptive neurones in rat dorsal horn. *Pain*, **24**, 211.

Dubner R. et al. (1984). Neural circuitry mediating nociception in the medullary and spinal dorsal horns. *Adv. Pain. Res. Ther.* **6**, 151.

Duggan A.F., North A. (1984). Electrophysiology of opioids. *Pharm. Rev.*, **35**.

Yaksh T., Noueihed R. (1985). The physiology and pharmacology of spinal opiates. *Ann. Rev. Pharm.*, **25**, 433.

Supraspinal Opioids

Basbaum A.I., Fields H.L. (1984). Endogenous pain control system. *Ann. Rev. Neurosci.*, **7**, 309.

Dickenson A.H., Le Bars D. (1987). Supraspinal morphine and descending inhibitions acting on the dorsal horn of the rat. *J. Physiol.*, **384**, 81.

Fitzgerald M. (1986). Monoamines and descending control of nociception. *TINS*, 51.

Le Bars D., Dickenson A.H., Besson J.M. (1983). Opiate analgesia and descending control system. *Adv. Pain. Res. Ther.*, **5**, 341.

Release of Opioids

Millan M.J. (1986). Multiple opioids systems and pain. *Pain*, **27**, 303.

Watkins L., Mayer D.J. (1982). Organization of opiate and non opiate pain control systems. *Science*, **216**, 1185.

51. Adrenergic Receptors

A. Adams

Nomenclature
The dual receptor theory
   α-receptor agonists
   α-receptor antagonists (α-blockers)
   β-receptor agonists
   β-receptor antagonists
   Dobutamine
Properties of adrenergic receptors
   α_1 and α_2-adrenergic receptors
   β_1 and β_2-receptors
Problems and possibilities of adrenergic
   receptor classification
Dopamine adrenergic receptors
The concept of presynaptic adrenergic
   receptors
   Presynaptic α-adrenergic receptors and the
     negative feed-back system
   Presynaptic β-adrenergic receptors and the
     positive feed-back system
   Presynaptic α and β-adrenergic receptors
     and the two feed-back systems

Receptor theory dates back to the work of Newport Langley (1852–1925) and Paul Ehrlich (1854–1915) in the early part of this century. The last two decades in pharmacology have been described as the age of the receptor and the receptor concept has been indispensable for discussing and understanding the mode of action of drugs. The rapid growth in understanding of adrenergic receptors, especially at the molecular level, over the last 10 years has been mainly due to the introduction of radiolabelled adrenergic ligands (i.e. molecules which specifically bind to one site on a protein or nucleic acid) of high specific activity that recognize and bind to tissue receptors, as well as to the availability of numerous selective agonists and antagonists.

Receptor pharmacology is based on the principle that communication between cells in the living organism is carried out by chemical messengers. The tissue, such as a nerve ending or a gland from which the messenger has orginated, releases a specific chemical substance called a transmitter or hormone. This transmitter is carried by the blood or other tissue to the cell that is going to respond. Only cells that have the proper receptor can respond to the appropriate transmitter.

The receptor has two main characteristics. First, it has an affinity for the molecular shape and conformation of the transmitter. This results in binding between the transmitter and the receptor and this binding is unique for each transmitter. Second, binding may trigger a response of the tissue.

However, chemicals other than the natural transmitters can also act at these receptors. Some are *agonists*, i.e. the binding to the receptor triggers a response in the tissue. But others are blocking agents, i.e. the binding is not followed by a response, but agonists *are prevented from* binding. In other words, these are blocking agents or *anti-agonists* or antagonists.

The existence of a noradrenergic mechanism in central vasomotor control has been suggested. In the central nervous system (CNS) there are several transmitters and associated receptors and their exact mode of action has not been fully elucidated. The noradrenalin terminal systems which innervate the nucleus and tractus solitarius, the dorsal motor nucleus of the vagus and the lateral sympathetic column are likely to be involved as they are important autonomic nuclei.

In the periphery there are only two neurotransmitter systems, the adrenergic system and the cholinergic system. In addition, there are receptors for histamine, serotonin, dopamine and angiotensin.

The chemical analogues of the transmitter compounds may have a variety of pharmacodynamic actions. Some compounds are agonists but can be either more potent or less potent than the real transmitter. Other compounds will bind to the receptor to produce a purely blocking action so that the receptor is rendered inactive. Some compounds act in a much more selective manner and act only on certain types of receptor. These actions can be either as agonists or as antagonists.

NOMENCLATURE

Sir Henry Dale in 1933 used the adjectives 'adrenergic' to designate nerve fibres that release the sympathetic transmitter and 'cholinergic' to designate those that release acetylcholine. These terms have also come to describe the receptors on which the corresponding neurotransmitters act. The words 'adrenergic receptor' are often telescoped into adrenoreceptor or adrenoceptor.

Dale found that ergot possessed certain properties which blocked the motor response in structures with a sympathetic innervation which were stimulated by adrenaline, whereas the inhibitory response was not blocked. The significance of these observations was not fully appreciated for many years due to uncertainties about the nature of the transmitter substance released by sympathetic nerves and that the effects of sympathetic stimulation are so diverse.

The catecholamines possess some of the most widespread and potent effects of all the various endogenous hormones and exogenous drugs. All the naturally occurring catecholamines, adrenaline, noradrenaline and dopamine, seem to function as neurotransmitters. They have important physiological and biological effects both in the CNS and in the periphery.

The adrenergic receptors are the site of action of the sympathetic neurotransmitter. The adrenal medullary hormone, adrenaline, also acts on these receptors but is a weaker agent than noradrenaline.

THE DUAL RECEPTOR THEORY

It was suggested in 1948 by Ahlquist that there were in fact two adrenergic receptors, alpha (α) and beta (β). Hence, adrenergic agonists could be classed as either α-agonists or β-agonists. At that time certain drugs were already known as sympatholytics—these are the α-adrenergic receptor blocking drugs (Fig. 51.1).

Ahlquist's main conclusions were based upon a detailed comparison of the relative effectiveness of five sympathomimetic amines. He compared the effects of noradrenaline, adrenaline, isoprenaline, and

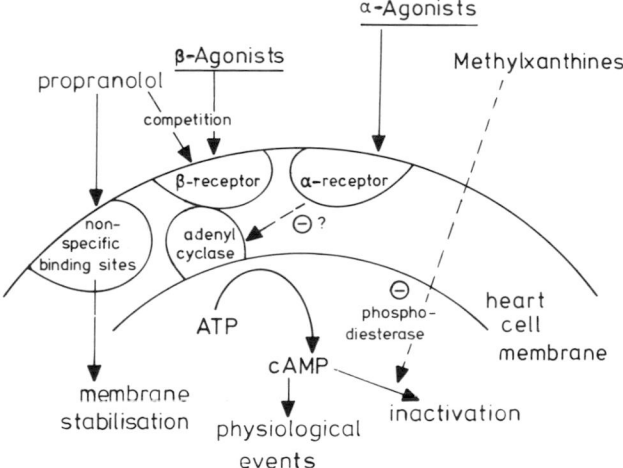

Fig. 51.1 α and β-receptors in cardiac muscle. β-agonists act on the β-receptor (a stereospecific receptor) in the heart cell membrane. α-agonists act through the α-receptor, methylxanthines mimic the effect of β-antagonists by inhibition of phosphodiesterase. (Reproduced with permission from L.H. Opie (1980)).

the methyl derivatives of noradrenaline and adrenaline, during experiments in dogs, cats, rabbits and rats. The various actions which he investigated included vasoconstriction and vasodilatation in different vascular beds, and the effects on the heart, uterus and intestine.

Ahlquist found that these various responses could be separated into two categories. In the first, adrenaline was the most effective compound and isoprenaline the least. These responses (such as vasoconstriction) were called α-adrenergic. In the other type of response the order was reversed, isoprenaline was the most active substance whereas noradrenaline was the least active. The second type of response was typified by the ability of the catecholamines to stimulate cardiac contractility. The response was called β-adrenergic (Table 51.1).

At the time Ahlquist performed his studies there were hardly any antagonist compounds available. However, ergotamine was available and when it was given it appeared to block the α but not the β-adrenergic effect. Subsequently, specific α-adrenergic blocking compounds were developed such as phentolamine and phenoxybenzamine.

Ahlquist's conclusions that there must be two main types of adrenergic receptor, α and β were strengthened when drugs such as pronethalol and propranolol were discovered which specifically blocked the β-adrenergic receptors. The location and density of the receptors and the nature and dose of the adrenergic stimulators to which they are exposed explain the range of physiological responses of the system. Although tissue may contain both kinds of receptor, in any given tissue one type of receptor is predominant and biases the effect of adrenergic stimulation in that tissue. Sympathetic effector cells may have α or β-receptors or both. The smooth muscle of blood vessels supplying skeletal muscles has β-receptors and α-receptors. These β-receptors are activated by low concentrations of adrenaline causing vasodilatation and the α-receptors are activated by adrenaline to cause vasoconstriction. When both types of receptor are activated in this tissue the response of α-receptors predominates.

α-receptors predominate in tissues which can exist for short periods with a reduction in blood supply (e.g. skin, kidney and the splanchnic bed). β-receptors predominate in muscle to ensure a good blood supply for activity. β-receptors also predominate in the heart so that when they are stimulated they cause an increase in the force and rate of cardiac contraction. Under conditions of great stress noradrenaline and adrenaline are released from the adrenal medulla to reinforce the actions of the sympathetic nervous system. The dominant secretion, which is adrenaline, differs from noradrenaline in having a greater β-receptor stimulating action. Adrenaline is also a powerful stimulator of α-receptors and vasoconstriction occurs in tisues in which this receptor is predominant. Specific blockade of α-receptors 'unmasks' the β-stimula-

TABLE 51.1
CLASSIFICATION OF ADRENERGIC RECEPTORS
(After Jenkinson, 1973 and Ahlquist, 1979)

System or tissue	Actions	Receptor	Comments
Cadiovascular			
Heart	Increased rate, force of contraction, conduction, and ventricular excitability	β	α-receptors may also have a minor role
Vessels	Constriction	α	The balance between constriction and dilatation varies in different beds. β-receptors predominate in the coronary arteries although α-receptors may also be present
	Dilatation	β	
Respiratory			
Tracheal and bronchial smooth muscle	Relaxation	β	α-receptors probably subserve contraction although the effect is small
Gut			
Longitudinal	Relaxation	α, β	Partly by a direct action on muscle (α and β) and partly by inhibition of the parasympathetic nervous system (α)
Sphincters	Constriction	α	
	Relaxation	β	
Other Smooth Muscle			
Uterus	Contraction	α	Depends on hormonal balance
	Relaxation	β	
Urinary bladder	Contraction (mainly trigone)	α	
	Relaxation (mainly detrusor)	β	
Splenic capsule	Constriction	α	
Iris	Pupillary dilation	α	
Skeletal Muscle			
	Changes in twitch tension	β	
	Increased release of acetylcholine	α	
	Increased glycogenolysis	β	
Adipose Tissue			
	Increased lipolysis	β	α-receptors may have a small inhibitory effect
Pancreas			
	Decreased insulin secretion	α	
	Increased insulin secretion	β	
Kidney			
	Increased plasma renin	β	

tory action of adrenaline; this is the basis of the 'adrenaline-reversal' phenomenon caused by ergot which Sir Henry Dale had noticed.

The development of the dual receptor theory directly or indirectly influenced many aspects of research: (1) it facilitated the development of more selective adrenergic agonists and antagonists; this in turn made available more pharmacological tools to probe control mechanisms in the body; (2) interest in receptors was rekindled in general and we now accept receptors for such diverse substances as serotonin, histamine, and morphine; the search for new transmitter chemicals has intensified; (3) it is now possible to separate drugs on the basis of whether they act on the receptor or on the biosynthesis, storage or release of the transmitter; (4) the β-adrenoceptor was one of the first receptors involved in the development of the second messenger concept (*see later*); (5) early studies on the β-receptor showed there are subtypes of this receptor, e.g. the β-receptors of the heart are different from those of the bronchi; (6) the effectiveness of β-blockade in essential hypertension has opened new areas of study, e.g. one possible mechanism of action of β-blockers in hypertension is the inhibition of renin release in the kidney; the angiotensin resulting from the renin is a likely cause of the elevated pressure.

α-Receptor Agonists

Adrenaline has the greatest affinity for α-receptors,

TABLE 51.2
RELATIVE ACTIVITIES OF CATECHOLAMINES ON ADRENERGIC RECEPTORS

Catecholamines	Alpha adrenergic receptors	Beta₁ adrenergic receptors	Beta₂ adrenergic receptors	Dopamine adrenergic receptors
Adrenaline	+ → + +	+ +	+ +	0
Noradrenaline	+ +	+ +	0	0
Isoprenaline	0	+ +	+ +	0
Dopamine	+ → + +	+ +	0	+ +
Dobutamine	+	+ +	+	0

followed by noradrenaline, dopamine, phenylephrine, metaraminol, methoxamine and ephedrine (Table 51.2). It must be remembered that noradrenaline and phenylephrine are effective β-receptor antagonists as well. Methoxamine is also a β-receptor antagonist although of lower potency (Fig. 51.2).

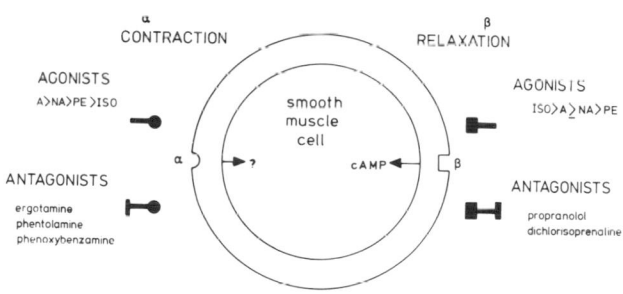

Fig. 51.2 α and β-adrenergic receptors in smooth muscle. The rank orders of agonists and antagonists are indicated, (A = adrenaline, NA = noradrenaline, PE = phenylephrine, ISO = isoprenaline). (Reproduced with permission from R.J. Lefkowitz (1978)).

Isoprenaline has a relatively high affinity for α-receptors. Its overall effect as an α-agonist, however, is low because the drug has a high affinity and potency on β-receptors as well. The net effect is the result of the combined α and β effect.

α-Receptor Antagonists (α-Blockers)

α-receptor blocking agents in descending order of affinity are: dihydroergotamine, phentolamine, phenoxybenzamine, ergotamine and tolazoline. The effects of substances such as phentolamine and tolazoline are readily reversible in experiments *in vitro* and are relatively short acting *in vivo*.

β-Receptor Agonists

The relative affinities of the β-agonists are isoprenaline, adrenaline, noradrenaline, dopamine (Table 51.2).

Isoprenaline is a potent drug in this category and it elicits responses from β-receptors in many tissues at very low concentrations indeed. However, the (−)-isomer can also activate α-receptors although much more higher concentrations are required to obtain a substantial response.

β-Receptor Antagonists

The first available agent of importance in this class was dichlorisoprenaline (DCIP). However, it is also a partial agonist, i.e. it shows intrinsic sympathomimetic activity (ISA) and it activates the receptors to such an extent that the drug is not only of no use in clinical therapeutics but its value in experiments *in vitro* is also somewhat doubtful.

The next drugs developed in this class were pronethalol and propranolol. Propranolol is largely without any ISA although some of the effects which have occasionally been reported from its use could be ascribed to β-receptor stimulation.

The development of selective antagonists which can block β-receptors in some tissues at lower doses than are required for others has been an important advance. This is called selectivity. For instance, practolol is much more effective against the actions of β-agonists on the heart than on vascular smooth muscle. This is an example of a drug showing cardiac selectivity. It is clinically important in the development of drugs without undesirable side-effects, such as bronchoconstriction.

More recently developed drugs which have partial agonist activity include acebutalol, alprenolol, oxprenalol and pindolol; these drugs cause a slight to moderate activation of the β-receptor, in addition to preventing the access of natural or synthetic catecholamines to the receptor sites (Fig. 51.3). Drugs with particular agonist activity, such as pindolol, cause less slowing of the resting heart rate than drugs without this property. On the other hand, the increase in heart rate with exercise or isoprenaline is decreased similarly by both types of β-blockers. An explanation for these findings is that the relative importance of the partial agonist effect of a drug like pindolol, as compared with its β-blocking action, is greatest when sympathetic tone is low and therefore is appreciated only in resting subjects. Studies in animals and human beings suggest that β-blockers with partial agonist

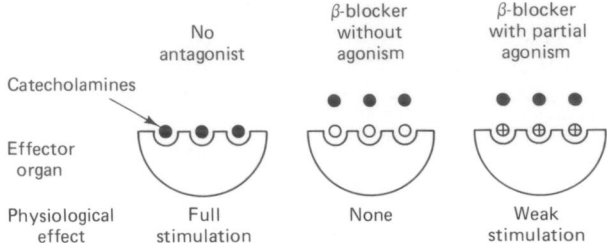

Fig. 51.3 Physiological effects of β-adrenergic blocking drugs with and without partial agonist activity, in the presence of circulating catecholamines. When circulating catecholamines (●) combine with β-adrenergic receptors, they produce a full physiological response. When these receptors are occupied by a β-blocker lacking partial agonist activity (○), no physiological effects from catecholamine stimulation can occur. A β-blocking drug with partial agonist activity (⊕) also blocks the binding of catecholamines to β-adrenergic receptors, but in addition the drug causes a relatively weak stimulation of the receptor. (Reproduced with permission from J. Koch-Weser (1983)).

activity may cause less depression of left ventricular function and intracardiac conduction than drugs lacking this property.

Dobutamine

Dobutamine is a drug which is chemically related to both dopamine and isoprenaline. Dobutamine is mainly a β_1-adrenergic agonist which produces positive inotropic and chronotropic effects on the heart, i.e. both the force of contraction and the heart rate are increased. However, in man the heart rate is little increased. Dobutamine has only a slight action on α-receptors, a slight action on β_2-receptors and no action on dopamine receptors.

PROPERTIES OF ADRENERGIC RECEPTORS

The precise location of adrenergic receptors within the cell is unknown. It is possible that the receptors are on the outer surface of the cell membrane because of the speed of onset of the actions of both α and some β-mediated effects. The exact nature of the adrenergic receptors is also unknown although investigations are being done to elucidate these problems. There is some evidence that some second messenger is involved in mediating α-adrenergic stimulated events. However, receptors on the cell surface are just the tip of the iceberg because on stimulation they trigger a cascade of biochemical events, first in the plasma membrane, and then in the interior of the cell. In many systems adrenergic receptors are able to transduce their messages through proteins in the plasma membrane that bind to guanine nucleotides. These transducing proteins then stimulate, or inhibit, effector systems such as adenylate cyclase, phospholipase A_2, phospholipase C, or ion channels. Depending on the subtype of adrenergic

receptor and the properties of the transducing and effector protein of the cell, second messengers such as cyclic-AMP, inositol triphosphate, diacylglycerol, and arachidonic acid and its many metabolites are either generated or prevented from forming. In addition, stimulation of adrenergic receptors can produce changes in intracellular ions, in particular, calcium. These second messengers then initiate numerous complex intracellular biochemical reactions to produce a physiological response characteristic of the target cell. Stimulation of the β-adrenergic receptor causes the activation of intracellular adenylate cyclase. This enzyme catalyses the formation of cyclic-AMP which in turn activates the contractile and metabolic mechanisms in the cell. This mechanism is not unique for β-adrenergic receptors since most hormones use the same system.

α_1 and α_2-Adrenergic Receptors

Adrenergic receptors exist as two pharmacologically distinct types designated α_1 and α_2 and it has been suggested that these receptors mediate cell activity through different mechanisms, α_1-effects being due to elevation of intracellular Ca^{2+} and α_2-effects to inhibition of adenylate cyclase. It should be stressed that the use of these terms α_1 and α_2 implies no particular anatomical location but indicates the pharmacological specificity of the receptor in response to drugs.

β_1 and β_2-Adrenergic Receptors

There are at least two different types of β-adrenergic receptors. Type 1 is associated with cardiac stimulation and type 2 is associated with smooth muscle relaxation (bronchial and vascular smooth muscle). Some β-adrenergic receptor blockers can act selectively on β_1 rather than β_2-receptors. This is an advantage when a drug such as practolol is used rather than propranolol for a cardiac β-blocking action because it is safer when used in a patient with asthma. On the other hand, a β_2-agonist is preferred for the treatment of severe bronchial asthma because it will act selectively on the β_2-receptors rather than on the β_1-receptors and consequently will reduce the amount of cardiac stimulation.

The β-receptor is probably part of the adenylate cyclase system and situated on the cell membrane. There are several receptor sites associated with adenylate cyclase: one for the β-antagonist, one for glucagon, one for thyroid hormone and one for histamine. Each agonist, acting on its receptor site can activate adenylate cyclase to produce a cyclic form of adenosine monophosphate, (cyclic AMP or cAMP) from ATP. Cyclic AMP is the intracellular messenger of β stimulation.

β-receptor activation has been shown to increase cyclic AMP in both cardiac and smooth muscle. However, it is not clear why this should lead to an increase in cardiac contractility and heart rate on the one hand, but to relaxation and inhibition of electrical activity in the longitudinal smooth muscle of the intestine on the other hand.

PROBLEMS AND POSSIBILITIES OF ADRENERGIC RECEPTOR CLASSIFICATION

The pharmacological classification of adrenergic receptors has created an illusion of morphological reality in the minds of many people. Although the nature and localization of α and β receptors are unknown, many investigations have implied or assumed that functionally and morphologically distinct, well-defined static membrane structures exist. Studies which have attempted to isolate these structures have instead led to concepts of a more dynamic image of receptors at molecular level.

The active centre of the enzyme adenylate cyclase itself could be the place where the β-receptor relates. Another possibility is that the β-receptor is located on a regulatory subunit of adenylate cyclase.

Are the responses which are mediated by α-receptors due to underlying changes in cyclic AMP? One possibility is that the α effects may result from a *fall* in the level of cyclic AMP, the converse of the β effect. However, the question is unsettled: in some tissues the final response is a rise in levels of cyclic AMP rather than a fall as might have been expected.

Although the dual receptor theory of α and β receptors is an attractive and simple concept, the later separation of the β-receptors into β_1-receptors in the heart and β_2-receptors in smooth muscle has introduced some problems. This has risen because of significant overlaps between the β-receptor subgroups and by a lack of homogeneity amongst the α-adrenergic receptors of different tissues.

This note of caution is underlined by a realization that schemes for the classification of β sub-groups, e.g., into β_1 and β_2-receptors, from comparisons of *agonist* potencies are not totally consistent with the tentative classification based on experiments with *antagonists*. Furthermore, when the potency ratios of the optical isomers of various β-agonists and antagonists are compared there appear to be no differences between heart and bronchial muscle. A difference in potency would have been expected if the receptors in these muscle types differed appreciably.

DOPAMINE ADRENERGIC RECEPTORS

Dopamine is the immediate precursor of noradrenaline and is a transmitter in the central nervous system. In the periphery, dopamine has a variety of different actions. It is an α-receptor agonist, a β-receptor agonist and it can enter adrenergic nerve endings to displace stored noradrenaline. Dopamine acts on unique and specific receptors called dopamine (or dopaminergic) receptors to cause vasodilatation in the renal and mesenteric vessels. The classical adrenergic

properties, both α and β, are relatively weak in blocking responses of the dopamine receptors. However, the butyrophenones, such as haloperidol, and some of the phenothiazines are potent dopamine receptor blockers.

The pharmacological classification of dopamine receptors is controversial; as many as five classes have been proposed. There are two general categories: D-1 dopamine receptors mediate the stimulation of adenylate cyclase activity, while D-2 dopamine receptors are either unassociated with this enzyme or mediate its inhibition.

THE CONCEPT OF PRESYNAPTIC ADRENERGIC RECEPTORS

Presynaptic α-Adrenergic Receptors and the Negative Feed-Back System.

When the neurotransmitter is released following the arrival of nerve impulses it interacts with specific receptors located in the membrane of the postsynaptic effector cell and so triggers the typical response of the effector organ. Thus there may be a contraction or relaxation of smooth muscle, positive chronotropic or inotropic effects or secretion of salivary glands.

In the case of nerve endings, the presence of α-adrenergic receptors in the effector organ is an important site of loss of released transmitter. However, when the α-adrenergic receptors of the effector cell are occupied by a blocking agent (such as phentolamine) the transmitter which is released during nerve stimulation will not be able to combine with these receptors. Hence, in these circumstances some of the transmitter will 'overflow' into, say, the venous system. The fate or main sites of loss of noradrenaline (NA) released through nerve stimulation are shown in Fig. 51.4. These are: (1) recapture or reuptake of the released transmitter through uptake into the neurone again; (2) uptake of the NA into tissues other than neurones, (3) metabolism by monoamine oxidase (MAO), coupled with either aldehyde reductase or aldehyde dehydrogenase, and by catechol-o-methyl transferase, and (4) uptake into the receptors and other binding sites.

Thus an increase in the overflow of transmitter can result either from a blockage of one or more of the various sites of loss (Fig. 51.4), or from an actual increase in the amount of noradrenaline released.

The α-adrenergic receptors may be present in the outer surface of noradrenergic nerve endings. Presynaptic α-adrenergic receptors are involved and the release of noradrenaline is regulated through a negative feed-back system mediated by the neurotransmitter itself (Fig. 51.5). Once the noradrenaline, which has been released by nerve stimulation, has reached a threshold concentration in the synaptic cleft, it activates the presynaptic α-adrenergic receptors. This triggers a negative feed-back mechanism which inhibits further release of the transmitter. This negative feed-

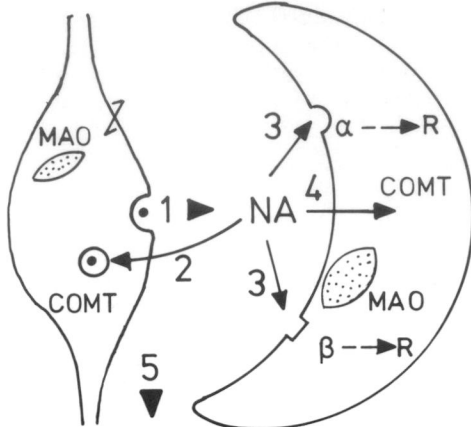

Fig. 51.4 The fate ('main sites of loss') of the transmitter during sympathetic nerve stimulation. 1. Total amount of transmitter released by nerve stimulation. 2. Noradrenaline (NA), recaptured by neuronal uptake, subsequently de-aminated or stored in vesicles. 3. Fraction of released transmitter available for activation of α or β-receptors, leading to response (R) of the effector organ. 4. Noradrenaline taken up for extraneuronal sites and subsequently metabolized, predominantly by catechol-o-methyltransferase (COMT). 5. 'Overflow' of noradrenaline into tissue fluids and bloodstream. (Reproduced with permission from S.Z. Langer (1977)).

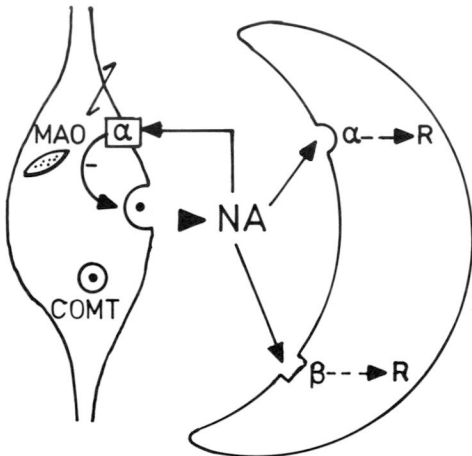

Fig. 51.5 Negative feed-back mechanism for noradrenaline released by nerve stimulation, mediated by presynaptic α-adrenergic receptors. Once noradrenaline (NA), released by nerve stimulation, reaches a threshold concentration in the synaptic cleft it activates presynaptic α-adrenergic receptors leading to an inhibition of transmitter release. The presynaptic negative feed-back mechanism is present both in tissues where the response (R) of the effector organ is mediated through α or β-receptors. (MAO = monoamine oxidase; COMT = catechol-o-methyltransferase). (Reproduced with permission from S.Z. Langer (1977)).

back mechanism operates by restricting the calcium available for the excitation-secretion coupling.

Although both the pre and postsynaptic α-adrenergic receptors are stimulated by α-receptor agonists and are blocked by β-receptor antagonists, it appears that the postsynaptic α-adrenergic receptors that mediate the responses of the effector organ, are not identical with the presynaptic α-adrenergic receptors which regulate the release of noradrenaline during nerve stimulation. Phenoxybenzamine is about thirty times more potent in blocking the *postsynaptic* α-adrenergic receptors (that mediate the responses of the effector organ) than it is in blocking the *presynaptic* α-receptors (that regulate the release of noradrenaline during nerve stimulation). Hence, the pre and postsynaptic adrenergic receptors are *not* identical, and it has been suggested that postsynaptic α-adrenergic receptors should be called α_1 and the presynaptic adrenergic receptors should be called α_2.

Presynaptic β-Adrenergic Receptors and the Positive Feed-Back System

A positive feed-back system has been suggested in noradrenaline nerve endings that is triggered through the activation of presynaptic β-adrenergic receptors. This is in addition to the presynaptic α-adrenergic receptor or negative feed-back system already described.

Activation of the positive feed-back system by β-adrenergic receptor agonists leads to an *increase* in transmitter release during nerve stimulation. The β_1 or β_2 nature of the presynaptic adrenergic receptors is somewhat controversial (Fig. 51.6). The release of additional transmitter which is triggered by the activation of presynaptic β-receptors may be mediated through a rise in the levels of cyclic AMP in noradrenergic nerve endings.

Presynaptic α and β-Adrenergic Receptors and the Two Feed-Back Systems

The autoregulation of noradrenaline release during nerve stimulation appears to be a function of the two presynaptic mechanisms already described.

The first mechanism is mediated by β-adrenergic receptors and is activated by low concentrations of noradrenaline, i.e., low frequencies of stimulation. The second mechanism is mediated through α-adrenergic receptors and is triggered when high concentrations of the transmitter are reached in the synaptic cleft and lead to inhibition of transmitter release (Fig. 51.7). The major regulatory mechanism for noradrenaline release by nerve stimulation under physiological conditions is believed to be mediated by presynaptic α-adrenergic receptors. This is concluded from the fact that the most pronounced increases in transmitter release are obtained when the presynaptic α-adrenergic receptors are blocked by drugs.

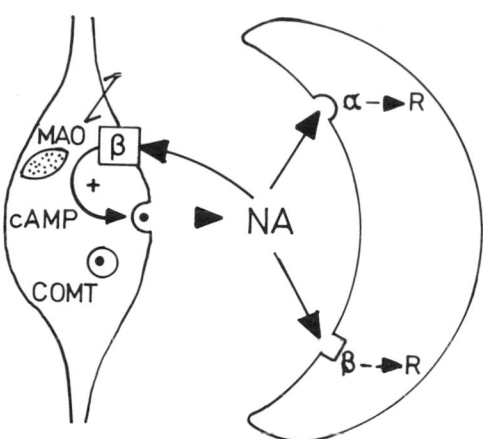

Fig. 51.6 Positive feed-back mechanism for noradrenaline (NA) released by nerve stimulation, mediated by β-adrenergic receptors. Noradrenaline released by low frequencies of nerve stimulation activates presynaptic β-adrenergic receptors. This effect appears to be mediated through an increase in the levels of cyclic AMP (cAMP) in noradrenergic nerve endings. The presynaptic positive feed-back mechanism is present both in tissue where the response (R) of the effector organ is mediated through α or through β-adrenergic receptors. (MAO = monoamine oxidase; COMT = catechol-o-methyltransferase). (Reproduced with permission from S.Z. Langer (1977)).

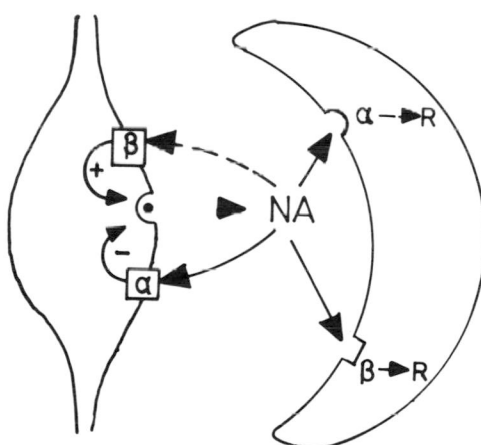

Fig. 51.7 The presynaptic α and β-adrenergic receptors and the autoregulation of noradrenaline (NA) release during nerve stimulation. When noradrenaline is released at low frequencies of nerve stimulation (i.e., there is only a low concentration of released transmitter in the synaptic cleft) the positive feed-back system (mediated by the presynaptic β-adrenergic receptors) is activated and leads to an increase in transmitter release. When the concentration of NA increases, a threshold is reached at which the negative feed-back mechanism (mediated by the α-adrenergic receptors) is triggered, leading to an inhibition of transmitter release. Both presynaptic feedback mechanisms are present in nerves, irrespective of the α or β nature of the receptors that mediate the response (R) of the effector organ. (Reproduced with permission from S.Z. Langer (1977)).

FURTHER READING

Ahlquist R.P. (1948). A study of the adrenotropic receptors. *Am. J. Physiol.*, **135**, 586.

Ahlquist R.P. (1973). Adrenergic receptors: a personal and practical view. *Perspectives Biol. Med.*, **17**, 119.

Ahlquist R.P. (1979). Adrenergic receptors and others. *Anesth. Analg.*, **58**, 510.

Ahlquist R.P. (1981). Adrenoceptors. In *Towards Understanding Receptors. Current Reviews in Biomedicine—1*. p.49. (Lamble J.W. ed.). Amsterdam: Elsevier.

Arbilla S., Langer S.Z. (1978). Differences between presynaptic and postsynaptic α-adrenoceptors in the isolated nictitating membrane of the cat: effects of metanephrine and tolazoline. *Br. J. Pharmacol.*, **64**, 259.

Bilezikian J.B. (1987). Defining the role of adrenergic receptors in human physiology. In *Adrenergic Receptors in Man*. p.37. (Insel P.A. ed.). New York: Marcel Dekker.

Black J.W., Pritchard B.N.S. (1973). Activation and blockage of β-adrenoceptors in common cardiac disorders. *Br. Med. Bull.*, **29**, 163.

Dale H.H. (1965). *Adventures in Physiology. With Excursions into Autopharmacology*. London: The Wellcome Trust.

Glynne A., Lucas R.A. (eds). (1978). *Proceedings of the European Dobutamine Symposium*. London: Eli Lilly.

Goldberg L.I. (1978). Recent advances in catecholamines. *Br. J. Clin. Pract. Symposium Supplement*, **32**, 1.

Iversen L.L. (1979). The chemistry of the brain. *Sci. Am.*, **241**, 118.

Jenkinson D.H. (1973). Classification and properties of peripheral adrenergic receptors. *Br. Med. Bull.*, **29**, 142.

Koch-Weser J. (1983). Pindolol: A new β-adrenoceptor antagonist with partial agonist activity. *New Engl. J. Med.*, **308**, 940.

Kunos G. (1976). Adrenoceptors. *Ann. Rev. Pharmacol. Toxicol.*, **18**, 291.

Langer S.Z. (1979). Presynaptic receptors and their role in the regulation of transmitter release. *Br. J. Pharmacol.*, **60**, 481.

Langer S.Z., Adler-Graschinsky E., Giorgi O. (1977). Physiological significance of alpha-adrenoreceptor—mediated negative feedback mechanism regulating noradrenaline release during nerve stimulation. *Nature*, **265 (5595)**, 648.

Langer S.Z., Shepperson N.B. (1984). Recent developments in vascular smooth muscle pharmacology: the postsynaptic α_2-adrenoceptor. In *Receptors, Again* p.60. (Lamble J.W., Abbott A.C., eds.). Amsterdam: Elsevier.

Leclerc G., Rouot B., Velly J., et al. (1981). β-adrenergic receptor subtypes. In *Towards Understanding Receptors. Current Reviews in Biomedicine—1* p.78. (Lamble J.W., ed.). Amsterdam: Elsevier.

Leff S.E., Creese I. (1984). Dopamine receptors re-explained. In *Receptors, Again*. p.119. (Lamble J.W., Abbott A.C., eds.). Amsterdam: Elsevier.

Lefkowitz R.J. (1978). Identification and regulation of adrenergic receptors. In *Psychopharmacology: A Generation of Progress*. (Lipton M.A., DiMascio A., Killam J.F., eds.). New York: Raven Press.

McGrath J.C. (1984). The variety of vascular α-adrenoceptors. In *Receptors, Again*. p.77. (Lamble J.W., Abbott A.C., eds.). Amsterdam: Elsevier.

Mennie A.T. (ed.). (1976). Dopamine hydrochloride. Proceedings of an International Symposium, London. *Proc. R. Soc. Med.*, **70**, Suppl. 2.

Nahorski S.R. (1981). Identification and significance of beta-adrenoceptor subtypes. In *Towards Understanding Receptors. Current Reviews in Biomedicine—1.* p. 71. (Lamble J.W., ed.). Amsterdam: Elsevier.

Opie L.H. (1980). Drugs and the heart. *Lancet*, **i**, 693.

Parascandola J. (1981). Origins of the receptor theory. In *Towards Understanding Receptors. Current Reviews in Biomedicine—1* (Lamble J.W., ed.). Amsterdam: Elsevier.

Schoken D.D. (1984). Adrenergic receptors of the placenta. In *Receptors, Again.* p. 49. (Lamble J.W., Abbott A.C., eds.). Amsterdam: Elsevier.

Venter J.C., Fraser C.M. (1984). The structure of α and β-adrenergic receptors. In *Receptors, Again.* p. 104. (Lamble J.W., Abbott A.C., eds.). Amsterdam: Elsevier.

52. Peripheral Cholinoceptors

W. C. Bowman

Sites and classification of peripheral cholinoceptors
Subtypes of cholinoceptors
Motor endplate nicotinic cholinoceptors
    Receptor structure and location
    Synthesis, degradation and down-regulation of endplate nicotinic receptors
    Denervated muscle
    Receptors in myasthenia gravis
    Receptor function
    Receptor desensitization
    Actions of receptor antagonists
Ganglionic nicotinic cholinoceptors
Muscarinic cholinoceptors

As long ago as 1878, Langley in Cambridge formulated the concept of receptors as a result of his experiments demonstrating the opposing actions of pilocarpine and atropine on salivary flow in the cat. He assumed that there was some substance in the physiological system with which atropine and pilocarpine were capable of forming compounds. Later, in 1905, he introduced the idea of a 'specific receptive substance' as the site of action of nicotine and curare in the myoneural junction. The actual term 'receptor' was first used around 1910 by Paul Ehrlich whose experiments led him to the idea, based on his experience of immunochemistry, that drugs act by combining with specific chemical groupings on larger molecules of cells. He called these groupings *receptors*, and he defined a receptor as 'that combining group of the protoplasmic molecule to which a foreign group, when introduced, attaches itself'.

As described below, some types of receptor have now been isolated in a pure form, but for many years, although an indispensable concept for discussion and for understanding mechanisms of action of neurotransmitters and drugs, they remained no more than hypothetical entities. A vast literature describes deductions concerning them based on pharmacological experiments in which mechanical cellular responses, many steps removed from the actual drug-receptor interaction, were measured. Studies of structure:action relations in such experiments, with both agonists and antagonists, have given some insight into the complementary nature of the binding groups that comprise the receptor recognition sites and have provided information for defining receptor types, including sub-types of receptors within a larger group. Related studies, initiated by Clark (1933, 1937) and Gaddum (1926, 1937), have allowed the derivation of mathematical descriptions of concentration-response relations based on and developed from the mass action law (Stephenson, 1956; Arunlakshana and Schild, 1959; Ariëns, 1964; van Rossum, 1966). Electrophysiological studies of the consequences of drug-receptor interactions, especially recordings of ionic conductance changes through single receptor-operated ion channels with a so-called patch clamp electrode, are the most fundamental receptor-mediated events that can presently be measured. Such measurements indicate that in some instances the interaction of an agonist molecule with one receptor recognition site facilitates further interactions, rather in the way that the binding of oxygen to haemoglobin facilitates the binding of more oxygen. This evidence of cooperativity in drug-receptor interactions necessitates some modifications of the more classical mathematical treatments; these modifications have been discussed by Colquhoun (1973) and Norman (1979).

Sites and Classification of Peripheral Cholinoceptors

The main pharmacological actions of the alkaloids muscarine (from the toadstool *Amanita muscaria*) and nicotine (from tobacco) have been known since the studies of Böhm and Langley respectively, and others, in the late 19th century. Dale (1914) noted that some effects of acetylcholine are reproduced by muscarine, whereas others are mimicked by nicotine, and accordingly he classified acetylcholine's actions as 'muscarine actions' and 'nicotine actions', the former being blocked by atropine and the latter by large doses of nicotine itself (we now know that tubocurarine is a preferable antagonist for nicotine actions). The adjectives *muscarinic* and *nicotinic* were soon coined, and since the agonist acetylcholine was the same in all cases, it was logical to infer that the two classes of actions are mediated by two different types of receptors, muscarinic actions via muscarinic cholinoceptors and nicotinic actions via nicotinic cholinoceptors. The main nicotinic cholinoceptors outside the brain and spinal cord are located on autonomic ganglion cells, adrenal medullary cells, and at the motor endplates of striated muscles. They are stimulated by acetylcholine released from preganglionic autonomic axons or from the axons of lower motoneurones. The main peripheral muscarinic cholinoceptors are located on smooth muscle cells, gland cells, and on cardiac cells (especially on the SA and AV nodes and on the atrial fibres). Most of the muscarinic cholinoceptors that are located on effector cells are those that are activated by acetylcholine released from postganglionic parasympathetic or cholinergic sympathetic axons, but there are exceptions. For example, most, and probably all, arterioles possess muscarinic receptors that respond to acetylcholine by an atropine-sensitive vasodilatation, yet it is unlikely that they all receive a cholinergic innervation.

More recent evidence has shown that, in addition to the aforementioned well documented sites, there are a number of other locations of peripheral cholinoceptor populations. These are enumerated below.

1. There is clear evidence that both parasympathetic and noradrenergic sympathetic nerve endings possess both muscarinic and nicotinic receptors (Rand and Varma, 1970; Hume et al., 1972; Fosbraey and Johnson, 1982). Activation of the muscarinic receptors inhibits transmitter release in response to nerve impulses, whereas activation of the nicotinic receptors has the opposite effect. At parasympathetic nerve endings these receptors are presumably activated by acetylcholine released from the same or from neighbouring axons of the same type; they may mediate feed-back modulatory roles on transmitter turnover. Receptors on nerve terminals that are activated by the same transmitter as that released from the nerve terminals are termed 'autoreceptors'.

Where there is a dual innervation by sympathetic and parasympathetic systems (e.g. the heart), the cholinoceptors on noradrenergic nerve endings appear to be activated by acetylcholine released from branches of the postganglionic parasympathetic axons (Levy and Blatberg, 1976; Shepherd et al., 1978). There are often inhibitory adrenoceptors on the parasympathetic nerve endings as well, but adrenoceptors are outside the scope of this section. The result is that each branch of the autonomic system, as well as modifying the activity of the effector cell in its specific way, can also inactivate the opposing innervation.

2. There is increasing evidence that somatic motor nerve terminals possess nicotinic autoreceptors that function in a positive feedback mechanism that helps to mobilize acetylcholine within the nerve endings.

During high frequencies of stimulation (above 1 Hz) some of the released acetylcholine acts on the postjunctional receptors to effect transmission, and some acts on the prejunctional receptors to enhance the mobilization of transmitter into the readily releasable situation. Hence, availability of transmitter matches the demand for it. Block of the postjunctional receptors impairs transmission, whereas block of the prejunctional receptors (e.g. by tubocurarine) means that availability of transmitter can no longer keep up with the demand when the traffic of nerve impulses is high. Consequently the contractions rapidly wane in amplitude during the repetitive stimulation, i.e., the well-known tetanic fade and train-of-four fade (for a review *see* Bowman et al., 1986).

There may also be an additional and separate population of nicotinic receptors on some non-myelinated part of the motor nerve endings, stimulation of which gives rise to repetitive activity in the motor nerves, which may be transferred to the muscle. Excessive activation of these receptors may depolarize the terminals and block transmission. One of the functions of acetylcholinesterase at the neuromuscular junction may be to protect the nerve endings from this type of re-excitation by the released transmitter (for reviews *see* Miyamoto, 1978; Bowman et al., 1986). The physiological function of these receptors, if any, is uncertain. There is even controversy as to their existence, some workers believing that the neural activity is initiated, not by acetylcholine directly, but by K^+ released from the postjunctional membrane as a consequence of postjunctional activity (Hohlfeld et al., 1981).

There may also be muscarinic receptors on somatic motor nerve endings, activation of which modulates acetylcholine release, although there is disagreement about the direction of this modulation. According to Das et al., (1978) and Ganguly and Das (1979), stimulation of prejunctional muscarinic receptors increases acetylcholine release but Abbs and Joseph (1980) found the opposite effect. Inhibition of transmitter release is the usual consequence of presynaptic muscarinic receptor stimulation at other synapses, and it seems unlikely that the neuromuscular junction would differ. The *Torpedo* electric organ is in many respects similar to the mammalian neuromuscular junction, and the evidence for presynaptic inhibitory muscarinic receptors in the electric organ is convincing (Dowdall et al., 1982). It may be, however, that there are two groups of prejunctional muscarinic receptors, one of which facilitates and the other inhibits transmitter release (Wessler et al., 1987, 1988).

3. The main cholinoceptors responsible for transmission through autonomic ganglia are the nicotinic cholinoceptors that may be blocked by, for example, hexamethonium or trimetaphan. These receptors mediate the fast synaptic potential that triggers off propagating action potentials in the postganglionic axons. However, the ganglionic response in sympathetic ganglia is usually more complex than this. In some

sympathetic ganglia, the initial fast depolarization is followed by a wave of hyperpolarization that has its origin in small dopaminergic interneurone-like cells called, because of their histochemical properties, small intensely fluorescent cells (SIF cells). SIF cells are located within sympathetic ganglia. They are activated by acetylcholine acting on muscarinic receptors and they give rise to the hyperpolarization by releasing dopamine on to the cell bodies of the postganglionic noradrenergic neurones. For a summary of the evidence *see* Greengard and Kebabian (1974). The physiological function of the SIF cells is not clear, although they obviously exert a negative modulating influence on postsynaptic excitability. In addition, there is a population of muscarinic cholinoceptors on the ganglion cells that modulates the so-called M-current. (The 'M' refers to the association with muscarinic receptors). The M-current is carried by outward flowing K^+ ions passing through a particular class of voltage-sensitive K^+ channels in the membrane of the ganglion cells. In frog ganglion cells, for example, it is switched on progressively between -70 mV and 0 mV. It flows continuously and forms a major component of the steady membrane conductance, tending always to increase the membrane potential and therefore to act as a braking current. Acetylcholine, acting on muscarinic receptors, inhibits the M-current by causing the closure of the K^+ channels, thereby causing a slow membrane depolarization which may not directly activate the cell, but which may facilitate the cell's response to signals mediated through nicotinic receptors (*see* Brown, 1984; Brown et al., 1986). M-currents are not confined to nervous structures; for example, they have been demonstrated in gastric smooth muscle cells (Sims et al., 1986).

4. Many sensory nerve endings possess nicotinic cholinoceptors, and injected acetylcholine produces an afferent discharge of impulses (Paintal, 1964). It is unlikely that these cholinoceptors play any physiological role in sensory transduction.

The sites of the peripheral cholinoceptors referred to above are illustrated in the diagram of Fig. 52.1. As a general rule, peripheral nicotinic receptors in vertebrates mediate excitation, whereas peripheral muscarinic receptors may mediate excitation (e.g. the gut) or inhibition (e.g. the heart) depending on the tissue.

SUBTYPES OF CHOLINOCEPTORS

Although the concept of two broad classes of cholinoceptors—muscarinic and nicotinic—remains useful, it is clear that there are subgroups of receptor types within each main group. Thus, the methonium series of compounds (Paton and Zaimis, 1949) serves to point up the difference between ganglionic and neuromuscular (or motor endplate) nicotinic receptors, the former being selectively blocked by hexamethonium (C6) and the latter selectively stimulated by the depolarizing drug decamethonium (C10). Accordingly,

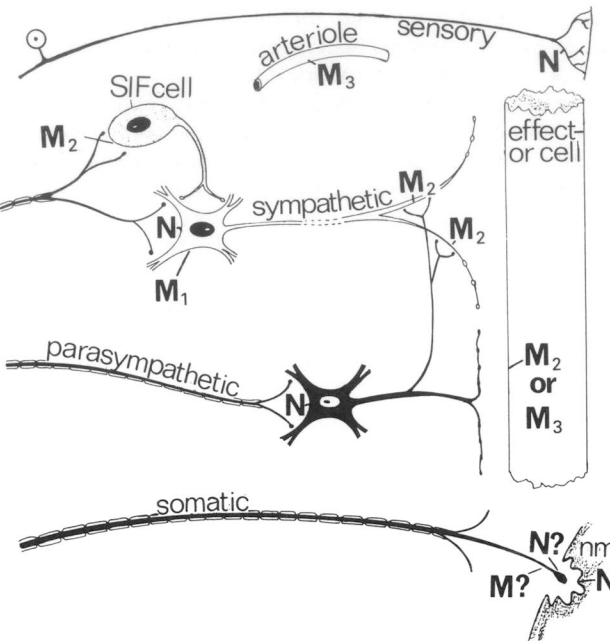

Fig. 52.1 The sites of peripheral muscarinic (M) and nicotinic (N) cholinoceptors. SIF cell small intensely fluorescent cell acts as an inhibitory interneurone within the ganglion; when activated releases dopamine on to the ganglion cell. nmj: neuromuscular junction. Subtypes of muscarinic receptors are indicated. Nicotinic receptors too are of different subtypes but have not yet been named. The existence of muscarinic and nicotinic receptors on somatic motor nerve terminals is not yet proven.

Brown (1979) describes the two subclasses as 'nicotinic C6 receptors' and 'nicotinic C10 receptors' respectively. The relative absence of ganglion blocking activity of the neuromuscular blocking drugs gallamine and pancuronium also emphasizes the difference, and certain toxins obtained from venoms (notably α-bungarotoxin which selectively blocks motor endplate nicotinic cholinoceptors, and kappa bungarotoxin and surugatoxin which block ganglionic nicotinic receptors) do likewise. These toxins are referred to again below. The nicotinic receptors postulated to be present on motor nerve terminals and to be responsible for facilitating transmitter mobilization have not yet been adequately categorized. However, there is preliminary evidence that they may represent a third subtype. They differ from motor endplate cholinoceptors in that they are insensitive to α-bungarotoxin, and they differ from ganglionic receptors in that they are insensitive to trimetaphan. Possibly they resemble some of the nicotinic cholinoceptors present on presynaptic nerve terminals in the brain.

Muscarinic cholinoceptors also appear not to be a homogeneous group (*see* Birdsall and Hulme, 1985 and Mitchelson, 1988, for discussion). Although all muscarinic receptors are stimulated by muscarine and acetylcholine, and blocked by atropine, it has long been evident that cardiac muscarinic receptors differ from muscarinic receptors on smooth muscle and gland cells. Thus, certain neuromuscular blocking drugs, amongst them gallamine (Riker and Wescoe, 1951) and pancuronium (Saxena and Bonta, 1970), block cardiac muscarinic receptors in doses much smaller than those necessary to block other visceral and glandular muscarinic receptors. This cardiac effect and consequent vagal blocking action of some neuromuscular blocking drugs contributes to their tendency to produce tachycardia. (For a review, *see* Marshall, 1980). The observation that gallamine selectively blocks cardiac muscarinic receptors does not in itself prove that the recognition sites of these receptors are of a different subtype. In fact it has been shown, more recently, that gallamine does not combine with the acetylcholine-binding site, that is with the receptor proper, but rather with a second and distinct binding site on the receptor complex. When drugs bind to this second site, they allosterically impair the binding of acetylcholine to the conventional site (Birdsall et al., 1985). Although the early observation with gallamine does not do more than provide a clue to the possibility that there are different muscarinic receptor subtypes, it does indicate that there are differences in receptor complexes as a whole, for not all muscarinic receptors are allosterically modified by gallamine. Those that are so modified by gallamine include the muscarinic receptors on SIF cells and those on autonomic nerve endings that negatively modulate transmitter release, as well as those in the heart (both myocardium and conducting tissue).

The next historical clue to the possibility that there are different subtypes of muscarinic receptors arose from the observation that certain muscarinic agonists, in particular those designated McN-A-343 (Roszkowski, 1961) and AH 6405 (Marshall, 1970), stimulated muscarinic receptors on sympathetic ganglion cells to cause an atropine-sensitive rise in blood pressure. Other muscarinic agonists known at the time (e.g. acetylcholine, methacholine, carbachol) produced a fall in blood pressure through relaxation of arteriolar smooth muscle. In more recent years, a large amount of work has been done in attempts to characterize fully the subtypes of muscarinic receptors, and to produce selective agonists and antagonists for them. Such selective drugs would have obvious therapeutic potential. An important observation arising from these studies is that the muscarinic antagonist drug pirenzepine shows high affinity for some muscarinic receptors and low affinity for others. On these grounds, some workers have designated only two subtypes of muscarinic receptors, those for which pirenzepine shows high affinity being designated M1, and the rest M2. However, most workers would agree that division into only two subtypes is an oversimplification. Table 52.1 indicates three subtypes, and this too is undoubtedly an oversimplification. The matter is extremely complex, and the reader is referred to reviews on the subject (Birdsall et al., 1985; Mitchelson, 1988), and the proceedings of two symposia (Hirschowitz et al., 1987; Levine et al., 1986) for further information and discussion. In some instances, it seems that different forms of receptor involve the same basic binding subunit but its binding characteristics are modulated in

TABLE 52.1

SOME PROPERTIES OF PERIPHERAL MUSCARINIC RECEPTOR SUBTYPES

	M_1	M_2	M_3
Relative by selective competitive antagonist	Pirenzepine	Methoctramine	Silahexocyclium
Relative by selective agonists	McN-A-343	Bridged propargyl esters of arecaidine	*cis*-3-acetoxy-*S*- methyl-thiane
Effect of gallamine at allosteric site	Weak	Potent	Weak
Receptor response coupling mechanism	Phosphoinositol lipid breakdown → closure of K^+-M channels	Inhibition of adenylate cyclase → opening of membrane K^+ channels	Phosphoinositol lipid breakdown → release of bound Ca^{2+}, and extra Ca^{2+} influx
Examples of tissue location and effect	Sympathetic ganglia (slow depolarization through closure of K^+-M channels) Ganglia or myenteric plexus of stomach (release of gastric acid)	Heart (bradycardia); SIF cells (release dopamine); possibly nerve terminals (inhibit transmitter release)	Smooth muscle (contraction); endothelium of arteries (release of EDRF); salivary and lacrimal glands (secretion)

Data obtained from literature reviewed by Birdsall and Hulme (1985) and Mitchelson (1988), and from proceedings of international symposia edited by Hirschowitz et al. (1984) and Levine et al. (1986).

different ways by their local environment, and they can be interconverted by various environmental modifications (Birdsall et al., 1979).

Neurotransmitters in general, including acetylcholine, do not readily penetrate cell membranes, yet responses to them are relatively rapid in onset (especially when nicotinic receptors are involved), and so it has long been assumed that receptors for neurotransmitters are constituents of the plasma membranes of postsynaptic or effector cells with their specific recognition and binding sites on the outside surface of the membrane. In accordance with the concept of outwardly orientated recognition and binding sites, both skeletal and smooth muscle fibres have been shown to respond only to the external application of acetylcholine to the receptor regions (del Castillo and Katz, 1955; Purves, 1974).

MOTOR ENDPLATE NICOTINIC CHOLINOCEPTORS

Refined electrophysiological analysis of the consequences of drug-receptor interactions together with the use of advanced biochemical, immunological and electronmicroscopical techniques and recombinant DNA technology have led to the isolation, purification and characterization of motor endplate type nicotinic cholinoceptors to an extent that far outstrips the study of any other kind of receptor. Studies of these cholinoceptors have been greatly aided by two important zoological contributions: the presence of a rich source of nicotinic cholinoceptor material of the motor endplate type in the electric organs of the electric eel (*Electrophorus electricus*) and the electric rays (principally *Torpedo marmorata* and *Torpedo californica*), and the ability of α-toxins from certain Elapid snakes (notably cobra toxin from the Thailand cobra and α-bungarotoxin from the Taiwan banded krait) to bind selectively and relatively irreversibly with this type of cholinoceptor. Progress has been such that it has proved possible for purified cholinoceptors to be isolated and then inserted into synthetic lipid membranes where they retain their sensitivity and responsiveness to acetylcholine (Boheim et al., 1981). In addition functional receptors, and even hybrid receptors formed from component parts of receptors from more than one species, have been induced to develop in toad egg cells, which normally do not possess cholinoceptors, by injecting the appropriate messenger RNAs obtained from electric organs or muscle.

Receptor Structure and Location

The early studies were carried out on acetylcholine receptors from the electric organs of electric eels and rays. Each receptor consists of five protein subunits or protamers, which span the membrane from side to side (Kistler et al., 1982). Two of the subunits designated α (alpha), are identical and have molecular weights of 40 000 daltons. The other three are slightly larger, and are designated $β$ (beta, MW 49 000), $γ$ (gamma, MW 60 000) and $δ$ (delta, MW 67 000). Each type of subunit is encoded by a different gene, although they are similar in overall structure and have homologous stretches where they are nearly the same, amino acid by amino acid. The five subunits are arranged in a cylinder around a central pore which functions as a cation channel when the receptor is activated. The structure of the receptor complex may therefore be represented as $α_2βγδ$. In fact, in the electric fish and probably in other species, the receptor *in situ* exists as a dimeric structure, the two monomeric forms being connected by a disulphide bond between the $δ$ subunits. It might be represented thus: $α_2βγδ$-S-S-$δγβα_2$.

Each subunit consists of a chain of amino acids, twisted into a helix, that crosses the membrane five times from one side to the other. Four of the membrane spanning regions are hydrophobic and form strong attachments to the lipids of the membrane. The fifth has one hydrophilic and three hydrophobic faces (i.e., it is amphipathic, having both hydrophilic and hydrophobic regions). The hydrophilic face of each subunit lines the pore in the centre of the complex, making it possible for cations surrounded by water molecules to pass through when the ion channel is in its open state (Stevens, 1985). The mammalian receptor, especially the fetal form, is almost certainly closely similar to that of the electric fish. However, whereas the fetal calf receptor resembles that of the electric fish, the adult bovine receptor contains, in place of the $γ$-subunit, a subunit designated $ε$ (epsilon). The $ε$-subunit has only 53% homology with the $γ$-subunit sequence, and it contains more acidic and fewer basic amino acids than the $γ$-subunit (Takai et al., 1985; Mishina et al., 1986). The mRNA encoding the $ε$-subunit becomes prominent soon after birth. In some way the newly arrived motor nerve terminals that come to innervate the muscle fibres, switch on expression of the gene encoding the $ε$-subunit while switching off expression of that encoding the $γ$-subunit. Figure 52.2 is a diagrammatic representation of an adult mammalian receptor complex.

The two α-subunits each carry a single recognition site that exhibits mutually exclusive binding for nicotinic agonists such as acetylcholine, carbachol, and succinylcholine, reversible antagonists such as tubocurarine, and irreversible antagonists such as α-bungarotoxin. The recognition or binding site is associated with the adjacent disulphide cross-linked cysteine residues (Cys 192 and Cys 193) in the extracellular portion of the protein of the α-subunits. Although the two α-subunits and the two binding sites are identical, the environment of the one differs from that of the other because the adjacent protamers differ (Fig. 52.2), and this may affect the binding characteristics. The essential presence of a positively charged centre in the molecules of acetylcholine and analogues of it, indicates that a negatively charged subsite (the anionic site) is a component of the receptor recogni-

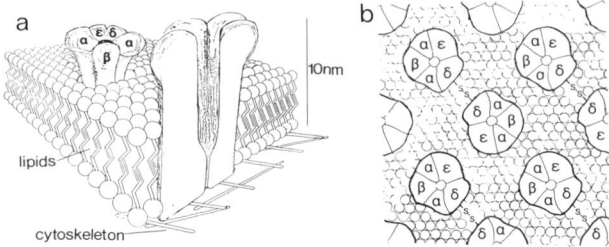

Fig. 52.2 (a) Diagram of a portion of a mature mammalian postjunctional motor endplate membrane showing two receptor complexes embedded in and spanning the bimolecular lipid layer. The two α subunits and the *β*, *δ* and ε subunits are labelled. These surround a central ion channel. The acetylcholine recognition sites are located on the α subunits, one on each. **(b)** Receptors in surface view. The receptors are drawn as dimeric structures linked in pairs by disulphide bonds that connect the two *δ*-subunits. (Reproduced with permission from Bowman W.C. *The Pharmacology of Neuromuscular Function* 2nd edn. London: Butterworth, in press).

tion site. This is presumed to be the locus of ion-pair formation between the receptor and the quaternary ammonium group of cholinoceptor agonists and antagonists. The high proportion of glutamate and aspartate residues present in purified cholinoceptor protein, suggests that dissociated carboxylate groups of these amino acids might constitute the negatively charged anionic site. The anionic site has strictly defined stereochemical characteristics, as extensive structure: action studies with agonists and antagonists show (for reviews, *see* Stenlake, 1979, 1980).

Karlin and his colleagues (for a review, *see* Karlin et al., 1973) studied the effects of substances that interact with SH groups (e.g. p-chloromercuribenzoate) and S-S groups (e.g. dithiothreitol) on receptor function. Their results provided an early indication that there are one or more SH groups in the receptor, although such groups did not appear to be part of the acetylcholine recognition site. An S-S group appeared to lie about 1 nm from the anionic site, and although it is probably not directly involved in ligand recognition and binding, reduction of this group profoundly alters the specificity of the receptor, presumably by altering its structure. Circumstantial evidence suggests that a hydrophobic bonding site lies between the anionic site and the disulphide group. Such a site would repel the OH group of substances such as choline. The effect might contribute to the lack of agonist potency of this alcohol in comparison with that of acetylcholine as well as with that of the ethyl (or propyl) trimethylammonium ion.

In a normal innervated muscle fibre, the postjunctional receptors are essentially restricted to the crests of the junctional folds of the motor endplate membrane where they are held in fixed clusters by the cytoskeleton. The density of receptors at the crests is over 5000/μm² and there are many millions of receptors at each endplate.

Synthesis, Degradation and Down-Regulation of Endplate Nicotinic Receptors

Most of the available information about receptor synthesis and degradation has been derived from studies on embryo skeletal muscle fibres grown in culture, but confirmatory evidence has been obtained in studies on denervated adult muscles. Much of the evidence has been comprehensively reviewed by Fambrough (1979) and references to the original work are contained in his review. In both embryo fibres and in denervated fibres, receptors are abundantly present over the whole area of cell membrane. It should be pointed out that activation of a muscle by its motor nerve restricts the acetylcholine-sensitive area of muscle fibre membrane essentially to the junctional region and it also depresses the turnover of receptors. However, the mechanisms underlying the synthetic and catabolic processes, as distinct from their rates, appear to be the same irrespective of innervation. The roles of the motor nerve in receptor localization and characteristics are referred to again below.

Acetylcholine receptors are synthesized intracellularly by a process that takes only about 15 min. The synthesis probably involves the assembly of a mannose-containing carbohydrate core which is linked to a phospholipid carrier (dolichol pyrophosphate). On completion, the carbohydrate cores are transferred to asparagine residues of polypeptide chains to form receptors. Receptor synthesis can be inhibited both by compounds that impair carbohydrate synthesis (e.g. tunicamycin, 2-deoxyglucose, D-glucosamine, donazonoreucine) and by compounds that impair protein synthesis either directly (e.g. puromycin, cycloheximide) or indirectly through inhibiting RNA synthesis (e.g. actinomycin D).

The newly synthesized acetylcholine receptors constitute an intracellular pool which is held in the membranes of the Golgi apparatus and the postGolgi vesicles. Within about 3 h each newly synthesized receptor is inserted into the plasma membrane: the order of insertion of receptors is apparently that in which they were synthesized. The rate of insertion is about 90 /(μm² · h). Incorporation of new receptors into the plasma membrane is unaffected by inhibition of protein synthesis, by cytochalasins (which disrupt microfilaments), and by variations either in membrane potential or in external calcium ion concentration. The process appears to be dependent on metabolic energy production, since it is blocked by inhibitors of ATP synthesis and is slowed or blocked by a fall in temperature. Activation of adenylate cyclase with the production of cyclic adenosine 3,5-monophosphate may be an essential trigger that initiates the synthesizing mechanism. The process is slowed but not blocked by colchicine which may indicate that it is partly dependent on functional microtubules.

Acetylcholine receptors in the membranes of cultured muscle fibres have an average lifetime of 17 h. The kinetics of breakdown indicate a random mechanism: that is to say that the most recently synthesized receptors are just as likely to be degraded as are any others. The mechanism of degradation appears to involve ATP-dependent movement of the receptor to the inside of the cell where proteolytic destruction occurs in lysosomes.

When a nerve fibre grows to make contact with a muscle fibre, a well-defined basement membrane appears between the two cells at the junction. Acetylcholine receptors cluster in the muscle fibre membrane beneath the basement membrane and become fixed in herring-bone arrays at the crests of the junctional folds. The proteins of the cytoskeleton act in concert with a heparin sulphate proteoglycan of the basement membrane to initiate clustering of the receptors and anchor them to the cytoskeleton (Froehner, 1986). At the same time, in some as yet unknown way, nerve activity, together with activation of the muscle fibre membrane, increases the stability of the junctional receptors so that their lifetimes extend to many days or weeks, and inhibits the synthesis of extrajunctional receptors (Kuromi, 1987). Since the extrajunctional receptors have a lifetime of only 20 h or so, extrajunctional regions of membrane quickly become virtually receptor-free and the chemosensitive region is thus effectively confined to the motor endplate membrane. Inhibition of the synthesis of extrajunctional receptors may depend upon activation of guanylate cyclase and the intracellular production of cyclic guanosine monophosphate.

The response of many cells to excessive action of a specific agonist is to reduce the number of, that is down-regulate, the membrane receptors for that agonist. The receptors are internalized and destroyed, but as yet little is understood about the factors that control the down-regulation. The motor endplate membrane is no exception; excessive transmitter action consequent upon prolonged treatment with anticholinesterase drugs has been shown to cause a reduction in the number of cholinoceptors (Chang et al., 1973; Gwilt and Wray, 1986). Down-regulation of endplate cholinoceptors may play a part in the temporary diminishing effectiveness of anticholinesterase treatment that often occurs in patients with myasthenia gravis.

Denervated Muscle

When a muscle fibre is denervated, the former endplate region retains its receptors for many days or weeks and may acquire more. The brake on receptor synthesis in extrajunctional regions of membrane is removed, and new receptors are rapidly synthesized and inserted into all regions of the membrane. The increase in the number of receptors is responsible for the increased sensitivity of chronically denervated muscle to acetylcholine and related agonists. (*See* Rash et al., 1978 and Fambrough, 1979). The receptors outside the junction are to some extent physiologically, pharmacologically and immunologically different from those at the motor endplate. In fact they resemble fetal receptors in their turn-over time and electrophysiological properties.

Receptors in Myasthenia Gravis

Simpson (1960) first suggested that myasthenia gravis is an autoimmune disease after noting that it often occurs in conjunction with other diseases of autoimmune aetiology. More recent evidence has confirmed the autoimmune nature of myasthenia gravis. Antibodies to acetylcholine receptor protein are present in the serum of patients with myasthenia gravis. Appropriate electronmicroscopical techniques indicate that the antibodies combine with the acetylcholine receptors and in so doing destroy the crests of the junctional folds of the postjunctional endplate membrane. This degenerative process is associated with the loss of 70–90% of the functional acetylcholine receptors. (For references and detailed discussion *see* Rash et al., 1978; Fambrough, 1979; Drachman et al., 1979; Vincent, 1980).

Receptor Function

Comprehensive descriptions of receptor function are given in the reviews by Ginsborg and Jenkinson (1976), Dreyer (1982) and Colquhoun (1986).

Receptor activation by acetylcholine or a related nicotinic agonist occurs in response to binding of molecules at both recognition sites on the α-subunits. The two sites exhibit positive cooperativity; that is to say that binding of an agonist molecule at one site facilitates binding of a second molecule at the other. Occupation of the two recognition sites by agonist molecules induces a conformational change in the protein of the α-subunits, and it is envisaged that a concerted transition between the subunits then occurs with the result that the cation channel opens (Taylor and Sine, 1982). The conformational change induced in the receptor associated protein is believed to result in the opening of a channel that allows small cations (Na^+, K^+, Ca^{2+}) to flow along their concentration gradients. At the neuromuscular junction, the membrane potential, the equilibrium potentials for the various ions, and the concentrations of those ions dictate that the main change induced by the opening of the receptor-operated ion channels is an influx of Na^+. The activated receptor complex may be depicted as in Fig. 52.3. The net inward Na^+ current occurs through a large number of receptor channels and depolarizes the membrane at the endplate region.

When acetylcholine or a related agonist is added to the solution bathing a muscle fibre, a depolarization of the endplates is readily recorded with an intracellular microelectrode. Careful recording shows, however, that the depolarization is not steady. Rather, it consists of minute fluctuations about the mean response. Katz and Miledi who first described the phenomenon with acetylcholine called it 'acetylcholine noise'. A convincing amount of evidence

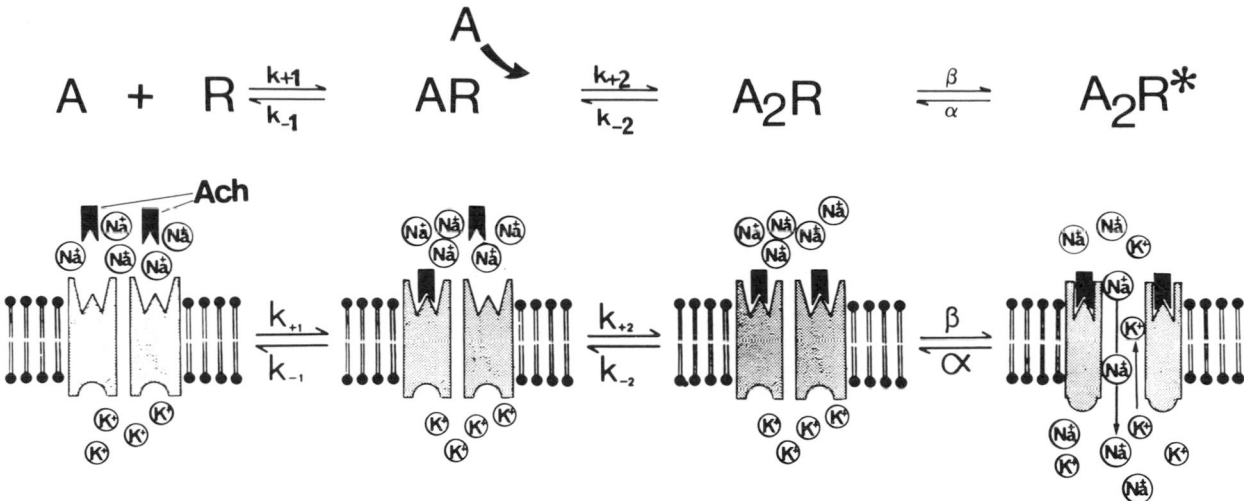

Fig. 52.3 Diagram of the interaction of acetylcholine (Ach) with endplate cholinoceptors. Two acetylcholine molecules combine with the recognition sites of the receptor and induce a conformational change that results in the opening of a cation channel allowing the diffusion of Na^+ and K^+. The combination of the first Ach molecule facilitates combination with the second (positive cooperativity). The interaction is represented by the reaction equation at the top in the conventional way. The acetylcholine molecules and their recognition sites are drawn much larger than to scale. k_{+1}, k_{-1}, k_{+2}, k_{-2}, etc. α and β are rate constants for the forward and backward reactions. A = acetylcholine, R = receptor and R^x = receptor with open ion channel. (Reproduced with permission from Bowman W.C. *The Pharmacology of Neuromuscular Function*, 2nd edn. London: Butterworths, in press).

indicated that the noise reflects the moment to moment fluctuations in the number of ion channels that are opened by the agonist. Refinements of the techniques for studying these elementary molecular events include the use of a voltage clamp apparatus which fixes the membrane potential at a level chosen by the experimenter so that depolarization cannot occur. The apparatus, virtually instantaneously, both generates and measures the amount of current needed to fix the voltage, and this current is proportional to the number of open ion channels. Factors governing the transition between open and closed states of the channels may also be studied by producing a large and abrupt perturbation in the conditions that determine the equilibrium (e.g. jumps in membrane potential), and then following the rate at which the system re-approaches equilibrium (relaxes). In a further refinement of the voltage clamp technique known as patch clamp analysis, measurements on single ion channels have been made (Fig. 52.4). These show that each channel produces a brief pulse of current with a rectangular form. Mathematical analysis of results obtained from all these types of experiment have provided detailed information about ion channel function. Thus, for example, at room temperature, acetylcholine causes the ion channels in a frog muscle endplate at its normal resting membrane potential to open for periods of about 1 ms (i.e. the mean ion channel open time is 1 ms) which allows the net entry of about 10^4 cations giving an elementary current of about 2 pA. Each open channel has a mean conductance (γ) of about 30 picosiemens (pS).

The corresponding variables for an ion channel in an adult mammalian muscle endplate are an elementary current of about 3.5 pA, a single channel conductance of about 60 pS, and a mean open time of 5–10 ms.

Each quantum of acetylcholine (i.e. supposedly the amount released from one vesicle to produce a miniature endplate potential) causes the opening of about 1700 ion channels, and at the peak of an endplate potential about 340 000 channels are open.

Channel opening time is dependent on membrane potential (there is an e-fold change for about 100 mV), possibly because the channel gating mechanism involves a rotating dipole so that the ease with which it opens and closes depends on the electric field. Channels close more rapidly when the membrane is depolarized, and *vice versa*. Thus, the depolarization associated with an action potential will hasten channel closing, and presumably hasten the removal of acetylcholine from its receptor, thereby rendering it susceptible to hydrolysis by acetylcholinesterase. It seems clear that, *in vivo*, any one acetylcholine molecule persists long enough to act on only one receptor complex before being destroyed by acetylcholinesterase. With a patch clamp electrode it can be seen that an increase in the concentration of acetylcholine, or other agonist, causes an increase in the frequency of channel opening, but does not modify the basic elementary event. When cholinesterase is inhibited, transmitter acetylcholine is allowed to make multiple interactions with the cholinoceptors before escaping by diffusion from the junctional cleft.

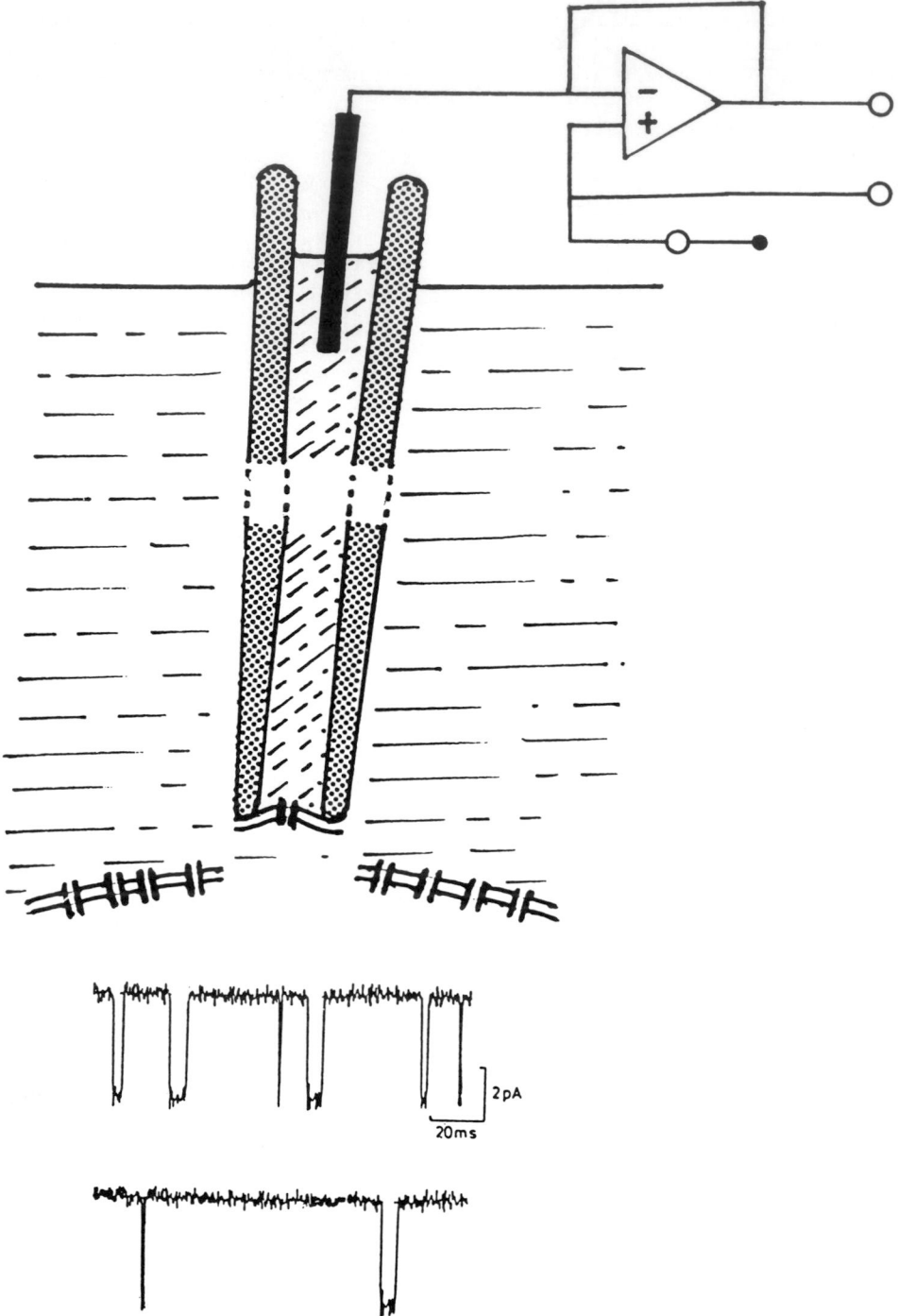

Fig. 52.4 Diagrammatic representation of a patch clamp technique (inside-out patch). The electrode tip is represented as enclosing only one receptor complex. Typical records are shown below: above with acetylcholine alone in the pipette; the downward deflections are of uniform amplitude but of different durations: below with acetylcholine and tubocurarine together in the pipette; the shape of the pulses of current have not changed but their frequency is reduced. (Reproduced with permission from Bowman W.C. *The Pharmacology of Neuromuscular Function*, 2nd edn. London: Butterworths, in press).

Different agonists give rise to different channel opening times. For example, carbachol produces shorter and suberylcholine longer channel open times than does acetylcholine (Colquhoun, 1979; Wray, 1980).

The interaction between acetylcholine (Ach), or any other cholinomimetic agonist, with its receptors can be expressed as illustrated in Fig. 52.3.

Acetylcholine receptors in fetal muscle and in denervated muscle have mean open times 2–4 times longer, and single channel conductances somewhat less, than those in adult innervated muscle. Since the main difference between adult and fetal receptors seems to be the substitution of the γ-subunit by the ε-subunit, it appears that the ε-subunit may influence conductance and be responsible for the fast type of channel gating. This has been confirmed in experiments in which hybrid receptors have been induced to develop in toad oocytes. Experiments currently in progress in Japan and other countries involve the extraction of messenger RNAs that specify individual receptor subunits from the muscles of different species—say calf (the endplates of which possess adult type receptors), fetal calf, and torpedo. By injecting the appropriate mRNAs into toad oocytes, acetylcholine receptors are induced to develop in the membrane, and their electrophysiological properties may be examined with a patch clamp system. By comparing the properties of hybrid receptors which differ from true receptors by only one type of subunit, the functions of the various subunits may be determined. This type of work (*see*, for example, Sakmann et al., 1985; Mishina et al., 1986) is in its infancy, but already there is evidence that both the δ- and the ε-subunits determine the channel closing step, whereas the α-subunit influences channel opening and agonist dissociation.

The functioning of the postjunctional motor endplate receptors may be summarized as follows. Acetylcholine molecules, released from the nerve endings in response to a nerve impulse, bind (about once each) with their receptors on the α-subunits. The binding induces a conformational change that results in the opening of a cation channel in the activated receptor complex. A brief rectangular pulse of inward cationic current (mainly Na^+) is permitted to flow. Many elementary current pulses summate to produce the endplate current. The endplate current depolarizes the endplate membrane so that there is a voltage drop across the endplate. This is the endplate potential, which, once it reaches a critical threshold, triggers off an all-or-nothing action potential that passes around the muscle fibre membrane to activate the contractile process.

Receptor Desensitization

When acetylcholine or another agonist is applied to the motor endplates for prolonged periods, the endplate membrane does not remain at the level of depo-larization initially produced. Instead the response declines to reach a steady level which may be only a very small fraction of the original effect; that is, the membrane potential may return virtually to its resting level despite the continued application of the agonist. Although the membrane potential may recover to normal, neuromuscular transmission remains blocked throughout the drug application (Thesleff, 1955). The waning response is said to be caused by receptor desensitization; it has been studied in some detail by refined electrophysiological techniques, and is fully discussed by Ginsborg et al. (1976), Zaimis and Head (1976), Bowman (1980), Colquhoun (1986) and Karlin et al. (1986) where references to the original work are quoted. A scheme that, though oversimplified, qualitatively accounts for many of the properties of desensitization, is shown in Fig. 52.5.

Several factors influence the rate of desensitization. Some agonists are more effective in producing it than others and it occurs more readily in the muscles of some species than in those of others. Even within the same species (frog), different types of muscle exhibit differences in desensitization. Some procedures or agents slow the rate or reduce the extent of desensitization produced by a given agonist. These include a fall in temperature, lack of Ca^{2+}, and drugs, including nystatin and adrenaline. Others hasten the rate of desensitization. These include membrane hyperpolarization, proadifen (SKF 525A), chlorpromazine, procaine, pentobarbitone, caffeine and halogenated anaesthetics.

The precise physical nature of the change that constitutes desensitization is not yet known, although there is some evidence that phosphorylation of the receptor proteins may be part of the mechanism. Elucidation of the mechanism is important, since it will provide a clearer picture of the channel gating or channel opening mechanism. Although it is possible to produce receptor desensitization by excessive nerve stimulation, the conditions have to be abnormal, and it seems probable that the phenomenon has no relevance to the physiological transmission mechanism. It may, however, have pharmacological relevance to the action of depolarizing neuromuscular blocking drugs, the so-called phase 2 block.

Actions of Receptor Antagonists

The main clinically used drugs of this type are tubocurarine, metocurine, alcuronium, gallamine, pancuronium, vercuronium, pipecuronium and atracurium. They have affinity for the recognition sites of the acetylcholine receptors but are incapable of producing the conformational change in the receptor protein that constitutes opening of the ion channel; that is to say, they are devoid of the property called 'efficacy' and act merely to impede the access of acetylcholine to the receptors. Occupation of only one of the two binding sites on a receptor complex by a blocking drug is sufficient to reduce greatly the probability that acetyl-

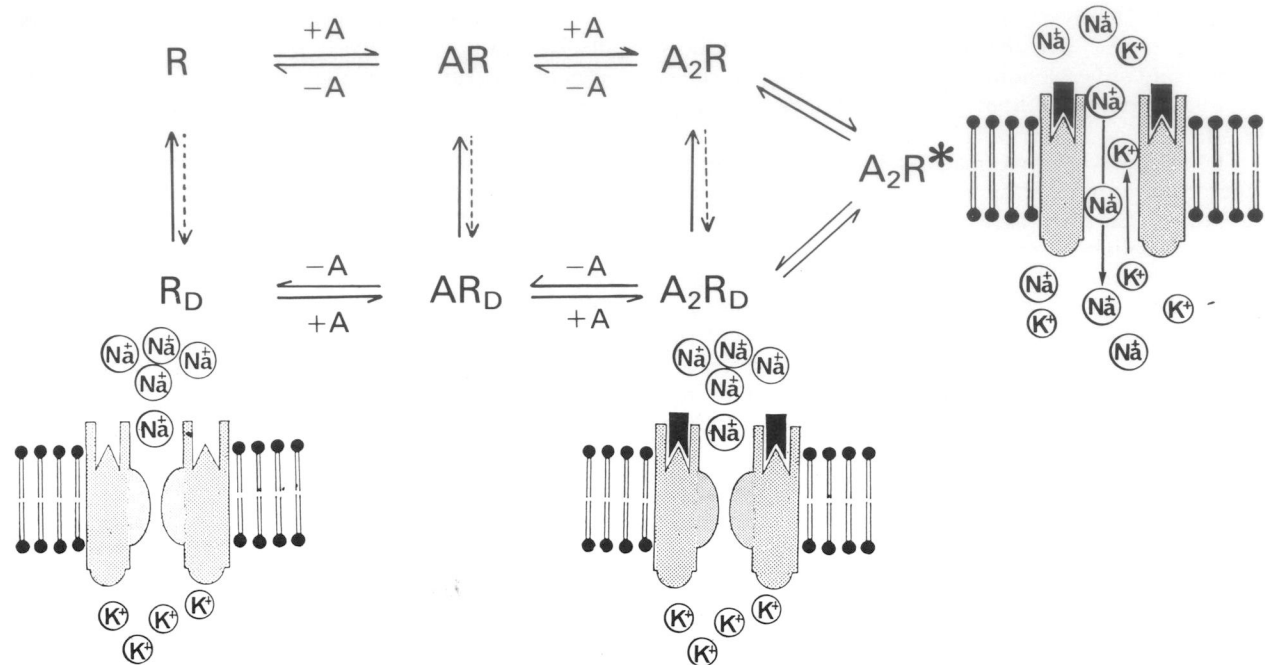

Fig. 52.5 Equation representing receptor activation and desensitization. The top row leading to A_2R^* is the same as in Fig. 52.3. R_D represents a desensitized receptor channel. Pictorial representations of A_2R, A_2R_D and R_D are included. Fig. 52.3 should be consulted for further information concerning the meaning of the symbols and diagrams. (Reproduced with permission from Bowman W.C. *The Pharmacology of Neuromuscular Function*, 2nd edn. London: Butterworths, in press).

choline will open the ion channel, since acetylcholine is most effective when it interacts with both binding sites. Studies of individual receptor function with a patch clamp electrode show that, in the presence of both acetylcholine and a nondepolarizing blocking drug of the reversible type, there is no change produced by the blocking drug in the individual channel open times nor in the shape or size of the elementary currents. The only effect is a reduction in the frequency of channel opening (*see* Fig. 52.4). Consequently, the sum of the elementary events constituting the endplate current (epc) is reduced in amplitude (but not changed in shape), and the reduced epp may fail to reach the threshold necessary to trigger the action potential and subsequent contraction so that muscle paralysis results.

The molecules of the blocking drug react dynamically with the receptor recognition sites, repeatedly associating with and dissociating from them. If this were not so, patch clamp recording would detect no response at all to acetylcholine in the presence of an effective concentration of blocking drug, rather than merely a reduction in the frequency of channel opening. Since the interaction is a dynamic one, it is possible to restore the frequency of opening to the initial level, simply by increasing the concentration of acetylcholine in the pipette. This kind of dynamic interaction with the receptor, coupled with the mutual antagonism between agonist and antagonist is charac-

teristic of block by competition, and indeed nondepolarizing blocking drugs of this type are often called competitive blocking drugs. It is, however, difficult to be certain that drugs of this type fulfil, at the neuromuscular junction, all of the strict criteria characteristic of competitive antagonists (Colquhoun, 1986).

α-bungarotoxin, and other α-toxins from the venoms of Elapid snakes, resemble the clinically used nondepolarizing drugs in that they bind in a highly selective way to the recognition sites of the motor endplate cholinoceptors. They differ from the clinically useful drugs, however, in that the binding is irreversible. Hence, an effective concentration of α-bungarotoxin totally abolishes the effect of acetylcholine in a patch clamp system, and an increase in the concentration of acetylcholine does not restore receptor activity.

Ion Channel Block

Refined electrophysiological techniques, including patch clamp recording, indicate that many drugs are capable of entering the open ion channels at the endplate and thereby occluding them (Adams, 1976; Wray, 1980; Dreyer, 1982; Lambert et al., 1983). Such drugs include barbiturates, some local anaesthetics, calcium channel blocking drugs, and some antibiotics. Inactivation of channels in this way accounts for the synergism at the neuromuscular junction between such drugs and neuromuscular blocking drugs. There are alternative mechanisms through which other drugs may impede channel opening and thereby potentiate neuromuscular blocking drugs (Dreyer, 1982). For example, some drugs (certain local anaesthetics and tricyclic antidepressants are examples) may alter channel properties by combining with the closed form of the receptor at a site other than the acetylcholine binding site, and inhalation anaesthetics may modify channel function by dissolving in the surrounding membrane lipids.

Surprisingly perhaps, under appropriate experimental conditions, neuromuscular blocking drugs may also enter and plug ion channels that have already been opened by acetylcholine. The extent, if any, to which this may occur clinically is not known. It seems that if it does occur it will only do so at the top of the dose range. It is, however, important that anaesthetists should bear the possibility in mind. Ion channel block with neuromuscular blocking drugs is use-dependent. It is therefore more likely to occur with increase in the frequency of channel opening by acetylcholine or with an increase in the number of open channels. Consequently, anticholinesterase drugs, through their action in causing acetylcholine accumulation, may actually enhance, rather than reverse, ion channel block. With a high dose of neuromuscular blocking drug some receptor recognition sites will be blocked and some ion channels will be blocked. An anticholinesterase overcomes the block at the former but may enhance that at the latter, so that the overall effect is small. It is a well-known clinical observation that neostigmine fails to reverse an excessively deep neuromuscular block produced by tubocurarine and related drugs, and ion channel block may partly account for its apparent paucity of effect.

GANGLIONIC NICOTINIC CHOLINOCEPTORS

A great deal less is known about the structure and formation of ganglionic nicotinic receptors than about those at the motor endplate, although it is generally believed that they function in an essentially similar way. One of the problems has been that, although snake toxins such as α-bungarotoxin bind to ganglia, they do not block ganglionic transmission, and the binding sites do not appear to be the cholinoceptors (see, for example, Brown, 1979). Surugatoxin, extracted from the Japanese ivory mollusc (*Babylonia japonica*), binds selectively to ganglionic nicotinic cholinoceptors but the dissociation rate is too fast to allow its effective use as a ligand analogous to that of α-bungarotoxin at endplate cholinoceptors (Brown et al., 1976). Attempts to synthesize irreversible ligands for ganglionic nicotinic cholinoceptors have also, so far, been unproductive.

The recent discovery of two hitherto unknown toxins that bind to ganglionic nicotinic receptors—kappa bungarotoxin and kappa flavitoxin from the venoms of the Taiwan banded krait and the red headed krait respectively (Chiappinelli, 1983; Chiappinelli et al., 1987)—may provide more useful agents for studying these receptors.

In an electrophysiological study of rat parasympathetic ganglia, Ascher et al. (1979) provided evidence for two types of ganglion blocking action. Perhaps surprisingly, the more traditional ganglion blocking drugs, tubocurarine and hexamethonium, apparently acted mainly by blocking agonist-opened ion channels, whereas trimetaphan, mecamylamine and surugatoxin blocked mainly in the expected way, by combining with the receptor recognition sites and thereby preventing binding of agonist molecules.

MUSCARINIC CHOLINOCEPTORS

As in the case of ganglionic cholinoceptors, muscarinic receptors have not yet been isolated. Responses to muscarinic receptor activation by agonists are considerably slower in onset than are responses to nicotinic receptor activation, probably at least partly because in many cases muscarinic responses are mediated by second messengers, such as the products of phosphorylated inositol lipid breakdown, rather than the direct opening of receptor-operated ion channels.

Paton and Rang (1965) set the stage for the study of receptor-ligand binding in their classical examination of the interaction of ^{3}H-atropine with muscarinic receptors of intestinal smooth muscle. ^{3}H-Benzetimide has also been used (Beld and Ariens, 1974). Antagonists specially synthesized for receptor-binding studies of this type include ^{3}H-quinuclidinyl benzilate (Yamamura and Snyder, 1974), and ^{3}H-benzilylcholine mustard which binds covalently to the alkylates and the receptor (Gill and Rang, 1966; Fewtrell and Rang, 1973). Two effective photoaffinity ligands (azido-N-methyl-4-piperidyl benzilate and p-azidoatropine methyl iodide) have also been synthesized (Sokolovsky, 1987). These have the advantage that their binding is completely reversible until photoactivation occurs. In general, the problem is that as well as the relatively small number of high affinity binding sites that constitute the receptors, there are also a large number of non-specific binding sites that may account for a high proportion of the total binding. Common techniques to obviate this problem are to measure, by liquid scintillation counting, the uptake of the labelled drug in the absence and in the presence of a receptor specific concentration of an agonist or antagonist. Subtracting the one from the other, gives the specific receptor bindings. An alternative method is to make use of the stereospecificity of the muscarinic receptor compared with the lack of stereospecificity of other binding sites. The total binding of a pharmacologically active isomer is compared with the non-specific binding of the pharmacologically inactive stereo isomer. Benzetimide provides an example of a drug that has been used in this way. (+)-Benzetimide (called dexetimide) is the pharmacologically active muscarinic receptor antagonist, while (−)-benzetimide, although it combines with the non-specific binding sites, does not block the muscarinic receptors.

On the basis of binding studies with benzilylcholine mustard, it has been calculated that there are about 200 specific binding sites (receptors) per μm^2 of intestinal smooth muscle cell (Fewtrell et al., 1973). From this figure, and estimates of the maximum increase in membrane conductance produced by carbachol, it appears that the conductance per site is between 10^{-1} and 5×10^{-1} pS. Autoradiography of preparations treated with labelled antagonists may in the future provide information on the detailed localization of muscarinic receptors in the cell membrane, but at present the spatial resolution of the method is inadequate.

The binding of benzilylcholine mustard to muscarinic cholinoceptors (unlike that of α-bungatotoxin to endplate cholinoceptors) is lost completely when the material is solubilized with non-ionic detergents. Furthermore, the binding material is much more firmly attached to the smooth muscle membrane, than is bound bungarotoxin to the endplate or electroplax membrane (Fewtrell et al., 1973; Fewtrell, 1976). Consequently, analysis of the structure of muscarinic receptors lags behind that of endplate nicotinic receptors.

Traditionally in pharmacology, receptors are classified according to the order of potency of agonists and the affinity constants of antagonists; that is to say, they are classified in terms of the characteristics of their recognition or binding sites, and not in accordance with the mechanisms that couple agonist binding to cellular response. Nevertheless, in many instances it happens that different receptor subtypes do trigger off different coupling mechanisms, and this often seems to be the case with subtypes of muscarinic receptors. M_1 receptor activation mediates the closure of $K^+(M)$ channels, as already mentioned. The mechanism through which this occurs involves activation of a GPT-binding protein, and possibly the subsequent generation of diacylglycerols and activation of protein Kinase C (Brown et al., 1989). M_{II} receptor activation leads to inhibition of adenylate cyclase. The role of β-adrenoceptors in stimulating the activity of adenylate cyclase is described in Chapter 51. Adenylate cyclase catalyses the production of cyclic AMP from ATP, and the cyclic AMP then acts to phosphorylate protein kinases that in turn trigger off various cellular processes. M_2 receptors are generally coupled to adenylate cyclase *via* an inhibitory GTP-binding protein. Hence, adenylate cyclase activity is curtailed and the cellular content of cyclic AMP falls. The fall in cyclic AMP concentration means that the specific protein kinases revert to their dephosphorylated, inactive form. Consequently, the relevant cellular activities are inhibited; for example, there is a negative inotropic

effect on the atria, and transmitter release at some synapses and neuroeffector junctions is negatively modulated. M_3 receptor activation is often coupled to the membrane enzyme phospholipase C. As with adenylate cyclase, GTP-binding proteins are involved. Activation of phospholipase C causes it to catalyse the breakdown of inositol phospholipids in the inner leaflet of the cell membrane. Inositol phosphates and diacylglycerol are released as second messengers and, among other actions, these cause the release of Ca^{2+} from the smooth endoplasmic reticulum and enhance Ca^{2+} influx through the cell membrane. The increased cellular concentration of Ca^{2+} then acts to bring about the cellular response, for example, contraction of smooth muscle.

The action of muscarinic agonists on arteries, and probably arterioles, is a special case worthy of emphasis. Muscarinic receptors are located both on the smooth muscle, where they mediate vasoconstriction, and on the endothelium where, indirectly, they mediate vasodilatation. In the intact healthy vessel, the endothelium receptors are the most susceptible to interaction with muscarinic agonists because the smooth muscle receptors are largely masked. Hence, the normal response to acetylcholine, or other muscarinic agonists, is vasodilatation. Activation of the muscarinic receptors on the endothelial cells causes the release from those cells of a labile vasodilator factor known as endothelium-derived relaxing factor (EDRF). The mechanism underlying release is Ca^{2+}-dependent and may involve breakdown of inositol phospholipids. Furchgott and his co-workers were the first to discover and describe the origins of EDRF and the dependence on it of the vasodilator action of acetylcholine (Furchgott and Cherry, 1984). EDRF (or at least one of them; there may be several) has now been identified, with reasonable certainty, as nitric oxide anion (Palmer et al., 1987), the same substance that is released from the so-called 'nitro vasodilator drugs' such as sodium nitroprusside. Nitric oxide penetrates the membranes of the smooth muscle cells where it stimulates the activity of cytosolic guanylate cyclase. This enzyme catalyses the formation of cyclic GMP from GTP, and the cyclic GMP triggers a cascade of events that brings about relaxation of the smooth muscle, and hence vasodilatation.

Generally speaking, with some exceptions, arteries and arterioles do not receive a cholinergic innervation so that it might be supposed that this vasodilator mechanism might have pharmacological but no physiological or pathological relevance. However, recent evidence suggests that acetylcholine may be present in endothelial cells, along with other vasodilator substances that are EDRF-dependent. It may therefore be that these substances play a role in maintaining the patency of blood vessels, and this raises the possibility that damage to the endothelium may lead to loss of dilator factors and to exposure of those muscarinic receptors on the smooth muscle cells that mediate vasoconstriction.

REFERENCES

Abbs E.T., Joseph D.N. (1981). The effects of atropine and oxotremorine on acetylcholine release in rat phrenic nerve-diaphragm preparation. *Br. J. Pharmacol.*, **73**, 481.

Adams P.R. (1976). Drug blockade of open end-plate channels. *J. Physiol.*, **260**, 531.

Ariëns E.J. (ed.) (1964). *Molecular Pharmacology*, Vol. 1. New York: Academic Press.

Arunlakshana O., Schild H.O. (1959). Some quantitative uses of drug antagonists. *Br. J. Pharmacol.*, **14**, 49.

Ascher, P., Large, W.A., Rang H.P. (1979). Studies on the mechanism of action of acetylcholine antagonists on rat parasympathetic ganglion cells. *J. Physiol.*, **295**, 139.

Beld A.J., Ariëns E.J. (1974). Stereospecific binding as a tool in attempts to localize and isolate muscarinic receptors II. Binding of (+)-benzetimide, (−)-benzetimide and atropine to a fraction from bovine tracheal smooth muscle and to bovine caudate nucleus. *Eur. J. Pharmacol.*, **25**, 203.

Birdsall, N.J.M., Bernie C.P., Burgen A.S.V., et al. (1979). Modulation of the binding properties of muscarinic receptors: evidence for receptor-effector coupling. In *Receptors: Neurotransmitters and Peptide Hormones*, p. 107. (Kuhar M.J., Enna S.J., Pepeu G., eds.). New York: Raven Press.

Birdsall N.J.M., Hulme E.C. (1985). Multiple muscarinic receptors; further problems in receptor classification. In *Trends in Autonomic Pharmacology*, Vol. 3, p. 17. (Kalsner S., ed.). London: Taylor & Francis.

Boheim G., Hanke W., Barrantes F.J. (1981). Agonist-activated ionic channels in acetylcholine receptor reconstituted into planar lipid bilayers. *Proc. Natl. Acad. Sci., USA*, **78**, 3586.

Bowman W.C. (1980). *Pharmacology of Neuromuscular Function*. Bristol: John Wright & Sons.

Bowman W.C., Harvey A.L., Gibb A.J., et al. (1986). Prejunctional actions of cholinoceptor agonists and antagonists, and of anticholinesterase drugs. In *New Neuromuscular Blocking Agents*. Chapter 5, Handb. Exp. Pharmac., Vol. 79, p. 141. (Kharkevich D.A., ed.). Berlin: Springer-Verlag.

Brown D.A. (1979). Neurotoxins and the ganglionic (C6) type of nicotinic receptor. In *Advances of Cytopharmacology*, Vol. 3, p. 225. (Ceccarelli B., Clementi F., eds.). New York: Raven Press.

Brown D.A. (1984). Muscarinic excitation of sympathetic and central neurones. In *Subtypes of Muscarinic Receptors*, p. 32. (Hirschowitz B.I., et al., eds.). Trends Pharmac. Sci. Supplement.

Brown D.A., Gahwiler B.H., Marsh S.J., et al. (1986). Mechanisms of muscarinic excitatory synaptic transmission in ganglia and brain. In *Subtypes of Muscarinic Receptors*, II, p. 66. (Levine R.R., et al., eds.). Trends Pharmac. Sci. Supplement.

Brown D.A., Garthwaite J., Hayashi E., et al. (1976). Actions of surugatoxin on nicotinic receptors in the superior cervical ganglion of the rat. *Br. J. Pharmacol.*, **58**, 157.

Brown D.A., Marrion N.V., Smart T.G. (1989). On the transduction mechanism for muscarine-induced inhibition of M-current in cultured rat sympathetic neurones. *J. Physiol.*, **413**, 469.

del Castillo J., Katz B. (1955). On the localization of acetylcholine receptors. *J. Physiol.*, **128**, 157.

Chang, C.C., Chen T.F., Chuang S.T. (1973). Influence of chronic neostigmine treatment on the number of acetylcholine receptors and the release of acetylcholine from the rat diaphragm. *J. Physiol.*, **230**, 613.

Chiappinelli V.A. (1983). Kappa bungarotoxin: a probe for the neuronal nicotinic receptor in the avian ciliary ganglion. *Brain Res.*, **277**, 9.

Chiappinelli V.A., Wolf, K.M., DeBin J.A., et al. (1987). Kappa flavitoxin: isolation of a new neuronal nicotinic receptor antagonist that is stucturally related to kappa-bungarotoxin. *Brain Res.*, **402**, 21.

Clark A.J. (1933). *Mode of Action of Drugs on Cells*. London: Arnold.

Clark A.J. (1937). General pharmacology. *Handbuch extp Pharmak.*, **4**.

Colquhoun D. (1973). The relation between classical and cooperative models for drug action. In *Drug Receptors*. p. 149. (Rang H., ed.). London: Macmillan.

Colquhoun D. (1979). The link between drug binding and response: theories and observations. In *The Receptors: A Comprehensive Treatise*. (O'Brien R.D., ed.). New York: Plenum.

Colquhoun D. (1986). On the principles of postsynaptic aciton of neuromuscular blocking agents. In *New Neuromuscular Blocking Agents*. Chapter 3, Handb. Exp. Pharmac., Vol. 79, p. 59. (Kharkevich D.A., ed.). Berlin: Springer-Verlag.

Dale H.H. (1914) The action of certain esters and ethers of choline, and their reaction to muscarine. *J.Pharmacol. Exp. Ther.*, **6**, 147.

Das M., Ganguly D.K., Vedasiromoni J.R. (1978). Enhancement by oxotremorine of acetylcholine release from the rat phrenic nerve. *Br. J. Pharmacol.*, **62**, 195.

Dowdall M.J., Golds P.R., Strange P.G. (1982). Characterization of presynaptic muscarinic autoreceptors in *Torpedo* electric organ. In *Presynaptic Receptors*, p. 103. (de Belleroche J., ed.). Chichester: Ellis Horwood.

Drachman D.B., Pestrouk A., Stanley E.F. (1979). Pathogenesis of myasthenia gravis as a disorder of acetylcholine receptors. In *Neurotoxins: Tools in Neurobiology*, p. 237. *Advances in Cytopharmacology*, Vol. 3. (Ceccarelli B., Clementi F., eds.). New York: Raven Press.

Dreyer F. (1982). Acetylcholine receptor. *Br. J. Anaesth.*, **54**, 115.

Fambrough D.M. (1979). Control of acetylcholine receptors in skeletal muscle. *Physiol. Rev.*, **59**, 165.

Fewtrell C.M.S. (1976). The labelling and isolation of neuroreceptors, *Neuroscience*, **1**, 249.

Fewtrell C.M.S., Rang H.P. (1973). The labelling of cholinergic receptors in smooth muscle. In *Drug Receptors*, p. 211. (Rang H.P., ed.). London: Macmillan.

Fosbraey P., Johnson E.S. (1982). Presynaptic muscarinic receptors for acetylcholine on cholinergic neurones in the guinea-pig ileum. In *Presynaptic Receptors*, p. 75. (de Belleroche J., ed.). Chichester: Ellis Horwood.

Froehner S.C. (1986). The role of the postsynaptic cytoskeleton in AchR organisation. *Trends Neurosci.*, **7**, 37.

Furchgott R.F., Cherry P.D. (1984). The muscarinic receptor of vascular endothelium that subserves vasodilation. In *Subtypes of Muscarinic Receptors* (Hirschowitz B.I. et al., eds.). Trends Pharmac. Sci., Supplement.

Gaddum J.H. (1926). The actions of adrenaline and ergotamine on the uterus of the rabbit. *J. Physiol.*, **61**, 141.

Gaddum J.H. (1937). The quantitative effects of antagonistic drugs. *J. Physiol.*, **89**, 7P.

Ganguly D.K., Das M. (1979). Effects of oxotremorine

demonstrate presynaptic muscarinic and dopaminergic receptors on motor nerve terminals. *Nature*, **278**, 645.

Gill E.W., Rang H.P. (1966). An alkylating derivative of benzilylcholine with specific and long-lasting parasympatholitic activity. *Mol. Pharmac.*, **2**, 284.

Ginsborg B.L., Jenkinson D.H. (1976). Transmission of impulses from nerve to muscle. In *Neuromuscular Junction*. (Zaimis E., ed.). *Handb. Exp. Pharmac.*, **42**, 229.

Greengard P., Kebabian J.W. (1974). Role of cyclic AMP in synaptic transmission in the mammalian peripheral nervous system. *Fed. Proc.*, **33**, 1059.

Gwilt M., Wray D. (1986). The effect of chronic neostigmine treatment on channel properties in the rat neuromuscular junction. *Br. J. Pharmacol.*, **88**, 25.

Hirschowitz B.I., Hammer R., Giachetti A., et al. (eds.) (1984). *Subtypes of muscarinic receptors. Trends Pharmac. Sci.*, Suppl. Amsterdam: Elsevier.

Hohlfeld R., Sterz R., Peper K. (1981). Prejunctional effects of anticholinesterase drugs at the endplate mediated by presynaptic acetylcholine receptors or by postsynaptic potassium efflux. *Pflugers Arch. Ges. Physiol.*, **391**, 213.

Hume W.R., de la Lande I.S., Waterson J.G. (1972). Effect of acetylcholine on the response of the isolated rabbit ear artery to stimulation of the perivascular sympathetic nerves. *Eur. J. Pharmacol.*, **1**, 227.

Karlin A., Cowburn D.A., Reiter M.J. (1973). Molecular properties of the acetylcholine receptor. In *Drug Receptors*. p. 193. (Rang H.P., ed.). London: Macmillan.

Karlin A., Kao P.N., Di Paula M. (1986). Molecular pharmacology of the nicotinic acetylcholine receptor. *Trends Pharmacol. Sci.*, **7**, 304.

Kistler J., Stroud R.M., Klymkowsky M.W., et al. (1982). Structure and function of an acetylcholine receptor. *Biophys. J.*, **37**, 371.

Kuromi H. (1987). Mechanism of acetylcholine receptor accumulation at the nerve-muscle junction during development. *Asia Pacific J. Pharmacol.* **2**, 195.

Lambert J.J., Durant N.N., Henderson E.G. (1983). Drug-induced modification of ionic conductance at the neuromuscular junction. *Ann. Rev. Pharmacol. Toxicol.*, **23**, 505.

Levine R.R., Birdsall N.J.M., Giachetti A., et al. (eds.). (1986). *Subtypes of Muscarinic Receptors II. Trends Pharmac. Sci.* Suppl. Amsterdam: Elsevier.

Levy M.N., Blatberg B. (1976). Effect of vagal stimulation on the overflow of norepinephrine into the coronary sinus during cardiac sympathetic nerve stimulation in the dog. *Circ. Res.*, **38**, 31.

Marshall I.G. (1980). Actions of non-depolarizing neuromuscular blocking agents at cholinoceptors other than at the motor endplate. In *Curares and Curarization*. p. 257. Amsterdam: Excerpta Medica.

Marshall R.J. (1970). A new muscarinic agent: 1,4,5,6-tetrahydro-5-phenoxypyrimidine (AH 6405). *Br. J. Pharmacol.*, **39**, 191P.

Mishina M., Takai T., Imoto K., et al. (1986). Molecular distinction between fetal and adult forms of muscle acetylcholine receptor. *Nature*, **321**, 406.

Mitchelson F. (1988). Muscarinic receptor differentiation. *Pharmacol. Therap.*, **37**, 357.

Miyamoto M.D. (1978). The actions of cholinergic drugs on motor nerve terminals. *Pharmacol. Rev.*, **29**, 221.

Norman J. (1979). Drug-receptor reactions. *Br. J. Anaesth.*, **51**, 595.

Paintal A.S. (1964). Effects of drugs on vertebrate mechanoreceptors. *Pharmacol. Rev.*, **16**, 34.

Palmer R.M.J., Ferrige A.G., Moncada S. (1987). Nitric oxide release accounts for the biological activity of endothelium-derived relaxing factor. *Nature*, **327**, 524.

Paton W.D.M., Rang H.P. (1965). The uptake of atropine and related drugs by intestinal smooth muscle of the guinea-pig in relation to acetylcholine receptor. *Proc. Roy. Soc. B.*, **163**, 1.

Paton W.D.M., Zaimis E. (1949). The pharmacological actions of polymethylene bistrimethylammonium salts. *Br. J. Pharmacol.*, **4**, 381.

Purves R.D. (1974). Muscarinic excitation: a microelectrophoretic study on cultured smooth muscle cells. *Br. J. Pharmacol.*, **52**, 77.

Rand M.J., Varma B. (1970). The effect of cholinomimetic drugs on responses to sympathetic nerve stimulation and noradrenaline in the rabbit ear artery. *Br. J. Pharmacol.*, **38**, 758.

Rash J.E., Hudson C.S., Ellisman M.H. (1978). Ultrastructure of acetylcholine receptors at the mammalian neuromuscular junction. In *Cell Membrane Receptors for Drugs and Hormones. A Multidisciplinary Approach.* p. 47. (Straub R.W., Bolis K., eds.). New York: Raven Press.

Riker W.F., Wescoe W.C. (1951). The pharmacology of Flaxedil with observations on certain analogs. *Ann. NY Acad. Sci.*, **54**, 373.

van Rossum J.M. (1966). Limitation of molecular pharmacology. Some implications of the basic assumptions underlying calculations on drug-receptor interactions and the significance of biological drug parameters. *Adv. Drug Res.*, **3**, 189.

Roszkowski A.P. (1961). An unusual type of sympathetic ganglionic stimulant. *J. Pharmacol. Exp. Ther.*, **132**, 156.

Sakmann B., Methfessel C., Mishina M. (1985). Role of acetylcholine receptor subunits in gating of the channels. *Nature*, **318**, 538.

Saxena P.R., Bonta I.L. (1970). Mechanism of selective cardiac vagolytic action of pancuronium bromide. Specific blockade of cardiac muscarinic receptors. *Eur. J. Pharmacol.*, **11**, 332.

Shepherd J.T., Lorenz R., Tyce G.M., et al. (1978). Acetylcholine-inhibition of transmitter release from adrenergic nerve terminals mediated by muscarinic receptors. *Fed. Proc.*, **37**, 191.

Simpson J.A. (1960). Myasthenia gravis: a new hypothesis. *Scot. Med. J.*, **5**, 419.

Sims S.M., Singer J.J., Walsh J.V. (1986). A mechanism of muscarinic excitation in dissociated smooth muscle cells. In *Subtypes of Muscarinic Receptors II, Trends Pharmac. Sci.*, p. 28. Amsterdam: Elsevier.

Sokolovsky, M. (1987). Photoaffinity labelling of muscarinic receptors. *Pharmacol. Ther.*, **32**, 285.

Stenlake J.B. (1979). Molecular interactions at the cholinergic receptor in neuromuscular blockade. *Prog. Med. Chem.*, **16**, 257.

Stenlake J.B. (1980). Neuromuscular blocking agents. In *Alfred Burger's Medicinal Chemistry*. 4th edn. (Wolff M.E., ed.). New York: Wiley-Interscience.

Stephenson R.P. (1956). A modification of receptor theory. *Br. J. Pharmacol.*, **11**, 379.

Stevens C.F. (1985). AchR structure: a new twist to the story. *Trends Neurosci.*, **8**, 1.

Takai T., Noda M., Mishina M., et al. (1985). Cloning, sequencing and expression of cDNA for a novel subunit of acetylcholine receptor from calf muscle. *Nature*, **315**, 761.

Taylor P., Sine S.M. (1982). Ligand occupation and the

functional states of the nicotinic-cholinergic receptor. *Trends Pharmacol. Sc.*, **3**, 197.

Thesleff S. (1955). The effects of acetylcholine, decamethonium and succinylcholine on neuromuscular transmission in the rat. *Acta Physiol. Scand.*, **34**, 386.

Vincent A. (1980). Immunology of acetylcholine receptors in relation to myasthenia gravis. *Physiol. Rev.*, **60**, 756.

Wessler I., Karl M., Mai M., et al. (1987). Muscarinic receptors on the rat phrenic nerve, evidence for positive and negative muscarinic feedback mechanisms, *Naunyn-Schmeid. Arch. Pharmacol.*, **335**, 605.

Wessler I., Diener A., Offermann M. (1988). Facilitatory and inhibitory muscarinic receptors on the rat phrenic nerve: effects of pirenzepine and dicyclomine. *Naunyn-Schmied. Arch. Pharmacol.*, **338**, 138.

Wray D. (1980). Noise analysis and channels at the post-synaptic membrane of skeletal muscle. *Drug Res.*, **24**, 9.

Yamamura H.I., Snyder S.H. (1974). Muscarinic cholinergic receptor binding in the longitudinal muscle of the guinea-pig ileum with ^{3}H-quinuclidinyl benzilate. *Mol. Pharmacol.*, **10**, 861.

Zaimis E., Head S. (1976). Depolarizing neuromuscular blocking drugs. In *Neuromuscular Junction. Handb. Exp. Pharmac.*, Vol. 42, p. 365. (Zaimis E., ed.). Berlin: Springer-Verlag.

53. Central Nervous System Transmitters
T. W. Stone

Excitation and inhibition
   Neurotransmitters
   Dicarboxylic amino acids
   Inhibitory amino acids
   Amines
   Acetylcholine
   Peptides
   Purines
   Gangliosides
   Cotransmission
   Synaptic transmitters and
     neuropharmacology

The vast majority of neurones in the central nervous system of vertebrates including Man appear to interact by means of chemical neurotransmission. In principle the process is similar to that seen at peripheral sites such as the neuromuscular junction and autonomic neuroeffector systems in that neurotransmitters are synthesized, usually in the cell body, and transported to nerve terminals where they are stored in synaptic vesicles. Upon invasion of the nerve terminal by an action potential the influx of calcium which accompanies the depolarization triggers the fusion of synaptic vesicles with the terminal membrane and the contents of this synaptic vesicle are expelled by exocytosis into the synaptic region. Electron micrographs of synapses in the central nervous system show that a significant proportion do exist as closely apposed cellular membranes with a narrow synaptic cleft between them (Shepherd, 1979). This is especially true, for example, of synapses onto the dendrites and dendritic apparatus (spines) of pyramidal cells in the cerebral cortex. In some regions such as the cerebellum, groups of synapses are enmeshed in a glial network to form complex systems in which the entire complex or glo-merulus (Shepherd, 1979) is protected from surrounding influences, and transmitters released by the component synapses do not gain access to the surrounding extracellular fluid.

Many systems of neurones, particularly those releasing amines as neurotransmitters, resemble the peripheral autonomic neurones in their morphology in that varicosities occur at intervals along the terminal branches of projecting neurones and the amines are released not into a narrow synaptic cleft but into a relatively voluminous perisynaptic region or space (Moore and Bloom, 1978).

EXCITATION AND INHIBITION

Broadly speaking neurotransmitters in the central nervous system may produce either excitation (usually depolarization) of neurones or inhibition (usually hyperpolarization). A common method for producing depolarization is to increase cation conducting channels within the neuronal membrane. The increased influx of sodium, potassium and calcium causes a reduction in membrane potential as happens at the endplate of the neuromuscular junction (Eccles, 1964).

Inhibitory neurotransmitters on the other hand usually hyperpolarize neurones by increasing permeability to chloride or potassium. In the latter case the increased efflux of potassium moves the membrane potential towards the potassium equilibrium potential of around $-100\,mV$. If the chloride permeability is increased however, there may be no obvious change of membrane potential since the chloride equilibrium potential is normally close to the resting potential. The effective increase in chloride permeability is still inhibitory however, because the increased membrane conductance effectively short circuits the membrane making depolarizing agents less effective (Eccles, 1964).

Neurotransmitters

The major distinction between synaptic transmission in the central nervous system and that in the peripheral nervous system is that in the former case there is a much larger number of neurotransmitter candidates. Some of the major classes of suggested compounds will be discussed briefly in the following paragraphs.

Dicarboxylic Amino Acids

Simple amino acids are probably used by a higher proportion of CNS synapses than any other chemical (Hicks et al., 1987). The major excitatory transmitter candidates are glutamic acid and aspartic acid. Since both compounds are an important part of normal cellular metabolism the evidence for a neurotransmitter function has come primarily from the demonstration that high affinity binding sites exist in localized regions of the central nervous system. These binding sites show a broadly similar pharmacology to the excitatory responses of neurones studied electrophysiologically, and are therefore often assumed (with little supporting evidence) to represent binding to functional receptor molecules. The application of glutamate or aspartate to neurones causes a general increase of cation excitability to produce depolarization in most cases. Indeed very few neurones have ever been detected in the CNS which do not respond to glutamate or aspartate. The released amino acids are believed to be removed rapidly from the receptors by an uptake process which transports them into glial cells and nerve terminals. In glial cells glutamate is metabolized to glutamine which is then transported into adjacent neurone terminals for reuse as glutamate.

There are several receptor types sensitive to glutamate and aspartate which have been classified on the basis of the agonists which preferentially activate them (Stone and Burton, 1988). These agonists do not normally occur in mammals and include N-methyl-D-aspartate (NMDA) quisqualic acid and kainic acid. The three receptor types are pharmacologically distinct although the NMDA receptor has been studied most in recent years because of the development of selective antagonists at this site. Each of the three primary agonists produces excitation by increasing cation conductance although the NMDA receptors operate channels which are selectively blocked by magnesium ions (Nowak, et al., 1984; Mayer and Westbrook, 1987). The result of this is that the NMDA channels are difficult to open at normal physiological magnesium concentrations unless the cell is previously depolarized to remove the magnesium ion blockade.

This voltage dependent block of NMDA operated channels has led to a variety of speculative proposals for the physiological function of these receptor types when mediating responses to glutamate and aspartate. Under normal circumstances it is proposed that synapses release glutamate or aspartate which produce a small degree of depolarization by activating kainate and/or quisqualate receptors. However, under conditions where there is a large amount of activity in amino acid releasing neurones the greater depolarization produced initially by quisqualate and kainate receptors will relieve the voltage dependent block of NMDA operated channels allowing activation of the NMDA receptors to become synergistic with activation of the quisqualate and kainate sites. The overall effect is a disproportionate depolarization of the neurone when the activity of incident neurones is high. This in turn has led to the suggestion that this mechanism may be important in epileptic situations where a triggering epileptic focus causes high neuronal activity increasing activation of the NMDA receptors and causing an NMDA mediated sustained excitation of neuronal activity. This would explain why NMDA receptor blocking agents are able to diminish or prevent seizures caused by a variety of chemical compounds as well as in genetically epilepsy prone rodents and primates (Stone et al., 1988).

A second relevance of the NMDA mechanism may be in long-term potentiation, a phenomenon in the hippocampus which is thought to be related to the formation of long-term memory traces in certain cells. The potentiation of synaptic activity which results from a brief high frequency tetanus to certain pathways in the hippocampus can be prevented again by NMDA antagonists, and it is interesting to note that the same antagonists have marked effects on certain forms of spatial learning ability.

Among the compounds which have marked NMDA antagonist properties are the dissociative anaesthetics such as phencyclidine and ketamine (Stone et al., 1988; Mayer et al., 1987). These compounds do not appear to block the NMDA receptor itself, but block the ionic channels opened by NMDA receptor activation. A recent discovery is that micromolar amounts of glycine are needed for activation of the NMDA receptor complex. Glycine binds at a strychnine-resistant site within the ionic channel.

Many neurones in the central nervous system are thought to release these amino acid transmitters including most corticofugal neurones projecting to the striatum, spinal cord and brain stem as well as ascending projections and projections to the cerebellum. Two of the pathways most clearly linked with amino acid transmission are the climbing fibre and mossy fibre inputs to the cerebellum.

There is still much interest in other possible endogenous compounds which may act at the amino acid receptors since the evidence for glutamate and aspartate themselves is still far from complete. Recent interest has been expressed in homocysteic acid and quinolinic acid both of which are found within the brain and which appear to be selective agonists for the NMDA population of receptors. Interest in these substances has grown recently not only because of the potential involvement in epilepsy, learning, and memory as noted above, but also because of the possible involvement in the cell death which occurs in degenerative diseases of the CNS such as Huntington's disease and possibly Alzheimer's disease (Stone et al., 1987; 1988).

Inhibitory Amino Acids

Whereas glutamate and aspartate are dicarboxylic acids the monocarboxylic acids, gamma-amino-butyric acid (GABA) and glycine are the predominant inhibitory transmitters in the CNS. Glycine is especially concerned with inhibition in the spinal cord where it mediates postsynaptic inhibition of neurones by increasing potassium and chloride permeabilities. GABA on the other hand (which is synthesized by decarboxylation of glutamate) is more important at higher levels of the central nervous system such as the striatum, cerebellum and cortex where its main effect is to increase chloride permeability. The localization of pathways involving either of these compounds has again been based partly on the existence of high affinity binding sites for the amino acids or stable analogues, or the distribution of uptake sites into presynaptic terminals (Curtis and Johnson, 1974).

The monocarboxylic or basic amino acids produce inhibition of neurones by increasing the potassium or chloride permeabilities. This often causes hyperpolarization, though this is not essential to the inhibitory action which can also result from the increased total membrane conductance. This 'short circuit' effect reduces the efficacy of excitatory inputs to the cell. GABA can also produce a presynaptic inhibition of neurotransmitter release, possibly acting at a population of receptors which can be activated by baclofen. These 'GABA-B' receptors appear to be widely distributed in the CNS but most especially in the spinal cord and cerebellum. Their existence may explain the antispastic properties of baclofen in motor disorders.

Selective antagonists are available for both inhibitory amino acids, thus facilitating the experimental study of their involvement in synaptic physiology. GABA-A responses can be blocked by bicuculline and picrotoxin, and glycine can be blocked by strychnine. As might be expected all these antagonists are convulsants as they suppress the inhibitory tone in the CNS normally preventing the excessive firing of neurones.

In addition, many compounds which have sedative or anaesthetic actions on the CNS may potentiate the actions of these inhibitory compounds. The most notable examples are barbiturates which greatly increase the conductance change produced by activation of GABA receptors. Similarly a number of benzodiazepines such as diazepam are thought to act primarily by stabilizing the GABA receptor/ion channel complex, thus prolonging conductance changes and neuronal inhibition.

Amines

A variety of primary amines are strongly favoured as neurotransmitter candidates in the CNS. These include noradrenaline (Moore and Bloom, 1979) and its precursor dopamine (Moore et al., 1978), 5–hydroxy-tryptamine (5HT) and histamine. Both noradrenaline and 5HT originate in cell groups in the brainstem which project fairly widely into the higher parts of the central nervous system. The major sites of origin are the locus coeruleus for noradrenaline containing neurones and the raphé nuclei for 5HT. The amines are released rather diffusely into a perisynaptic region and probably do not act as rapid, fast acting synaptic transmitters like the amino acids. Rather their action is likely to be that of a longer term modulator of cell excitability or even that of a modulator of responses to other neurotransmitters. Like the amino acids all the amine transmitters are removed from the extracellular space by uptake (transport) processes. Within the nerve terminals some of the amine may then be destroyed by monoamine oxidase, while some may be recycled into synaptic vesicles for reuse.

Dopamine is released from groups of neuronal cell bodies in the brain stem, those in the ventral tegmentum, and pars compacta of the substantia nigra (Moore et al., 1978). These dopaminergic neurones project to the mesolimbic system and striatum respectively. It is in the striatum that the dopaminergic terminals compete with cholinergic interneurones to determine the final activity of efferent neurones. Any loss of the dopaminergic projection, as in Parkinson's disease, results in an imbalance between this inhibitory dopamine and excitatory cholinergic balance and the resultant change in efferent neurone activity is a primary cause of some symptoms of Parkinson's disease.

Projection of all three amines to the limbic system areas such as hippocampus, amygdala, nucleus accumbens and olfactory tubercle are involved intimately in the control of mood and the expression of emotion. Dopamine has been linked primarily with these phenomena, and many of the tranquilizing or neuroleptic drugs currently in clinical use are active by virtue of a modification of dopaminergic function. However, there is increasing evidence that the noradrenaline and 5HT systems are also affected by these drugs and may contribute significantly to the normal control of mood and emotion.

Acetylcholine

Acetylcholine undoubtedly is a neurotransmitter in the CNS though at relatively few sites. The most obvious site is the synapse between recurrent motor neurone collaterals and interneurones within the spinal cord known as Renshaw cells. In addition, there are cholinergic neurones within the cerebellum, thalamus and striatum, the latter region containing intrinsic cholinergic neurones which have been referred to above. There are also regions of the septum which project cholinergic neurones into the hippocampus and these are probably involved in the control of learning and memory. They may explain for example the amnesic effects of certain anticholinergic drugs such as scopolamine.

A large cholinergic nucleus also exists in the nucleus basalis of Meynert, the major projection from which ascends to the cerebral cortex. This projection has become of great interest with the proposal that Alzheimer's disease involves a degeneration of the nucleus basalis neurones and thus the secondary loss of cholinergic input into the neocortex (Coyle et al., 1983).

Peptides

A large number of peptides have now been described in the central nervous system which have potent effects on central neurones but which have not been classified as neurotransmitters according to the various criteria developed for more classical compounds such as acetylcholine. These peptides are therefore referred to by the rather vague term 'neuroactive' peptides and include some compounds which have other functions elsewhere in the body. For example some gastrointestinal hormones such as vasoactive intestinal polypeptide (VIP), cholecystokinin (CCK) and, substance P, as well as neurotensin, somatostatin and others exist in discrete regions of the CNS which can be correlated to a limited extent with the existence of a high sensitivity of neurones to the compounds (Gregory, 1982). There are also hypothalamic releasing hormones such as thyrotrophin releasing hormone, somatostatin, corticotrophin releasing hormone and hormones from the neurohypophysis such as vasopressin and oxytocin which have some features of neurotransmitters. In all, some 50 or 60 peptides have been suggested to have major effects on central neurones either as neurotransmitters or as neuromodulators (Iversen, 1984).

The term neuromodulator perhaps requires explanation. A neuromodulator is conceived as a compound which may or may not have direct effects of its own on neurones in the CNS but whose primary effect is to modify the sensitivity of neurones to other agents. This may occur acutely, that is, the presence of the peptide or other neuromodulator may modify the sensitivity of a cell to a second compound applied simultaneously, or it may take the form of a long-term up or down-regulation in the number of receptors for the primary transmitter. The main difficulties in assessing the precise function of peptides is that the methods for their detection are often inadequate to demonstrate that their release is related to neuronal depolarization and that until very recently no compounds were available which selectively antagonized the activation of peptide receptors. This situation is now beginning to change with the growth of commercial interest in peptide analogues. The use of antagonists to block activation of synaptic pathways and to modify gross animal behaviour is likely to yield more definitive information on their physiological roles as neurotransmitters or neuromodulators within the next 10 years.

Purines

Like the amino acids, purines such as adenosine and ATP are an important part of normal cellular metabolism but there is now a great deal of evidence to suggest that these compounds can be released in order to modify cellular activity either as neurotransmitters or neuromodulators. ATP was the first compound to be proposed as a neurotransmitter of non-cholinergic nerves in the peripheral nervous system (Burnstock, 1972) and recent electrophysiology has supported this view with the use of selective desensitizing agents and antagonists. Such work has not yet been performed in the central nervous system although there is evidence for actions of ATP on central neurones which are not explicable in terms of this nucleotide's metabolism to adenosine. It may be that ATP has a specific function in the central nervous system distinct from other purine molecules.

Adenosine however, has a much clearer and more widespread role (Stone, 1989). Adenosine can be released from most tissues when they are activated and appears to act as a negative feedback modulator of tissue activity. In many cases the release of adenosine occurs in proportion to the imbalance between the metabolic demand being placed upon a tissue by its activation and the supply and availability of nutrients, particularly oxygen, to that tissue. Thus a large increase of neuronal activity in a region of the CNS, while nutrient supply remains unchanged, will result in an efflux of adenosine. The functions of adenosine which combat the increased activity are then many. Firstly, the purine can inhibit the release of neurotransmitters from the impinging neurones possibly by reducing calcium influx into the terminal (Stone, 1981). Secondly, adenosine can have direct inhibitory effects on the tissues including both smooth muscle and neurones in the central nervous system where it appears to increase potassium permeability, thus causing hyperpolarization. Thirdly adenosine can modify the sensitivity of cells to conventional neurotransmitters, thus acting like a neuromodulator as defined above. Acting in this way adenosine has been shown to modify the sensitivity of neurones to acetylcholine and amine neurotransmitters, though its effects on other neuroactive compounds have not yet been studied in detail.

Gangliosides

There are undoubtedly many other classes of compounds within the central nervous system which influence neuronal activity and synaptic transmission. These include lipids, prostaglandins, gangliosides and probably others. The latter compounds, the gangliosides, have recently become of particular interest because not only can they modify the sensitivity of cells to classical transmitters but they also seem to promote the growth and regeneration of neurones in the central nervous system (Rahmann, 1985). This led to some speculation that there may be a relationship between the two phenomena; commercial interest in the synthesis of ganglioside analogues is partly a result of this suggestion. It should be emphasized however, that there is no evidence that gangliosides or prostaglandins for that matter are stored in synaptic vesicles or released in a transmitter-like, calcium-dependent fashion. They may release more slowly into the extracellular space in association with the general turnover and metabolism of cells.

Cotransmission

Some neurones appear to contain more than one of the neurotransmitter substances mentioned above. Refined histochemical techniques and an examination of release has now confirmed the fact that a proportion of neurones throughout the CNS contain two or more such agents and these can be released, or their concentrations modified in parallel, by appropriate stimuli. The simultaneous release process is referred to as cotransmission (Hokfelt, 1984). The hypothalamic hormone thyrotrophin releasing hormone (TRH) is, for example, colocalized and coreleased with 5HT, while the opioid peptides (the enkephalins) seem to be colocalized and released along with noradrenaline and CCK is colocalized with dopamine. Some pairs of peptides such as somatostatin and neuropeptide Y are localized within the same groups of neurones in the striatum. Cotransmission, however, is not restricted to peptides since there is much evidence for a cotransmitter role of ATP and noradrenaline or acetylcholine, at least at peripheral nervous system terminals (Campbell, 1987). This is less clear for the central nervous system although recent evidence supports the view that this phenomenom may exist at certain sites in the CNS (Hokfelt et al., 1986).

The function of cotransmission is not yet clear although it is generally assumed that the presence of a longer term neuromodulator compound, usually a peptide, will act to modify the sensitivity of neurones to the primary transmitter in a manner which is related to the degree of neuronal activity and therefore modulator release. A high degree of neuronal activity for example may cause the accumulation of the peptide cotransmitter which is responsible for the decrease in receptor number or down regulation which occurs as a result of that activity.

Some of these cotransmitter substances may be of clinical or commercial relevance. The coexistence of CCK and dopamine for example in terminals of the nigro-striatal tract has resulted in interest in the synthesis of CCK analogues which may be able to increase the number of dopamine receptors and therefore the overall function of the dopaminergic pathway.

Synaptic Transmitters and Neuropharmacology

It should be clear from the above discussion that a number of centrally active drugs are known to act on transmitter receptors or on the synthesis and release of neurotransmitters. Some anticonvulsants may well interfere with the actions or release of excitatory amino acids (Croucher et al., 1982) while dissociative anaesthetics block their effects, and it has been commented that barbiturates and benzodiazepines potentiate the action of inhibitory amino acids such as GABA (Skolnick and Paul, 1982). Currently, there is a great deal of interest in the possibility that the purines are involved in the action of benzodiazepines or barbiturates since the latter compounds displace purines from their binding sites in the brain. Xanthines such as caffeine and theophylline are also moderately potent antagonists of adenosine, being more effective in this regard than as inhibitors of phosphodiesterase. Most of the stimulant actions of xanthines on the CNS are probably the result of adenosine antagonism (Synder, 1985). It is thus worth considering the possibility that xanthine related drugs or beverages may be contraindicated in states of CNS hyperexcitability or during the induction of anaesthesia.

Antidepressant compounds almost invariably interact primarily with the amine systems, though different groups of compounds act with greater facility on one or other of the noradrenergic, dopaminergic and 5-hydroxytryptaminergic neurone groups. It is likely that there is a great deal of cross talk between these amine systems and that there is also considerable non-selectivity in the action of some compounds developed primarily with one amine system in mind. Some of the most potent antidepressants in current clinical use actually inhibit the uptake of 5-hydroxytryptamine in the acute phases following their administration but this is unlikely to account for the delay witnessed before clinically antidepressant action is noted. The clinical action is more readily correlated with a down-regulation of catecholamine β-receptors.

The neuroleptic agents such as phenothiazines and butyrophenones are excellent antagonists of dopamine receptors of which there are two varieties. The blockade of dopamine receptors in both the limbic system, where the neuroleptic action is presumably mediated, and at the nigro-striatal terminals, provides an adequate explanation for the development of motor dyskinesias and related motor deficits following chronic administration of these compounds. There is probably a compensatory up-regulation of dopamine receptors following chronic blockade which accounts for this phenomenon.

REFERENCES

Burnstock G. (1972). Purinergic nerves. *Pharmacol. Rev.*, **24**, 509.

Campbell G. (1987). Co-transmission. *Ann. Rev. Pharmacol.*, **27**, 51.

Coyle J.T., Price D.L., DeLong M.R. (1983). Alzheimer's disease: a disorder of cortical cholinergic innervation. *Science*, **219**, 1184.

Croucher M.J., Collins J.F., Meldrum B.S. (1982). Anticonvulsant action of excitatory amino acid antagonists. *Science*, **216**, 899.

Curtis D.R., Johnston G.A.R. (1974). Amino acid transmitters in the mammalian CNS. *Ergebn. Physiol.*, **69**, 97.

Eccles J.C. (1964). *The Physiology of Synapses*. Berlin: Springer.

Gregory R.A. (ed.) (1982). Regulatory peptides of gut and brain. *Br. Med. Bull.*, **38**, 219.

Hicks T.P., Lodge D., McLennan H. (eds.). (1987). *Excitatory Amino Acid Transmission*. New York: A.R. Liss.

Hokfelt T. (1984). Chemical anatomy of the brain. *Science*, **225**, 1326.

Hokfelt T., Fuxe K., Pernow B. (1986). Co-existence of neuronal messengers: a new principle in chemical transmission. *Progr. Brain Res.*, **68**.

Iversen L.L. (1984). Amino acids and peptides: fast and slow chemical signals in the nervous system. *Proc. Roy. Soc.*, **B221**, 245.

Mayer M.L., Westbrook G.L. (1987). The physiology of excitatory amino acids in the vertebrate CNS. *Progr. Neurobiol.*, **28**, 197.

Moore R.Y., Bloom F.E. (1978). Central catecholamine neuron systems; anatomy and physiology of the dopamine systems. *Ann. Rev. Neurosci.*, **1**, 129.

Moore R.Y., Bloom F.E. (1979). Central catecholamine neuron systems: anatomy and physiology of the norepinephrine and epinephrine systems. *Ann. Rev. Neurosci.*, **2**, 113.

Nowak L., Bregestovski P., Ascher P., et al. (1984). Magnesium gates glutamate-activate channels in mouse central neurones. *Nature*, **307**, 462.

Rahmann H. (ed.) (1985). *Gangliosides and Modulation of Neuronal Function*. Berlin: Springer.

Shepherd G.M. (1979). *The Synaptic Organization of the Brain*. Oxford: O.U.P.

Skolnick P., Paul S.M. (1982). Benzodiazepine receptors in the CNS. *Int. Rev. Neurobiol.*, **23**, 103.

Snyder S.H. (1985). Adenosine as a neuromodulator. *Ann. Rev. Neurosci.*, **8**, 103.

Stone T.W. (1981). Physiological roles for adenosine and ATP in the nervous system. *Neuroscience*, **6**, 523.

Stone T.W. (1989). Purine receptors and their pharmacological potential. *Adv. Drug Res.*, **18**, 291.

Stone T.W., Connick J.H. Winn P., et al. (1987). Endogenous neurotoxic agents. *CIBA Found. Symp.*, **126**, 204.

Stone T.W., Burton N.R. (1988). NMDA receptors and ligands in the vertebrate CNS. *Progr. Neurobiol.*, **30**, 333.

54. The Pharmacology of Local Anesthetic Agents

B. Covino

Pharmacodynamic aspects
Pharmacokinetic aspects
Systemic toxicity of local anesthetic agents
Summary

Chemical compounds that demonstrate local anesthetic activity usually possess an aromatic end, an amine end, and an intermediate chain (Fig. 54.1). Those agents which possess an ester link between the aromatic portion and the intermediate chain are referred to as amino esters and include procaine, chloroprocaine and tetracaine. Local anesthetics with an amide link between the aromatic end and the intermediate chain are referred to as amino amides and include lidocaine, mepivacaine, prilocaine, bupivacaine and etidocaine. The ester and amide compounds differ with regard to their chemical stability, degradation and potential for inducting allergic type reactions. The ester agents are less stable chemically than the amide drugs. The amino esters are hydrolyzed in plasma by the enzyme cholinesterase, whereas the amide compounds undergo enzymatic degradation in the liver. Para-aminobenzoic acid which is one of the metabolites of ester type compounds can cause allergic type reactions in a small percentage of the general population. The amino amides are not metabolized to para-aminobenzoic acid and are rarely associated with allergic reactions.

PHARMACODYNAMIC ASPECTS

Local anesthetic agents differ in terms of their intrinsic potency, onset and duration of anesthetic activity (Covino and Vassallo, 1976; De Jong, 1977; Covino, 1986). These anesthetic properties are essentially determined by physicochemical characteristics which are related to the chemical structure of the specific agent (Fig. 54.1). The physicochemical properties which essentially determine anesthetic activity are lipid solubility, protein binding, and pK_A. A comparison of homologous chemical compounds demonstrates the relationship between structure, physicochemical properties and anesthetic activity. Within the ester series of agents, tetracaine essentially differs from procaine by the addition of a butyl group to the aromatic end of the molecule. As a result tetracaine is considerably more lipophilic and more highly protein bound than procaine. Within the amide series bupivacaine differs from mepivacaine by the addition of a butyl group to the amine end of the molecule which renders bupivacaine more lipophilic and more protein bound than mepivacaine. Etidocaine is a

| Agent | Chemical configuration | | | Physicochemical properties | | | | Pharmacological properties | | |
	Aromatic lipophilic	Intermediate chain	Amine hydrophilic	Molecular weight (base)	pK (25°C)	Partition coefficient	Per cent protein binding	Onset	Relative potency	Duration
Esters										
Procaine				236	8.9	0.02	6	Slow	1	Short
Tetracaine				264	8.5	4.1	76	Slow	8	Long
Chloroprocaine				271	8.7	0.14	—	Fast	1	Short
Amides										
Prilocaine				220	7.9	0.9	55	Fast	2	Moderate
Lidocaine				234	7.9	2.9	64	Fast	2	Moderate
Mepivacaine				246	7.6	0.8	78	Fast	2	Moderate
Bupivacaine				288	8.1	27.5	96	Moderate	8	Long
Etidocaine				276	77	141	94	Fast	6	Long

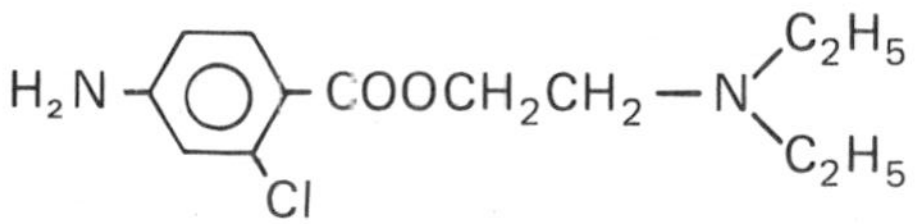

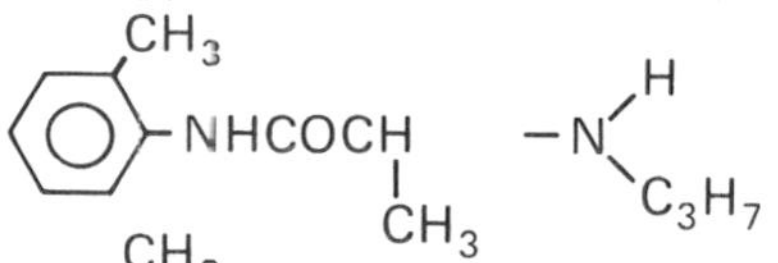

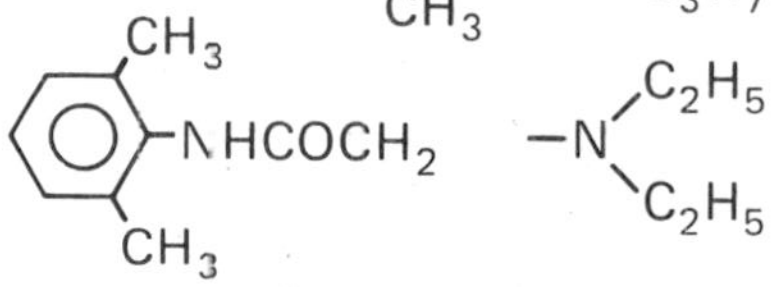

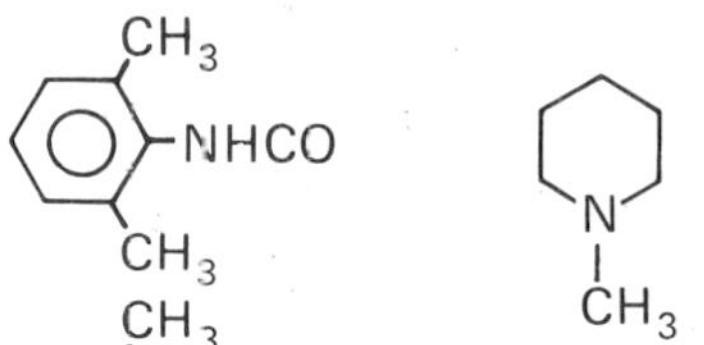

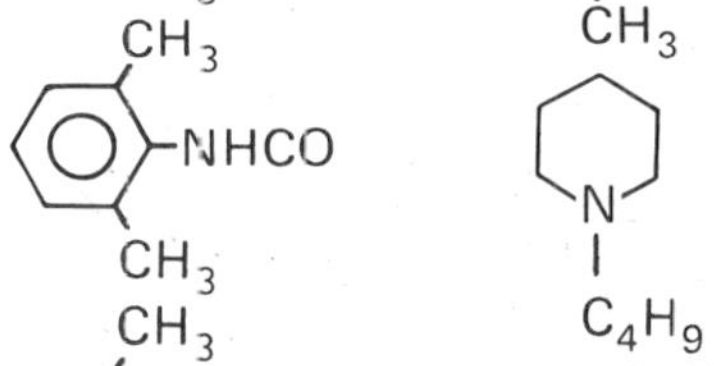

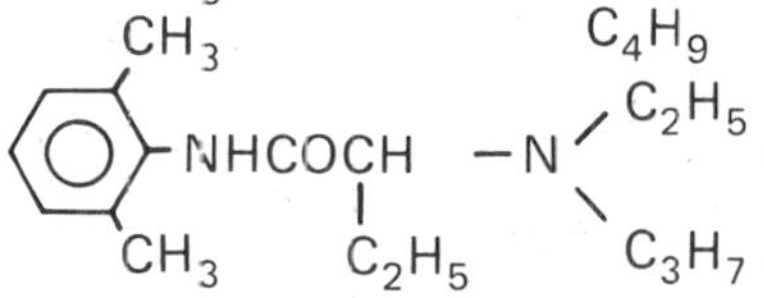

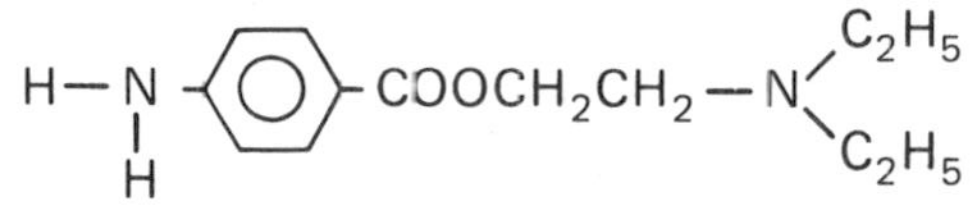

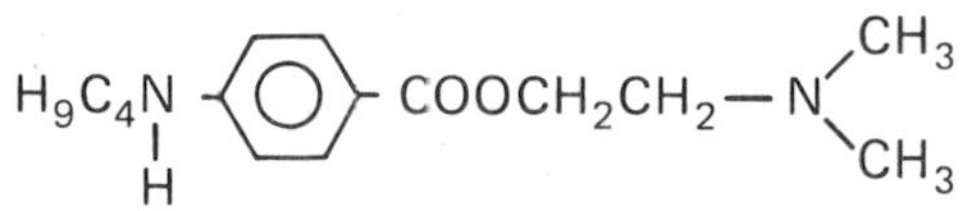

Fig. 54.1 Chemical structure, physicochemical and pharmacological properties of local anesthetic agents.

derivative of lidocaine which differs by substitution of a propyl group for a N ethyl group on the amino nitrogen, and addition of an ethyl group to the α carbon in the intermediate chain. As a result, etidocaine is markedly more lipid soluble and more highly protein bound than lidocaine.

Lipid solubility appears to be the primary determinant of intrinsic anesthetic potency, whereas protein binding regulates the duration of anesthetic activity (*see* Fig. 54.1). Chemical compounds which are highly lipophilic will penetrate the nerve membrane more easily, such that less molecules are required for conduction blockade. Local anesthetic agents are believed to bind to a receptor protein in the sodium channel. Highly bound drugs will remain at the receptor site for a prolonged period of time, resulting in an extended duration of anesthetic activity.

The pK_A of a chemical compound represents the pH at which the ionized and nonionized forms are in complete equilibrium. The uncharged form of the local anesthetic agent diffuses most readily across the nerve sheath and nerve membrane, and so determines the onset of action. The percentage of a specific local anesthetic drug present in the base form is inversely proportional to the pK_A of that agent. For example, 35% of mepivacaine, lidocaine, prilocaine and etidocaine which possess a pK_A of approximately 7.7 exists in the base form when injected into tissue with a pH of 7.4. On the other hand, tetracaine possesses a pK_A of 8.6 such that only 5% is present in a nonionized form at a tissue pH of 7.4. As a result, agents such as lidocaine, mepivacaine, prilocaine and etidocaine show a rapid onset of action, whereas tetracaine, which possesses a high pK_A, has a slow onset time.

In vivo vascular absorption of local anesthetic agents will decrease the number of anesthetic molecules available for conduction blockade, and decrease the apparent anesthetic potency and duration of action of a specific compound. In the concentrations commonly employed for regional anesthesia, most local anesthetics except cocaine appear to be vasodilators. The relative degree of vasodilatation produced by different local anesthetic drugs may vary. For example, lidocaine is basically a more potent local anesthetic than mepivacaine. However, in man little difference in the relative anesthetic potency of lidocaine and mepivacaine exists and the duration of mepivacaine is somewhat longer than that of lidocaine due to the greater degree of vasodilatation produced by lidocaine.

On the basis of differences in structure and physicochemical properties, the various agents may be classified as follows: (1) agents of low anesthetic potency and short duration of action; procaine and chloroprocaine. (2) agents of intermediate anesthetic potency and duration of action; lidocaine, mepivacaine and prilocaine. (3) agents of high anesthetic potency and prolonged duration of action; tetracaine, bupivacaine and etidocaine. In terms of onset of action, chloroprocaine, lidocaine, mepivacaine, prilocaine and etido-caine possess a relatively rapid onset of action. Bupivacaine is intermediate in terms of onset of anesthesia, while procaine and tetracaine possess a slow onset of action.

PHARMACOKINETIC ASPECTS

The absorption of local anesthetics varies as a function of site of injection, dosage, addition of a vasoconstrictor agent, and the specific agents employed (Tucker, 1986). Absorption occurs most rapidly after intercostal nerve blockade, followed by injection into the caudal canal, lumbar epidural space, brachial plexus and sciatic femoral sites, and subcutaneous tissue. For example, the intercostal administration of 400 mg of lidocaine without epinephrine results in an average peak venous plasma level of approximately 7 µg/ml, while the same dose of lidocaine employed for brachial plexus block yields a mean maximum blood level of approximately 3.5 µg/ml.

The blood level of local anesthetic agent is related to the total dose of drug administered rather than the specific volume or concentration of solution employed. A linear relationship tends to exist between the amount of drug administered and the peak anesthetic blood level. For example, the maximum blood level of lidocaine increases from approximately 1.5 µg/ml to 4 µg/ml as the total dose administered into the lumbar epidural space is raised from 200–600 mg. Depending on the site of administration, a peak blood level of 0.5–2.0 µg/ml is achieved for each 100 mg of lidocaine or mepivacaine which is injected.

Addition of a vasoconstrictor to local anesthetic solutions decreases the rate of absorption of certain agents from various sites of administration. 5 µg/ml of epinephrine (1:200 000) significantly reduces the peak blood levels of lidocaine and mepivacaine, irrespective of the site of administration. Epinephrine will significantly decrease the peak blood levels of prilocaine, bupivacaine, and etidocaine achieved after peripheral nerve blocks, but has less influence on the absorption of these drugs following lumbar epidural administration.

The rate and degree of vascular absorption varies between agents. Lidocaine and mepivacaine are absorbed more rapidly than prilocaine, while bupivacaine is absorbed more rapidly than etidocaine. The lower blood levels of prilocaine probably reflect its tendency to produce less vasodilatation than lidocaine or mepivacaine. The lower peak blood levels of etidocaine compared to bupivacaine may be related to the greater lipid solubility and uptake by peripheral fat of etidocaine.

Following absorption from the injection site, local anesthetic agents distribute throughout total body water. An initial rapid disappearance from blood (α phase) occurs which is related to uptake by rapidly equilibrating tissues, i.e., tissues with a high vascular perfusion. A secondary slower disappearance rate (β phase) reflects distribution to poorly perfused tissues

TABLE 54.1
PHARMACOKINETIC PROPERTIES OF AMIDE LOCAL ANESTHETIC AGENTS

	Lidocaine	Mepivacaine	Prilocaine	Bupivacaine	Etidocaine
V_d (L)	212	150	380	209	666
$T_{1/2}\alpha$ (seconds)	57	43	29	162	129
$T_{1/2}\beta$ (minutes)	96	114	93	210	156
Cl (L/min)	0.95	0.78	2.84	0.47	1.22
Hepatic % extraction	63	52	189	31	81

V_d = Volume of distribution
$T_{1/2}\alpha$ = Distribution half-life
$T_{1/2}\beta$ = Elimination half-life
Cl = Clearance

and metabolism and excretion of the compound. The disappearance rate of prilocaine is significantly more rapid than that of lidocaine or mepivacaine. (Table 54.1). The rate of tissue redistribution for these latter two agents is similar. Similarly, the α and β half-lives of etidocaine are significantly shorter than those of bupivacaine, which indicates a more rapid rate of tissue redistribution and metabolism for etidocaine. Although all tissues will take up local anesthetics, the highest concentrations are found in the more highly perfused organs, such as lung and kidney. The greatest percentage of an injected dose of a local anesthetic agent distributes to skeletal muscle due to the large mass of this tissue in the body.

The metabolism of local anesthetic agents varies according to their chemical classification (Tucker and Mather, 1979). The ester or procaine-like agents undergo hydrolysis in plasma by the enzyme, pseudo-cholinesterase. Chloroprocaine shows the most rapid rate of hydrolysis ($4.7\,\mu mol/(ml \cdot h)$) compared to procaine ($1.1\,\mu mol/(ml \cdot h)$) and tetracaine ($0.3\,\mu mol/(ml \cdot h)$). Less than 2% of unchanged procaine is excreted, while approximately 90% of para-aminobenzoic acid, which is the primary metabolite of procaine, appears in urine. On the other hand, only 33% of diethylaminoethanol, the other major metabolite of procaine, is excreted unchanged.

The amide or lidocaine-like agents undergo enzymatic degradation primarily in the liver. Prilocaine undergoes the most rapid rate of hepatic metabolism. Lidocaine, mepivacaine, and etidocaine are intermediate in terms of rate of degradation, while bupivacaine is metabolized most slowly. The metabolism of the amide-type agents is more complex than that of the ester drugs. The complete metabolism for all the amide compounds has not been elucidated. Lidocaine which has been studied most extensively undergoes primarily oxidative de-ethylation to monoethylglycinexylidide, followed by a subsequent hydrolysis to hydroxy-xylidine. Less than 5% of unchanged amide-type drugs is excreted into the urine. The major portion of an injected dose appears in the form of various metabolites. For example, 73% of lidocaine can be accounted for in human urine by hydroxy-xylidine.

The renal clearance of the amide agents is inversely related to their protein-binding capacity. Prilocaine, which has a lower protein-binding capacity than lidocaine has a substantially higher clearance value than lidocaine. Renal clearance is also inversely proportional to the pH of urine, suggesting urinary excretion by nonionic diffusion.

SYSTEMIC TOXICITY OF LOCAL ANESTHETIC AGENTS

The central nervous sytem appears to be particularly susceptible to the systemic actions of local anesthetic agents (Scott, 1986). Initially, local anesthetic agents produce signs of CNS excitation. Human volunteers receiving intravenous infusions of local anesthetics describe feelings of lightheadedness and dizziness followed frequently by visual and auditory disturbances such as difficulty in focusing, and tinnitus. Other subjective CNS symptoms include disorientation and occasional feelings of drowsiness. Objective signs of an excitatory CNS effect include shivering, muscular twitching and tremors. Ultimately, generalized convulsions of a tonic-clonic nature occur. If a sufficiently large dose of a local anesthetic agent is administered systemically, the initial signs of CNS excitation are rapidly followed by a state of generalized CNS depression. Seizure activity ceases and respiratory depression and ultimately respiratory arrest occur.

In general, the dose of local anesthetic agents administered intravenously and the blood level of these various agents at which signs and symptoms of CNS excitation and overt convulsions occur are directly related to the intrinsic anesthetic potency of the agent (Covino, 1987). For example, in cats procaine was least potent in terms of CNS activity. A dose of approximately 35 mg/kg was required to cause convulsions. On the other hand, bupivacaine was the most potent agent studied in terms of CNS activity with convulsions occurring at a mean dose of 5 mg/kg. Lidocaine, mepivacaine and prilocaine were agents of intermediate potency with regard to the dose required to produce convulsive activity. Comparison of the intrinsic anesthetic potency of these local anesthetics indicates that a correlation dose exist between the ability of the compounds to suppress conduction in peripheral nerve and the ability to cause CNS excitation (Fig. 54.2).

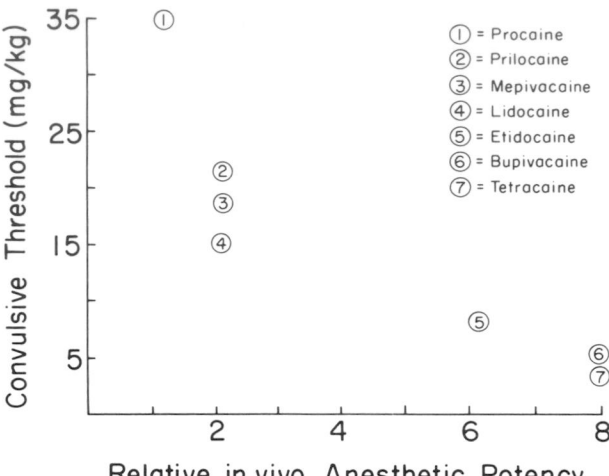

Fig. 54.2 Relationship between convulsive dose in cats and dogs and *in vivo* anesthetic potency of various local anesthetic agents.

Local anesthetic agents can also produce profound effects on the cardiovascular system (Reiz and Nath, 1986). The systemic administration of these agents can exert a direct action both on cardiac muscle and on peripheral vascular smooth muscle. In general, the cardiovascular system appears to be more resistant to the effects of local anesthetic agents than the central nervous system. Studies in dogs and sheep have indicated that doses of local anesthetic agents which cause significant cardiovascular effects are approximately three times higher than the dose of these agents which will have distinct effects on the central nervous system. The sequence of cardiovascular events that usually occurs following the systemic administration of local anesthetic agents is as follows; at relatively nontoxic blood levels of these agents, either no change or a slight increase in blood pressure may be observed. The slight increase in blood pressure may be related to a modest increase in cardiac output and heart rate which have been seen in some animal preparations and is believed due to an enhancement of sympathetic activity by these agents. In addition, the direct vasoconstrictor action of local anesthetics on certain peripheral vascular beds at low concentrations may be responsible in part for a slight increase in systemic blood pressure. As the blood level of local anesthetic agents approaches toxic concentrations, a fall in blood pressure is usually the first sign of a systemic effect on the cardiovascular system. The initial hypotension appears to be related to the negative inotropic action of these agents which results in a decrease in

cardiac output and stroke volume. If the amount of local anesthetic administered is excessive, then a profound and irreversible state of cardiovascular depression occurs which is related not only to the negative inotropic action of the local anesthetics, but also to the profound peripheral dilatation that these agents can produce due to their direct relaxant effect on vascular smooth muscle. At high concentrations the depressant effect of these agents on the excitability of cardiac tissue will also become evident as a decrease in sinus rate and AV conduction block. Ultimately, the combined peripheral vasodilatation, decreased myocardial contractility and depressant effect on rate and conductivity will lead to cardiac arrest and circulatory collapse.

In general, a relationship exists between the potency of various agents as local anesthetic drugs, and their depressant effect on the cardiovascular system (Fig. 54.3). In recent years there has been some suggestion that the more potent highly lipid soluble and highly protein bound local anesthetic agents such as bupivacaine may be relatively more cardiotoxic than the less potent, less lipid soluble and protein bound local anesthetics, such as lidocaine. A decreased margin of safety exists between the dose of bupivacaine to cause CNS toxicity and the dose to cause cardiovascular toxicity, as compared to lidocaine. Also, pregnant animals appear to be more sensitive to the cardiotoxic effects of bupivacaine than nonpregnant animals. In addition, it has been reported that bupivacaine can induce cardiac arrhythmias in various animal species, whereas no such changes were observed with lidocaine.

SUMMARY

The clinically useful local anesthetic agents can be divided chemically into the amino esters e.g., procaine, chloroprocaine and tetracaine, and the aminoamides, eg., lidocaine, mepivacaine, prilocaine, bupivacaine and etidocaine. Pharmacologically, these agents can be categorized as agents of low potency and short duration of action, e.g., procaine and chloroprocaine; agents of intermediate potency and duration of action, e.g., lidocaine, mepivacaine and prilocaine; and agents of high potency and long duration, eg., tetracaine, bupivacaine and etidocaine.

The pharmacological profile of local anesthetics is primarily related to their physicochemical properties. Lipid solubility and protein binding appear to be the primary determinants of potency and duration of action. The pK_A of the various agents will influence the onset of conduction blockade.

The systemic toxicity of local anesthetics involves mainly the central nervous system and cardiovascular system. All local anesthetics can induce convulsions at high doses followed by CNS depression. This class of agents can also cause myocardial depression and peripheral vasodilatation leading to profound hypotension and cardiac arrest. The more potent agents such

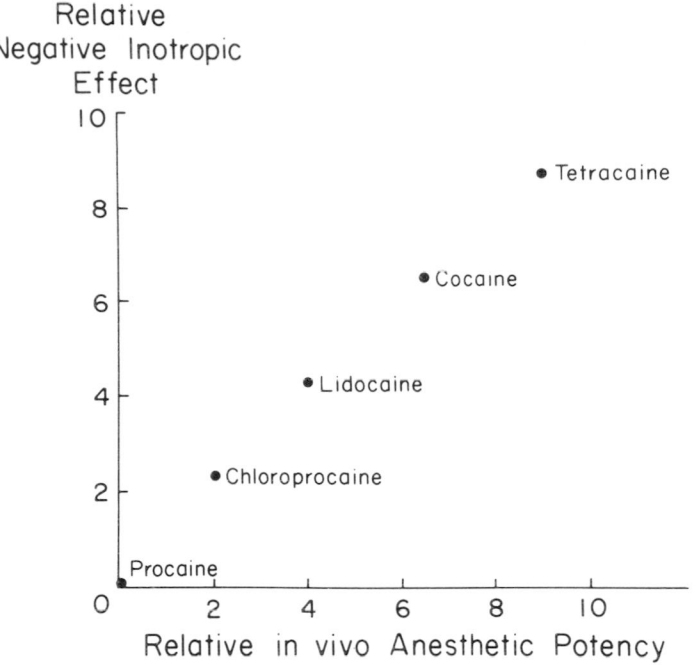

Fig. 54.3 Relationship between myocardial depressant effect in dogs and *in vivo* anesthetic potency of various local anesthetic agents.

as bupivacaine appear to be relatively more cardiotoxic than the less potent agents such as lidocaine.

The toxicity of local anesthetics is related to the blood level of the specific agent. The blood level of local anesthetics, in turn, is determined by their rate of vascular absorption and the rate of tissue redistribution and metabolism. The rate of absorption is a function of the site of administration, dosage, addition of a vasoconstrictor and specific agent employed. Among the amino amides prilocaine shows the most rapid rate of tissue redistribution and hepatic metabolism. In the amino ester group, chloroprocaine undergoes the most rapid rate of hydrolysis in plasma.

REFERENCES

Covino B.G., Vassallo B.G. (1976). *Local Anesthetics: Mechanism of Action and Clinical Use*. New York: Grune & Stratton.

Covino B.G. (1986). Pharmacology of local anesthetic agents. *Br. J. Anaesth.*, **58**, 701.

Covino B.G. (1987). Toxicity and systemic effects of local anesthetic agents. In *Local Anesthetics*. (Strichartz G.R., ed.). Berlin, Heidelberg: Springer-Verlag.

De Jong R.H. (1977). *Local Anesthetics* (2nd edn.). Springfield: Charles C. Thomas.

Reiz S., Nath S. (1986). Cardiotoxicity of local anesthetic agents. *Br. J. Anaesth.*, **58**, 736.

Scott D.B. (1986). Toxic effects of local anesthetic agents on the central nervous sytem. *Br. J. Anaesth.*, **58**, 732.

Tucker G.T. (1986). Pharmacokinetics of local anesthetics. *Br. J. Anaesth.*, **58**, 717.

Tucker G.T., Mather L.E. (1979). Clinical pharmacokinetics of local anesthetics. *Clin. Pharmacokinetics*, **4**, 241.

55. Hypersensitivity to Drugs and Other Substances

M. Fisher and C. Hirschman

THE RELEVANCE OF HYPERSENSITIVITY TO ANAESTHETIC DRUGS

The Boston Collaborative Drug Surveillance Programme determined the incidence of severe anaphylactoid reactions during anaesthesia as 1:4395 general anaesthetics, with confidence limits of 1:980 to 1:20 000, (Beard and Jick, 1985) and most published figures are within these limits. This may be compared to an incidence of anaphylaxis of 6:10 000 hospitalized patients (Porter and Jick, 1977) suggesting that even with the increase in anaesthetic reactions that was believed to occur during the 1970's, anaesthetic drugs are inherently safer than drugs overall. Indeed, only one study of anaesthetic mortality has implicated such reactions as a significant factor (Utting et al., 1979).

Terminology

The terminology regarding anaphylactoid reactions during anaesthesia is confusing and may contribute to the morbidity and mortality. The terms 'anaphylactic, reaginic, antibody mediated', 'hypersensitive' and 'allergic' should strictly only be used when true IgE mediated reactions are proven. The synonymous 'allergoid', 'pseudoallergic', and 'anaphylactoid', should be reserved for clinical situations in which there is no proof of an immune basis. The inherent danger in this terminology, is the assumption that if the reaction is not labelled anaphylactic, it is of the nonimmune type and the drug can safely be given again. It is absolutely vital to appreciate that the terms 'allergoid', 'pseudoallergic' and 'anaphylactoid' imply that no immune basis has been established. In many cases, this means that either nobody has looked for an antibody or looked with inappropriate technology. With the increasing use of the term 'anaphylaxis' to describe non-antibody mediated events such as exercise anaphylaxis and vibration anaphylaxis the use of the term to describe a clinical syndrome is now accepted (Sheffer, 1985). In this review the term clinical anaphylaxis (CA) will be used to describe reactions.

Drugs dissolved in the solvent Cremophor EL carry an unacceptably high risk of severe anaphylactoid reactions and have largely been withdrawn. With the exception of cremophor-based drugs, we believe that the risk of a severe CA, in a patient with no past history of such a reaction, is not a rational basis for drug selection. Virtually every drug used in anaesthesia has produced a severe CA. The incidence of severe CA is not related to the direct histamine releasing properties of the drug. Rather, the quantity of the drug used in a region appears to be the most significant factor in the incidence of reactions to the drug.

Muscle relaxant drugs are the most common cause of severe reactions during anaesthesia. Reactions to the newer relaxants vecuronium and atracurium were described soon after their introduction into clinical practice. The likelihood of reactions to a muscle relaxant is related to frequency of use rather than intrinsic danger or the histamine releasing ability of the drug, although pancuronium appears safer than other relaxants.

The incidence of reactions to colloids has been the subject of bitter debate raising important questions as to their safety. Half-life is probably a more important criterion for colloid selection than reaction rate, as all colloids carry similar risks of CA (Ring and Messmer, 1977). All synthetic blood volume replacement solutions cause more reactions than lactated Ringer's solution, but are safer than blood. They rarely, if ever, produce reactions in shocked patients.

PREDICTING THE PATIENT AT RISK

All published studies show an increased incidence of a history of allergy, atopy and asthma in patients who have experienced severe anaphylactoid reactions during anaesthesia, when compared to patients who undergo uneventful anaesthesia. Such information has led some authors to postulate that the presence of a history of atopy, with or without an elevated IgE level, may have predictive value in the selection of drugs to minimize the risk of a severe allergic reaction. This is not true. The predictive value of such a history is shown in Table 55.1, and the value is low due to the low prevalence of the disorder (Fisher et al., 1987).

Neither pretreatment nor diagnostic intradermal

TABLE 55.1

PREDICTIVE VALUE OF A HISTORY OF ALLERGY, ATOPY OR ASTHMA IN PREDICTION OF RISK OF CLINICAL ANAPHYLAXIS
DURING ANAESTHESIA.

Incidence Parameter	1:500				1:20 000			
	Allergy	Atopy	Both	Asthma	Allergy	Atopy	Both	Asthma
Sensitivity %	44.9	33.04	23.79	18.91	44.9	33.04	23.79	18.91
Specificity %	85.1	91.5	93.6	95.9	85.1	91.5	93.6	95.9
Positive predictive value %	0.6	0.77	0.71	0.92	0.01	0.02	0.02	0.02
Negative predictive value %	99.9	99.9	99.9	99.9	1	1	1	1
False alarm rate %	99.7	99.6	99.6	99.5	99.99	99.98	99.98	99.98
False reassurance rate %	.07	.07	.09	.09	0	0	0	0

Reproduced by permission of The Editor, *British Journal of Anaesthesia.*

testing is totally reliable in preventing reactions, leaving the problem that even if the high risk patient is identified, little could be done regarding absolute identification of the agent likely to produce a reaction. Moreover, the absence of previous exposure does not preclude a reaction being immunological in origin, and therefore attributing a reaction to a particular drug on the basis of previous exposure is not valid. For the muscle relaxants, true IgE mediated reactions have been demonstrated on first exposure (Fisher, 1980). It is postulated, but not proven, that such patients were sensitized by other chemicals, which crossreacted with the muscle relaxants.

THE MECHANISM OF THE REACTIONS

There is disagreement among workers about the mechanism of the various types of reactions. No one mechanism seems to account for all reactions. Further, it is unlikely that a single mechanism is responsible for all the clinical manifestations in a single reaction, although this is likely in minor reactions and has been demonstrated in reactions to haemaccel (gelatin solution) in volunteers (Lorenz et al., 1982). The complement system, the hypersensitivity mediators and the cellular components of the immune system are intimately linked at many levels. An isolated biological defence mechanism becoming harmful to the host would be a most unusual event in nature. The physical properties of solutions may be responsible for nonimmunological reactions.

Direct Histamine Release

High concentrations of many induction agents, muscle relaxants, narcotics and colloid solutions produce histamine release in nonallergic subjects.

Although recent articles appearing in the anaesthesia literature implicate histamine release as a significant mechanism for hypotension produced by these drugs, we seriously question that histamine release *per se* is responsible for a major portion of severe cardiovascular effects of these drugs.

The histamine released presumably originates from mast cells and basophil granules, which contain other vasoactive substances. Furthermore, mast cells and basophil degranulation may be accompanied by release of rapidly synthesized mediators, such as eicosanoids and bradykinin. These other mediators, whose plasma levels do not necessarily parallel those of histamine, may be responsible for more of the cardiovascular effects associated with mast cell degranulation than with the histamine itself. Both morphine and curare in particular have multiple direct effects on the vasculature which could well account for much of the hypotension.

In an editorial by Beavan (1981), it was stated that 'increases of 2–5 ng/ml of histamine are invariably associated with tachycardia, widespread flushing and urticaria and increases above 5 ng/ml with severe hypotension'. A recent study with histamine infusion demonstrated a 30% increase in pulse pressure (usually reflecting diastolic hypotension) at mean histamine plasma levels at 2.5 ng/ml. However, since massive quantities of histamine (500 000 ng infused over thirty minutes) had to be infused in one arm, to achieve plasma histamine concentrations of 2.5 ng/ml in the opposite arm, the effective histamine level in the central circulation must have been in excess of the 2.5 ng/ml measured. Furthermore, a study by Atkins et al. (1982) measuring histamine levels during antigen aerosol challenge showed peak histamine levels ranging from 18–60 ng/ml in five out of six subjects without significant haemodynamic abnormalities. The sixth patient who became hypotensive had a peak plasma level of 80 ng/ml. Similarly, during a study of immunotherapy for insect hypersensitivity, insect venom increased plasma histamine into the 2–10 ng/ml range without eliciting hypotension. Three patients with plasma histamine levels above 10 ng/ml (two above 50 ng/ml) were severely hypotensive. Therefore, the relationship between magnitude of histamine release and magnitude of hypotension appears unpredictable. Furthermore, although changes in histamine level following morphine have shown some correlation with decreases in systemic vascular resistance (but not hypotension), this in no way implies causation.

If histamine is important in producing hypotension, one ought to be able to block the hypotension by histamine receptor antagonists. A study attempted this and claimed success (Philbin et al., 1981). However, close examination of their data reveals an increase in heart rate and blood pressure in patients receiving diphenhydramine and a diphenhydramine-cimetidine combination to values above the control levels. If this new (and more appropriate) baseline is used for comparison, then morphine following placebo produced a 29% two minute blood pressure decrease, morphine following diphenhydramine produced at 29% decrease, and morphine following combined treatment with diphenhydramine and cimetidine produced a 25% decrease in mean blood pressure. Thus, the actual decrease in blood pressure in all groups was similar. Further, Mongur and Whelan (1953), showed that d-tubocurarine was unlikely to release sufficient histamine to cause a severe cardiovascular reaction.

The magnitude of histamine release appears to be related to the volume, concentration and rate of administration of the drug. While minor reactions due to direct histamine release are very common, the incidence of severe reactions is rare. Many very potent histamine releasers in common use, such as morpine, d-tubocurarine and papaveretum rarely produce severe reactions, while drugs which are poor histamine releasers (Althesin, suxamethonium and alcuronium) are common aetiological agents. Direct histamine release may certainly cause reactions of minor and intermediate severity, particularly when high concentrations and rapid infusions are used in patients who have cardiovascular disease.

Drugs which release histamine from mast cells and basophils are also suspected of producing bronchospasm in humans. There is even less compelling evidence showing a relationship between histamine release and bronchospasm, than that linking hypotension and histamine. In histamine infusion studies neither has the airway resistance been measured, nor the bronchospasm mentioned as a symptom, even at the highest concentrations infused. Crago et al. (1972) found that airway resistance was higher in normal subjects paralysed with d-tubocurarine, than with pancuronium, while Simpson et al. (1985) failed to find a significant difference.

In conclusion, a demonstration of histamine release by a drug *in vitro* or even *in vivo* is not proof that all or any clinical signs attributed to the drug are causally related to the histamine *per se*. However, classes of patients (atopic) exist that demonstrate greater 'histamine releasability' than nonatopic—(Laxenaire et al., 1982) and patients with airway hyper-reactivity demonstrate extreme airway sensitivity to many mediators including histamine (Spector, 1983). In such patients, histamine releasing drugs may be contraindicated, even though there is no evidence in the literature suggesting or proving that appropriate doses of histamine releasing drugs cause a higher incidence of significant adverse effects or more severe reactions in atopic compared to nonatopic patients.

Type I Hypersensitivity

A variety of mechanisms, some presumably unrelated to hypersensitivity, account for many adverse drug reactions but the incidence of true type I hypersensitivity is not known. The evidence of intradermal testing, passive transfer testing, basophil and leucocyte histamine release, (Vervloet et al., 1979, 1983; Fisher 1980, 1981; Youngman et al., 1983; Laxenaire et al., 1982), radioimmunoassay (Baldo and Fisher, 1983a) and inhibition of radioimunoassay (Baldo and Fisher, 1983b) suggest that IgE antibodies play an important role in a considerable number of anaesthetic reactions. Apart from intradermal testing, which may be a demonstration of increased direct histamine release, antibodies can be demonstrated in less than 60% of reactions. This may reflect a nonimmunological basis of the reaction, or the low sensitivity of the tests. The lack of previous exposure in many reactions and the small size of the molecules involved also suggest that true allergy is unlikely. Recent studies have shown, however, that muscle relaxant can bind to IgE directly. The substituted ammonium groups on muscle relaxants, appear to be important as the sensitizing agent (Baldo and Fisher, 1983a). They have bivalent groups less than 20 Å apart, which make them antigenic. Although the demonstration of an antibody after a reaction to a drug is not proof of a cause and effect relationship when a life threatening reaction, clinically resembling anaphylaxis, occurs immediately after an appropriate dose of a drug, the demonstration of an IgE antibody to the drug strongly suggests such a relationship. With dextrans, the situation is even more confused. Dextran-reactive IgM antibodies may be demonstrated, but many patients who react do not have such antibodies and many patients with antibodies do not react (Hedin et al., 1976). IgE antibodies to thiopentone have recently been demonstrated in patients reacting to thiopentone (Harle et al., 1986).

Complement Activation

Watkins et al., (1976) have shown activation of the classical and alternative pathways of complement during severe reactions to induction agents, while Brown et al., (1981) have demonstrated complement activation during a reaction to a local anaesthetic. Furthermore a complement dependent IgE antibody to protamine has been demonstrated after a reaction to protamine (Lakin et al., 1978). Watkins (1982) postulates two mechanisms by which reactions to anaesthetic drugs can occur. Activation of the classical complement pathway (usually on second exposure) by an undefined immune complex and non-specific or nonimmunological activation of the alternative pathway. Both mechanisms could be involved in reactions occurring on either first or subsequent exposure. In contrast (Radford et al., 1982) showed that all patients reacting to althesin on first exposure had alternative pathway activation and all patients reacting on second exposure had classical pathway activation. The reason for the differing results of the two groups is probably related to the handling of specimens after the reaction as activation occurs *in vitro* if specimens are not carefully transported. Alternative pathway activation may be associated with chronic disease or sepsis and lead to reactions involving structurally different drugs on different occasions (Watkins et al., 1978). However, significant complement activation has been clearly noted in uneventful anaesthesia (Haslam et al., 1980). It is highly likely that this is an independent mechanism as Watkins (1982) postulates, but it is unclear whether it is a cause and effect mechanism or an epiphenomenon in all cases. Complement activation is an important component of aggregate anaphylaxis.

Other Mechanisms

There are a considerable number of other mechanisms which produce the symptoms of anaphylaxis. The kallikrein/kinin system may be activated by plasma protein solutions; the eicosanoid system may be activated by aspirin. Platelet and leukocyte antibodies may produce reactions to blood. Alterations in osmolality of the blood due to mannitol or contrast media, or the alveolar fluid due to nebulized water may produce symptoms. Protamine is an excellent example of the multiple ways in which a single compound may produce reactions. IgE and IgG complement dependent antibodies have been detected in immediate reactions, rapid infusion produces direct vasodilatation. Delayed pulmonary oedema by an unknown mechanism has also been attributed to protamine.

Cross-Sensitivity

Cross-sensitivity occurs between cremophor based drugs, local anaesthetics, including amide and ester groups (Incaudo, et al., 1978), and muscle relaxants (Vervloet, et al., 1979, 1983). Suxamethonium, decamethonium, and gallamine; and alcuronium and d-tubocurarine commonly show cross-sensitivity, with some patients showing sensitivity to all the relaxants tested. Cross-sensitivity between muscle relaxant drugs has been confirmed in *in vitro* IgE radioimmunoassay inhibition studies using sera from patients who experienced severe anaphylactoid reactions to muscle relaxants.

CLINICAL FEATURES

The increase in cases of clinical anaphylaxis in operating rooms presented us with a unique opportunity to study in detail the clinical events which occur. The patients in the operating room are usually naked, monitored, and in the presence of at least one medical observer, which provides better opportunity for accurate observation than clinical anaphylaxis occurring in hospital wards or in the community.

Organ System Involvement

In 206 patients, the involvement of organ systems is shown in Table 55.2. Cardiovascular collapse was the most common severe feature occurring in 90% of patients. Seventeen patients had a single organ system involved, cardiovascular collapse in twelve, angioneurotic oedema in three, and bronchospasm in two.

The clinical features are related to smooth muscle contraction, vasodilatation and increased capillary permeability. Cardiac effects are primarily related to vasodilatation and plasma loss. The role of the heart as a target organ in anaphylaxis is disputed. While animal models and *in vitro* studies of human cardiac muscle show effects on conduction, force of contraction and coronary blood flow, there is little evidence of cardiac failure in humans. In a study of 186 patients with anaphylactic cardiovascular collapse, Fisher (1986) found that serious arrhythmias and cardiac failure rarely occurred except in patients with primary cardiac disease. We documented primary cardiac failure in only two patients with normal hearts suggesting that such failure is rare.

The assessment of cardiac function is complicated by the secondary effects of acidosis, hypoxaemia, high intrathoracic pressure, and the effects of compensatory endogenous catecholamine and therapeutic exogenous catecholamine levels.

Treatment

The optimum treatment of clinical anaphylaxis is not known, and controlled trials are impossible. Fortunately, there is a pleasing correlation between the cellular effects of drugs such as adrenaline and aminophylline which raise intracellular levels of cyclic 3–5 AMP and the repeated (anecdotal) demonstration of efficacy of these drugs in the majority of patients.

The use of animal models has limited application in the study of the treatment of clinical anaphylaxis in man. Firstly, many species respond predictably with a response usually involving a single organ system. Further, the mechanism of inducing clinical anaphylaxis influences the pathological features. The optimum treatment for clinical anaphylaxis is not known.

Sympathomimetic Drugs

Most reviewers, since the 1930's, state that adrenaline is the drug of choice in anaphylaxis. It is usually effective whether given intramuscularly or intravenously.

Two criticisms of adrenaline in therapy have appeared in the literature. Barach et al. (1984) noted

TABLE 55.2
THE FREQUENCY OF CLINICAL FEATURES IN 206 PATIENTS WITH SEVERE ANAPHYLACTOID REACTIONS
DURING ANAESTHESIA.

Clinical feature	Induction agents	Muscle relaxants	Other drugs
Number of patients	44	115	47
Cutaneous features			
Rash	6	9	6
Urticaria	4	9	13
Generalized Flush	22	47	25
Bronchospasm			
Transient	7	26	8
Severe	3	17	5
Cardiovascular			
Tachycardia	41	103	39
Bradycardia	2	8	7
Other arrythymia	4	13	9
Hypotension	41	106	41
Vasodilatation	38	99	37
Vasoconstriction	0	5	0
Pulmonary oedema	0	4	5
Angioneurotic oedema	7	38	8
Generalized oedema	4	10	3
Gastrointestinal features	9	11	3

the risk of arrhythmias, especially in those patients receiving halothane. Induced ventricular fibrillation was precipitated by the combination of adrenaline and halothane in four patients (Fisher, 1986). This is not a contraindication to the drug, but an indication that great care should be exercised. In non-monitored patients, adrenaline should be given intramuscularly and in monitored patients, infused cautiously. Hamberger et al. (1980) showed that the endogenous catecholamine response in anaphylaxis induced in dogs was greater than the effect of 0.5 mg of adrenaline by injection, and suggested there was no value in administering the drug. However, Worstman et al. (1984) showed, in cardiac arrest patients, that the administration of adrenaline led to an increase in serum levels, to levels greater than those produced by endogenous catecholamines, suggesting that the cumulative effect is important. Irrespective of postulates based on animal studies, there is little question in the literature that adrenaline is effective in ameliorating both bronchospasm and cardiovascular collapse.

Volume Replacement

The crystalloid *versus* colloid controversy has raged since the 1950s and we have no wish to fuel the topic further. In some patients with anaphylactic cardiovascular collapse, haemo-concentration is associated with poor perfusion and haemoglobin levels, which can be restored by colloid, but not crystalloid infusion, suggesting that colloid solutions are the treatment of choice. The theoretical criticism that these solutions carry the risk of anaphylaxis does not appear valid. These patients are in shock and therefore producing catecholamines and steroids, and in addition, are likely already to have released most of their mediators of anaphylaxis.

External Cardiac Massage

The most common error in the management of the early cases in our series and in the literature was the failure to use adrenaline and replace volume. The most common error in the later cases in our series, and in the literature, was the failure to institute external cardiac massage in patients without blood pressure, but with benign arrhythmies. It cannot be overemphasized that external cardiac massage is indicated for problems of flow, not electrical activity.

Management of Bronchospasm

This is the most difficult clinical feature to treat. The common characteristic of the patient who dies with bronchospasm was that not all possible therapeutic manoeuvres were attempted, although it cannot be categorically stated that outcome would have been influenced. Adrenaline and aminophylline infused intravenously in association with nebulized β stimulants are the initial treatment of choice. Well documented successes with less common treatments, such as volatile anaesthetics, ketamine, infiltration of the lung hilum with local anaesthetic and cardiopulmonary bypass have been described. While not drugs of first choice there are anecdotal reports of some improvement in patients with H_1 and H_2 blockers.

Corticosteroids

It has not been possible to study the effects of corticosteroids on experimental anaphylaxis in man, although corticosteroids clearly protect against lethal anaphylaxis in the mouse and rabbit but not in the guinea pig. There is also some evidence that corticosteroids reduce the incidence and severity of radio contrast media reactions (Greenberger et al., 1981).

The immediate reaction involving IgE dependent mast cell mediator release manifested by airway smooth muscle constriction, increased permeability and mucous secretion may not be altered acutely by corticosteroids (Schleimer, 1985). However, this immediate reaction may be followed by a more delayed one in which steroids profoundly reduce inflammatory cell infiltrates, inhibit many target tissue responses and potentiate the smooth muscle and inflammatory cell responses to catecholamines. Steroids also inhibit arachidonic acid metabolite release, but the significance of it is presently unclear. Because there is little risk to the short-term use of steroids and potential benefit, we advocate their use in the treatment of acute anaphylaxis in humans, especially in cases poorly responsive to other treatments, and in cases in which bronchospasm is a prominent feature.

DIAGNOSIS

After a life-threatening reaction, two priorities exist.

1. to identify the drug responsible
2. to determine which other drugs are safe for subsequent anaesthesia.

The only reliable and readily available method for this is intradermal testing, which has been successfully used by a number of workers. Although the method has been criticized by some workers, the criticisms have not been supported by data. The mechanism responsible for the positive tests is disputed (Watkins, 1982). In practical terms, however, if a strict protocol is adhered to, intradermal testing often provides reliable information as to the drug responsible. Indeed, if more than one drug is used and intradermal tests are negative, no other test currently available, has so far, determined the responsible drug. Intradermal testing is of no value in reactions to contrast media or colloids (Fisher 1981), or in minor or type IV reactions. With local anaesthesia it is only valuable as part of progressive challenge.

The measurement of sequential changes in complement activation gives information that a reaction has probably occurred. Although usually obvious clinically, such demonstration is useful in confirming a reaction in a patient with a single clinical feature.

Further, the demonstration of alternate pathway activation may suggest that a patient is likely to react to structurally unrelated drugs. Changes in IgE levels have been used to suggest a type I hypersensitivity mechanism. It is our belief that the plasma loss and volume replacement, which occurs in anaphylactoid reactions make measurement of levels of any substance of very dubious value. Leucocyte histamine release (Vervloet et al., 1979, 1983), basophil degranulation (Laxenaire et al., 1982), passive transfer testing (Fisher, 1980, 1981; Laxenaire et al., 1982), and radioimmunoassay (Baldo and Fisher, 1983a, b) all remain the province of specialist laboratories and give information about mechanisms, rather than information about the drug responsible.

After further evaulation, however, some of these methods may be of value for the identification of patients with allergies to specific drugs. Before that can occur, it will be necessary to examine thoroughly relationships between clinical data on the one hand and laboratory test results on the other. When true IgE-mediated allergic drug reactions are suspected, efforts should be made to correlate results of skin testing with both leukocyte histamine release findings and the presence of drug-specific IgE antibodies.

FOLLOW UP

Second anaphylactoid reactions usually occur because of inadequate investigation or follow up, or failure to appreciate cross-sensitivity. However, patients with alternate complement activation may react to structurally unrelated drugs, and even if the agent responsible is known, subsequent safety cannot be absolutely guaranteed.

The principles of safe future management of these patients are:

1. The reaction should be investigated by every means available.
2. The reaction should be explained to the patient and the patient given a letter stating the drugs given, the nature of the reaction, the results of investigations, and the conclusion. The details of subsequent anaesthesia should be recorded in the letter.
3. The patient should be encouraged to wear a warning bracelet.
4. Subsequent anaesthesia should be administered in a hospital with full resuscitation facilities by a qualified anaesthetist.
5. Alternative techniques, such as regional block and volatile induction, should be considered.
6. Alternative drugs to those incriminated or used previously should be chosen, if possible.
7. An intravenous line should be inserted preoperatively and monitoring commenced prior to induction. Drugs should be given slowly or by infusion. Adrenaline should be drawn up prior to commencement.

REFERENCES

Atkins P.C., Rosenblum F., Dunsky E.H., et al. (1982). Comparison of plasma histamine levels and symptoms and cyclic nucleotides after antigen and methacholine in man. *J. Allergy Clin. Immunol.*, **66**, 478.

Baldo B.A., Fisher M.M. (1983a). Anaphylaxis to muscle relaxant drugs cross reactivity and moleular basis of bindings of IgE antibodies detected by radioimmunoassay. *Mol. Immunol.*, **20**, 1393.

Baldo B.A., Fisher M.M. (1983b). Detection of serum IgE antibodies that react with alcuronium and tubocurarine with life threatening reactions to muscle relaxant drugs. *Anaesth. Int. Care.*, **11**, 194.

Barach E.M., Nowak R.M., Lee T.G., et al. (1984). Epinephrine for treatment of anaphylactic. *J. Am. Med. Assoc.*, **251**, 2118.

Beard K., Jick H. (1985). Cardiac arrest and anaphylaxis with anaesthetic agents. *J. Am. Med. Assoc.*, **254**, 2742.

Beaven M.A. (1981). Anaphylactoid reactions to anesthetic drugs (editorial). *Anesthesiology*, **55**, 3.

Best N., Teissner B., Grudzinskas J.G., et al. (1983). Classical pathway activation during an adverse response to protamine. *Br. J. Anaesth.*, **55**, 1149.

Brown D.T., Beamish D., Wildsmith J.A.W. (1981). Allergic reaction to an amide anaesthetic. *Br. J. Anaesth.*, **53**, 435.

Casale T.B., Bowman S., Kaliner M. (1984). Induction of human cutaneous cell degranulation by opiates, endogenous opioid peptides. Evidence for opiate and nonopiate receptor participation. *J. Allergy Clin. Immunol.*, **73**, 775.

Crago R.R., Bryan A.C., Laws A.K., et al. (1972). Respiratory flow resistance after curare and pancuronium measured by forced oscillations. *Can. Anaesth. Soc. J.*, **19**, 604.

Doenicke A. (1980). Pseudo-allergic reactions due to histamine release during intravenous anaesthesia. In *Pseudoallergic Reactions 1. Genetic Aspects and Anaphylactoid Reactions*, pp. 224–250. (Dukor P., Kallos P., Schlumberger H.D., et al., eds.). Basel: Karger.

Ebertz J.M., Hermens J.M, McMillan J.C., et al. (1986). Functional differences between human cutaneous mast cells and basophils: a comparison of morphine-induced histamine release. *Agents and Actions*, **18**, 455.

Fisher M.McD. (1980). Reaginic antibodies to anesthetic drugs. *Anesthesiology*, **52**, 318.

Fisher M.McD. (1981). The diagnosis of acute anaphylactoid reactions to anaesthetic drugs. *Anaesth. Intens. Care*, **9**, 235.

Fisher M.McD. (1986). Anaphylactic cardiovascular collapse: clinical observations on pathophysiology and treatment. *Anaesth. Intens. Care*, **14**, 17.

Fisher M.McD., Outhred A., Bowey C.J. (1987). Can clinical anaphylaxis to anaesthetic drugs be predicted from allergic history? *Br. J. Anaesth.* **59**, 690.

Flacke W., Gillis R.A. (1968). Impulse transmission via nicotinic and muscarinic pathways in the stellate ganglion. *J. Pharmacol. Exp. Ther.*, **163**, 266.

Greenberger P.A., Patterson R., Simon R., et al. (1981). Pretreatment of high risk patients requiring radiocontrast media studies. *J. Allergy Clin. Immunol.*, **67**, 185.

Hamberger B., Fredholm B.B., Farnebo L.O. (1980). Anaphylaxis and plasma catecholamines. *Life Sci.*, **26**, 1465.

Harle D.G., Baldo B.A., Smal M.A., et al. (1986). Detection of thiopentone-reactive IgE antibodies following anaphylactoid reactions during anaesthesis. *Clin. Allergy*, **16**, 493.

Haslam P.J., Townend P.J., Branthwaite M.A. (1980). Complement activation during cardiopulmonary bypass. *Anaesthesia*, **35**, 22.

Hedin H., Richeter W., Ring J. (1976). Dextran-induced anaphylactoid reactions in man. *Intern. Arch. Appl. Immunol.*, **52**, 145.

Hermans J.M., Ebertz J.M., Hanifin J.M., et al. (1985). Comparison of histamine release in human skin mast cells induced by morphine, fentanyl, and oxymorphone. *Anesthesiology*, **62**, 124.

Hirshman C.A., Edelstein R.A., Ebertz J.M., et al. (1985). Thiobarbiturate-induced histamine release in human skin mast cells. *Anesthesiology*, **63**, 353.

Incaudo G., Schatz M., Patterson R., et al. (1978). *J. Allergy Clin. Immunol.*, **56**, 339.

Lakin J., Blocker T., Strong D., et al (1978). Anaphylaxis to protamine sulphate mediated by a complement dependent IgE antibody. *J. Allergy Clin. Immunol.*, **61**, 102.

Laxenaire M.C., Moneret-Vautrin D.A., Boileau S., et al. (1982). Adverse reactions to intravenous agents in anaesthesia in France. *Klin. Wochenschr.*, **60**, 1006.

Lewis T. (1927). *The Blood Vessels of the Skin and their Responses*. London: Shaw and Sons.

Lorenz W. (1983). Hypersensitivity reactions induced by anaesthetic drugs and plasma substitutes: influence of paradigms on incidence and mechanisms. In *Immunotoxicology*, pp. 283–305. (Gibson G.G., Hubbard R., Parke D.V., eds.). London: Academic Press.

Lorenz W., Doenicke A., Meyer R., et al. (1972). Histamine release in man by propanidid and thiopentone: pharmacological effects and clinical consequences. *Br. J. Anaesth.*, **44**, 355.

Lorenz W., Neugebauer E., Schmal A. (1982). Le dosage de l'histamine plasmatique lors de reactions anaphylactoides che le sujet anesthesie. *Annales Française Anesthesie et Reanimation*, **1**, 271.

Mongur, J.L., Whelan R.F. (1953). Histamine release by adrenaline and d-tubocurarine in the human subject. *J. Physiol.*, **120**, 156.

North F.C., Kettelkamp N., Hirshman C.A. (1987). Comparison of cutaneous and *in vitro* histamine release by muscle relaxants. *Anesthesiology*, **66**, 543.

Philbin D.M., Moss J., Akins C.W., et al. (1981). The use of H_1 and H_2 histamine antagonists with morphine anesthesia: a double-blind study. *Anesthesiology*, **55**, 292.

Porter J., Jick H. (1977). Drug related deaths among medical inpatients. *J. Amer. Med. Assoc.*, **237**, 879.

Radford S.G., Lockyer J.A., Simpson P.J. (1982). Immunological aspects of adverse reactions to althesin. *Br. J. Anaesth.*, **54**, 469.

Ring J., Messmer K. (1977). Incidence and severity of anaphylactoid reactions to colloid volume substitutes. *Lancet*, **1(8009)**, 466.

Schleimer R.P. (1985). The mechanism of anti-inflammatory steroid action in allergic diseases. *Am. Rev. Pharmacol. Toxicol.*, **25**, 381.

Sheffer A.L. (1985). Anaphylaxis. *J. Allergy Clin. Immunol.*, **75**, 227.

Simpson D.A., Wright D.J., Hammond J.E. (1985). Influence of d-tubocurarine, pancuronium and atracurium on bronchomotor tone. *Br. J. Anaesth.*, **57**, 753.

Spector S.L. (1983). Bronchial inhalational challenges with aerosolized bronchoconstrictive substances. In *Provocat-*

ive Challenge Procedures: Bronchial, Oral, Nasal and Exercise, Vol. 1, pp. 137–177. (S.L. Spector, ed.). Boca Raton: CRG Press.

Utting J.E., Gray T.C., Shelley F.C. (1979). Human misadventure in anaesthesia. *Can. Anaesth. Soc. J.*, **26**, 472.

Vervloet D., Arnaund A., Vellieux P., et al (1979). Anaphylactic reactions to muscle relaxants under general anaesthesia. *J. Allergy Clin. Immunol.*, **63**, 348.

Vervloet D., Senft M., Dugue P., et al. (1983). Anaphylactic reactions fo modificd fluid gelatins. *J. Allergy Clin. Immunol.*, **71**, 535.

Ward J.M., McGrath R.L., Weil J.V. (1972). Effects of morphine on peripheral vascular response to sympathetic stimulation. *Am. J. Cardiol.*, **29**, 659.

Watkins J., Padfield A., Alderson J.D. (1978). Underlying immunopathology as a cause of adverse responses to two intravenous anaesthetic agents. *Br. Med. J.*, **1**, 1180.

Watkins J., Salo M. (1982). Trauma Stress and Immunity in Anaesthesia and Surgery. London: Butterworths.

Watkins J., Udnoon S., Appleyard T.N., et al. (1976). Identification and quantitation of hypersensitivity reactions to intravenous anaesthetic agents. *Br. J. Anaesth.*, **48**, 457.

Worstman J., Frank S., Cryer P.E. (1984). Adrenomedullary response to maximal stress in humans. *Am. J. Med.*, **77**, 779.

Youngman P.R., Taylor K.M., Wilson J.D. (1983). Anaphylactoid reactions to neuromuscular blocking agents: A commonly undiagnosed condition? *Lancet*, **ii**, 597.

56. Metabolism and Toxicity of Inhaled Anesthetics

J. Baden

Drug metabolism
 Enzyme induction
Metabolism of individual inhaled anesthetics
 Halothane
 Enflurane
 Isoflurane
 Nitrous oxide
Toxicity
 Halothane
 Enflurane
 Isoflurane
 Nitrous oxide

The inhaled anesthetics, with the possible exception of nitrous oxide, are metabolized in the body. In this respect, they are entirely similar to the numerous chemicals (xenobiotics) that arc taken up by the body but are not used for the generation of energy or for other normal cellular processes. In general, metabolism is an important defence against accumulating toxic levels of chemicals that otherwise could not easily be excreted by the liver or kidneys. Inhaled anesthetics, however, do not depend on the liver or kidneys for their excretion but rather are excreted unchanged by the lungs; their metabolism serves mainly to increase the chance of toxicity.

DRUG METABOLISM

Drug metabolism occurs predominantly in the liver and to a lesser extent in other organs such as the lung and kidney. Two broad phases are recognized. Phase

1 consists of oxidation, reduction or hydrolysis reactions that produce more water-soluble but not necessarily less toxic compounds than the parent drug. Phase 2 consists of conjugation reactions that tend to produce less toxic and often more water-soluble compounds than the parent drug. Products from phase 1 reactions may be subject to phase 2 reactions.

The two phases of drug metabolism are controlled by different enzyme systems. Phase 1 enzymes are mainly membrane bound. The most important enzymes for anesthetic metabolism are in the P-450 or mixed-function oxidase system. This NADPH-dependent electron transport chain is located primarily in smooth endoplasmic reticulum and to a much lesser extent in nuclear membrane. Cytochrome P-450 is a heme-containing enzyme that is central to the system's catalytic activity. Other enzymes in the system include NADPH-dependent cytochrome P-450 reductase, NADPH-dependent cytochrome b_5 reductase and cytochrome b_5. A greatly simplified scheme of cytochrome P-450-mediated hydroxylation is shown in Fig. 56.1. The cycle starts with the formation of a cytochrome P-450-drug complex (step a). This complex accepts an electron from NADPH

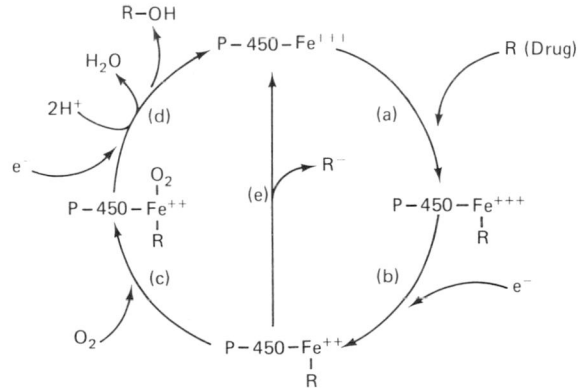

Fig. 56.1 Simplified cytochrome P-450-mediated pathway for drug metabolism.

whereupon the Fe^{3+} in cytochrome P-450 is reduced to Fe^{2+} (step b). The reduced cytochrome complex then combines with a molecule of oxygen (step c). After addition of another electron and an internal re-arrangement of charge (step d), an oxygen atom is added to the drug and the complex decomposes with release of the hydroxylated drug and regenerated (Fe^{3+}-containing) cytochrome P-450. Step d involves several intermediate steps. An interesting additional pathway (step e), that is thought to operate during metabolism of drugs like halothane, is the direct transfer of an electron from the reduced complex to the drug (Brault, 1985).

Some phase 1 enzymes are not associated with the cytochrome P-450 system. For example, the mixed-function amine oxidase system is also located in smooth endoplasmic reticulum and catalyzes many oxidation reactions, especially those involving nitrogen and sulphur containing compounds. In addition, several oxidation enzymes such as monoamine and diamine oxidases and alcohol dehydrogenase are found in the soluble fraction of the cell. With the exception of methoxyflurane, the inhaled anesthetics are not metabolized by these other phase 1 enzyme systems (Wang et al., 1986).

Phase 2 or conjugation reactions are syntheses that often involve the transfer of a compound from its activated form to the xenobiotic or drug. The most frequently encountered example and one that is typical of this class of reactions is the conjugation of a drug with glucuronic acid. It is catalyzed by uridine diphosphate (UDP)-glucuronyltransferase, which is tightly bound to the smooth endoplasmic reticulum.

UDP-glucuronic acid + ROH

$$\xrightarrow{\text{UDP-glucuronyltransferase}} \text{RO-glucuronic acid} + \text{UDP}$$

Addition of the glucuronic acid to the drug (R) may be to groups other than -OH, such as -COOH, $-NH_2$ and -SH groups. These are not present on inhaled anesthetics but may be acquired as a result of phase 1 reactions. The resultant glucuronide is more water soluble because it contains a polar sugar moiety.

Enzyme Induction

A variety of factors can affect drug metabolism. They include, age, sex, nutritional status, pregnancy, disease processes, especially of the liver, and genetic factors. In addition, certain drug-metabolizing activities of the endoplasmic reticulum can be increased or decreased by specific foreign chemicals. Most commonly, such chemicals are enzyme inducers, that is, they increase the rate of synthesis of metabolizing enzymes without increasing the rate of degradation. Two main classes of enzyme inducers represented by phenobarbitone and 3-methylcholanthrene are found. They differ in the pattern of membrane-bound enzymes that they induce. There are many examples in

general medical practice in which enzyme induction alters the therapeutic efficacy or degree of toxicity of a drug. In contrast, although increased metabolism of some currently used inhaled anesthetics may occur following enzyme induction, the clinical consequences are minimal.

METABOLISM OF INDIVIDUAL INHALED ANESTHETICS

Only metabolism of the most widely used inhaled anesthetics, halothane ($CF_3CHClBr$), enflurane (CHF_2-O-CF_2CHClF), isoflurane (CHF_2-O-$CHClCF_3$) and nitrous oxide (N_2O) will be described in this brief overview. Historical and experimental anesthetics and those of limited clinical use are described in other sources (Cohen and Van Dyke, 1977; Plummer et al., 1982b; Baden and Rice, 1986).

Halothane

Recent experiments indicate that about 45% of an absorbed dose of halothane is metabolized and that metabolism plays a more important role in the drug's elimination than was previously recognized (Carpenter et al., 1986). Most metabolism occurs via an oxidation pathway (Fig. 56.2) that results in the

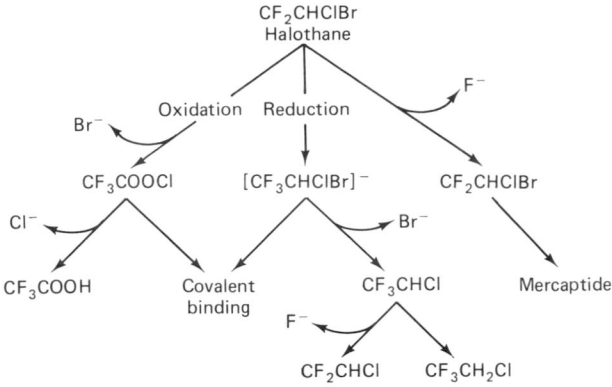

Fig. 56.2 Halothane metabolic pathway.

formation of trifluoroacetic acid, and chloride and bromide ions. These end-products are excreted in the urine as sodium salts (Rehder et al., 1967). Trifluoroacetyl chloride is a reactive intermediate metabolite.

Halothane is also metabolized to a small extent by a reductive pathway (Fig. 56.2). The reductive metabolism is accentuated in experimental animals by hypoxia (Cousins et al., 1979; Ross et al., 1979; McLain et al., 1979; Jee et al., 1980) and is presumed to proceed via a cytochrome-P450 catalyzed one or two-electron reduction of the halothane molecule. The end-products of reductive metabolism are bromide and fluoride ions and two volatile compounds, difluoro-chloroethylene and trifluorochloroethane (Mukai et al., 1977; Cousins et al., 1979; Sharp et al., 1979). In addition, difluorochlorobromoethylene has been identified as a urinary mercaptide (Cohen et al., 1975). Free radicals are produced during the metabolism of halothane (Plummer et al., 1982a) and may have a role in the production of halothane-associated hepatitis, a subject that will be discussed in the toxicity section. Enzyme inducing agents increase reductive metabolism and hepatotoxicity in experimental animals (Reynolds and Moslen, 1977; Cousins et al., 1979; Jee et al., 1980) but there is little evidence that they play a similar role in man.

Enflurane

Enflurane is oxidatively metabolized by the cytochrome-P450 system. Estimates of the absorbed dose metabolized range from about 2.5%-8.5% (Chase et al., 1971; Carpenter et al., 1986). Initial oxidation may occur at either the chlorofluoromethyl or the difluoromethyl carbon (Fig. 56.3).

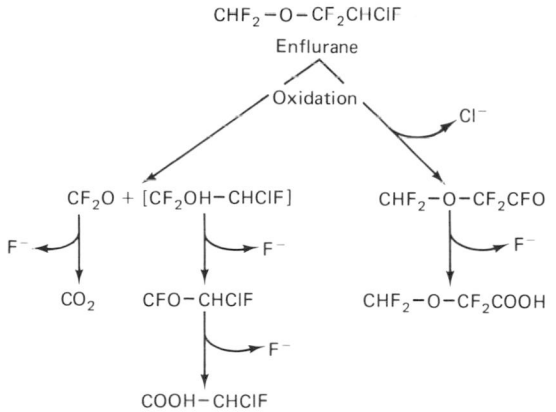

Fig. 56.3 Enflurane metabolic pathway.

Predictions based on molecular theory indicate that oxidation at the chlorofluoromethyl carbon would be the preferred pathway (Loew et al., 1974). The isolation of moderate amounts of difluoromethoxydifluoroacetic acid in rat liver and human urine but only trace amounts of chlorofluoroacetic acid support the prediction (Burke et al., 1981). Reductive metabolism does not occur. The effects of enzyme induction on enflurane defluorination are interesting. The classic inducing agents, phenobarbital and 3-methylcholanthrene, do not increase production of inorganic fluoride in experimental animals or in man (Barr et al., 1974; Dooley et al., 1979; Van Dyke, 1983; Pantuck et al., 1985). Compounds containing the hydrazine moiety, however, such as the antituberculous drug isoniazid, are able to induce enflurane defluorination (Rice et al., 1980).

Isoflurane

Isoflurane, a pentafluorinated methyl ethyl ether, is an isomer of enflurane. Only 0.2% of an absorbed dose is oxidatively metabolized and, thus, it is the least metabolized of all the fluorinated anesthetics (Holaday et al., 1975). The principal metabolites of isoflurane are trifluoroacetic acid, fluoride ions and chloride ions. Cleavage occurs predominantly at the ether linkage and proceeds along either of two pathways with subsequent release of fluoride ions from the one-carbon fragments (Fig. 56.4). Like enflurane, isoflurane does

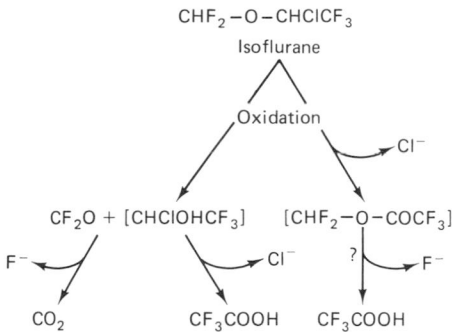

Fig. 56.4 Isoflurane metabolic pathway.

not undergo reductive metabolism. Enzyme induction occurs in rats pretreated with phenobarbitone and other drugs, and results in increased production of inorganic fluoride (Rice et al., 1983; Bradshaw and Ivanetich, 1984). There is no evidence, however, that similar increased defluorination occurs in surgical patients who are taking enzyme inducing agents (Mazze et al., 1974).

Nitrous Oxide

There is no evidence that nitrous oxide is metabolized by mammalian tissues. Intestinal bacteria of rat and man, however, can reductively metabolize nitrous oxide *in vitro* (Hong et al., 1980). The reaction probably occurs via a single electron transfer process that results in hydroxyl radicals and molecular nitrogen (Fig. 56.5).

$$N_2O \xrightarrow{e^-} [N_2O] \longrightarrow \cdot OH + OH^- + N_2$$

Fig. 56.5 Proposed nitrous oxide metabolic pathway in bacteria.

TOXICITY

Toxicity of inhaled anesthetics can be acute or chronic. Acute toxicity occurs after a single administration or after several administrations within a 24 hour period. Classic examples in anesthetic practice include polyuric renal failure after methoxyflurane anesthesia and massive hepatic failure after halothane anesthesia. Chronic toxicity requires repeated exposure to the anesthetic for months to years. The neurotoxicity seen in abusers of nitrous oxide is one

TABLE 56.1
MECHANISMS OF ANESTHETIC TOXICITY

1. Intracellular accumulation of toxic end-products

2. Covalent binding of reactive intermediates to cellular macromolecules

3. Formation of haptens that initiate an immunological reaction

4. Physicochemical reaction of nitrous oxide with vitamin B_{12}

example. Regardless of the type of toxicity, a limited number of mechanisms are recognized (Table 56.1). In the following sections, toxicity of the four commonly used inhaled anesthetics noted above will be described.

Halothane

Halothane Hepatitis

Hepatitis is by far the most important toxic effect of halothane. Many reviews about it have been published, including those by Strunin (1977), Brown (1981) and Neuberger and Kenna (1987) and only the most salient features will be described here.

The incidence of massive hepatic necrosis following halothane administration is low, about 1 in 35 000 (Bunker et al., 1969). Nevertheless, in Britain, some investigators regard it as the commonest cause of iatrogenic induced fulminant hepatic failure (Neuberger et al., 1987). Lesser degrees of liver damage probably occur much more often. There are several factors which appear to predispose an individual to halothane hepatitis: namely, obesity, female sex, older age, previous allergic history and previous halothane anesthesia. Some long-held clinical beliefs, however, are now thought to be false. For example, halothane hepatitis was once thought to be extremely rare in children but is now known to occur moderately often in this group (Neuberger et al., 1987).

The low incidence of halothane hepatitis and the lack of a suitable animal model have made the elucidation of its etiology a difficult and controversial task. Two main theories have been proposed. The first is that a toxic metabolite formed during halothane's biotransformation is directly responsible for the hepatic damage. The discovery of a reductive pathway of halothane metabolism added considerable weight to the theory. This pathway produces reactive intermediates that are capable of binding to liver macromolecules and presumably of causing hepatocyte dysfunction and death. In many animal models, low oxygen tension and enzyme induction exacerbate the reductive pathway and result in increased concentrations of free radicals, increased convalent binding of metabolites and more severe liver damage (Widger et al., 1976; Reynolds et al., 1977; Plummer et al.,

1982a). It is unknown whether such animal models in which hepatic necrosis can be produced so reliably are relevant to the human condition which occurs so sporadically. Those who believe that a direct parallel exists between animal and human liver damage have suggested that a pattern of enzymes that favour the reductive pathway of halothane metabolism occurs in a minority of individuals (Brown and Geha, 1983). If other factors are present such as hypoxia or retention of toxic metabolites from a prior halothane anesthetic, severe liver damage may occur. No evidence has been gathered in man to support this theory. The second main theory, which has been extensively discussed (Neuberger et al., 1987), is that halothane hepatitis is an immune mediated phenomenon. It also depends on the metabolism of halothane, but in this case, reactive metabolites bind to cellular macromolecules to generate unusual antigens that are recognized as foreign by the body. The unusually high prevalence of nonspecific rashes, arthralgias, peripheral eosinophilia and auto-antibodies seen in patients after halothane hepatitis favor an immunological etiology. Additionally, there is evidence that specific antibodies and lymphocytes that are cytotoxic to halothane sensitized hepatocytes are present in patients who develop halothane hepatitis but not in those who develop other types of liver damage (Vergani et al., 1980; Neuberger et al., 1983). Many questions must be answered, however, before an immunological mechanism can be definitely implicated. For example, what is the nature of the antibodies and how are they generated? Even an immunological mechansm of halothane hepatitis may depend on an idiosyncratic pathway of metabolism.

Other Toxicity

There is no convincing evidence that halothane produces serious toxicity in other organ systems. Furthermore, it is not a chemical teratogen or carcinogen (Wharton et al., 1979; Baden et al., 1979) and is not a mutagen in mammalian cells (Basler and Röhrborn, 1981).

Enflurane

Nephrotoxicity

Because of the release of moderate amounts of inorganic fluoride (F^-) during the metabolism of enflurane, questions about its nephrotoxic potential have been raised. Theoretically, the risk should be much less than with methoxyflurane because of enflurane's lower rate of metabolism and lower lipid solubility. Results from human studies indicate that this is the case. In surgical patients receiving enflurane exposures averaging 2.7 MAC-hours, peak serum F^- levels averaged only 22.2 µmol/L and no renal impairment was observed (Cousins et al., 1976). In volunteers, 9.6 MAC-hours of enflurane produced peak levels of only 33.6 μmol/L and no clinically significant renal impairment (Mazze et al., 1977). The levels of F⁻ observed are well below 50–80 μmol/L at which clinically significant, but minimal, renal insufficiency is seen with methoxyflurane. Thus, enflurane appears to be safe for the majority of patients. Even patients with mild to moderate renal insufficiency appear to suffer no additional renal impairment if enflurane rather than halothane is used as part of their anesthetic regimen (Mazze et al., 1984). Patients on enzyme inducing drugs such as phenobarbitone and ethanol also do not develop renal impairment after enflurane anesthesia (Dooley et al., 1979). The only patients who have levels of F⁻ in the potentially toxic range after enflurane anesthesia are about 50% of those who are chronically treated with isoniazid (Mazze et al., 1982). Unlike patients who have similar peak levels of F⁻ after methoxyflurane, however, these patients do not develop clinically significant renal impairment. The reason is that levels peak earlier and fall quicker after enflurane than after methoxyflurane exposure because of enflurane's lower lipid solubility. Thus, the kidney is exposed to much lesser amounts of F⁻.

Other Toxicity

Enflurane-induced hepatotoxicity has occasionally been reported (Lewis et al., 1983) but generally discounted for lack of convincing evidence. Even if one accepted the reports as real, the incidence would be less than one case per 2 million administrations. There is no evidence for other specific organ toxicity, mutagenicity, teratogenicity or carcinogenicity.

Isoflurane

Its low rate of metabolism and the lack of any known toxic metabolites has led to the hope that isoflurane would be without toxic effects. Indeed, this appears to be the case; after at least 100 million administrations around the world, no significant evidence for acute or chronic toxicity has been reported.

Nitrous Oxide

The disruptive effect of nitrous oxide on vitamin B_{12} and folate metabolism has been well described (Chanarin, 1980; Nunn, 1987). Its biochemical basis is oxidation of the cobalt in vitamin B_{12} and the subsequent irreversible inactivation of methionine synthase. This cytosolular enzyme catalyzes the conversion of methyltetrahydrofolate and homocysteine to tetrahydrofolate and methionine (Fig. 56.6). Failure to produce these products has a number of biochemical consequences including reduced synthesis of DNA and proteins. The clinical syndrome that follows is essentially the same as that seen in pernicious anemia; there is megaloblastic hemopoiesis and subacute combined degeneration of the cord.

The inhibition of methionine synthase is both rapid and long-lasting. Within one hour of exposure to high concentrations (50–70%) of nitrous oxide in rats (Deacon et al., 1980) and mice (Koblin et al., 1981), the enzyme is almost completely inactivated. Recovery of activity takes 3–4 days because oxidation of the covalently bound vitamin B_{12} is irreversible and new enzyme must be synthesized. Human methionine synthase is inactivated more slowly (Koblin et al., 1982). Nevertheless, after several hours of routine anesthesia at least 50% of activity is lost. The decrease of thymidine synthesis takes somewhat longer to develop but also lasts several days. Experimental data suggest that there is a threshold concentration between 500–1000 ppm (0.05–0.1%) below which

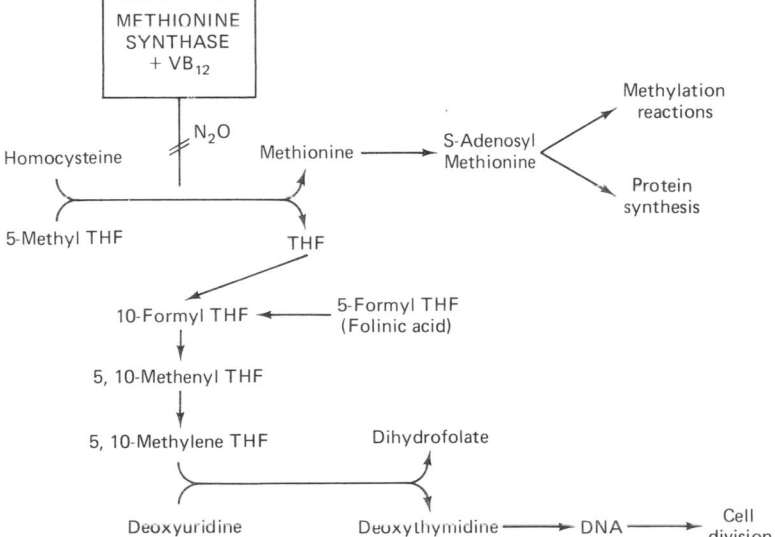

Fig. 56.6 Simplified vitamin B_{12} and folate pathways affected by nitrous oxide.

nitrous oxide has no biochemical effect (Sharer et al., 1983). The shortest exposure time required to produce megaloblastic hemopoiesis varies among patients and perhaps depends on their general state of health. In healthy patients undergoing routine surgery, mild megaloblastic bone marrow changes are not seen after 6 h but are seen after about 12 h of exposure to 50% nitrous oxide; after 24 h of exposure, changes are marked (O'Sullivan et al., 1981). Limited evidence suggests that nitrous oxide produces bone marrow changes earlier in seriously ill patients (Amos et al., 1982), though, this remains to be confirmed in controlled studies. Evidence also suggests that the bone marrow changes are preventable by pretreating patients with large doses of folinic acid (O'Sullivan et al., 1981).

The neurologic disease, subacute combined degeneration of the spinal cord, develops in those who chronically abuse nitrous oxide or in those rare individuals who work for many months in an environment grossly contaminated with the gas (Sahenk et al., 1978; Layzer, 1978). The most likely mechanism is a lack of methionine which results in an interference in myelin production (Scott et al., 1981). Dental personnel who are occasionally exposed to greater than 1000 ppm waste nitrous oxide in poorly ventilated dental suites for long periods may be particularly at risk. On the other hand, operating room personnel are almost never exposed to such conditions and would not be expected to have problems. Epidemiologic surveys confirm that dental but not operating room personnel have a higher incidence of neurologic disease (Brodsky et al., 1981) although exposure to waste nitrous oxide has not definitely been shown to be the cause.

The reproductive toxicity which follows nitrous oxide exposure has been reviewed recently (Baden, 1985). When high concentrations (50–75%) are administered continuously to pregnant rodents for at least 24 hours during organogenesis, the rates of resorptions (equivalent to spontaneous abortions in humans) and congenital anomalies are increased markedly. Exposure either to lesser concentrations or for shorter periods usually does not result in adverse effects. No equivalent human data are available. The assumption has been made that nitrous oxide's effects on vitamin B_{12} and folate metabolism are responsible for the adverse reproductive effects in experimental animals. Recent evidence casts some doubt on that hypothesis (Fujinaga et al., 1987), although data are too preliminary to draw firm conclusions.

REFERENCES

Amos R.J., Amess J.A.L., Hind C.J., et al. (1982). Incidence and pathogenesis of acute megaloblastic bone marrow change in patients receiving intensive care. *Lancet*, **2**, 835.

Baden J.M. (1985). Mutagenicity carcinogenicity, and teratogenicity of nitrous oxide. In *Nitrous Oxide N_2O*. (Eger E. I, II., eds.). New York: Elsevier.

Baden J.M., Mazze R.I., Wharton R.S., et al. (1979). Carcinogenicity of halothane in Swiss/ICR mice. *Anesthesiology*, **51**, 20.

Baden J.M., Rice S.A. (1986). Metabolism and toxicity of inhaled anesthetics. In *Anesthesia, Vol. 1*. 2nd edn. (Miller R.D., ed.). New York: Churchill Livingstone.

Barr G.A., Cousins M.J., Mazze R.I., et al. (1974). A comparison of the renal effects and metabolism of enflurane and methoxyflurane in Fischer 344 rats. *J. Pharm. Exp. Ther.*, **188**, 257.

Basler A., Röhrborn G. (1981). Lack of mutagenic effects of halothane in mammals *in vivo*. *Anesthesiology*, **55**, 143.

Bradshaw J.J., Ivanetich K.M. (1984). Isoflurane: a comparison of its metabolism by human and rat hepatic cytochrome P-450. *Anesth. Analg.*, **63**, 805.

Brault D. (1985). Model studies in cytochrome P-450-mediated toxicity of halogenated compounds: radical processes involving iron porphyrins. *Environ. Health Perspect.*, **64**, 53.

Brodsky J.B., Cohen E.N., Brown B.W., Jr., et al. (1981). Exposure to nitrous oxide and neurologic disease among dental professionals. *Anesth. Analg.*, **60**, 201.

Brown B.R. Jr. (1981). Hepatotoxicity of halogenated inhalation anesthetics. In *Anesthesia and the Patient with Liver Disease*. Vol. 4. (Brown B. R., ed.). Philadelphia: F.A. Davis.

Brown B.R., Geha D.C. (1983). Inhalation anesthetics and hepatic injury. In *Complication in Anesthesiology*. (Orkin F.K., Cooperman L.H., eds.). Philadelphia: Lippincott.

Bunker J.P., Forrest W.H., Mosteller F., et al. (1969). *The National Halothane Study*. Maryland: National Institute of General Medical Sciences.

Burke T.R., Branchflower R.V., Lees D.E., et al. (1981). Mechanism of defluorination of enflurane. Identification of an organic metabolite in rat and man. *Drug Metab. Disposition*, **9**, 19.

Carpenter R.L., Eger E.I., Johnson B.H., et al. (1986). The extent of metabolism of inhaled anesthetics in humans. *Anesthesiology*, **65**, 201.

Chanarin I. (1980). Cobalamins and nitrous oxide: a review. *J. Clin. Pathol.*, **33**, 909.

Chase R.E., Holaday D.A., Fiserova-Bergerova V., et al. (1971). The biotransformation of Ethrane in man. *Anesthesiology*, **35**, 262.

Cohen E.N., Trudell J.R., Edmunds H.N., et al. (1975). Urinary metabolites of halothane in man. *Anesthesiology*, **43**, 392.

Cohen E.N., Van Dyke R.A. (1977). *Metabolism of Volatile Anesthetics: implications for Toxicity*. Menlo Park: Addison-Wesley.

Cousins M.J., Greenstein L.R., Hitt B.A., et al. (1976). Metabolism and renal effects of enflurane in man. *Anesthesiology*, **44**, 44.

Cousins M.J., Sharp J.H., Gourley G.K., et al. (1979). Hepatotoxicity and halothane metabolism in an animal model with application for human toxicity. *Anaesth. Intens. Care*, **7**, 9.

Deacon R., Lumb M., Muir M., et al. (1980). Selective inactivation of vitamin B_{12} in rats by nitrous oxide (N_2O). In *Vitamin B_{12}*. (Zagalak B., Friedrich W., eds.). Berlin: Walter de Gruyter.

Dooley J.R., Mazze R.I., Rice S.A., et al. (1979). Is enflurane defluorination inducible in man? *Anesthesiology*, **50**, 213.

Fujinaga M., Baden J.M., Yhap E.O., et al. (1987). Reproductive and teratogenic effects of nitrous oxide, isoflurane, and their combination in Sprague-Dawley rats. *Anesthesiology*, **67**, 960.

Holaday D.A., Fiserova-Bergerova V.I., Latto I.P., et al. (1975). Resistance of isoflurane to biotransformation in man. *Anesthesiology*, **43**, 325.

Hong K., Trudell J.R., O'Neil J.R., et al. (1980). Metabolism of nitrous oxide by human and rat intestinal contents. *Anesthesiology*, **52**, 16.

Jee R.C., Sipes I.G., Gandolfi A.J., et al. (1980). Factors influencing halothane hepatotoxicity in the rat hypoxic model. *Toxicol. Appl. Pharmacol.*, **52**, 267.

Koblin D.D., Waskell L., Watson J.E., et al. (1982). Nitrous oxide inactivates methionine synthetase in human liver. *Anesth. Analg.*, **61**, 75.

Koblin D.D., Watson J.E., Deedy J.E., et al. (1981). Inactivation of methionine synthetase by N_2O in mice. *Anesthesiology*, **54**, 318.

Layzer R.B. (1978). Myeloneuropathy after prolonged exposure to nitrous oxide, *Lancet*, **2**, 1227.

Lewis J.H., Zimmerman H.J., Ishak K.G., et al. (1983). Enflurane hepatotoxicity. A clinico-pathologic study of 24 cases. *Ann. Intern. Med.*, **98**, 984.

Loew G., Motulsky H., Trudell J., et al. (1974). Quantum chemical studies of the metabolism of the inhalation anesthetics methoxyflurane, enflurane, and isoflurane. *Mol. Pharm.*, **10**, 406.

Mazze R.I., Calverley R.K., Smith N.T. (1977). Inorganic fluoride nephrotoxicity: prolonged enflurane and halothane anesthesia in volunteers. *Anesthesiology*, **46**, 265.

Mazze R.I., Hitt B.A., Cousins M.J. (1974). Effect of enzyme induction with phenobarbital in the *in vivo* and *in vitro* defluorination of isoflurane and methoxyflurane. *J. Pharm. Exp. Ther.*, **190**, 523.

Mazze R.I., Sievenpiper T.S., Stevenson J. (1984). Renal effects of enflurane and halothane in patients with abnormal renal function. *Anesthesiology*, **60**, 161.

Mazze R.I., Woodruff R.E., Heerdt M.E. (1982). Isoniazid-induced enflurane defluorination in humans. *Anesthesiology*, **57**, 5.

McLain G.E., Sipes I.G., Brown B.R. (1979). An animal model of halothane hepatotoxicity: roles of enzyme induction and hypoxia. *Anesthesiology*, **51**, 321.

Mukai S., Morio M., Fujii K., et al. (1977). Volatile metabolites of halothane in the rabbit. *Anesthesiology*, **47**, 248.

Neuberger J.M., Gimson A.E.S., Davis M., et al. (1983). Specific serological markers in the diagnosis of fulminant hepatic failure following halothane anaesthesia. *Br. J. Anaesth.*, **55**, 15.

Neuberger J., Kenna J.G. (1987). Halothane hepatitis: a model of immune mediated drug hepatotoxicity. *Clin. Sci.*, **72**, 263.

Nunn J.F. (1987). Clinical aspects of the interaction between nitrous oxide and vitamin B_{12}. *Br. J. Anaesth.*, **59**, 3.

O'Sullivan H., Jannings F., Ward K., et al. (1981). Human bone marrow biochemical function and megaloblastic hematopoiesis after nitrous oxide anesthesia. *Anesthesiology*, **55**, 645.

Pantuck E.J., Pantuck C.B., Ryan D.E., et al. (1985). In-

hibition and stimulation of enflurane metabolism in the rat following a single dose or chronic administration of ethanol. *Anesthesiology*, **62**, 255.

Plummer J.L., Beckwith A.L.J., Bastin F.N., et al. (1982a). Free radical formation *in vivo* and hepatotoxicity due to anesthesia with halothane. *Anesthesiology*, **57**, 160.

Plummer J.L., Cousins M.J., Hall P.M. (1982b). Volatile anaesthetic metabolism and acute toxicity. In *Reviews on Drug Metabolism and Drug Interactions*. Vol. IV. (Beckett A.H., Temple P., eds.). London: Freund.

Rehder K., Forbes J., Alter H., et al. (1967). Halothane biotransformation in man. A quantitative study. *Anesthesiology*, **28**, 711.

Reynolds E.S., Moslen M.T. (1977). Halothane hepatotoxicity: enhancement by polychlorinated biphenyl pretreatment. *Anesthesiology*, **47**, 19.

Rice S.A., Dooley J.R., Mazze R.I. (1983). Metabolism by rat hepatic microsomes of fluorinated ether anesthetics following ethanol consumption. *Anesthesiology*, **58**, 237.

Rice S.A., Sbordone L., Mazze R.I. (1980). Metabolism by rat hepatic microsomes of fluorinated ether anesthetics following isoniazid administration. *Anesthesiology*, **53**, 489.

Ross W.T., Daggy B.P., Cardell R.R. (1979). Hepatic necrosis caused by halothane and hypoxia in phenobarbital-treated rats. *Anesthesiology*, **51**, 327.

Sahenk Z., Mendell J.R., Couri D., et al. (1978). Polyneuropathy from inhalation of N_2O cartridges through a whipped-cream dispenser. *Neurology*, **28**, 485.

Scott J.M., Wilson P., Dinn J.J., et al. (1981). Pathogenesis of subacute combined degeneration: a result of methyl group deficiency. *Lancet*, **8**, 334.

Sharer N.M., Nunn J.F., Royston J.P., et al. (1983). Effects of chronic exposure to nitrous oxide on methionine synthase activity. *Br. J. Anaesth.*, **55**, 693.

Sharp J.H., Trudell J.R., Cohen E.N. (1979). Volatile metabolites and decomposition products of halothane in man. *Anesthesiology*, **50**, 2.

Strunin L. (1977). Postoperative hepatic dysfunction. In *The liver and Anaesthesia*. Vol. 3 (Strunin L., ed.). London: W.B. Saunders Company.

Van Dyke R.A. (1983). Enflurane, isoflurane and methoxyflurane metabolism in rat hepatic microsomes from ethanol-treated animals. *Anesthesiology*, **58**, 221.

Vergani D., Mieli Vergani G., Alberti A., et al. (1980). Antibodies to the surface of halothane altered rabbit hepatocytes in patients with severe halothane associated hepatitis. *New Engl. J. Med.*, **303**, 66.

Wang S., Rice S.A., Serra M.T., et al. (1986). Purification and identification of rat hepatic cytosolic enzymes responsible for defluorination of methoxyflurane and fluoroacetate. *Drug Metab. Dispos.* **14**, 392.

Wharton R.S., Wilson A.I., Mazze R.I., et al. (1979). Fetal morphology in mice exposed to halothane. *Anesthesiology*, **50**, 41.

Widger L.A., Gandolfi A.J., Van Dyke R.A. (1976). Hypoxia and halothane metabolism *in vivo*: release of inorganic fluoride and halothane metabolite binding to cellular constituents. *Anesthesiology*, **44**, 197.

57. Drug Trials and Statistical Validation

Ian Power and A. A. Spence

This chapter is about the collection and analysis of information for the purposes of research and development, including audit, in clinical practice. For many years the mainstay of research in anaesthesia has been the *clinical trial* in which an arrangement is contrived to observe perhaps two, often small, groups of subjects who are assumed to differ in only one respect—exposure or lack of exposure to the factor under investigation. The commonest example is a drug trial. Superficially attractive, this approach is increasingly under scrutiny because of the difficulty in being quite sure that no other factor can influence the outcome; that is, the study is properly *controlled*.

EPIDEMIOLOGY

In recent years the development of computers has made it possible for large numbers of observations on or characteristics of patients to be stored and analysed easily, and this has led to the development of epidemiological studies. *Epidemiology* is the study of a population as it is; thus there is no manipulation of the conditions as in a clinical trial. Epidemiological studies may consider a *population*, that is, everyone known to exist in a particular defined category. For example the MRC sponsored study on the health of women doctors in the UK 1976–86 (Spence, 1987)

sought to study all women in the hospital service under the age of 40 years at the time of recruitment.

Sometimes information derived from a whole population is unnecessary or difficult or expensive to obtain and an appropriate fraction or *sample* of the population is taken instead.

Epidemiological studies allow us to calculate the *incidence* or *prevalence* of a disorder or problem. Incidence is the rate of occurrence—a measure of the emergence of new cases. Prevalence is a measure of the occurrence in a population.

We can say that the incidence of suxamethonium apnoea is approximately 1 in 3 000 adults who received the drug. If we know how many patients in the population have atypical pseudocholinesterase, that is an expression of the prevalence of that state.

Incidence is affected by preventive measures or increased causation of a particular disorder. Prevalence is influenced by a recovery or death.

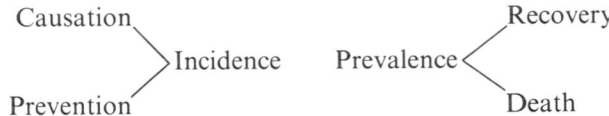

Epidemiological studies are increasingly applied to *audit* of clinical practice—a measure of the quality of a process or outcome. Audit is regarded as an important component of *quality assurance* in medicine, a term which denotes the steps that are taken, usually by the medical profession itself, to define and maintain standards below which no practitioner will fall and which are recognized as being in the public interest.

Cohort Studies

A group of individuals (cohort) considered to be subject to an influence or risk are reviewed in comparison with a control group, similar in every respect to the cohort except that they are not subject to the risk factor. For example, the well known UK study of smoking in doctors (Doll and Peto, 1976) compared mortality in smokers and non-smokers over 20 years. It was assumed that in other respects (social class and environmental influences) the two groups were the same. Thus differences in disease patterns were considered to reflect the effect of cigarette smoking.

Cohort studies may be *cross-sectional*—the cohort and the control group are examined at a single point in time—or *longitudinal* in which the study is conducted over a period of time with continuous interval observations. Both cross sectional and longitudinal studies can be illustrated by the long-running issue as to whether or not the operating room as a working environment is hazardous to health, particularly as regards reproductive outcome. Various cross sectional studies in the 1970s (Tannenbaum and Goldberg, 1985) suggested that there may be a variety of risks, notably an increase in the reporting of spontaneous abortion by those who were exposed to the operating room environment. The United Kingdom MRC study referred to above, is a longitudinal study which appears to be showing that the early anxieties may have been ill founded. Among possible explanations for the apparent discrepancy is the fact that cross sectional studies call for a very high standard of information gathering, since there may not be the opportunity to make further enquiries of the cohort after the initial collection of information has been made. Confounding variables (discussed in greater detail in the section on clinical trials) may be crucial. Information gathering on spontaneous abortion, for example, must take account of a wide variety of factors which are thought to influence the risk of abortion: maternal age, smoking and alcohol habit, previous obstetric history etc. Where cohort studies depend on individuals providing information on a questionnaire, involving the need to recall information that is several years old, there is a strong possibility of bias. Axelsson and Rylander (1982) provided convincing evidence that the recall of miscarriages in a postal questionnaire among anaesthetists differed from the information already held in an occupational health record. The titling or explanation given at the outset of a postal enquiry may bias responses (Vessey, 1978) because it may induce antagonism or motivation differentially among the respondents. The use of checklists to stimulate the memory of respondents is well known to produce a greater yield or reporting than will occur if a questionnaire simply offers a space for open recall.

Case Control Studies

These set out to examine a group of patients with a specified disease or characteristic and a control group deemed suitable for comparison. Let us assume access to a large file of accurate records regarding the outcome from spinal (subarachnoid) anaesthesia. From this we might choose to select *cases* of severe headache as a postoperative complication. For control purposes we will take all patients receiving spinal anaesthesia (Table 57.1).

TABLE 57.1

	Total on file	Headache
	30 000	98
Age (*years*)		
mean	48	32
s.d.	6.3	4.3
range	16–87	18–62
Females	18 320	76
Males	11 780	22

Applying statistical tests to these data, and indeed simply looking at them, it emerges that the mean age of those who suffer headache is significantly less than that for the whole group and the problem appears to be much more common in women than in men. From such data it would seem reasonable to conclude that young women are a high risk group in relation to spinal headache. This assumes, however, that no other important factor has been overlooked.

THE CLINICAL TRIAL

Clinical trials can be considered under the following headings:

1. The Hypothesis.
2. Experimental Design.
3. Presentation and statistical analysis of results.

The Hypothesis

At the centre of any clinical trial is an idea, or hypothesis, which is under scrutiny. The formulation, investigation and resultant modification of this idea is discussed in this section. The process used to examine an hypothesis is the *experimental method* of scientific investigation.

The Idea and the Hypothesis

A clinical trial (concerning a drug for example) may be precipitated by a question arising from published literature, scientific meetings, informal discussions, a problem encountered in practice, or perhaps even inspiration. Many published trials nowadays are set up by the pharmaceutical company concerned, as part of their programme of research and also to satisfy drug regulatory authorities. The idea constructed as a statement forms the initial hypothesis for the study. One necessary qualification of an hypothesis is that it is open to analysis and testing by scientific methods.

The Testing of an Hypothesis by the Experimental Method

The experimental method was developed by Claude Bernard as a counter to the school of thought which had proposed that advancement in scientific knowledge was made only from deduction on the basis of known facts. Such reasoning tended to produce little advancement and much sterile discussion.

In the experimental method, deduction from a known body of knowledge is only an initial stage which provides ideas which can then be tested by the practical step of performing an experiment and observing and analysing the results. The experiment is designed to test the hypothesis. Depending on the result, the hypothesis is rejected, modified, or retained for further examination.

The experiment, therefore, is central to this method. It must be designed, executed, and analysed correctly. It is possible to confuse the issue by asking either such complicated or so many questions in the experiment that the answer cannot be recognized from the results. Therefore the experimental design should be as simple as possible. Careful observation and recording of the results is also essential for the success of this method.

A necessary attribute of an experiment is that it's method be known, and that the results are reproducible, allowing independent verification of the findings by other investigators.

The experimental method is therefore a continuing process whereby hypotheses are proposed, experiments performed, results observed and analysed, and further hypotheses evolved.

Drug Trials

The application of such a scientific method to clinical investigations may not always appear easy. Hence the need for a clear understanding of the hypothesis. For example, if a new agent is being assessed as a possible analgesic its effect may be compared with that of an active agent. The hypothesis to be tested would be that the active agent would have greater effect than the placebo.

The importance of understanding this is reflected in the terminology used in the statistical analysis of clinical trials. The basis of most statistical testing in this situation is an estimation of the probability of the *null hypothesis* occurring. The null hypothesis in the analgesic study would be that *there is no difference between the new drug and the placebo*. The original idea that *the new agent is more potent than a placebo* would form the *alternate hypothesis*.

If the statistical test applied indicated that the probability of the null hypothesis occurring was unlikely according to predetermined criteria, (usually less than five times in a hundred), then the null hypothesis would be rejected in favour of the alternate hypothesis.

The example given was a simple one, but there is often a tendency to be unclear over the main point of the investigation and therefore to neglect the initial step of defining the hypothesis to be examined. Unfortunately this may lead to complicated statistical tests being applied to results in a vain attempt to find an answer to an undefined question.

EXPERIMENTAL DESIGN

The analysis of results from a trial is confused by the sources of variability encountered in clinical studies. This variability may make conclusions from the study difficult to obtain, and may indeed confound the whole investigation. Observer and subject bias can also invalidate a study if not accounted for.

These problems and the measures used to minimize them are described under the following headings.

1. Sources of variability
2. Confounding factors
3. The design of trials
4. Bias

Sources of Variability

a. Subject
b. Environmental

The variability encountered in drug trials can be attributed to two main sources: the variable response shown by different individuals to a drug—*subject*, and the variability introduced by practical aspects of the experimental design—*environmental*. The factors involved in each group are listed in Table 57.2.

TABLE 57.2

Subject	Environmental
Age	Time of observation
Sex	Apparatus
Weight	Method of drug administration
Intelligence	
Personality	
Motivation	
Disease states	
Other drug therapy	

Subject Variables

In a clinical study the subjects can be expected to differ in their response to a drug for various reasons. For example, if the trial concerned the effect of an agent on arterial pressure, then individuals of different ages may be expected to have varying responses. Similarly, an investigation of an analgesic agent would have to take into account the age and sex of the subjects since each of these factors is considered to affect pain tolerance. The weight of the patient may affect the subject's response in a fixed dose study. Intelligence, personality, and motivation are of importance in many studies, especially those concerning the individual's feelings, as in the production of anxiolysis. In the same manner the presence of disease states and drug therapies may modify the individual's response to many trial drugs.

Environmental Variables

Practical aspects of a study may also introduce variability. For example, in studies of postoperative analgesia it is obviously necessary to make observations on the effect of treatment at comparable times in the postoperative period. Equipment used to measure the response to a drug may be associated with inherent errors, as in the recording of arterial pressure. In addition, if different drugs in a trial are given by various routes or regimens this is obviously a source of variability in response.

If, in a drug study, the subject and environmental factors happened to have equal effect on the groups of subjects studied, then the scatter of the results would be increased and conclusions more difficult to make.

However, if these factors were unevenly spread between groups then the implications for the study would be much more serious (*see below*).

Confounding Factors

Confounding factors may be considered as sources of variability which are not spread equally through the groups of subjects being investigated. In this case, instead of making the conclusions more difficult to arrive at, they may invalidate, or confound, the investigation.

Consider a trial to investigate the potency of an analgesic in the postoperative period. The drug is given to one group of patients (A) and the analgesic potency compared with that of a standard drug administered to another group (B). Later it emerges that A are predominantly elderly males, whereas B comprises mainly of young females. The two groups are obviously not comparable.

The Design of Trials

a. The control of variables
b. The controlled clinical trial
c. Two-sample designs
d. Randomization

It is the purpose of the design of drug studies to reduce the effect of the factors described above, and to prevent any from confounding the study.

The Control of Variables

Individual variables can be reduced in magnitude by controlling their appearance in the study. For example, the effect of age can be reduced by only including patients of a certain age range in the study. This will not remove the effect of age, but diminish it. In the same way, the effect of weight can be controlled, but other subject variables, such as personality, are more difficult to control. Often, particularly when small numbers are studied, failure to elicit full information about the subjects conceals critical factors which could invalidate the whole exercise.

This form of control can only be taken so far, otherwise the trial is comprised of very artificial groups of subjects making it difficult to extrapolate results from them to the general population.

The Controlled Clinical Trial

In most drug trials the effect of a new drug is compared to a *control* drug. The control may be a standard, established agent, or a placebo. The advantage of including a control is that the trial becomes a comparison between two agents, the effect of one of which is presumed to be known.

Such drug trials are carried out according to strict plans. In the design of the plan the effect of environmental variables must be minimized.

Two-Sample Designs

Controlled trials where a study drug is compared with a control drug can be carried out in various ways.

- Within patients: repeated measurements
- Between patients: matched pairs, independent groups

Within Patient Comparisons. In the *repeated measurements design* the patient receives both drugs in a random order, and so the effects of both are assessed on the same individual. This is a very attractive design, because the patient acts as his own control, and the subject variables discussed previously are reduced to a minimum. This design, however, cannot be applied easily in anaesthesia. For example, it would be impossible to apply this to a new intravenous induction agent unless the patient had to undergo more than one anaesthetic.

Between Patient Comparisons. The *matched pairs design.* Certain of the subject variables described above are selected and pairs of patients matched according to them. Each member of the pair receives either the trial or the control drug. Observations on members of the pair should be close together in time. This design seeks to reduce the influence of subject variables, but it may not be as effective as the repeated measurements design. The investigators choose the variables to match, and the assumption is made that they have identified the important factors.

In the *independent groups design* the trial agent and the control are investigated in two completely separate groups of patients in which no matching has taken place. Apart from those which are specifically included or excluded in the plan (inclusion or exclusion criteria) the individual sources of variability are not dealt with and larger numbers of subjects are required for this method. However, because of the ease of application in clinical trials this is the most commonly used two-sample trial design. This method relies upon the *random allocation* of subjects to the two treatments to avoid confounding factors.

Randomization is the process by which the subjects in a drug trial are allocated to either receive the study drug or the control, and the allocation is governed by chance. The randomization may be done in many ways including the tossing of a coin, or specially designed tables of random numbers may be used. The purpose of randomization is to ensure that confounding factors do not occur in a trial by promoting even spread of subject variables in the study groups.

Bias

One major factor which can easily invalidate a drug study is the presence of bias. This can either be on the part of the subject or the investigator.

The subject taking part in a study may develop bias for or against the trial agent. One understandable reason is a natural mistrust of *new* drugs. For this reason, the trial is enhanced if the subject does not know whether the trial or the control agent is being administered. This is known as a *single blind* study.

The investigators bias may include the natural enthusiasm for the discovery of new, more efficient treatments. In addition, if the observer knows which agents are being administered then he might draw conclusions from the first few cases in a study which bias his approach to the rest of the trial. If possible, it is best if neither the subject nor the observer knows the nature of the drug administered, that is, the study is *double blind*.

PRESENTATION AND STATISTICAL ANALYSIS OF RESULTS

1. Measurement
2. Raw data
3. Descriptive statistics
4. Inferential statistics

Measurement

The measurement of biological events is not done on one scale. Some events are simply classed, with no relationship between the classes, others are recorded on precise scales with known units and an exact zero point. An understanding of the *level of measurement* used is required for the correct statistical analysis of collected data.

Levels of Measurement
Nominal. The lowest level. Events are simply classed and there is no relationship between the classes other than they are different.

Ordinal. Events are classed according to a system which denotes ranking between classes. In addition to a difference between groups, there is a relationship of order.

Interval. Data has all the characteristics of the ordinal scale, the difference between two numbers is constant and there is an arbitrary unit of measurement.

Ratio. A scale with all the characteristics of being interval, but which in addition has as it's origin a true zero point.

Raw Data

The data collected in a study should be formulated and presented in such a fashion that it is immediately accessible to analysis by others. Summary, or descriptive, statistics are useful, but they should not replace the hard data. However, it is not always necessary to present a long list of figures. By preparing

tables and diagrams, the information can be given in a palatable manner. The discipline of presenting results in a communicative way benefits the investigator as much as others, in that it is often at the stage of careful consideration of the raw data that points leading to important conclusions are recognized.

Descriptive Statistics

Descriptive statistics are used to summarize data. A necessary part of this is a description of the central tendency of the data, and of the variability around this.

Description of Central Tendency
Mean, median, and mode. The *mean* is the arithmetic sum of all the observations divided by their number.

When all the observations are ranked, the *median* is the observation which has half the observations above and half below it. If the number of observations is an even number then the median lies half way between the two middle ranks.

The *mode* is the most commonly occurring observation. In a small sample the mode may not be very useful, but with large numbers of observations the mode can be a useful indicator of the centrality of data.

The choice between these indicators is based on the distribution of the data collected. If the data is symmetrically distributed than the mean, median, and mode will lie very close together, and in that case the mean is probably the best to quote. In asymmetrical, or skewed, data the mode may be useful, but the median is usually the best indicator of the central tendency of the data.

Measures of Dispersion
The Range and Interquartiles. In describing a set of numbers it is useful to state the range of values from the lowest to the highest. The *range*, however, gives very little information about the spread of the data. The *interquartile* range, which embraces 25–75% of values, may give additional information.

The Variance. To indicate the variability of the figures around a mean, it could perhaps by considered useful to subtract the mean from all the individual figures, sum this (denoted Σ) and divide by the number of observations (N) producing a *mean variation*, but if this was done the result would always be zero.

Mean variation =
$$\frac{\Sigma \text{ (each observation} - \text{the mean)}}{N} = 0$$

However if the differences from the mean were all squared, summed, and divided by the number of figures, we would have a *mean squared variation* which would indicate the variability of the observations around the mean. This mean squared variation is a useful indicator of spread of data and is termed the *variance*.

$$\text{Variance} = \frac{\Sigma \, (\text{each observation} - \text{the mean})^2}{N}$$

The square root of the variance is the *standard deviation* and is often denoted by σ.

$$\text{Standard deviation} \, (\sigma) = \sqrt{\text{Variance}}$$

Neither the variance nor the standard deviation have units, but it is obvious that a large spread of data around the mean will be associated with a large variance and standard deviation.

The choice between these measures of dispersion depends on the nature and distribution of the data. If the level of measurement is at least interval and the distribution is symmetrical, then the variance and standard deviation are appropriate. If, however, the level of measurement is less than interval or the distribution asymmetrical, then the range or the interquartiles should be used.

The Normal Distribution

The *normal distribution* is symmetrical, or bell shaped, and is characteristic of much biological information (e.g. the distribution of height in the population).

Many of the assumptions inherent in *parametric* statistical tests are based on this distribution. Such tests should not be used for data which is not normally distributed. *Nonparametric* statistical tests make fewer assumptions, are known as *distribution free* statistics, and can be applied to data without consideration of the distribution.

Inferential Statistics

Having constructed an experiment, carried it out, collected and summarized the data, the question then remains of whether any apparent differences between the experimental groups are true differences (due to the experimental conditions) or the result of subject and environmental variability. Inferential statistical tests are applied to the results to indicate whether there is a difference between the groups.

The Null Hypothesis

In order to determine whether we have found a difference between two treatments, we first construct an hypothesis which states that there is no real difference and that any observed differences are due to chance variation—the *Null Hypothesis* (H_o). The *Alternate Hypothesis* H_A is that there is indeed a difference and this will be accepted if H_o is rejected.

Significance Testing (α, β Errors and Power)

Having constructed the null hypothesis we apply a statistical test to the data which will indicate the probability (P value) of the differences between the experimental groups being due to chance variations. If this probability is high then H_o is accepted. If the calculated probability is low then H_o is rejected in favour of the alternate hypothesis.

The level of probability at which H_o is rejected is known as the *significance level*, α, and this is set by the investigators. This may be one in ten ($P_{0.1}$), or one in twenty ($P_{0.05}$), or less.

An often accepted level of significance is a P value of 0.05, which means that the null hypothesis will be rejected if the statistical test indicates that the differences between the experimental groups would be expected to occur, by chance, less often than one in twenty times (e.g. calculated P of less than 0.05). Inherent in this argument is the chance or error, α *error*, that the observed differences will occur by chance once in twenty times and that the H_o could therefore be wrongly rejected.

$$\alpha \text{ error—}H_o \text{ wrongly rejected.}$$

The obvious way to reduce the α error is to increase the significance level, α, to 0.01, or 0.001. However this increases the possibility of missing differences in treatment when they are in fact present, denoted β *error*.

$$\beta \text{ error—}H_o \text{ wrongly accepted.}$$

The *power* of a test is the ability to recognize a difference between groups when it is present. For a given α level the power of a study can be increased by making more observations. Tables exist which indicate the numbers of observations required to give a certain power assuming an α level, and these should be consulted at the design stage of an investigation (*see* Gore and Altman, 1982, pp. 6–8).

It is important to understand that statistical tests do not prove or disprove either the null or the alternate hypotheses. All that is examined is the likelihood of the null hypothesis occurring by chance.

Choosing the Appropriate Statistical Test

Parametric or Nonparametric Data?

In the first instance, the level of measurement of the data will determine whether parametric tests can be applied (Table 57.3).

TABLE 57.3

Level of measurement	Statistical tests
Nominal	Nonparametric
Ordinal	Nonparametric
Interval	Parametric and nonparametric
Ratio	Parametric and nonparametric

TABLE 57.4

	Advantages	Disadvantages
Parametric	Increased power	Normal distribution More calculations
Nonparametric	All levels of measurement Distribution free Easy calculations	Power less than parametric tests

Beyond this consideration the two types of tests have various advantages and disadvantages (Table 57.4). Much biological data lends itself to analysis by nonparametric statistics. In addition the problem of lower power can be compensated for by increasing the number of observations.

Paired or Unpaired Data?

A distinction must be drawn between data which is paired (within patients or matched pairs) and that which is unpaired (between patients, unmatched). Different statistical tests are applied to paired and unpaired data (Table 57.5).

The appropriate test can then be applied to the data. This will produce a *test statistic* which can be used to calculate a probability value, P. This calculated P value can then be compared with expected P values from statistical tables taking account of the significance level, α H$_o$ can then be accepted or rejected accordingly.

Confidence Levels or Hypothesis Testing?

Recently there has been a move away from simply reporting the results of statistical analyses as *significant* or *not significant*. Rather the reporting of the difference between mean values from experimental groups together with *confidence intervals* (usually at the 95% level) for that difference has been encouraged (Gardiner and Altman, 1986). This usually applies to data analysed by parametric statistics, but confidence intervals can be calculated for some non-parametric analyses (Campbell and Gardner, 1988).

The Process of Inferential Statistical Analysis can be Summarized

1. State the null (H$_o$) and alternate hypotheses.
2. Set the significance level (α).
3. Select and apply the appropriate statistical test for the data and experimental design to obtain the test statistic.
4. Calculate the P value for the test statistic.
5. If this P value is less than the expected P value obtained from statistical tables, reject H$_o$ and accept the alternate hypothesis. If the calculated P is equal to or greater than the expected value, accept H$_o$.
6. If appropriate calculate confidence intervals.

FURTHER READING

Abramson J.H. (1984). *Survey methods in Community Medicine*. 3rd edn. Edinburgh: Churchill Livingstone.

Armitage P., Berry G. (1987). *Statistical Methods in Medical Research*. Oxford: Blackwell Scientific.

Axelsson G., Rylander R. (1982). Exposure to anaesthetic gases and spontaneous abortion. Response bias in a postal questionnaire study. *Int. J. Epidemiol.*, **11**, 250.

Bailar II. J.C., Mosteller F. (1986). Medical uses of statistics. *New Engl. J. Med.*

Buring J.E., Hennekens C.H., Mayrent S.L., et al. (1985). Health experiences of operating room personnel. *Anesthesiology*, **62**, 325.

Campbell M.J., Gardner M.J. (1988). Calculating confidence intervals for some non-parametric analyses. *Br. Med. J.*, **296**, 1454.

Delbecq A.L., Van de Ven A.H. (1971). A group process model for problem identification and program planning. *J. Appl. Behav.*, **7**, 466.

Doll R., Peto R. (1976). Mortality in relation to smoking: 20 years observations made on male British doctors. *Br. Med. J.*, **2**, 1525.

Fowkes F.G.R. (1982). Medical audit cycle. A review of methods and research in clinical practice. *Med. Educat.*, **16**, 228.

Gardner M.J., Altman D.G. (1986). Confidence intervals rather than P values: estimation rather than hypothesis testing. *Br. Med. J.*, **292**, 746.

Gore S.M., Altman D.G. (1982). Statistics in practice. *Br. Med. J.* (publication).

TABLE 57.5

Level of measurement	Nonparametric		Parametric	
	Unpaired	Paired	Unpaired	Paired
Nominal	Chi-square		—	—
Ordinal	Mann-Whitney U test	Wilcoxon signed ranks test	—	—
Interval	as above		Unpaired t test	Paired t test
Ratio	as above		as above	

Greene J., D'Oliveria M. (1982). *Learning to Use Statistical Tests in Psychology*. Milton Keynes: Open University Press.

Hamilton M. (1974). *Lectures on the Methodology of Clinical Research*. Edinburgh: Churchill Livingstone.

Lunn J.N. (ed.). (1984). *Quality of Care in Anaesthetic Practice*, London: London Royal Society of Medicine.

Lunn J.N. (ed.). (1986). *Epidemiology in Anaesthesia*. p. 168. London: Edward Arnold.

Medico-Pharmaceutical Forum (1987). *Clinical trials*. Report of the working party on clinical trials of the Medico-Pharmaceutical Forum.

Miller J. (1984). Experimental design and statistics, In *New Essential Psychology*, 2nd edn. (P. Herriot ed.). London, New York: Methuen.

Royal College of Physicians. (1984). *Guidelines on the Practice of Ethics Committees in Medical Research*.

Siegel S. (1956). *Nonparametric Statistics*. New York: McGraw-Hill.

Spence A.A. (1987). Environmental pollution by inhalation anaesthetics. *Br. J. Anaesth.*, **59**, 103.

Tannenbaum T.N., Goldberg R.J. (1985). Exposure to anaesthetic gases and reproductive outcome. A review of epidemiologic literature. *J. Occup. Med.*, **27**, 659.

58. Methods of Drug Analysis
V. Marks

Concept
Principles
Choice of drugs to be monitored
Indications for measuring drugs in blood
Timing
   Choice of body fluid
Methods of measurement
   Immunoassay
   Radioreceptor assays
   High performance liquid chromatography (HPLC)
   Gas-liquid chromatography (GLC)
   High-performance thin layer chromatography (HP-TLC)
   Bioassay

Drugs play a central role in the practice of modern medicine, as they have done since the beginning of time. Without them surgery, as we know it, would be impossible and treatment of nonsurgical diseases would be extremely limited. It cannot be denied, however, that drugs, even when not deliberately abused, are, at the present time, amongst the commonest causes of illness, or at least discomfort, leading to admission to the medical wards of hospitals. This is nothing new, however, for according to William Seward, an 18th century wit and friend of Dr. Samuel Johnson 'A doctor is defined to be a man whom we hire for the purpose of telling stories in the chamber of a sick person till nature effects a cure or his medicine kills the patient'.

There is a growing body of evidence that, for most drugs, their therapeutically desirable effects depend more upon their concentration in the blood than upon the dose administered (Koch-Weser, 1972, 1975; Marks et al., 1973). Likewise, virtually all drugs that benefit patients carry with them the risk of producing toxic effects—which are both predictable and dose dependent—as well as certain others which are unpredictable and nondose dependent, i.e. they are idiosyncratic. There is still comparatively little that can be done to prevent the latter but, by careful monitoring of blood drug levels the ill effects of many potentially toxic, but clinically useful, drugs can be minimized without reducing the dose to such low levels as to make them ineffective.

CONCEPT

The idea that the treatment of disease by drugs might be improved by measuring their concentration in the blood and adjusting the dosing regime in order to bring the concentration within a predetermined or optimum range is a comparatively new one. In its present form it dates back no further than to the early 1970s (Koch-Weser 1972; Marks et al., 1973) and owes its growth to the confluence of several conceptual and technological advances which have themselves appeared only during the past couple of decades. Of these developments the most important are:

1. The emergence from the age old disciplines of pharmacy, materia-medica and academic pharmacology of an entirely new one—that of clinical pharmacology. A further development has been the emergence of clinical pharmacokinetics as a speciality (Halkin, 1984).
2. An interest in, and understanding of, the biochemistry of xenobiotics and drug metabolism.
3. The discovery of genetics as a major determinant of drug metabolism and responsiveness in man.
4. The application, to clinical medicine, of a number of analytical techniques capable of measuring blood drug levels at therapeutic concentrations.

It is not intended to consider either pharmacokinetics or drug metabolism in detail here since these topics have been excellently reviewed by others. Nevertheless it will be necessary to highlight some of the most salient points.

PRINCIPLES

Most drugs, excluding those used in anaesthetics and dermatology, are taken orally and absorbed through the gut into the hepatic venous portal system. Many bind, to some extent reversibly, to plasma proteins and varying amounts are rapidly removed from the circulation by metabolism, mainly by the liver, or through filtration by the kidney. Drugs that remain in the circulation unbound to protein sooner or later come into equilibrium with the interstitial fluid and eventually bind to receptors on the surface of the cells where they exert their effect. The strength of the stimulus received by the cell is therefore, far removed from the only quantifiable variable in drug therapy— the dose of drug that is actually administered. It should therefore cause no surprise that, in general, there is only a poor correlation between the dose of a drug administered and the clinical effect it produces. Put differently, a dose of drug that in one subject might be totally ineffective—because most of it had already been removed from the circulation before it came into contact with its target cells—could in another subject produce serious toxic effects.

Possible reasons for this poor correlation between dosage and therapeutic efficacy have only recently received the attention they undoubtedly deserve. The most important are given in Table 58.1. Poor bioavail-

TABLE 58.1

Reasons for poor correlation between drug dosage and therapeutic effectiveness

Inappropriate drug for patient's condition, i.e. wrong diagnosis
Poor bioavailability or absorption of drug
Genetic differences in metabolism (pharmacogenetics)
Acquired differences in rates of elimination
Differences in tissue responsiveness

ability is no longer the problem it was at the beginning of the present era when it was responsible for many large scale disasters, such as those involving digoxin (Beller et al., 1971), or near disasters, such as those involving phenytoin. The improvement has come about largely because drug licensing authorities have insisted upon bioequivalence studies being performed on all new preparations and formulations of established drugs before they are released onto the market.

Another reason for divergence between blood drug concentrations and biological effectiveness is the development of tolerance at the cellular level. This is seen more with some drugs, e.g. morphine, than with others, e.g. bromocriptine, and does not effect all actions equally. Bromocriptine, for example, retains its therapeutic efficacy indefinitely, without any increase in dosage, even though its initially undesirable side-effects may have disappeared completely. Cross

tolerance between totally different classes of drugs, e.g. alcohol and barbiturates, is another cause of discrepancy between blood drug levels and therapeutic effect when they might otherwise be expected to exist.

The theoretical basis for therapeutic drug monitoring rests upon three premises:

1. Therapeutic response to a drug correlates better with its concentration in blood than with the dose administered. This is clearly inapplicable to drugs which are either not absorbed when given orally, e.g. cholestyramine, or which exert their effect wholly or mainly at their site of application, e.g. topical steroids
2. There exists an optimum therapeutic range within which the majority of patients experience clinical benefit with a minimum of toxic or unpleasant side effects.
3. That, by adjusting the dose and timing of drug administration on the basis of the blood drug level—and in accordance with pharmacokinetic principles—a better therapeutic outcome can be achieved than by the exercise of sound clinical judgement alone.

These premises have so far been established for only a very small number of drugs and in some cases they are known to be invalid. Drugs whose effects are mediated by irreversible reactions or by denaturation of intracellular proteins, e.g. monoamine-oxidase inhibitors, or by depletion of stored materials, e.g. reserpine, belong to this latter category.

Inherent in the concept of therapeutic drug monitoring as a clinically useful activity is the assumption that the blood drug concentration reflects its concentration at the cell surface. This is not necessarily true if, for example, the blood supply to the tissues is impaired. Thus, in the case of badly perfused cancers treated with short-lived antitumour agents, toxic concentrations of the drug may occur in the patients own tissues, as reflected in the venous blood level, whilst only ineffectively low drug concentrations are achieved within the tumour itself. In other situations much of the drug present in the circulation may be protein bound and consequently unavailable to the tissues. In such cases the total blood drug concentration may be a poor indicator of its concentration at the cell surface. For this reason some authorities advocate measurement of dialysable, ultrafilterable or 'free', rather than total, plasma drug levels. This idea has not gained widespread acceptance, however, and the data base against which to interpret the results is not yet available.

CHOICE OF DRUGS TO BE MONITORED

Many drugs are now amenable to measurement in any reasonably well equipped clinical laboratory and some can be measured in the clinic or at the patients bedside (Mould and Marks, 1988). For only a small number of drugs, however, has it been shown unequi-

TABLE 58.2

OPTIMUM THERAPEUTIC CONCENTRATION IN PLASMA OF DRUGS FOR WHICH TDM HAS BEEN ESTABLISHED AS VALUABLE

	Mass units	*SI units* **
Anticonvulsants		
Carbamazepine*	Steady state 4–12 mg/L	15–46 µmol/L
Ethosuximide*	Steady state 40–100 mg/L	280–700 µmol/L
Phenytoin*	Steady state 10–20 mg/L	40–80 µmol/L
Antidepressants		
Imipramine*	Steady state > 100 µg/L	More than 350 nmol/L
Lithium	—	0.5–1.2 mmol/L 12 h after last dose
Nortriptyline*	Steady state 50–150 µg/L	190–570 nmol/L
Antibiotics		
Amikacin*	Peak 15–25 mg/L; trough <4–6 mg/L	
Gentamicin*	Peak 4–12 mg/L; trough <2 mg/L	
Kanamicin*	Peak 20–25 mg/L; trough <4–6 mg/L	
Tobramicin*	Peak 4–10 mg/L; trough <2 mg/L	
Antitumour		
Methotrexate*	Less than 4.5 mg/L 24 h after i.v. dosing	Less than 10 µmol/L 24 h after i.v. dosing
Cardioactive		
Digitoxin*	Steady state 10–30 µg/L	13–40 nmol/L
Digoxin*	Steady state 1–2 µg/L	1.3–2.6 nmol/L
Lignocaine*	Steady state 2–5 mg/L	8–20 µmol/l
Procainamide*	Steady state 4–10 mg/L	16–40 µmol/L
Miscellaneous		
Theophylline*	Steady state 10–15 mg/L	55–85 µmol/L
Cyclosporine*	?	?

* For most of the drugs for which therapeutic monitoring has been established as useful, simple-to-use homogenous immuno-assay kits are available commercially.

** The Association of Clinical Biochemists has recommended (Ratcliffe and Worth, 1986) that the SI system should, where possible, be used for reporting drug concentration in biological fluids.

vocally to be worthwhile doing so. These are listed in Table 58.2. Only for them have 'optimum therapeutic ranges' been established with sufficient rigour to justify their use by busy practicing clinicians who have no intention of using their data for anything more than treating patients. The list of drugs for which there are suggestive but far from conclusive data is very much longer and growing, but will receive no further consideration here even though it possibly includes some—such as cyclosporine and amiodarone—that will become routinely assayed within a few years from now. The difficulty at this stage is to know which will and which will not do so.

INDICATIONS FOR MEASURING DRUGS IN BLOOD

The general indications for measuring the concentration of a drug in blood include the investigation of its pharmacokinetics, protein binding bioavailability and the comparability of drug preparations, as well as for clinical control of drug therapy and detection of drug abuse. There are, however, a number of specific clinical indications which apply to a greater or lesser extent to all of the drugs for which therapeutic drug monitoring is indicated.

1. **Failure of expected therapeutic response.** The commonest reason for this is non-compliance (Pearson, 1982) but others include reduced bioavailability due, for example, to unsuspected poor intestinal absorption; more rapid elimination by metabolism than usual, possibly secondary to enzyme induction by another drug or even the drug itself; reduced access to the drug's site of action and tissue or organ unresponsiveness.

2. **Guide to dosage of drugs used for prophylaxis.** Ordinarily drugs are given to alleviate symptoms or correct physical signs. When however, they are given to people at high risk of developing a disease or recurrence, e.g. depression, there may be no other way of ensuring that an optimum blood drug concentration has been achieved than by measuring it. This indication is especially important when there is coexisting disease, such as hepatic or renal impairment, which alters the drug's ordinary pharmacokinetics so as to render the usual guidelines on dosage inappropriate. This is particularly important in the case of treatment with anti-arrhythmic drugs, such as lignocaine, whose plasma half-life may be greatly prolonged by poor liver perfusion consequent upon the very myocardial infarction for which treatment is being given.

3. **Individualization of treatment where no simpler method exists.** It has long been customary to adjust treatment continuously with antidiabetic drugs, e.g. glibenclamide, in order to achieve a satisfactory lowering of blood glucose concentration. Similarly, doses of anticoagulants such as warfarin, are adjusted in order to maintain prothrombin times to within well defined limits; indeed without such controls it is doubtful whether treatment with this class of drug would be considered ethical. For many drugs, however, no such simple markers exist, yet the consequences of both under and overtreatment can be disastrous. Antibiotics such as gentamicin, probably provide the best example of drugs falling into this category. Others include theophylline and phenytoin.

4. **Differentiation of drug toxicity from the effects of undertreatment.** This is the main reason for measuring plasma digoxin concentrations since, contrary to common belief, no optimum therapeutic range has been established for this drug. In clinical practice, the symptoms of digoxin overdose may be extremely difficult to distinguish from those consequent upon a resurgence of the heart failure for which the drug was prescribed in the first place, and is generally caused by noncompliance. Since treatment of over and underdigitalization is so very different, an accurate differential diagnosis before treatment is commenced is essential and justifies urgent plasma digoxin assay.

5. **During clinical trials.** This is one of the most important of all indications for measuring blood drug levels and equating them with clinical improvement or the appearance of toxicity. Assay permits the trialist to assess the drug's clinical efficacy and optimum mode of usage more thoroughly than may otherwise be possible, and to establish whether routine monitoring is likely to have a place in the regular treatment of patients with the drug in the future. Moreover, during the first few months after a drug's general release onto the market, measurement of its concentration in blood serves to identify those patients who, for one reason or another, cannot eliminate it from their bodies at the normal rate and consequently are at special risk from its toxic effects.

TIMING

As drugs are usually administered intermittently, their concentration in blood is subject to fluctuations. Therapeutic responses to drugs which act upon the patient's own tissues rather than upon micro-organisms or tumour cells usually correlate better with steady-state rather than with peak or trough plasma levels. Toxic effects on the other hand often relate more closely to peak than to steady-state plasma drug levels.

The steady-state concentration is an hypothetical rather than real concentration (Duthie and Nimmo, 1987) and corresponds to the concentration achieved after 5–6 doses of the drug given at regular intervals of not more than the biological half-life of the drug. In this hypothetical steady-state situation there is little or no redistribution of drug between the various body compartments and elimination by metabolism or excretion exactly equals that provided by drug dosage. Once the steady-state has been reached the size and timing of the fluctuations about the mean blood level are determined by the mode of delivery, bioavailability and interval between dosing, as well as by the pharmacokinetics of the drug itself. The optimum therapeutic range for most drugs for which it has been determined, relates to the blood concentration immediately preceding the next scheduled dose or to a sample of blood collected at a defined time after the last dose. Because of the relatively long interval between altering the dose of a drug and attainment of a new steady-state little clinical importance can be attached to blood drug measurements which are made less than 4–5 half-lives after making a dosage change. This fact is often insufficiently appreciated by clinicians unfamiliar with the principles of pharmacokinetics which can be crudely defined as what people do to drugs in contrast to pharmacodynamics, which is what drugs do to people.

Choice of Body Fluid

Most assays for therapeutic drug monitoring are performed on blood plasma or serum. There is however, a growing tendency to use saliva, especially for children who, unlike adults, prefer spitting to giving blood. The use of saliva for therapeutic drug monitoring (TDM) is limited to drugs, such as theophylline, in which partition between plasma and saliva is solely on the basis of their concentration in plasma and not upon such variables as rate of saliva flow and from which salivary gland the saliva originated. Claims that salivary drug concentrations, because they correlate better with 'free' than with total plasma drug concentrations, are more clinically relevant have not been established unequivocally and the data upon which to build such an opinion do not yet exist.

Breath, which should in theory be an ideal medium upon which to carry out measurements of volatile drugs, has no clinical value except in a research environment. The main reason for this is its impracticability. Whilst the concentration of a volatile drug in alveolar air is more or less in equilibrium with its concentration in blood plasma the same relationship does not hold for expired air which consists of a mixture of alveolar and dead space air of variable composition. This fact is allowed for in breath alcohol measurements made for forensic purposes but even so it still creates certain problems (Simpson, 1987). The difficulty created by variable mixing can, to a certain extent, be overcome by the use of a rebreathing technique but the use of breath drug measurements has not found favour except for research and law-enforcement purposes.

METHODS OF MEASUREMENT

Various techniques have been employed for measuring the concentration of drugs in body fluids for clinical purposes. Immunoassays in one form or another are undoubtedly the most important and played a seminal role in the establishment of (TDM) as a clinically practicable procedure. Much of our pharmacokinetic knowledge, on the other hand, and the principles upon which TDM depends were obtained from studies using standard physicochemical techniques. They are still used in some laboratories but are generally demanding of both time and analytical skills.

Immunoassay

The introduction of immunoassay for the measurement of drugs in blood, more than anything else, made the concept of therapeutic drug monitoring a practical rather than theoretical proposition. Although for clinical use, the original radioimmunoassay techniques have now largely given way to procedures which are easier to perform but conceptually more complex (Collins, 1985), they remain the method of choice during the developmental phase of a drug assay or when very low concentrations (i.e. below 1 nmol/L) are expected to be encountered.

Few drugs are naturally immunogenic but most can be rendered so by conjugating them to proteins by any one of many different procedures, each of which has its own advantages and disadvantages (Marks et al., 1974). Conjugation makes it possible to produce specific drug-binding antibodies which are the most important of the three key reagents required for any immunoassay, the other two being appropriate standards and a label. The label must be capable of being measured by a physicochemical technique.

The principles of immunoassay in general, and of those used for the measurement of drugs in biological fluids in particular, have been extensively reviewed (Marks et al., 1980). Many of the newest techniques are covered by patents and are available only as kits from their manufacturers.

Immunoassay kits are available for most of the drugs listed in Table 58.2. They seldom require the use of apparatus that is not generally available within any well equipped laboratory and several manufacturers are now making preprogrammed microprocessor-controlled instruments designed specifically and exclusively for use with their reagents.

Of the three key reagents common to all immunoassay methods, it is the antibody that confers sensitivity and specificity; the label—which can be a radioactive isotope, an enzyme, a fluorophore, a chemi or bioluminescent label, a drug-protein, or drug-latex particle conjugate—determines what apparatus must be used to measure the size of the signal. Most of the drug immunoassays available commercially and many of those developed by researchers themselves can be performed without pretreatment of the specimen (i.e. on unextracted samples) and are both rapid and simple to perform provided the manufacturer's instructions are followed.

In radioimmunoassay the drug (analyte) present in a sample at unknown concentration is allowed to compete with a known, constant amount of radiolabelled analyte for a limited number of antibody-binding sites. At equilibrium both the labelled and the unlabelled drug exist either bound to antibody or unbound (i.e. 'free'). Since binding is competitive, the amount of labelled drug bound to the antibody is inversely proportional to the amount of native (unknown) drug present. The 'bound' and 'free' labels are separated by any of a number of different techniques. The amount of drug present in the original sample can then be computed from a standard curve prepared by treating known standards in exactly the same way as the samples using either the 'free' or the 'bound' counts, whichever is the more convenient or appropriate (Teale, 1978).

As radioimmunoassays require separation of the bound from the free fractions, they are often referred to as heterogeneous assays and demand considerably more expertize for their performance than so-called homogeneous assays. In these the nature of the signal emitted by the antibody-bound label is different (and can therefore, be distinguished) from that emitted by the free label. Consequently, physical separation of the two components is not necessary and the whole reaction, from the addition of sample to the reagents to making the final physicochemical measurement, can be carried out in a single tube.

The so-called homogeneous immunoassay techniques are currently the most popular method for making blood drug measurements and are generally very simple to perform. They usually require a plasma or serum sample of 100 µl or less and involve only the addition to it of one, two or rarely three reagents in an orderly and timed sequence. Results become available within 1–3 min of commencing the assay.

The most serious objection to the use of immunoassays is their susceptibility to interference by metabolites of the drug itself or its analogues. Thus most immunoassays for morphine, but not all, react to a greater or lesser extent with one or both of its glucuronides as well as with the native drug. This failing renders immunoassays, unless they are combined with a separation technique such as HPLC, unsuitable for toxicological diagnosis or for making measurements on samples of blood collected from subjects in whom doubt exists as to the exact nature of the drug being used. When used with HPLC, however, immunoassays acquire a sensitivity and specificity possessed by few other techniques apart from mass spectrometry.

Radioreceptor Assays

If the antibodies used in a competitive radioimmuno-assay are replaced by drug receptors prepared from sonicated cells by centrifugation, so-called radioreceptor assays (RRA) can be developed. These have different specificities but similar sensitivities to those of a radioimmunoassay developed against the same drug (Tune, 1984). Radioreceptor assays utilize a radioactive—usually tritiated—preparation of the drug as tracer which competes not only with the native drug but also with its active (and possibly inactive, blocking) metabolites for the limited number of binding sites provided by the receptors available. Because of the uncertainty attending the exact nature of the compounds capable of binding to drug receptors, results obtained with radioreceptor assays must be interpreted with caution. Indeed, results obtained by these methods and those using more conventional methods (e.g. GLC, HPLC and immunoassay) do not always correlate very closely. Nevertheless, used prudently, RRA is a valuable addition to the research analyst's armamentarium.

High Performance Liquid Chromatography (HPLC)

The theory underlying the principles of HPLC is complex and its exposition would be out of place here. Further information can be found in standard texts (Koenigsberger, 1978). In general, HPLC provides an opportunity for separating into its constituents a complex mixture of compounds on the basis of their individual physicochemical properties and measuring each one of them as they emerge from the column by one of the many techniques available. The most commonly employed detection and quantification systems at the present time include visible, ultraviolet and infrared absorptiometry and fluorescence, and electrochemical detection.

So-called 'normal phase' HPLC columns, employing silica gel as the support medium, for example, allow for early elution of the nonpolar (i.e. lipid-soluble) native drug in a rapidly moving nonpolar solvent system; the generally more polar metabolites elute somewhat later. By changing the nature of the support medium and/or solvent pH, temperature, etc., different patterns can be obtained and the most useful chosen for regular use depending upon the purpose for which the chromatography is being performed.

What is generally referred to as reverse phase HPLC is much more commonly used for making drug measurements than is 'normal phase' chromatography (Drayer, 1984). Reverse phase HPLC depends upon the use of nonpolar support columns and polar solvents (of which those containing methanol or acetonitrile are the most common) to effect elution. These columns have a high resolving power, and the weak surface energies of the nonpolar support medium plus the polar nature of the mobile phase permits rapid analysis of underivatized drugs (and their metabolites).

For straightforward therapeutic drug monitoring, where interest centres entirely upon one substance, conditions which permit rapid throughput without sacrifice of sensitivity or specificity will generally be selected; if the purpose is, however, to study not only the native compound but also it metabolites and/or the presence of other compounds of interest, operating conditions will be adjusted accordingly.

The advantages of HPLC are its wide applicability to analysis whereby it can be used for compounds of almost every kind; a reduced need for pre-purification and derivatization (although advantage can, where necessary or desirable, be taken of both); amenability to automation; and finally, the preservation (rather than the destruction) of the specimen, permitting identification to be carried out upon it if necessary. Collection of the individual fractions as they emerge from the column for subsequent analysis by immunoassay or mass spectrometry provides an opportunity for even greater specificity and sensitivity than can be achieved by virtually any other analytical technique.

HPLC is technically demanding; though much less so than formerly. It is comparatively robust and new methods are generally easier to develop than with many other techniques making it an excellent tool for anyone wishing to study drug disposition within the body. The apparatus is necessarily large and neither it, nor the methodology, is well suited to decentralized clinical usage, for which immunoassay, in one form or another, is the method of choice.

The sensitivity of HPLC depends upon the quality of apparatus used—especially the pumps. The general proposition that the better the equipment the more it costs is as true of HPLC as with any other technology. Probably the most important single factor is the nature and reliability of the detector and its suitability for the drug in question. The most commonly used detectors employ visible or ultraviolet light absorption (UV detection) but greater sensitivity can often be obtained by using fluorimetric or electrochemical detection when the substances being measured have the appropriate physicochemical attributes (Moore et al., 1984). By means of such instrumentation sensitivity equal to, or surpassing, that of GLC can often be obtained.

Gas-Liquid Chromatography (GLC)

GLC has the sensitivity necessary to make it suitable for measuring all but the most potent drugs provided they are volatile, or can be rendered so by simple pre-column or on column derivatization and are stable at temperatures up to about 200°C. Many of the problems encountered in the early days of GLC have been surmounted by improvements in the equipment, the nature and reliability of the chromatographic columns, the detectors and the extraction procedures. Further details can be found in standard texts (Chakraborty and Lynaugh, 1978; Agurell and Lindgren, 1981).

Capillary columns which permit almost unlimited separation of individual constituents of complex mixtures of compounds are now available for use with most conventional GLC instruments and by appropriate choice of detector, for example flame ionization (general purpose), nitrogen amplified flame ionization, electron capture and even mass spectrometry (GC-MS), the sensitivity of GLC can be arranged so that it is capable of measuring specific compounds in solution, provided they have the correct physico-chemical properties, down to concentrations of 1 nmol/L or less.

The introduction of automatic sampling, temperature programming and microprocessor-controlled data handling has gone a long way towards removing the tedium formerly associated with this technique which is still, however, relatively capital and labour intensive. It is also relatively slow, time consuming and more suitable for batch than single sample analysis. Thus, like other chromatographic techniques, GLC is more suited to investigative or research work involving the detection, identification and/or measurement of drugs in biological fluids than to therapeutic drug monitoring when simplicity, availability and speed are at a premium (Marks, 1985).

High-Performance Thin Layer Chromatography (HP-TLC)

The comparatively new technique of HP-TLC may begin to play a role in the quantification of drugs of clinical interest now that sensitive and robust reflectance absorptiometers are available for use in conjunction with exquisitively fine thin layer chromatographic plates. It is unlikely, however, that HP-TLC will ever become a serious rival to immunoassay or GLC for clinical therapeutic drug monitoring although it may find a role in the detection and/or quantification of drug abuse and in polypharmacy.

Bioassay

Bioassays of one sort or another, were until the advent of immunoassay techniques, the principal method for measuring antibiotics and antitumour agents in biological fluids. Although sensitive and reliable when only one drug is present, bioassays are generally too labour intensive, time consuming and slow to yield clinically useful information. Moreover they are affected by the presence, in the sample, of substances (including other antibiotics) which possess similar biological (i.e. antibacterial) properties to the drug under investigation. This can be both advantageous when, for example, the drug itself is a mixture of substances rather than a pure compound (e.g. bleomycin) and disadvantageous when, for example, only one of a couple of antibiotics is nephro- or ototoxic but both are antimicrobial in the assay system. Radioreceptor assays are a special kind of 'bioassay' and are considered separately.

Near Patient Testing

Within the past few years solid phase reagents, also known as reagents on a stick, which are suitable for making blood drug measurements in the clinic, operating theatre, or even at the patient's bedside, have become available (Mould et al., 1988). They require only a minimum of skill and apparatus in order to obtain a result of sufficient accuracy upon which to base a clinical decision.

Simple quality assurance procedures must, however, be followed as with all other near patient testing techniques (Marks, 1988). In addition care must be taken to ensure that the units used for reporting the results are those with which the user is familiar. Various types of units are used by the different reagent manufacturers but there is growing acceptance amongst the international medical community for the view that the concentration of drugs in biological units, like that of other analytes, should be expressed in molar rather than mass units (Baron, 1986; Ratcliffe and Worth, 1986).

Interpretation

Nowhere in the whole of clinical medicine is the concept of the 'normal (or reference) range' more scientifically inappropriate yet so clinically necessary as in therapeutic drug monitoring. The range of plasma concentrations of a drug below which the number of subjects deriving no benefit from it, and above which the incidence of undesirable side effects becomes unacceptably high, is best referred to as the 'optimum therapeutic range'. For some drugs e.g. lithium used for prevention of recurrent depression, the optimum therapeutic range may be the only guide to correct dosing whilst for others, e.g. digoxin, it does no more than facilitate distinction between symptoms caused by underdosing from those caused by overdosing.

Derivation of an optimum therapeutic range is a lengthy procedure involving detailed serial observation of many patients and correlating the blood drug levels measured on numerous occasions with eventual clinical outcome. This is, however, only a retrospective study. Confirmation of the value of the tentative optimum therapeutic range so obtained, requires a prospective study. In such studies the benefits of using the tentative range to modulate treatment *versus* clinical judgement without access to blood drug measurements are compared. At the present time prospective studies in which use of a suggested optimum therapeutic range has been shown unequivocally to improve clinical outcome are limited and available for only a small range of drugs (Table 58.2).

Analytical technology is no longer the limiting factor to the extension of therapeutic drug monitoring. Instead it is the clinical value of the analytical data since, until an optimum therapeutic range has been established, the results are virtually worthless, except for research purposes. That it is not easy to determine an optimum therapeutic range is exemplified by the problems encountered by clinical pharmacologists and transplant surgeons (Wadhwa et al., 1987) in establishing an optimum therapeutic range for cyclosporine. All authorities are agreed that cyclosporine, which is an extremely useful but toxic drug that has revolutionized the outcome of transplant surgery should be monitored during use by measuring its concentration in blood in order to achieve maximum efficacy. The difficulty is that despite intensive investigation no plasma cyclosporine concentration has been identified below which clinical effectiveness is usual but toxicity rare.

How data derived from therapeutic drug assays can or should be used for the better management of patients is still an unsettled question since optimum use implies possession of knowledge of not only the pharmacokinetics of the individual drug (see additional reading list), but also of its pharmacodynamics and drug relationships. This is the reason why many clinicians resort to obtaining help in interpretation from clinical pharmacists or pharmacologists, where they exist or clinical biochemists where they do not, as being the individuals most likely to have the knowledge to make assay results interpretable and the basis for therapeutic action. The increasing availability of small mobile computer modules programmed with the appropriate drug pharmacokinetic algorithms will also go some of the way to overcoming the problem of interpretation in the future. This will become increasingly important as the list of drugs for which drug assays become desirable, and the facilities for making them outside the laboratory increases (Mould et al., 1988).

REFERENCES

Agurell S., Lindgren J.E. (1981). Gas-chromatography—mass spectrometry in drug level analysis. In *Therapeutic Drug Monitoring* pp. 110–130. (Richens A., Marks V., eds.), Edinburgh: Churchill Livingstone.

Baron D.N. (1986). Use of molar units for drugs and toxins? *Br. Med. J.*, **293**, 2.

Beller G.A., Smith T.W., Abelmann W.H., et al. (1971). Digitalis intoxication. A prospective clinical study with serum level correlations. *New Engl. J. Med.*, **284**, 989.

Chakraborty J., Lynaugh N. (1978). Gas-liquid chromatography-mass spectrometry. In *Scientific Foundations of Clinical Biochemistry*, vol. 1. pp. 144–165. (Williams D., Nunn R.F., Marks V., eds.). Oxford: Heinemann Medical.

Collins W.P. (1985). *Alternative Immunoassays*. Chichester: John Wiley.

Drayer D.E. (1984). Reversed phase length performance liquid chromatography: optimizing peak resolution. In *Proceedings of the Second World Conference on Clinical Pharmacology and Therapeutics*. pp. 809–819. (Lemberger L., Reidenberg M., eds.). Bethesda: American Society of Pharmacology and Experimental Therapeutics.

Duthie J.R., Nimmo W.S. (1987). Steady state pharmacology. In *Drugs in Anaesthesia: mechanisms of action*. pp. 428–440. (Feldman S.A., Scurr C.F., Paton Sir W., eds.). London: Edward Arnold.

Halkin H. (1984). Principles of clinical pharmacology IV. Bedside clinical pharmacology and consultation. In *Proceedings of the Second World Conference on Clinical Pharmacology and Therapeutics*. pp. 31–37. (Lembeger L., Reidenberg M.M., eds.). Bethesda: American Society for Pharmacology and Experimental Therapeutics.

Koch-Weser J. (1972). Serum drug concentrations as therapeutic guides. *New Engl. J. Med.*, **287**, 227.

Koch-Weser J. (1975). The serum level approach to individualization of drug dosage. *Eur. J. Clin. Pharmacol.*, **9**, 1.

Koenigsberger R. (1978). High performance chromatography.In *Scientific Foundations of Clinical Biochemistry*, Vol. 1 pp. 165–185. (Williams D.L., Nunn R.F., Marks V., eds.). Oxford: Heinemann Medical.

Marks V. (1985). Therapeutic drug monitoring. In *Clinical Biochemistry Nearer the Patient*. pp. 190–194. (Marks V., Alberti K.G.M.M.). Edinburgh: Churchill Livingstone.

Marks V. (1988). Essential considerations in the provision of near-patient testing facilities. *Ann. Clin. Biochem.*, **25**, 220.

Marks V., Lindup W.E., Baylis E.M. (1973). Measurement of therapeutic agents in blood. In *Advances in Clinical Chemistry*, Vol. 16, pp. 47–109. New York: Academic Press.

Marks V., Morris B., Teale D. (1974). Pharmacology. *Br. Med. Bull.*, **30**, 80.

Marks V., Mould G.P., O'Sullivan M.J.O., et al. (1980). Monitoring of drug disposition by immunoassay. In *Progress in Drug Metabolism*, Vol. 5, pp. 255–310. (Bridges J.W., Chasseaud L.F., eds.). Chichester: John Wiley.

Moore R.A., Baldwin D., McQuay H.J., et al. (1984). HPLC of morphine with electrochemical detection: analysis in human plasma. *Ann. Clin. Biochem.*, **21**, 125.

Mould G., Marks V. (1988). The use of solid-phase chemistry in therapeutic drug monitoring. *Clin. Pharmacokin.*, **14**, 65.

Pearson R.M. (1982). Who is taking their tablets? *Br. Med. J.*, **285**, 757.

Ratcliffe J.G., Worth H.G. (1986). Recommended units for reporting drug concentrations in biological fluids. *Lancet*, **i**, 202.

Simpson G. (1987). Accuracy and precision of breath-alcohol measurements for a random subject in the post-absorptive state. *Clin. Chem.*, **33**, 261.

Sansom L.N. (1980). Introductory pharmacokinetics. *Clin. Biochem. Rev.*, **1**, 36.

Teale J.D. (1978). Radioimmunoassay. In *Scientific Foundations of Clinical Biochemistry*, Vol. 1, pp. 299. (Williams D.L., Nunn R.F., Marks V., eds.). Oxford: Heinemann medical

Tune L. (1984). Radioreceptor assays in clinical medicine: focus on serum anticholinergic drug concentration measurements. In *Proceedings of the Second World Conference on Clinical Pharmacology and Therapeutics* pp. 836. (Lemberger L., Reidenberg M., eds.). Bethesda: American Society of Pharmacology and Experimental Therapeutics.

Wadhwa N.K., Schroeder T.J., Pesce A.J., et al. (1987). Cyclosporine drug interactions: a review. *Therap. Drug. Mon.*, **9**, 399.

FURTHER READING

La Du B.N., Mandel H.G., Way E.L. (eds.). (1971). *Fundamentals of Drug Metabolism and Drug Disposition*. Baltimore: Williams and Wilkins.

Moyer T.P., Boeckx R.L. (eds.). (1982). *Applied Therapeutic Drug Monitoring*, Vol. 1: Fundamentals. Washington: The American Assoc. for Clinical Chemistry.

Richens A., Marks V. (eds.). (1981). *Therapeutic Drug Monitoring*. Edinburgh: Churchill Livingstone.

Widdop B. (ed.). (1985). *Therapeutic Drug Monitoring*. Edinburgh: Churchill Livingstone.

Taylor W.J., Finn A.L. (1981). *Individualizing Drug Therapy: Practical applications of drug monitoring*. Vols. 1, 2 and 3. New York: Gross, Townsend, Frank.

SECTION 4
ANAESTHETIC APPARATUS AND MONITORING

59. Anaesthetic Breathing Systems
W. Bruce

The modern anaesthetic machine is usually equipped with calibrated rotameters and accurate vaporizers in order to supply known flows and concentrations of oxygen and anaesthetic gases and vapours. This anaesthetic mixture is then delivered to the patient by means of an anaesthetic breathing system. The anaesthetic breathing system is that part of the delivery apparatus between the fresh gas outlet from the anaesthetic machine, or other gas source and the patient connection, including inspiratory and expiratory pathways. The patient connection will usually be a facemask, endotracheal tube or catheter mount.

Anaesthetic breathing systems have been used since the introduction of inhalational anaesthetic agents into medicine in the 1840's. The earlier systems often used elaborate combinations of breathing hoses, vaporizing chambers, reservoir bags and valves or stopcocks relying upon air as the carrier gas. Modern anaesthetic breathing systems still utilize combinations of many of these components. Unfortunately many of these modern systems rely upon combinations of components arranged for reasons of convenience and ease of access rather than function or efficiency. As will be discussed later in the chapter the choice of breathing system and the conditions of use can greatly alter the composition of the gas mixtures breathed by the patient.

CLASSIFICATION

Differing classifications of anaesthetic breathing systems abound and much confusion exists as to the application of older terminology such as 'open', 'semi-open', 'semi-closed' and 'closed'. McMahon (1951) classified the Mapleson systems with high fresh gas flow as 'open', whereas Moyers (1953) classifies the same systems as 'semi-open' with high fresh gas flow, but 'semi-closed' at low fresh gas flow. Conway (1970) classifies them as 'semi-closed' and Baraka (1977) classifies them as 'semi-open' (with reservoir bag). It is difficult, in view of this confusion, to persevere with a classification based upon these terms.

An alternative classification can be used, based upon the geometry of the systems. All devices used to deliver anaesthetic gas mixtures to a patient can be classified as: anaesthetic breathing systems, insufflation devices or vaporizing devices. Insufflation devices, which provide a 'one-way' flow of gases towards the patient without providing a facility (e.g., reservoir) for inspiration or a pathway for expiration, and vaporizing devices, which can be directly applied to the patient e.g., Schimmelbusch mask, should no longer be described as anaesthetic breathing systems and will not be discussed further.

GENERAL PRINCIPLES

Anaesthetic breathing systems can then be divided into:

1. Systems which utilize carbon dioxide absorption. These systems, the most commonly used of which is the circle absorption system, direct expired gases through a carbon dioxide absorption chamber. Provided oxygen is added to the system these gases can then be reinhaled without adverse physiological effects.
2. Rebreathing systems. These are systems in which there is no physical separation of inspired and expired gases. Therefore, under conditions of relatively low fresh gas flow into the system or patient hyperventilation, rebreathing of carbon dioxide containing gases is made possible. This group of systems contains the six systems classified by Willis et al. (1975), together with some recent modifications of these and the circle system without absorber.
3. Nonrebreathing systems. These systems use one-way or nonrebreathing valves to direct and separate inspired and expired gases. They can be used with continuous-flow or intermittent-flow anaesthetic machines or as a 'draw-over' system e.g., Triservice system. They are also commonly used as resuscitation devices e.g., Ambu and Laerdal systems.

Rebreathing

When a subject is able to inspire into his alveolar

space a portion of his alveolar expirate rebreathing is said to exist. A necessary result of such rebreathing is that the gas inspired by the subject will contain a higher concentration of carbon dioxide and possibly water vapour and a lower concentration of oxygen and anaesthetic gas than present in fresh gas. The alveolar concentration of any gas (FA_{gas}) is determined by: the rate of uptake of the gas from, or excretion into the alveolar space ($\dot{V}_{gas}$), the level of alveolar ventilation ($\dot{V}_A$), and the mean inspired concentration of the gas (FI_{gas}). Mathematically this can be expressed as:

$$FA_{gas} = \frac{\dot{V}_{gas}}{\dot{V}_A} + FI_{gas}$$

The normal response to rebreathing in conscious or lightly anaesthetized subjects is an increase in minute ventilation with little or no change in alveolar CO_2 or oxygen concentrations. If the ability to increase ventilation is blocked as in mechanically ventilated subjects or in subjects given powerful respiratory depressants then the predominant effect of rebreathing will be an increase in alveolar CO_2 concentration and a reduction in alveolar oxygen concentration. Clinically significant rebreathing is said to occur when the criteria described by Kain and Nunn (1968) have been satisfied:

1. An increase of at least 10% in minute ventilation in the presence of an unchanged or raised arterial CO_2 tension.
2. An increase of at least 0.7 kPa in arterial CO_2 tension in the presence of an unchanged minute ventilation.
3. An increase of at least 5% in minute ventilation in the presence of an increase of at least 0.3 kPa in arterial CO_2 tension.

Most investigators accept alveolar or end-tidal CO_2 tensions as approximating to arterial CO_2 tensions for application of these criteria. It must be stressed that the changes in minute ventilation and alveolar CO_2 concentrations induced by rebreathing may take time to reach a new equilibrium. One reason for this is the quantity of CO_2 stores (15–20 L) in the body and the buffering systems available.

In the case of anaesthetic breathing systems which have efficient CO_2 absorption, alveolar CO_2 concentration will be determined only by CO_2 production and alveolar ventilation. However, in breathing systems which allow rebreathing, the alveolar CO_2 concentration will be determined by CO_2 production, alveolar ventilation and the inspired CO_2 concentration. The inspired CO_2 concentration will be determined by the system geometry and the fresh gas flowrate. It is common practice to describe the efficiency of the various rebreathing systems in terms of the fresh gas flow rate necessary to prevent rebreathing.

The consequences of rebreathing include, not only changes in alveolar gas composition, but also the physiological sequelae of these changes. Elevated arterial CO_2 tension is associated with: increased cardiac output, increased cerebral blood flow, a respiratory acidosis with compensatory hyperventilation, a shift to the right of the oxygen dissociation curve and an increase in the extracellular potassium concentration. With increasing arterial CO_2 tensions, sympathetic stimulation occurs causing alterations of regional blood flow with reduced splanchnic, hepatic and renal blood flow, probably secondary to increased vascular resistances within these circulations. Pulmonary vascular resistance is also sensitive to elevated alveolar CO_2 concentration with a resultant increase in pulmonary vascular resistance and also an increase in bronchial smooth muscle tone (Sykes 1987). Rebreathing during spontaneous ventilation should be avoided and during mechanical ventilation if rebreathing is allowed then some degree of hyperventilation should be planned to achieve normocapnia.

Resistance and Work of Breathing

All confined pathways for the flow of gas offer some resistance to flow. The resistance of any apparatus will be greatly affected by those parts of it with the smallest internal diameter, and the characteristics of any valves used. In smooth straight tubes gas flow will be laminar at low flow rates and so resistance to flow will be inversely proportional to the fourth power of tube radius and directly proportional to tube length, gas flow rate and gas viscosity. Turbulent flow can be induced by changes in tube diameter and by changes in direction of flow and resistance to flow will then be inversely proportional to the fifth power of the radius and directly proportional to the square of volume flow and gas density. Gas flow in anaesthetic breathing systems is often in a transitional form between laminar and turbulent flow making predictions of gas flow characteristics difficult.

Although anaesthetized patients retain some ability to compensate for added resistance to breathing by increasing inspiratory muscle tension a reduction in ventilation is a common sequel to increased inspiratory resistance (Nunn and Ezi Ashi, 1961). Increased expiratory resistance is usually well-tolerated, although high levels of expiratory resistance will initiate active expiration. Campbell et al. (1959) found that active expiration was not required to overcome expiratory pressures up to $10 \, cmH_2O$. Large changes in alveolar pressure may also have an adverse effect on the cardiovascular system.

If resistance to breathing is increased, then the work of breathing must also be increased. Studying resistance to breathing in terms of the pressure drop across a breathing system at a constant flow ignores the fact that breathing systems have an elastic resistance to flow as well as a frictional component. This elastic resistance will be determined by the distensible components of the breathing system and the changing nature of flow within the system. This problem can be overcome by applying simulated or real ventilation to breathing systems and analysing pressure volume loops. The additional work of breathing imposed by the systems will be equal to the area of the pressure-volume loop. Barnes et al. (1977) used simulated ventilation and Kay et al. (1983) used both simulated and volunteer ventilation to investigate the additional work of breathing imposed by several breathing systems. All the systems studied increased the work of breathing with the additional expiratory work exceeding additional inspiratory work. Increasing the fresh gas flow rate into the system resulted in an increase in expiratory work. Of the commonly used systems the circle absorption system imposes the highest additional inspiratory work and the Bain system at high fresh gas flow rates imposes the highest additional expiratory work. Some degree of expiratory resistance and positive end-expiratory pressure may however be beneficial in preventing early airway closure and alveolar collapse.

Heat and Moisture Conservation

There is now little dispute that breathing dry gases at room temperature for long periods of time under anaesthesia is harmful. Chalon et al. (1972) demonstrated that ciliated respiratory mucosal cells were destroyed when exposed to dry anaesthetic gases for long periods. Ciliary function ceases, mucous clearance reduces and postoperative pulmonary complications are increased. Body temperature decreases at a faster rate under anaesthesia when dry anaesthetic gases are breathed. There are many methods available to reduce this problem including the use of the circle absorption system or rebreathing systems to provide more humid, warmer gases. It has been recommended that an optimal water content of inspired gases should exceed 23 mg/L. Only two anaesthetic breathing systems have been shown to approach this level of humidification—the circle absorption system and the Bain system using mechanical ventilation and ventilation/fresh gas flow ratio of 3:1.

Components

Anaesthetic breathing systems are combinations of several of the following: breathing hoses, reservoir bags, adjustable pressure limiting valves (APL), exhaust or 'pop off' valves, unidirectional valves, CO_2 absorbers, connectors and adaptors, Vaporizers are often incorporated into the breathing system and bacterial filters are commonly used. The design and manufacture of these components is usually governed by international and/or regionally accepted standards.

Whilst 22 mm diameter corrugated black antistatic rubber breathing hoses are still used in many departments, increasing use has been made of 22 mm diameter corrugated plastic hoses. The hoses are designed to prevent kinking when wound into a 50 mm internal diameter spiral. Plastic hoses however are more prone to kinking than rubber hoses. The volume per unit length of both types of hose is about 400–450 ml/m. Both types of breathing hoses are relatively non-compliant with approximate compliances of rubber hoses 1 ml/(m·cmH$_2$O) and plastic hoses 0.3–0.8 ml/(m·cmH$_2$O) (Russell 1983). Plastic hoses unfortunately form pinholes more commonly than rubber hoses thus making system pressure checks more important. Plastic hoses also tend to slip off connections more easily than rubber hoses and do not stand autoclaving, although many departments reuse plastic hoses after pasteurizing. Resistance to gas flow through breathing hoses is minimal with a pressure gradient at 30 L/min flow of less than 0.15 cmH$_2$O/m. Plastic breathing hoses are lighter than rubber hoses, and are less likely to pull on conical fittings and less force is applied to the patient connection. They are transparent, and they absorb less volatile anaesthetic agent than rubber hoses.

Reservoir bags are usually made of rubber or neoprene although plastic bags are also available. They function as reservoirs of gas in the breathing system to compensate for breathing system volume changes caused by a constant fresh gas flow but a variable extraction from (inspiration) and addition to the system (expiration). The reservoir facilitates the delivery of gas despite brief but high peak flow rates. It also serves to facilitate manual or assisted ventilation, provides a monitor of respiration, and provides a pressure limiting function with the bags designed to distend enormously when subjected to pressures above 50–60 cmH$_2$O without increasing pressure above this (Parmley et al., 1972). Plastic reservoir bags are less compliant and pressures of 150 cmH$_2$O are possible. If a breathing system does not include a compliant reservoir bag then some form of pressure release valve should be incorporated into the system to prevent patients being exposed to pressures in excess of 50–60 cmH$_2$O.

Adjustable pressure limiting valves (APL valves) are designed to vent excess gas from the breathing system. The APL valves in common use are variable orifice, variable resistance devices. Modern APL valves include a facility for scavenging. Most APL valves are of similar design to the Heidbrink valve consisting of a light disc held onto a circular knife edge by a light spring with tension in the spring adjusted by a screw thread. The opening pressure of these valves should be high enough (approximately 0.5 cmH$_2$O) to allow distension of the reservoir bag but once open the valve should not provide excessive resistance to flow. Nott et al. (1977) found that at 30 L/min gas flow 44% of Heidbrink type valves had resistances above that suggested as an acceptable maximum by Nunn (1969) i.e. 3 cmH$_2$O pressure drop at 30 L/min flow. The newer valves designed for use with scavenging systems all provided less resistance than this maximum.

Unidirectional valves are mainly used in circle

absorption systems to control the direction of flow without providing significant resistance to flow. Low resistance is achieved by making the valve area as large as possible and the valve disc as light as possible. Discs are often made of mica and have an opening pressure less than $0.5\,cmH_2O$ with a pressure drop of less than $1\,cmH_2O$ at $30\,L/min$ when dry. Care must be taken to maintain the valve in a horizontal position.

Connectors are designed to join two or more components with an airtight seal. Adaptors, which are specialized connectors designed to establish functional continuity between otherwise incompatible components may be required. All connections between components of modern adult anaesthetic breathing systems are achieved with 22 mm or 15 mm male to female fittings. Fittings are conical with a 1 in 40 taper and are commonly constructed of plastic. Unfortunately connectors are a frequent site of disconnection and a failsafe method of connection of components has yet to be described. Connectors are also a potential cause of turbulent gas flow and subsequently higher resistance.

SYSTEMS UTILIZING CARBON DIOXIDE ABSORPTION

Carbon dioxide absorption has been used in anaesthetic practice since John Snow used potassium hydroxide during chloroform anaesthesia (Snow 1858). Aqueous sodium hydroxide was later used to absorb carbon dioxide by Jackson in the United States (Jackson 1915). During World War 1 granular forms of gas absorbents were developed for use in gas masks and in 1924 Waters described his 'to and fro' absorption system (Waters 1924).

Brian Sword is credited with introducing the circle absorption system into anaesthesia (Sword 1930) and various modifications have been used since (*see* Fig. 59.1). Techniques using low fresh gas flows into the circle absorption system became popular with the introduction of cyclopropane in the 1930s. In recent years, the circle absorption system is still most commonly used with fresh gas flows of 4–8 L/min. With better monitoring equipment, the high cost of the more modern volatile anaesthetic agents and concern about environmental pollution, interest in using lower fresh gas flows remains. The circle absorption system is today, the most commonly used anaesthetic breathing system in the world.

Absorbents

The circle absorption system relies upon either soda lime or barium hydroxide lime to absorb carbon dioxide. Modern soda lime contains approximately 80% calcium hydroxide, 4% sodium hydroxide, 1% potassium hydroxide with water making up the remainder. In addition, small amounts of indicator and hardeners (silica and kieselguhr) are present. Barium hydroxide

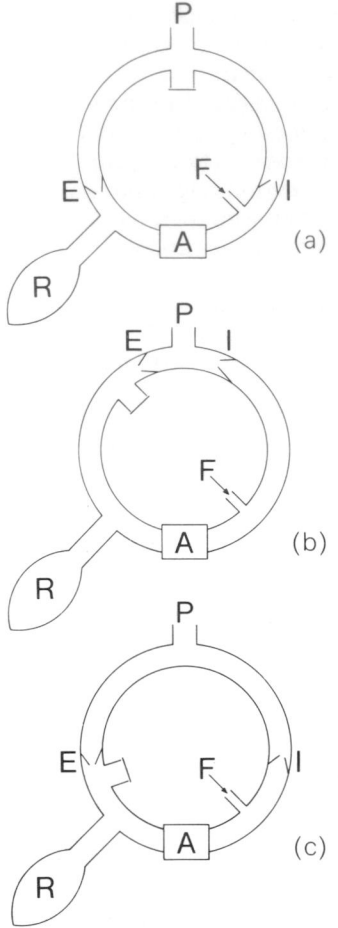

Fig. 59.1 Three different circle system arrangements. (a) Overflow close to patient. Efficiency high during spontaneous ventilation but low in controlled ventilation. (b) Overflow and unidirectional valves close to patient. Efficiency high during both spontaneous and controlled ventilation. (c) Overflow remote from patient. Efficiency during spontaneous ventilation less than system (a) but equal to system (b) during controlled ventilation. A = absorber; F = fresh gas inlet; P = patient; R = reservoir bag; E and I = unidirectional valves.

lime on the other hand, contains 20% barium hydroxide and 80% calcium hydroxide as well as an indicator. No hardeners are necessary as barium hydroxide and water form an octahydrate crystal with sufficient hardness to stop dust formation and ensuring a more stable water content.

The water content of granular absorbents is essential because the chemical reactions involved in absorbing carbon dioxide take place in solution. The overall reaction of carbon dioxide with soda lime is:

$$2CO_2 + 2H_2O \rightarrow 2H_2CO_3$$
$$2H_2CO_3 + 2NaOH + Ca(OH)_2 \rightarrow CaCO_3 + Na_2CO_3 + 4H_2O$$

In soda lime, the carbonic acid reacts with sodium or potassium hydroxide to form intermediate carbonates which then react with calcium hydroxide to form calcium carbonate with an equilibrium favouring calcium carbonate stability.

The absorbent capacity of soda lime is 25.1 L of carbon dioxide per 100 g and for barium hydroxide lime is 27.1 L of carbon dioxide per 100 g (Spain, 1981). However, indicator change and a rise in inspired carbon dioxide levels will normally have occurred after absorption of 9–19 L of carbon dioxide per 100 g of soda lime. The chemical reactions involved in carbon dioxide absorption in soda lime are exothermic (13 700 calories per mole CO_2 absorbed) and produce water. Fortunately, these properties can be used to advantage.

Carbon dioxide absorbents will also absorb small amounts of anaesthetic vapours and gases. There is a potential, but unsubstantiated risk that patients susceptible to malignant hyperthermia or hepatotoxicity may develop problems if exposed to absorbents contaminated with, for example, halothane. Halogenated anaesthetic vapours are more readily absorbed by dry soda lime than by wet soda lime.

Degradation of halogenated anaesthetic agents occurs in the absorbent with the production of potentially toxic products. Degradation will occur more rapidly at higher temperatures. One example of this type of reaction is the degradation of trichlorethylene in the presence of warm soda lime to produce dichloracetylene. Apart from being spontaneously combustible this product has been implicated as a cause of cranial nerve lesions and as a possible cause of death following trichlorethylene anaesthesia using a circle absorption system. No halogenated anaesthetic agent is totally resistant to degradation in soda lime and the more modern agents, isoflurane and I-653 both produce small quantities of fluoroform when exposed to dry soda lime (Eger and Strum, 1987).

When carbon dioxide absorbents are handled roughly (particularly soda lime) the resultant dust may be harmful to the respiratory tract or cause facial burns (Lauria, 1975). This is less of a problem with the circle absorption system than older absorption systems, e.g., the Waters 'to and fro' system.

Function of the Circle System

In the presence of efficient CO_2 absorption in a circle system, gas inspired by a subject will be free of CO_2 and fresh gas flow will not affect CO_2 homeostasis. The important variables to consider here are inspired and alveolar concentrations of oxygen and anaesthetic agent. At high fresh gas flows expired gas will tend to be flushed from a circle absorption system and inspired and fresh gas will have the same composition. As fresh gas flow is reduced from these high levels an increasing proportion of the inspirate will be made up of expired gas from which CO_2 has been removed. This expired gas will also differ from fresh gas in oxygen and anaesthetic agent concentrations, these differences being determined by the rate of uptake of

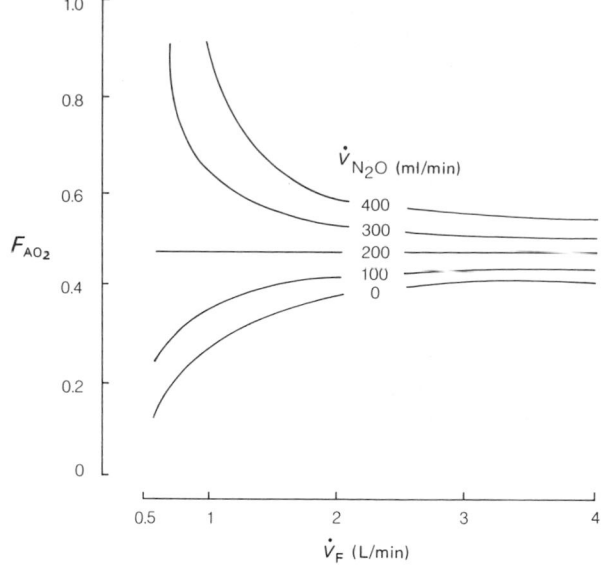

Fig. 59.2 Variations of F_{AO_2} with fresh gas flow ($\dot{V}_F$) and nitrous oxide uptake $\dot{V}_{N_2O}$ in a circle system. An oxygen uptake of 200 ml/min, a carbon dioxide excretion of 160 ml/min and an F_{ACO_2} of 0.05 are assumed.

oxygen and anaesthetic agent by the subject. The efficiency of the system in conserving fresh gas and minimizing rebreathing at relatively high fresh gas flows will be a function of the geometry of the system (Eger and Ethans, 1968)—see Fig. 59.1 and 59.2. Economy of fresh gas requires that the reservoir bag and the subject should be on opposite sides of both the expiratory and inspiratory unidirectional valves and that the overspill valve must not be between the subject and the inspiratory unidirectional valve (Eger, 1974). The composition of inspired gas will also be influenced by the degree of mixing of fresh and expired gases in the system, and this may be affected by the respiratory pattern or mode of ventilation (Schoonbee and Conway, 1981). As fresh gas flow approaches basal levels the geometry of the system plays a diminishing part in determining function.

At fresh gas flows equal to gas uptake from the circle system, the limiting situation is reached. At this point fresh gas flow will contain only enough oxygen to satisfy the subjects metabolic demands and enough anaesthetic agent to satisfy the uptake of anaesthetic agent by the subject and the components of the system as well as that agent degraded within the system by soda lime. As fresh gas flows are reduced to basal levels several practical considerations become vital.

1. The system must be free of leaks. This can only be ensured by rigorous preanaesthetic checks and continued vigilance.
2. There must be accurate monitoring of gas mixtures within the system. Inspired oxygen concentration and inspired or end-expired anaesthetic vapour concentration must be monitored.

3. There must be efficient CO_2 absorption. This can only be demonstrated with certainty by monitoring inspired CO_2 concentration.
4. Rotameters must be accurate at low flow levels.
5. There must be an adequate source of anaesthetic vapour to the system. It is possible to achieve a high concentration of anaesthetic vapour in the fresh gas flow by using a 'bubble through' vaporizer. However the commonly used vaporizers, e.g., Fluotec Mk III will not be able to deliver an adequate mass of anaesthetic vapour for smooth induction of anaesthesia with fresh gas flow at basal levels. Delivery of adequate amounts of anaesthetic vapours to the system can be achieved by using a low resistance vaporizer inside the circle (e.g., Goldman vaporizer) or by direct injection of liquid anaesthetic agent into the expiratory limb of the system using a glass syringe and optimally a syringe driver. Vaporizers used inside the circle system will deliver more anaesthetic agent at higher levels of ventilation whereas vapour delivery from vaporizers used outside the circle is dependent upon fresh gas flow. Most vaporizers used inside the circle system have minimal temperature compensation and with prolonged use water vapour within the circle will tend to condense in the cool liquid anaesthetic and potentially reduce the output.

The obvious danger with the use of in-circle vaporizers is overdosage of anaesthetic vapour. As this situation will generally cause a degree of hypoventilation in those subjects breathing spontaneously the potential for serious overdosage is higher when subjects are mechanically ventilated. Accurate prediction of vapour concentrations within the system using either in-circle or out-of circle vaporizers is impossible at basal fresh gas flows, so monitoring of vapour concentration is necessary.

Having a source of anaesthetic vapour within the circle enables the anaesthetist to alter the concentration of anaesthetic vapour rapidly. Relying upon a vaporizer in the fresh gas line when basal flows of perhaps 200 ml of oxygen are used limits significantly both the rate of delivery of anaesthetic vapour to the system and the possible rate of change of anaesthetic vapour concentration within the system. The rate of change of anaesthetic vapour concentration within the circle will be determined by the circle system volume, fresh gas flow rate and net gas uptake and can be expressed in terms of a time constant:

$$\text{Time constant} = \frac{\text{Circle system volume}}{\text{Fresh gas flow—net gas uptake}}$$

The time constant will be prolonged if the circle system has a large volume, if fresh gas flow is low or if net gas uptake is relatively high. For example in a circle system of 5 L volume with a fresh gas flow of 250 ml/min and a net gas uptake of 200 ml/min the time constant will be 100 min, but at 5 L/min fresh gas

flow the time constant will be slightly greater than 1 min.

Since, at basal fresh gas flow into the circle system, gases will tend to mix uniformly it is then possible to mathematically predict inspired and alveolar concentrations of oxygen and anaesthetic agent for any known value of uptake of oxygen and anaesthetic agent at known levels of ventilation (Conway, 1980). Figure 59.2 shows the results of such calculations when nitrous oxide and oxygen are supplied to a circle system as a 50:50 mixture and at flows from 500 ml/min to 4 L/min. A constant oxygen consumption of 200 ml/min and a constant ventilation to produce an alveolar CO_2 concentration of 5% have been assumed. As fresh gas flow falls so alveolar oxygen levels fall when anaesthetic uptake is low in relation to oxygen consumption, and rise when anaesthetic uptake is high. These changes are slight when fresh gas flow is high, but become increasingly marked as fresh gas flow approaches basal levels. As alveolar oxygen levels rise so alveolar nitrous oxide levels must fall. The use of low fresh gas flow at times when anaesthetic uptake is high may lead to an inadequate alveolar concentration of anaesthetic agent.

This illustrates an important problem of low flow anaesthetic breathing systems—the increasing influence of gas uptake upon gas concentrations within the system as fresh gas flow is reduced towards basal levels. Anaesthetic uptake will vary during exposure with initially high levels of uptake falling towards zero as equilibrium is approached. The closest approximation (Lowe, 1979) available for the rate of uptake of anaesthetic vapour ($\dot{V}_{AN}$) in adult man at time t after the start of administration is:

$$\dot{V}_{AN} = k \cdot t^{-1/2} \text{ ml/min}$$

where k has a value of 1000 for nitrous oxide (Severinghaus, 1954) and of 55 for halothane (Lowe, 1979). This formula suggests that for halothane, uptake after 20 min would be greater than 12 ml vapour per min and after 1 h uptake would be a little over 7 ml/min.

Rapid uptake of anaesthetic agent following induction will present problems where out-of circle vaporizers are used and two methods are available to overcome this. Either fresh gas flows into the system can be increased for the first 15–20 min (Conway, 1983) or the system can be primed with vapour-rich fresh gas (Lowe, 1979).

Another problem encountered when using the circle system at basal fresh gas flow is nitrogen accumulation within the system. The body contains approximately 1 L of dissolved nitrogen and 2 L of nitrogen in the FRC. This will potentially dilute the gases within the system. This probably can be overcome by using a period of high fresh gas flow at induction of anaesthesia using oxygen or oxygen/nitrous oxide. The majority of the nitrogen contained within the FRC will be 'washed out' by this technique in 2–5 min (Lowe and Ernst, 1981). Following this denitrogenation some nitrogen will undoubtedly leave the dissolved body stores and enter the system. Barton and Nunn (1975) found that this produced a nitrogen concentration of less than 4% within the system after one hour.

Advantages of the Circle Absorption System

1. **Economy.** Using basal gas flows a considerable cumulative saving can be demonstrated even allowing for the cost of monitoring equipment and absorbent. Nunn (1979) estimated a saving of some 78 cents (US)/h using a basal flow system opposed to a system, using halothane, consuming 7 L/min. Obviously this saving will be greater when using enflurane or isoflurane. Virtue (1979) estimated a savings of $5.00 (US)/h when enflurane anaesthesia was used. Bengstrom et al. (1988) found that average drug costs per hour of anaesthesia (including intravenous drugs) using isoflurane/N_2O/O_2 in a circle absorption system were approximately $9.00 (US) using fresh gas flows of 3–6 L/min, and $5.00 (US) using low flow. Obviously the economic advantage may be more significant in underdeveloped countries. Another consideration is that newer agents being developed will probably be more expensive than isoflurane.

2. **Conservation** of heat and moisture. Absorption of CO_2 liberates water and heat resulting in a higher water content of inspired gases and some warming of those gases. There will obviously be some cooling of gases in the inspiratory tubing between the absorber and the patient, but gases reaching the patient will still be warmer and wetter than fresh gas. As fresh gas flow into the circle system increases so more expired gas will be vented from the system reducing the amount of CO_2 absorbed and thus heat and moisture production within the system.

3. **Pollution** of both the workplace and the atmosphere is minimized. Doubt still surrounds claims that pollution of the operating suite with anaesthetic gases may produce a higher incidence of female infertility, spontaneous abortion and fetal abnormalities as well as poor cognition, performance and malaise. Nitrous oxide has been shown to inactivate methionine synthetase in concentrations exceeding 1000 parts per million and the toxicity of lower concentrations of nitrous oxide has yet to be determined (*see* Nunn and Chamarin, 1985). It is agreed however that a reduction in operating suite pollution from anaesthetic agents is a worthwhile goal and in the USA the National Institute for Occupational Safety and Health (NIOSH) recommends nitrous oxide levels be kept below 25 parts per million and halogenated agent levels less than 1 part per million. Efficient scavenging, efficient air conditioning and the use of the circle system with low fresh gas flows will achieve a reduction in pollution. However, relying upon scavenging or air conditioning to reduce pollution whilst high fresh gas flows are used will usually ensure that more waste anaesthetic gases are 'dumped' into the atmo-

sphere where there is evidence of ozone breakdown by chlorofluorocarbons. Whilst the anaesthetic contribution to chlorofluorocarbon pollution may be small it is a contribution which can be reduced.

3. **Education.** The technique of using the circle system with low fresh gas flow provides the anaesthetist with a more intimate knowledge of the patient's metabolism and oxygen demands. Oxygen utilization will be the inflow rate necessary to maintain a constant end expired reservoir bag volume with the expiratory valve closed.

Disadvantages of the circle absorption system with low fresh gas flows include the necessary monitoring equipment, the fact that the system is bulky and has more components than the more simple systems, the slow rate of change of gas composition and the necessary extra vigilance. The system also offers a higher resistance to breathing than many of the simpler systems (Kay et al., 1983) and attempts have been made to reduce the inspiratory resistance using a circulator (Revell, 1959) and a fresh gas driven venturi (Neff et al., 1968).

The majority of anaesthetists are reluctant to use the circle system at basal fresh gas flow probably because of unfamiliarity, some of the mentioned disadvantages, worries about nitrogen accumulation, and the need for more frequent 'fine-tuning'. Many will wish to use nitrous oxide and this adds some complexity at low flows. Multiple techniques have been described to allow nitrous oxide use at low gas flow involving denitrogenation, high initial gas flows for 15–20 min (Virtue, 1974) followed by a gas flow of 500 ml/min ($F_1O_2 = 0.6$) or using a primed circuit adding oxygen at basal flow and titrating the nitrous oxide flow to produce an oxygen concentration of 30–40%.

The safest way of using nitrous oxide during low flow techniques is to start with a period of high nitrous oxide-oxygen flows and then reduce flow towards the values suggested by Virtue (1974) with inspired oxygen concentration subsequently controlled by suitable monitoring. During the course of administration nitrous oxide inflow will need to be gradually and continuously reduced as nitrous oxide uptake declines (Conway, 1983).

Use of the circle absorption system at higher fresh gas flows (3–6 L/min) is common practice and at these flows there may still be slight advantages over many of the rebreathing systems and nonrebreathing systems in terms of economy, heat and moisture conservation and lower pollution. At these high flows CO_2 absorbent will tend to last longer as gas vented from the system will contain alveolar gas prior to exposure to absorbent. At a fresh gas flow of 3 L/min, provided oxygen concentration is monitored, nitrous oxide can be used safely. Tec type out-of circle vaporizers will be able to deliver enough anaesthetic vapour to satisfy patient uptake without the necessity to monitor vapour concentration within the system, the majority of rotameters found on anaesthetic machines will be accurate, the time constant of the system should not exceed 2 min, there will be considerable conservation of heat and moisture, and pollution and cost will be reduced in comparison to rebreathing systems. The anxieties of many anaesthetists about using the circle system at low fresh gas flow will also be relieved at this flowrate. There can be little justification for using flows higher than this for the duration of anaesthesia.

REBREATHING SYSTEMS

Mapleson (1954) described and analysed five feasible ways, denoted from A-E in which a source of fresh gas, mask, reservoir bag, expiratory valve and length of wide bore tubing could be arranged to administer gases to a subject. Willis et al. (1975) later added the F system to the original five arrangements (Fig. 59.3).

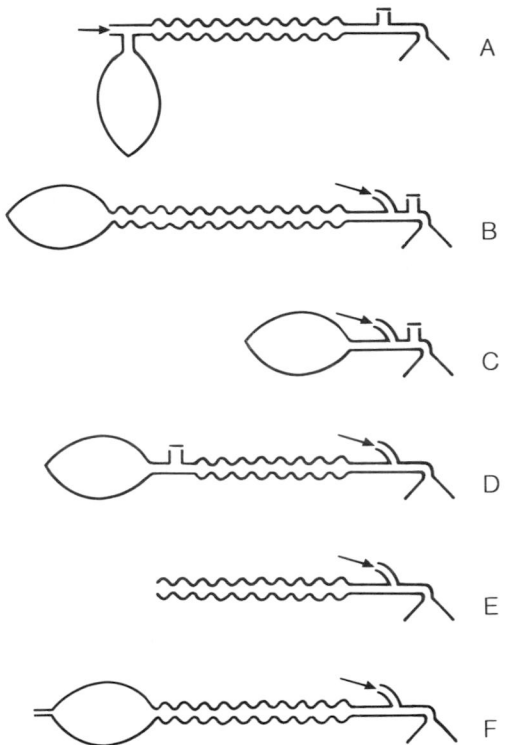

Fig. 59.3 Six rebreathing anaesthetic systems (Reproduced with permission from Willis et al., 1975).

The A system is the Magill attachment, the B and C systems have mixed behaviour and the D, E and F systems can all be regarded as T-pieces. Several other systems are now included in the rebreathing group including further modifications of the Mapleson systems, systems combining several Mapelson systems, and also the circle system without absorber.

The Mapleson A System

This system was first used by Sir Ivan Magill in the 1920s and is still commonly referred to as the Magill

attachment. Mapleson (1954) published the first formal analysis of the system and concluded from this theoretical approach that during spontaneous ventilation a fresh gas flow equal to the subjects alveolar ventilation should ensure that all gas breathed by the subject should have the same composition as fresh gas. When used during spontaneous respiration (Fig. 59.4) the APL valve is closed at the beginning of

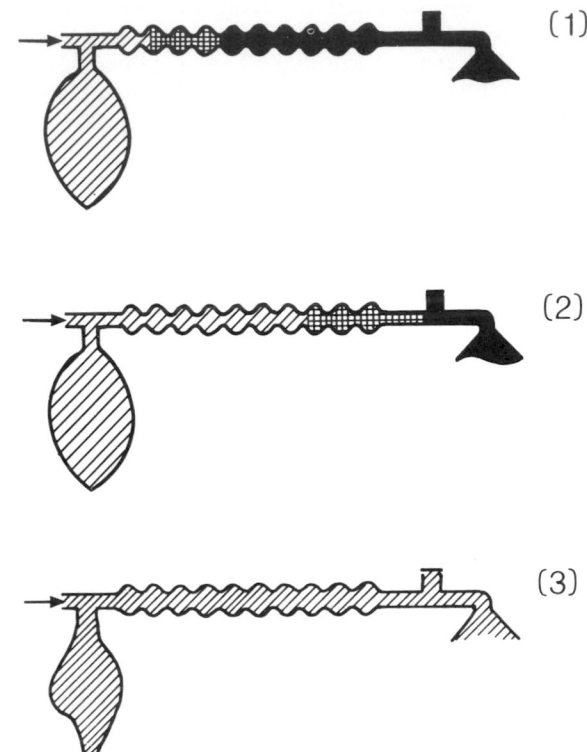

Fig. 59.4 The Mapleson A system during spontaneous ventilation. In (1) during expiration the reservoir bag fills as both fresh gas and the patient's expirate, including dead space (hatched) and alveolar gas (dark) enter the system. In (2) as expiration proceeds alveolar gas is vented from the system and dead space gas is 'pushed' towards the APL valve by the fresh gas flow. Inspiration is then able to proceed with minimal rebreathing of alveolar gas (3).

expiration then as expiration proceeds fresh gas enters the system at the reservoir end and dead space gas and alveolar gas will enter the wide bore tubing from the subject end. As expiration proceeds further the reservoir bag will fill with fresh gas and dead space and alveolar gas will then be pushed towards an open expiratory valve by the continuing fresh gas flow. At the most efficient fresh gas flow all alveolar gas will be vented from the system leaving only dead space gas and fresh gas within the system.

This descripton assumes there is no longitudinal mixing of gases within the system, that the wide bore tubing of the system will accommodate the subjects tidal volume without alveolar gas reaching the reservoir bag and that there is a stable respiratory pattern. It would also be necessary then to have a sharp, well maintained demarcation between dead space and alveolar gas during expiration but it can be seen in Fig. 59.5 that the CO_2 content of expired gas does not

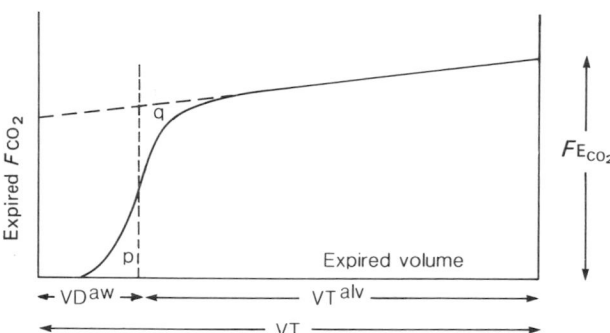

Fig. 59.5 Assessment of anatomical dead space using expired CO_2 concentration. When area p equals area q then VD will equal anatomical dead space. Note that CO_2 appears in the expired gas before all the dead space gas is expired and there is a steady rise in expired CO_2 towards the end of expiration. (Modified with permission from Nunn, 1977, p. 217.)

yield a vertical line at the dead space—alveolar gas interface and that alveolar gas is not of uniform composition as shown by a gradual rise in CO_2 concentration during expiration. Conway et al. (1976) found that there was longitudinal gas mixing within the system and that if a volume of fresh gas equal to the alveolar expirate was supplied to the system during a respiratory cycle the small degree of mixing would result in a small amount of CO_2 containing gas remaining in the system and forming the first part of the succeeding alveolar inspirate. As this CO_2 containing gas is rebreathed in early inspiration, the minimum inspired CO_2 may still be zero in the presence of significant rebreathing.

Clinical studies by Kain et al. (1968) in patients and Norman et al. (1968) and Conway et al. (1976) in volunteers showed that a fresh gas flow of 70% of minute ventilation could prevent rebreathing with the Mapleson A system during spontaneous ventilation. An accurate prediction of fresh gas flow requirements of the A system will therefore rely upon prediction of minute ventilation. Because of the variable nature of minute ventilation, it is recommended that a higher than minimum fresh gas flow be used. Fresh gas flow in the order of 80–90% of predicted minute ventilation (Conway, 1983) should allow an adequate margin of safety, such that rebreathing is unlikely.

The Mapleson A system at low fresh gas flow (i.e. below alveolar ventilation) behaves in a way that results in alveolar CO_2 concentration is determined by fresh gas flow and CO_2 production and being independent of alveolar ventilation as predicted by

Mapleson (1958) and Conway et al. (1976). Conway also predicted that an increase in ventilation caused by rebreathing will increase CO_2 production and may allow alveolar gas to enter the reservoir bag, turning the system into a 'mixing device' with high CO_2 concentrations throughout the system.

During controlled ventilation with the Mapleson A system the efficiency changes dramatically. The APL valve will vent gases during inspiration and much of this vented gas will be fresh gas. Several clinical studies using the Mapleson A system during controlled ventilation have been carried out. Sykes (1959) suggested that the necessary fresh gas flow to avoid rebreathing was impractically high. Marshall and Henderson (1968) were able to produce a reduction in arterial CO_2 tension in all patients studied at 10 L/min fresh gas flow. They found that the system was more efficient at higher tidal volumes. Obiaya and DaKouraju (1976) found normocarbia easy to achieve at 9 L/min fresh gas flow. Theoretically, efficiency during controlled ventilation will be improved by venting as much gas as possible from the system during early inspiration, i.e. using a decelerating flow inspiratory pattern as well as a large tidal volume. There is no doubt however that the Mapleson A system is less efficient and less predictable during controlled ventilation than during spontaneous ventilation and is best avoided for prolonged controlled ventilation.

Recent Modifications of the Mapleson A System

Some of the disadvantages of the classical Mapleson A system are limited access to the expiratory valve which is at the patient connection and difficulty in scavenging. Lack (1976) overcame these problems by developing a system with the expiratory valve at the machine end of the system and using a coaxial hose (Fig. 59.6). A noncoaxial version of this system is also

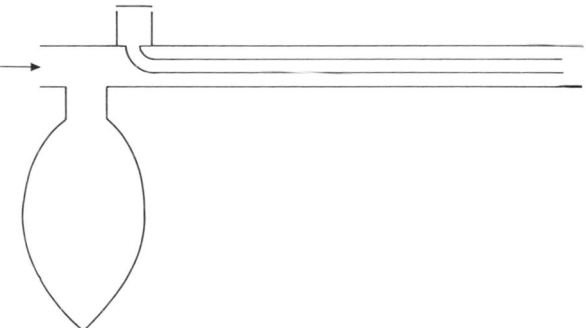

Fig. 59.6 Schematic representation of the coaxial Lack system. Outer tube diameter is 28 mm with 14 mm diameter inner tube.

available. The Lack system has a large diameter outer tube 2.8 cm in diameter with an inner tube of 14 mm internal diameter and is 1.5 metres long. Using an outer tube of this dimension has lowered the inspiratory resistance with the inner tube in place to less than the inspiratory resistance of the classical Mapleson A system (Kay et al., 1983). Expiratory resistance was found to be acceptable by Nott et al. (1977) at 1.35 cmH$_2$O for a 30 L flow. Clinical studies have shown the Lack system to function as a Mapleson A system with fresh gas flows of minute ventilation or less needed to prevent rebreathing (Millar, 1987), Nott et al., 1982). Barnes et al., 1980 however found evidence of rebreathing at fresh gas flows equal to minute ventilation while Humphrey (1982) found the Lack system to be more efficient than the Magill system. A fresh gas flow of 80–90% of minute ventilation is therefore recommended. The noncoaxial form of this system can also be expected to have similar requirements.

Miller (1979) described a valveless Mapleson A configuration system which he named the preferential flow system and a later comparison with a Magill system during spontaneous ventilation showed that both systems function efficiently with rebreathing being detectable at approximately 60–80% of minute ventilation Miller and Couper (1983).

Voss (1985) described the first 'enclosed' Mapleson A system (Fig. 59.7) and suggested that during spon-

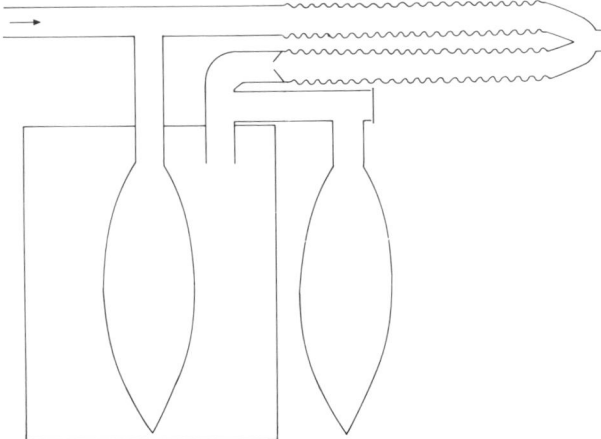

Fig. 59.7 Enclosed Magill Anesthestic Breathing System. During spontaneous ventilation this system will behave like a classical Mapleson A. During controlled ventilation pressure around the inspiratory reservoir bag will serve to squeeze the inspiratory reservoir bag and close the expiratory unidirectional valve. During expiration alveolar gas and some deadspace gas will be vented hence maintaining efficiency.

taneous ventilation fresh gas flow should equal minute ventilation. This was further supported by Bruce and Soni (1989). The most impressive benefit of this system is that during controlled ventilation with this system the expiratory one-way valve will remain closed during inspiration and hence a high proportion of vented gas will be alveolar gas. In theory ventilation need only equal alveolar ventilation. The result

will be a much more easily predictable Pa_{CO_2} than with the T-piece system where a very large minute ventilation is necessary to produce similar predictability. In practice it is found that during the initial part of expiration when controlled ventilation is used, some anatomical dead space gas is also vented and unless the expiratory one- way valve is weighted or a flow restrictor (i.e. resistance) is used in the expiratory limb, then a fresh gas flow of 80–90% of minute ventilation should be used. Miller and Miller (1958) described a similar system and together with the enclosed preferential flow system categorized these systems as enclosed afferent reservoir breathing systems. They found that during mechanical ventilation these systems were more efficient than the Mapleson D (Bain) system.

Other attempts have been made to modify Mapleson A systems during controlled ventilation. Carden (1972, 1974) used a length of Penrose drain at the end of a corrugated hose to replace the expiratory valve. He was able to pinch off the drain with each manual ventilation allowing easy control of Pa_{CO_2} in both children and adults at fresh gas flows equal to predicted minute ventilation. Jonsson has also described a valve which will close during inspiration whether ventilation is controlled or spontaneous.

The Mapleson B and C Systems

In theory during spontaneous ventilation these two systems should have identical fresh gas flow requirements. The fresh gas flow rate should supply a volume equal to the alveolar portion of each breath between commencement of inspiration and the early part of expiration when the alveolar gas arrives at the expiratory valve. This flow will usually be slightly greater than minute ventilation. Any CO$_2$ containing gas that passes the fresh gas inlet will be in a blind limb and will contribute to rebreathing, hence even slight changes in tidal volume may precipitate rebreathing. When the Mapleson C system is used for controlled ventilation all expired gas will mix in the reservoir bag with fresh gas entering during expiration. During inspiration this mixture, together with inflowing fresh gas will both enter the lungs and be ventilated. Normocapnia should result if both ventilation and fresh gas flow are 50% greater than resting minute volume. During controlled ventilation with the B system, the corrugated tubing may act as a reservoir for fresh gas flowing during any end-expiratory pause and lesser levels of fresh gas flow and ventilation may be required than with the Mapleson C system.

The Mapleson D, E and F Systems

These systems are geometrically T-pieces at the subject end and only really differ in the way that they vent gases. The first T-piece was described by Ayre in 1937. During spontaneous ventilation as long as fresh gas flow exceeds peak inspiratory flow, rebreathing will not occur in these systems. However peak inspiratory flow in many subjects may exceed 20 L/min and many anaesthetic machines will be unable to deliver such high flows; apparatus resistance at this high fresh gas flow must also be considered. A compromise can be achieved taking into consideration the character of inspiratory flow. Figure 59.8 shows a representative

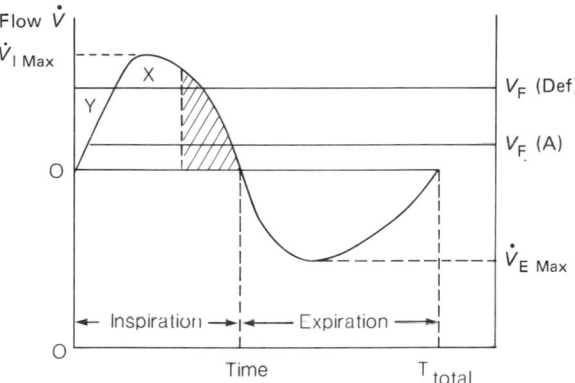

Fig. 59.8 Illustration of a representative respiratory flow wave form during halothane anaesthesia. The vertical broken line during inspiration divides inspiration into alveolar volume and dead space (hatched). At fresh gas flow $V_F(D)$ when area Y equals area X then no rebreathing should occur. Fresh gas flow $V_F(A)$ for a Mapleson A system to avoid rebreathing is also shown. Modified with permission from L.O. Johnsson and H. Zetterstrom, 1985.)

respiratory flow pattern with the vertical broken line during inspiration dividing the area under the curve (inspired volume) into alveolar volume and dead space volume (hatched area). If fresh gas flow is maintained at $\dot{V}_F(D)$ then initially this flow will exceed inspiratory flow resulting in excess volume (Y) collecting in the reservoir limb. When inspiratory flow exceeds fresh gas flow, then volume Y will also be inspired and as long as volumes X and Y are equal, significant rebreathing should not occur. This fresh gas flow will usually be at least twice the minute ventilation. For comparison the fresh gas flow requirement for a Mapleson A system ($\dot{V}_F(A)$) has also been drawn in.

Maximal efficiency of these systems will be achieved when there is minimal longitudinal mixing in the system and when the respiratory flow pattern is optimized. Mapleson (1954) predicted that an end-expiratory pause would allow some accumulation of fresh gas at the subject end of a T-piece and improve efficiency. Byrick and Janssen (1980) found that enflurane anaesthesia provided a larger end-expiratory pause during spontaneous ventilation than halothane anaesthesia and this was reflected in lower fresh gas flow requirements. Johnsson and Zetterstrom (1985) found that an end-expiratory pause was rarely demon-

strable when using halothane anaesthesia. Mapleson also suggested that a higher peak inspiratory flow rate might be associated with more entrainment from the expiratory limb.

The Bain system (Bain and Spoerel, 1972) is now the most commonly used T-piece system for adults. It is a coaxial Mapleson D system (Fig. 59.9) with a 22 mm internal diameter outer tube and a 7 mm in-

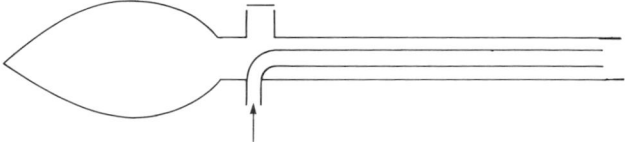

Fig. 59.9 Schematic representation of the Bain coaxial anaesthetic system. The outer tube is 22 mm diameter with the inner tube being approximately 7 mm.

ternal diameter inner tube and is 1.8 m long. Without a reservoir bag it will be a coaxial Mapleson E system and with an open tailed reservoir bag, a coaxial Mapleson F system. Bain described several advantages of this system including its light weight, ease of use with one tube, adaptability to all types of anaesthetic procedures, usefulness in all age groups and ease of scavenging. Defects or dislocation of the inner tube of the Bain system may cause significant rebreathing.

Suggested fresh gas flow rates for the T-piece systems and Bain system during spontaneous ventilation vary enormously in the published studies. In an early review of T-pieces Harrison (1964 a, b) concluded that a fresh gas flow of 2.5–3 times the minute volume was required to prevent rebreathing. Bain et al. (1972) suggested fresh gas flow rates of 5.5–7 L/min during spontaneous ventilation for the Bain system. Conway et al. (1977) suggested that a fresh gas flow of three times the minute ventilation would prevent rebreathing. Rose et al. (1978) using a lung model found that at the fresh gas flow rates suggested by Bain and Spoerel dangerous hypercarbia could result in situations involving limited respiratory compensation, high CO_2 production or an increase in physiological or aparatus dead-space. Further studies by Ungerer (1978), Nott et al. (1977) and Humphrey (1982) suggest high fresh gas flows of greater than twice the minute ventilation are necessary to prevent significant rebreathing. The exact figure will be determined by the inspiratory flow pattern, dead space—tidal volume ratio and the relative durations of inspiration and expiration. These fresh gas flows will often result in a high expiratory resistance.

During controlled ventilation with T-piece systems some rebreathing is usually anticipated and these systems are capable of producing normocarbia with fresh gas flows slightly less than predicted minute ventilation, There is however a necessity to ventilate at a minute ventilation of approximately twice the predicted minute ventilation before alveolar CO_2

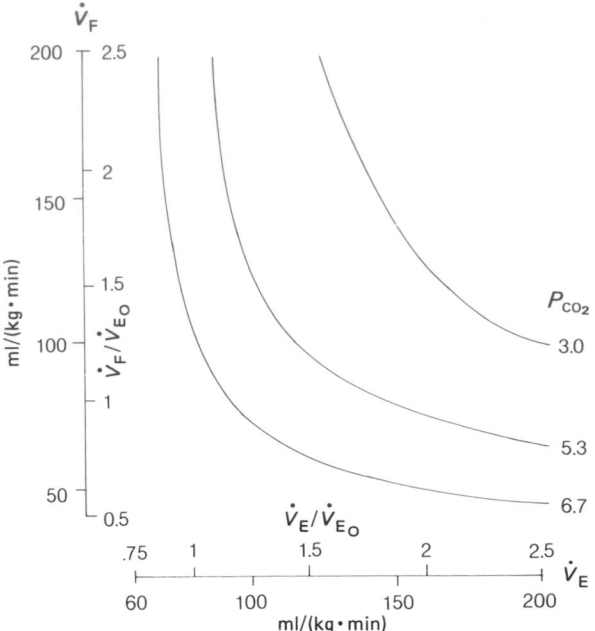

Fig. 59.10 Fresh gas and ventilatory requirements for three levels of P_{CO_2} during controlled ventilation with a T-piece. $\dot{V}_F$ is at ATPD and $\dot{V}_E$ at BTPs and both are expressed as fractions of resting minute volume and in ml/(kg·min) (assuming a V_{CO_2} of 2.2 ml/(kg·min). The CO_2 isopleths are for a P_{CO_2} of 3, 5.3 and 6.7 kPa (22.5, 40 and 50 mmHg).

becomes relatively insensitive to changes in ventilation. Figure 59.10 shows the fresh gas and ventilation levels needed to produce various alveolar CO_2 levels, assuming a simple square wave inspiratory flow pattern. Flows are expressed both as fractions of resting minute volume and in ml/kg for an assumed CO_2 production of 2.2 ml/(kg·min) STPD. It can be seen that if ventilation is high $F_A CO_2$ is fresh gas flow dependent, whilst the converse applies when fresh gas flow is high.

Clinical studies by Bain and Spoerel (1973) and Henville and Adams (1976) have found that normocarbia can be achieved in the majority of patients using fresh gas flows of 70 ml/(kg·min). Caution however must be exercised when using T-piece systems during controlled ventilation in patients who have an abnormal CO_2 production. Body temperature, age, metabolic disturbances, pregnancy, sepsis and stress are all known to affect the CO_2 production. An accurate prediction of fresh gas flow requirements will need to take these factors into account. If control of alveolar CO_2 is important, then monitoring end-tidal CO_2 concentration is the best guide.

Combined Systems

Waters (1961) described an anaesthetic breathing system that could be converted from a Mapleson A to a Mapleson D system by rotation of a lever and adjustment of a valve. Since then several systems have been described (Manicon and Schoonbee, 1976; Salkield, 1985; Burchett and Bennett, 1985; Humphrey et al.,1986). These systems are designed to allow the use of a Mapleson A system for spontaneous ventilation and can be converted to T-pieces for controlled ventilation. In theory fresh gas flow requirements for these systems are less than minute ventilation for spontaneous and controlled ventilation. In practice these systems have been shown to function efficiently in each mode. Indeed Humphrey et al. (1986) recommends that a fresh gas flow rate of only 50 ml/(kg·min) will avoid rebreathing in the Humphrey ADE system in the A mode during spontaneous ventilation. Bradley et al. (1985) found no difference between a similar system (the multicircuit system) and a traditional Mapleson A during spontaneous ventilation. The potential for malposition of the controlling levers of these systems does exist.

Hafnia Modifications

In these systems the expiratory valve of a conventional Mapleson A, B, C or D system is replaced by a device which withdraws gas from the system at a flow equal to fresh gas flow (Christensen et al, 1978; Thomsen and Jorgensen, 1976). The virtues of the Hafnia system are easy control of scavenging and reduction in resistance. The claim that as gas is removed from the system continuously these systems need the same fresh gas flow for spontaneous and controlled ventilation does not bear close scrutiny. This is only true if the characteristics of the respiratory waveform and degree of gas mixing in the system are the same with both modes of ventilation, and this is certainly not so. There are no differences in performance between the Hafnia T-piece systems and conventional T-pieces. The Hafnia A system requires higher flows than the conventional system during spontaneous breathing, but is more efficient than its conventional counterpart during controlled ventilation.

Circle Systems without Absorbers

When the absorber is removed from a circle system, a rebreathing system is produced. Normocapnia can be produced with moderate levels of fresh gas flow if ventilation is adequately high and this system has been advocated for controlled ventilation. Sujwa and Yamamura (1970) suggested fresh gas flows in the order of 60 ml/(kg·min) with a ventilation of thrice normal. Scholfield and Williams (1974) set fresh gas flow to the subject's predicted alveolar ventilation and used a minute volume two to four times this value. Carbon dioxide levels with these systems depend upon CO_2 output, fresh gas flow and ventilation and are also influenced by geometry of the system and the degree of mixing. Snowdon et al. (1975) demonstrated marked differences in performance of circle systems without absorbers and with different sites of entry of fresh gas. Schoonbee et al. (1981) have found that mixing in the system, and therefore its performance, could be greatly modified by changes in respiratory frequency. Gaseous homeostasis appears to be less predictable and more variable with the circle system without an absorber than with other methods of hyperventilation and deliberate rebreathing.

NONREBREATHING SYSTEMS

Nonrebreathing systems are not used commonly in routine hospital anaesthetic practice. However they have been found to be invaluable for use in situations outside the operating suite.

Low resistance, draw-over vaporizers and the use of ventilation devices, e.g. Oxford Inflating Bellows allow general anaesthesia to be conducted with or without controlled ventilation. Oxygen can be added to the gas inlet if necessary.

Many different designs for the valves of such systems are available (Sykes, 1959) and they are most conveniently used in modifications of the Mapleson A or C rebreathing systems where they replace the expiratory valve. Under ideal circumstances a nonrebreathing system will allow full control over the inspired atmosphere when fresh gas flow is equal to minute volume, the valve merely increasing apparatus dead space by 10–15 ml. In practice, reflux of expired gas into the inspiratory limb often occurs due to sluggish closure or inefficient seating of the valve. This reflux will usually consist of dead space gas. Sticking of the expiratory mechanism of the valve during spontaneous breathing can lead to air being inhaled, whilst in controlled ventilation some slipping of gas through the valve may occur early in inspiration leading to a reduced tidal volume. Life threatening malfunction of these valves does occur (Munford, in press).

During spontaneous breathing with a nonrebreathing system, serious dysfunction of the valve can occur if there is even a small discrepancy between fresh gas inflow and minute ventilation. If fresh gas supply is deficient, the reservoir bag of the system will become depleted of gas, limiting and finally preventing inspiration. An excess supply of fresh gas will raise pressure in the inspiratory reservoir; this will eventually cause the valve to jam in the inspiratory position and prevent expiration. It is usual in these systems to supply a small excess of fresh gas over minute ventilation and incorporate some form of overflow valve in the inspiratory limb to prevent pressure rising. The Ambu E valve is designed to leak when pressure on its inspiratory side rises gradually.

REFERENCES

Adams A.P. (1976). Anaesthetic ventilators and associated breathing circuits. *Br. J. Clin. Equip.*, **1**, 13.

Atkinson R.S. (1960). Trichlorethylene anesthesia. *Anesthesiology*, **21**, 67.

Ayre P. (1937). Anaesthesia for intracranial operations; a new technique. *Lancet*, **1**, 561.

Bain J.A., Spoerel W.E. (1972). A streamlined anaesthetic system. *Canad. Anaesth. Soc. J.*, **19**, 426.

Bain J.A., Spoerel W.E. (1973). Flow requirements for a modified Mapleson D system during controlled ventilation. *Canad. Anaesth. Soc. J.*, **20**, 629.

Baraka A. (1977). Functional classification of anaesthesia circuits. *Anaesth. Intens. Care*, **5**, 172.

Barnes P.K., Browne, C.H.W., Conway C.M. (1977). The work of ventilating semi-closed rebreathing systems. *Br. J. Anaesth.*, **49**, 1173.

Barnes P.K., Conway C.M., Purcell G.R.G. (1980). The Lack anaesthetic system. *Anaesthesia*, **35**, 393.

Barnes P.K., Seeley H.F., Gothard J.W.W., et al. (1976). The Lack anaesthetic system: an assessment during spontaneous ventilation. *Anaesthesia*, **31**, 1248.

Barton F., Nunn J.F. (1975). Totally closed nitrous oxide/oxygen anaesthesia. *Br. J. Anaesth.*, **47**, 350.

Bengstrom J.P., Sanander H., Stengvist O. (1988). Comparison of costs of different anaesthetic techniques. *Acta Anaesth. Scand.*, **32**, 33.

Bradley J.P., Marsland A.R., Massang J.R. (985). The multi circuit system. A study during spontaneous ventilation in awake volunteers using the Mapleson A mode. *Anaesth. Intens. Care*, **13**, 158.

Bruce W.E., Soni N.C. (1989). Preliminary evaluation of the enclosed Magill breathing system. *Br. J. Anaesth.*, **62**, 144.

Burchett K.R., Bennett J.A. (1985). A new coaxial breathing system. A combination of the benefits of Mapleson A, D and E systems. *Anaesthesia*, **40**, 181.

Byrick R.J. (1980). Respiratory compensation during spontaneous ventilation with the Bain circuit. *Cand. Anaesth. Soc. J.*, **27**, 96.

Byrick R.J., Janssen E.G. (1980). Respiratory waveform and rebreathing in T-piece circuits. A comparision of enflurane and halothane waveforms. *Anesthesiology*, **53**, 371.

Campbell E.J.M., Freedman S., Smith P.S., et al. (1959). Sensitivity of conscious human subjects to added external elastic impedance to breathing. *J. Physiol.*, **150**, 9.

Carden E. (1972). A new and highly efficient circuit for paediatric anaesthesia. *Canad. Anaesth. Soc. J.*, **19**, 572.

Carden E. (1974). Efficient positive pressure ventilation with a modified Magill circuit in adults. *Canad. Anaesth. Soc. J.*, **21**, 242.

Chalon J., Ali M., Turorf H. (1981). *Humidification of Anaesthetic Gases*. Springfield III: Charles C. Thomas.

Chalon J., Loew D.A.Y., Malebranche J. (1972). Effects of dry anaesthetic gases on tracheobronchial ciliated epithelium. *Anesthesiology*, **37**, 338.

Christensen K.N., Thomsen A., Hansen O., et al. (1978). Flow requirements of the Hafnia modifications of the Mapleson circuits during spontaneous respiration. *Acta Anaesth. Scand.*, **2**, 27.

Chu Y.K., Rah K.H., Boyan C.P. (1977). Is the Bain breathing circuit the future anaesthetic system? An evaluation. *Anaesth. Analg. Curr. Res.*, **56**, 84.

Conway C.M. (1970). Anaesthetic circuits. In *Scientific Foundations of Anaesthesia* (Scurr C., Feldman S., eds.). Philadelphia: Davis.

Conway C.M. (1980). Alveolar oxygen concentration during use of a circle system with carbon dioxide absorption. *Br. J. Anaesth.*, **52**, 233.

Conway C.M. (1983). Anaesthetic breathing systems. *Br. J. Anaesth.*, **57**, 649.

Conway C.M., Davis F.M., Knight H.J., et al. (1976). An

experimental study of gaseous homeostasis and the Magill circuit using low fresh gas flows. *Br. J. Anaesth.*, **48**, 447.

Conway C.M., Seeley H.F., Barnes P.K. (1977). Spontaneous ventilation with the Bain anaesthetic system. *Br. J. Anaesth.*, **49**, 1245.

Eger E.I. (1974). *Anaesthetic Uptake and Action*. Baltimore: Williams & Wilkins.

Eger E.I., Ethans C.T. (1968). The effect of inflow, overflow and valve placement on economy of the circle system. *Anesthesiology*, **29**, 93.

Eger E.I., Strum D.P. (1987). The absorption and degradation of isoflurane and I 653 by dry soda lime at various temperatures. *Anesth. Analg.*, **66**, 1312.

Harrison G.A. (1964a). Ayre's T-piece: A review of its modifications. *Br. J. Anaesth.*, **36**, 115.

Harrison G.A. (1964b). The effect of respiratory flow pattern on rebreathing in the T-piece system. *Br. J. Anaesth.*, **36**, 206.

Henville J.D., Adams A.P. (1976). The Bain anaesthetic system: an assessment during controlled ventilation. *Anaesthesia*, **31**, 247.

Holmes C. McK., Spears G.F.S. (1977). Very-nearly-closed-circuit anaesthesia; a computer analysis. *Anaesthesia*, **32**, 846.

Humphrey D. (1982). The Lack Magill and Bain anaesthetic breathing systems. *J. Roy. Soc. Med.*, **75**, 513.

Humphrey D., Brock-Utne J.G., Downing J.W. (1986). Single lever Humphrey A,D,E, low flow universal anaesthetic breathing system. *Can. Anaesth. Soc. J.*, **33**, 698.

Jackson D.E. (1915). A new method for the production of general analgesia and anesthesia with a description of the apparatus used. *J. Lab. Clin. Med.*, **1**, 1.

Johnsson L.O., Zetterstrom H. (1985). Flow pattern and respiratory characteristics during halothane anaesthesia. *Acta Anaesth. Scand.*, **29**, 309.

Kain M.L., Nunn J.F. (1968). Fresh gas economies of the Magill circuit. *Anesthesiology*, **29**, 964.

Kay B., Beatty P.C.W., Healy T.E.J., et al. (1983). Change in the work of breathing imposed by five anaesthetic breathing systems. *Br. J. Anaesth.*, **55**, 1239.

Lack J.A. (1976). Theatre pollution control. *Anaesthesia*, **31**, 259.

Lauria J.I. (1975). Soda lime dust contamination of breathing circuits. *Anesthesiology*, **42**, 628.

Lowe H.J. (1979). The anaesthetic continuum. In *Low Flow and Closed System Anaesthesia* (Aldrete J.A., Lowe H.J., Virtue R.W., eds.). New York: Grune & Stratton.

Lowe H.J., Ernst E.A. (1981). *The Quantitative Practice of Anesthesia. Use of Closed Circuit*. Baltiore: Williams and Wilkins.

Manicom A.W., Schoonbee C.G. (1976). The Johannesburg A-D circuit switch: a valve device for converting a coaxial Mapleson D into a coaxial Mapleson A system. *Br. J. Anaesth.*, **51**, 1185.

Mapleson W.W. (1954). The elimination of rebreathing in various semiclosed anaesthetic systems. *Br. J. Anaesth.*, **26**, 323.

Mapleson W.W. (1958). Theoretical considerations of the effect of rebreathing in two semiclosed anaesthetic systems. *Br. Med. Bull.*, **14**, 64.

Marshall M., Henderson G.A. (1968). Positive pressure ventilation using a semiclosed system: a reassessment. *Br. J. Anaesth.*, **40**, 265.

McMahon J. (1951). Rebreathing as a basis for classification of inhalational techniques. *J. Am. Assoc. Nurse Anesthetists*, **19**, 133.

Millar S.W., Barnes P.K., Soni N. (1987). Comparison of the Magill and Lack anaesthetic breathing systems in anaesthetised patients. *Br. J. Anaesth.*, **59**, 930.

Miller D.M. (1979). A new universal anaesthetic system using a preferential flow T-piece. *S. Afr. Med. V.*, **55**, 721.

Miller D.M., Couper J.L. (1983). Comparison of the fresh gas flow requirements and resistance of the Preferential Flow System with those of the Magill System. *Br. J. Anaesth.*, **55**, 569.

Miller D.M., Miller J.C. (1958). Enclosed afferent reservoir breathing systems. *Br. J. Anaesth.*, **60**, 469.

Moyers J. (1953). A nomenclature for methods of inhalation anaesthesia. *Anesthesiology*, **14**, 609.

Neff W.B., Burke S.F., Thompson R. (1968). A venturi circulator for anaesthetic systems. *Anesthesiology*, **29**, 838.

Norman J., Adams A.P., Sykes M.K. (1968). Rebreathing with the Magill attachment. *Anaesthesia*, **23**, 75.

Nott M.R., Norman J. (1978). Resistance of the Heidbrink type expiratory valves. *Br. J. Anaesth.*, **50**, 477.

Nott M., Walters F., Norman. J. (1977). A comparison of the Lack and Bain semiclosed circuits in spontaneous respiration. *Br. J. Anaesth.*, **49**, 512.

Nott M.R., Walters F.J.M., Norman J. (1982). The Lack and Bain systems in spontaneous respiration. *Anaesth. Intens. Care*, **10**, 333.

Nunn J.F. (1966). *Applied Respiratory Physiology*. 1st edn., p. 83. London: Butterworths.

Nunn J.F. (1977). *Applied Respiratory Physiology*, 2nd edn. London: Butterworth.

Nunn J.F. (1979). Potential Economics of Using Closed Circuit Anesthesia. In *Low Flow and Closed System Anaesthesia* (Aldrete J.A., Lowe H.J., Virtue R.W., eds.). New York: Grune and Stratton.

Nunn J.F., Chamarin I. (1985). Nitrous oxide inactivates methionine synthetase. In *Nitrous Oxide* (Eger E.I., ed.). London: Edward Arnold.

Nunn J.F., Ezi-Ashi T.I. (1961). The respiratory effects of resistance to breathing in anaesthetized man. *Anesthesiology*, **22**, 174.

Nunn J.F., Newman H.C. (1964). Inspired gas, rebreathing and apparatus dead space. *Br. J. Anaesth.*, **36**, 5.

Obiaya M.O., DaKouraju P. (1976). Magill circuit and controlled ventilation. *Can. Anaesth. Soc. J.*, **23**, 135.

Parmley J.B., Tahir A.H., Dascomb H.E., et al. (1972). Disposable versus reusable rebreathing circuits: advantages, disadvantages, hazards and bacteriological studies. *Anesth. Analg. Curr. Res.*, **51**, 888.

Revell D.G. (1959). An improved circulator for closed circle anaesthesia. *Can. Anaesth. Soc. J.*, **6**, 104.

Rose D.K., Byrick R.J., Froese A.B. (1978). Carbon dioxide elimination during spontaneous ventilation with a modified Mapleson D system: studies in a lung model. *Canad. Anaesth. Soc. J.*, **25**, 353.

Salkield I.A. (1985). The multi circuit system: description of a device providing several Mapleson functions. *Anaesth. Int. Care*, **13**, 153.

Scholfield E.J., Williams N.E. (1974). Prediction of arterial carbon dioxide tension using a circle system without carbon dioxide absorption. *Br. J. Anaesth.*, **46**, 442.

Schoonbee C.G., Conway C.M. (1981). Factors affecting carbon dioxide homeostasis during controlled ventilation with circle systems. *Br. J. Anaesth.*, **53**, 471.

Severinghaus J.W. (1954). The rate of uptake of nitrous oxide in man. *J. Clin. Invest.*, **33**, 1183.

Snow J. (1858). *On Chloroform and Other Anaesthetics*, edited by B.W. Richardson. London: Churchill.

Snowdon S.L., Powell D.L., Fadl E.T., et al. (1975). The circle system without absorber: use with controlled ventilation. *Anaesthesia*, **30**, 323.

Spain J.A. (1981). Cost of delivery of anesthetic gases re-examined III. *Anesthesiology*, **55**, 711.

Spoerel W.E., Aitken R.R., Bain J.A. (1978). Spontaneous respiration with the Bain breathing circuit. *Can. Anaesth. Soc. J.*, **25**, 30.

Sujwa K., Yamamura H. (1970). The effect of gas inflow on the regulation of CO_2 levels with hyperventilation during anaesthsia. *Anesthesiology*, **33**, 440.

Sword B.C. (1930). The closed circle method of administration of gas anaesthesia. *Curr. Res. Anaesth. Analg.*, **9**, 198.

Sykes M.K. (1959). Non-rebreathing valves. *Br. J. Anaesth.*, **3**, 450.

Sykes M.K. (1987). Essential monitoring. *Br. J. Anaesth.*, **57**, 901.

Thomsen A., Jorgensen S. (1976). The Hafnia circuit. *Acta Anaesth. Scand.*, **20**, 395.

Ungerer M.J. (1978). A comparison between the Bain and the Magill anaesthetic systems during spontaneous breathing. *Can. Anaesth. Soc. J.*, **25**(2), 122.

Virtue R.W. (1974). Minimal flow nitrous oxide anaesthesia. *Anesthesiology*, **40**, 196.

Virtue R.W. (1979). Low flow anesthesia: advantages in its clinical application, cost and ecology. In *Low Flow and Closed System Anesthesia* (Aldrete J.A., Lowe H.J., Virtue R.W., eds.). New York: Grune and Stratton.

Voss T.J.V. (1985). The ultimate circuit: or—not another circuit? *Anaesth. Intensive Care*, **13**, 98.

Waters D.J. (1961). A composite semiclosed anaesthetic system suitable for controlled or spontaneous respiration. *Brit. J. Anaesth.*, **33**, 417.

Waters R.M. (1924). Clinical scope and utility of carbon dioxide filtration in inhalational anesthesia. *Anesth. Analg.*, **3**, 20.

Willis B.A., Pender J.W., Mapleson W.W. (1975). Rebreathing in a T-piece: volunteer and theoretical studies of the Jackson-Rees modification of Ayre's T-piece during spontaneous respiration. *Br. J. Anaesth.*, **47**, 1239.

60. The Design and Calibration of Anaesthetic Vaporizers
John A. Bushman

Classification of vaporizers
  Volatile agents
  Temperature changes
  Fluctuations in pressure
  Contamination
  Draw-over vaporizers
  Calibration of vaporizers

TABLE 60.1

Agent	s.v.p. 20°C	% of 1 Atmos	Maintenance %
Diethyl ether	440	57	5–15
Halothane	243	32	0.5–2
Isoflurane	238	31	1–2.5
Enflurane	175	23	1.5–3
Trichloroethylene	60	7	1–1.5
Methoxyflurane	23	3	0.25–1

expressed as a % of 760 mmHg and the concentration of the agent required for the maintenance of anaesthesia.

From this table it is evident that the design of the proportionating valve for a particular agent is such that the vaporizer can produce a clinically useful range of vapour concentrations for that agent.

An anaesthetic vaporizer is a device designed to deliver a controlled amount of anaesthetic vapour to the inspired gas flow. This is normally expressed as a percentage of saturated vapour added to the gas flow. The saturated vapour pressure at room temperature (s.v.p. at 20°C) of all the volatile anaesthetic agents currently in use is greater than that required to anaesthetize a patient. For this reason the essential feature of a vaporizer is a proportionating system which determines the ratio between the volume of gas which passes through the vaporizer and the volume which bypasses the vaporizer before it reaches the patient circuit.

Table 60.1 shows for a number of volatile agents, the s.v.p. in mmHg at 20°C, the s.v.p. at 20°C

CLASSIFICATION OF VAPORIZERS

There have been a number of attempts to classify vaporizers. The variety of types available makes an adequate classification difficult. Dorsch and Dorsch (1975) suggested the following classification:

1. Method of regulating the output concentration
   a. variable bypass
   b. measured flow
2. Method of vaporization
   a. flow over
      i with wick
      ii without wick
   b. bubble through
   c. flow over or bubble through

3. Location
   a. outside the breating circuit
   b. inside the breathing circuit
4. Temperature compensation
   a. none
   b. by supplied heat
   c. by flow alteration (manual or automatic)
5. Specificity
   a. agent specific
   b. multiple agent

The simplest form of vaporizer, the plenum vaporizer (from the Latin, 'a space filled with matter') is shown in Fig. 60.1. The simplest vaporizer in use of

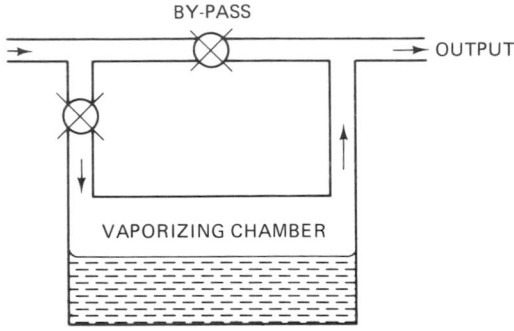

Fig. 60.1 Simple plenum vaporizer.

this type is the Goldman (1962). The advantages of such a vaporizer are that it is small and relatively inexpensive and can be used outside or within a circle system. It would be classified as a variable bypass, flow over without wick, in or out of circuit, no temperature compensation and multiple agent type.

One early common form of this type of simple apparatus was the Boyle vaporizer shown in Fig. 60.2. This apparatus was in use in this form in 1930, though Boyle had been developing the idea since 1918 (Boyle, 1918). As in the case of the Goldman, as the temperature of the agent fell so did the concentration of the agent leaving the vaporizer. The degree of the saturation of the gas passing out of the bottle was not only dependent on the position of the plunger but also on the gas flow through the device. For this reason it was not possible to calibrate the vaporizer, and the position of the controls was determined by clinical judgement. This type of vaporizer would be classified as a variable bypass, flow over or bubble through, out of circuit, no temperature compensation and multiple agent type.

Volatile Agents

Developments in vaporizers since the Boyle vaporizer have attempted to overcome these defects. In the more modern type of vaporizer, the manufacturer has tried

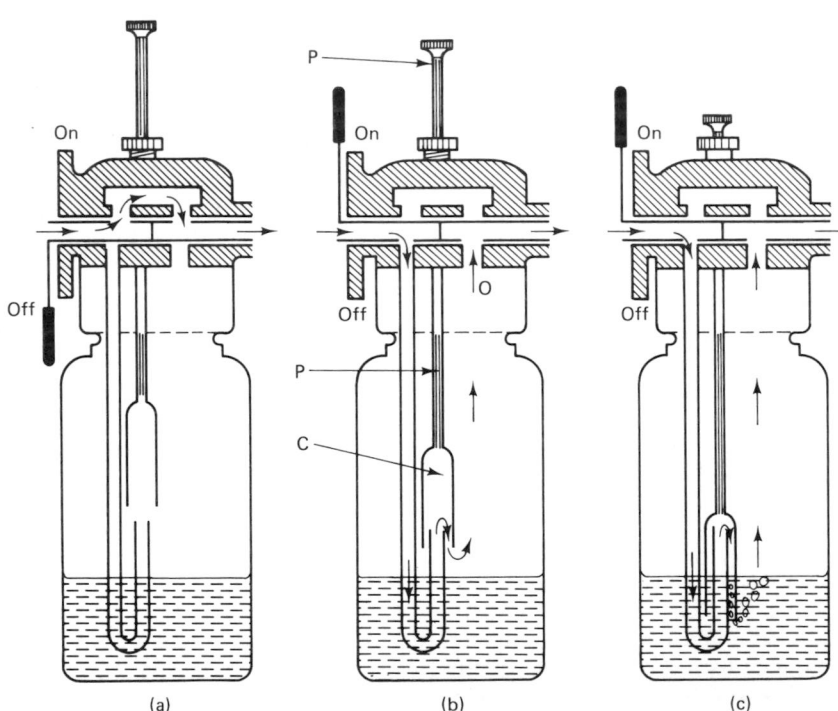

Fig. 60.2 Three diagrams of the Boyle's vaporizer showing (a) the control lever in the 'off' position, (b) the control lever fully 'on' and the cowl C lowered so as to cause the gases to impinge on the surface of the liquid, and (c) the cowl C further lowered so as to cause the gas to bubble through the liquid. (Reproduced with permission from Ward (1987) in *Anaesthetic Equipment: Physical Principles and Maintenance*, p. 83. London: Bailliere Tindall).

to design the chamber so that the gas leaving it is always fully saturated with the vapour before it rejoins the bypassed gas stream, despite changes in the flow rate delivered to the vaporizer. This is normally achieved by ensuring that the gas travels a labyrinthine path through the chamber which is lined with wicks saturated by the volatile agent. The long path length increases the surface area of the liquid and the wicks minimize the effect of the level of the liquid in the chamber (Fig. 60.3).

A volatile liquid vaporizes by losing molecules from its surface. The molecules leaving the liquid are those having a sufficient velocity to overcome the intermolecular Van der Waals forces between the molecules. The result is a decrease in the mean kinetic energy within the liquid and therefore the temperature of the liquid falls. This in turn reduces the vapour pressure of the liquid. The rapidity of the fall in temperature is dependent on a number of factors which include the heat of vaporization of the liquid, the specific heat of the material forming the walls of the vaporizer and the

specific heat of the liquid. It should be noted that if the temperature of the liquid is raised its s.v.p. will increase until at the boiling point of the liquid, its s.v.p. will equal one atmosphere pressure.

The heat of vaporization of a liquid is defined as the number of calories required to evaporate 1 g of liquid. As a general rule the more volatile the liquid the lower is the number of calories required.

The specific heat of a substance is defined as the amount of heat required to raise the temperature of 1 g of the substance by 1°C. The optimum material would therefore have a high density and a high specific heat. Copper is a frequently used material for the bodies of vaporizers as it has a high density and a reasonably high specific heat. Brass is also a favoured material as it can be machined easily and then plated to make it resistant to corrosion.

The same argument applies to the ideal characteristics of the volatile agent. Ideally this should have a high density and a high specific heat in order to minimize temperature changes during vaporization.

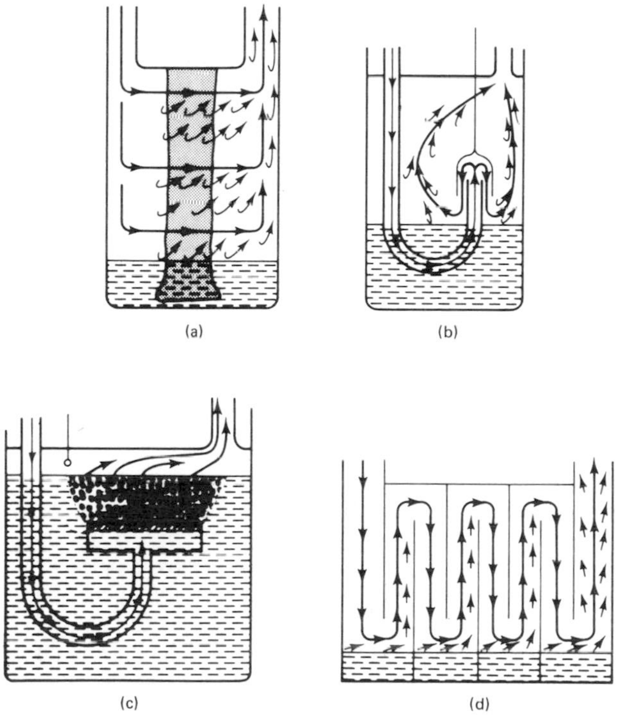

Temperature Changes

In modern vaporizers compensation for temperature changes is achieved by one of two means. It can be

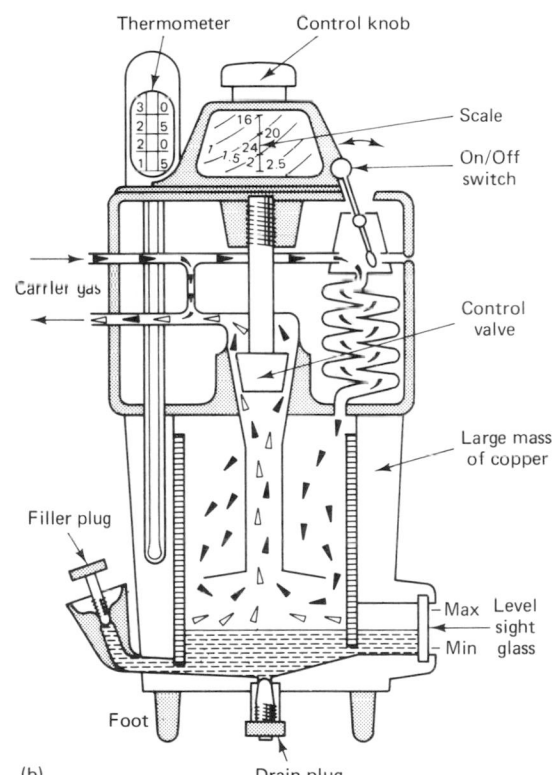

Fig. 60.3 Methods of increasing the vaporization rate in a vaporizer. (a) The liquid anaesthetic agent is drawn up a wick, thus presenting a greater surface area for vaporization. (b) The mixed gas flow is directed onto the surface of the liquid anaesthetic agent by cowl. (c) The mixed gases are broken up into a large number of small bubbles which pass through the liquid anaesthetic agent, thus presenting the maximum possible surface area to the liquid. (d) A series of baffles repeatedly redirect the mixed gas flow onto the surface of the liquid anaesthetic agent. (Reproduced with permission from Ward (1987) in *Anaesthetic Equipment: Physical Principles and Maintenance*. p. 80. London: Bailliere Tindall).

Fig. 60.4 The Dräger Vapor temperature indicated, level compensated vaporizer. Working principles. Note the large mass of copper, which acts as a heat sink. (Reproduced with permission from Ward (1987) in *Anaesthetic Equipment: Physical Principles and Maintenance*. London: Bailliere Tindall).

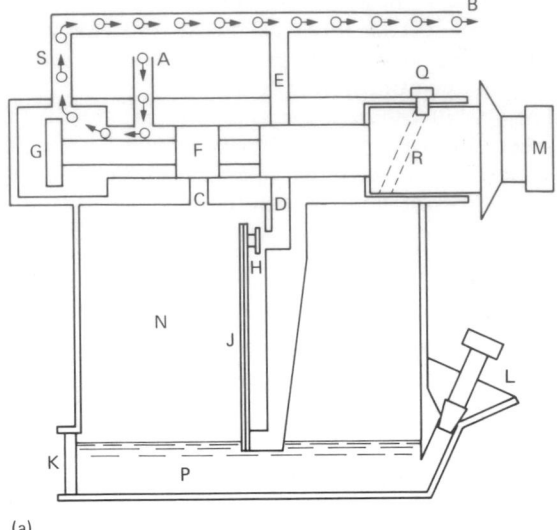

(a)

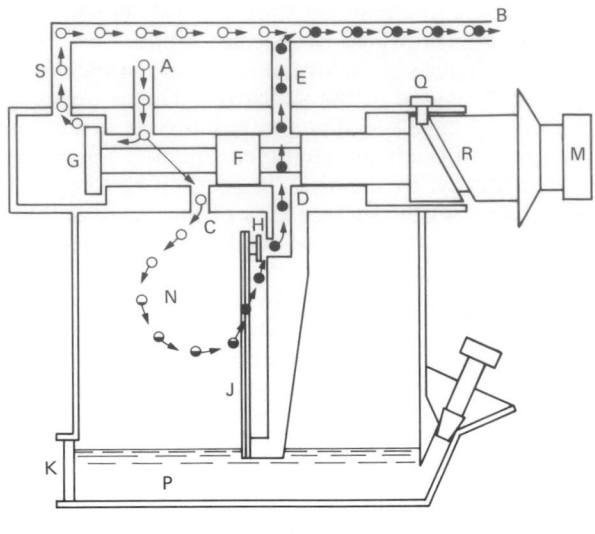

(b)

Fig. 60.5 The Fluotec (Mark 2) shown diagrammatically at (a) in the 'off' position and at (b) in the open or any calibrated position. In (a) metered gas enters at A and as shown by the arrows it meets the spindle F, goes through the by-pass valve G, along the port S to B and thence to the patient. None of the gas can enter or leave the vaporizing chamber N as ports C and D are closed by spindle F. Rotation of the control M causes the spindle F to move to the right by virtue of the spiral groove R. (Note: In the actual vaporizer this groove R consists of a straight keyway type groove running into a spiral groove but for this explanation we shall consider it as a simple spiral). As the spindle F moves to the right the ports C and D are opened, and the opening of the by-pass port C is considerably reduced. This results in the 'open' position.

In (b) rotation of the control dial M adjusts the opening of the port G which splits the gas flow between the vaporizing chamber N and the diluting gas passing along S, thus altering the percentage of the mixed gases. The amount of 'Fluothane' picked up in the vaporizing stream will vary with the temperature of the 'Fluothane'. The 'Fluothane' temperature will vary, either due to variation of room temperatures or to the cooling which takes place when 'Fluothane' is vaporized. To compensate for this, the valve H is controlled by a bimetallic strip J and opens automatically when the temperature falls, and closes when the temperature rises. At a given dial setting, therefore, the mixed percentage issuing at B is independent of room temperature or previous use of the FLUOTEC. (Reproduced with permission from Dorsch and Dorsch (1980) in *Understanding Anaesthesia Equipment: Construction, Care and Complications*, p. 6. Baltimore: The Williams & Wilkins Co).

done manually by fitting a thermometer so that it is immersed in the liquid agent and then calibrating the proportionating control for both temperature and percentage. In the majority of modern vaporizers it is done automatically by having a second proportionating valve within the body of the vaporizer which is controlled thermostatically. An example of the first design is the 'Vapor' vaporizer by Dräger. This is shown in Fig. 60.4. Note the thermometer and the combined temperature and concentration markings on the control valve. The rate of the change in temperature within the vaporizer is minimized by making its body from copper. The 'Vapor' would be classified as variable bypass, flow over wick, out of circuit, temperature compensated by flow alteration (manual) and agent specific.

In the earlier automatically temperature controlled vaporizers, the temperature compensating valve was situated in the liquid volatile agent. The essential component of such a valve is a bimetallic strip. As the name suggests this is made of two strips of metal bonded together. The metals chosen have different coefficients of expansion so that a change in temperature from that at which they were bonded causes the

strip to bend. An example of this type of vaporizer is the 'Fluotec' Mark 2 and a cross-section of this is shown in Fig. 60.5. Also note in this figure the long path taken by the gas in the chamber as it passes the walls covered with wicks saturated by the agent. Despite these efforts to ensure that the gas in the chamber was fully saturated, the 'Fluotec' Mark 2 showed a wide variation in the concentration of vapour it produced at low flow rates. These variations are shown in Fig. 60.6. Note the marked rise in the concentration at around 1 L/min, followed by a fall at a flow of less than 500 ml/min.

Because of the composition of the bimetallic strip, it is chemically active and prone to corrosion in a mixture of oxygen and volatile agent. In order to overcome this problem most manufacturers now site the temperature compensating valve in the gas stream which bypasses the chamber containing the volatile agent. An example of this type of vaporizer is the 'Fluotec' Mark 3, a cross-section of which is shown in Fig. 60.7. Note in this figure that in addition to the

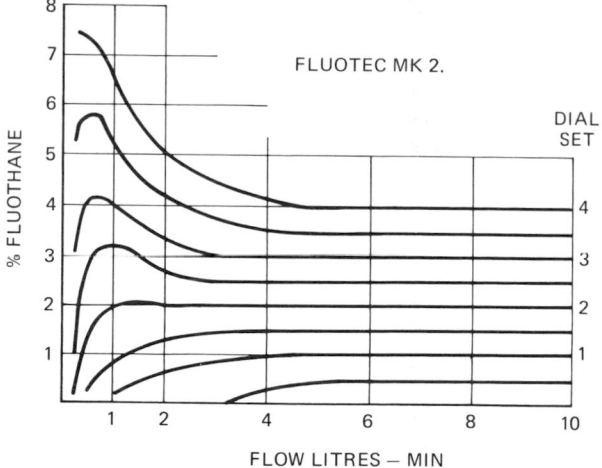

FLUOTEC MK 2.

DIAL SET

Fig. 60.6 The Fluotec Mark 2. Before leaving the works, each Fluotec is carefully checked for accuracy of calibration over a range of gas flows. A typical set of results is given showing the increased output percentage at the low flows referred to earlier. All Fluotec Mark 2 Vaporizers are fitted with a tag on which this same typical performance is illustrated. By reference to this chart the actual delivered percentage at any dial setting for gas flows below 4 L/min can quickly be found. As an example, let us say that the dial is set for 3½% and that the gas flow is 1 L/min. Reference to the chart will show that the actual delivered percentage is slightly over 5%. It should also be noted that at 250 ml/min there is available a range of concentrations from 0% at the 2% dial setting to 7½% at the 4% dial setting. There is ample adjustment between these two dial positions for choosing the concentration required. With gas flows above 4 L/min, the actual concentration delivered corresponds with the dial setting. (Reproduced with permission from Dorsch and Dorsch (1980) in *Understanding Anaesthesia Equipment: Construction, Care and Complications*, p. 8. Baltimore: The Williams & Wilkins Co).

features of the Mark 2, a copper helix has been introduced to increase the temperature stabilization and increase the length of the path traversed by the gas. Copper has a high thermal conductivity and this ensures that the temperature of the bimetallic strip is in equilibrium with the temperature of the wicks. Compared to the Mark 2 this vaporizer has greatly improved the performance at low flow rates, as illustrated in Fig. 60.8. This type of vaporizer would be classified as variable bypass, flow over wick, out of circuit temperature compensated by flow alteration (automatic) and agent specific.

Fluctuations in Pressure

The use of the plenum type vaporizer with some ventilators caused problems. This was due to the pumping effect caused by fluctuations in pressure within the vaporizer chamber as described by Hill and Lowe (1962). The fluctuations were due to the pressure

required to inflate the bellows of some ventilators during the expiratory phase of the patient. When the ventilator cycles to the inspiratory phase, the pressure in the vaporizer chamber will fall to the patient's airway pressure. During this phase vapour may leave the vaporizer by its inlet port in addition to that leaving via its outlet port. This effect is shown in the top section of Fig. 60.9. One solution was to lengthen the inlet port so that vapour did not reflux into the fresh gas flow. This situation is shown in the bottom half of Fig. 60.9. The simpler method now adopted by most manufacturers is to pressurize the backbar of the anaesthetic machine to a pressure greater than that required to operate any ventilator which is likely to be attached. This keeps the pressure of the gases in the backbar constant and thus prevents back flow from the inlet port of a vaporizer into the fresh gas flow.

Contamination

A further problem can arise if two or more vaporizers are in series with each other on the backbar of the anaesthetic machine. If two vaporizers are in use at the same time the downstream vaporizer will be contaminated by the vapour from the upstream vaporizer. To achieve a given concentration, agents with a low volatility require a greater proportion of the fresh gas flow to pass through the vaporizer than is needed in the case of a more volatile agent. Thus contamination can be minimized by having the less volatile agent in the upstream vaporizer. When using agents with similar boiling points the less potent should be in the upstream vaporizer so that any contamination will have the minimum effect on the patient when the downstream vaporizer is used on its own. The risk of contamination can be removed if vaporizers incorporating an interlock system are used. This system positively prevents more than one vaporizer being on at any time. One such system is that used in the Tec 4 vaporizers made by Ohmeda. A diagram of this system is shown in Fig. 60.10.

The Foregger Copper Kettle

The proportionating system in all the vaporizers dealt with so far has been a single valve which determines the splitting ratio. An alternative method is to supply an accurately measured flow of fully saturated vapour to the fresh gas flow. This type of vaporizer is usually referred to as a 'copper kettle' (Morris, 1952) after the first system of this type marketed by the Foregger Company. A cross-section of this vaporizer is shown in Fig. 60.11. The British equivalent of this type of vaporizer was the Halox made by the British Oxygen Company (Young, 1966). This is shown in Fig. 60.12 and its connection to the anaesthetic machine is shown in Fig. 60.13. The great advantage of this type of vaporizer is that it can supply adequate quantities of vapour to a closed circuit even at basal flows. This is frequently not possible with vaporizers designed

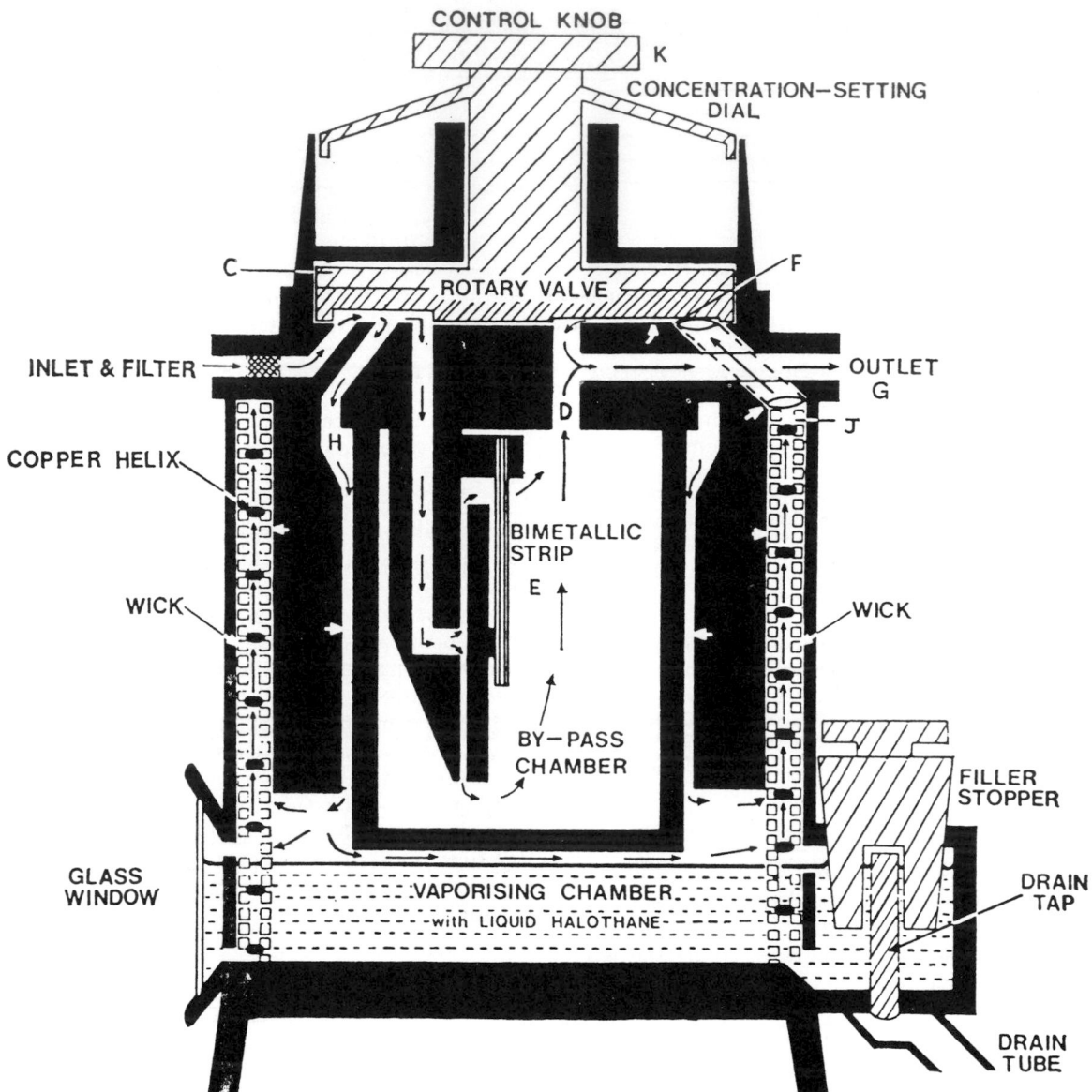

Fig. 60.7 Cross-section of a Mark 3 Fluotec vaporizer.

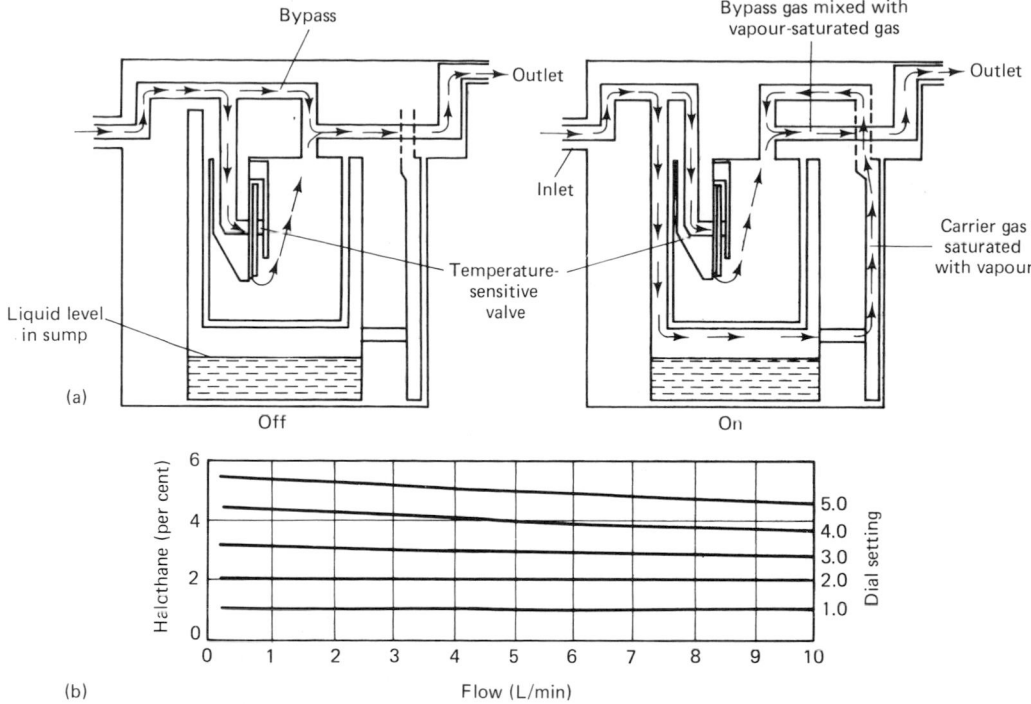

Fig. 60.8 (a) The Fluotec Mark 3 vaporizer, which operates in much the same way as the Mark 2, but incorporates several refinements. Working principles (for simplicity, the control valve has been omitted). In the 'off' position, the carrier gas passes through two passages, a simple bypass and a second bypass in which the flow is regulated by a temperature-sensitive valve. In the 'on' position, the first bypass is closed but the second remains open, and the gas also passes through a passage leading to the vaporization chamber, the valve for which is opened to a degree according to the vapour concentration required. Note that in this vaporizer the carrier gas passing through the vaporization chamber is fully saturated owing to the large area of wicks from which the liquid evaporates. The pathway by which the vapour-laden gas leaves the vaporization chamber may be in the form of a relatively long tube to help overcome the 'pumping effect'. (b) Performance characteristics. (Reproduced with permission from Ward (1980) in *Anaesthetic Equipment: Physical Principles and Maintenance*. p. 87. London: Bailliere Tindall.)

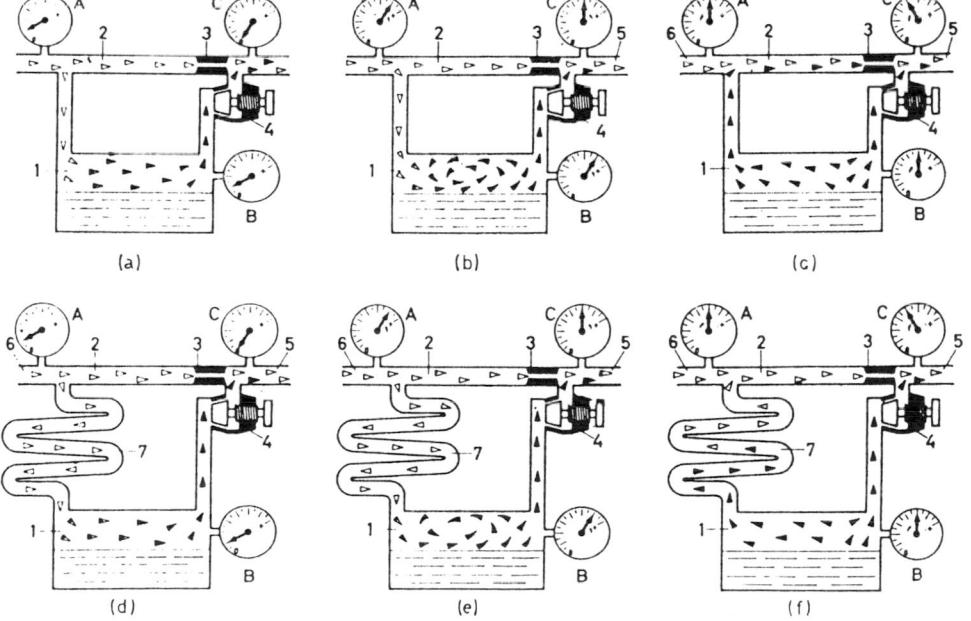

Fig. 60.9 a, b, c. The release of positive pressure from the vaporizing chamber allows vapour to rejoin the bypass from the normal inlet to the chamber; (d) this effect is eliminated by the use of a long inlet pipe to the vaporizing chamber.

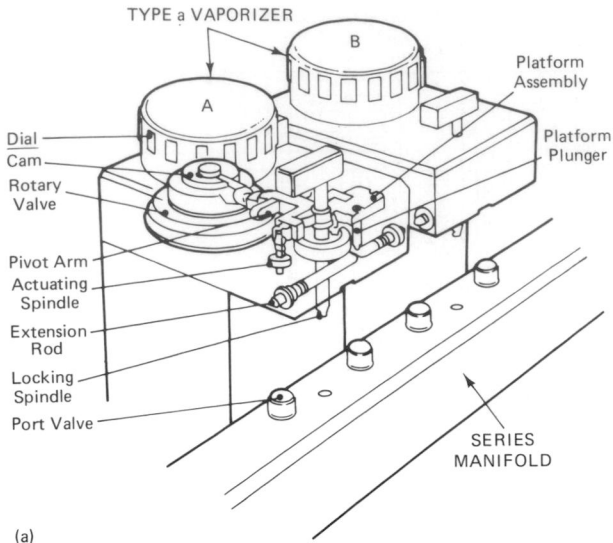

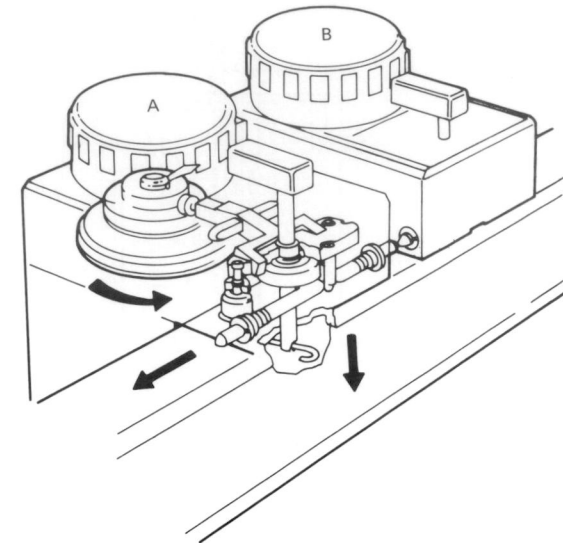

Fig. 60.10 (a) The Tec 4 vaporizer. The interlock mechanism comprises a cam which is located on the drive spindle between the rotary valve and the control dial, a cam follower located on a pivot arm and a platform assembly which is free to move up or down the spindle. Thus the cam moves simultaneously when the control dial is operated. The locking lever is interconnected with the control dial such that the dial cannot be turned until the vaporizer is 'locked' in position on the manifold. The cam follower is arranged to rise up or down on the incline on the contact face of the cam when the control dial is rotated. This movement is transmitted by the pivot arm to the platform assembly. Two actuating spindles are located on the underface of the platform which seal the adjacent face to prevent a gas leakage. These spindles are aligned with the valve ports on the manifold. The single downward movement of the platform has a dual role: 1) The actuating spindles open the manifold port valves. 2) The plunger on the platform causes the extension rods to be extended and thereby prevent an adjacent vaporizer from being turned 'on'.

(b) Vaporizer A is locked on manifold with dial ON. Cam is rotated so that pivot arm moves platform assembly downwards. Downward action of platform causes plunger to extend the rods to preclude turning ON vaporizer B. Actuating spindles open port valves so that carrier gas can flow through vaporizer. Vaporizer B is locked on manifold, dial OFF, extension rods retracted. (Reproduced with permission from Dorsch and Dorsch (1980) in *Understanding Anaesthesia Equipment: Construction, Care and Complications*, p. 5. Baltimore: The Williams & Wilkins Co).

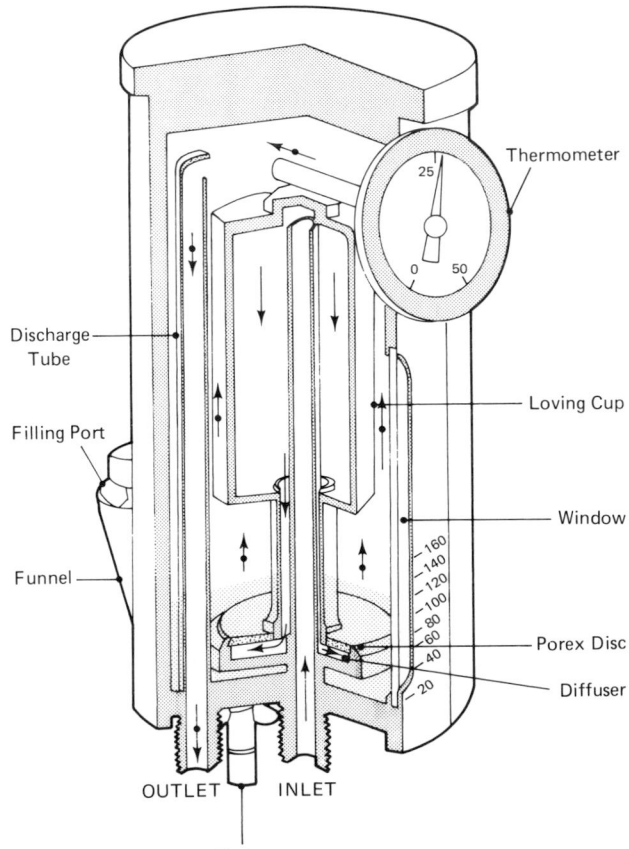

Fig. 60.11 Copper kettle vaporizer. The redesigned version with the filling port at the side to prevent overfilling. *See* text for details. (Redrawn courtesy of Foregger, Division of Air-products and Chemicals Inc. p. 105 London: Bailliere Tindall).

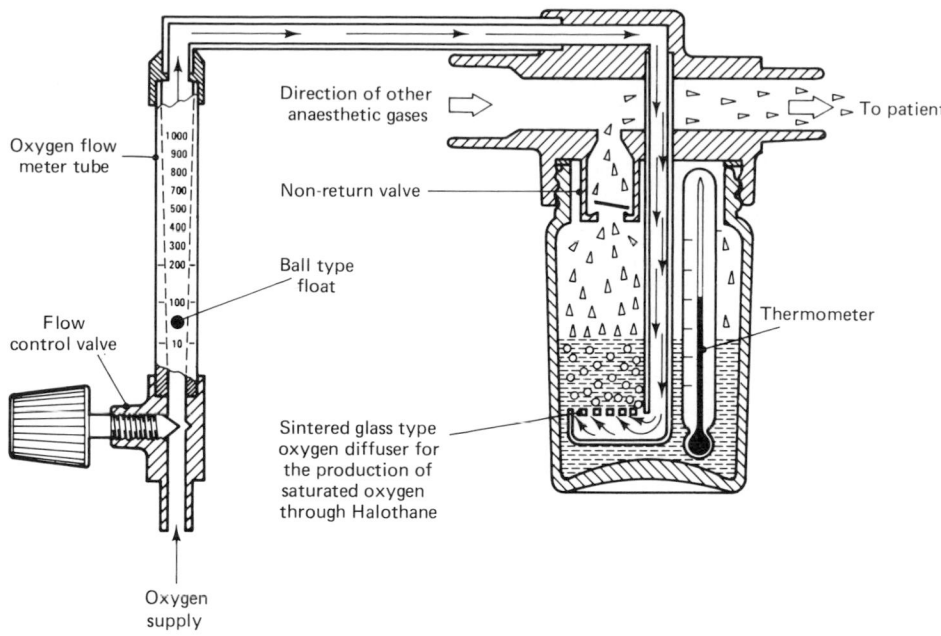

Oxygen flow
meter tube

Flow
control valve

Ball type
float

Direction of other
anaesthetic gases

Non-return valve

To patient

Thermometer

Sintered glass type
oxygen diffuser for
the production of
saturated oxygen
through Halothane

Oxygen
supply

Fig. 60.12 The Halox vaporizer (Reproduced with permission from Ward (1987) in *Anaesthetic Equipment: Physical Principles and Maintenance*. p. 95. London: Bailliere Tindall).

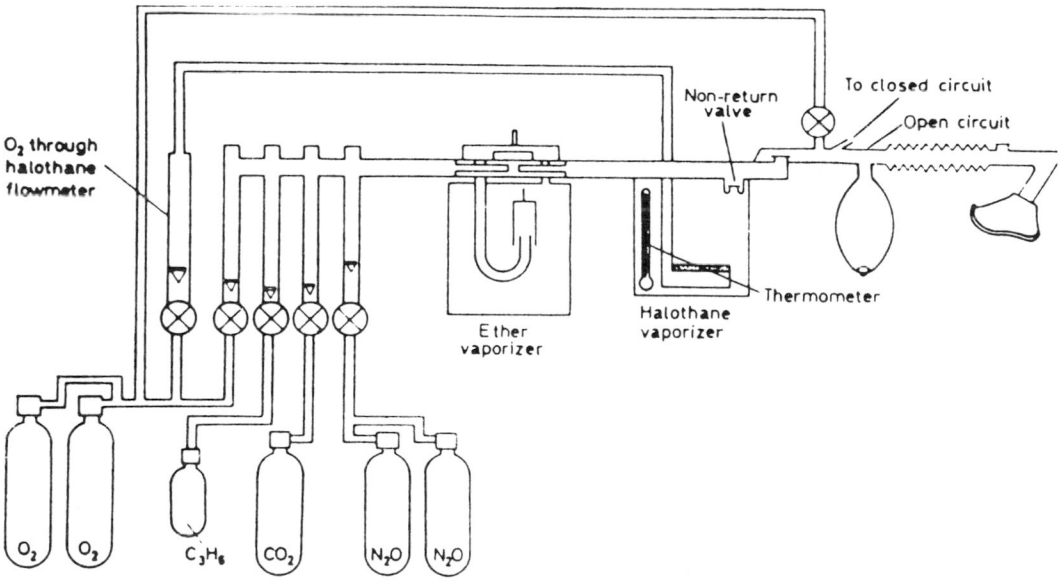

O₂ through
halothane
flowmeter

Non-return
valve

To closed circuit

Open circuit

Ether
vaporizer

Halothane
vaporizer

Thermometer

O₂   O₂   C₃H₆   CO₂   N₂O   N₂O

Fig. 60.13 The connection of a Halox vaporizer to the manifold of a Boyle anaesthetic machine.

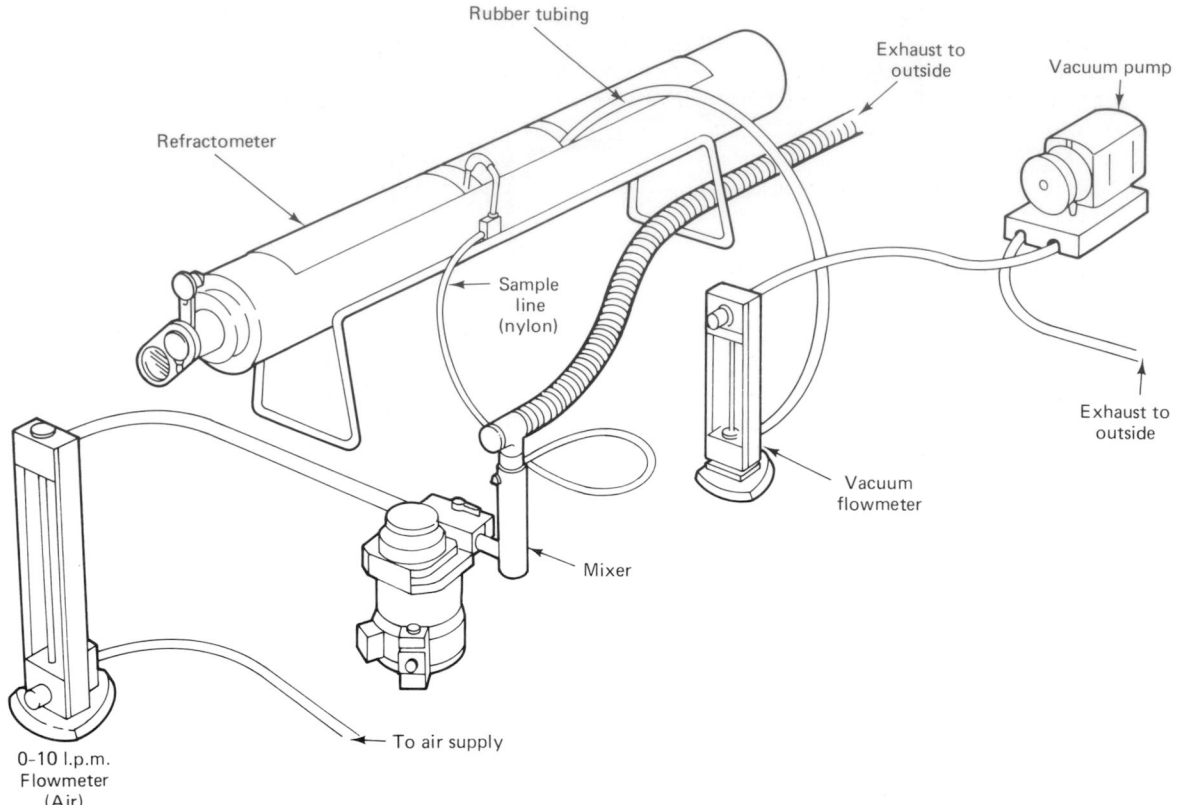

Fig. 60.14 A refractometer. General arrangement for room temperature (22°C) test.

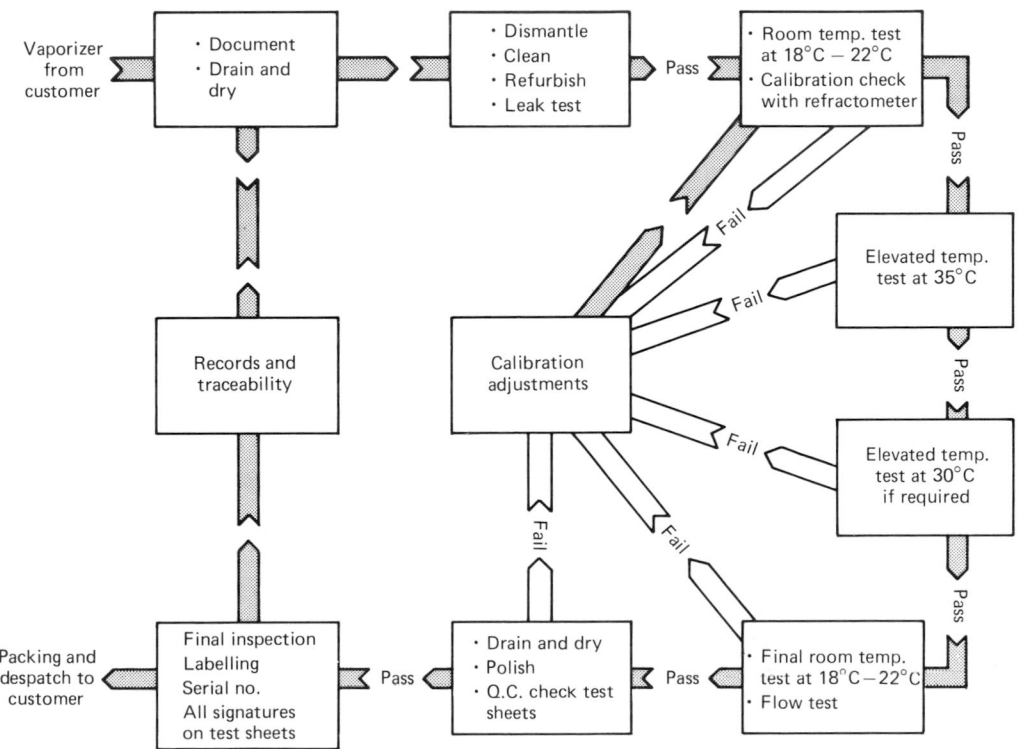

Fig. 60.15 Tec vaporizer standard service centre procedure.

specifically for semi-closed circuits. These vaporizers would be classified as measured flow, bubble through, out of circuit and without temperature compensation. The Foregger copper kettle is not agent specific but the Halox was designed specifically for use with halothane. The calculation of the settings to give a required concentration at a given temperature is not difficult but is certainly tedious. This is particularly so if the calculation needs to be repeated throughout the anaesthetic as conditions change and the temperature of the agent falls. The Halox is supplied with a slide rule in order to ease this problem. If the density of the volatile agent is known it is possible to calculate the mass of the agent delivered to the circuit from the s.v.p. of the agent and the flow rate through the kettle, as demonstrated by Collis (1966); Jennings et al., (1967).

Draw-over Vaporizers

Apart from the Goldman, the vaporizers discussed so far have been designed for use out of the patient circuit. Draw-over vaporizers are intended for use in anaesthetic circuits and require different characteristics, the most important of which is a low resistance to flow. A particularly successful example of this type is the EMO (Epstein, Macintosh, Oxford) draw-over vaporizer made by Penlon (Epstein and Macintosh, 1956). The temperature stability of the vaporizer is enhanced by an integral water reservoir with a capacity of 1.25 L. This is classified as a variable bypass, flow over wick, in circuit, temperature compensated and agent specific. The EMO is made for a number of different agents including diethyl ether, halothane, chloroform, trichloroethelene and the azeotrope ether-halothane.

The Blease Universal vaporizer is of interest as it can be used as a plenum type or as a draw-over vaporizer. (Merrifield et al., 1967). It can also deal with a number of different agents as the proportionating valve can be replaced by one designed for use with a particular agent. A potential disadvantage is that a valve inappropriate for the agent may be used in error. Comment has also been made as to the accuracy of the vaporizer when used in certain conditions. (Schreiber and Weis, 1965).

Calibration of Vaporizers

In order to calibrate a vaporizer, the manufacturer must obtain the refractive index of the agent at various concentrations from the agent manufacturer. This is then used to calibrate the vaporizer with a refractometer (Edmondson, 1957). The figure for the refractive index of the vapour at various percentages is supplied by the manufacturer of the volatile agent.

The arrangement of the apparatus is shown in Fig. 60.14. Note the use of a nylon sample tube to ensure that the sample arriving at the refractometer is the same as that leaving the vaporizer. The flow through the refractometer is as close as possible to atmospheric pressure. The standard test procedure adopted by Ohmeda, who make the TEC series of vaporizers is shown in Fig. 60.15. Newly manufactured vaporizers would begin the test procedure with the first of the room temperature tests. Hulands and Nunn (1970) describe how a portable refractometer can be used to check the calibration of a vaporizer on site, though possibly not to the level of accuracy guaranteed by the manufacturer.

Other methods of checking the accuracy of a vaporizer are by ultraviolet analysers, infrared analysers or gas chromatography. All the above methods require the calibration of a vapour of known concentration. This can be obtained from an accurate recently serviced vaporizer, such as the 'Vapor' by Dräger or from known vapour mixtures prepared in cylinders under pressure as decribed by Hill (1961).

REFERENCES

Boyle H.E.G. (1918). Nitrous oxide-oxygen-ether outfit. *Proc. Roy. Soc. Med.*, **II, I.** (Anaesth Sect.) 30.
Collis J.M. (1966). Concentration graphs for the Halox vaporizer. *Anaesthesia*, **21**, 558.
Dorsch J.A., Dorsch S.E. (1975). *Understanding Anaesthesia Equipment: Construction, Care and Complications.* Baltimore: Williams and Wilkins.
Edmonson W. (1957). Gas analysis by refractive index measurement. *Br. J. Anaesth.*, **29**, 570.
Epstein H.G., Macintosh R. (1956). An anaesthetic inhaler with automatic thermo-compensation. *Anaesthesia*, **11**, 83.
Goldman V. (1962). The Goldman vaporizer Mark 2. *Anaesthesia*, **17**, 537.
Hill D.W. (1961). Production of accurate gas and vapour mixtures. *Br. J. Appl. Phys.*, **12**, 410.
Hill D.W., Lowe H.J. (1962). Comparison of concentrations of Halothane in closed and semi-closed circuits during controlled ventilation. *Anesthesiology*, **23**, 291.
Hulands G.H., Nunn J.F. (1970). Portable interference refractometers in anaesthesia. *Br. J. Anaesth.*, **42**, 1051.
Jennings A.M.C., Taylor T.H., Young J. (1967). Nomograms for the Halox vaporizer. *Br. J. Anaesth.*, **39**, 598.
Merrifield A.J., Hill D.W., Smith K. (1967). Performance of the Portablease and the Fluoxair portable anaesthetic equipment with reference to use under adverse conditions. *Br. J. Anaesth.*, **39**, 50.
Morris L.E. (1952). A new vaporizer for use with anaesthetic agents. *Anesthesiology*, **13**, 587.
Schreiber P., Weis K.H. (1965). Konzentrationsmessungen mit dem Gardner-Universal-Verdamper. *Anaesthetist.*, **14**, 289.
Young J. (1966). The practical use of the Halox vaporizer. *Anesthesia*, **21**, 551.

61. Ventilators and Humidifiers

John A. Bushman

THE EARLY YEARS

As long ago as 1555 Vesalius was aware that the ventilation of the lungs was essential to life. He demonstrated that with artificial ventilation he could maintain the life of a tracheotomized dog whose thorax had been opened. Hooke (1667) demonstrated the use of bellows to ventilate the lungs, though he failed to demonstrate his belief that this also supported the circulation. In 1806 the Royal Humane Society adopted the bellows as the preferred method for the ventilation of the lungs in the treatment of the nearly drowned. Leroy (1827) was the first to point out the hazards of the barotrauma resulting in the rupture of the lungs. The technique fell into disrepute because it was not possible to measure or control the inflation pressure. Matas (1899) used O'Dwyer's (1885) blind intubation apparatus to ventilate a patient's lungs during an operation on the chest wall. The difficulties of blind intubation and the danger of barotrauma continued to cause problems and when Sauerbruch (1904) claimed that these could be overcome with his 'differential method' of ventilation many in Europe abandoned intermittent positive pressure ventilation. In America, Meltzer and Auer (1909) persisted with periodic insufflation of the lungs. Following this work Elsberg (1910) designed his own apparatus and used the Kirstein pattern of laryngoscope designed under the direction of Chevalier Jackson (1913). Despite the teachings of Sauerbruch,

Lawson and Sievers working in Leipzig developed a pump for positive pressure artificial ventilation. Mastery of the technique of endotracheal intubation developed slowly. Because of the lack of skilled endoscopists Green and Janeway evolved a series of head boxes within which the pressure could be cycled over a wide range of inspiratory times, expiratory times and pressures. Later Janeway (1913) invented a machine which would synchronize with the patient's spontaneous respiratory effort, thus producing the first respiratory assistor.

The treatment of poliomyelitis was the next great challenge for artificial ventilation. A common ventilator of the time, the Pulmotor, was reported to cause rupture of the lungs, the stomach or the oesophagus. To overcome this problem Drinker and Shaw (1929) invented the tank ventilator which became known as the 'iron lung'. This became freely available to any hospital in the British Empire by the generosity of Lord Nuffield. Under the overall guidance of Professor Macintosh and his department at Oxford, anesthetists became the clinicians who best understood the apparatus and so began the anaesthetist's involvement in intensive care.

THE EVOLUTION OF THE VENTILATOR

The development of the modern ventilator did not begin until the end of World War I when Giertz (1916), formerly as assistant to Sauerbruch, demonstrated that rhythmic inflation of the lungs produced results superior to insufflation. This gave added impetus to the development of the endotracheal tube and Frenckner (1934) produced a series of endotracheal and endobronchial tubes to be used with an air driven ventilator. Working with Anderson et al., (1940), an engineer from the Aga company and Crafoord (1938), a thoracic surgeon, Frenckner's ventilator was launched as the 'Spiropulsator' in 1940. Thus the concept of Intermittent Positive Pressure Ventilation (IPPV) was firmly launched. For the history of the development of ventilators readers are referred to Mushin et al. (1980), Hayes (1982) and Bernsten et al. (1986).

CLASSIFICATION OF VENTILATORS

There are at least sixty ventilator manufacturers operating in Europe and the United States of America and many of these produce more than one machine. Although a fully comprehensive classification of all the various ventilators in production is theoretically possible, it would be both clumsy and confusing. The classification given here attempts to describe simply the mode of operation of any machine currently available and to give an indication of the type of ventilatory problem for which it is most suited. The classification is based on that of Collis and Bushman (1966).

The Power Source

In order to function, a ventilator requires a source of power to move gases into the patient's lungs. The power can be derived from the energy of compressed gases or from some external source such as an electric motor, which then drives a compressor to provide a source of pressure.

Those machines using the energy stored in compressed gases can always be used for ventilation, even in the absence of cylinders, provided a suitable compressor is available, i.e. they can be converted to use an external power source. The compressor however must be of the type which does not contaminate the air (e.g. with oil) if it is used to ventilate the patient's lungs (Bushman and Clark, 1967).

Ventilators using external power as the primary source can entrain any gases supplied to them and are therefore independent of pressurized supplies. Some machines which are dependent on the energy of compressed gases economize in the use of the pressurized supply by employing a venturi device (injector) to entrain other gases (e.g. room air) at ambient pressure. This arrangement is economical but the proportion of the gas entrained is reduced as back pressure builds up. The final composition of the gas delivered to the patient is therefore unknown, although it usually lies within certain specified limits. An additional disadvantage is that the venturi is a noisy device.

Energy is also required to cycle a ventilator i.e., to change the ventilator from the inspiratory phase to the expiratory and back again into the inspiratory phase. This power may come from the main supply source or may require an independent source. Examples of the latter system are the Siemens-Elema 'Servo' Ventilator, the Engstrom ECS 2000 ventilator and the 'Sheffield Infant' ventilator. In these the primary power is supplied by the compressed gases but power from the mains drives the electronic timing circuits and the valves controlling inspiration and expiration. This type of ventilator will cease to function if either power source fails.

Parameters of Ventilation

There are five main parameters involved in ventilation. These are:

1. Minute volume
2. Tidal volume
3. Ventilatory rate
4. End inspiratory pressure
5. Lung compliance

These parameters are related as follows:

Minute volume = Rate × Tidal volume . . . (1)
Tidal volume = Pressure × Compliance . . . (2)

Although the compliance may change it is not under the control of the operator. There are thus four variables which may be controlled and these are subject to the restrictions given above, so there are only two independent variables. It follows from equation (2) that if either the tidal volume or the pressure is set then the other is determined by the compliance.

Therefore arbitrary values can be assigned to any two of the four controlled ventilatory parameters, except both tidal volume and pressure at the same time. The remaining two parameters will be uniquely determined by equations (1) and (2). In addition to assigning arbitrary values to some parameters it is common to limit the range of other parameters. This is most commonly done in the setting of a maximum value for the end inspiratory pressure, which in turn will limit the tidal volume for a given compliance.

Cycling Parameters

Cycling is the process of terminating one phase of ventilation and commencing the next. There are therefore two points in each ventilatory cycle when this occurs, once from inspiration to expiration and once from expiration to inspiration. In ventilation the important factor is determining when cycling occurs and there are three means by which this can be achieved:

1. Time cycling, i.e. cycling occurs after a certain preset time has elapsed
2. Volume cycling, i.e. cycling occurs when a certain volume has been delivered to the patient
3. Pressure cycling, i.e. cycling occurs when a certain pressure has been reached.

The actual mechanism of cycling is purely technical and some ventilators may have two methods available at any one time. This is common in pressure cycled machines where expiration to inspiration is initiated by the patient taking a breath, 'patient triggering'. Should the patient not make an inspiratory effort within a preset time than an override comes into action and cycles the machine back into inspiration.

Flow Characteristics

The pressure flow pattern of gases entering the patient's lungs during inspiration depends on the characteristics of both the patient and the ventilator. Ventilators can be divided into two classes according to their flow characteristics, namely:

1. Pressure generators
2. Flow generators

In pressure generators a certain pattern of pressure is applied to the inspired gases and this is relatively independent of any flow which results. The applied pressure is usually within the normal physiological limits required to ventilate the lungs, i.e. usually not in excess of $40 \, cmH_2O$. The end inspiratory pressure is largely determined by the pressure setting on the machine.

In flow generators a certain pattern of flow is produced which is relatively independent of the resistance to that flow. The applied pressure is normally well in excess of that required to ventilate the lungs, i.e. usually in excess of $500 \, cmH_2O$. The resistance encountered to the flow and the total compliance will determine the pressures in the airways.

These two types can be readily distinguished by considering the effect of a severe obstruction to the flow of gas. In a pressure generator the pressure developed follows the prescribed pattern of the machine but in the flow generator the pressure will immediately rise to the maximum of which the machine is capable. Harm to the patient is prevented by limiting the maximum inspiratory pressure to some reasonable value.

Minute Volume Dividers and Non-minute Volume Dividers

These are two important groups of machines and the use of each type has physiological consequences with regard to the treatment of the patient. The distinction between the two types is no longer as rigid as it was. A number of machines now on the market, which are primarily minute volume dividers, behave as non-minute volume dividers if the patient triggers the machine from expiration to inspiration. Examples of this type of machine are described in the section of modern ventilators.

Minute Volume Dividers

In this group of machines the minute volume is one of the directly assigned parameters. First, and most obviously, they deliver the assigned minute volume regardless of the manipulation of any other controls on the machine. It is common practice to vary the minute volume by a control external to the ventilator, e.g. by adjusting rotameters on an anaesthetic machine or a pump supplying the ventilator. This means that even if a patient trigger device is incorporated, the machine is still controlling the ventilation and not assisting it. If the patient triggers the machine from expiration to inspiration this will only have an effect on the respiratory rate. The minute volume will remain as it was before, set by the rotameters. As the patient has no control over his minute volume he can do nothing to lower or raise his P_{CO_2}. The only way in which the patient can increase his minute volume in such a machine is to entrain air into the system by his own inspiratory effort. Most time cycled and volume cycled machines are minute volume dividers.

Secondly, as has been pointed out above, once the minute volume has been set it is only possible to set one other parameter, the others being uniquely determined by this setting. In the majority of machines the parameter set is either the rate or the tidal volume. The compliance will then determine the end inspiratory airway pressure and the pressure limiting valve, if fitted, may be set to limit the pressure to just above that required to ventilate the lungs.

Thirdly, minute volume dividers cannot compensate for leaks in the circuit and the minute volume received by the patient will be reduced by the amount of the leak.

Non-minute Volume Dividers

In non-minute volume dividers there are four parameters, any two of which can be set. These are airway pressure, flow rate, tidal volume and respiratory rate. The minute volume will be uniquely determined by the assigned parameters. It should be appreciated that although minute volume, tidal volume, ventilatory rate and pressure are fundamental to the description of a ventilator, they are frequently not set as such on any particular machine. For instance ventilatory rate is often determined by controls which actually adjust the inspiratory and expiratory times. These in turn may be controlled by the pressure at which the machine cycles. The majority of pressure cycled machines are non-minute volume dividers.

As has been shown earlier, if the pressure is fixed so is the tidal volume for any given value of compliance (*see* Equation 2 *above*). The compliance however is not normally known and therefore although the tidal volume is determined its actual value is unknown and has to be measured. Similarly if the tidal volume is assigned, the pressure will be determined by the compliance, therefore the pressure must be measured in order to determine the compliance and so complete the description of ventilation.

In practice it is convenient if the fundamental parameters can be set by the use of calibrated controls rather than by adjustment of uncalibrated knobs, the function of which may not be clear and which may possibly interact with each other.

Additional Features Considered Desirable in Modern Ventilators

The majority of modern ventilators capable of supplying Continuous Mandatory Ventilation (CMV) have one or more additional features which allow the IPPV to be tailored to the particular requirements of the individual patient. The correct use of these features depends on an understanding of how they will affect the ventilation perfusion ratio. The majority of patients requiring IPPV have either predominantly a ventilatory defect or a perfusion defect. The aim in the use of the features dealt with below is to aid the more severe of the defects. This must be done with caution as ventilation is added at the expense of perfusion and *vice versa*.

Negative End Expiratory Phase (NEEP)
The use of NEEP during IPPV lowers the mean intrathoracic pressure and reduces the deleterious effect of

positive intrathoracic pressure on venous return to the thorax. The beneficial effect of NEEP is only seen clearly in shocked hypovolaemic patients, i.e. it aids perfusion. If used incautiously it causes peripheral atelectasis, i.e. a decrease in ventilation. This will ultimately cause an increase in pulmonary vascular resistance.

Positive End Expiratory Pressure (PEEP)

PEEP increases the volume of the lung potentially available for gas exchange. It probably does this by the recruitment of gas exchange airspaces and the prevention of terminal airway collapse (Falke et al. 1972). Because PEEP raises the mean intrathoracic pressure it tends to reduce the cardiac output. The effect is seen immediately following the addition of PEEP but in a normovolaemic patient some compensation occurs and the cardiac output returns to near normal. This compensation does not occur in shocked hypovolaemic patients and in these patients the use of PEEP may well be fatal.

Mandatory Minute Volume (MMV)

When using MMV the minute volume is set to the minimum required to ensure the patient's blood gases remain within satisfactory limits and the number of mechanical tidal volumes supplied by the ventilator is reduced as the patient breathes spontaneously. As the patient's efforts increase so he will wean himself off the ventilator. The method assumes that the patient's requirement for oxygen and his carbon dioxide production remain constant.

Intermittent Mandatory Ventilation (IMV)

This, like MMV is used on patients who have the ability to perform some spontaneous ventilation. In IMV the minimum number of tidal volumes per minute is set on the ventilator. The circuit is continuously purged with a high gas flow, usually with some degree of Continuous Positive Airway Pressure (CPAP), so the inspiratory effort made by the patient is minimized.

Continuous Positive Airway Pressure (CPAP)

CPAP is a valuable adjunct to IMV as it improves oxygenation and reduces the inspiratory effort required by the patient. It is particularly valuable in the treatment of chest injuries. These patients, after an initial period of ventilation, may do well on CPAP alone.

EXAMPLES OF SOME MODERN VENTILATORS

The choice of ventilators dealt with in this section is intended to be representative of their type and includes a cross section of those most likely to be found in use in the United Kingdom.

The 'Amsterdam Infant' Ventilator
(Fig. 61.1)

This compact ventilator is a sophisticated electronic 'thumb' acting on the end of an Ayres 'T' piece. The ventilator is supplied with a constant flow of gas from a high pressure source.

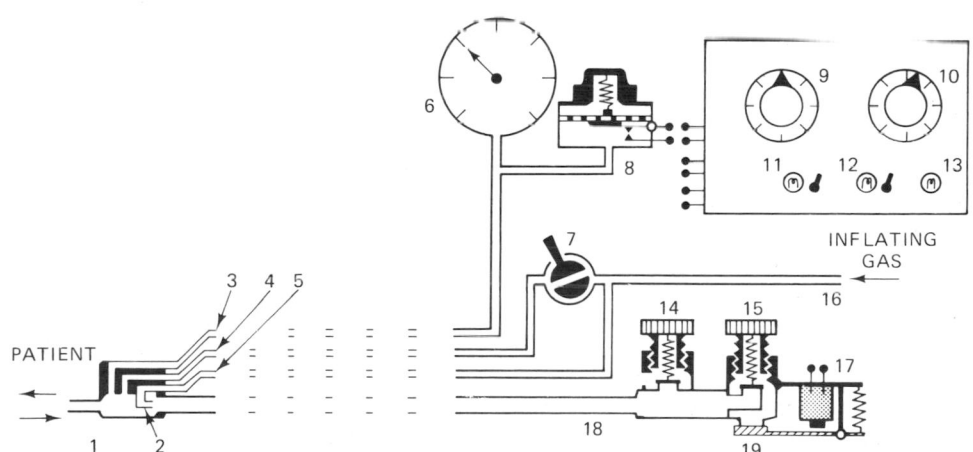

Fig. 61.1 Diagram of the 'Amsterdam Infant' ventilator Mark 2. 1 = connector block; 2 = jet of injector; 3 = manometer tube connection; 4 = direct supply tube to airway; 5 = injector jet connection; 6 = manometer; 7 = trigger sensitivity/expiratory pressure control; 8 = patient trigger mechanism; 9 = I:E ratio control; 11 = mains on/off switch; 12 = trigger switch; 13 = inspiratory phase indicator lamp; 14 = positive pressure safety valve; 15 = positive end-expiratory pressure valve; 16 = inflating gas inlet; 17 = solenoid; 18 = expiratory tube; 19 = solenoid-operated valve. (Reproduced with permission from Mushin et al., 1980 *Automatic Ventilation of the Lungs*, 3rd edn., Fig. 16.2. Oxford: Blackwell Scientific Publications.)

Description

The inflating gas flows continuously, at a rate determined by one or more rotameters, through valve (7) to the connector block (1). When the valve (19) is closed the patient's lungs will be inflated by the fresh gas flow. When the valve is opened the expiratory phase commences and the patient's airway will fall to a pressure determined by the setting of the PEEP valve (15) and the setting of the valve (7), the latter determining the amount of negative pressure produced by the venturi in the mixing block. The expiratory valve (19) is controlled by the solenoid (17) which is driven by a timing circuit which determines the number of times the valve opens and closes in a minute. This is set by control (10) and can be varied between 20 and 60 breaths per minute. The setting of the rotameters determines the inspiratory flow rate. The ratio between the time the valve (19) is closed and the time it is open, i.e. the Inspiratory Expiratory ratio (the I:E ratio), is set by the control (9). A trigger mechanism (8) allows triggering of the ventilator in response to an inspiratory effort from the patient, the trigger sensitivity being set by the valve (7).

Functional Analysis

This ventilator is classified as a time cycled flow generator which behaves as a minute volume divider until the patient triggers the machine when it then behaves as a non-minute volume divider.

The Bennet MA1 Ventilator
(Fig. 61.2)

This versatile ventilator is operated by electronically controlled solenoid valves. An integral compressor ventilates the patient with air which can be enriched with oxygen. A heated humidifier and a nebulizer are part of the inspiratory circuit.

Description

During inspiration the air compressor (49) delivers air to the injector (43) at a pressure of about $120\,cmH_2O$ via the energized solenoid valve (44). The entrained air pressurizes the chamber (39) via the 'Peak flow' control (41) and so drives the contents of the concertina bellows (38) into the patient at a flow rate determined by control (41). At the same time the two capsule valves (36) and (1) are inflated. Valve (36) prevents gas leaving the chamber (39) and valve (1) prevents gas leaving the patient. The weighted valve (32) is also open allowing gas to leave the spirometer bellows (31) which collapses under its own weight. As the concertina bag (38) is driven upwards by the high pressure in the chamber (39) the potentiometer (40) is rotated. This forms part of a feedback mechanism with the 'normal volume' control (63) and when the volume set on this control is reached the solenoid valve (44) is turned off and the ventilator cycles to the expiratory phase. Inspiration may also be terminated if the setting of the 'normal pressure limit' control (14) is exceeded.

With the solenoid valve (44) de-energized air from the compressor (49) will flow to the injector (42) and the resulting pressure will close the diaphragm operated valve (17) thus preventing the reflux of gas from the inspiratory circuit. Due to the fall in pressure from the venturi (43) the capsule valves (1) and (36) will collapse. Gas then flows out of the patient to fill the spirometer bellows (31) and the concertina bag (38) will fill via the one-way valve (18). Note that the speed of gas leaving the patient can be regulated by the 'expiratory resistance' control (34). This controls the speed at which the pressure in capsule valve (1) falls to atmospheric pressure. The ratio between the amount of air to that of oxygen filling the bag is determined by the 'oxygen percentage' control (23). Air will enter the system via the one-way valve (19) and the filter (20). Oxygen enters the system via the diaphragm operated demand valve (26). Note the oxygen excessive pressure alarm contacts (22) and the oxygen failure alarm contacts (21) forming part of the oxygen supply system.

There are two important attachments to the basic ventilator. The first is a negative pressure attachment (51–55) which replaces the spirometer (31). The negative pressure is supplied during the expiratory phase by the injector (55) due to the de-energization of the solenoid (44). The negative pressure achieved is determined by the 'negative pressure' control (54). The negative pressure achievable is limited by the valve (52) to $-9\,cmH_2O$.

The second attachment is a PEEP valve (56–57) and can be fitted as an alternative to the negative pressure attachment. During the expiratory phase the chamber (56) can be pressurized by the regulator (57) thus controlling the deflation of the capsule valve (1), the PEEP produced being dictated by the pressure set in the chamber (56).

Cycling from expiration to inspiration may occur after a fixed time or due to the patient triggering the ventilator, the respiratory rate being set by the frequency control (66) and the trigger by the 'sensitivity' control (13).

One further facility the ventilator has is the ability to give the patient a number of single or multiple sighs over a period of time. The number of sighs is set by the 'sigh per hour' and 'multiple sigh' controls (69). The sigh volume is set by the control (64) and the sigh pressure limit by control (15).

Functional Analysis

The ventilator requires an electrical supply to provide power for the air compressor. In addition it requires oxygen if the air with which the patient will be ventilated requires enrichment with oxygen.

The ventilator is normally cycled from inspiration to expiration after a preset volume has been delivered

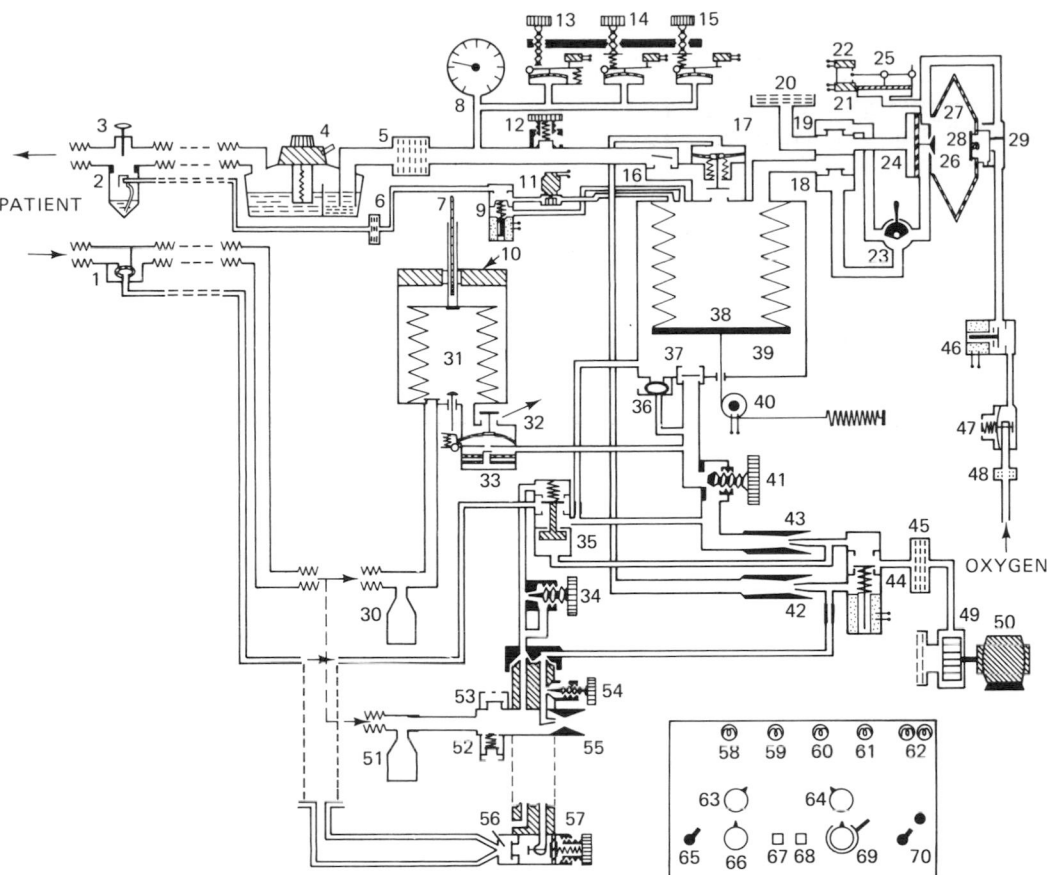

Fig. 61.2 Diagram of the Bennett MA1 ventilator. 1 = capsule valve; 2 = nebulizer; 3 = thermometer; 4 = humidifier; 5 = filter; 6 = filter; 7 = engraved rod; 8 = manometer; 9 = solenoid valve; 10 = on/off switch for expired volume alarm; 11 = compressor for nebulizer; 12 = safety valve; 13 = 'sensitivity' control; 14 = 'normal pressure limit' control; 15 = 'sigh pressure limit' control; 16 = one-way valve; 17 = diaphragm operated valve; 18 = one-way valve; 19 = one-way valve; 20 = filter; 21 = oxygen failure alarm contacts; 22 = excessive pressure alarm contacts; 23 = 'oxygen percentage' control; 24 = diaphragm; 25 = oxygen alarm unit; 26 = diaphragm operated valve; 27 = 'accumulator'; 28 = one-way valve; 29 = valve; 30 = water trap; 31 = spirometer; 32 = weighted valve; 33 = diaphragm; 34 = 'expiratory resistance' control; 35 = valve; 36 = capsule; 37 = one-way valve; 38 = concertina bag; 39 = chamber; 40 = potentiometer; 41 = 'peak flow' control; 42 = injector; 43 = injector; 44 = solenoid valve; 45 = filter; 46 = solenoid valve; 47 = pressure regulator; 48 = filter; 49 = air compressor; 50 = electric motor; 51 = water trap; 52 = negative pressure safety valve; 53 = one-way valve; 54 = negative pressure control; 55 = injector; 56 = chamber; 57 = PEEP control; 58 = 'assist' warning lamp; 59 = 'pressure' warning lamp; 60 = 'ratio' warning lamp; 61 = 'sigh' indicator lamp; 62 = 'oxygen' indicator and warning lamps; 63 = 'normal volume' control; 64 = 'sigh volume' control; 65 = main on/off switch; 66 = frequency control; 67 = 'manual normal' press button; 68 = 'manual sigh' press button; 69 = 'sigh per hour' and 'multi-sigh' controls; 70 = nebulizer on/off switch. (Reproduced with permission from Mushin et al., 1980. *Automatic Ventilation of the Lungs*, 3rd edn., Fig. 22.2. Oxford: Blackwell Scientific Publications.)

but it may also be pressure cycled. Cycling from expiration to inspiration is by time or the patient triggering the machine.

While cycled by volume and time the ventilator behaves as a minute volume divider. However if the patient triggers the ventilator it will behave as a non-minute volume divider and the patient will determine his own minute volume as long as it remains higher than that determined by the volume and time settings.

Because of the high pressure supplied by the injector (43) to the chamber (39) the ventilator is classified as a flow generator.

The Bird Mk8 Series 1 Ventilator
(Fig. 61.3)

This machine is now quite old but there are still many in use and though simple in operation it has all the

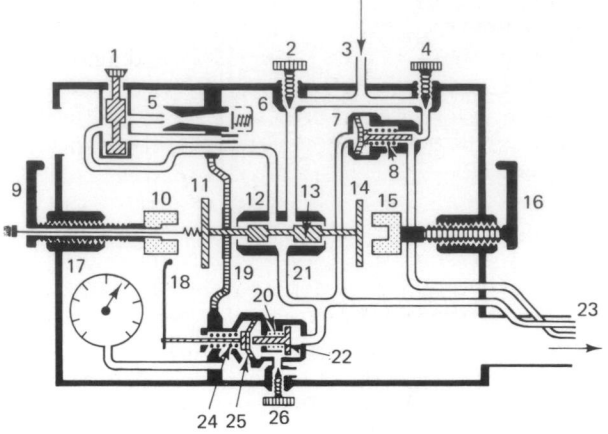

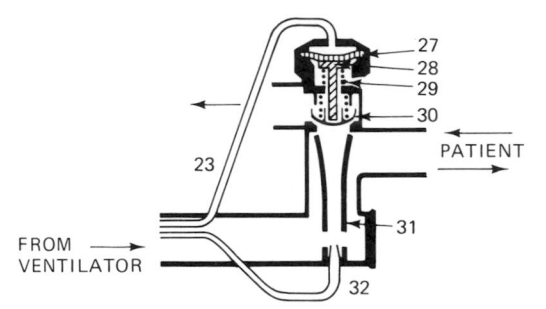

Fig. 61.3 Diagrams of the Bird Mark 8 ventilator (first generation) and expiratory valve assembly. 1 = 'air-mix' control; 2 = 'inspiratory time flowrate' control; 3 = driving-gas inlet; 4 = 'negative pressure generator' control; 5 = injector; 6 = one-way valve; 7 = main chamber; 8 = piston; 9 = 'inspiratory effort' control; 10 = magnet; 11 = soft-iron plate; 12 = outlet; 13 = ceramic sliding valve; 14 = soft-iron plate; 15 = magnet; 16 = 'inspiratory pressure limit' control; 17 = manometer; 18 = striking arm; 19 = diaphragm; 20 = spring; 21 = outlet; 22 = piston; 23 = small-bore tube; 24 = spring; 25 = diaphragm; 26 = 'expiratory time' control; 27 = diaphragm; 28 = push rod; 29 = spring; 30 = expiratory valve; 31 = injector; 32 = small-bore tube. (Reproduced with permission from Mushin et al., 1980. *Automatic Ventilation of the Lungs*, 3rd edn., Figs. 24, a, b, Oxford: Blackwell Scientific Publications.)

features of a gas powered, pressure cycled, non-minute volume divider which may act as a flow generator or a pressure generator.

Description

The ventilator consists of a green plastic box which is divided into two halves by a wall. Set in this wall is a venturi injector (5) and a diaphragm (19). The right half of the box is connected to the patient circuit. The left half is at atmospheric pressure. Attached to the diaphragm is a rod connected to a spool valve (12 and 13). Soft-iron discs are attached to each end of the rod. Oxygen at 300–380 kPa (45–55 lbf/in²) enters the

ventilator at (3). When the ventilator is turned on both halves of the box are at atmospheric pressure and the rod and its attachments are moved to the right. The oxygen supply will flow through the flow rate control (2), through the spool valve (13), to the outlets (12) and (21). Outlet (12) is connected to the 'air-mix' control (1) and outlet (21) is connected via the fine bore tubing (23) to the expiratory valve. When pressure is high in outlet (21) the expiratory valve will be held closed. With the 'air-mix' control pushed in (off) the oxygen passes unmixed into the right hand half of the box, and hence to the patient. If the control is pulled out (on) the oxygen passes through the injector (5) and entrains air from the left half of the box which is injected into the right half. This is connected to the patient's upper airways and so forms a closed system. As oxygen or an air-oxygen mix flows into this system the pressure will rise, inflating the patient's lungs. As the pressure rises in the right side of the box so will the force tending to push the diaphragm to the left. Eventually the pressure will be high enough to pull the soft-iron disc (14) away from the magnet (15) and the diaphragm, spool valve, rod and discs will flip to the left. The pressure required to cycle the ventilator at the end of inspiration depends on the proximity of the magnet (15) to the soft-iron disc (14). This distance is adjustable by the rotation of the 'inspiratory pressure limit' control (16). The movement of the spool valve cuts off the high pressure oxygen supply and the expiratory valve opens as the high pressure in (23) via (21) falls to atmospheric pressure.

During the inspiratory phase the line (21) has also pressurized the pistons (8) and (22). Piston (8) shuts off the high pressure supply from (4), the 'negative pressure generator' control. If this control is open during the expiratory phase the injector (31) will be energized and a negative pressure expiratory phase will be generated. Piston (22) is part of the 'expiratory time' control. During the inspiratory phase the piston (22) forces the striking arm (18) to the left. During the expiratory phase the spring (24) pushes the striking arm back to the right at a speed controlled by the valve (26) which allows the gas behind the diaphragm to escape. As the striking arm (18) pushes against the disc (11) it will eventually overcome its attraction to the magnet (10). More commonly this ventilator is cycled by the patient's own inspiratory effort. This will reduce the pressure in the right side of the box and so tend to pull the diaphragm to the right, so cycling the ventilator back into the inspiratory phase. The inspiratory effort required by the patient is determined by the distance between the magnet (10) and the soft-iron disc (11), the distance being controlled by rotation of the 'inspiratory effort' control (9).

Functional Analysis

With the 'air-mix' control pushed in (off) the machine will act as a flow generator as the energy available to inflate the lungs comes directly from the high pressure gas supply. With the control pulled out (on) the operation of the machine is more complex and difficult to predict. This is because the venturi is affected by back pressure due to the rising pressure in the right side of the box as the patient's lungs are inflated. This effect is exaggerated if the 'inspiratory time flow rate' control (2) is partially closed. Therefore when the air-mix is turned on it is impossible to ventilate patients requiring high inflation pressures at low flow rates.

The Manley Ventilator
(Fig. 61.4)

This basic ventilator, manufactured by Blease Medical Equipment, is driven solely by the fresh gas flow delivered to the ventilator and thence to the patient. This may be air and oxygen or a mixture of anaesthetic gases and vapours as the machine is equally suitable for ward or anaesthetic use. The machine produces a considerable back pressure to the fresh gas which needs to be at a pressure of at least 35 kPa (5 lbf/in^2). There is no provision for patient triggering.

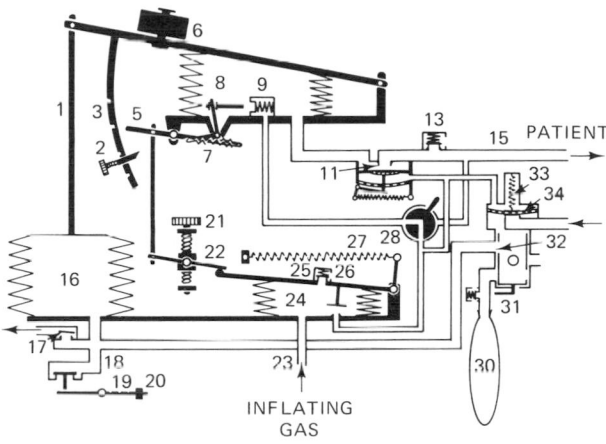

Fig. 61.4 Diagram of the Manley ventilator model MN2. 1 = rod; 2 = adjustable stop; 3 = arm; 5 = lever; 6 = movable weight; 7 = click mechanism; 8 = main concertina bag; 9 = valve; 11 = inspiratory valve; 13 = safety valve; 15 = inspiratory tube; 16 = negative pressure concertina bag; 17 = one-way valve; 18 = weighted air inlet valve; 19 = lever; 20 = counterweight; 21 = 'inspiratory phase' control; 22 = lever; 23 = inflating gas inlet; 24 = small concertina bag; 25 = top-plate of concertina bag (24); 26 = safety-valve; 27 = spring; 28 = 'manual/automatic' tap; 30 = reservoir bag; 31 = 'manual/automatic/negative pressure' tap; 32 = port; 33 = spring; 34 = diaphragm of expiratory valve. (Reproduced with permission from Mushin et al., 1980. *Automatic Ventilation of the Lungs*. 3rd edn., Fig. 61.2. Oxford: Blackwell Scientific Publications.)

Description
During the inspiratory phase the small bellows (24) fills with fresh gas flow via the connection (23). The spring (27) maintains the pressure in this bellows to

around 150 cmH$_2$O. The valve (9) in the main bellows is closed so the pressure generated in the small bag (24) keeps the expiratory valve (34) closed against the pull of the spring (33). The same pressure holds open the inspiratory valve (11) and the contents of the main bellows (8) is driven into the patient at a pressure dictated by the position of the weight (6). The maximum pressure attainable is limited by the safety valve (13) to 35 cmH$_2$O. During this time the small bellows (24) continues to fill and will eventually move the lever (22), the position of which is set by the 'inspiratory phase' control (21). The motion of the lever (22) will reset the toggle mechanism comprising (5), (7) and (8) and this will open the valve (9) and the contents of the small bellows (24) will flow rapidly into the main bellows (8). The resulting drop in pressure behind the diaphragms of the inspiratory (11) and expiratory (34) valves will cause the former to close and the latter to open. The fresh gas flow will continue to fill the main bellows (8) via the small bellows (24), the 'manual/automatic' tap (28) and the valve (9). The expiratory phase is terminated when the adjustable stop (2) on the arm (3) resets the toggle mechanism (5), (7) and (8). This allows the valve (9) to close. As a result the pressure rises behind the inspiratory (11) and expiratory valve (34) diaphragms, which open and close respectively and the machine cycles into the inspiratory phase.

The ventilator can be supplied with or without an expiratory negative phase attachment. The diagram shows this facility and its action is self evident.

It should be noted that in order to turn the machine from automatic to manual operation requires the movement of both the 'manual/automatic' tap (28) and 'manual/automatic/negative pressure' tap (31).

Functional Analysis
As the highest pressure the ventilator can generate is 40 cmH$_2$O it is defined as a pressure generator, though for a number of reasons this pressure does not remain constant throughout the inspiratory phase. The 'Brompton Manley' is essentially the same machine but the addition of a spring and a heavier weight (6) raises the pressure in the bellows (8) to 70–80 cmH$_2$O and so it should be regarded as a flow generator.

Although this is an apparently simple machine there has been much semantic discussion as to the best method of classifying the way it cycles. The machine is clearly a minute volume divider, the minute volume being set by the rotameters supplying the machine with fresh gas. Time and volume are therefore interdependent. The point at which the machine cycles, is dictated by the resetting of the toggle mechanism (5), (7) and (8). This resetting occurs whenever either the bellows (8) or the small bellows (24) reach a volume which resets the toggle mechanism. So far as the actual mechanism of cycling is concerned it would be correct to regard the ventilator as being volume cycled. However it can be argued logically that it is the fresh gas flow rate that determines the time taken for a bellows to fill to a given volume and therefore the ventilator is time cycled. The reader may feel that a classification which adds to understanding by describing a mechanism may be preferable to one that demonstrates an individual's ability for logical argument.

The Siemens-Elema 'Servo' 900 Ventilator
(Fig. 61.5)

The basic mechanics of this versatile ventilator are very simple. Its versatility is dependent on ingenious electronic control circuits which modify its basic mechanical properties. The ventilator requires an electricity supply and an inflating gas in order to operate.

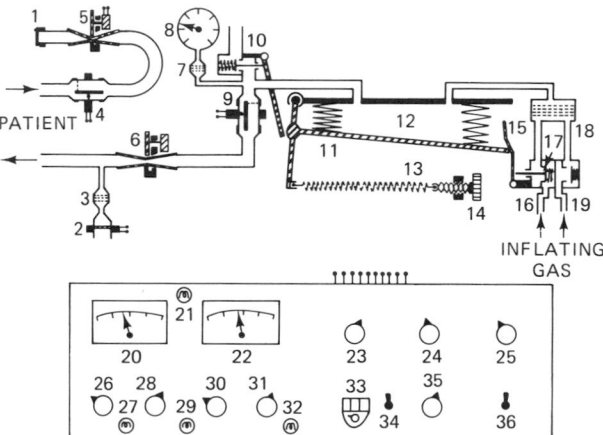

Fig. 61.5 Diagram of the Siemens-Elema 'Servo' 900 ventilator . 1 = one-way valve; 2 = pressure transducer; 3 = filter; 4 = expiratory flow sensor; 5 = expiratory valve; 6 = inspiratory valve; 7 = filter; 8 = working pressure gauge; 9 = inspiratory flow sensor; 10 = safety-valve; 11 = pivoted baseplate; 12 = concertina bag; 13 = spring; 14 = preset working-pressure control; 15 = lever; 16 = high pressure gas inlet; 17 = valve; 18 = filter; 19 = low pressure gas inlet; 20 = 'expired minute volume' meter; 21 = mains indicator lamp; 22 = 'airway pressure' meter; 23 = 'breaths/min' control; 24 = 'inspiratory time %' control; 25 = 'pause time % control; 26 = 'expired minute volume lower limit' warning control; 27 = expired minute volume warning lamp; 28 = 'expired minute volume upper limit' warning control; 29 = 'airway pressure lower limit' warning lamp; 30 = 'airway pressure lower limit' warning control; 31 = 'airway pressure upper limit' warning control; 32 = 'airway pressure upper limit' warning lamp; 33 = 'preset inspiratory minute volume' control and indicator; 34 = waveform selection switch; 35 = 'maximum expiratory flow' control; 36 = 'sigh function' control. (Reproduced with permission from Mushin et al., 1980. *Automatic Ventilation of the Lungs*, 3rd edn., Fig. 85. 2. Oxford: Blackwell Scientific Publications.)

Description
The inflating gas or gases fill the bellows (12) against a pressure supplied by the spring (13). The tension in the spring, and hence the pressure in the bellows can be regulated by the preset working-pressure control (14) within a range $10–100\,cmH_2O$, the pressure set being indicated on the working-pressure gauge (8). The inflating gas can enter the bellows (12) by one of two routes. The low pressure gas inlet (19) is designed to accept flows from rotameters, as is the case if the ventilator is used in anaesthesia. The high pressure gas inlet is designed to work from direct connection to pipelines. This inlet is opened if the bellows (12) is less than half full. Over filling of the bellows is prevented by the opening of the safety valve (10).

Inspiration commences when the electronically controlled inspiratory valve (6) opens, the expiratory valve (5) being closed. The volume and pressure of the resulting flow of gas to the patient is measured by the inspiratory flow sensor (9) and by the pressure transducer (2), and is indicated on the 'airway pressure' meter (22). The inspiratory valve (6) is able to control the flow of gas dynamically, its performance being controlled by the waveform selection switch (34) working in a feedback circuit in conjunction with the flow sensor (9). The setting of the 'preset inspiratory minute volume' (33) controls and indicates the tidal volume. At the end of a time dictated by the settings of the 'breaths/min' (23), 'inspiratory time %' (24) and the 'pause time' (25), the ventilator cycles to the expiratory phase. The inspiratory valve (6) closes and the expiratory valve (5) opens, the expiratory flow rate being measured by the expiratory flow sensor (4) and indicated on the 'expired minute volume' meter (20). The expiratory valve also can be dynamically controlled and works in conjunction with the expiratory flow sensor (4) and the 'maximum expiratory flow' control (25). Note that the pressure transducer (2) on the inspiratory side is downstream from the inspiratory valve (6) so is able to measure the pressure in the circuit during the expiratory phase.

Functional Analysis
If the pressure in the bellows (12) is only a little above the final airway pressure the ventilator acts as a pressure generator. If the pressure in the bellows is considerably greater than the final airway pressure then the machine acts as a flow generator.

The machine is cycled from inspiration to expiration by time as outlined above. Also in theory it can be pressure cycled by setting the 'airway pressure upper limit' control (31) but this produces an alarm signal and is not the intended use of this control. The machine is cycled from expiration to inspiration by time or by patient triggering.

If the fresh gas supply is delivered from rotameters via the low pressure gas inlet (19) the machine behaves as a minute volume divider. If supplied from a pipeline via the high pressure gas inlet (16) it will behave as a minute volume divider unless the patient triggers the machine, in which case the patient will dictate the minute volume so long as it remains in excess of that set on the ventilator.

The Possible Future Development of Ventilators

The single most predictable factor determining the future development of ventilators is that the cost of machined components will increase and the cost of electronic components will decrease. This will encourage manufacturers to develop machines with the minimum number of mechanical components which can be controlled by electronics. There are a number of advantages to the user as a result of this approach. One such advantage is that it is possible to site the mechanical part of the ventilator, which is small, close to the patient while the controlling electronics can be more conveniently sited on the anaesthetic machine. It will also be possible to control the ventilator with a signal from another piece of apparatus such as a carbon dioxide analyser, thus allowing the possibility of closed loop control. It is likely that the key components of these machines will be critical orifices controlled by high speed pneumatic valves. A number of these machines exist either in prototype or on the drawing board. These machines will be very versatile as they are relatively unconstrained by mechanical limitations but their development costs are high. It remains to be seen if the savings in manufacturing costs can be passed on to the consumer.

HUMIDIFICATION

Water evaporates to form water vapour. In doing so the partial pressure of water vapour in the gases above the surface of the water is increased. This process continues until the gases above the water are saturated with water vapour. The saturated water vapour pressure at body temperature (37°C) is 47 mmHg. One of the more important functions of the upper respiratory tract is the humidification of the inspired air. By the time this reaches the bronchi in a person breathing normally it is close to being saturated with water vapour. This is not the case in a patient who is intubated and ventilated with pipeline gases as the normal humidification area has been bypassed and the gases are dry. Dalhamn (1956), Chalon et al. (1972) and Forbes (1974) have shown that under these conditions the activity of the cilia is depressed as is the transport of mucous and the clearance of foreign material. Patients who are intubated and ventilated with dry gases should therefore have some form of humidification incorporated in the ventilatory circuit. Opinions vary as to the period of ventilation that makes this requirement mandatory but it is likely that all patients would benefit from humidification though it is infrequently done in the operating theatre. For patients in an ITU having longterm respiratory support the need for humidification is clear.

The Classification of Humidifiers

Humidifiers can be divided into three main categories:

1. Heated water vapour generators
   a. Heated water bath humidifiers.
   b. Bubble humidifiers.
2. Jet nebulizer humidifiers.
   a. Main stream.
   b. Side stream.
3. Ultrasonic humidifiers.

1) Heated Water Vapour Generators
a) Heated Water Bath Humidifiers. The principle of this type of humidifier is to raise the saturated water vapour pressure in the inspired gas as it passes over the surface of heated water. The temperature of the water in the bath is normally kept at a temperature which ensures that the temperature of the gas when it reaches the patient is at, or only slightly below, body temperature. The temperature of the inspired gas is measured at the end of the inspiratory circuit at the attachment to the patient by a thermistor. This is part of a feedback circuit which regulates the heating of the bath to keep the temperature as measured by the thermistor at 37°C. If the ambient temperature is low then this will necessitate the water bath being several degrees higher than body temperature. Due to the fall in temperature as the humidified gas passes to the patient, water will condense out of the inspired gas onto the walls of the inspiratory tubing. The tubing can be considered as an extension of the water bath ensuring the gas remains fully saturated as it passes to the patient. A disadvantage of this simple system is that the inspiratory tubing will eventually become full of water which may then be driven into the patient by the ventilator. The amount of condensation can be reduced by lagging the tubing to the patient and can be prevented by heating the tubing to ensure the temperature of the gas does not fall as it passes to the patient.

b) Bubble Humidifiers. This is an extension of the heated water bath humidifier which is suitable for the humidification of gases from a high pressure source. In order to increase the surface area available the incoming dry gas is driven through a fine porous plate under the surface of the liquid. The gas emerges as a large number of very small bubbles which then rise slowly through the warm water to become saturated.

2) Jet Nebulizers
These employ the Bernouilli principle. In 1738, Bernouilli formulated the laws which apply to fluids flowing through pipes with varying diameters. He demonstrated that the pressure in such a system would be at its lowest where the speed of the fluid was greatest. About sixty years later Venturi designed the injector which bears his name and demonstrated that a marked fall in pressure occurred at the point of the maximum constriction in a pipe. Using such a system, a gas flow can be made to entrain a liquid. In a humidifier the venturi is designed to ensure that many very small droplets of water are formed, many small

enough to form a stable colloid with air. This formation of fine droplets greatly increases the surface area of the entrained water and so increases the rate of vapour formation. The fact that the smaller particles form a colloid ensures that they are carried into the upper airways where their evaporation rate is increased due to the rise in temperature. Because some of the water will enter the lung in a liquid phase rather than a gaseous phase this method of humidification is ideal for medication.

Nebulizers can be of two types:

a) Main Stream Nebulizers. These are situated in the tubing of the inspiratory circuit in such a way that the droplets they produce are introduced directly into the fresh gas flow to the patient. This makes them ideal for the administration of drugs to the upper airway.

b) Side Stream Nebulizers. These are connected to the inspiratory circuit by a 'T' piece so that only the smaller more stable particles reach the circuit to be carried to the patient. These smaller particles have greater penetration into the depths of the lung but less of the droplets formed are carried into the lung.

3) Ultrasonic Humidifiers

These humidifiers consist of a rapidly vibrating plate onto which water is dripped. The plate consists of a piezoelectric crystal which is caused to vibrate by a high frequency alternating current at about 5 MHz. The resulting energy transferred to the water drops causes them to break up into minute droplets which form a colloid with the inspired gas thus ensuring that the droplets are carried into the depths of the lungs. There are two important points to bear in mind when using this type of humidifier. These small droplets can be highly irritant and this form of humidification may thus be unsuitable for conscious spontaneously breathing patients. Secondly it is possible to carry large amounts of water into the lungs and possibly overload the patient's circulation.

REFERENCES

Anderson S., Crafoord C., Frenckner P. (1940). A new and practical method of producing rhythmic ventilation during positive pressure anaesthesia with: description of the apparatus. *Acta Otolaryngol. Scand.*, **28**, 95.

Bernsten A.D., Skowronski G.A., Oh T.E. (1986). New generation ventilators. *Anaesth. Intens. Care*, **14**, 293.

Bushman J.A., Clark P.A. (1967). Oil mist hazard and piped air supplies. *Br. Med. J.*, **2**, 588.

Chalon J., Loew D.A.Y., Malebranche J. (1972). Effect of dry anaesthetic gases on tracheobronchial ciliated epithelium. *Anesthesiology*, **37**, 338.

Collis J.M., Bushman J.A. (1966). An assessment of ten lung ventilators. World Med. Electron., **4**, 134; **4**, 166; **4**, 199.

Crafoord C. (1938). On the technique of pneumonectomy in man. *Acta Chirurgica Scand.*, Suppl. **54**.

Dalhamn T. (1956). Mucous flow and ciliary activity in the trachea of healthy rats and rats exposed to respiratory irritant gases. *Acta Physiol. Scand.* Suppl. **36**, 123.

Drinker P., Shaw L. (1929). An apparatus for the prolonged administration of artificial respiration. *J. Clin. Invest.*, **7**, 229.

Elsberg C.A. (1910). Clinical experiences with intratracheal insufflation (Meltzer) with remarks of the value of the method for thoracic surgery. *Ann. Surg.*, **52**, 23.

Falke K.J., Pontoppidan H., Kumar A., et al. (1972). Ventilation with positive end expiratory pressure in acute lung disease. *J. Clin. Invest.*, **51**, 2315.

Forbes A.R. (1974). Temperature, humidity and mucous flow in the intubated trachea. *Br. J. Anaesth.*, **46**, 29.

Frenckner P. (1934). Bronchial and tracheal catheterization. *Acta Otolaryngol. Scand.*, Suppl. **20**, 100.

Giertz J.H. (1916). Studier Ofver tryckdifferensandning (rytmisk luftenblasning) vid intrathoracala operationer. *Uppsala Lakaref*, **22**, 1.

Hayes B. (1982). Ventilation and ventilators. *J. Med. Eng. Tech.*, **6**, 177.

Hooke R. (1667). An account of an experiment made by R. Cooke of preserving animals alive by blowing through their lungs with bellows. *Phil. Trans. R. Soc.*, **2**, 539.

Jackson C. (1913). The technique of insertion of intratracheal insufflation tubes. *Surg. Gynecol. Obstet.*, **17**, 507.

Janeway H.H. (1913). Intratracheal anaesthesia. *Ann. Surg.*, **58**, 927.

Leroy J. (1827). Recherches sur la l'asphyxie. *J. Physiol. Exp. Path.*, **7**, 45.

Matas R. (1899). On the management of acute traumatic pneumothorax. *Ann. Surg.*, **29**, 409.

Meltzer S.J., Auer J.L. (1909). Continuous respiration without respiratory movements. *J. Exp. Med.*, **11**, 622.

Mushin W.W., Rendell-Baker L., Thompson P.W., et al. (1980). *Automatic Ventilation of the Lungs*. Oxford: Blackwell Scientific Publications.

O'Dwyer J. (1885). Two cases of croup treated by tubage of the glottis. *N. Y. Med. J.*, **42**, 605.

Sauerbruch F. (1904). Zur Pathologie des offenen Pneumothorax und die Grundlagen meines Verfahrens zu seiner Ausschaktung. *Mitteilungen aus den Grenzgebieten der Medzin und Chirurgie*, **13**, 399.

62. Explosions
J. Blackburn

Source of ignition
Prevention
Conclusions

Anaesthetic fires and explosions occur infrequently because of the widespread use of intravenous agents, halothane and other noninflammable inhalational agents, and improved safety precautions in modern anaesthetic practice. However, a potentially explosive mixture is present if ether, cyclopropane, ethyl chloride or ethylene are administered, and the use of hyperbaric oxygen for the treatment of various disorders has created a new fire hazard. In addition, it has been shown by Cameron and Ingram (1971) that surgical drapes will burn readily if they are ignited while oxygen and nitrous oxide enriched gases are vented underneath them.

Three conditions are required for the production of a fire or explosion:

1. the presence of a flammable agent
2. a gas which supports combustion (such as oxygen or nitrous oxide)
3. a source of ignition of sufficient energy.

Table 62.1 shows the limits of flammability of some anaesthetic agents (Coward and Jones, 1952; Mushin and Jones, 1987).

TABLE 62.1

Drug	Air %	Oxygen %	Nitrous oxide %	Density (Air = 1)
Diethyl ether	1.8 to 36	2.1 to 82	1.5 to 24	2.56
Divinyl ether	1.7 to 27	1.8 to 85	1.4 to 25	2.42
Ethyl chloride	4.0 to 15	4.0 to 67	2.1 to 33	2.23
Cyclopropane	2.4 to 10	2.4 to 63	1.6 to 30	1.45
Ethylene	2.8 to 28	2.9 to 80	1.9 to 40	0.97

Trichloroethylene, halothane, enflurane, isoflurane and methoxyflurane are normally considered to be noninflammable, as flammable concentrations cannot be obtained from vaporizers under clinical conditions.

Combustion is initiated by supplying 'activation energy', in some form, to heat the mixture above its ignition temperature. This increases the energy of the molecular collisions occurring in the mixture, and initiates the chemical reaction. Vigorous oxidation, which can occur in flammable anaesthetic mixtures when the activation energy is supplied, leads to the production of heat and light. Flames produced by oxidation may be static, like a candle flame, or may

travel through the mixture. If the rate of combustion is very fast the temperature rises rapidly and the flame travels with high velocity through the mixture, producing shock waves. The rapid rise in pressure causes additional heating and an explosion occurs. Such explosions may result in severe injury or death of the patient or theatre personnel.

If the mixture contains very little of the flammable agent, then a flame cannot travel away from the source of ignition, because relatively few molecules react per unit volume, and insufficient heat is produced to raise the temperature of adjacent areas of the mixture above their ignition temperature. Also, in mixtures with a high concentration of the flammable agent, heat production is low because there is insufficient oxygen to react with the agent and the mixture does not burn.

In general, the agents shown in Table 62.1 burn with a static or travelling flame when mixed with air in suitable proportions, but explode when mixed with oxygen, nitrous oxide, or nitrous oxide/oxygen mixtures.

Most flammable anaesthetic agents mixed with air ignite at about 400°C, although suitable mixtures of diethyl ether with air may ignite at only 200°C, when a cool flame can travel slowly through the mixture and may ignite an additional explosive mixture some distance away. When mixed with oxygen the minimum ignition temperature is about 350°C.

In general, an explosive mixture with oxygen requires about 1 microjoule of energy to ignite it, this is 1/100th of the energy required to ignite a mixture with air.

The characteristics of the source of ignition are important. The faster the energy is supplied to the mixture from the ignition source and the smaller the volume to which it is supplied, the lower will be the minimum ignition energy.

In practice, flammable concentrations of anaesthetic agents are not often found. Coste and Chaplin (1937) have demonstrated that the mixture obtained 5 cm away from the mask of a patient anaesthetized with open ether was nonflammable. A sample of gas taken 2.5 cm above a pool of ether ignited (ether concentration 2.12%), but a sample taken 20 cm above the ether did not burn (ether concentration 0.19%) and the ether could not be ignited by a gas flame 8 cm above the pool. This work has been extended by Vickers (1970) who analysed gas mixtures at various distances from the expiratory valve of an anaesthetic circuit. Ether 15% at 8 L/min, or cyclopropane 50% at 1 L/min was discharged into still air in a room. At the closest sampling point 10 cm lateral to the expiratory valve, the concentration of ether or cyclopropane was never higher than 90% of the lowest explosive concentration for the gas mixture in use. Furthermore, the concentration of flammable agent decreased very rapidly as distance from the outlet valve increased.

It would therefore appear that the 'zone of risk' as

originally defined was unnecessarily wide and that: 'an area extending for 25 cm around any part of the anaesthetic circuit, or the gas paths of an anaesthetic apparatus should be regarded as a zone of risk' (Recommendations of the Association of Anaesthetists of Great Britain and Ireland, 1971). Full precautions should be taken against all sources of ignition within this zone.

A British Standard has been prepared (British Standards Institution, 1979), some of the recommendations are summarized as follows:

1. **'Anaesthetic-proof category G' equipment.** The equipment should not have a surface temperature of more than 90°C and must not produce sparks with sufficient energy to ignite a mixture of ether and oxygen. The electrical supply should be less than 24 V a.c. or 50 V d.c. The equipment should be marked with a green band containing the symbols 'APG'. This equipment can be used within an 'enclosed medical gas system' (in practice the anaesthetic breathing circuit, including the patient's respiratory tract) and within 5 cm of places where gas leaks can occur from such a system.
2. **'Anaesthetic-proof' equipment.** The surface temperature of this equipment should be less than 150°C and sparks produced should have insufficient energy to ignite a mixture of ether and air. The equipment should be marked with a green dot containing the symbols AP. The equipment can be used within 5–25 cm of an 'enclosed medical gas system'.
3. **Other equipment.** Equipment used outside the 25 cm zone of risk can be of normal construction.

Some concern has been expressed about explosion risks following the administration of flammable agents which are then discontinued. Vickers (1965) has used ether or cyclopropane with oxygen for induction and intubation. The patient was subsequently ventilated with a nonexplosive mixture using a semi-open circuit and the gas mixture at the expiratory valve was found to be nonexplosive within three minutes of discontinuing the explosive agent in the case of ether and one minute in the case of cyclopropane. Thus it would seem appropriate that full precautions against explosions should be taken in anaesthetic rooms and operating theatres, but that they are unnecessary in recovery rooms, intensive care units, or other locations.

SOURCE OF IGNITION

1. Static electricity. This is an important cause of anaesthetic explosions, and sparks which occur on connecting or disconnecting the breathing circuit are particularly dangerous.
2. Electric arcs from diathermy, switches, motors, faulty apparatus and short circuits.

3. Hot filaments of endoscope bulbs and cautery, open flames or fires and lasers.

A spark is an efficient ignition source as the gas is heated to a high temperature. Anaesthetic mixtures with air cannot be ignited by sparks arising from the discharge of static electricity as insufficient energy is supplied to initiate combustion, but explosive anaesthetic mixtures with oxygen can be ignited in this way. However, diathermy, electric motors, switches and other devices can arc repeatedly so that considerable energy can be supplied which may ignite any suitable gas mixture.

PREVENTION

Explosions can be prevented (a) by avoiding flammable anaesthetic agents, particularly when mixed with oxygen, (b) by rendering explosive mixtures non-flammable, (c) by eliminating all sources of ignition.

1. If air is used instead of oxygen, flammable anaesthetic mixtures will burn but not explode.
2. Efficient air conditioning of the operating theatre will reduce the concentration of flammable mixture in the atmosphere, and 15–20 air changes per hour are recommended. As all the flammable anaesthetic agents except ethylene are heavier than air (*see* Table 62.1), air should be extracted near floor level, preferably near the anaesthetic machine. The use of closed circuit systems will also limit the escape of flammable agents (HMSO, 1956).
3. Diluents such as nitrogen or helium (Stephens and Bourne, 1960; Hingson, 1958) and energy-absorbing substances may be added to anaesthetic mixtures. When either nitrogen or helium are used the oxygen concentrations of the inspired gas mixture may have to be reduced to unacceptably low levels.
4. Sources of ignition should be eliminated wherever possible.

a) Static electricity is difficult to eliminate completely, but a number of precautions should be taken.

(i) Earthing. If every piece of equipment in an operating theatre was connected directly to earth through a low resistance pathway, static charges would leak to earth and would not accumulate. However, in this situation, if faults develop in electrical apparatus, theatre personnel and patients may run the risk of electrocution. If a piece of equipment was not effectively grounded and its case became live, then anyone connected through a low resistance pathway to earth who touched the faulty apparatus would experience a severe electric shock, as a large current could flow through the body to earth. In practice, a compromise is reached whereby static charges are dissipated by providing a resistance path to earth of 50 kΩ–100 MΩ. This reduces the risk of electrocution, by limiting the current which can flow to earth.

(ii) Materials which readily acquire static charge, like nonconducting rubbers, wool, nylon and many other plastics are avoided. Antistatic rubber is used for face masks, tubing, footwear, trolley wheels and most other purposes. Details of the test procedures and resistance limits are given in Health Technical Memorandum No. 1 (1977) and British Standards Institution (1979). In general, electrical resistance of most materials should be 50 Ω–1 MΩ, but after use the upper acceptable limit is increased to 100 MΩ. Endotracheal tubes need not be made of conducting material since, when in use, they are covered with a conducting film of water that prevents the accumulation of static charges. Also, drip sets and diathermy quivers are not made of conducting material.

(iii) New floors should be made of conducting material with the following electrical resistance (Health Technical Memorandum No. 2, 1977): Upper Limit: The resistance between 2 electrodes of area 25 cm² each weighing 1 kg placed on the floor 60 cm apart should not exceed 2 MΩ on average and all areas tested should have resistances of less than 5 MΩ. For existing floors the limits are 20 MΩ and 50 MΩ respectively. Lower Limit: using the above electrodes, the average resistance should not be less than 50 kΩ and all areas tested should have a resistance of more than 20 MΩ.

(iv) If possible, relative humidity should not be allowed to fall below 50%. The generation of static electricity is more difficult under conditions of high humidity as the surface film of moisture will conduct away static charges to earth.

(v) Radioactive sources can be used to ionize the air in a localized area and so dissipate any static charges.

(b) **Electric arcs** are capable of igniting anaesthetic agents mixed with air, oxygen or nitrous oxide.

The diathermy is used routinely during surgery and is, of course, a good ignition source. If the gut is opened using diathermy, small explosions due to the ignition of hydrogen sulphide, methane or hydrogen may occur. Similar explosions could occur during laparoscopy if nitrous oxide was used for distending the abdomen and the bowel perforated by diathermy.

Switches on electrical equipment used close to anaesthetic apparatus should be of the sparkless locking variety, but wall-mounted switches and socket outlets can be of normal construction regardless of fixing height (Department of Health and Social Security, 1969).

Intrinsically safe electrical circuits have been developed, where it is possible to arrange that an arc which might occur has insufficient energy to ignite an explosive mixture. The current flowing in an intrinsically safe circuit is usually limited by a series resistor, so that ignition cannot occur under most fault conditions. These circuits are only suitable for small battery-operated devices such as endoscopes.

(c) **Cautery or open flames** should not be allowed within the zone of risk in the presence of explosive anaesthetic mixtures and, for additional safety, endoscope bulbs should be battery-operated and under-run so that overheating or bursting of the bulb cannot occur.

CONCLUSIONS

Prevention of anaesthetic explosions is of paramount importance and it is essential that appropriate safety measures are enforced. On the other hand, it is important that the subject is viewed in perspective and that unnecessary precautions, which may jeopardize the patient in other ways, are avoided.

During the last ten years in Great Britain, no anaesthetic explosion attributable to static electricity have been reported to the Department of Health and Social Security. This is due partly to the widespread use of nonflammable agents and also to the use of antistatic rubber and other precautions. The use of antistatic rubber in the anaesthetic breathing circuit is of particular importance, as otherwise sparks may occur when parts of the circuit are connected or disconnected.

It appears that only sources of ignition in close proximity to the anaesthetic circuit, conducting airways and the lungs are likely to cause explosions. In an adequately air-conditioned theatre, flammable gas mixtures are rapidly diluted by room air and become nonexplosive. Thus, electrical apparatus used at a normal distance from the patient or the anaesthetic machine can be regarded as safe, particularly if it is operated above floor level. This includes nonspark proof ECG and X-ray machines. Wall-mounted switches and socket outlets in anaesthetizing areas need no longer be of the sparkproof locking variety, which have plugs which are not interchangeable with those in general use.

The Recommendations of the Association of Anaesthetists of Great Britain and Ireland (1971) concerning explosion hazards have been published, based on the work of Vickers (1965, 1970) and the British Standards Institution (1979) have laid down specifications for the safety of medical electrical equipment. These recommendations cover the 'Zone of Risk' and antistatic precautions not only in operating theatres, but in recovery rooms, X-ray departments and other sites in which anaesthetics are not normally given.

REFERENCES

British Standards Institution (1979). *Specification for Safety of Medical Electrical Equipment*. **BS5724** Part 1.

Cameron B.G.D., Ingram G.S. (1971). Flammability of drape materials in nitrous oxide and oxygen. *Anaesthesia*, **26**, 281.

Coste J.H., Chaplin C.A. (1937). An investigation into the risks of fire or explosion in operating theatres. *Br. J. Anaesth.*, **14**, 115.

Coward H.F., Jones G.W. (1952). *Limits of Flammability of Gases and Vapours.* US: Bur. Mines, Bull. No. **503**.

Department of Health and Social Security (1969). *Switches and Socket-outlets in Anaesthetising Areas.* **G/H39/6**. London: HMSO.

Health Technical Memorandum No. 1 (1977). *Anti-static Precautions: Rubber, Plastics and Fabrics.* London: HMSO.

Health Technical Memorandum No. 2 (1977) *Anti-static Precautions: Flooring in Anaesthetising Areas.* London: HMSO.

Hingson R.A. (1958). The Western Reserve anesthetic machine, oxygen-inhalator and resuscitator, *J. Am. Med. Ass.*, **167**, 1077.

HMSO (1956). *Report of a Working Party on Anaesthetic Explosions, including Safety Code for Equipment and Installations.* London: HMSO.

Mushin W.W., Jones P.L. (1987). *Physics for the Anaesthetist*, 4th edn. Oxford: Blackwell Scientific Publications.

Recommendations of the Association of Anaesthetists of Great Britain and Ireland (1971). Explosion hazards. *Anaesthesia*, **26**, 155.

Stephens K.F., Bourne J.G. (1960). Anaesthesia for mass casualties. *Lancet*, **ii**, 481.

Vickers M.D. (1965). Duration of the explosion hazard following induction with ether or cyclopropane. *Anaesthesia*, **20**, 315.

Vickers M.D. (1970). Explosion hazards. *Anaesthesia*, **25**, 482.

FURTHER READING

Vickers M.D. (1978). Fire and explosion hazards in operating theatres. *Br. J. Anaesth.*, **50**, 659.

63. Patient Monitoring for Routine Anesthesia

R. Rubsamen, C. Cook and R. Kitz

Towards a standard for patient monitoring
The Harvard standards for patient monitoring
  Validation of the Harvard standards
  Beyond minimal monitoring
Blood pressure
  Accuracy of blood pressure determination
ECG
Ventilation and circulation monitoring
Temperature measurement
Summary

The primary monitor for all anesthetics is the anesthetist. What we address in this chapter is the minimal monitoring configuration which he or she should have available during the administration of all anesthetics. We describe the development of the Harvard standards for patient monitoring during anesthesia. Subsequently, we discuss some of the clinical considerations surrounding the use of the recommended monitoring modalities.

TOWARDS A STANDARD FOR PATIENT MONITORING

Prior to 1986, no university or official organization of anesthetists in the US had endorsed a recommendation for the minimal monitors to be used during administration of anesthesia. However, the indirect construction of such a standard began in 1973 consequent to medical malpractice litigation. In that year, the first of a series of four court cases was tried in California addressing the question of constant pulse monitoring. In the first case, the plaintiff asserted that constant pulse monitoring by the anesthetist would have prevented or reduced patient injury during a postpartum tubal ligation (Alameda County Superior Court). The jury accepted the view of the expert witness for the patient-plaintiff who stated that the due care standard for the community was constant pulse monitoring for all general anesthetics, no matter how brief. In fact, an informal survey done at the time suggests that although constant pulse monitoring was the *preferred* practice in the community it was not commonly observed (Rubsamen, 1986). No legal precedent could be set by such a decision, but the message sent to the anesthesia community was clear: failure to use constant pulse monitoring during anesthesia incurred the risk of legal liability. By the mid 1970's, after all four of these cases had been decided in favor of the patient-plaintiff, constant pulse monitoring for all anesthetics, regardless of how brief, became the standard of practice throughout California. Court decisions rather than medical considerations dictated the modification of practice patterns.

While the court system continued to exert its influence on the practice of anesthesia in California and other jurisdictions, it was not followed by a national effort to articulate a standard of monitoring for anesthesia. Leaders in anesthesia risk analysis, however, had recognized decrements in vigilance as an important component of anesthetic misadventures.

Cooper et al. (1978), reported a series of anesthetic critical incidents in Boston area hospitals during the late 1970s. They noted that simple errors occurred frequently but were typically of little consequence because they were discovered and corrected by the vigilant anesthetist before an untoward event took place. Cooper (1984) stated that 'most analyses of collections of cases of anesthetic mishaps, malpractice claims, or deaths strongly implicate failures in vigilance as a primary cause of injury'. He went on to note the importance of monitoring as a vigilance aid, alerting the anesthetist to potential problems at the time they developed. The concept of monitoring as a vigilance aid suggests that a monitor can be thought of in two different ways: a *vigilance monitor* which typically interacts with the anesthetist via an alarm to indicate a *change* in patient vital signs, and a *data acquisition monitor* which the anesthetist uses occasionally to acquire *specified numerical data* to better direct therapeutic intervention. Assuming that lapses in vigilance are responsible for most anesthesia morbidity and mortality, *vigilance monitoring* suggests a solution.

Emphasizing the importance of rapid recognition of a change in clinical state during anesthesia Philip and Raemer (1985), recommended an *optimal anesthesia monitoring array* maximizing the attributes of effectiveness, noninvasiveness, manageability and economy. Arguing that employing an optimization algorithm to find the ideal combination of monitors for anesthesia would be impractical, they presented a 'best guess' of an ideal array consisting of six respiration and five circulation monitors.

THE HARVARD STANDARDS FOR PATIENT MONITORING

In order to improve patient care and, secondarily, to reduce malpractice claims, respresentatives from the nine hospitals affiliated with Harvard Medical School formulated standards for minimal monitoring for all anesthetics performed within these institutions. Acknowledging the paucity of experimental data to guide the formulation of standards, the committee used several factors as criteria for monitor selection including availability, cost, simplicity and intraoperative distracting influence. The sensitivity, specificity and predictability of candidate monitors were also evaluated. In its selection of monitoring modalities, the committee also considered the influence of 'reasonable care' standards resulting from relevant court decisions (Eichorn et al., 1986).

The full standards are shown in Fig. 63.1. The most important requirement is listed first, i.e., the anesthetist must be present during the administration of the entire anesthetic. Note the requirement for *continuous monitoring* of ventilation and circulation. Qualitative techniques are acceptable here because it is *vigilance*

monitoring which is being required for these parameters.

Validation of the Harvard Standards

Data from The Harvard Teaching Hospitals suggests a decrease in accidents and associated death rate among ASA I and II patients following the adoption of the Monitoring Standards. However, this decrease is not statistically significant (Table 63.1).

There is no firm data to show that requiring anesthetists to monitor their patients more intensively has decreased the incidence of patient injury. There is, however, considerable optimism in this regard. Pierce (1988) has noted that medical malpractice insurance carriers have lowered their rates to subscribers because of the declining number of claims over the past several years. Whether or not this decline is due to the use of more monitoring cannot be shown. Nevertheless, he notes that the Joint Underwriters Association has offered a 20% reduction in malpractice premiums to Massachusetts anesthetists who agree to use pulse oximetry and capnography in conjunction with all anesthetics.

Beyond Minimal Monitoring

We have decribed a minimal monitoring standard for routine anesthesia. Clearly, more monitoring will be required for the more complex cases. Since each monitoring modality carries with it a risk, we must judiciously select each additional monitoring technique that we wish to employ. At first, it would seem that essentially noninvasive monitors carry no additional risk. However, even a truly 100% noninvasive monitor (which in fact may not exist) giving a false reading may indirectly cause injury by precipitating an inappropriate intervention by the anesthetist. In general, it is intuitively clear that there is an optimum number of monitors for a given case and that as the complexity of the case increases, this optimal number may also increase.

As Fig. 63.2 illustrates, a theoretical benefit/risk ratio begins at near zero when no monitors are employed because benefit is zero while risk is finite. As the number of monitors used increases, benefit and risk increase together until they reach some optimum at the peak of the curve. The descending limb of the curve represents increasing risk from additional monitoring with decreasing benefit. As this qualitative diagram is meant to show, the curves for sicker patients will be displaced to the right where the optimum number of monitors will be higher than for healthy patients undergoing anesthesia for routine surgery. The selection of each monitor for a given patient requires an understanding of the indications and liabilities of each. A discussion of each of the basic monitoring modalities outlined in the Harvard standard follows.

These standards apply for any administration of anesthesia involving department of anesthesia personnel and are specifically referable to preplanned anesthetics administered in designated anesthetizing locations (specific exclusion administration of epidural analgesia for labor or pain management). In emergency circumstances in any location, immediate life support measures of whatever appropriate nature come first with attention turning to the measures described in these standards as soon as possible and practical. These are minimal standards that may be exceeded at any time based on the judgment of the involved anesthesia personnel. These standards encourage high-quality patient care, but observing them cannot guarantee any specific patient outcome. These standards are subject to revision from time to time, as warranted by the evolution of technology and practice.

Anesthesiologist's or Nurse Anesthetist's Presence in Operating Room

For all anesthetics initiated by or involving a member of the department of anesthesia, an attending or resident anesthesiologist or nurse anesthetist shall be present in the room throughout the conduct of all general anesthetics, regional anesthetics, and monitored intravenous anesthetics. An exception is made when there is a direct known hazard, eg. radiation, to the anesthesiologist or nurse anesthetist, in which case some provision for monitoring the patient must be made.

Blood Pressure and Heart Rate

Every patient receiving general anesthesia, regional anesthesia, or managed intravenous anesthesia shall have arterial blood pressure and heart rate measured at least every five minutes, where not clinically impractical.*

Electrocardiogram

Every patient shall have the electrocardiogram continuously displayed from the induction or institution of anesthesia until preparing to leave the anesthetizing location, where not clinically impractical.*

Continuous Monitoring

During every administration of general anesthesia, the anesthetist shall employ methods of continuously monitoring the patient's ventilation and circulation. The methods shall include for ventilation and circulation each, at least one of the following or the equivalent †:

For ventilation -- Palpation or observation of the reservoir breathing bag, auscultation of breath sounds, monitoring of respiratory gases such as end-tidal carbon dioxide, or monitoring of expiratory gas flow. Monitoring end-tidal carbon dioxide is an emerging standard and is strongly preferred.

For Circulation -- Palpation of a pulse, auscultation of heart sounds, monitoring of a tracing of intra-arterial pressure, pulse plethysmography / oximetry, or ultrasound peripheral pulse monitoring.

It is recognized that brief interruptions of the continuous monitoring may be unavoidable.

Breathing System Disconnection Monitoring

When ventilation is controlled by an automatic mechanical ventilator, there shall be in continuous use a device that is capable of detecting disconnection of any component of the breathing system. The device must give an audible signal when its alarm threshold is exceeded. (It is recognized that there are certain rare or unusual circumstances in which such a device may fail to detect a disconnection.)

Oxygen Analyzer

During every administration of general anesthesia using an anesthesia machine, the concentration of oxygen in the patient breathing system will be measured by a functioning oxygen analyzer with a low concentration limit alarm in use. This device must conform to the American National Standards Institute No. Z.79.10 standard.*

Ability to Measure Temperature

During every administration of general anesthesia there shall be readily available a means to measure the patient's temperature.

Rationale -- A means of temperature measurement must be available as a potential aid in the diagnosis and treatment of suspected or actual intraoperative hypothermia and malignant hyperthermia. The measurement monitoring of temperature during *every* general anesthetic is not specifically mandated because of the potential risks of such monitoring and because of the likelihood of other physical signs giving earlier indication of the development of malignant hyperthermia.

*Under extenuating circumstances the attending anesthesiologist may waive this requirement after so stating (including the reasons) in a note in the patient's chart.

†Equivalence is to be defined by the chief of the individual hospital department after submission to and review by the department heads, Department of Anesthesia Harvard Medical School, Boston.

Fig. 63.1 Standards for patient monitoring during anesthesia at the Harvard Medical School Teaching Hospitals, adopted March 25, 1985; revised July 3, 1985.

TABLE 63.1

ACCIDENT AND DEATH RATE AMONG ASA I AND II PATIENTS BEFORE AND AFTER ADOPTION OF
MONITORING STANDARDS AT THE HARVARD TEACHING HOSPITALS

Dates	*ASA I & II anesthetics*	*Intraoperative accidents*	*Associated deaths*
1/76–6/85	757 000	10 (1/75 700)	5 (1/151 400)
Standards adopted 7/85 7/85–12/87	260 000	1 (1/260 000)*	0 (0)*

* = Not significant

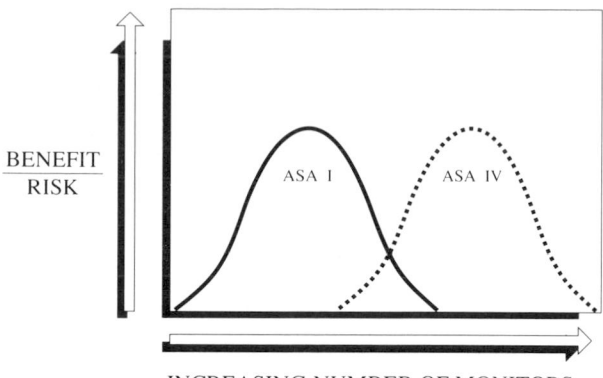

BENEFIT RISK

ASA I   ASA IV

INCREASING NUMBER OF MONITORS

Fig. 63.2 Qualitative representation of benefit risk ratio as a function of the level of monitoring. The benefit/risk ratio is shown as a theoretical function administration of an anesthetic.

BLOOD PRESSURE

Accuracy of Blood Pressure Determination

Through the normal course of the administration of many anesthetics the patient's blood pressure can be expected to change. This fact alone explains the keen interest with which the anesthetists approach intraoperative blood pressure measurement. The search for a gold standard for blood pressure measurement, however, has only served to demonstrate that blood pressure is a function of the way it is measured (Bruner et al., 1981a).

Noninvasive blood pressure monitoring (i.e., through the use of a blood pressure cuff) is the most commonly employed method of intraoperative blood pressure determination. With an appropriately sized cuff, one can expect to obtain a measurement in rough agreement with a simultaneously obtained intra-arterial value (Geddes and Whistler, 1977). Three basic techniques are recognized for determination of blood pressure by cuff: auscultation, oscillometry and occlusion of an intra-arterial pressure waveform measured distal to the cuff site.

The von Recklinghausen Oscillotonometer is a specialized device designed to facilitate the determination of noninvasive blood pressure through the observation of needle bounce (Silvay and Griffin, 1984). Although this instrument is no longer in common use, automatic devices for the noninvasive determination of blood pressure rely on the same basic principle. Instead of relying on a human observation of an oscillating needle, these devices use an on-board computer to analyse transduced pressure impulses transmitted back from a partially inflated cuff bladder. An internal program interprets these oscillations in a predetermined way in order to derive a numerical value for the patient's blood pressure. How accurate is such a technique?

Yelderman and Ream (1979) compared blood pressure determinations obtained with a cuff using an oscillometric technique with simultaneously determined intra-arterial pressure measured in the contra-lateral radial artery. They determined that the minimum cuff pressure for maximum needle oscillation yields a mean blood pressure determination accurate to within 1.4 torr when considering a series of pooled samples. In contrast, they found that the accuracy of any individual determination using this technique was somewhat less than 14 torr (1 torr is equal to 1 mmHg or 0.133 kPa).

Instruments for the automatic determination of blood pressure typically display systolic and diastolic as well as mean pressure. If the only parameter being assessed is cuff pressure oscillation, how is this done? A general answer to this question is not forthcoming because the algorithms used by these machines are proprietary. However, Hutton et al. (1984), reported that the Dinamap 845 automatic noninvasive blood pressure recorder determines systolic and diastolic pressure at the cuff pressures where the oscillations begin to increase and stop decreasing in amplitude, respectively. They state that the device reports mean pressure at a point where pressure oscillations are at a maximum.

Is there a general way that noninvasive blood pressure data, obtained by oscillometry or auscultation, can be related to directly measured (i.e., by intra-arterial cannulation) blood pressure? In an extensive review of the world literature, Bruner points out that studies comparing noninvasively measured to directly measured blood pressure can be grouped into two categories: those that find close correlation between the two and those that do not, and concludes that indirect measurement of blood pressure by auscultation and oscillometry are relying on flow related phenomena (Bruner et al., 1981b). In contrast, the direct measurement of blood pressure by an intra-arterial cannula is a pressure-dependent technique. Therefore measurements by the two different techniques cannot be expected to correlate in a predictable fashion.

Clearly, precise correlation between noninvasive and direct blood pressure measurements is not essential for vigilance blood pressure monitoring. During the administration of an anesthetic we are more interested in blood pressure changes than in an absolute determination of the patient's blood pressure at any given time.

At first, one might assume that accuracy considerations would vanish if all patients were monitored with intra-arterial pressure cannulae. In fact, precise blood pressure determination of directly-measured blood pressure is complicated both by the methodology used to make direct blood pressure measurements and by problems with defining what constitutes the systolic blood pressure component of the arterial pressure waveform.

It is not the purpose of this brief review to consider all theoretical aspects of invasive blood pressure measurement. However, there are two points about which the clinician should be aware in order to properly interpret hemodynamic waveform data in the operating theatre or the intensive care unit. The first point is that *reflection* constitutes an important component of the arterial pressure waveform.

To understand this, consider that the human arterial tree consists of vessels which progressively decrease in diameter as one moves distally from the aortic root. At each point in the system where a large vessel is connected to a smaller one, an impedance mismatch occurs which produces a reflection of the propagated arterial waveform back to its point of origin. Changes in the impedance of this system by the induction of anesthesia may produce profound changes in the appearance of the radial arterial pressure waveform without changing centrally measured root pressure.

A simple experiment may make this concept less abstract. Bruner (1978) describes augmentation of systolic pressure seen on a radial arterial tracing when a cuff proximal to the cannula site is partially inflated. He explains this phenomenon as the result of introducing a proximal reflector which intercepts the reflection initiated at the impedance mismatch distal to the cannulation site, and reflects this back again to the cannula, resulting in a summing effect. Figure 63.3 illustrates this point.

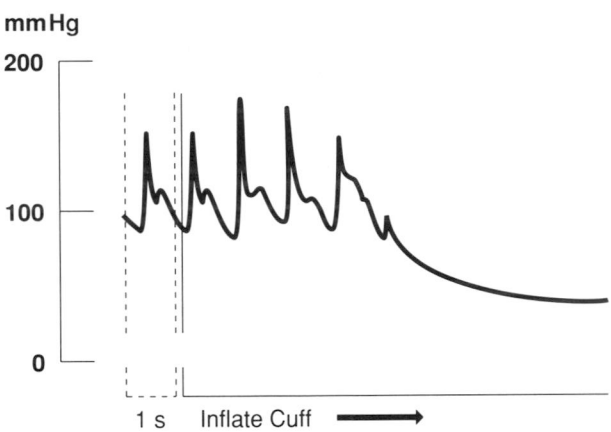

Fig. 63.3 Radial arterial pressure vs. time. Systolic pressure as recorded from a radial artery is seen to increase as a proximal blood pressure cuff is partially inflated. (Redrawn with permission from Bruner et al., 1981. Comparison of direct and indirect methods of measuring arterial blood pressure, Part I. *Med. Instrum*, **15**, 4.)

This experiment argues strongly that pressure wave reflection in the arterial system does in fact take place. What is the clinical relevance of this observation? Consider the awake, anxious patient prior to the induction of anesthesia with an arterial cannula in place. If one notes the systolic blood pressure and then induces anesthesia one may be under the impression that a major fall in blood pressure has taken place (Fig. 63.4). In fact, the disappearance of the

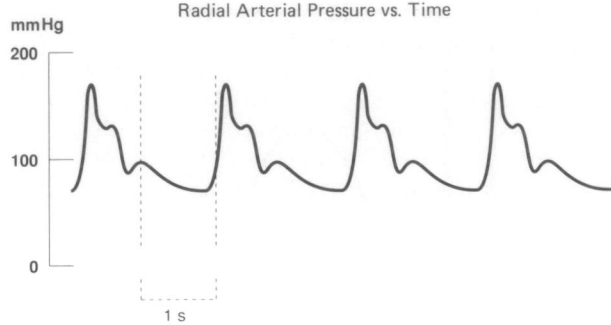

10.15 a.m. Awake, apprehensive

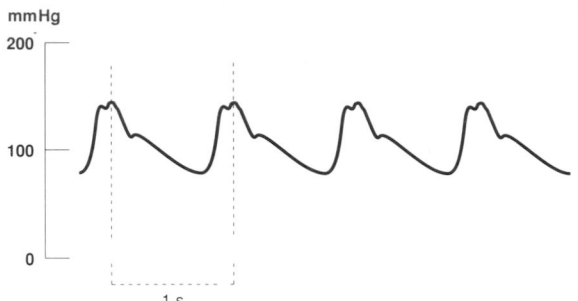

11.45 a.m. Anesthesia, superficial surgery

Fig. 63.4 Radial arterial pressure vs. time. Changes in systemic vascular tone occurring with induction of anesthesia cause a disappearance of the systolic pressure peak. (Redrawn with permission from Bruner et al., 1981. Comparison of direct and indirect methods of measuring arterial blood pressure, Part I. *Med. Instrum.*, **15**, 8.)

prominent peak may be primarily due to loss of reflection of pressure waves from the lower body to the upper extremity cannula.

It is important to recognize that the prominent overshoot peak seen in the preinduction figure contributes relatively little to the total area under the arterial pressure curve. If one realizes that mean pressure is proportional to the integral (i.e. the area) of the arterial pressure waveform, then following mean pressure rather than systolic pressure may provide a more realistic view of central arterial pressure during periods of changes in the impedance of the systemic arterial tree.

The second important clinically relevant point regarding the methodology of direct blood pressure measurement is the *frequency response* of the measuring system. Most clinically employed pressure transducer systems consist of a strain gauge connected to an arterial cannula via a column of fluid contained in a semirigid tube of arbitrary length. Such a system has a resonant frequency at which passive amplification of pressure waves travelling through the system will occur. The problem occurs when the resonant frequency of the measuring system is close to that of one or more of the components of the arterial pressure waveform. This will result in the amplification of that component more than the other components.

Taking an hypothetical example, consider the relatively high frequency first peak component of the arterial pressure waveform. If the resonant frequency of the transducer system is close to that of this peak, it will be preferentially amplified. The definitive technical solution to this problem would be to have a system with absolutely flat frequency response. One way to do this would be to place the strain gauge directly in the artery. Something very close to this is achieved in pressure measuring devices using optically based pressure measurement technology contained within the arterial cannula. Such a system eliminates the need for a hydraulic system to conduct the pressure waveform from the artery to an external transducer.

Unfortunately, the indwelling arterial transducer described is expensive and not in common clinical use. An alternative approach is to again rely on mean blood pressure as the clinical guide. Following mean pressure will de-emphasize the contribution of the narrow, high frequency initial first peak component of the arterial pressure waveform.

Clearly there are direct risks associated with methods of blood pressure determination. The occurrence of compartment syndrome from the application of a blood pressure cuff has been described (Celoria et al., 1987). Case reports of thrombosis associated with arterial cannulation also appear in the literature. There is, however, no data available on the possible indirect risks of blood pressure monitoring resulting from interpretation errors. We have discussed the difficulty of comparing noninvasive with direct blood pressure data. We have outlined the problems with deriving numerical values for blood pressure based on arterial pressure waveforms. These facts suggest to us that the notion of a true blood pressure may not be obtainable. Therefore basing an intraoperative therapeutic intervention strategy on a single blood pressure reading is a less robust approach than treating a blood pressure trend consisting of a series of points, all obtained by the same technique.

ECG

The electrocardiogram in the general operating theatre is a vigilance monitor. Equipment for monitoring the intraoperative ECG typically displays one lead and is specifically designed to alert the anesthetist to changes heralding ischemia or a change in rhythm.

As there is a high degree of electrical noise present in the surgery suite, ECG monitors typically contain filters designed to block artifactual signals from blending with the displayed signal. Artifact is distinguished from the ECG signal by frequency. In order to block the typically high frequency artifact component, the monitor must subject all incoming signals to low-pass filtering.

This approach is far different from that employed by static, 12 lead ECG machines typically used by cardiologists. In the latter systems, little or no filtering is

employed because large amounts of artifact (usually from electrocautery) are not present in the environments where diagnostic ECG equipment is customarily employed.

The consequence of this is that the filtered waveform present on the operating theatre ECG screen may look different from a record obtained simultaneously on a 12 lead diagnostic electrocardiograph. The most clinically significant manifestation of this difference occurs in the ST segment where ST changes may artifactually appear on the monitor with a low-pass filter at the input. These changes act to elevate or depress the ST segment thus mimicking ischemia or concealing real ischemia by offsetting true ST changes back toward the baseline (Arbeit et al., 1970).

The solution to this problem is to recognize that artifactual ST changes can occur and to realize that some monitoring equipment allows the front end filtering to be selectively removed if desired. If such an option exists, we believe that it should always be placed in the *no filter* mode, sometimes also referred to as the *diagnostic* mode. Dealing with more electrical noise on the ECG tracing in exchange for an unbiased view of ST segment changes is a small price to pay.

VENTILATION AND CIRCULATION MONITORING

Pulse oximetry allows the anesthetist to monitor the final common pathway of ventilation and circulation: the delivery of oxygenated blood to the periphery. This technique is especially important because it is noninvasive and provides single parameter output which is intuitively easy to interpret.

The importance of this modality as an early detector of ventilation problems cannot be overemphasized. Newbower et al. (1960) describe 62 breathing circuit disconnects in a retrospective study of 790 critical incidents associated with the administration of anesthesia. Pulse oximetry was not in use at that time. The most common pivotal factor in initial discovery of the disconnect was a change in heart rate and or blood pressure (26% of total). Indeed, they report that detection of a breathing circuit disconnection was slow enough in 50% of the cases to allow at least some changes in vital signs.

Decreases in hemoglobin oxygen saturation measured by pulse oximetry have been shown to precede changes in vital signs or skin color (Brooks and Gravenstein, 1985). Pulse oximetry is clearly capable of providing a valuable early warning for ventilation problems.

The term *pulse oximeter* was originally used by Dr. William New, an anesthetist and engineer, to describe a device designed by his group for measuring hemoglobin oxygen saturation on a beat to beat basis. His device was the first to use solid state sensor technology at the patient's finger thus eliminating the need for cumbersome fiber optic cables. Many derivative instruments have been subsequently developed and pulse oximetry is now commonplace in US operating rooms.

A pulse oximeter assumes that the transduced flow wave is produced by arterial blood and that when no flow is measured only venous blood is present. The absorbance of the vascular bed during each of these components of the pressure wave is measured at two wavelengths. The hemoglobin oxygen saturation is then calculated using data originally derived experimentally from a set of healthy subjects (Yelderman and Cornman, 1983).

The designers of pulse oximeters are therefore assuming that patients being monitored have normal hemoglobin. Thus one cannot assume that the oxyhemoglobin dissociation curve can be used in all cases to derive P_{O_2} from the displayed oxygen saturation. This does not effect the pulse oximeter's superb ability to accurately display trends in oxygen saturation so important to the anesthetist. Decreases in saturation can therefore be detected quickly and their causes rectified before the situation becomes acute.

The measurement of end tidal CO_2 provides another opportunity to detect and correct ventilation problems early. In addition, end tidal CO_2 monitoring provides a reliable estimate of arterial P_{CO_2} (Weinger and Brimm, 1987) thus allowing this important metabolic parameter to be assessed in real time.

Using an end-tidal CO_2 monitor in every case allows endotracheal placement of the breathing tube to be verified and provides an opportunity to detect ventilation problems before any change in oxygen saturation takes place. Potential drawbacks of routine end tidal CO_2 monitoring also need to be considered.

End tidal CO_2 monitors work by passing a beam of infrared light through the gases in the breathing circuit. Some function by drawing a sample from the breathing circuit into the instrument itself. Others place the beam path at the breathing circuit. In both cases, the opportunity for patient cross-contamination exists unless all parts in contact with vapor are disposable. In addition, the introduction of an additional connection in the breathing circuit provides another opportunity for disconnection.

We have found that the high level of condensation produced by humidification systems produces a high failure rate in end tidal CO_2 monitors. This phenomenon is observed with side stream devices which draw their sample from the breathing system as well as instruments which mount the optical path device on the breathing system.

Side stream end tidal CO_2 monitors vary in the amount of gas drawn from the breathing system for analysis. The amount drawn away may interfere with the administration of closed circuit anesthesia. In addition, the sampling interval of side stream systems may be too long for use with the rapidly breathing infant. Displayed values for end tidal CO_2 may therefore represent averages taken over an unspecified number of breaths.

End-tidal CO_2 (E_tCO_2) can also be measured by mass spectrometers which draw samples from the breathing system. A mass spectrometer has the added advantage of being able to display the concentration of most anesthetic agents. Using a more expensive technology than the infrared based E_tCO_2 units, mass spec instruments are typically shared between operating rooms through the use of sample multiplexing. In this scheme, a valve mechanism local to a centrally placed mass spec device sequentially scans a bank of narrow bore flexible tubes each emanating from a different breathing circuit. During each scan interval, a quantum of gas is drawn from a breathing circuit via the typically long connecting tube. This is quickly analyzed and the results are electronically transmitted back to the originating operating theatre.

As a result of sample multiplexing, the anesthetist does not receive breath-to-breath data. Instead, data from one breath only every few minutes is available. An important use of end tidal CO_2 monitoring is the rapid detection of ventilation problems. The response time is often extended by critical minutes if a sample multiplexed mass spec system is used to derive end tidal CO_2 data. Two recent technological developments have improved this situation. First, recognizing the importance of breath-to-breath display of E_tCO_2, at least one manufacturer of sample multiplexed systems has added an inline, continuous infrared based E_tCO_2 system superimposed on the mass spec system. A more robust solution to the problem of intermittent display of mass spec data is the development of portable, stand alone mass spec units designed for use in the operating theatre in a continuous side stream mode. Such instruments are currently offered by at least three companies.

The measurement of inhalation anesthetic concentration through the use of infrared technology is possible, and designers of infrared E_tCO_2 equipment are incorporating this capability into their equipment. It remains to be seen if this approach will reduce the demand for mass spec in the clinical setting.

TEMPERATURE MEASUREMENT

The final modality addressed in the Harvard standards for patient monitoring is thermometry. Specifically, a readily available means for the measurement of patient temperature is mandated.

The role of temperature measurement in the diagnosis of malignant hyperthermia is clear. Equally apparent is the need for continuous temperature measurement in the patient undergoing a long abdominal procedure involving the extensive exposure of viscera. In fact, temperature loss prior to incision can be significant. In a study of intraoperative temperature changes in adults aged 20–85 years, Morris (1971) has shown that the greatest drop occurred in the first hour of anesthesia. He notes that during this period the temperature gradient between the patient and the operating theatre is greatest. He hypothesizes that prepping a large area of exposed skin with alcohol and ether in a cold room explains the observed 0.5–1.3°C decrease during the first hour of anesthesia.

It is well recognized that heat loss occurs rapidly in infants and children owing to their increased surface area to volume ratio. However, in adults heat loss during surgery occurs more rapidly with increasing age. Goldberg and Roe (1966) have examined intraoperative heat deficit in a group of patients of differing ages. Their results show that patients greater than 60 years old undergo a rate of heat loss twice that of patients 20–39 years old during procedures of similar length. This increased heat deficit in the elderly was found to be independent of body surface area and operation type. This study underlines the need for close temperature monitoring in this age group.

Many instruments are available for the intraoperative measurement of temperature. Severinghaus (1959) has demonstrated a significant temperature gradient between the esophagus and the rectum during induced hypothermia and subsequent rewarming in dogs and humans. No patient in his study showed a consistent agreement between rectal and esophageal temperature to within 0.7°C. He concludes that a thermocouple placed in the lower esophagus below the auricle reflects central arterial blood temperature more accurately than a rectally placed probe.

Commercial instruments exist for the measurement of central temperature through the use of a tympanic membrane probe. In a review of the literature regarding the use of these devices by Reitan and Barash (1984), the remarkable accuracy of temperature measurement via the tympanic membrane is noted. The studies reviewed showed a 0.1°C correlation between thermocouples placed in the lower esophagus and at the tympanic membrane. However, Reitan and Barash (1984) also found a 2–4% reported incidence of external auditory canal bleeding in most series. In addition, they found two reported cases of tympanic membrane rupture from probe placement during routine surgery.

Another noninvasive temperature measurement modality is made possible by liquid crystal technology. Flexible plastic strips containing liquid crystals display temperature through color changes. The strips have an adhesive backing and are easily applied to the forehead. This technique has been found unsatisfactory for the accurate detection of fever in an outpatient setting (Lewit et al., 1982).

Lees et al. (1978) have found liquid crystal thermometry a useful method for following temperature trends in patients under anesthesia. Specifically, they studied the effectiveness of the technique for detecting intraoperative hyperthermia and noted a several degree difference between esophageal and the cooler skin temperature measured by the liquid crystal strip. However, the relationship between the two techniques was linear over the range studied (34–39°C esophageal). The temperature strips were found to require 60 s to undergo a 1.1°C transition over the entire operating range.

Because of the linear relationship between esophageal temperature and forehead temperature measured with the liquid crystal technique and the rapid response time of the liquid crystal strip method, Lees et al. (1978) concluded that liquid crystal skin thermometry is an acceptable screening technique for the detection of intraoperative hyperthermia. They did not study the ability of this technique to linearly follow intraoperative hypothermia. However, they recommend a practice of switching to a core temperature measurement technique if a significant increase or decrease in temperature is noted on the cutaneously applied liquid crystal device.

This technique of thermometry may serve as an adequate vigilance monitor assuming willingness to immediately switch to an esophageal temperature probe if a cutaneous temperature change is detected. It is standard practice to rely on esophageal thermocouple measurement in cases where the need for close temperature monitoring is anticipated.

SUMMARY

The standards for patient monitoring during anesthesia at Harvard Medical School represent the first specific guidelines for intraoperative patient monitoring ever published in the US. These standards are minimal and represent a set of vigilance monitors designed to help prevent untoward events from occurring during the administration of routine anesthesia. Each of these monitoring modalities is briefly discussed. It is understood that the recommended monitoring configuration is minimal and that the decision to escalate the level of monitoring will be made by the anesthetist on a case by case basis. Finally, the anesthetist is the ultimate patient monitor. The introduction of advanced monitoring equipment into the operating theater should not and must not interfere with the ability of the anesthetist to apply his or her clinical judgment.

REFERENCES

Alameda County Superior Court #419901.

Arbeit S.R., Rubin I.L., Gross H. (1970). Dangers in interpreting the electrocardiogram from the oscilloscope monitor. *JAMA*, **211**, 453.

Brooks T.D., Gravenstein N. (1985). Pulse oximetry for early detection of hypoxemia in anesthetized patients. *J. Clin. Monitoring*, **1**, 135.

Bruner J.M.R. (1978). *Handbook of Blood Pressure Monitoring*. PSG Publishing Co.

Bruner J.M., Krenis L.J., Kunsman J.M. (1981a). Comparison of direct and indirect methods of measuring arterial blood pressure, Part III. *Med. Instrum.*, **15**, 4.

Bruner J.M., Krenis L.J., Kunsman J.M. (1981b). Comparison of direct and indirect methods of measuring arterial blood pressure, Part I. *Med. Instrum.*, **15**, 8.

Celoria G., Dawson J., Teres D. (1987). Compartment syndrome in a patient monitored with an automated blood pressure cuff. *J. Clin. Monitoring*, **3**, 139.

Cooper J.B. (1984). Toward prevention of anesthetic mishaps. *Int. Anesthesiol. Clin.*, **22**, 167.

Cooper J.B., Newbower R.S., Long C.D., et al. (1978). Preventable anesthesia mishaps—a study of human factors. *Anesthesiology*, **49**, 399.

Eichorn J.H., Cooper J.B., Cullen D.J., et al. (1986). Standards for patient monitoring during anesthesia at Harvard Medical School. *JAMA*, **256**, 1017.

Geddes L.A., Whistler B.S. (1977). The error in indirect blood pressure measurement with the incorrect size of cuff. *Am. Heart J.*, **93**, 4.

Goldberg M., Roe C.F. (1966). Temperature changes during anesthesia and operations. *Arch. Surg.*, **93**, 365.

Hutton P., Dye J., Prys-Roberts C. (1984). An assessment of the Dinamap 845. *Anesthesia*, **39**, 261.

Lees D.E., Schuette W.S., Bull J.M., et al. (1978). An evaluation of liquid-crystal thermometry as a screening device for intraoperative hyperthermia. *Anesth. Analg.*, **57**, 669.

Lewit E.M., Marshall C.L., Salzer J.E. (1982). An evaluation of a plastic strip thermometer. *JAMA*, **247**, 321.

Morris R. (1971). Operating room temperature and the anesthetized, paralyzed patient. *Arch. Surg.*, **102**, 95.

Newbower R.S., Cooper J.B., Long C.D. (1980). Failure analysis—the human element. In *Essential Noninvasive Monitoring in Anesthesia*. pp. 269–281. (Gravenstein J.S., Newbower R.S., Ream A.K., et al., eds.). New York: Grune and Stratton.

Philip J.H., Raemer D.B. (1985). Selecting the optimal anesthesia array. *Med. Instrum.*, **19**, 122.

Pierce E.C. (1988). Monitoring instruments have significantly reduced anesthetic mishaps. *J. Clin. Monitoring*, **4**, 111.

Reitan J.A., Barash P.G. (1984). Noninvasive monitoring. In *Monitoring in Anesthesia*. 2nd edn. pp. 141–144. (Saidman L.J., Smith N.T., eds.) New York: Butterworth.

Rubsamen D.S. (1986). The standard of care and where it comes from. *Sem. Anesth*, **5**, 237.

Severinghaus J.W. (1959). Temperature gradients during hypothermia. *Ann. New York Acad. Sci*, **80**, 515.

Silvay G., Griffin R. (1984). The history and development of cardiovascular monitoring during anesthesia. *Mount Sinai J. Med*, **51**, 560.

Yelderman M., Cornman J. (1983). *Real Time Oximetry, Computing in Anesthesia and Intensive Care*. pp. 328–341. (Prakash O., ed.). Boston: Martinus Nijhoff.

Yelderman M., Ream A.K. (1979). Indirect measurement of mean blood pressure in the anesthetized patient. *Anesthesiology*, **50**, 253.

Weinger M., Brimm J. (1987). End-tidal carbon dioxide as a measure of arterial carbon dioxide during intermittent mandatory ventilation. *J. Clin. Monitoring*, **3**, 73.

64. Computers and the Anesthetist

M. Harmel and J. Leslie

Historical perspectives
Current computers
    Analog computers
    Digital computers
Computer languages
Utilization in anesthesia
    Monitoring
    Anesthetic records
    Data collection and retrieval
    Drug delivery systems
    Computer aided instruction
Future applications and development
    Hardware
    Networking
    Artificial intelligence
Summary
Glossary

Historical Perspectives

The abacus, the first digital computer, came into being over 2500 years ago, and is still being used today. As society became more complex and the population grew and began to aggregate in cities, the need for mechanical assistance in calculation became insistent. However, it was not until the seventeenth century that the stimulus to create a machine for the purpose of assistance and precision in calculation became forceful enough to result in the design of an arithmetic machine. It was to Schickard in Germany and Pascal in France that we owe this device.

As so often happens, advances were slow in the beginning for it was not until 1694 that an effective calculating machine was made by Leibniz. While variations and innovations occurred over the next 150 years, the next real contribution came from the eccentric genius, Charles Babbage, in England. He designed and had built a 'difference engine' which was capable of handling polynominals, by the method of differences. Attempts at making a larger difference engine and then an analytical engine were never brought to fruition. Remarkably, the British government supported this endeavor with substantial monies. Meanwhile, calculating machines were refined and improved, but the challenges inherent in the processing and analysis of massive amounts of data, both in science and government, could not be met. In the US the explosive growth of the population reflected in the census, made this abundantly clear. It was Herman Hollerith who brought the punch card, originated by Jacquard to help automate the operation of his looms, and the electric tabulator to the rescue. The role of the punch card was intimately linked with the ultimate development of the electronic computer.

Computer development in the twentieth century was almost entirely confined to the US. In the thirties collaboration between the General Electric Company and the Massachusetts Institute of Technology resulted in the A–C differential analyser for estimating the generation and distribution of electric power. This was soon followed by the general purpose differential analyser of Vanevar Bush which was principally used to construct firing tables for the prediction of trajectories for the artillery. Two analysers, one at the ballistics research center in Aberdeen and the other at the Moore School of Engineering of the University of Pennsylvania, became linked for this purpose in the event of war. Government funding and the interest of John Mauchly and J. Presper Eckert at the Moore School, led to the highly secret project which resulted in the creation of ENIAC, the first digital computer. (Goldstine, 1972; Shurkin, 1984).

In the intervening forty years we have witnessed phenomenal technological advances in the design of computers. The more recent advent of microprocessors and electronic miniaturization have brought computers into the fabric of everyday life. First utilized in hospital management, and now invading all branches of medicine, the computer and its applications have become part and parcel, if not yet essential, to anesthetic practice and research. It will be the purpose of this chapter to review the ultilization of this twentieth century behemoth as it affects all phases of anesthesia; machines, monitoring, education, data management and the implications for the future of the anesthetist and the computer. To aid readers in understanding many important terms and definitions of computer terminology, a glossary is included at the end of the chapter which defines the terms found in bold letters within the text of this chapter.

CURRENT COMPUTERS

The computer was originally designed to store and manipulate numbers and solve complex equations efficiently. (Goldstine, 1972). The rapid advances in electronic technology have led to major changes and improvements in the **hardware** structure of computers and **software** development. For both the analog or digital computers, much of the hardware design is essentially the same; they differ, however, in the form in which information is received, processed and displayed. Digital computers deal with discrete numbers and analog computers with continuously varying signals.

Analog Computers

An analog signal is a variable signal that changes continuously over time, as exemplified by fluid pressure waves or the electroencephalogram. An important component of an analog device is the transducer that converts a constantly varying signal into analog electrical signals which are measured and displayed as 'real time' output signals. Perhaps the most common analog **input device** in anesthesiology is the pressure transducer which easily **interfaces** with a computer for transfer and analysis of pressure wave information.

Most analog computers have been replaced with analog-to-digital convertors. These convertors quantify the analog signal at specified times to generate a digital number to represent the time specific data. Multiplexing is the process of controlling several analog-to-digital convertors to permit the device to output several parameters almost simultaneously, as many modern monitoring devices perform.

Digital Computers

Digital computers receive some form of numerical input, perform calculations or manipulations of the data, and return the results or information determined by the retrieval and processing steps. These functions are the processes of information:

- Input
- Storage
- Processing
- Calculation
- Output

Interestingly, there have been very few significant changes since the basic design of ENIAC, the electronic computer of Mauchly and Eckert (Goldstine, 1972). There have been however, significant changes in complexity, speed, efficiency, size, input and output interfaces, and cost. Figure 64.1 is a diagrammatic representation of the basic components of a digital computer system.

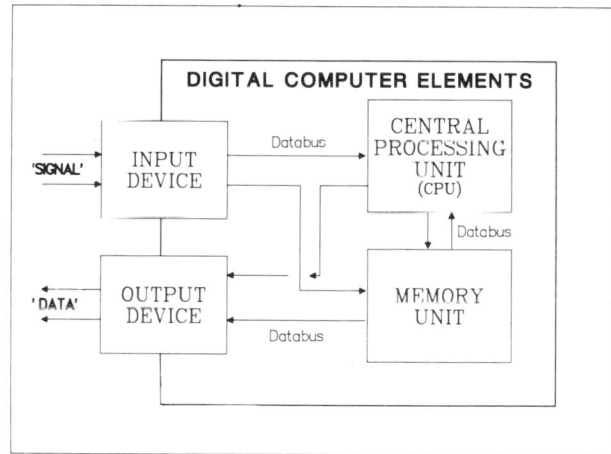

Fig. 64.1 Representation of the basic components of a digital computing device. Each component's function is described in more detail within the text.

InputOutput (I/O) Devices

Input/output (I/O) devices are the interface between the processing unit of the computer and the operating environment or personnel utilizing the device. These include many devices such as the keyboard, monitor, terminal, printer, tape, plotter, and the now familiar 'light pens' and 'mouse' driven systems. Ideally, the 'man-machine interface' should be simple, legible, compatible, and accessible. The major improvements in these devices have centred on providing I/O devices that are more 'user friendly'.

Memory

Each character of information is stored electronically as a series of binary numbers, zeros or ones (**bits**), which represent electronic 'on' or 'off' switching. A group of eight bits has been designated a **byte**. It is possible to express any information in a set or series of bytes that permit storage, processing, and retrieval of the information by appropriate I/O devices. The I/O devices and processing rules or logic which the processing unit utilizes, may be written as strings of zeros and ones. This is known as **machine language** or machine code. **Assembly language** consists of symbols which represent specific series of the on-off signals for the bit storage areas of the computer. An **assembler** then converts these **programming** symbols into the zeros and ones which the **central processing unit** (CPU) receives and processes.

The key to the speed of the modern computer comes from the present bit switching speed (on or off) of several million times/s. Modern microcomputers have **memory** capacities measured in megabytes or gigabytes, with each bit only micrometers in size. The intrinsic or local computer memory is in two forms:

1. Read-Only Memory (ROM), consists of a set of bytes which usually cannot be changed or erased by the computer and represents permanently stored information.
2. Random Access Memory (RAM), another form of memory storage, is the computer's byte information storage into which new instructions or data are temporarily stored, processed, and then returned to the appropriate interface.

Other important forms of remote or mass memory storage include the floppy diskette, the hard disk, magnetic tape, digital tape, and more recently optical storage diskettes.

All of the memory units as well as the I/O devices are managed by the control unit of the computer. The control unit initiates the **program** directing the computer, places the instructions in memory, obtains the needed data from the specific input devices, directs the processing by the CPU, and then sends the results to the appropriate **output device**. The CPU is central to the process of information retrieval, storage and mathematical processing.

COMPUTER LANGUAGES

The CPU must rely on an appropriate set of instructions (in the machine code of bits) to be utilized by its very high speed binary adding device in performing all the calculations. These step by step instructions of electronic switching of the storage bits are the series of commands forming the **algorithm** or computer **program**. The 'higher level languages' (BASIC, COBOL, FORTRAN, PASCAL, C, FORTH, etc.) consist of more complex programming symbols or terms that simplify the process of writing the program algorithm by utilizing quasi-English instructions which are easier for the programmer to comprehend than machine language for the process of actually writing the program. These language commands and the series of programmed instructions must first, however, be converted back into a string of machine codes before the computer can 'understand' and utilize the instructions. This language conversion is performed by an **interpreter** program or a **compiler**. Different compilers exist in order to produce unique machine code instructions for various computer hardware and CPUs.

UTILIZATION IN ANESTHESIA

Monitoring

The modern physiologic monitoring device is a microprocessor driven computer interfaced with increasingly sophisticated electronic or electromechanical sensors. The level of monitoring required in the management of patients has undergone a significant increase (Beneken and Blom, 1983). For a variety of reasons, it is no longer sufficient to utilize a chest stethoscope with a blood pressure cuff alone in physiologic monitoring, not the least of which in the US for example, is the medicolegal climate. The electronic revolution has impinged on the instrumentation available to monitor the cardiovascular, respiratory, nervous and neuromuscular systems and in consequence, a myriad of devices have been made available with which the anesthetist feels he or she cannot do without. These instruments have added significantly to the cost of an anesthetic and presumably to patient safety through vigilant microprocessor driven monitors combined with alarms (Brown et al., 1984). The construction of physiologic monitoring devices is a straightforward problem (Burton et al., 1980). The required components and their overall function within the monitoring environment are illustrated in Fig. 64.2. Specialized monitors for varied purposes may be improved by making appropriate changes in the basic components interacting with the CPU or in the programs directing the CPU. The actual devices for physiologic monitoring may be packaged individually (i.e. electrocardiogram, pulse oximeter, etc.) or combined for multiple display of analog and/or digital format.

Anesthetic Records

It has been estimated that 6% of the anesthetic time is

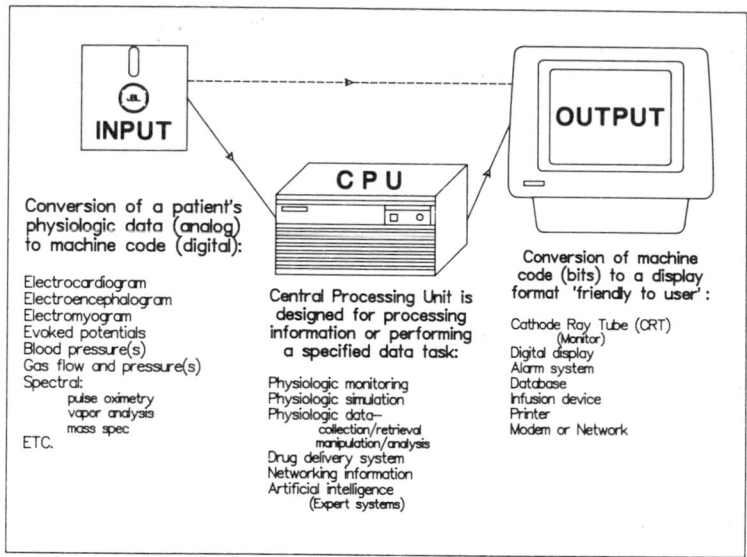

Fig. 64.2 Comparison of the components of a standard digital computer with the medical computing devices in current use for patient care.

related to the accurate recording of events on the medical record (Boquet et al., 1980). The record has always been a subject of veracity and reliability. Often the physiologic data is postscripted, especially during induction and assuredly in the face of untoward events (Wiener and Weil, 1978). The online recording of physiologic data has been a reality for almost two decades (Block et al., 1985; Mitchell et al., 1981; Burton et al., 1980; Olsson 1983; Wiener et al., 1978). However, the ready acceptance of an objective record has been hindered by the cost of systems, a reluctance to be dependent for this vital information on a machine and/or computer, and the question of reliability. Several systems beginning with the DAME at Duke University, the CICRAM at San Diego, and CARR at Emory University have assayed the feasibility of this objective (Burton et al., 1980; Mitchell et al., 1981; Frazier et al., 1982; Block et al., 1985). While the online real-time recording has proceeded well, the entry of non-physiologic information has, for the time, precluded a facile computer generated record. So far drug and event entry has been a combination of terminal and handwritten entries. Specialized interfaces have also been utilized to improve the process of such data entry including specialized keypads (Baetz et al., 1977), bar code readers (Block et al., 1981), virtual speech recognition units or SRUs (Doddington and Schalk, 1981), and the modern computer light pens and touch screens. Indeed, within the past few years, several commercial systems have now become available.

The Ohmeda system records realtime data from the Modulus II monitoring systems and prints these values on an anesthesia record. The system also provides a separate I/O touch panel keyboard display

screen for the user to input data such as drug selection and dosing. The Datascope version of a record keeper also provides a processing unit to interface with their monitors to process and reformat the digital data to be recorded onto a standardized anesthesia record form. There are no means of inputting any non-physiologic data, however, and these must be hand written.

Perhaps the most advanced computerized record generating system now available, the Dräger Model 3 anesthesia machine, contains multiple CPUs for not only displaying the physiologic analog data on a CRT but also generating the anesthesia record. The unit requires additional input from the clinician for the recording of intravenous drugs but the record can be formatted to write the physiologic values onto the anesthetist's record format of choice. Another interesting system available, CARIN, developed for the Macintosh computer, will interface with numerous monitoring devices and produce a standard anesthesia record on the computer screen and print the record in six colors. The CARIN system is also capable of recording some of the physiologic and anesthetic record information in a database format (Leslie, personal communication).

Data Collection and Retrieval

The initial attempt at data collection, retrieval and analysis was in the Department of Anesthesiology at the University of Wisconsin in Madison. Residents transferred database information to punch cards which were then sorted annually and a report rendered (Harmel, personal communication). However, even today with the advanced technology available, few Departments collect data other than for individual study protocols. The over-riding consideration in establishing a general database system is cost of hardware, software and especially personnel.

However, in an effort to implement such a system, the Cardiac Anesthesia Division of the Department of Anesthesiology at Duke University has developed a comprehensive database which is derived from the patient's history and the anesthetic record. This information provides an ongoing data collection which is then analysed and provides insights into clinical care and management (Leslie, personal communication). The power and ease of retrieval and analysis of information for retrospective studies which may influence clinical care is profound.

Drug Delivery Systems

Not only have computers become an integral element of anesthetic monitoring, they also control many modern drug-delivery systems (Brown et al., 1984). The earliest reported attempt at a machine controlled delivery system was in the early 1950's with barbiturates (Soltero et al., 1951). This failed because of hardware inadequacies. The advent of the microprocessor controlled infusion device has brought numerous successful drug infusion systems (Suppan, 1977; Reves et al., 1978; Wiener et al., 1978; Cooper et al., 1978a; Fukui and Smith, 1981; Brown et al., 1984).

Perhaps the most famous of the interactive anesthesia delivery systems is the Boston Anesthesia System (BAS) (Cooper et al., 1978a). This represented, at least in the late 1970's, a major innovation in anesthetic delivery by a system utilizing digital gas flow controls, solidstate pressure transducers, and a specialized anesthetic gas injector system all under microprocessor control. Other systems have also been developed by the anesthetists at the University of Arizona, the University of Utah and the University of Alabama to mention only a few (Brown et al., 1984). Many of the principles and solutions to design problems perfected by these groups are now found in the modern commercially available anesthetic machines. It is important to distinguish between two types of computer controlled drug delivery systems: open loop versus closed loop. The basic differences are illustrated in Fig. 64.3. The most common system in current use is the open loop delivery system. Many adjuvant anesthetic drugs such as sodium nitroprusside are currently administered utilizing microprocessor controlled infusion pumps. These pumps deliver drug at a user determined value. More sophisticated pumps are digital computing devices that perform and also monitor the drug infusion process. These devices monitor the infusion pressure, tabulate the volumes infused, perform selftests, monitor for air bubbles in the lines, and even notify the user of a malfunction utilizing specialized alarm systems.

To utilize closed loop computer drug administra-

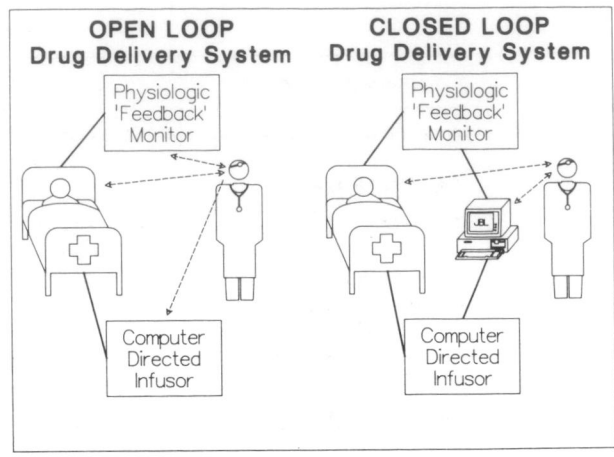

Fig. 64.3 Graphic representation of the principles of open loop versus closed loop drug delivery systems. Note especially the role of the anesthetist in the two different drug delivery systems.

tion systems, the computer must receive input from sensors monitoring the patient and the expected physiologic responses to the drug administered. It has now been possible to utilize computer modeling to develop a pharmacokinetic model of a drug administered to a patient based upon expected absorption, distribution, metabolism, and clearance of the drug (see Table 64.1.). Variations of these parameters are utilized to model the administration of the drug in different patients by refining the drug administration algorithm on a realtime basis as the patient reacts to the drug (Reves et al., 1978). The predicted blood levels of the drugs have been very accurate when compared to measured blood levels; however, with fixed algorithm predictions, interpatient variability remains a problem (Alvis et al., 1985). Closed loop drug delivery systems are already in trials utilizing monitored patient variables (electromyogram) to permit the computer to utilize 'adaptive control' of the drug infusion with the anesthetist determining the start and stop timepoints for muscle relaxation (Quill, Duke University, personal communication).

Computer Aided Instruction

Computer-aided instruction (CAI) and learning (CAL) programs have been developed during the past decade. As early as 1975, Attia et al. demonstrated that CAI could improve the learning experience of first month anesthesia residents as compared to standard 'textbook only' techniques. Kenney and Schmulian (1979) in Glasgow demonstrated the effectiveness of CAL when compared to a traditional lecture format. However, the acceptance of these modalities has been slow. Indeed software has been limited but several representative examples of CAL programs currently available are listed in Table 64.1. The man-

TABLE 64.1

Computer program title	Purpose	Source
Arterial blood gases	Blood gas simulations and interpretations	Williams and Wilkins
ACIDBAS.BAS		Univ. Maryland
ANSIM	Inhalation anesthetic uptake simulation	Univ. Maryland
Closed system anesth.		Univ. Maryland
Closed circuit anesth.		Washington Univ.
GAS MAN		Addison-Wesley
GUS (Gas Uptake Sim.)		Univ. North Carolina
MAC MAN		Univ. Maryland
DRUGDOSE.BAS	Calculations of drug and anesthetic doses	Univ. Maryland
Pediatric Drugs		Duke University
Pancuronium DOS 3.3	Simulates pharmacokinetics	Washington Univ.
Pancuronium Simulation		Univ. Maryland
Arrhythmias Tutorial	Diagnosis and management simulations	Williams and Wilkins
CPR Training		Washington Univ.
Cardiac Arrest		Washington Univ
Computer CPR Training		Univ. Maryland
Computer-Assisted ACLS		Columbia Univ.
Anesthesiology Review		Glaxo
Endotracheal intubation	Assisted instruction	Ohio State Univ.
Insertion of Swan-Ganz		Temple University

* Composite list of Computer-Aided Instruction (CAI) programs currently utilized in anesthesia training programs. Several other computer programs not listed here are discussed in more detail in the section on computer aided instruction or in the annotated bibliography.

machine interface is still perhaps the most important factor in this process (Becker, 1987). With the newer generation being 'bred' to use the computer, this barrier may disappear but for the moment general acceptance has been slow (Kearsley, 1987).

CAL programs can be in the simple form of tutorials, like an electronic textbook, with increased viewer interest generated by the 'electronic medium' and employing the unique computer displays of information and graphics, (Holley and Heller, 1981; Philips 1987). The tutorials may also be in an interactive format through questions and answers. Repetitive question and answer tutorials may be considered electronic drills which focus on specific areas programmed to repeat questions in areas of poor performance (Attia et al., 1975). These drills may take the form of computer games to maintain user interest and attention. Finally, the CAL programs may model a clinical situation which permits the users to 'practice' at their own speed (Table 64.1.). With complete patient safety, programs may simulate a variety of clinical anesthetic problems ranging from pharmacologic management of hemodynamic instability to predictive simulations of narcotic blood levels. These teaching simulations are also available for the inhalational anesthetics with such computer programs as Gas Man or ANSIM (Philip, 1987).

FUTURE APPLICATIONS AND DEVELOPMENT

Hardware

While invasive monitoring is currently widely applied, especially in anesthesia for cardiovascular surgery and in patients with cardiovascular instability, the proliferation of noninvasive devices has been a direct result of the microprocessor; automatic blood pressure determinations, pulse oximetry, newer capnography, the processed electroencephalogram, evoked potential monitoring, respiratory function monitoring, neuromuscular monitoring are all current and functioning. The integration and refinement of these modalities will proceed pari passu with the advances in computer technology. Already, such techniques as intraoperative transesophageal echocardiogram (TEE), intraoperative MUlti-GAted scanner (MUGA), intraoperative cerebral blood flow counter, Positron Emission Tomography (PET) scanner and Magnetic Resonance Imaging (MRI) are being investigated (Cahalan et al., 1987). Raman spectroscopy may provide a cheaper, simpler and more reliable anesthetic and respiratory gas monitoring than mass spectroscopy (Van Wagenen et al., 1986). These techniques are only viable because of the computer, and the implications for anesthesiology and the anesthetist are profound.

Networking

Networking is the linking together of a number of computers in a communication network, permitting the transfer of information between them. The increase in computer power plus the reduction in cost as the technology develops will make the anesthetic work station the hub of such a network linking peripheral area activities (i.e. laboratories, X-ray, blood bank, etc.) to the operating room. The first attempt to do this in the operating theatre on a reasonable trial basis was the DAME system (Duke Automatic Monitoring Equipment) in which general purpose computers designed for physiologic monitoring, were linked with a data manager, the anesthetic record printed by the data manager at the remote station, and in addition all computers could communicate with each other via the manager, as shown in Fig. 64.4. In the course of its history, over 20 000 records were generated but the experiment did not reach its potential. The man-machine interface proved to be a substantial barrier for data and drug entry, and the records were never programmed for analysis by the host computer. However, with the direction of computer power and sophistication, especially in speech recognition units where drug data and events may be entered online and input from an electronic anesthetic machine, a complete objective record is entirely possible. Such records may then be subjected to programmed statistical analysis, quality assurance documentation and a variety of other programmed analyses which may assess physiologic response to the pharmacologic manipulations.

The inclusion of other hospital information systems within a network including the anesthesia systems, may permit significant improvements in efficiency and safety in clinical care. Networks have already made it possible for the surgeon's office to enter patient scheduling information. Laboratory values, diagnostic studies, concurrent medications, potential drug interactions, and standardized 'protocols' are also available for networking. Much may depend on the institutional interest and support in determining how rapidly and how complete such systems will be in utilization at various institutions.

Artificial Intelligence

The term 'artificial intelligence' (A.I.) was first introduced in 1956 by John McCarthy. Computer-based A.I. models have been designed, written, tested, and are used in some areas of clinical medicine today (Shortliffe, 1987). Anesthesiology, with its growing dependence on computer based monitoring and drug-delivery systems, is one of the specialities where computer technology is particularly suited to test A.I. applications (Miller, 1983). Computer based A.I. systems have been developed to aid in clinical drug therapy, interpret patient laboratory data, and critique the patient anesthetic management plan. Several systems currently in use and potentially relevant to the anesthetist are listed in Table 64.2.

A subroutine of A.I. is the 'Expert System' (Waterman, 1986). The knowledge of an expert is utilized to format a **knowledge base** which is coupled with an

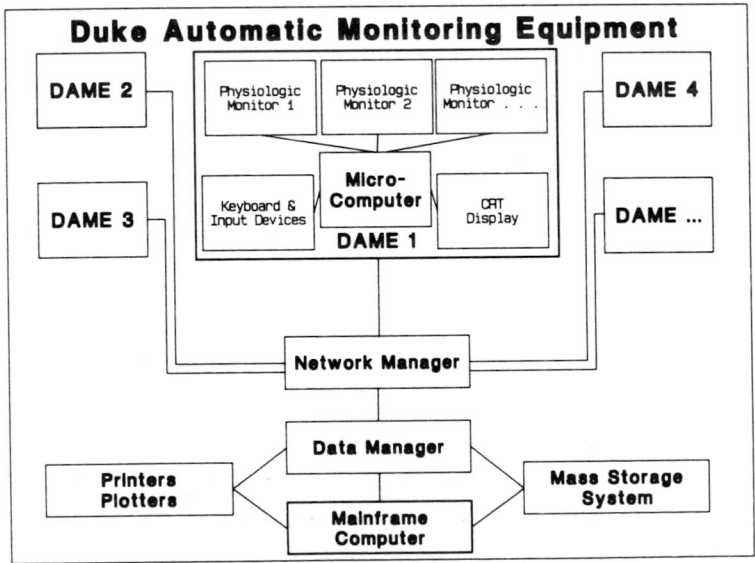

Fig. 64.4 Model diagram of the Duke Automatic Monitoring Equipment (DAME) from Duke University Department of Anesthesiology. The system demonstrates the principles of system design for integrated physiologic monitoring, computerized record generation, networking, and potential operating theater database systems.

TABLE 64.2

Expert systems (A.I.)	Purpose and source
DXplain	Assist in general medical diagnosis. J. Amer. Med. Assoc. 1987; 258: 67–74
VQ-ATTENDING	Critique ventilation management. Int. J. Clin. Monit. Comput. 1986; 2: 135–142
PROTIS	Aid in management of diabetes. Press Med. 1985; 14: 2085–2088
ONCOCIN	Chemotherapy protocol advisor. Ann. Int. Med. 1985; 103: 928–936
CADIAG-I	Aid in general medical diagnosis. Comput. Biol. Med. 1985; 15: 315–335
MED-I	Aid in diagnosis of chest pain. Klin. Wochenschr. 1985; 63: 511–517
DRUG INTERACTIONS	Critique combination drug therapy. Proc. First Conf. Art. Intell. Appl. 1984
HT-ATTENDING	Aid in hypertension therapeutics. Comput. Biomed. Res. 1984; 17: 38–54
ATTENDING	Critique anaesthetic management plans. Anesthesiology 1983; 58: 362
PUFF	Pulmonary function test interpretation. Comput. Biomed. Res. 1983; 16: 199–208
INTERNIST-I	Aid in general medical diagnosis. N. Engl. J. Med. 1982; 307: 468–476

Composite list of presently available Artificial Intelligence (A.I.) or 'Expert System' computer programs written in areas of potential interest to the anesthetist. These computer applications are discussed in more detail in the A.I. section and in the annotated bibliography.

inference engine to create two of the three components of an expert system. The third element of the system is an interface (I/O device) to permit the user to direct the system and it's goals. These components are shown in Fig. 64.5. Each component of the hardware is similar to the basic units of the digital computer, but such systems require much larger, faster CPU's and memory storage units. The programming languages utilized for A.I. systems are unique however.

One of the earliest model systems, MYCIN, was produced at Stanford University, utilizing rules and 'packets' of knowledge assembled from numerous experts (Buchanan and Shortliffe, 1984). MYCIN aids in the differential diagnosis of infections, and has performed well in comparison with recognized experts in this area of diagnosis. The most comprehensive system in anesthesiology is ATTENDING, written and maintained at Yale University (Miller, 1983).

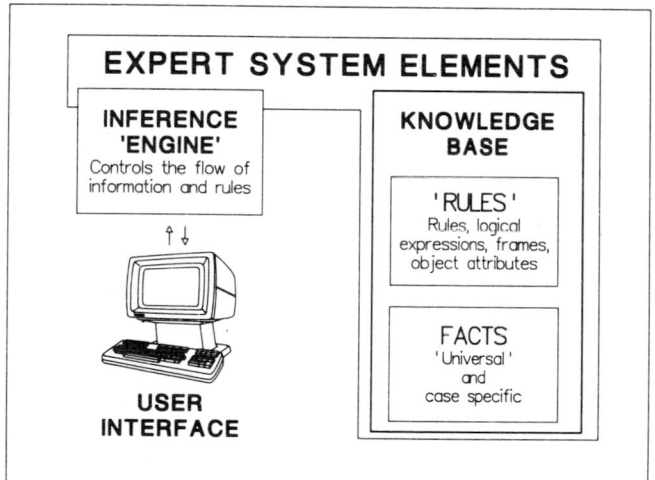

Fig. 64.5 Graphic representation of the basic components of a simplified Expert System designed to utilize the principles of artificial intelligence in the potential medical care delivery areas.

ATTENDING requires the input of information concerning the patient's medical history, the planned surgical procedure, and the anesthetist's proposed anesthetic management plan. The A.I. system then 'critiques' the proposed plan in English prose by reviewing potential benefits and risks as well as other potential anesthetic management plans. The critique details the agents and techniques chosen for premedication, induction, intubation, and maintenance of either general or regional anesthesia. The anesthesia group at Yale has continued to expand and revise this system (Miller, 1986). Several reviews of the concepts of such systems, the inherent problems, and the potentials of future expert systems in medicine are available (Clancey and Shortliffe, 1984; Waterman, 1986; Kearsley, 1987; Shortliffe, 1987).

SUMMARY

There can be little doubt that computers have become an integral part of the practice of modern anesthesia. Computers provide almost error free online data display and analysis (Block et al., 1985). They are tireless in these repetitive tasks and eternally vigilant. Their ability to store massive amounts of data and provide for retrieval and analysis of this information can be a sound basis for decisions and programs which have the potential to greatly enhance the safe management of clinical anesthesia (Olsson, 1983). So insidiously have the microprocessor and the computer invaded our practice that in the near future it may be unthinkable, if not outright malpractice, not to have certain computerized devices routinely available to monitor all patients (i.e. pulse oximeter, capnograph, etc.) (Eichhorn et al., 1986).

The technological advances in computer design and power, and reduction in costs now force serious consideration to the incorporation of the objective computerized record into anesthetic practice. With this step, the establishment of useful databases for retrieval and analysis of patient information becomes a reality that may have a significant impact on the conduct of anesthesia.

There still remains the fact that while intuitively we assume that on-line monitoring and objective records will lead to 'better and safer' anesthesia, there is to date no hard data to prove this assumption. There is no argument that can contest the cost effectiveness of pencil and paper, a chest stethoscope and blood pressure cuff in the hands of an alert and vigilant anesthetist. But lack of vigilance and human error do exist and play a significant role in anesthetic mishaps, possibly accounting for two-thirds of such incidents (Cooper et al., 1978 b; 1984). To reduce error, and to substitute inexorable distraction free operation, is the objective of computer technology applied to anesthesia. There is no question that the computer today can offer these advantages for a price. However, there still remain several problems. It is imperative that the computer systems employed in the practice of anes-

thesia function efficiently, and, above all, accurately, as the cost of a complete back-up system would be prohibitive; it is necessary to provide a friendlier interface and overcome the present barriers of communication via a terminal no matter how simplified; to make appropriate choice in input and output display that meets the needs for the decision process inherent in anesthetic management; these items must be solved if the computer and the anesthetist are to have a sound marriage. The technology is here; its refinement and adaptation to medical and anesthetic practice is a matter of time and prejudice.

GLOSSARY

Algorithm—a sequence of step-by-step instructions providing the details for the computer to perform a specific task. A term used to describe the program format for many common series of computer instructions.

Analog Computer—a device which operates on data or information received in analog form.

Analog-to-digital Converter (A/D)—a device which measures a voltage and then displays that measurement as a discrete number (digit).

ASCII—(American Standard Code for Information Interchange) an internationally accepted format of data representation utilizing a byte code for character representations. The combination of 7 bits, with an optional parity code (for a total of 8 bits per character) yields a possible 256 different values for a series of bytes.

Assembler—a system that will convert various program language commands and instructions into machine code that is executable by the specific computer or operating system for which the assembler was written.

Assembly language—a set of computer specific programming instructions that are converted into machine code for execution by the computer.

BASIC—the anagram for the programming language developed as Beginners All-purpose Symbolic Instruction Code.

Baud—a measure of the speed of transmission of digital data where one baud is equal to one bit per second. The term was derived from the name of J.M.E. Baudot, a pioneer in the field of telegraphy in the late 1800's.

Binary code—the symbolic representation of information which the computer utilizes for the format of storage. The smallest unit of storage is the bit.

Bit—the smallest unit of electronic information storage utilized by the computer as either 'on' (one) or 'off' (zero). It represents the conjunction of the words binary and digit.

Buffer—a section of RAM (Random Access Memory) that is used for the temporary storage of data.

Byte—a grouping of bits, generally eight, which represents the usual required storage size for a single character of information in a computer.

C—a high level language developed at Bell Laboratories.

Chip—a millimeter size rectangle of silicon onto which miniature electronic circuitry is etched.

COBOL—the anagram for the programming language developed as COmmon Business Oriented Language.

Compiler—a program which converts statements or symbols into machine language for execution by the computer.

CPU (Central Processing Unit)—the area or part of the computer hardware which performs all the mathematical processes of the computer.

Database—a collection of data (information) that is stored for later analysis or retrieval.

Databus—the hardware system which permits transfer of machine level information between the components of the system or between the various input and output devices.

Floppy disk—a piece of magnetic storage material in the shape of a small phonograph record encased in a protective sheath.

FORTRAN—the anagram for the programming language developed as FORmula TRANslation especially for highspeed numeric calculations.

Hardware—the actual physical components of a system that are assembled together to form the computer system (i.e. circuit boards, memory chips, wiring, etc.).

Inference engine—the programming commands within an expert system (A.I.) which control the strategy and methods of applying the rules to the information or facts being analysed.

Input device—a term describing any hardware system which permits transfer of information into a computer; i.e. keyboard, floppy disk, hard disk, 'mouse', digitizer, light pen, bar code reader.

Interface—the connection which permits intelligent communication between two devices or a device and a human operator as in a keyboard or monitoring screen.

Knowledge base—the part of an expert system (A.I.) which contains the set of rules or logical expressions describing the important relationships of the facts and information that the system is designed to consider.

Machine language—the bits of information utilized within a specific computer to represent the information being stored, processed, or transferred.

Megabyte (MB)—2^{20} or 1 048 576 bytes.

Memory—the information storage area of the computer or peripheral device where the numbers or characters are stored electronically as bits or combinations of bits.

Modem—(MOdulator-DEModulator) an electronic device that converts data within the computer to a format that can be transmitted over phone lines permitting computer to computer communication.

Output device—any hardware system that permits transfer of information from the computer to the user in an interpretable format; i.e. CRT, monitor, printer, synthesized voice.

Parallel—a method of connecting two devices which permits the simultaneous transmission of more than one bit between the two devices over more than one communication wire.

Peripheral device—a term referring to the input and output devices connected to the computer.

Program—a set or series of step-by-step instructions to the computer which instruct the control unit how to perform a specific task.

Software—the programs or electronic instructions which direct the computer hardware in task performance.

ANNOTATED REFERENCES

Alvis J.M., Reves J.G., Govier A.V., et al. (1985). Computer-assisted continuous infusions of fentanyl during cardiac anesthesia: Comparison with a manual method. *Anesthesiology*, **63**, 41.

> Presentation of a comparison of computer-assisted continuous infusion (CACI) versus a manual method demonstrating improvements in hemodynamic stability with fewer hypertensive episodes or requirements for adjuvant drug interventions in the CACI group.

Attia R.R., Miller E.V., Kitz R.J. (1975). Teaching effectiveness: Evaluation of computer-assisted instruction for cardiopulmonary resuscitation. *Anesth. Analg*, **54**, 308.

Evaluation of the potential value, problems, and effectiveness of CAI in teaching clinical medicine such as CPR.

Baetz S.R., Schneider A.J., Fadel J. (1977). The anesthesia keyboard system: an improvement in anesthesia record keeping. Exhibit, Annual Meeting, *Am. Soc. Anesthesiol.*
Presentation of the initial trials at improving the physician-computer interface for the anesthetic record keeper with special keyboards.

Becker H.J. (1987). Using Computers for Instruction. *BYTE*, Feb.
This issue of the magazine contains numerous articles reviewing and detailing historic and current attempts with CAI in both medical and nonclinical areas of instruction. An excellent current review of ongoing CAI projects.

Beneken J.E.W., Blom J.A. (1983). An integrative patient monitoring approach. In *An Integrated Approach to Monitoring*. pp. 121–131. (Gravenstein J.S., Newbower R.S., Ream A.K. et al., eds.) Boston: Butterworths.
An early but timely review of the problems of patient monitoring and the relevant considerations in clinical monitoring design and utilization.

Block F.E., Burton L.W., Beddingfield S. (1981). A year's experience with bar codes. Presentation, Microcomputers in Anesthesiology Symposium, Biloxi, Miss.,
A review of the technology, interface techniques, and clinical experience with a bar-code reader for drug information entry into a computer generated record system, DAME (*see also* Block et al., 1985).

Block F.E., Burton L.W., Rafal M.D. et al. (1985). Two computer-based anesthetic monitors: the Duke automatic system and the microdame. *J. Clin. Monit. Comput.*, **1**, 30.
A review of the development, problems, success, and potential for the integrated computer monitoring and anesthetic record generating system.

Boquet G., Bushman J.A., Davenport H.T. (1980). The anesthetic machine: a study of function and design. *Br. J. Anaesth.*, **52**, 61.
A study and review of the time and manual performance duties of an anaesthetist during clinical care as relevant to the potentials for man-machine interfaces to improve patient care.

Brown B.R., Calkins J.M., Saunders R.J. (eds.). (1984). *Future Anesthesia Delivery Systems*. Philadelphia: F.A. Davis Co.
An excellent text reviewing all aspects of modern anesthetic delivery system design, development, and clinical applications.

Buchanan B., Shortliffe E. (1984). Rule-based expert systems: *The MYCIN Experiment of the Stanford Heuristic Programming Project*. Reading MA: Addison-Wesley.
A retrospective examination of MYCIN, one of the most extensive and successful projects applying artificial intelligence in the area of clinical medicine.

Burton L.W., Block F., Davis D., et al. (1980). The Duke Automatic Monitoring System (DAME) and the objective anesthesia record. Scientific Exhibit, Annual Meeting, Am. Soc. Anesthesiol.
Initial national exhibit of the integrated monitoring and anaesthetic recording system designed and built in the Department of Anaesthesia under the direction of Dr. Merel Harmel.

Cahalan M.K., Litt L.L., Botvinick E.H., et al. (1987). Advances in noninvasive cardiovascular imaging: implications for the anesthesiologist. *Anesthesiology*, **66**, 356.
An excellent review of many of the current noninvasive methods of assessment of cardiovascular function in the areas of echocardiography, nuclear medicine, and magnetic resonance imaging.

Clancey W.J., Shortliffe E.H. (eds.). (1984). *Readings in Medical Artificial Intelligence: The First Decade*. Reading, Mass: Addison-Wesley.
Painstakingly selected and presented in historical context, this collection presents some of the most complete and influential works done in artificial intelligence in medicine since 1971.

Cooper J.B., Newbower R.S., Kitz R.J. (1984). An analysis of major errors and equipment failures in anesthesia management: Considerations for prevention and detection. *Anesthesiology*, **60**, 74.
An excellent review of the subject and presentation of a study (1089 critical incidents) demonstrating areas of concentration which could potentially improve clinical care and reduce anesthetic related morbidity and mortality.

Cooper J.B., Newbower R.S., Long C.D., et al. (1978b). Preventable anesthesia mishaps: A study of human factors. *Anesthesiology*, **49**, 399.
A review of the factors which led to anesthetic mishaps and areas of potential improvement to provide safer patient care.

Cooper J.B., Newbower R.S., Moore J.W., et al. (1978a). A new anesthesia delivery system. *Anesthesiology*, **49**, 310.
Presentation of the Boston Anesthesia System (BAS), a microprocessor controlled anesthetic delivery system.

Doddington G.R., Schalk T.B. (1981). Speech recognition: turning theory into practice. *Spectrum*, **18**, 26.
A review of the problems, principles, current applications, and discussion of the potentials for this technology in computer-interfaces.

Eichhorn J.H., Cooper J.B., Cullen D.J. et al. (1986). Standards for patient monitoring during anesthesia at Harvard Medical School. *J. Am. Med. Assoc.*, **256**, 1017.
A report, and explanatory background information on the currently recommended patient monitoring standards during anesthesia at Harvard Medical School.

Frazier W.T., Paulsen A.W., Harbort R.A., et al. (1982). Integrated anesthesia delivery monitoring system with computer-assisted anesthesia record generation. Presentation, Annual Meeting, *Assoc. Adv. Med. Instrument.*
Presentation and discussion of the CARR system designed and built at Emory University for integrated physiologic monitoring and anesthetic record generation by computer control.

Fukui Y., Smith N.T. (1981). Interaction among ventilation, the circulation, and the uptake and distribution of halothane. Use of a hybrid computer model I. The basic model. *Anesthesiology*, **54**, 107.
An early model of the use of a computer generated simulation model of inhalational anesthetic uptake. Presents the principles of designing and implementing such a computer modeling system.

Goldstine H.H. (1972). *The Computer from Pascal to von Neumann*. Princeton: University Press, Princeton.

A comprehensive, entertaining, and well written review of the historical development of the modern computer.

Holley H.S., Heller F.N. (1981). The microcomputer in anesthesia education. *Anesthesiol. Rev.*, **8**, 29.
An review of the area of CAI and the demonstrated potential for CAI in learning anesthesia and clinical medicine.

Kearsley G. (1987). *Artificial Intelligence and Instruction*. Park Row Software, Reading MA: Addison-Wesley.
An up-to-date collection of largely original articles on the state-of-the-art in intelligent tutoring systems by many of the 'experts' the field of CAI.

Kenney G.N.C., Schmulian C. (1979). Computer-assisted learning in the teaching of anaesthesia. *Anaesthesia*, **34**, 159.
One of the initial studies documenting the potential benefit of learning anesthetic principles with the aid of CAI.

Miller P.L. (1983). Critiquing anaesthetic management: The 'ATTENDING' computer system. *Anesthesiology*, **58**, 362.
The article presenting the principles of the ATTENDING expert system, the earliest and most comprehensive A.I. system in anesthesia to date. A good, but brief review of expert system design principles and of the process of A.I. system implementation.

Miller P.L. (1986). Extending computer-based critiquing to a new domain: ATTENDING, ESSENTIAL-ATTENDING, and VQ-ATTENDING. *Int. J. Clin. Monit. Comput.*, **2**, 135.
An update on the original anesthetic management plan critiquing expert system. ATTENDING (*see* Miller, 1983), as well as a description of two additional A.I. systems recently developed at Yale University.

Mitchell M.M., Meathe E.A., Ozaki G.T., et al. (1981). Comprehensive Integrated Clinical/Research Anesthesia Monitor. Exhibit, Annual Meeting, *Am. Soc. Anesthesiol.*
Exhibition of the San Diego designed and built computer system for an integrated physiologic monitoring system combined with an anesthetic record generator.

Olsson G.L. (1983). An interactive information system for anaesthesia. In *Computing in Anaesthesia and Intensive Care*. pp. 86–95. (Prakash O., ed.). Boston: Martinus Nijkoff.
An excellent review of the field of microcomputers and physiologic monitoring with an emphasis on state-of-the-art systems and future design and development.

Philip J.H. (1987). Gas Man An example of goal oriented computer-assisted teaching which results in learning. *Inter. J. Clin. Monitor. Comput.*, (in press).
Presentation of a computer-simulation program of

uptake of inhalational anesthetics and the value of such CAI for improving resident learning and performance.

Reves J.G., Sheppard L.C., Wallach R., et al. (1978). Therapeutic uses of sodium nitroprusside and an automated method of administration. *Int. Anesthesiol. Clin.*, **16**, 51.
An original paper reviewing the principles of microprocessor-controlled drug adminstration and a presentation of a system designed and built to control hypertension with a closed-loop drug administration system.

Shortliffe E.H. (1987). Computer programs to support clinical decision making. *J. Am. Med. Assoc.*, **258**, 61.
An editorial briefly reviewing several key medical expert systems and the problems which such systems create. The author also discusses the limited success of medical A.I. and the problems which must be solved.

Shurkin J. (1984). *Engines of the mind: a history of the computer*. New York, London: W.W. Norton.
An excellent historical review of the landmark discoveries and developments leading to the modern computer.

Soltero D.E., Faulconer A., Bickford R.G. (1951). The clinical application of automatic anesthesia. *Anesthesiology*, **12**, 574.
Initial report of the closed-loop clinical administration of barbiturates utilizing feedback information from electroencephalogram monitoring.

Suppan P. (1977). Feedback monitoring in anesthesia: indirect measurement of arterial pressure and its use for the control of halothane anaesthesia. *Br. J. Anaesth.*, **49**, 141.
An example of the closed-loop drug administration technique for the control of the delivery of inhalational anesthesia in the clinical setting.

Van Wagenen R.A., Westenskow D.R., Benner R.E., et al. (1986). Dedicated monitoring of anaesthetic and respiratory gases by Raman scattering. *J. Clin. Monit.*, **2**, 215.

Waterman D.A. (1986). *A Guide to Expert Systems*. Reading, MA: Addison-Wesley.
In one comprehensive book, Waterman combines explanations of how expert systems work, why they are important, how to build one, how to gather knowledge from the experts, and potentially what a system can and cannot perform. Also contains an excellent bibliography of relevant papers in the area.

Wiener F., Weil M.H. (1978). Computer-based monitoring and data measurement in critical care. *Methods Inf. Med.*, **17**, 252.
A review of the principles of physiologic monitor networking and the presentation of one such system.

Index